Pitfalls in Histopathologic Diagnosis of Malignant Melanoma

Pitfalls in Histopathologic Diagnosis of Malignant Melanoma

A. BERNARD ACKERMAN, M.D.
Professor of Dermatology and Pathology
Director, Institute for Dermatopathology
Jefferson Medical College of
Thomas Jefferson University
Philadelphia, Pennsylvania

LORENZO CERRONI, M.D.
Assistant Professor of Dermatology
Department of Dermatology
University of Graz, Austria

HELMUT KERL, M.D.
Professor and Chairman
Department of Dermatology
University of Graz, Austria

With the assistance of
HANS-PETER SOYER, M.D.
Department of Dermatology
University of Graz, Austria

Drawings by
MARIO DI LEONARDO, M.D.
Department of Dermatology
Jefferson Medical College of
Thomas Jefferson University
Philadelphia, Pennsylvania

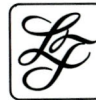

Lea & Febiger
PHILADELPHIA · BALTIMORE · HONG KONG
LONDON · MUNICH · SYDNEY · TOKYO

A WAVERLY COMPANY

1994

Lea & Febiger
Box 3024
200 Chester Field Parkway
Malvern, Pennsylvania 19355-9725
U.S.A.
(215) 251-2230

Executive Editor—John F. Spahr, Jr.
Project Editor—Dorothy DiRienzi
Production Manager—Thomas J. Colaiezzi

Library of Congress Cataloging-in-Publication Data
Ackerman, A. Bernard, 1936–
    Pitfalls in histopathologic diagnosis of malignant melanoma / A.
  Bernard Ackerman, Lorenzo Cerroni, Helmut Kerl.
      p.   cm.
    Includes index.
    ISBN 0-8121-1352-7
    1. Melanoma—Histopathology.   I. Cerroni, Lorenzo.   II. Kerl,
  Helmut.   III. Title.
    [DNLM: 1. Diagnostic Errors. 2. Histological Techniques.
3. Melanoma—diagnosis. 4. Skin Neoplasms—diagnosis.   WR 500
A182p]
RC280.M37A27   1993
616.99′47707583—dc20
DNLM/DLC
for Library of Congress   92-49579
    CIP

NOTE: Although the author(s) and the publisher have taken reasonable steps to ensure the accuracy of the drug information included in this text before publication, drug information may change without notice and readers are advised to consult the manufacturer's packaging inserts before prescribing medications.

Reprints of chapters may be purchased from Lea & Febiger in quantities of 100 or more. Contact Sally Grande in the Sales Department.

Copyright © 1994 by Lea & Febiger. Copyright under the International Copyright Union. All Rights Reserved. This book is protected by copyright. *No part of it may be reproduced in any manner or by any means without written permission from the publisher.*

PRINTED IN THE UNITED STATES OF AMERICA

Print number: 5 4 3 2 1

To the memory of Leon Ackerman who, for 50 years, invested nearly every fiber of his being in his cherished son BERNIE

For Gigi Cerroni who taught, by his generosity, love, and example, the lesson of how to be a human being to his son LORENZO

To the memory of Charlotte Kerl who was able to provide, under difficult circumstances, a full measure of parental devotion to her son HELMUT

Preface

Start out with the conviction that absolute truth is hard to reach in matters relating to our fellow creatures, healthy or diseased, that slips in observation are inevitable even with the best trained faculties, that errors in judgment must occur in the practice of an art which consists largely of balancing probabilities;—start, I say, with this attitude in mind, and mistakes will be acknowledged and regretted; but instead of a slow process of self-deception, with ever increasing inability to recognize truth, you will draw from your errors the very lessons which may enable you to avoid their repetition.
—William Osler

No cutaneous neoplasms are as vexing for diagnosis to histopathologists as malignant melanoma and its simulators, and none as grave in implications for misdiagnosis as malignant melanoma. If a malignant melanoma, removed incompletely, is interpreted incorrectly as a Spitz's nevus and left untreated, death from metastasis will be the likely result. Less grave, but serious nonetheless, is misreading a Spitz's nevus (or any other type of melanocytic nevus) as a malignant melanoma. Such a lesion usually is re-excised with lateral margins of several centimeters of normal skin and sometimes margins in depth that include fascia. In some instances, a skin graft is required to close the wound. Even regional lymph nodes may be extracted, all for a neoplasm that is entirely benign.

Nowhere, to our knowledge, can a histopathologist learn about pitfalls in histopathologic diagnosis of malignant melanoma in a way that is comprehensive, systematic, and effective. This volume endeavors to do that by alerting readers to a range of pitfalls in histopathologic diagnosis of malignant melanoma and instructing them in a method that enables pits to be avoided. The method utilizes repeatable criteria for histopathologic diagnosis of melanocytic neoplasms of all kinds based foremost on features of their architectural pattern, particularly their silhouette. Proper use of this method is demonstrated in a didactic introductory chapter that establishes firm, repeatable criteria for diagnosis of benign and malignant neoplasms of melanocytes.

Each of the 101 pitfalls that constitute the substance of this book focuses on a knotty problem in histopathologic diagnosis or differential diagnosis of malignant melanoma. Every pitfall is encompassed in four pages, each of which is designed to serve one or more particular purposes. The first page, always on the left-hand side, bears a large photomicrograph, taken at scanning magnification, which permits assessment of the architectural pattern of the melanocytic neoplasm under consideration. The facing page shows, at the top, the very same scanning photomicrograph that appears on the page opposite it, but much reduced in size. Beneath the photomicrograph taken at scanning magnification are two rows of three photomicrographs each, the first row "shot" at medium power and the second at high power. Boxes positioned in three separate loci on the "scanning" photomicrograph indicate the precise sites of each of the three photomicrographs taken at next higher magnification. At the bottom of the second page, a pivotal question asked repeatedly of every histopathologist is posed: "What is your diagnosis?" On the basis of the morphologic findings pictured, and those alone, a reader is challenged to make a specific diagnosis. When the page is turned, the same seven photomicrographs that appear on page two are shown again, but this time with numerous lead lines that call attention to histopathologic findings deemed to be important for rendering a specific diagnosis. Pertinent clinical information is provided in the upper left-hand corner of the page. Also on this third page is found an answer to the question asked on the previous page, i.e., a specific diagnosis couched in the language of clinical dermatology. On the facing page, the fourth and last, are listed both Criteria for Diagnosis and Pitfalls in Diagnosis of the melanocytic neoplasm that has been illustrated.

The organization of the text for each of the 101 pitfalls attempts to simulate the circumstance of a histopathologist at a microscope as he or she grapples with a perplexing problem in diagnosis of malignant melanoma or a simulator of it. Our strategem may at first seem diabolical. We hope to induce colleagues who use this book to fall headlong into every trap that we have set for them. The motive, however, is not malevolent. Every time a histopathologist falls into a pit, there follows inevitably the painful task of climbing out of it and, in the process, of re-assessing, modifying, and even abandoning long-held tenets that failed to prevent entrapment by that particular pit. In histopathology, as in the rest of life beyond a microscope, we learn best, and most, from our mistakes. Paradoxically, with a reflective turn of mind, the more mistakes we make, the more competent we become.

The histopathologic sections that form the basis of each of the pitfalls were not selected at random. We, the authors, also erred in no small number of them, and so did colleagues who sent them to us in consultation. We think that we profited from our mistakes and from repeated study of those sections, and we hope that readers will too.

Of the thousands of hours devoted to the preparation of this book, the authors spent hundreds of them working together in New York City and in Graz, and also at sites of national and international meetings in such disparate places as San Antonio and Poertschach, Atlanta and Florence. The work was as intense as it was joyful. In general, responsibility for the book may be attributed as follows: Bernie Ackerman spawned the idea and wrote the text, Lorenzo Cerroni "shot" nearly all of the photomicrographs and organized nearly all of the written and pictorial material, and Helmut Kerl not only contributed a critical mind to the text and a critical eye to thousands of photomicrographs, but also assembled the bibliography and acted as cement that held the project together. In short, we functioned as a team, and the results of that effort are both this book and even stronger friendships forged in the making of it.

New York, New York	A. BERNARD ACKERMAN, M.D.
Graz, Austria	LORENZO CERRONI, M.D.
Graz, Austria	HELMUT KERL, M.D.

Acknowledgments

We are indebted to:

Ivan Georgiev, who developed so expertly the thousands of photomicrographs that grace these pages.

Jim Harter, for lightning speed and daunting accuracy in the typing of countless drafts of the manuscript.

Emmilia Hodak and Ilana Avinoach, who assisted in the formulation of a classification of blue nevi.

The late Howard King, who designed the book in the fashion that he did everything, artistically, meticulously, and lovingly.

Mark V. Smith, who pursued with incredible tenacity the course of patients whose lesions are presented in these pages.

Technicians in the laboratories of dermatopathology at New York University School of Medicine and the Department of Dermatology of the University of Graz for preparing histopathologic sections of such superb quality.

Contents

I. Melanocytes in Normal Skin   1
   A. Cytologic Features   1
   B. Distribution   1
   C. Location   3

II. Nevi   3
   A. Definition   3
   B. Congenital Nevi   5
      1. Blue   10
      2. Non-blue   10
   C. Acquired Nevi   46
      1. Unna's Nevus   46
      2. Miescher's Nevus   46
      3. Spitz's Nevus   51
      4. Clark's Nevus   86

III. Melanomas   108
   A. Definition   108
   B. Principles   108
   C. Melanoma in Situ   110
   D. Desmoplastic Melanoma, Neurotropic Melanoma, and Melanoma with Neural Differentiation   120
   E. Thickness as a Measure of Prognosis   121

IV. Melanoma in Association with a Nevus   142

V. Regression of Melanoma   158

VI. Metastases of Melanoma to Skin   170

VII. Benign Simulators of Melanoma   182
   A. Melanocytic   182
      1. Spitz's Nevi   182
      2. Combined Nevi   183
      3. Persistent (Recurrent) Nevi   194
      4. Halo Nevi   194
      5. Ancient Miescher's and Unna's Nevi   199
      6. Congenital Nevi in Newborns and Infants   199
      7. Nevi on Genitalia of Young Adults   212
      8. Nevi on Palms and Soles   212
      9. Nevi in Association with Lichen Sclerosus et Atrophicus in Anogenital Region   212
      10. Junctional Nevi above Band of Melanophages   212
      11. Melanosis of the Genitalia   213
      12. Melanocytic Proliferation in the Epidermis above Some Intradermal Miescher's Nevi   213
      13. Melanocytic Proliferation in the Epidermis above Fibrous Papules of the Face   213
      14. Melanocytic Proliferation in the Epidermis of Severely Sun-Damaged Skin, Especially of a Face   213
      15. Melanocytic Proliferation in the Epidermis of Solar Lentigines   228
      16. Melanocytic Proliferation in the Epidermis of Normal Skin of an Eyelid   228
   B. Non-melanocytic   228

VIII. Confusing Concepts   248

Bibliography   263

IX. Pitfalls 1–101   267

Index   673

Key to Findings Identified by Leaders

collarette(s) = collarette(s) of adnexal epithelium

column(s) = column(s) of melanocytes

confluence = confluence of nests of melanocytes

cord(s) = cord(s) of melanocytes

dendrite(s) = dendrites of melanocytes

fascicle(s) = fascicle(s) of melanocytes

fascicles vary = fascicles of melanocytes vary in size and shape

globule(s) = dull pink globule(s) within the epidermis

junction = dermo-epidermal junction

maturation = maturation of melanocytes with progressive descent into the dermis, i.e., nuclei become smaller

melanocyte = neoplastic melanocyte

melanocytes equidistant = solitary melanocytes equidistant from one another

melanocytes not equidistant = solitary melanocytes not equidistant from one another

nest(s) = nest(s) of melanocytes

nests not equidistant = nests of melanocytes not equidistant from one another

nests vary = nests of melanocytes vary in size and shape

scatter = scatter of melanocytes throughout an epithelium, i.e., epidermal or adnexal

sheet(s) = sheet(s) of melanocytes

solitary melanocyte(s) = melanocyte(s) arranged as solitary unit(s)

solitary melanocytes predominate = melanocytes disposed as solitary units predominate over melanocytes arranged in nests

splaying = splaying of melanocytes among bundles of collagen

strand(s) = strand(s) of melanocytes

Although accurate clinical diagnosis of pigmented lesions* in the skin must take into account color and aspects of topography, the most important single criterion for precise clinical diagnosis of pigmented cutaneous lesions is silhouette. In fact, silhouette alone usually enables clinical differentiation of malignant melanomas** from nevi of all kinds. Although every clinical feature of a pigmented lesion in the skin should be noted and assessed in an attempt to come to a specific diagnosis of it, the most telling finding is silhouette. Assessment of silhouette also is the surest route to accurate diagnosis of proliferations of melanocytes when they are viewed through a conventional microscope.

The silhouette of any neoplasm is appraised best at scanning magnification. With scanning magnification histopathologists can diagnose nevi and melanomas of all kinds most reliably and differentiate nevi from melanomas. Pitfalls in diagnosis abound when high magnification is used in an attempt to accomplish that differentiation. Some Spitz's nevi, for example, may have many more atypical melanocytes, more strikingly atypical melanocytes, and more mitotic figures than many melanomas. There may be less nuclear atypia in some melanomas with neural differentiation than in some wholly benign ancient schwannomas. In sum, histopathologic diagnosis and differential diagnosis of melanocytic neoplasms are achieved best by judging their silhouettes at scanning magnification. Needless to mention, there are many exceptions to this "rule," just as there are to all "dicta" about morphologic diagnosis.

---

*A distinction between pigmented lesions and melanocytic lesions is an important one. Not all pigmented lesions are melanocytic, but most melanocytic lesions are pigmented. For example, tattoos, lesions of argyria, and plaques of Kaposi's sarcoma are pigmented, but they are not melanocytic. Tattoos may be black as a consequence of carbon, argyria is bluish gray because of silver, and plaques (as well as some patches and nearly all tumors) of Kaposi's sarcoma are purplish as a result of blood. In brief, pigmented lesions are not necessarily a reflection of the effects of an increased number of melanocytes. Even some lesions pigmented by melanin do not result from a proliferation of melanocytes, e.g., freckles, urticaria pigmentosa, and dermatofibromas, in each of which the epidermis is hyperpigmented, but the number of melanocytes is not increased notably. In contrast, melanocytic lesions such as nevi and melanomas are typified by proliferations of melanocytes. The vast majority of melanocytic lesions are pigmented clinically by melanin, but some, such as long-standing skin-colored intradermal types of Unna's nevi, reddish expressions of Spitz's nevi, and so-called amelanotic melanomas, including some desmoplastic melanomas, are devoid of brown or black color.

**Throughout this book, the term "melanoma" will be used as a synonym for malignant melanoma.

Only three diagnoses are available when a histopathologist assesses a proliferation of melanocytes in the skin: (1) nevus, (2) melanoma, and (3) melanoma in association with a nevus. If a histopathologist cannot make one of those three diagnoses, then the honest response, phrased in Old English, should be "Ic ne wat," i.e., "I don't know." No attempt should be made to maneuver behind hedges, euphemisms, and non-diagnoses like "active junctional nevus," "atypical melanocytic hyperplasia," "pagetoid melanocytic proliferation," "mild, moderate, and severe dysplasia," "borderline melanoma," and "minimal deviation melanoma." These phrases are evasions that do not communicate to a clinician, directly and forthrightly, whether the lesion under consideration is a nevus, a melanoma, or a melanoma in association with a nevus. Furthermore, they permit a histopathologist to sustain the delusion that a diagnosis actually is being made when, in truth, only an inadequate description, badly phrased, is being rendered.

I. Melanocytes in Normal Skin

A. Cytologic Features

Melanocytes may be distinguished from keratinocytes, which constitute the bulk of the epidermis, by the fact that (1) they are situated as solitary units at the dermo-epidermal junction or in the basal layer and that (2) they have smaller, darker nuclei that seem to be surrounded by clefts (Fig. 1). In fact, the clefts are not around the nuclei per se, but around a wisp of cytoplasm that surrounds the nuclei. In vivo, melanocytes have abundant cytoplasm, but when they are immersed in alcohols of various strengths during the stages through which specimens pass in processing, that cytoplasm shrinks markedly and gives melanocytes the appearance of being "clear cells." In actuality, melanocytes in histologic sections are not cells with clear cytoplasm, but cells whose shrunken cytoplasm is encircled by clefts.

B. Distribution

Melanocytes are present throughout the entire integument, but they are more populous in some regions than in others. For example, melanocytes are more numerous on the cheeks than on the trunk. The ratio of melano-

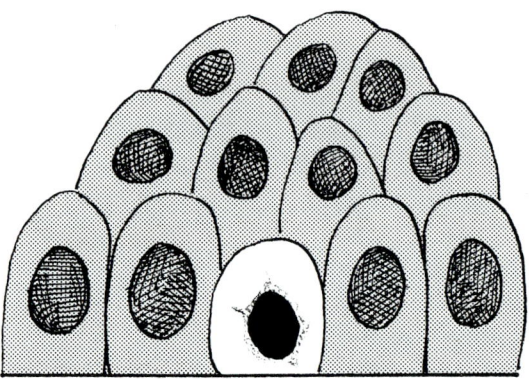

Fig. 1. A melanocyte in the basal layer surrounded partially by keratinocytes. The melanocyte is distinguished easily from the keratinocytes by its smaller, darker nucleus. Furthermore, as pictured, a melanocyte often is separated from keratinocytes by a prominent cleft.

cytes to keratinocytes at the base of the epidermis varies from about 1:4 to 1:10 depending on the region. With advancing age, the ratio shifts further in favor of keratinocytes. The relative number of melanocytes is the same for both sexes and for all races.

Differences in coloration among the races result, not from differences in the number of melanocytes, but from the activity of melanocytes as gauged by the rate at which they produce melanin and the amount of melanin that they make. Melanocytes of dark-skinned races make more melanin.

C. Location

Melanocytes in skin are situated mostly at the junctions of epidermis and dermis, upper part of follicular epithelium and dermis, and upper portion of intradermal eccrine duct and dermis, and in bulbs of hair follicles (Fig. 2). Melanocytes at the junction of epidermis and dermis give normal skin its color, described imprecisely as white, yellow, black, and red. Unlike melanocytes at the dermo-epidermal junction of normal skin, melanocytes in follicular bulbs are strikingly dendritic and, in persons with dark brown or black hair, heavily pigmented by melanin. Melanocytes in follicular bulbs are responsible for the color of hair in blonds, brunettes, and redheads, as well as in those whose hair is black.

Curiously, a melanoma never has been reported to have arisen from melanocytes in a follicular bulb, in contrast to the countless numbers of melanomas that have been known to develop from melanocytes positioned at the dermo-epidermal junction. The remaining melanomas, scant by comparison, begin in the dermis or subcutis of deep congenital nevi, in blue nevi, and from ectopic melanocytes in diverse viscera and in other recondite sites.

---

*The word "nevus" in this book is synonymous with "melanocytic nevus." The term "nevus cell" is not used because the cells that constitute a melanocytic nevus are melanocytes. The terms "nevus cell," "nevus-cell nevus," "nevocytic nevus," and "nevo-melanocytic nevus" are inaccurate and will not appear in these pages; only "melanocyte," "melanocytic nevus," and "nevus" will.

II. Nevi*

A. Definition

A nevus is merely a spot, but not every spot in the skin is a proliferation of melanocytes, e.g., spots formed by blood vessels such as port wine stains and spots entirely devoid of melanocytes as those in vitiligo. Not even all spots pigmented by melanin are proliferations of melanocytes, e.g., solar lentigines consist almost entirely of pigmented keratinocytes. Not every pigmented spot termed a "nevus," e.g., Becker's nevus, is truly a nevus of melanocytes. Becker's nevus, a hamartoma of epidermal, follicular, and smooth muscle components, is pigmented as a consequence of melanin within the epidermis, but is not associated with nests of melanocytes within the epidermis, the sine qua non for diagnosis of a junctional nevus.

The term "nevus" in classic pathology is a synonym for hamartoma, i.e., a condition in which elements present normally at a site are arranged faultily there. The term "nevus" in clinical dermatology and in dermatopathology, however, is not restricted to hamartomas like congenital melanocytic nevi, but is applied also to neoplasms such as acquired melanocytic nevi and to "nevus cells," which actually are melanocytes. If clinicians and histopatholgists are to employ the word "nevus" clearly and meaningfully, they must become sensitized to the indiscriminate application of that word to certain hamartomas, neoplasms, and cells (melanocytes) that constitute those hamartomas and neoplasms. Furthermore, it is mandatory that the designation "nevus" always be used with a modifier that will ensure precision, e.g., melanocytic nevus, epidermal nevus, nevus sebaceus, connective tissue nevus, nevus flammeus, nevus lipomatosis, Becker's nevus, Sutton's nevus, Werther's nevus.

Melanocytic nevi may begin and develop in two very different ways:

1. Proliferation of melanocytes first at the dermo-epidermal junction. The melanocytes proliferate first as solitary units and then in nests, i.e., three or more melanocytes per congregation. When nests of melanocytes are confined entirely to the epidermis (and epithelial structures of adnexa) and particularly to the dermo-epidermal junction, the condition is termed a "junctional nevus." When, in time, as new nests continue to originate at the dermo-epidermal junction and melanocytes of a junctional nevus descend

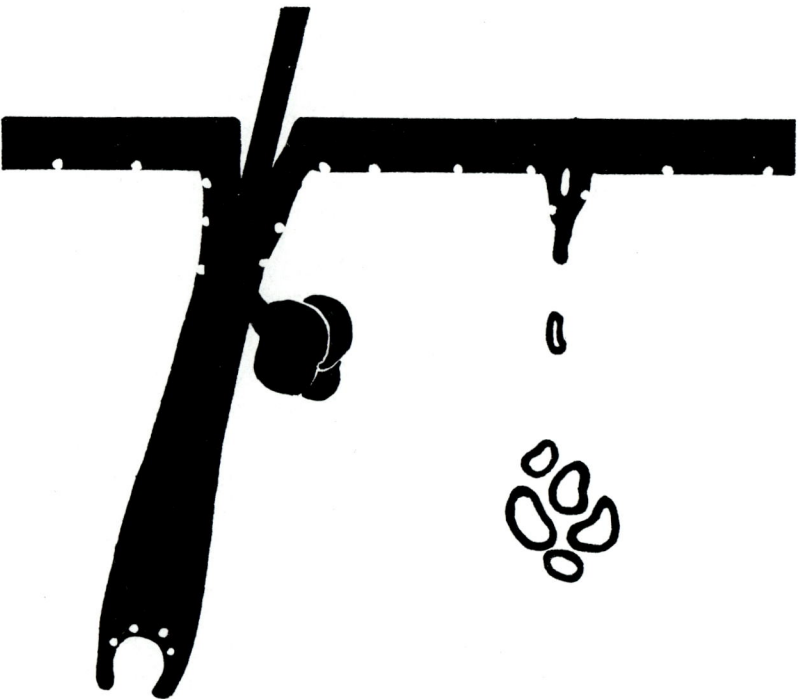

Fig. 2. Localization of melanocytes in normal skin. Melanocytes are found normally either in the basal layer of the epidermis or at the junction of the epidermis and dermis, the junction of the infundibular portion of hair follicles and the dermis, and the junction of the uppermost portion of eccrine dermal ducts and the dermis. Melanocytes also are present in bulbs near the base of follicles. Melanocytes at the dermo-epidermal junction are responsible for the color of skin, and melanocytes in follicular bulbs for the color of hair.

from the epidermis into the dermis, a compound nevus comes into being. Ultimately, when all of the melanocytes, arranged usually in nests, cords, and strands or a combination of them, are confined to the dermis, the nevus is designated intradermal (Fig. 3). This sequence unfolds in all four types of acquired nevi (Unna's, Miescher's, Spitz's, and Clark's) and in types of congenital nevi, other than blue nevi.* Ten cytologic types of melanocytes constitute acquired and congenital nevi (and melanomas, too): small round, large round, pagetoid, balloon, polygonal, oval, spindle, dendritic, wavy, and multinucleate (Fig. 4). Any of these cytologic types of melanocytes may monopolize a nevus or combine with other cytologic types within a nevus.

2. Proliferation of melanocytes mostly within the dermis from the outset. The epidermis usually is spared, some of the melanocytes within the dermis are bipolar dendritic and pigmented markedly by melanin (Fig. 5), and there are practically no discrete conventional nests of melanocytes, although there may be fascicles of melanocytes. This pattern is specific for blue nevi, which are congenital nevi. Although blue nevi generally are confined to the reticular dermis, melanocytes that compose them may be present in the subcutaneous fat and deeper and, uncommonly, even in the capsules of lymph nodes. The connective tissue in the dermis of blue nevi may be unaffected by the proliferation of melanocytes, or it may be collagenized strikingly, i.e., collagen bundles contiguous with dendritic melanocytes may be thickened markedly. Traditionally, blue nevi have been classified as either common or cellular, but that classification is flawed seriously. For example, the terms "common" and "cellular" are not contrasting ("common" should be apposed by "uncommon" and "cellular" by "acellular"). Furthermore, common blue nevi also are cellular, i.e., they comprise numerous deeply pigmented bipolar dendritic melanocytes. Last, several types of blue nevi cannot be categorized as either "common" or "cellular."

---

*The designations "acquired" and "congenital" are artificial even if they may be convenient for purposes of classification. Nevi named "congenital" usually, but surely not always, are visible readily on the skin at birth. Those termed "acquired" are not apparent at birth. The melanocytes that constitute the latter, however, must have been present in the skin from the time of parturition; almost certainly, those melanocytes did not migrate to the skin after birth. In that sense, "acquired" melanocytic nevi are actually tardive types of congenital melanocytic nevi. In any event, the classic "congenital" and "acquired" types of nevi differ from one another clinically, histopathologically, and biologically.

Parenthetically, blue nevi are not always blue clinically. Some are gray, others are black, and still others are brown. Only exceedingly rarely does a melanoma arise in a pre-existing blue nevus.

For practical purposes, blue nevi are found mostly in the skin, but they have been recorded also on the ocular, nasal, and oral mucous membranes, and in the lymph nodes, vagina, cervix, ovaries, prostate, spermatic cord, and maxillary sinus.

In conclusion, a melanocytic nevus is a proliferation of melanocytes that may be limited to the epidermis (junctional) or the dermis (intradermal) or be present at both sites (compound). Nevi may appear at sites other than the skin, such as conjunctiva, oral mucous membranes, and lymph nodes. Ten cytologic types of melanocytes are the building blocks of nevi. Because nevi are completely benign, they evolve for a time and then cease growing perceptibly. The clinical, histopathologic, and biologic attributes of nevi are diametric to those of melanoma.

B. Congenital Nevi

Congenital nevi tend to be larger, usually dramatically larger, than acquired nevus (Fig. 6). An exception is Clark's acquired nevus that may attain several centimeters in diameter in those rare individuals who have an impressive family history of melanoma or a personal history of one and sometimes several melanomas.

Attempts have been made to classify congenital nevi according to size, e.g., less than 1.5 cm for *small* congenital nevi, 1.5 to 19.9 cm for *intermediate* congenital nevi, and 20.0 cm or more for *large* congenital nevi. Thus far, efforts to classify congenital nevi by size have failed because the classification is arbitrary and not based upon correlation of clinical and histopathologic findings, or of those two findings with biologic considerations. We classify congenital nevi morphologically as blue and non-blue (Tables 1 and 2), and categorize them further as superficial and deep according to histopathologic attributes.

A classification of congenital nevi into blue and non-blue types turns upon definition of blue nevus, a determination that is arbitrary and imperfect. Two thorny problems that concern blue nevi can be expressed as questions: "What is a blue nevus?" and "Are blue nevi congenital, acquired, or both?"

Text continues on page 10

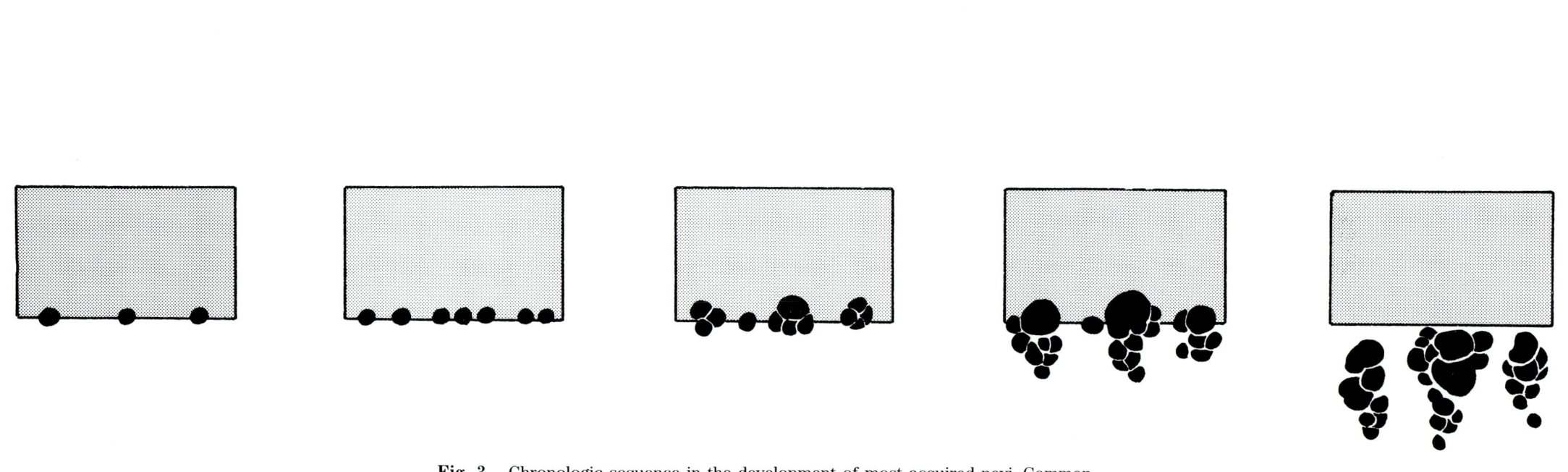

Fig. 3. Chronologic sequence in the development of most acquired nevi. Common acquired nevi, such as those named eponymically for Unna, Miescher, Spitz, and Clark, begin their development in normal skin *(extreme left)* where melanocytes are arranged as solitary units at the dermo-epidermal junction. In time, the melanocytes proliferate as solitary units at the dermo-epidermal junction, and some of them congregate into small nests that are present at the dermo-epidermal junction, but usually not above it (except for some Spitz's nevi). Later, nests of melanocytes at the dermo-epidermal junction enlarge, and some melanocytes disposed as solitary units and in nests there descend into the dermis. After many years, all of the melanocytes of the nevus have spilled into the dermis *(far right)*. Illustrated, in chronologic sequence, are melanocytes in normal skin, melanocytes in a simple lentigo, melanocytes in a junctional nevus, melanocytes in a compound nevus, and melanocytes in an intradermal nevus. As may be inferred, a simple lentigo is a stage in the evolution of a junctional nevus.

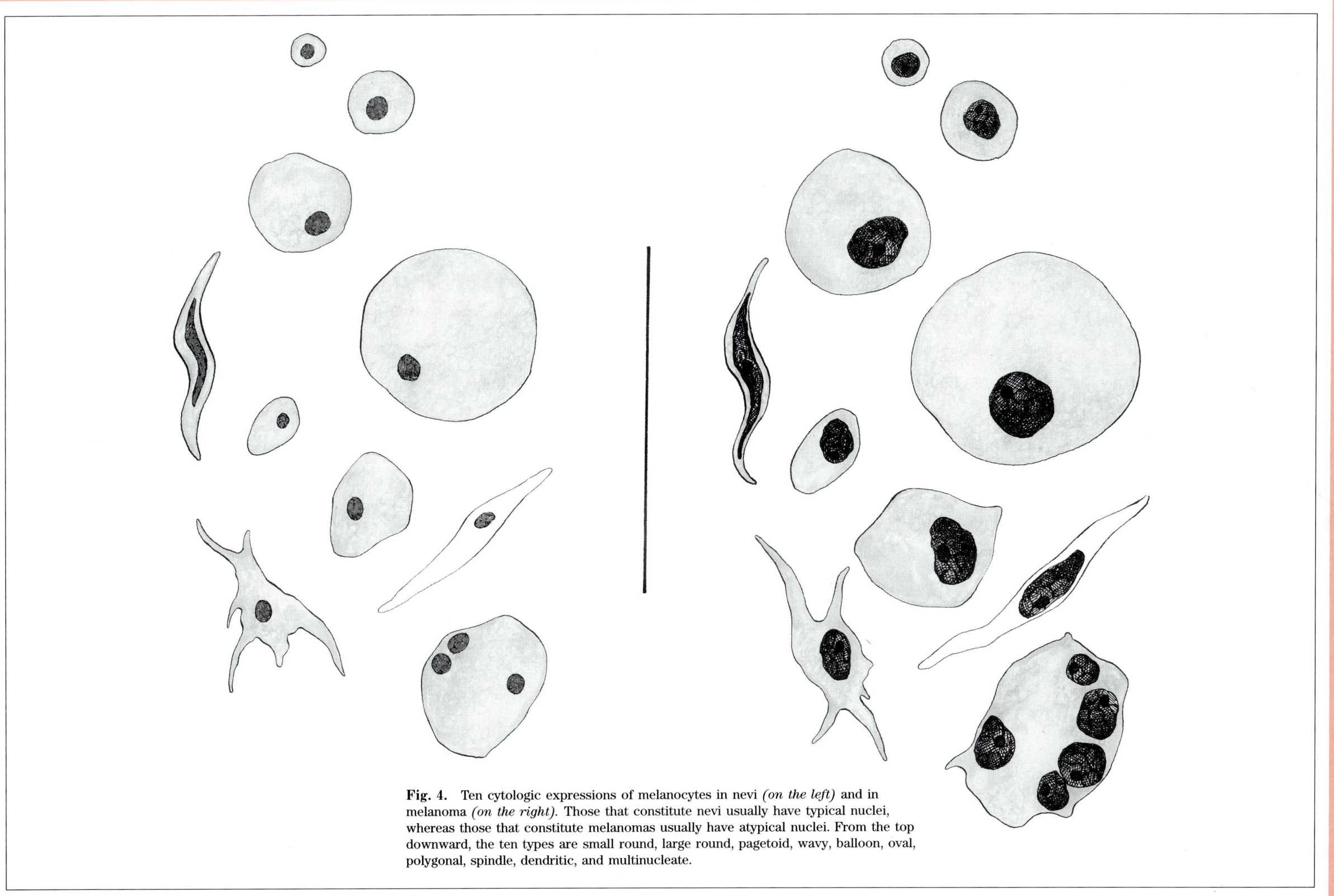

Fig. 4. Ten cytologic expressions of melanocytes in nevi *(on the left)* and in melanoma *(on the right)*. Those that constitute nevi usually have typical nuclei, whereas those that constitute melanomas usually have atypical nuclei. From the top downward, the ten types are small round, large round, pagetoid, wavy, balloon, oval, polygonal, spindle, dendritic, and multinucleate.

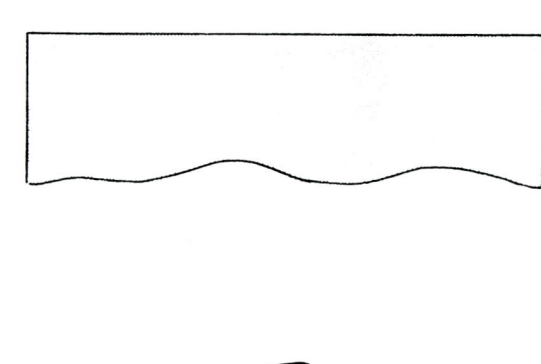
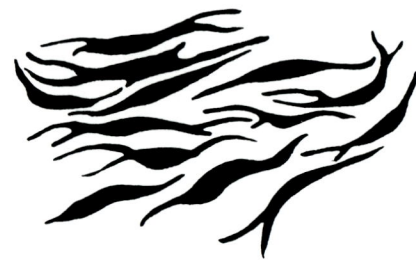

Fig. 5. Silhouette of one type of blue nevus. Blue nevi are congenital, usually tardive, and wholly intradermal. They do not progress from junctional to compound stages; in fact, there are no junctional nests. The melanocytes that constitute them reside in the dermis (and sometimes subcutaneous fat) from the outset and some of them are markedly pigmented, bipolar, and dendritic. Collagen bundles associated with a blue nevus may be unaffected by the proliferation of melanocytes, or they may be strikingly thickened. In short, the chronologic sequence of a blue nevus differs from that of Unna's, Miescher's, Spitz's, or Clark's nevus, as does the absence of discrete nests of melanocytes so characteristic of those four acquired nevi.

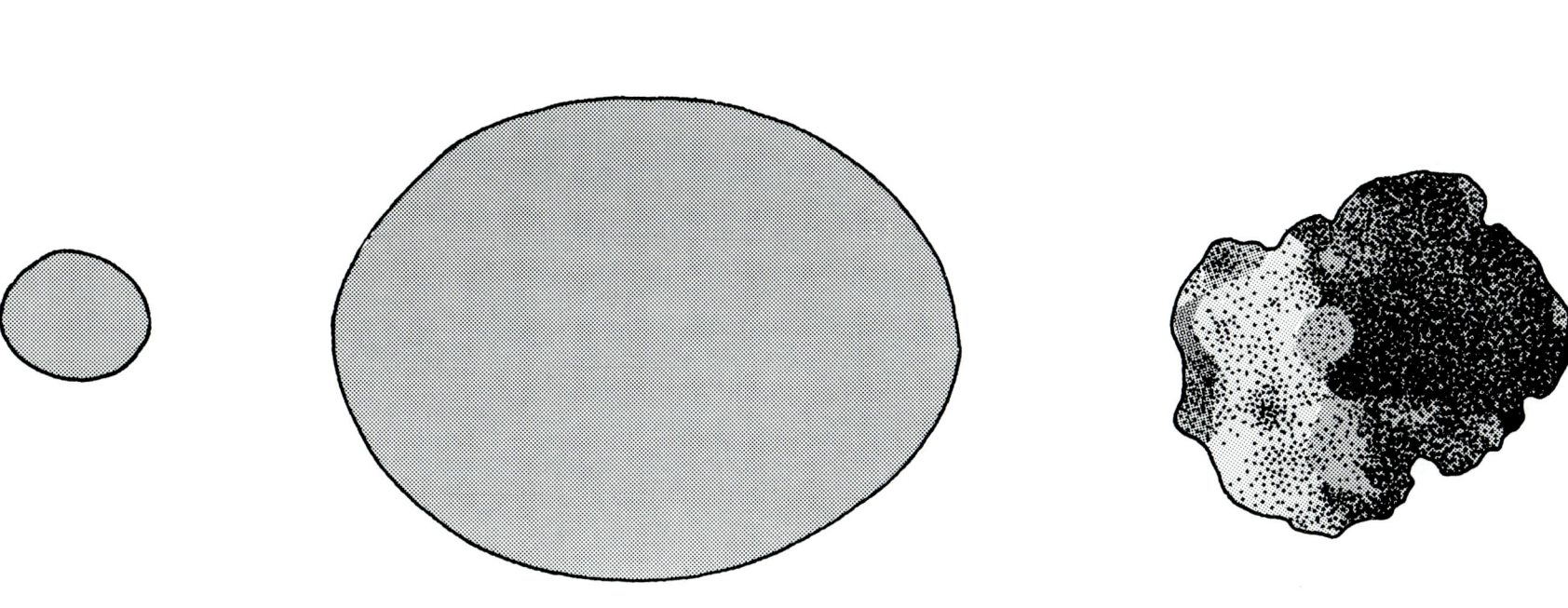

Fig. 6. Silhouettes and distributions of pigment in an acquired nevus, a congenital nevus, and a melanoma. In general, acquired nevi, as seen on the left, are small, symmetric, well-circumscribed with smooth margins, and uniform in pigment. In contrast, a superficial congenital nevus is usually larger than an acquired nevus, but it, too, is symmetric, well-circumscribed by smooth margins, and relatively uniform in color. An acquired melanocytic nevus often is ovoid, pyramidal, or otherwise geometric, and congenital nevi are even more varied in shape. In contrast to acquired and congenital nevi of all kinds, a melanoma is overtly asymmetric, circumscribed by scalloped, notched, or jagged borders, and variegated in color, ranging from fawn to black, from red to blue, and even white in foci. There are exceptions to each of these generalizations.

TABLE 1. Histopathologic Classification of Non-blue Congenital Nevi

A. Superficial
1. Angiocentric and adnexocentric distribution of melanocytes mostly
2. Melanocytes splayed focally between collagen bundles in the upper half of the reticular dermis

B. Deep
1. Melanocytes often in band-like distribution in the upper part
2. Diffuse distribution of melanocytes in the lower part throughout the reticular dermis at least

---

A blue nevus is a proliferation of melanocytes, some of which must be heavily pigmented, bipolar, and dendritic, in the reticular dermis and sometimes in the subcutaneous fat (and rarely as solitary units in the epidermis), but which do not form conventional nests of melanocytes.

Most blue nevi are acquired in the sense that they are not apparent clinically at birth. All blue nevi, however, must be congenital, i.e., the responsible melanocytes in the dermis (and subcutaneous fat) had to have been present at those sites in utero. Unlike those melanocytic nevi that begin with proliferation of melanocytes at the dermo-epidermal junction, from whence melanocytes presumably spill into the dermis, blue nevi do not develop at that junction. In fact, there are no nests of melanocytes at all within the epidermis of blue nevi. In short, so-called acquired blue nevi represent tardive forms, i.e., delayed manifestations, of congenital blue nevi. That conclusion seems to be particularly justified for those blue nevi known colloquially as nevi of Ota and Ito. About half of all nevi of Ota and Ito are present at birth, the others being delayed from weeks to decades before becoming apparent. Clinically and histopathologically, there are no differences between the congenital and "acquired" expressions of Ota's and Ito's nevi. Clinically, they are bluish patches, and histopathologically they consist of markedly pigmented, bipolar, dendritic melanocytes arranged entirely as solitary units and scattered widely throughout the dermis and sometimes the upper part of the subcutaneous fat.

TABLE 2. Histopathologic Classification of Blue Nevi

A. Superficial (with or without collagenization or neurotization)
1. Dendritic melanocytes
   a. Band-like, in tangles
   b. Wedge-shaped, in tangles
2. Predominantly dendritic melanocytes
   a. Band-like
   b. Wedge-shaped, diffuse and/or interstitial
3. Predominantly non-dendritic melanocytes
   a. Band-like, diffuse or fascicular
   b. Wedge-shaped, diffuse or fascicular

B. Deep (with or without collagenization or neurotization)
1. Dendritic melanocytes
   a. Multifocal, in tangles
   b. Multifocal, solitary units
2. Predominantly dendritic melanocytes
   a. Multifocal
   b. Bulbous
3. Predominantly non-dendritic melanocytes
   a. Multifocal
   b. Bulbous

All congenital nevi that do not fulfill histopathologic criteria for blue nevi qualify as non-blue congenital nevi. Both blue and non-blue congenital nevi may be classified further as superficial and deep types based upon observations made of them histopathologically, usually at scanning magnification (Tables 1, 2). In brief, when assessed at scanning power, most melanocytes in superficial congenital nevi are situated above the mid-reticular dermis (although some may be present focally in the lower half of the reticular dermis) (Figs. 7, 8). In deep congenital nevi, in contrast, melanocytes are present throughout the entire reticular dermis and often in widened septa in the subcutaneous fat (and, at times, in fat lobules, walls of large vessels, fascia, skeletal muscle, and even in deep tissues) (Figs. 9, 10). Sometimes, in deep congenital nevi, there may be only a sprinkling of melanocytes in the lower part of the reticular dermis and septa of the subcutaneous fat, but it is the extent of distribution of the melanocytes, not the quantity of them, that determines whether a congenital nevus is considered by us to be superficial or deep. Deep congenital nevi involve nearly the entire reticular dermis; superficial ones do not come close to that.

In addition to entirely different distributions of melanocytes in superficial and deep types of congenital nevi, the patterns formed by melanocytes in congenital nevi also are varied. In brief, those patterns in blue nevi can be described generally as band-like, wedge-shaped, multifocal (solitary units and in tangles), and bulbous. In contrast, melanocytes in non-blue

Text continues on page 15

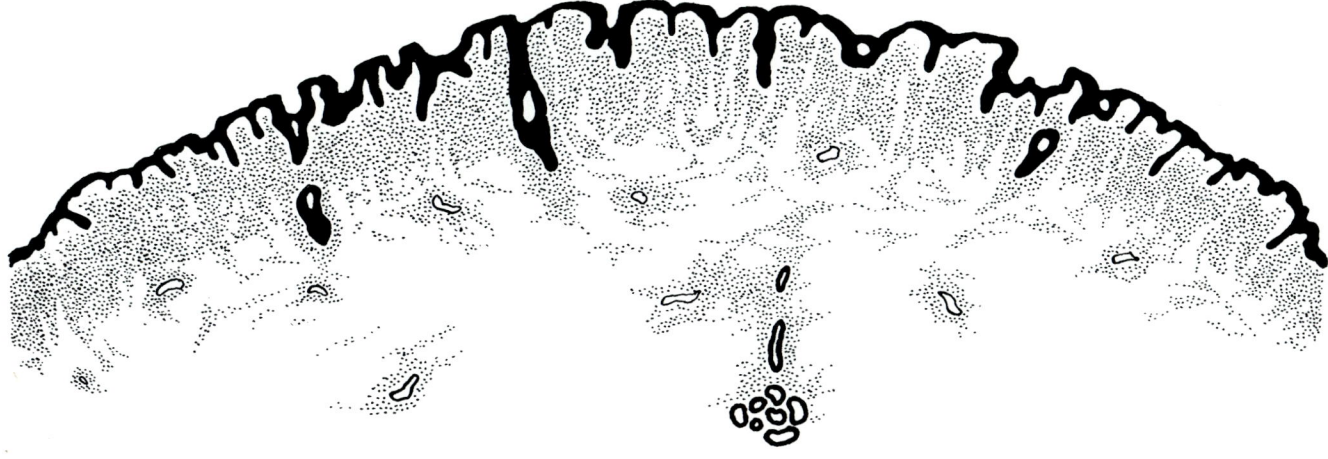

Fig. 7. Superficial congenital nevus (non-blue). This drawing depicts one of several histopathologic patterns of superficial congenital nevi. The lesion is broad, symmetric, and characterized by a band-like infiltrate of melanocytes in the upper part of the dermis and by melanocytes in the upper and mid-portion of the reticular dermis that are splayed between bundles of collagen, encircle blood vessels, and are arrayed around, and sometimes within, epithelial and non-epithelial structures of adnexa.

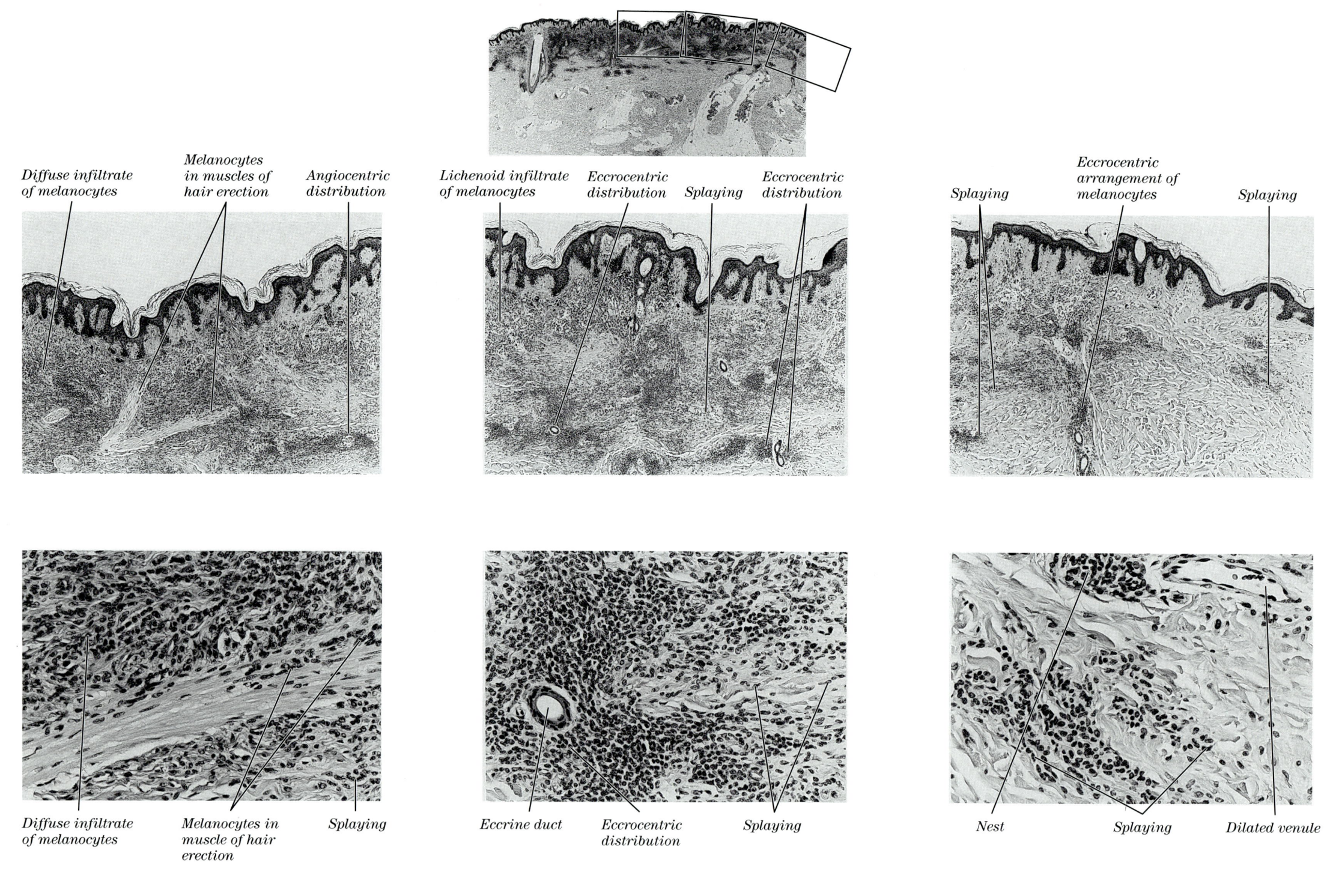

8 • Congenital Nevus *(superficial type)*

Criteria for diagnosis of this non-blue congenital nevus (superficial type)

This is a nevus because:

1. The neoplasm is relatively symmetric.
2. It is relatively well-circumscribed.
3. Melanocytes within the epidermis are situated at the dermo-epidermal junction, not above it.
4. There is maturation of melanocytes.

This is a non-blue superficial congenital nevus because:

1. Most melanocytes are positioned above the mid-reticular dermis.
2. Melanocytes in the reticular dermis are arrayed in angiocentric fashion.
3. Melanocytes in the reticular dermis are distributed in eccrocentric manner.
4. Some melanocytes arranged as solitary units are present within muscles of hair erection.
5. Melanocytes are splayed between collagen bundles in foci in the upper half of the reticular dermis.

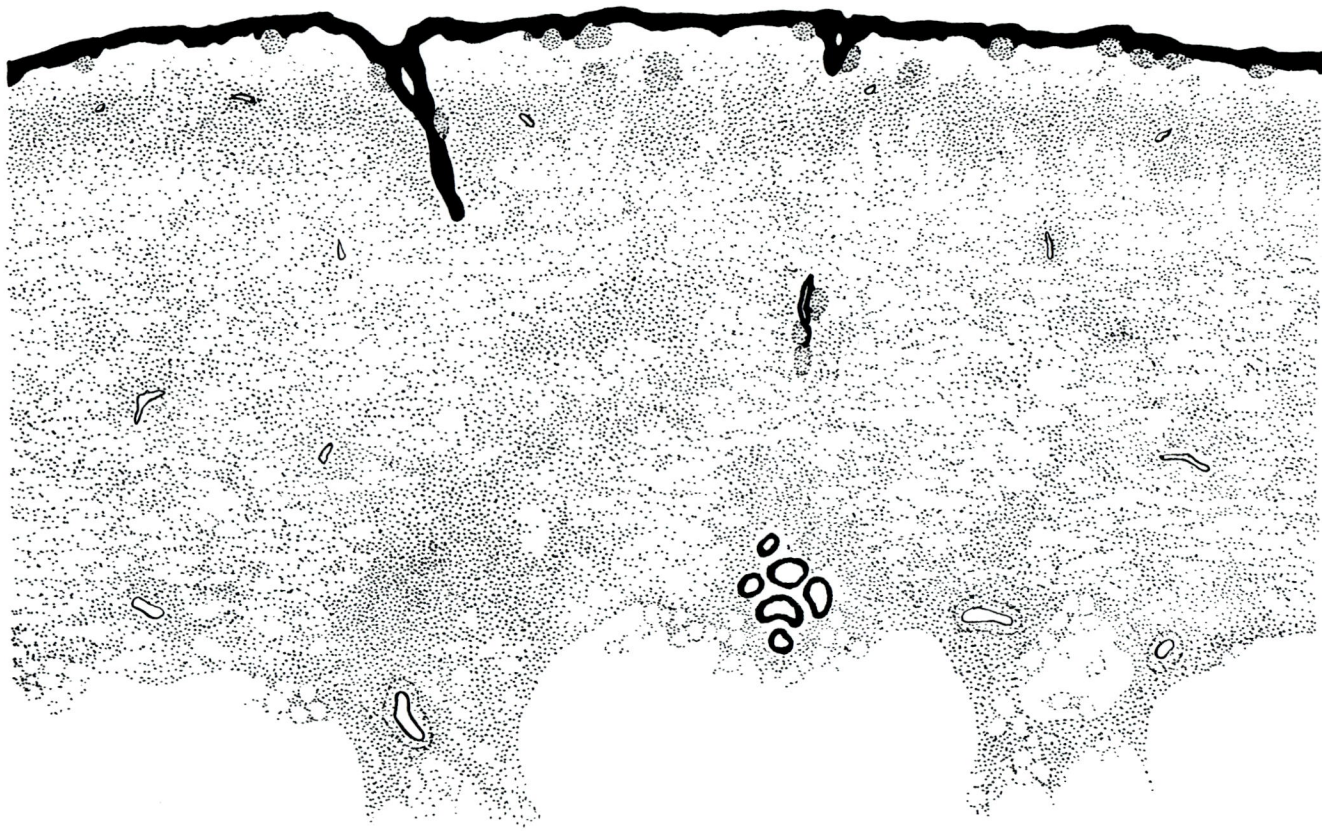

Fig. 9. Deep congenital nevus (non-blue). Histopathologically, this deep type of non-blue congenital nevus is characterized by a dense, diffuse infiltrate of melanocytes that extends throughout the entire reticular dermis and far into septa in the subcutaneous fat. Nests of melanocytes are situated at the dermo-epidermal junction and reach far down epithelial structures of adnexa, namely, hair follicles and eccrine ducts. Note the striking differences between a deep congenital nevus, such as this one, and the superficial congenital nevus shown in Fig. 7.

superficial congenital nevi are aligned along venules and along both epithelial and non-epithelial structures of adnexa (angio-adnexocentric pattern). Nests of melanocytes also are present within the substance of epithelial (e.g., sebaceous glands and eccrine ducts) and non-epithelial (e.g., nerve fascicles and muscles of hair erection) structures of adnexa (Fig. 11). In addition, some melanocytes nearly always are splayed in strands between bundles of collagen in discrete foci in the upper half of the reticular dermis. In contrast, melanocytes in non-blue deep congenital nevi are scattered diffusely throughout the entire reticular dermis and frequently throughout at least the upper part of fibrous septa in the subcutaneous fat. There are neither angio-adnexocentricity nor splaying of melanocytes in distinct foci within the reticular dermis. Melanocytes may be found in variable numbers within the walls of large vessels in the subcutaneous fat and as clusters in subendothelial position in lymphatics and smaller blood vessels within the dermis. Nests of melanocytes may pepper lobules in the subcutaneous fat. The proliferation of melanocytes within the epidermis, epithelial structures of adnexa, and non-epithelial structures of adnexa is nowhere near as striking as it is in superficial congenital nevi.

Histopathologic characteristics of superficial and deep types of non-blue congenital nevi correlate well with clinical attributes of those types. In general, superficial types are flattish, light brown, and devoid of a blanket of terminal hairs (although some may be papillated and terminal hairs may spring from them). Deep types are elevated, dark brown, and blanketed by dark terminal hairs. Superficial types tend to be smaller than deep types, but the former may be very large and the latter very small. The stereotype of the superficial type is nevus spilus (congenital speckled lentiginous nevus) and of the deep type giant hairy nevus. The latter, often grotesque, congenital nevus may be so widespread as to be nearly universal, it may cover part or all of an extremity (so-called garment nevi), and it may come in any size or shape, including tiny, as is the case for some "satellite" nevi. "Satellite" nevi are small, sometimes tiny congenital nevi of various shapes present in conjunction with a widespread giant hairy nevus. The histopathologic findings in all of these dark hairy congenital nevi, irrespective of size, are basically those of one pattern, i.e., deep type of non-blue congenital nevus.

Blue nevus was described first in 1906 by Max Tièche, then a student of Josef Jadassohn. It usually presents itself clinically as a macule that tends to become a papule and, episodically, a nodule. As has been stated already, patches of blue nevi in the forms of nevi of Ota and Ito may appear many years after birth on the face and trunk, respectively, although presence at birth is just as common. Presence at or near birth is the rule for mongolian spot (patch). A papule of a blue nevus characteristically is domed, sharply circumscribed, and bluish in most instances. At scanning magnification, the neoplasm, like benign neoplasms in general, is symmetric. A requisite for histopathologic diagnosis of blue nevus is the presence in the reticular dermis of some prominently pigmented, bipolar, dendritic melanocytes (Figs. 5, 12), although that criterion alone is not sufficient because melanocytes of that character may be noted infrequently in Spitz's nevi and invariably in "deep penetrating nevus." In some lesions, the dendritic melanocytes are the sole constituent of the nevus (Fig. 13); in others, oval melanocytes predominate overwhelmingly (Fig. 14), and in others still dendritic and oval melanocytes are present in about equal numbers. Presumably, oval melanocytes in a blue nevus are those that have lost their dendrites. Melanophages are invariable accompaniments of a blue nevus, but their numbers vary greatly. In some lesions, melanophages are so numerous that they obscure melanocytes. In blue nevi in general, epithelial and non-epithelial structures of adnexa are spared by the proliferation of melanocytes (Fig. 15). By convention, blue nevi in which markedly pigmented, bipolar, dendritic melanocytes predominate overwhelmingly have been designated "common," and those in which fascicles of oval melanocytes are dominant have been termed "cellular." As already has been stated, the appellations "common" and "cellular" not only are inaccurate, but also they fail to encompass many expressions of blue nevi.

The numerous histopathologic expressions of blue nevus are reflections of the cytologic type or types of melanocytes, number of melanocytes, presence or absence of collagenization (crowded thickened bundles of collagen in proximity with the proliferation of melanocytes) (Fig. 16), distribution of melanocytes in the epidermis, dermis, and subcutaneous fat, and arrangement of melanocytes either as solitary units, in fascicles, or both. Except for instances of combined blue nevi, i.e., a blue nevus concurrent with features of an Unna's, Miescher's, Spitz's, or Clark's nevus in a single biopsy specimen (Fig. 17), blue nevi do not contain discrete nests of melanocytes, unlike the situation in other types of nevi. Although one expression of blue nevus consists of oval melanocytes arranged in fascicles, and another of oval melanocytes in roundish aggregations that are encircled by a diffuse infiltrate of strikingly pigmented bipolar dendritic melanocytes, dis-

Text continues on page 32

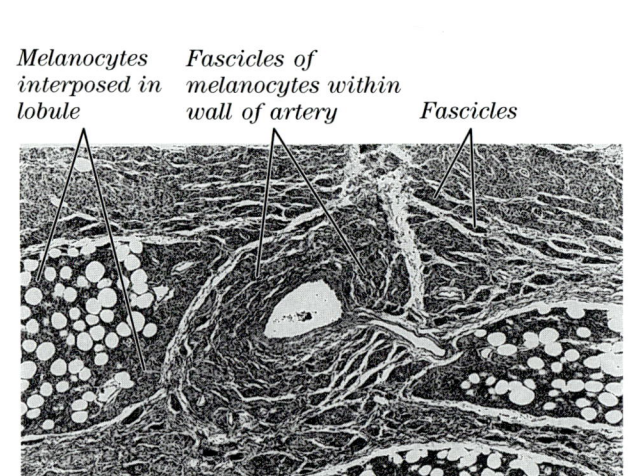

10 · Congenital Nevus *(deep type)*

Criteria for diagnosis of this non-blue congenital nevus (deep type)

This is a nevus because:

1. The neoplasm is relatively symmetric.
2. Melanocytes within the epidermis, both those arranged as solitary units and those in nests, are situated at the dermo-epidermal junction, not above it.
3. Melanin is distributed mostly in the upper portion of the lesion.
4. Melanocytes mature.

This is a non-blue deep congenital nevus because:

1. Monomorphous melanocytes are distributed diffusely throughout the reticular dermis and within septa and lobules of the subcutaneous fat.
2. The neoplasm is very broad.
3. Nests of melanocytes are present within the wall of a vein.
4. Signs of neural differentiation of melanocytes are present in the subcutaneous fat.

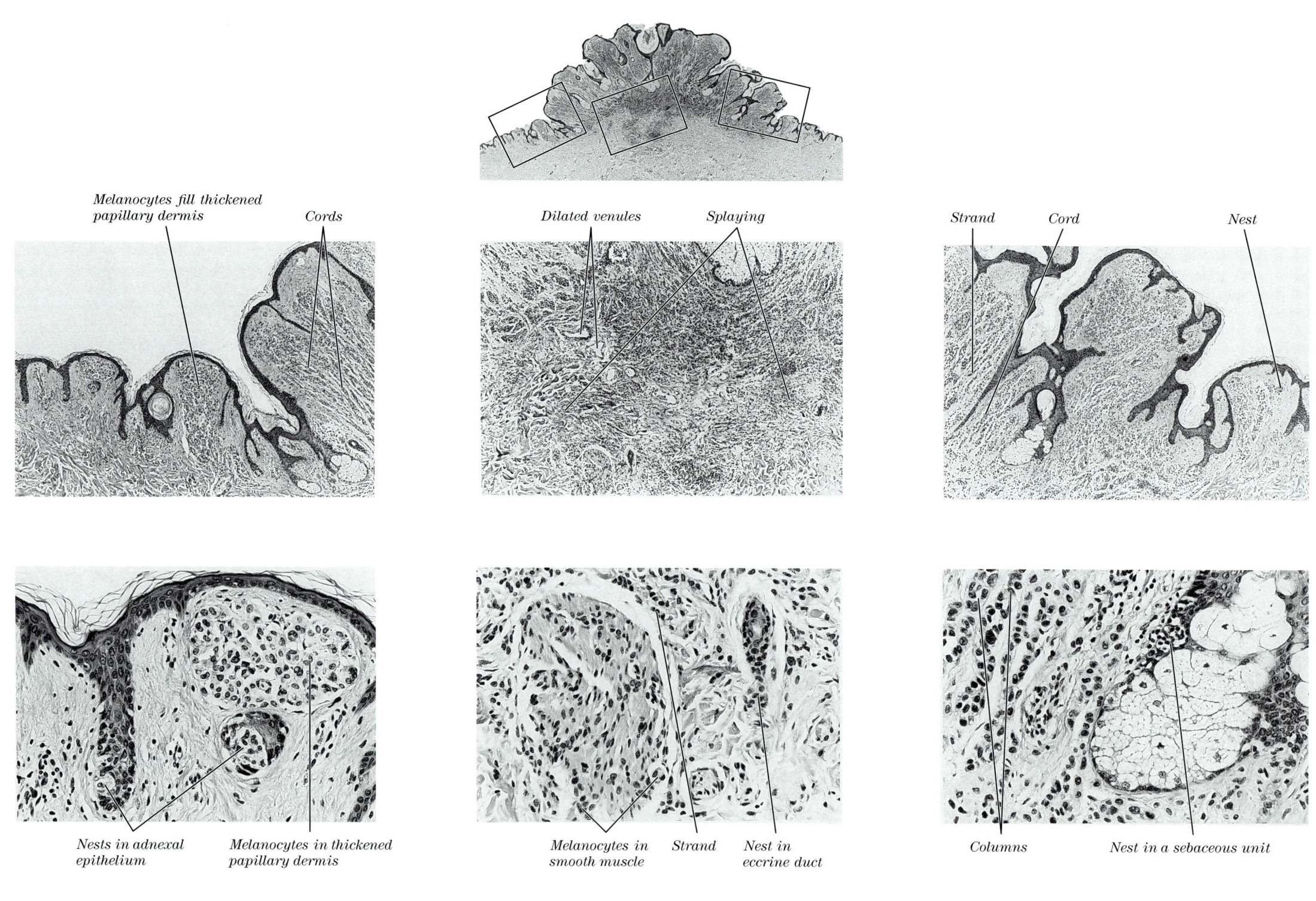

11 • Congenital Nevus *(superficial type)*

Criteria for diagnosis of this non-blue congenital nevus (superficial type)

This is a nevus because:

1. The neoplasm is symmetric.
2. It is well-circumscribed.
3. Melanocytes mature.
4. Nuclei of melanocytes are relatively uniform.

This is a non-blue superficial congenital nevus because:

1. Most melanocytes are situated above the mid-reticular dermis.
2. Some nests of melanocytes are housed within infundibula, sebaceous lobules, and eccrine ducts.
3. Melanocytes are arranged as solitary units within muscles of hair erection.
4. Melanocytes are splayed between collagen bundles in foci in the upper part of the reticular dermis.

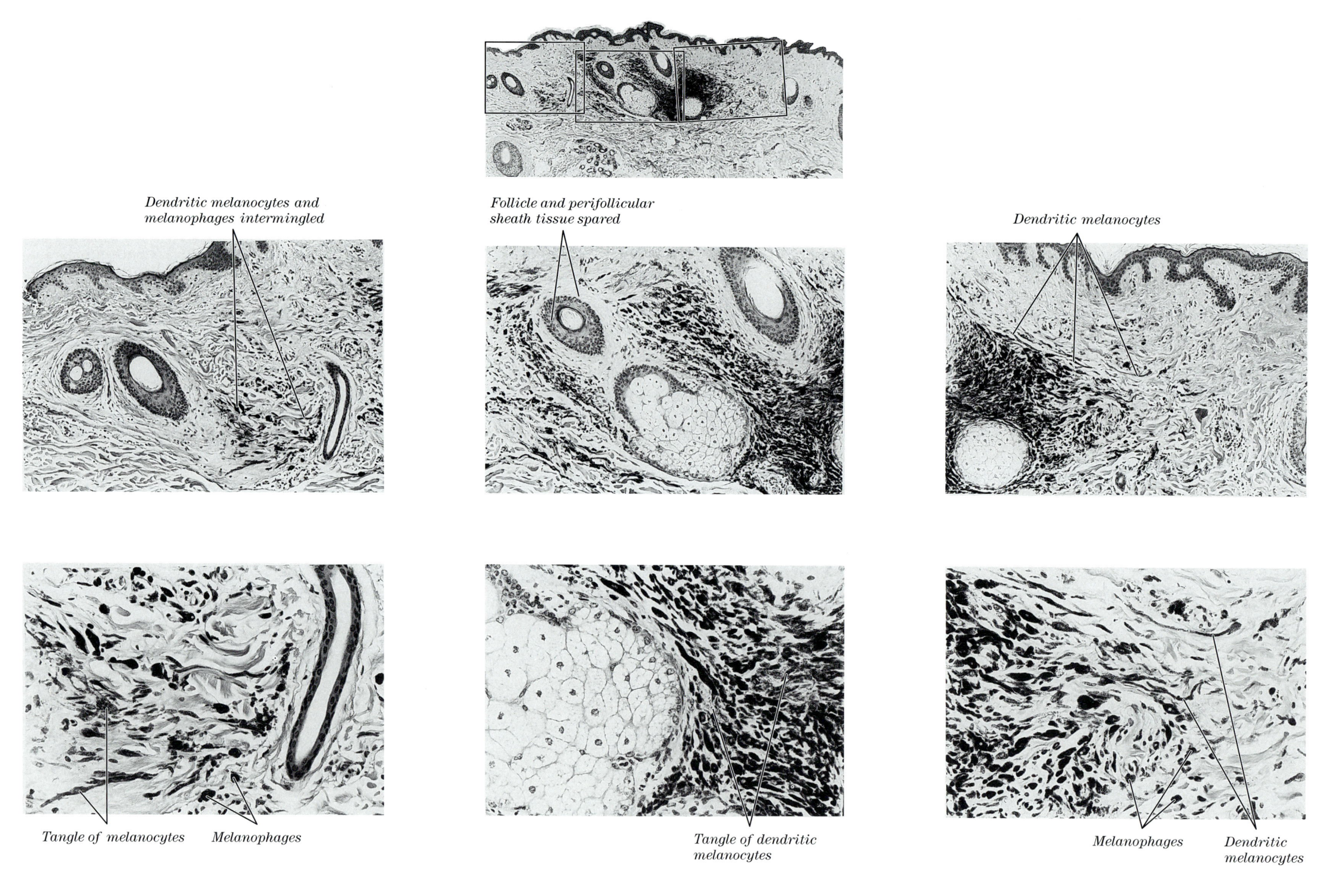

12 • Blue Nevus *(superficial dendritic type)*

Criteria for diagnosis of this blue nevus (superficial dendritic type)

This is a blue nevus because:

All of the neoplastic cells are markedly pigmented, strikingly bipolar, dendritic melanocytes.

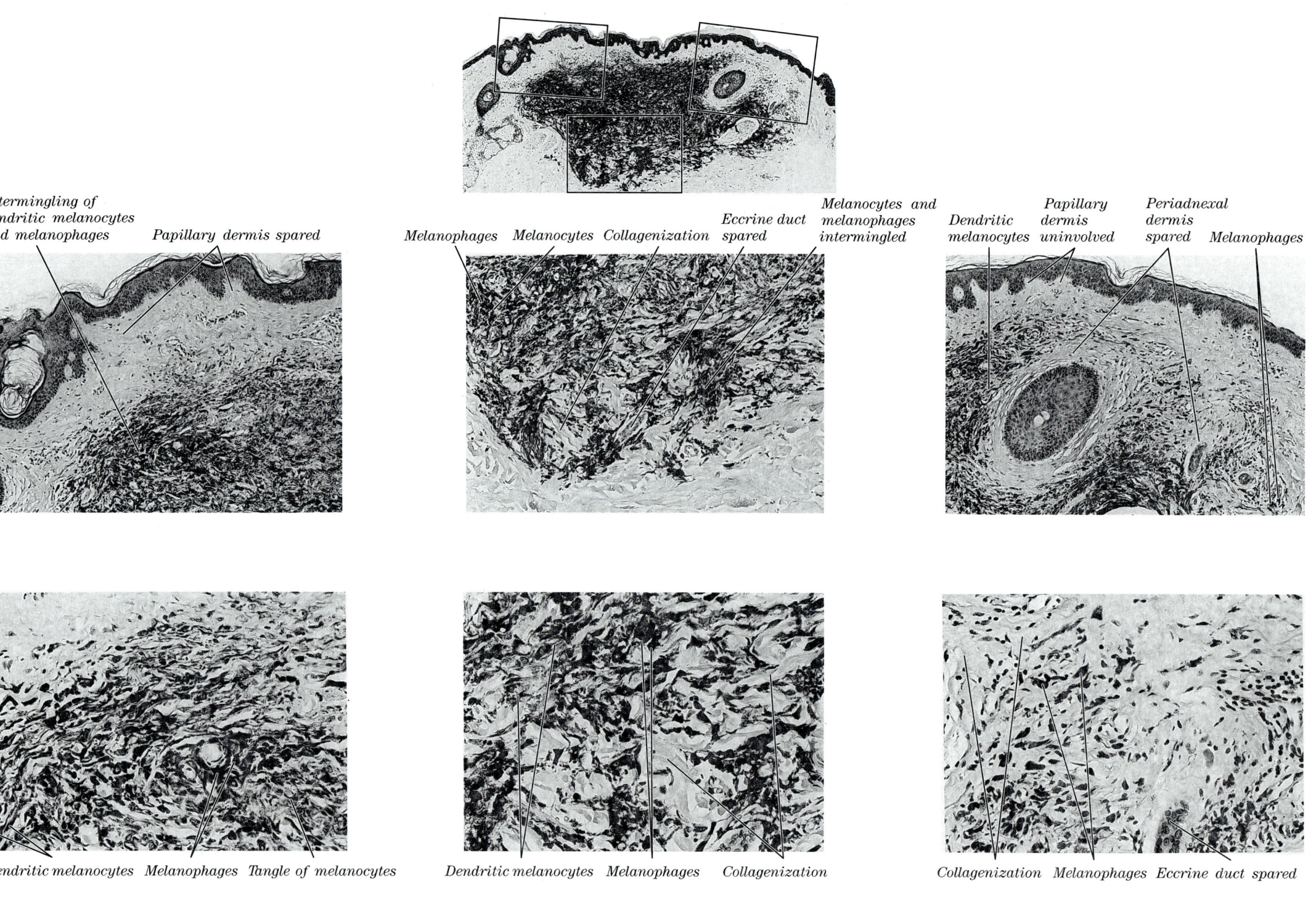

13 • Blue Nevus *(deep dendritic type)*

Criteria for diagnosis of this blue nevus (deep dendritic type)

1. Innumerable heavily pigmented bipolar dendritic melanocytes with typical nuclei are present throughout the dermis.
2. The neoplasm is well-circumscribed.
3. Neoplastic cells spare the epidermis.
4. Neoplastic cells spare epithelial and non-epithelial structures of adnexa.
5. Collagen bundles proximate to dendritic melanocytes are thickened.

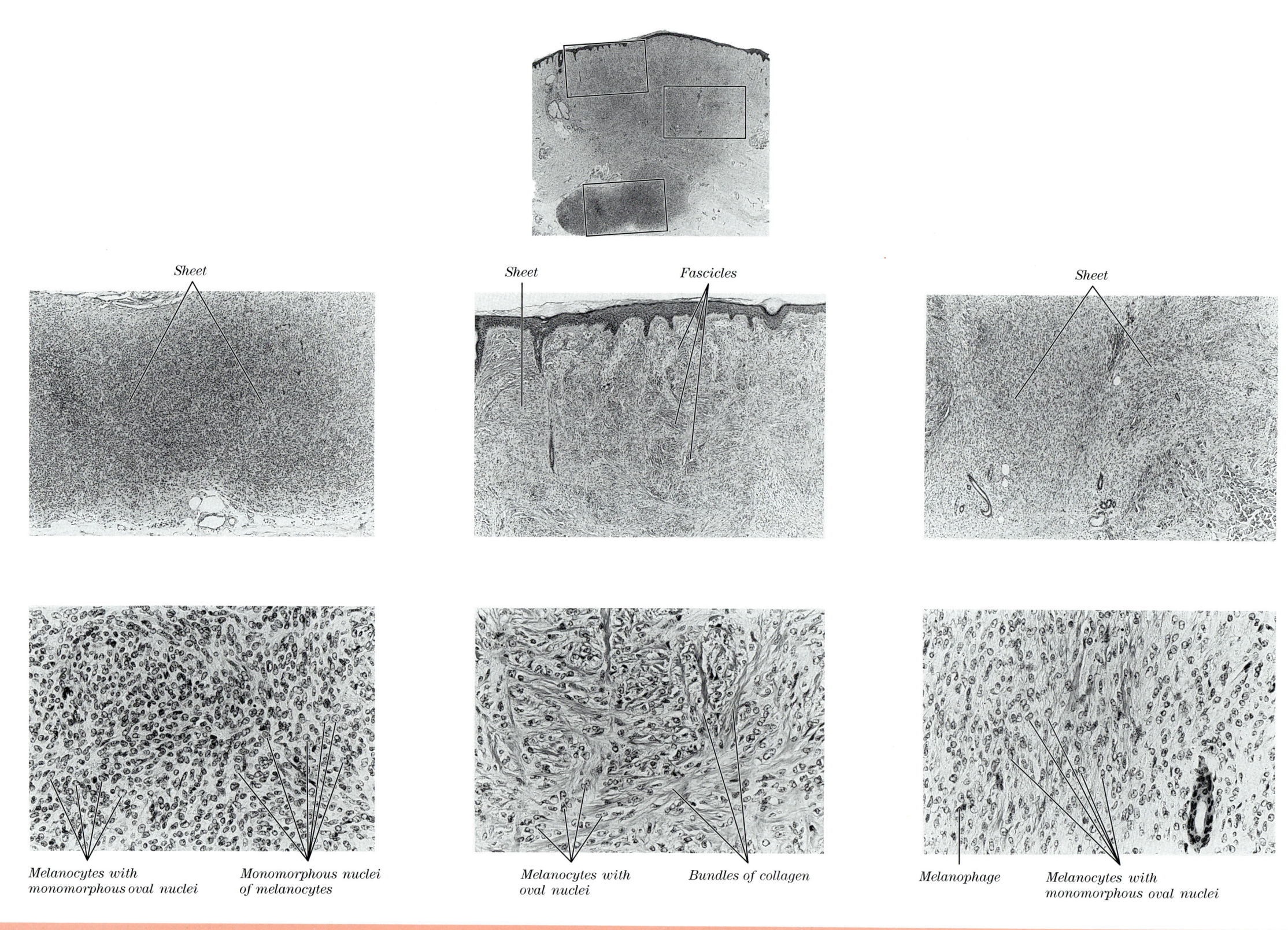

14 • Blue Nevus *(deep non-dendritic type)*

Criteria for diagnosis of this blue nevus (deep predominantly non-dendritic type)

This is a blue nevus because:

1. Some pigmented bipolar dendritic melanocytes are present within the benign proliferation of melanocytes.
2. There are no discrete nests of melanocytes in the dermis.
3. The epidermis is spared by the pathologic process.

This is a predominantly "oval-cell" type of blue nevus because:

Most melanocytes within this proliferation have an oval shape.

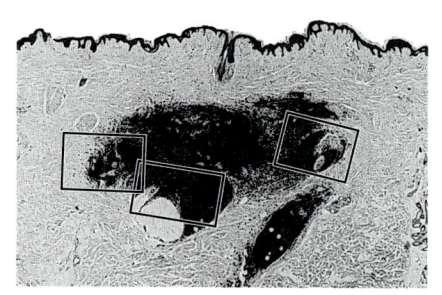

| Non-epithelial structures spared | Melanophages | Sheet of heavily pigmented melanocytes accompanied by melanophages | Sheet of dendritic melanocytes and melanophages | Dendritic melanocytes in a septum | Thickened bundles of collagen | Sheet of markedly pigmented dendritic melanocytes in concert with melanophages | Smooth muscle | Scattered pigmented dendritic melanocytes in muscles of hair erection | Many dendritic melanocytes and melanophages |

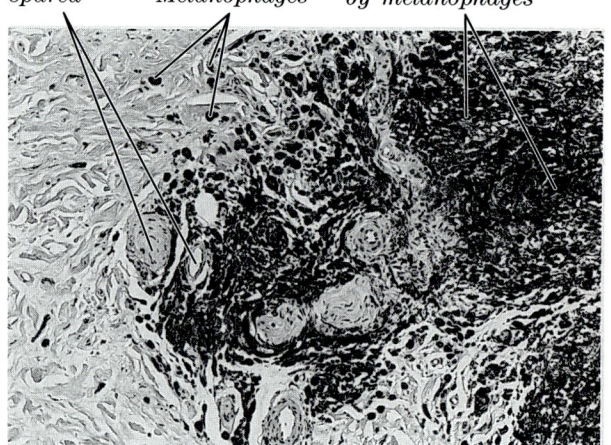
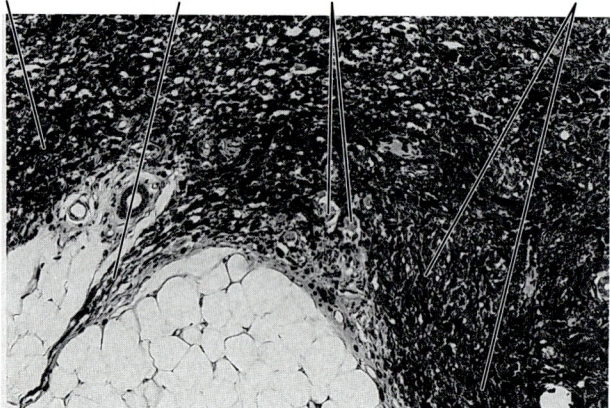
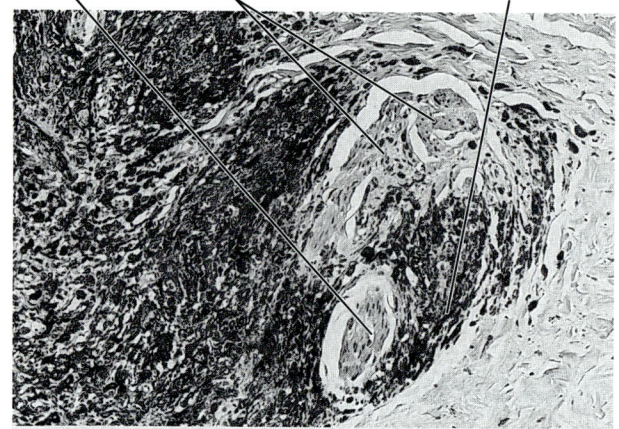

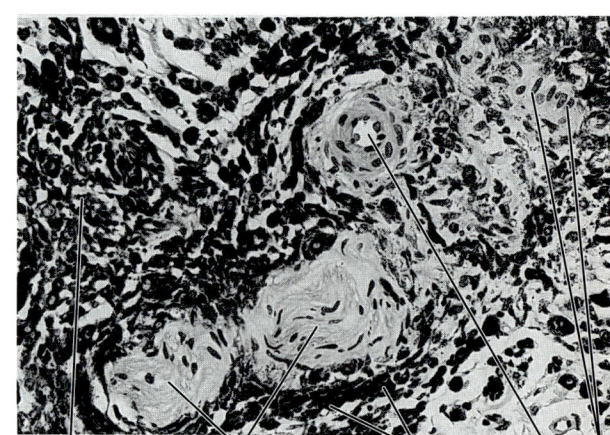
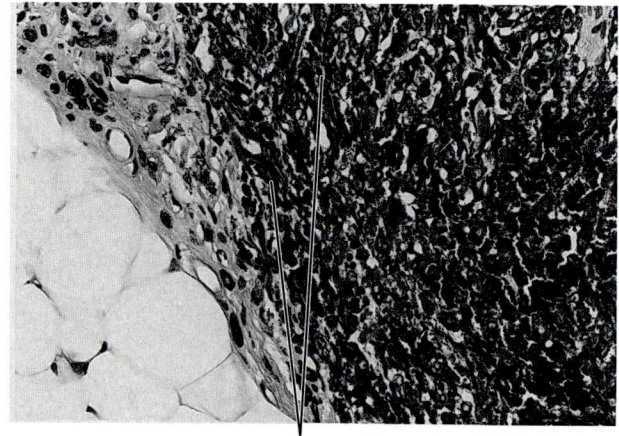
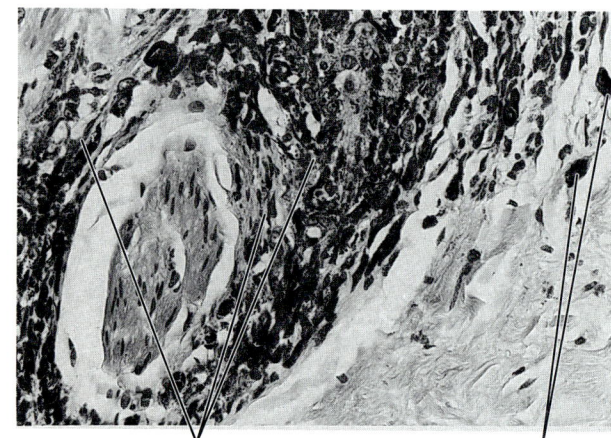

| Dendritic melanocytes | Nerve fascicles spared | Melanophages | Blood vessel | Oval melanocytes | Tangle of heavily pigmented dendritic melanocytes intermingled with melanophages | Dendritic melanocytes surround a muscle of hair erection | Melanophages |

15 · Blue Nevus (*deep dendritic type*)

Criteria for diagnosis of this blue nevus (deep dendritic type)

This is a nevus because:

1. The neoplasm is very small, approximately 3.0 mm in greatest diameter.

2. It has a wedge shape.

3. Neoplastic melanocytes spare epithelial and non-epithelial structures of adnexa.

4. Melanin in melanocytes and macrophages is distributed in relatively uniform fashion throughout the neoplasm.

This is a blue nevus because:

1. Heavily pigmented bipolar dendritic melanocytes predominate within the neoplasm.

2. Numerous melanophages are present in association with dendritic melanocytes.

3. The epidermis and epithelial structures of adnexa are spared.

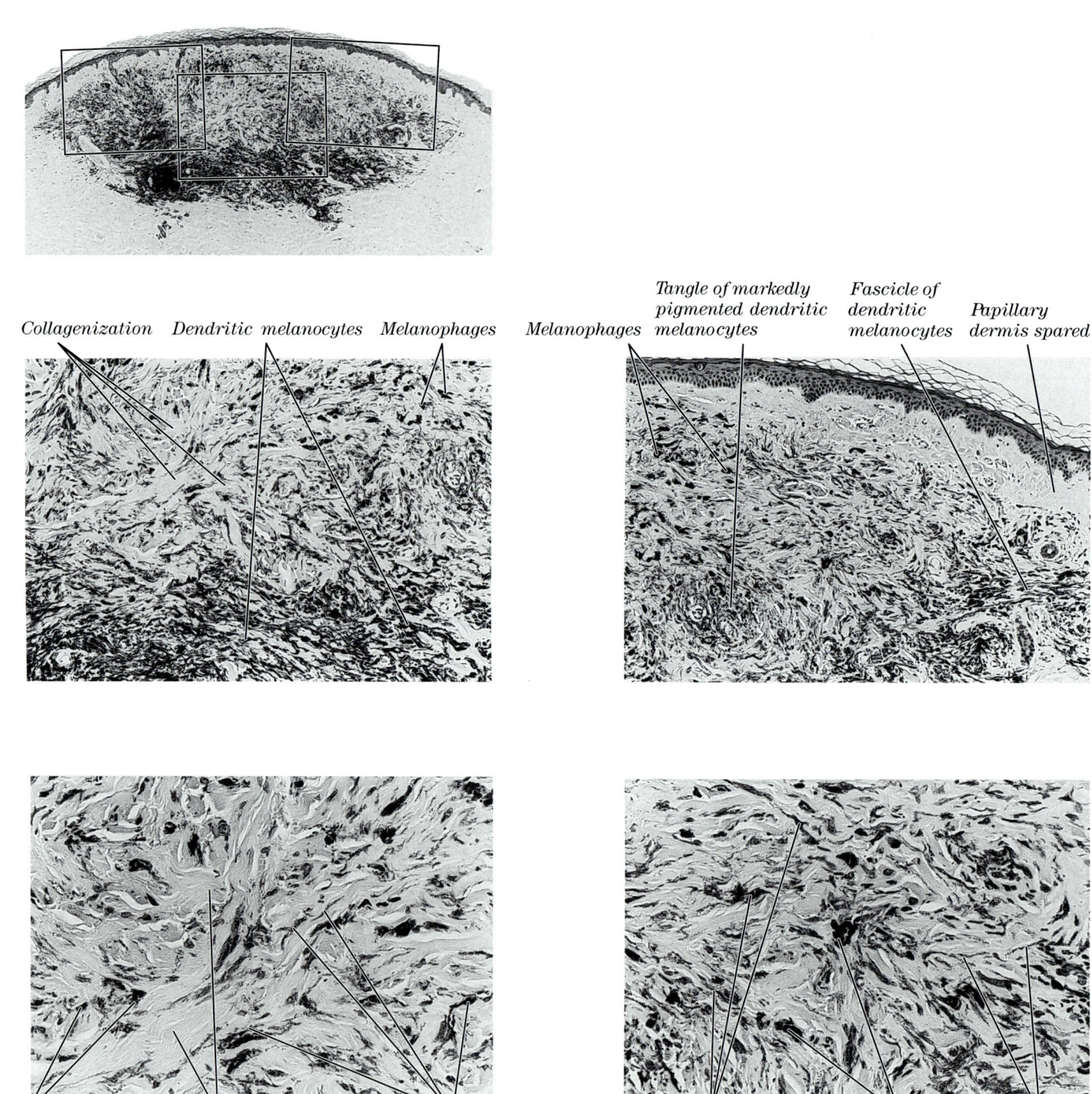

16 • Blue Nevus *(superficial dendritic type)*

Criteria for diagnosis of this blue nevus
(superficial predominantly dendritic type with extensive collagenization)

This is a blue nevus because:

1. Many of the melanocytes in this proliferation have markedly pigmented, extremely elongated, bipolar dendrites.
2. The epidermis and epithelial structures of adnexa are spared by the process.

This is a predominantly dendritic expression of blue nevus because:

Overtly dendritic melanocytes predominate within this proliferation, but melanocytes whose dendrites seem to be absent also are present.

Collagenization is apparent in the form of:

Markedly thickened bundles of collagen, arranged haphazardly, in concert with the proliferation of bipolar dendritic melanocytes.

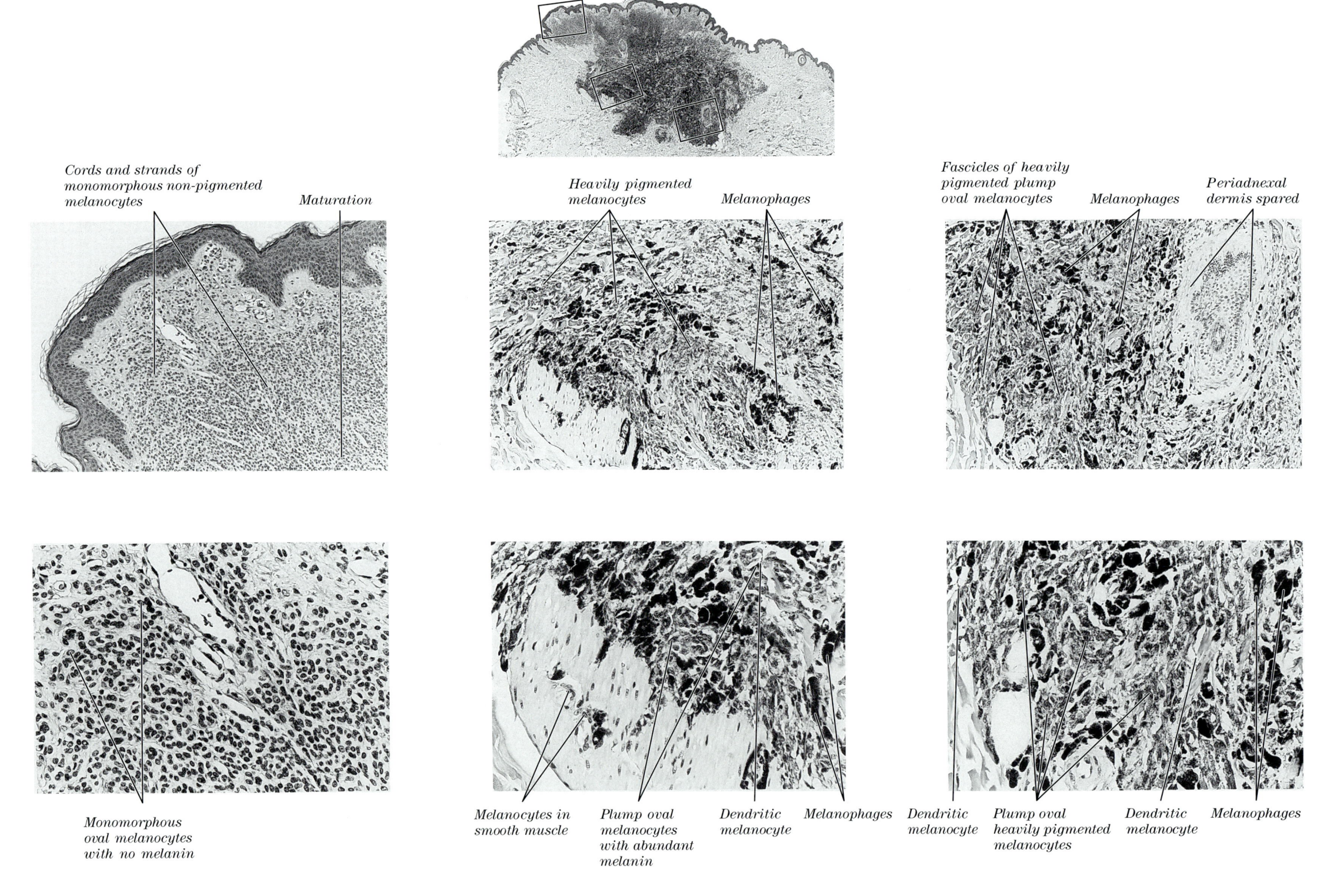

30 · 17 • Combined Nevus *(Clark's and blue)*

Criteria for diagnosis of this combined nevus (Clark's and blue)

This is a combined nevus because:

1. Relative symmetry obtains for both components of this melanocytic neoplasm, i.e., the heavily pigmented bipolar dendritic melanocytes in the reticular dermis and the relatively non-pigmented oval melanocytes in a thickened papillary dermis.

2. The vertical dimension of the heavily pigmented portion of the neoplasm almost equals that of the horizontal one.

3. Epithelial structures of adnexa are spared by the markedly pigmented portion of the neoplasm.

4. Melanin is distributed in relatively even fashion within neoplastic cells of the strikingly pigmented part of the neoplasm.

5. Nuclei of melanocytes are relatively monomorphous in the heavily pigmented component of the neoplasm.

6. No mitotic figures are present in neoplastic cells.

crete nests of melanocytes are not seen in blue nevi. Parenthetically, it is enigmatic that a congenital nevus, i.e., a blue nevus, comes to be found in association with an acquired nevus (Unna's, Miescher's, Spitz's, or Clark's). It seems reasonable to conclude that in these instances, both components of a combined nevus are congenital. In short, there are congenital analogues of each of the four major types of acquired nevi. In our estimation, virtually all combined nevi are congenital.

Uncommonly, solitary units of markedly pigmented dendritic melanocytes may appear in the epidermis above an intradermal blue nevus (Fig. 18). Because there are no nests of melanocytes, only individual melanocytes within the epidermis, this unusual expression of blue nevus does not qualify as a compound blue nevus. The presence of nests of melanocytes within both the epidermis and the dermis are requisite for identification of a compound nevus of any type. The intra-epidermal changes of the blue nevi under discussion resemble somewhat those of a labial lentigo with its darkly pigmented, strikingly elongated dendrites arranged as solitary units, rather than a junctional melanocytic nevus with its nests of melanocytes. To our knowledge, there is no authentic junctional or compound type of blue nevus. Virtually all blue nevi are mostly intradermal, although some of them also may be present in the upper part of the subcutaneous fat. Blue nevi may be classified histopathologically according to location of melanocytes, types of melanocytes, arrangement of melanocytes, and alterations of collagen, as shown in Table 2.

A blue nevus typified by scatter of bipolar dendritic melanocytes tends to involve the upper half of the dermis but, on occasion, may include the lower half of the dermis as well. Nearly all of the melanocytes in an early lesion are dendritic and unassociated with collagenization. In time, only melanocytes at the periphery of a lesion are dendritic, older ones toward the center being oval and associated with striking collagenization. In another type of blue nevus constituted of bipolar dendritic melanocytes arranged compactly, melanocytes replete with melanin are situated in the upper part of the reticular dermis where bipolar dendrites often are parallel to one another and to the skin surface. A variant that favors the face or upper part of the chest consists of markedly pigmented dendritic melanocytes arranged in a tangle at the top of the reticular dermis. No collagenization accompanies bipolar dendritic melanocytes in this type of blue nevus.

An uncommon type of blue nevus consists of prominent fascicles of oval melanocytes, with only a few bipolar dendritic melanocytes being present mostly at the periphery of the neoplasm. The fascicles intersect one another, fill the dermis, and extend into the upper part of the subcutaneous fat. Collagenization is not present.

Melanocytes in blue nevi may extend broadly and deeply (Fig. 19). Those findings are reflected clinically as patches rather than macules, and plaques and nodules rather than papules. Histopathologically, some blue nevi have a proclivity for involvement of the subcutaneous fat. When a blue nevus is "bottom-heavy" and occupies the subcutaneous fat extensively, almost certainly that nevus was visualized clinically at birth.

A distinctive type of blue nevus consists of darkly pigmented, bipolar dendritic melanocytes, accompanied by melanophages, scattered throughout the reticular dermis and often the septa in the upper part of the subcutaneous fat. The number of melanocytes is so few that usually they are not discernible at scanning magnification, although melanophages may be perceptible at that power. There are neither oval melanocytes arrayed as solitary units or in fascicles, nor signs of collagenization in these lesions. When this type of blue nevus appears as a bluish patch on a face, it is known popularly as nevus of Ota (Fig. 20), on the back as nevus of Ito, and over the sacrum as mongolian spot. That "spot" actually is a patch that is present nearly universally in dark-skinned peoples. Melanomas do not develop in mongolian spots and arise exceedingly rarely in nevus of Ito and very uncommonly in nevus of Ota, and then within the substance of the proliferation of dendritic melanocytes, not at the dermo-epidermal junction. Nevus of Ota also involves mucous membranes of the eye, nose, and mouth. As has been mentioned, about half of all nevi of Ota seem to be acquired at puberty or thereafter. The bluish patches are indistinguishable clinically and histopathologically from lesions of the condition that are present at birth. We consider the seemingly acquired nevus of Ota to be a tardive expression of a congenital nevus.

Less common than the bluish patches of blue nevi on the face and back and those over the sacrum constituted of scattered pigmented bipolar dendritic melanocytes is a bluish nodule or tumor that consists of a combination of discrete aggregations of oval melanocytes that are surrounded by innumerable bipolar dendritic melanocytes (Fig. 21). The latter are so darkly pigmented by melanin that they cause the aggregations of oval melanocytes to appear, at first glance, to be amelanotic. In fact, the oval melanocytes do contain melanin, but much less of it than the dendritic ones. The lesion, usually situated on a buttock, involves the entire reticular dermis and some of the subcutaneous fat. It tends to be vertically oriented vis-a-vis the epidermis, symmetrical, sharply circumscribed, and marked by smooth borders (Fig. 22). Colloquially, it is known as Masson's blue neuronevus, but, in actuality, it is simply a combination of "dendritic" and "nondendritic" blue nevus (Fig. 23); melanoma practically never develops within it.

Melanoma hardly ever occurs in association with any kind of blue nevus. If melanoma does develop in that circumstance, it should not be referred to as "malignant blue nevus," but as "melanoma." All malignant neoplasms of melanocytes are melanomas; the benign proliferations of melanocytes in which they arise are nevi. In short, there is no "malignant blue nevus," only melanoma in association with a blue nevus.

When melanomas arise in non-blue superficial congenital nevi, as they do uncommonly, the proliferation of melanocytes begins at the dermo-epidermal junction, just as it does in melanomas that develop de novo and in those that originate in acquired nevi. In contradistinction, melanomas that occur in deep congenital nevi, an event encountered exceedingly rarely, tend to arise within the substance of the nevus in either the dermis or the subcutaneous fat, rather than at the dermo-epidermal junction. As usual, there are exceptions to that rule, too, and, very rarely, a melanoma may start at the dermo-epidermal junction of a non-blue deep congenital nevus. Melanomas arise exceedingly rarely in blue nevi and then within the substance of the lesion, not at the dermo-epidermal junction.

In conclusion, there are two basic types of congenital nevi and they can be classified readily as blue and non-blue, and further as superficial and deep, based upon histopathologic differences that are apparent at scanning magnification. The two fundamental types and the two subdivisions of them not only are different from one another histopathologically, but also clinically and biologically. Last, it must be noted that each of the acquired types of nevus, i.e., Unna, Miescher, Spitz, and Clark, has a congenital analogue, that, although usually superficial, also may be deep. In a combined nevus with elements of Clark's nevus and blue nevus, it is likely that the entire nevus is congenital.

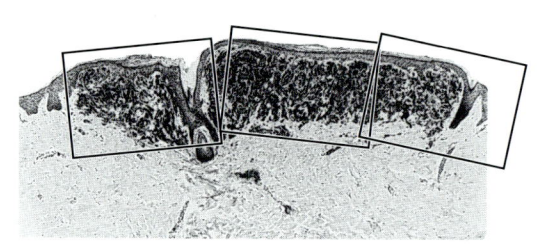

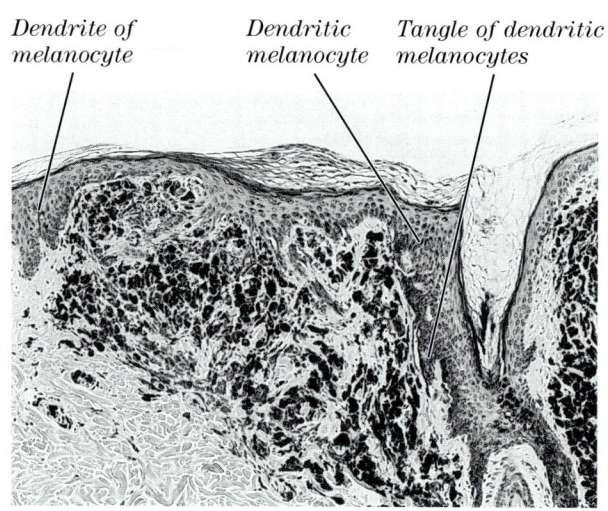
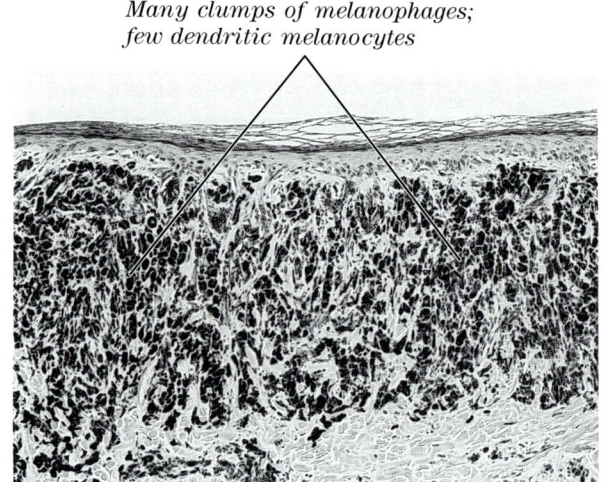
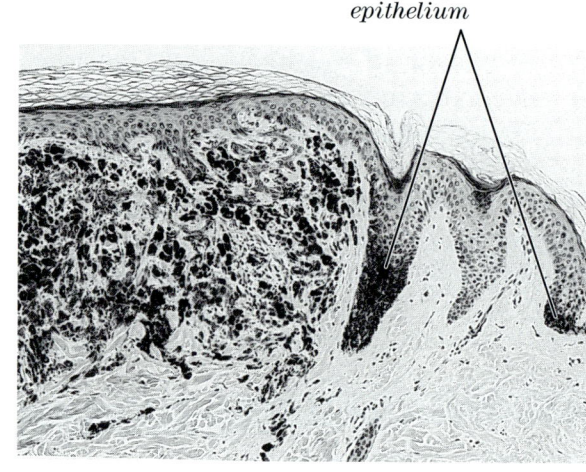

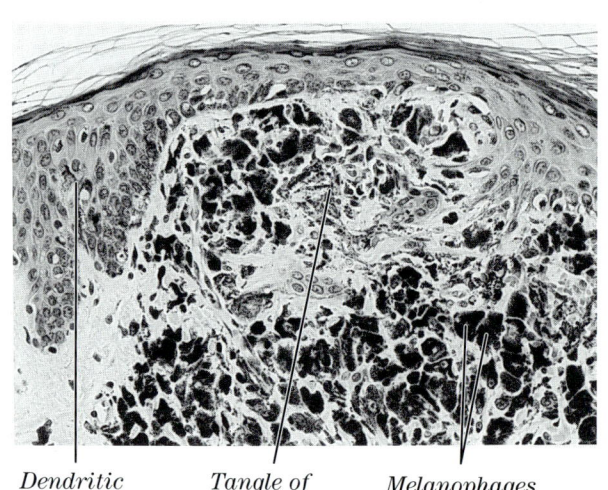
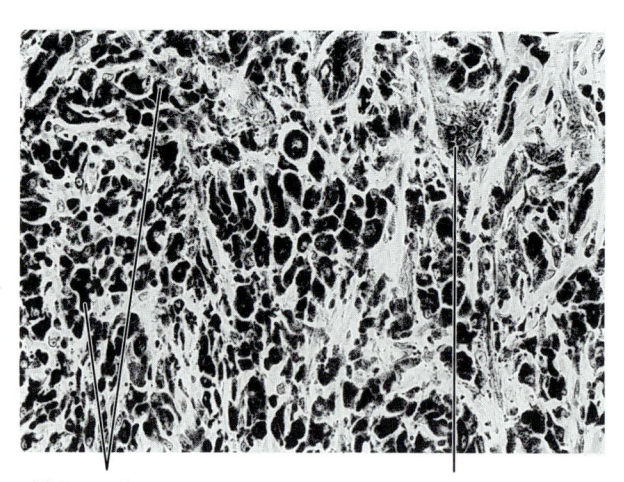
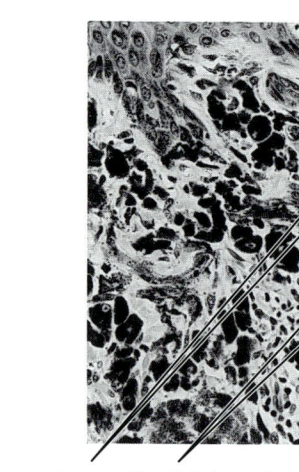
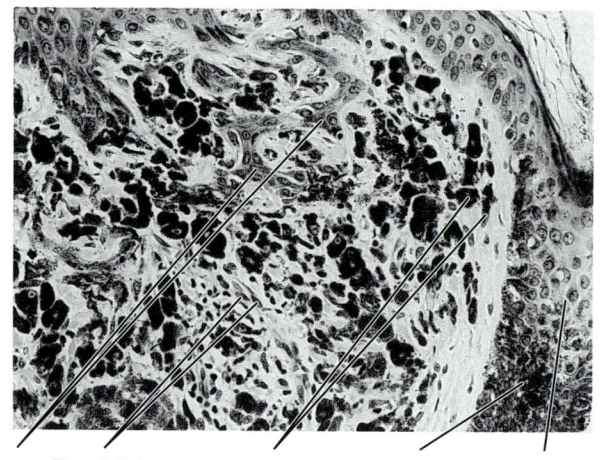

18 • Blue Nevus *(superficial dendritic type)*

Criteria for diagnosis of this blue nevus (superficial type with prominent intra-epidermal dendritic melanocytes)

This is a blue nevus because:

1. Heavily pigmented bipolar dendritic melanocytes are present within the dermis.

2. There are no discrete nests of melanocytes within the dermis or the epidermis.

This is not a compound nevus because:

Dendritic melanocytes within the epidermis are arranged as solitary units only, not in nests.

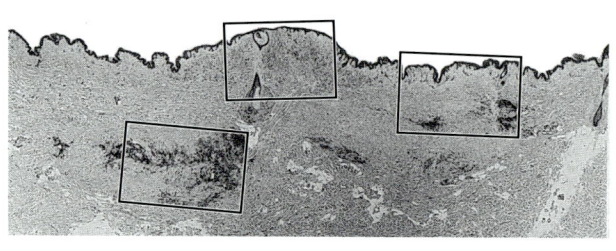

Dendritic melanocytes splayed between collagen bundles

Dendritic and oval melanocytes splayed between wiry collagen bundles *Melanophages*

Tangles of dendritic melanocytes

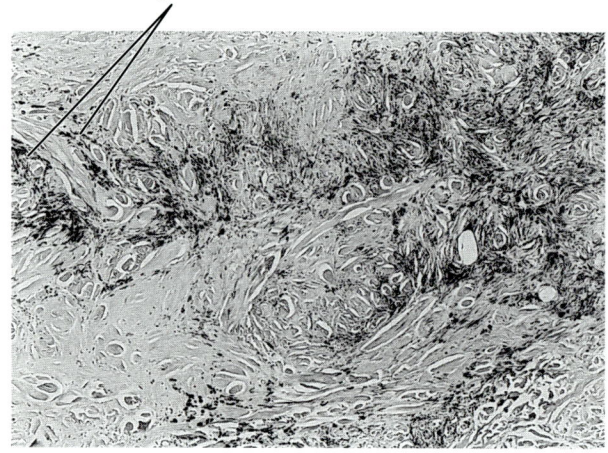
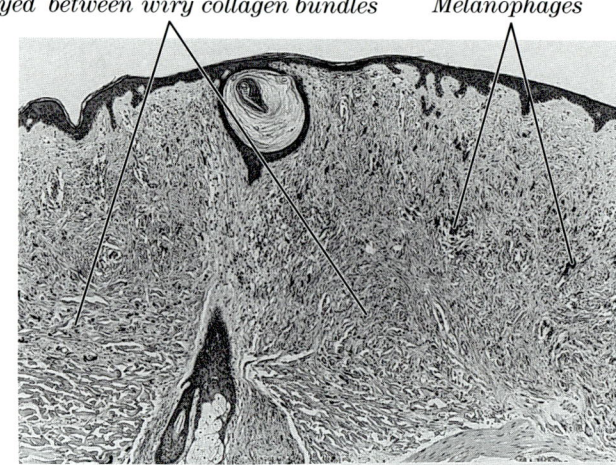
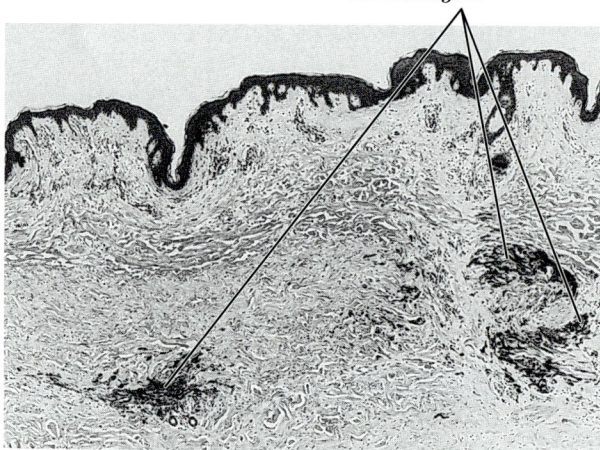

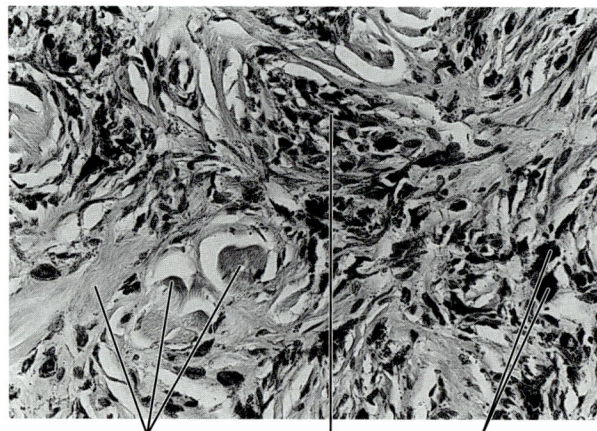
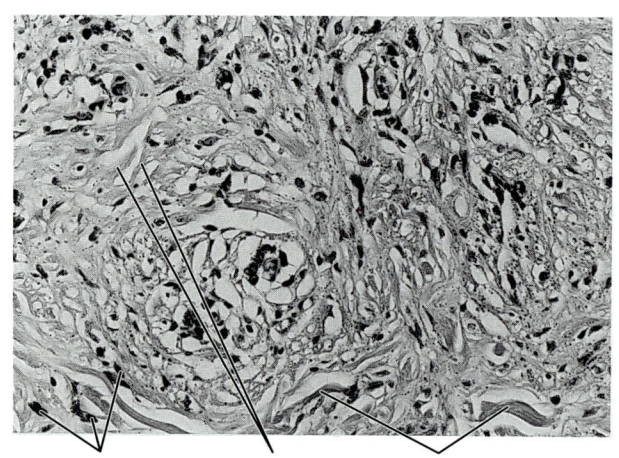
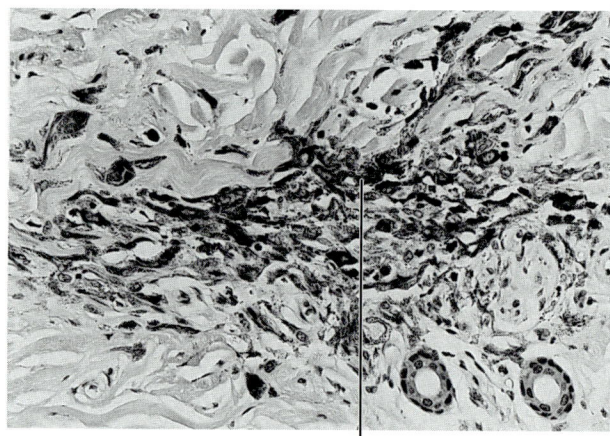

Thickened collagen bundles *Dendritic melanocytes* *Melanophages*

Oval melanocytes *Wiry collagen bundles* *Thick collagen bundles*

Tangle of dendritic melanocytes

19 · Blue Nevus *(deep dendritic type)*

Criteria for diagnosis of this
blue nevus (deep dendritic type)

This is a blue nevus because:

1. Strikingly dendritic, heavily pigmented, bipolar melanocytes are situated at the periphery of the neoplasm mostly.

2. Dendritic melanocytes are positioned between markedly thickened bundles of collagen.

3. No neoplastic cells are in mitosis.

4. Epithelial structures of adnexa are spared by the neoplasm.

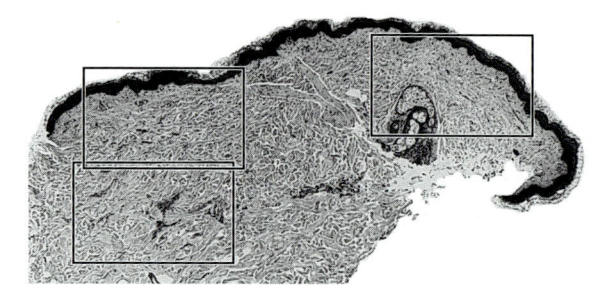

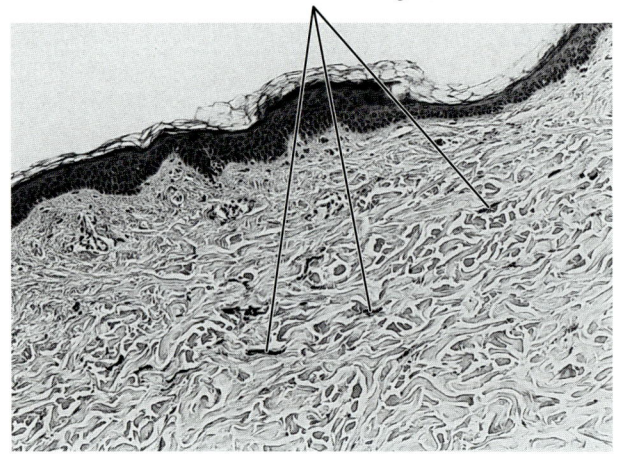
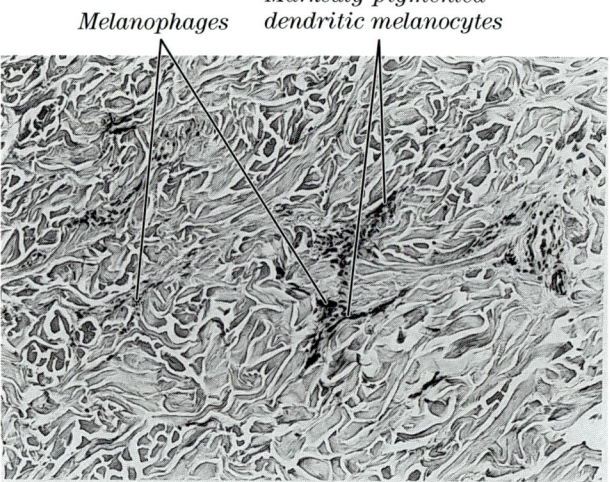
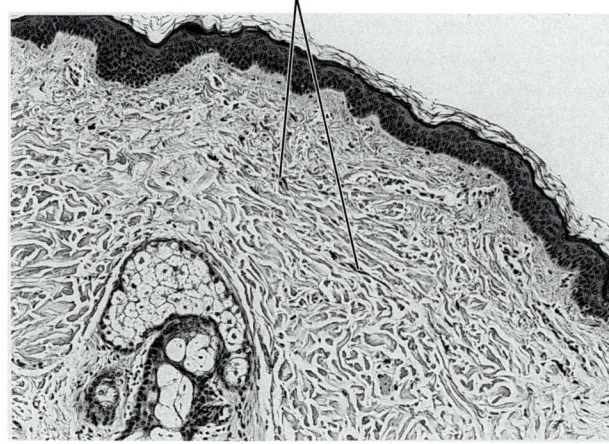

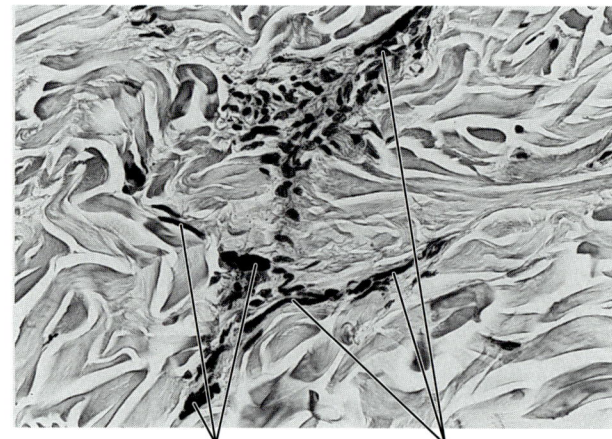
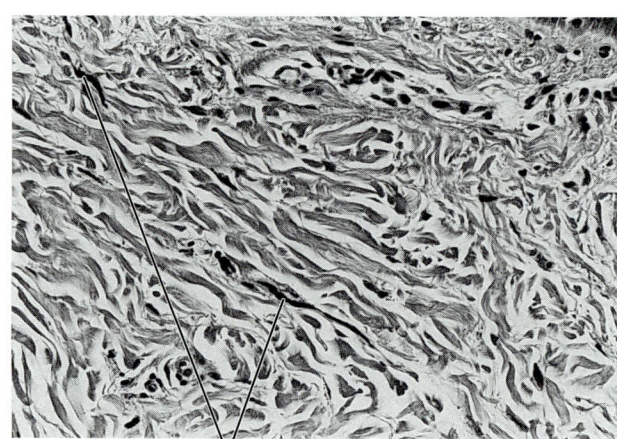

38 · 20 · Blue Nevus *(deep dendritic multifocal type)*

Criteria for diagnosis of this
blue nevus (deep dendritic multifocal type)

This is a blue nevus because:

Markedly pigmented bipolar dendritic melanocytes constitute the lesion.

This is a nevus of Ota because:

Dendritic melanocytes arranged as solitary units are scattered throughout the dermis.

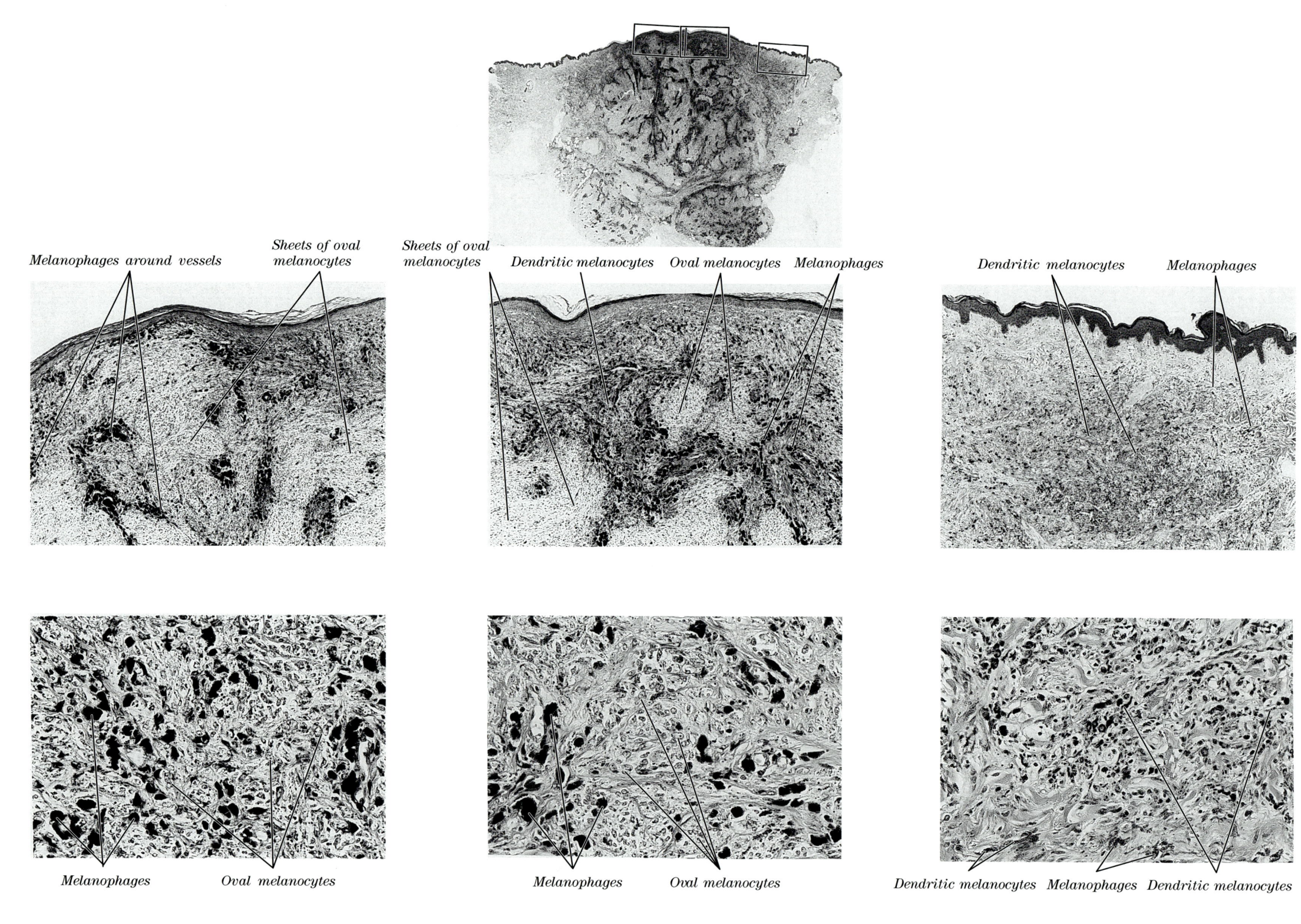

21 • Blue Nevus *(deep predominantly non-dendritic type)*

Criteria for diagnosis of this blue nevus (deep predominantly non-dendritic type)

This neoplasm is benign because:

1. It is vertically oriented.
2. It is relatively symmetric.
3. Its base is well-circumscribed by smooth-surfaced nodules.
4. Neoplastic melanocytes mature.
5. Neoplastic cells have monomorphous nuclei.

This is a blue nevus because:

Some melanocytes within the dermis have bipolar dendritic shapes and are heavily pigmented.

This is a Masson's type of blue nevus because:

There are two components of the lesion: fascicles of melanocytes with plump oval nuclei and relatively scant melanin within abundant cytoplasm, and heavily pigmented, bipolar, dendritic melanocytes that surround fascicles.

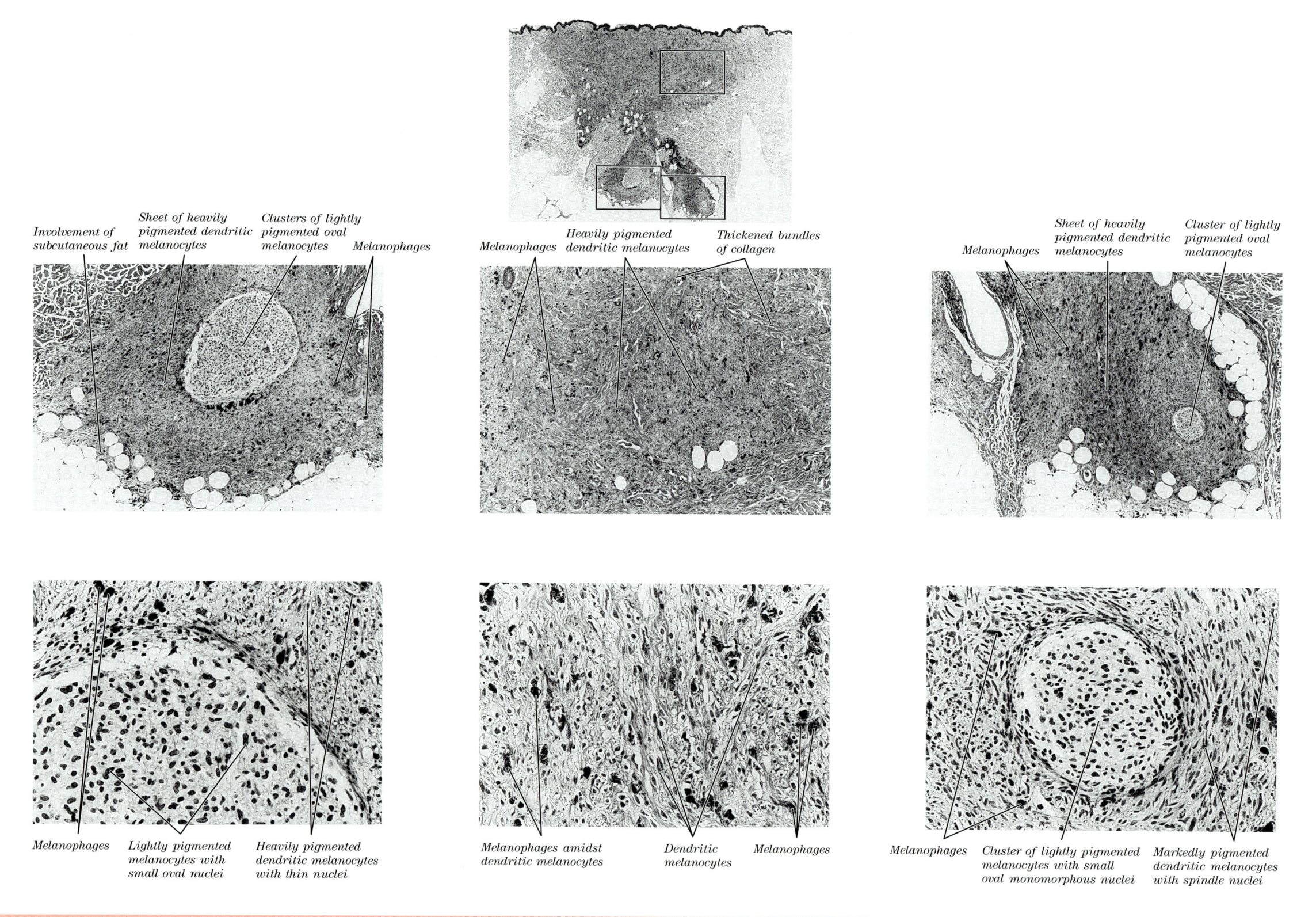

42 · Blue Nevus *(deep predominantly non-dendritic type)*

Criteria for diagnosis of this blue nevus (deep predominantly non-dendritic type)

This neoplasm is benign because:

1. It is oriented vertically.
2. It is somewhat wedge-shaped.
3. It is well-circumscribed.
4. Nuclei of melanocytes that constitute it are small and monomorphous.

This is a blue nevus because:

1. Bipolar dendritic melanocytes are present within the neoplasm.
2. The dendritic melanocytes are heavily pigmented by melanin.

This is a Masson's type of blue nevus because:

Within diffuse zones of strikingly pigmented dendritic melanocytes are discrete oval and round zones of lightly pigmented oval melanocytes.

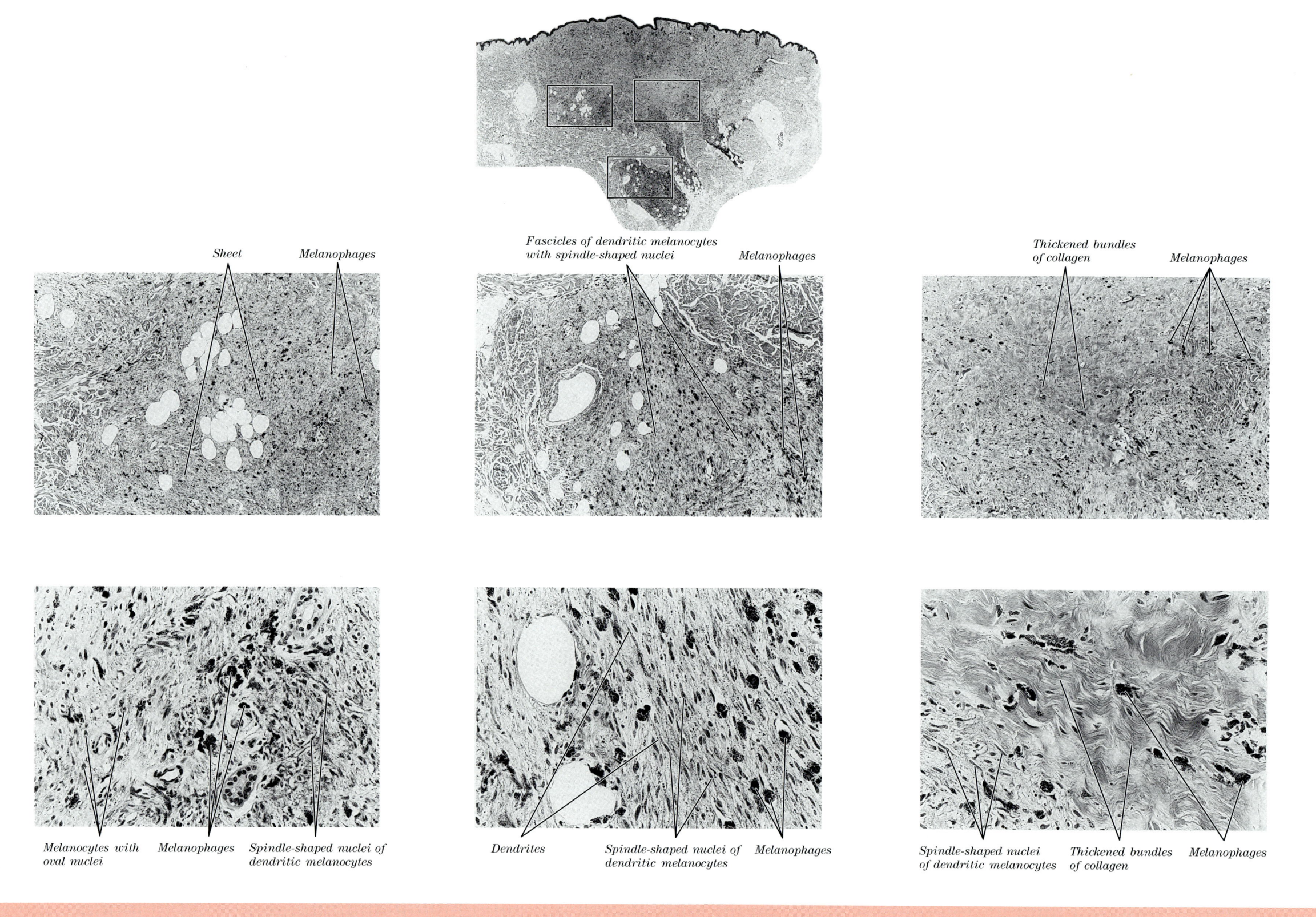

23 · Blue Nevus *(deep predominantly non-dendritic type)*

Criteria for diagnosis of this blue nevus (deep predominantly non-dendritic type)

This is a blue nevus because:

1. Neoplastic cells with markedly pigmented, strikingly elongated, bipolar dendrites are present.
2. There are no discrete nests of melanocytes.

The section comes from the same specimen as the section shown in Figure 22. The findings indicate that a Masson's blue neuro-nevus is truly a variant of blue nevus.

C. Acquired Nevi

Four types of common acquired nevi proceed in repeatable fashion through junctional, compound, and intradermal stages: Unna's, Miescher's, Spitz's, and Clark's. They can be differentiated readily from one another by architectural pattern (particularly silhouette), distribution of melanocytes, and cytologic character of melanocytes.

Clinically, each of the four types of common acquired nevi whose nests of melanocytes evolve from being entirely junctional to completely intradermal tends to be small, i.e., usually, but surely not always, less than 6.0 mm in diameter, symmetric, well-circumscribed, and relatively uniform in color, mostly in hues of browns, but sometimes of reds and even the cast of normal skin. Histopathologically, these nevi, in addition to being smallish, symmetric, and well-circumscribed, have in common maturation of individual melanocytes with progressive descent into the dermis (i.e., the deeper the melanocytes, the smaller their nuclei) and maturation of nests (the deeper the nests, the smaller they become). Within the epidermis, nests of melanocytes are relatively equidistant from one another, relatively uniform in size and shape, and discrete (i.e., they do not tend to confluence), and nests predominate over melanocytes arranged as solitary units. Melanocytes within nests are cohesive, and those arranged both as solitary units and in nests are situated at the dermo-epidermal junction and not above it. The upper portion of epithelial structures of adnexa may be affected by the proliferation of melanocytes in the same manner as the epidermis. Last, melanin is distributed symmetrically throughout these acquired nevi, both within melanocytes themselves and within melanophages.

It is because there are exceptions to each of these generalizations about histopathologic characteristics of acquired melanocytic nevi that pitfalls in diagnosis of them come to be.

1. Unna's nevus. Nevi that are polypoid or sessile, dome-shaped or papillomatous, and often mistaken clinically for acrochordons (skin tags) because they are mostly exophytic and soft are designated Unna's nevus by us because Paul Gerson Unna first described them, illustrated them, and named them "soft nevi" in 1896. They are found mostly on the trunk, arms, and neck, practically never on the legs. Most nevi of Unna's type are simply maleable excrescences. Histopathologically, Unna's nevi are characterized by being much more exophytic than endophytic, vastly intradermal, and composed of nests, cords, and strands of melanocytes (Figs. 24, 25). Nearly all the melanocytes in Unna's nevi are stationed in a tremendously thickened papillary dermis, but a few may extend just into the reticular dermis where they are not splayed in strands between bundles of collagen in distinct foci, unless that nevus is a congenital one. In sections from some specimens of Unna's nevi, small nests of melanocytes may be noted at the junction of dermis and epidermis, qualifying them as compound, rather than wholly intradermal, nevi.

The melanocytes in Unna's nevi usually are small and round or oval. Multinucleate melanocytes may be numerous or absent. The nuclei of those melanocytes are typical and none are in mitosis as a rule. Only uncommonly does a melanoma originate in a Unna's nevus, and when that happens, the malignant process begins at the dermo-epidermal junction.

In the course of many years, morphologic changes develop in the dermis of Unna's (and Miescher's) nevus that signify the neoplasm is long-standing. Those "aging" changes are "neurotization," i.e., formation of structures that resemble Meissner's corpuscles, adipose metaplasia expressed as variable numbers of adipocytes among the melanocytes of the nevus, and fibroplasia in the form of whorls of sclerosis around individual melanocytes of the nevus in the upper part of the dermis and of fibrosis that may replace much of the nevus. It may be that the number of multinucleate melanocytes also is a reflection of the age of a lesion, i.e., the more numerous the multinucleate cells, the older the nevus. Rarely, ancient Unna's nevi may exhibit atypical nuclei of melanocytes. Although this constellation of alterations indicates senescence of a nevus, they also are evidence that the nevus still exists. In short, nevi of all kinds may regress, but they do not disappear without a trace.

2. Miescher's nevus. This distinctive nevus occurs mostly on the face as a firm, nearly skin-colored or brownish hemispherule. Histopathologically, it is gently domed and predominantly endophytic, the neoplastic melanocytes tending to be arranged in a wedge and often extending from beneath the thinned papillary dermis to near the base of the reticular dermis and even just into the subcutaneous fat (Figs. 26, 27). The melanocytes are arranged in nests, cords, and strands. Melanin, when noticeable easily at scanning magnification, assumes an umbrella-like arc in the uppermost part of the nevus where it is lodged within melanocytes and within macrophages. Within the wedge formed by neoplastic melanocytes in the reticu-

Text continues on page 51

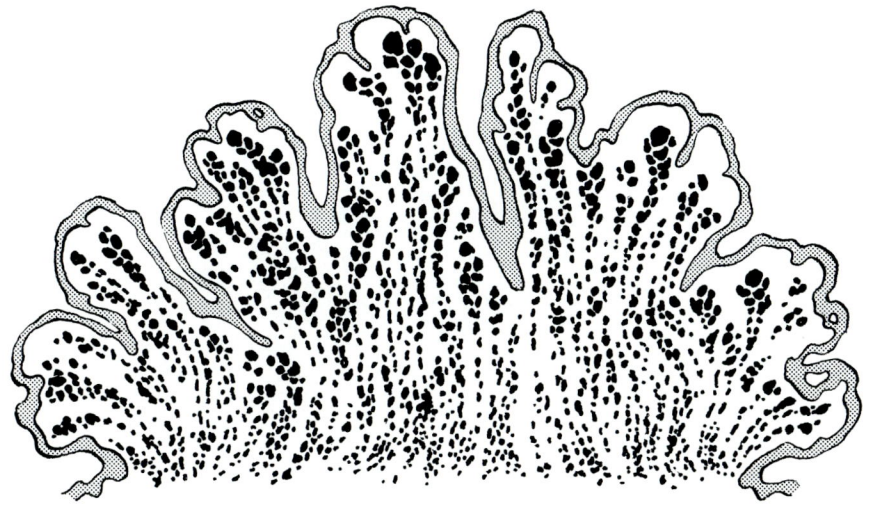

Fig. 24. Unna's nevus. This sessile nevus extends for a considerable distance above the skin surface, is mostly intradermal, and is associated with a pattern of orderly nests, cords, and strands of melanocytes within the exophytic papillary dermis. Clinically, such a lesion is soft and frequently resembles an acrochordon.

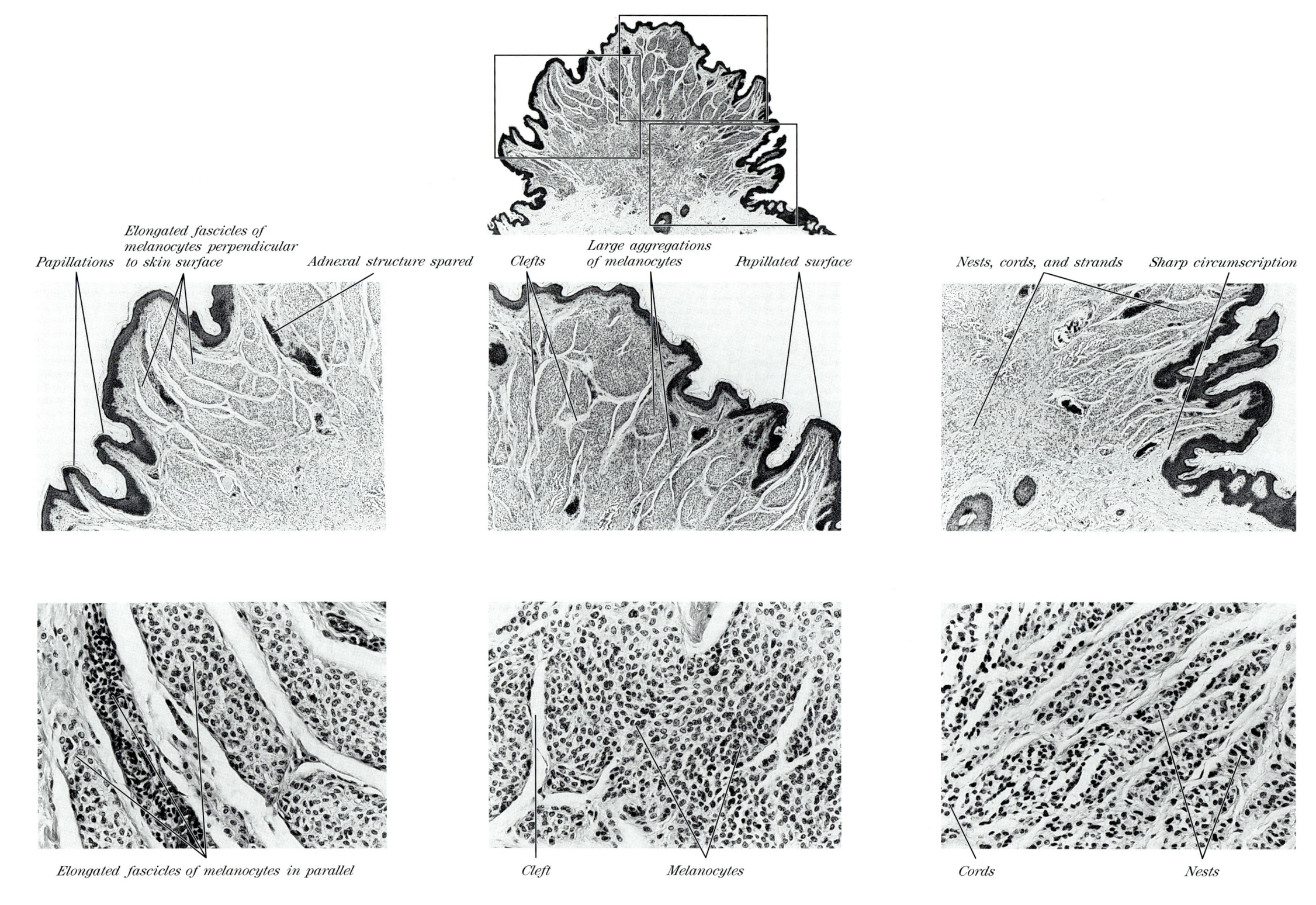

25 • Unna's Nevus

Criteria for diagnosis of this Unna's nevus (intradermal type)

This neoplasm is benign because:

1. It is symmetric.
2. It is well-circumscribed.
3. There is maturation of melanocytes.
4. Nuclei of melanocytes are small and monomorphous.

This is an Unna's nevus because:

1. The neoplasm is exophytic.
2. It is papillomatous.
3. It is confined to a markedly thickened papillary dermis.

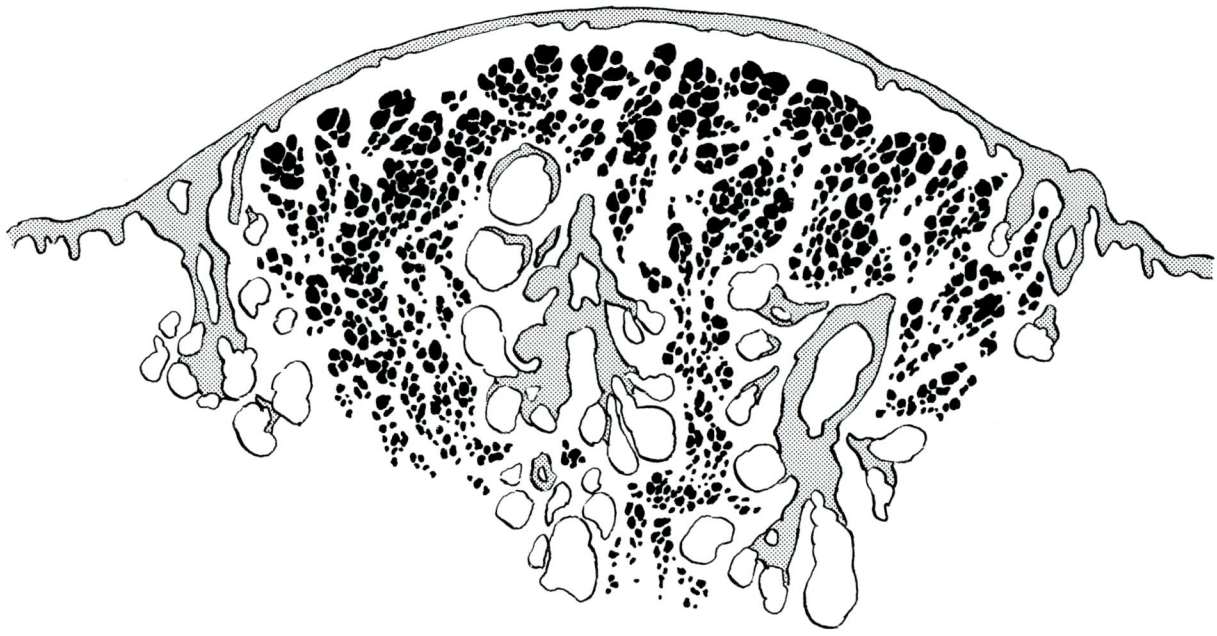

Fig. 26. Miescher's nevus. This domed and wedge-shaped melanocytic nevus is mostly endophytic, and the nests, cords, and strands of melanocytes that constitute it extend far into the reticular dermis. Nearly always it is situated on the face or scalp.

lar dermis, folliculo-sebaceous structures and specialized fibrous tissue that surrounds them are spared dramatically. Sometimes small nests of melanocytes are situated also at the dermo-epidermal junction, so that Miescher's nevi may be compound, as well as wholly intradermal. All Miescher's nevi, like all Unna's nevi, begin at the junction of epidermis and dermis, but they cannot be identified for what they are at that early stage, clinically or histopathologically, because the signs that give them their uniqueness are found in the dermis alone, i.e., dramatically exophytic in a thickened papillary dermis for Unna's nevus and strikingly endophytic and wedge-shaped in a reticular dermis for Miescher's nevus. Only Spitz's nevus can be identified accurately when it is still entirely junctional, and then on the basis of a distinctive pattern formed by nests of melanocytes and by keratinocytes in the epidermis, and characteristic cytopathologic findings of melanocytes there.

The signs of longevity mentioned in the histopathologic description of Unna's nevi, namely, neural differentiation (Fig. 28), adipose metaplasia, and fibroplasia (including collagenization) (Fig. 29), may all be seen in Miescher's nevi, too. In addition, rare examples of aged Miescher's nevi may display melanocytes with atypical nuclei.

This markedly endophytic type of acquired melanocytic nevus is named by us for Guido Miescher who, with von Albertini, published, in 1935, observations that focused attention on the dermal component of it. He designated melanocytes that constituted those intradermal nevi "types A, B, and C" on the basis of the appearances of the cells at different levels of the reticular dermis, the A type being highest, largest, and pigmented; the C type being lowest, smallest, and non-pigmented.

3. Spitz's nevus. Even though Sophie Spitz contended in her original article, published in 1948 and titled "Melanomas in Childhood," that the nevus that now bears her name was a true malignant melanoma in children, in later publications she, along with Arthur Allen, came to conclude that it actually was a distinctive type of nevus. Their publications set forth some criteria for diagnosis of that particular nevus which so often was and is confused histopathologically with authentic melanoma. By now it is an accepted tenet of dermatologists, pediatricians, and pathologists that the lesion described by Spitz is one type of nevus, not a melanoma, and that it may arise in adults as well as in infants and children.

Clinically, there are several variants of Spitz's nevus, but the two most common are a solitary reddish papule (usually in children) and a solitary brownish or black papule (usually in adults). Some Spitz's nevi in children, however, may be brown and some in adults pink. In children, nevi of Spitz's type favor the face, and in adults they incline to the trunk in men and to the legs in women. There are two congenital manifestations of Spitz's nevi: a cluster of pink, red, or brown papules atop a subtle fawn-colored patch (the agminated form) and many discrete, pink, red, or brown papules and nodules distributed widely and often unilaterally (the widespread form). Spitz's nevi are common in Caucasians, much less so in Asians, and rare in Africans.

Histopathologically, there are many morphologic expressions of Spitz's nevi, but they are united by a common denominator, i.e., some melanocytes with largish nuclei, abundant cytoplasm, and oval, spindle, round, or polygonal shapes (Fig. 30).*

Spitz's nevi, like Unna's, Miescher's, and Clark's nevi, begin at the dermo-epidermal junction (Fig. 31), become compound in time (Fig. 32), and end wholly intradermal (Fig. 33). They can be recognized histopathologically at each of these stages. In addition to the common denominators of large size of some melanocytes and characteristic shapes of melanocytes, junctional and compound types of Spitz's nevi usually are marked by distinctive architectural features: compact orthokeratosis, hypergranulosis, uneven, sometimes jagged, spinous-cell hyperplasia, clefts between elongated nests of melanocytes and adjacent keratinocytes, orientation of elongated nests of melanocytes perpendicular to the skin surface, dull pink globules (Kamino bodies) within the epidermis, and patchy lymphocytic infiltrates around venules throughout the nevus (Figs. 34, 35). Some examples of Spitz's nevus show edema and widely dilated venules in the upper part of the dermis.

Multinucleate melanocytes are common in Spitz's nevi and even may predominate within the epidermis or dermis in a given lesion (Fig. 36). Dendritic melanocytes are found frequently within the epidermis of Spitz's nevi in Asians (and in the rare lesions in Africans), but infrequently in Caucasians, except within the epidermis of the "pigmented spindle-cell" variant.

---

*An exception is the "pigmented spindle cell" variant of Spitz's nevus in which oval nuclei of melanocytes are not very large and cytoplasm not very abundant.

Text continues on page 67

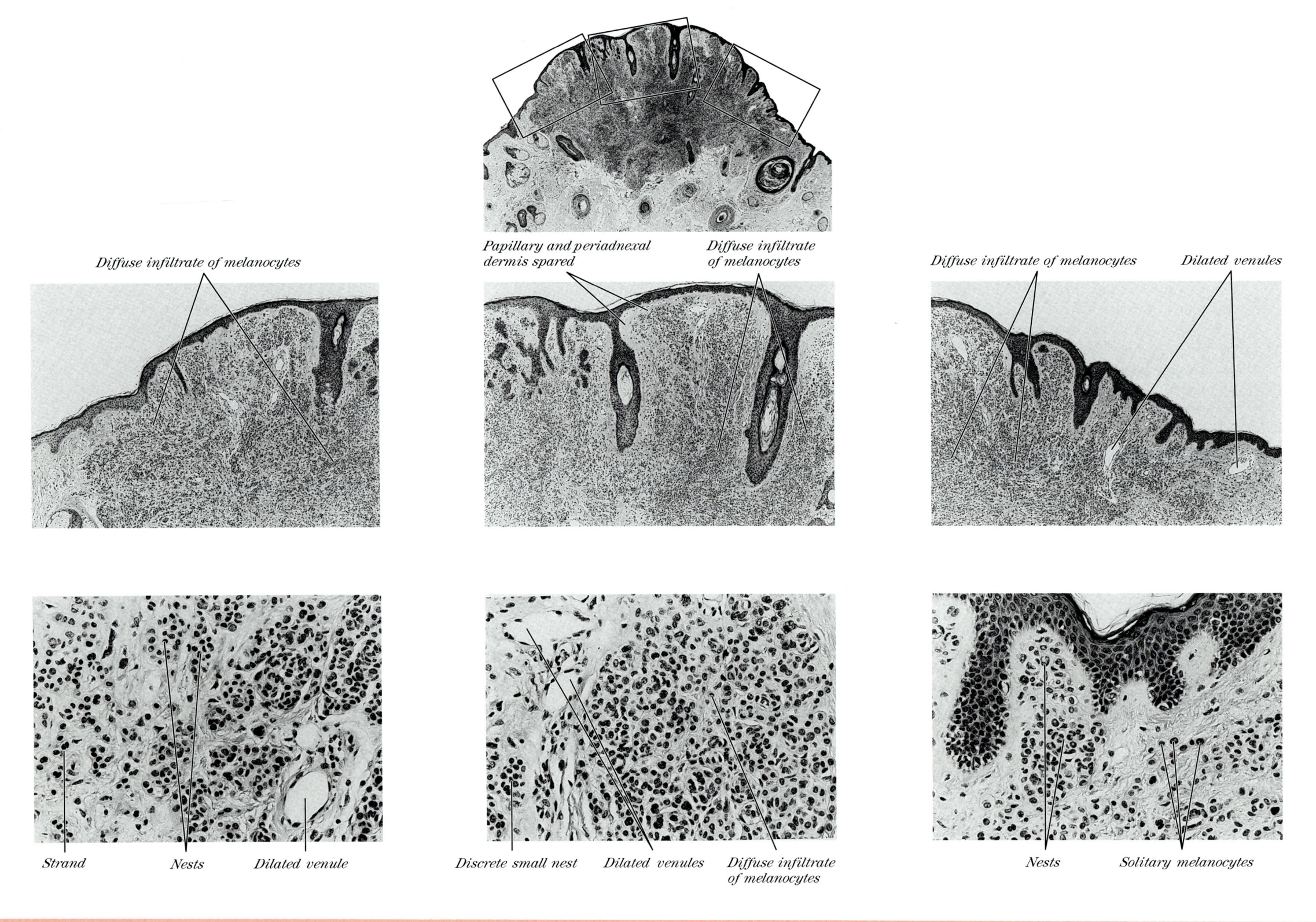

27 · Miescher's Nevus

Criteria for diagnosis of this Miescher's nevus

This lesion is benign because:

1. It is symmetric.
2. It is well-circumscribed.
3. It is wedge-shaped.
4. It spares epithelial structures of adnexa.
5. Melanocytes mature.
6. Melanocytes within the epidermis, arranged wholly as solitary units, are seated at the dermo-epidermal junction and not above it.

This is a Miescher's nevus because:

1. It is dome-shaped.
2. It is mostly endophytic.
3. It is wedge-shaped.
4. It is situated on a face, which is the usual site.

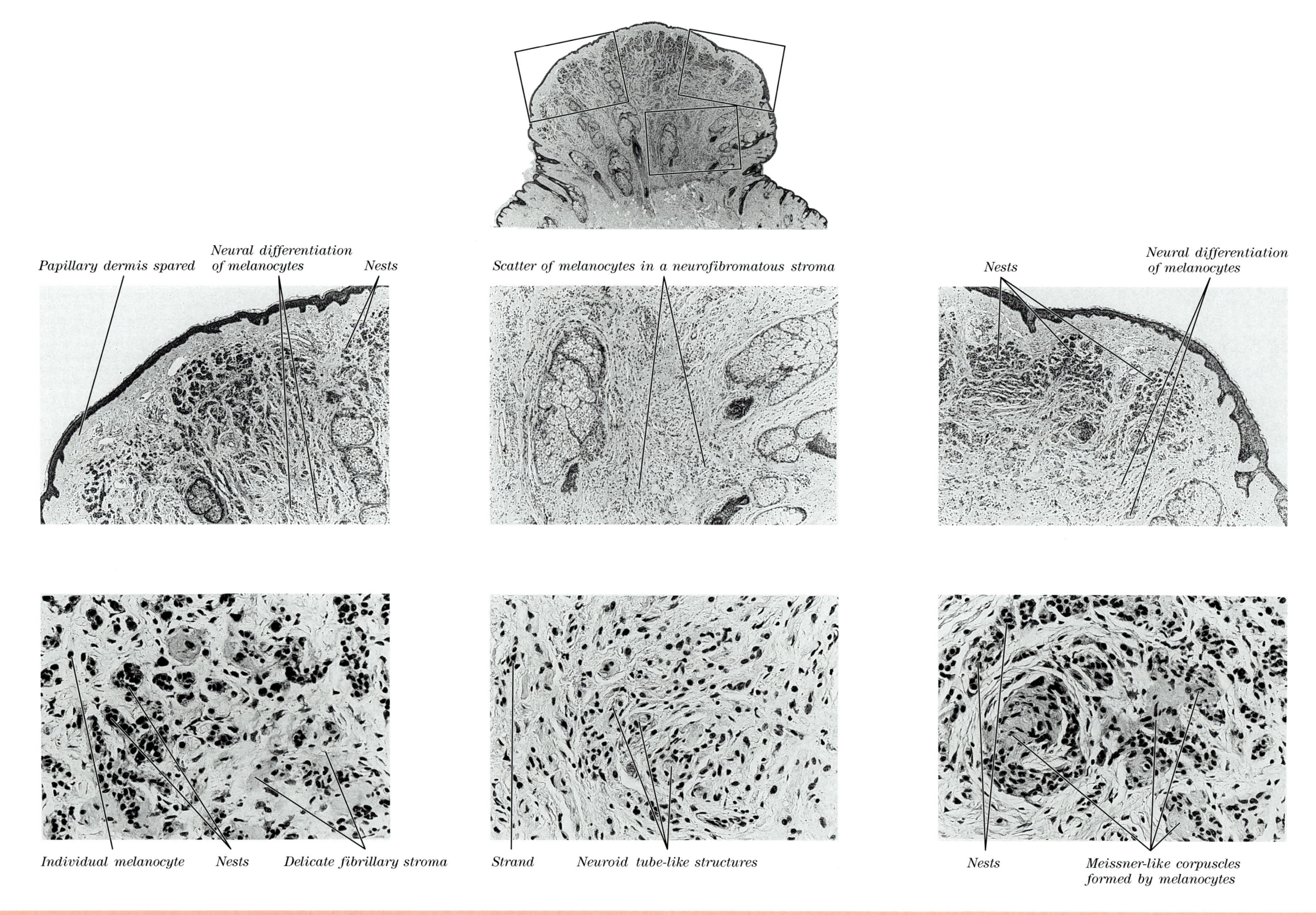

28 • Miescher's Nevus

Criteria for diagnosis of this intradermal type of Miescher's nevus (with neurotization)

This is an intradermal type of Miescher's nevus because:

1. It is dome-shaped.
2. It is mostly endophytic.
3. Neoplastic melanocytes extend well into the reticular dermis.
4. Meissner-like corpuscles, seen also in Unna's nevus, are apparent.
5. The lesion is on a face.

Signs of neurotization are:

Formation of structures that resemble Meissner's corpuscles.

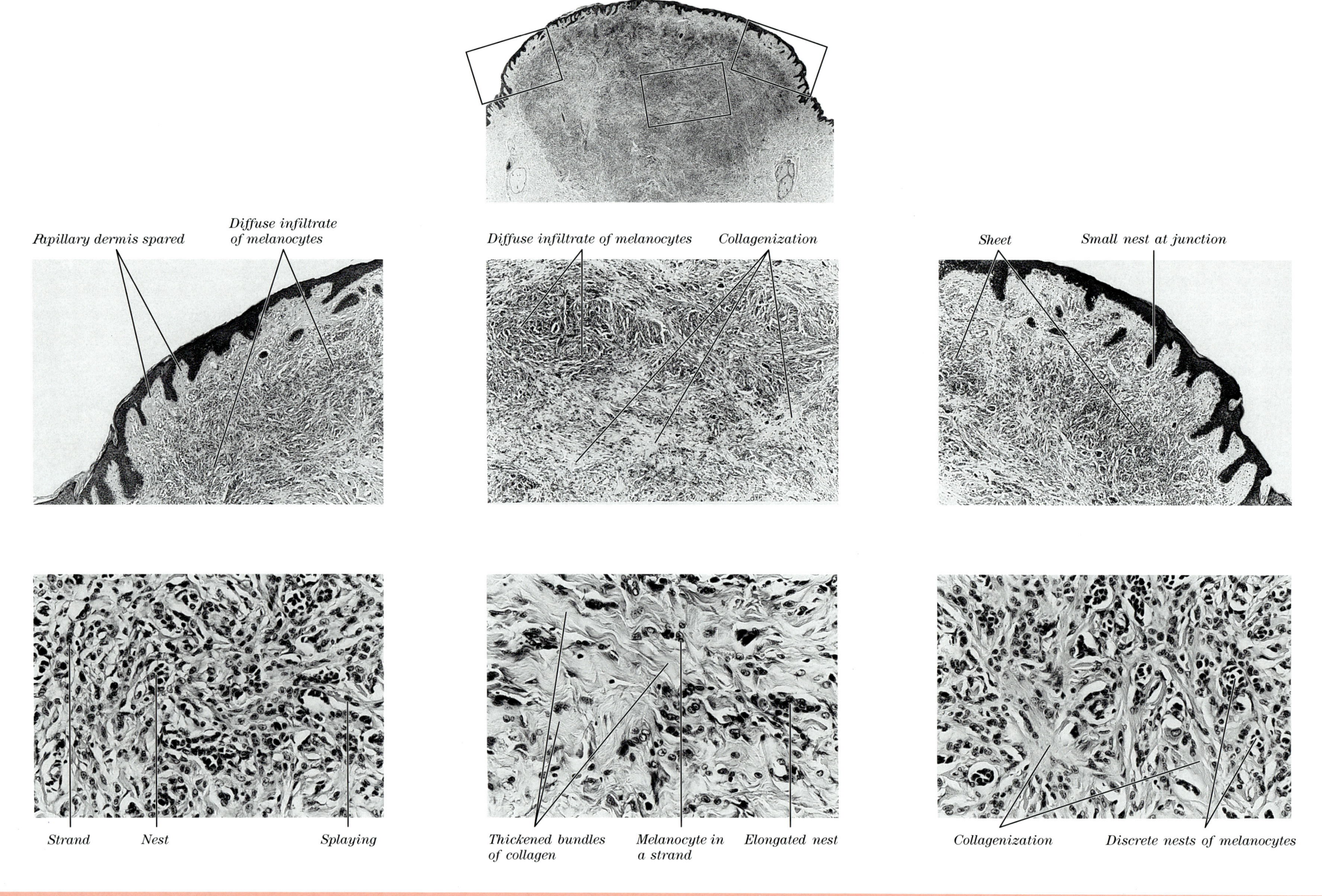

29 • Miescher's Nevus

Criteria for diagnosis of this intradermal type of Miescher's nevus (with collagenization)

This is a nevus because:

1. The neoplasm is symmetric.
2. It is well-circumscribed.
3. It is wedge-shaped.
4. Melanocytes mature.
5. Nuclei of melanocytes are relatively uniform.

This is a Miescher's nevus because:

1. The neoplasm has a dome shape.
2. It is mostly endophytic.
3. It is wedge-shaped.
4. Melanocytes extend far into the reticular dermis.

Signs of collagenization are:

Collagen bundles within the substance of the nevus are thickened markedly and arranged haphazardly.

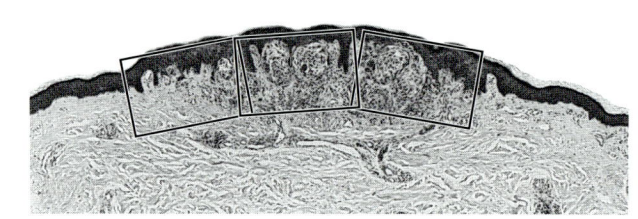

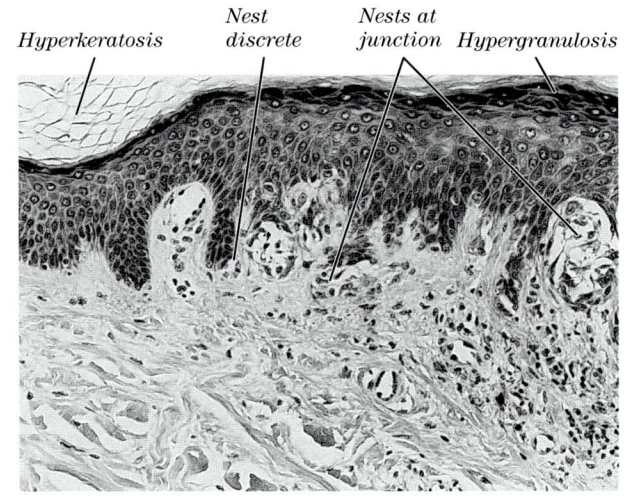
Hyperkeratosis · Nest discrete · Nests at junction · Hypergranulosis

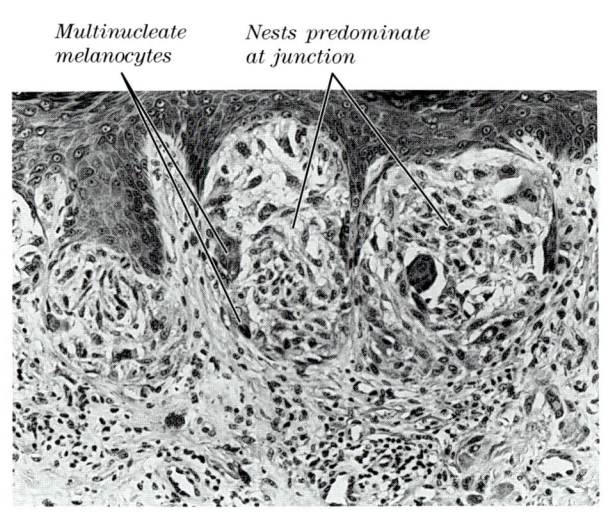
Multinucleate melanocytes · Nests predominate at junction

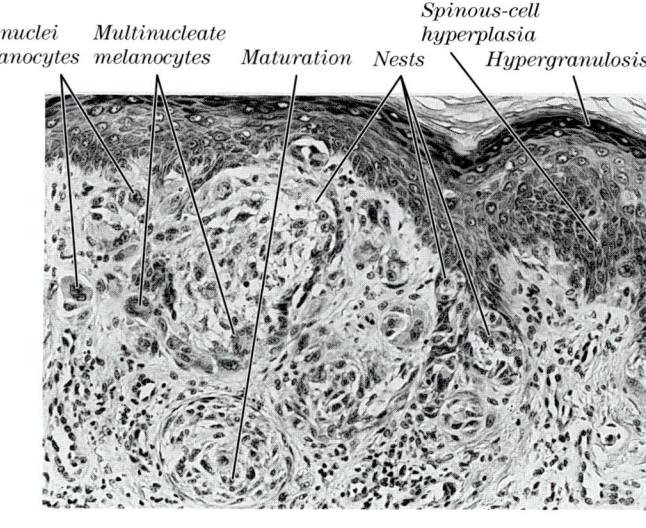
Large nuclei of melanocytes · Multinucleate melanocytes · Maturation · Nests · Spinous-cell hyperplasia · Hypergranulosis

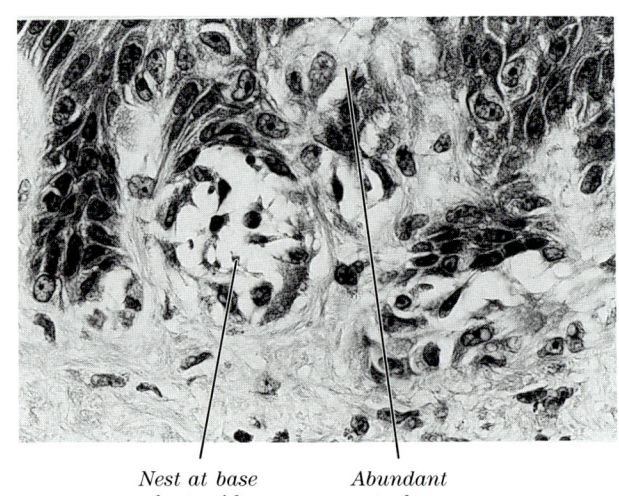
Nest at base of rete ridges · Abundant cytoplasm

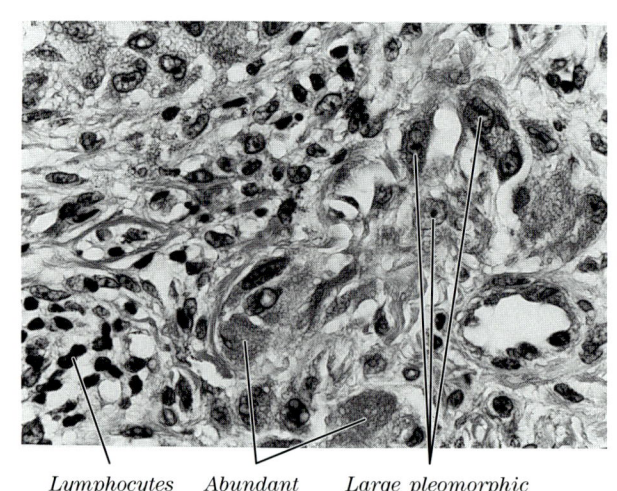
Lymphocytes · Abundant cytoplasm · Large pleomorphic nuclei of melanocytes

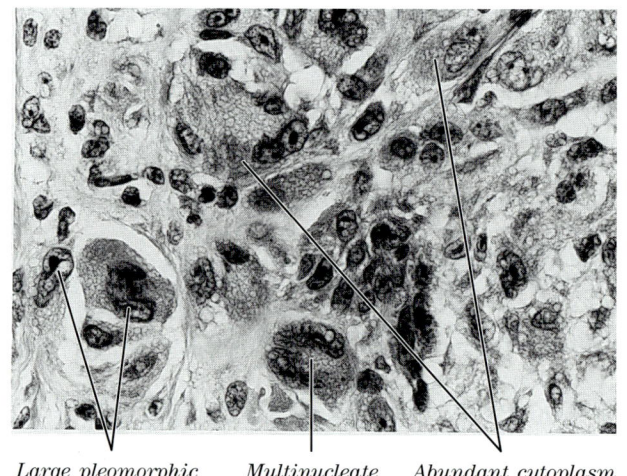
Large pleomorphic nuclei of melanocytes · Multinucleate melanocyte · Abundant cytoplasm of melanocytes

30 · Spitz's Nevus

Criteria for diagnosis of this Spitz's nevus (compound type)

This is a nevus because:

1. It is relatively symmetric.
2. It is well-circumscribed.
3. Most melanocytes within the epidermis are arranged in nests, rather than as solitary units.
4. Nests of melanocytes within the epidermis are situated mostly at the dermo-epidermal junction, not above it.
5. Melanocytes mature focally.

This is a Spitz's nevus because:

1. Many melanocytes have large nuclei, abundant cytoplasm, and oval, round, and polygonal shapes.
2. Numerous melanocytes are binucleate and multinucleate.
3. There are hyperkeratosis, hypergranulosis, and spinous-cell hyperplasia.
4. Patchy perivascular lymphocytic infiltrates are present throughout the lesion.

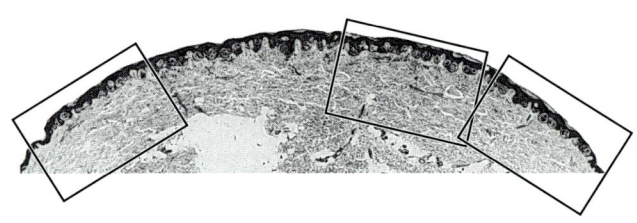

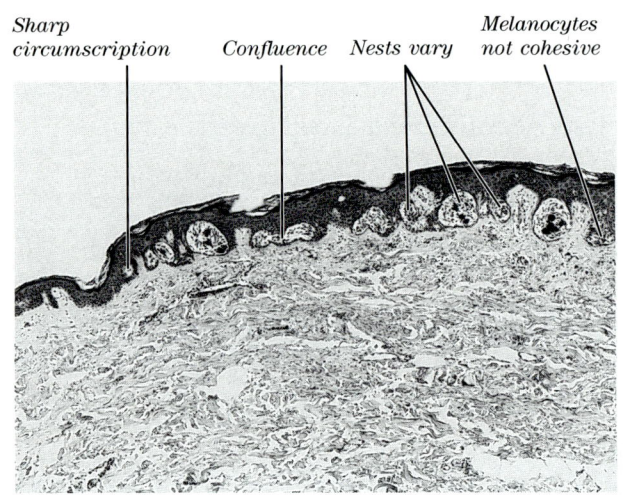

Sharp circumscription | Confluence | Nests vary | Melanocytes not cohesive

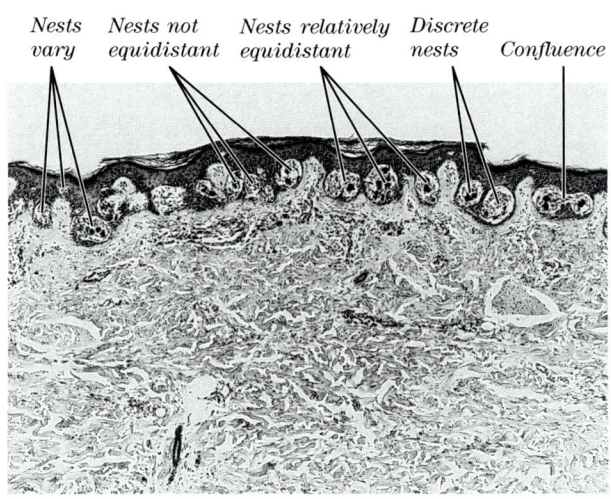

Nests vary | Nests not equidistant | Nests relatively equidistant | Discrete nests | Confluence

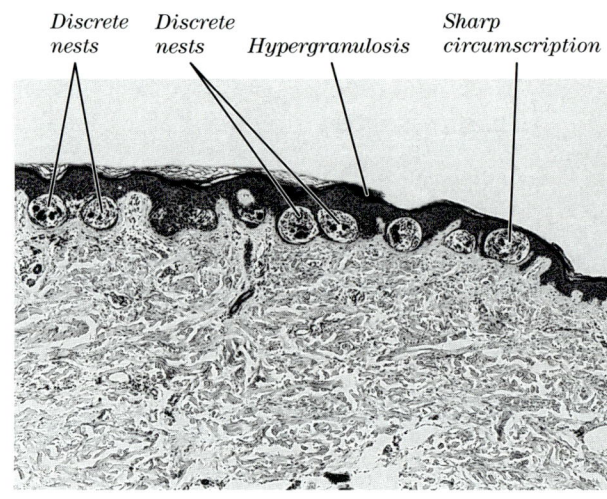

Discrete nests | Discrete nests | Hypergranulosis | Sharp circumscription

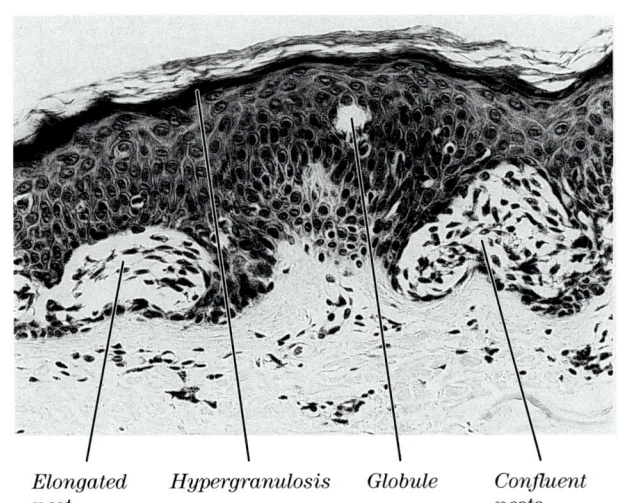

Elongated nest | Hypergranulosis | Globule | Confluent nests

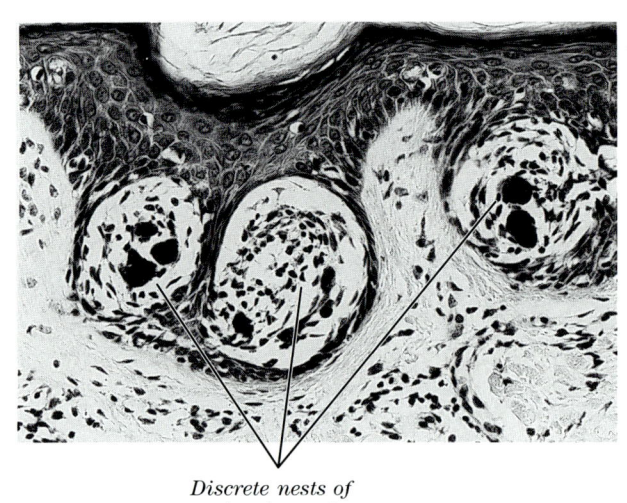

Discrete nests of oval melanocytes

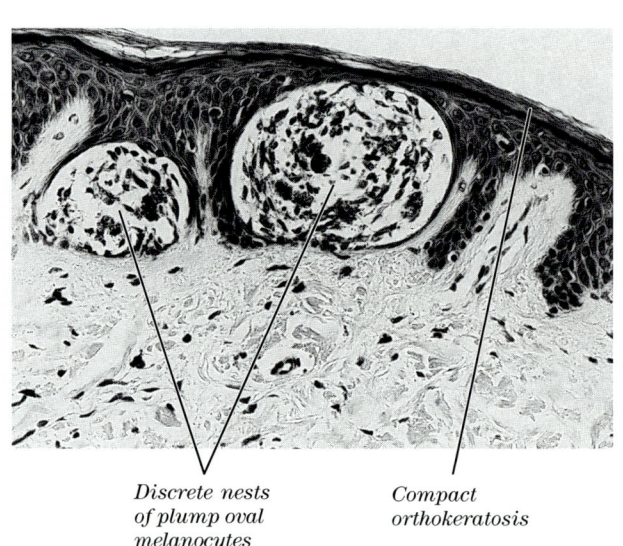

Discrete nests of plump oval melanocytes | Compact orthokeratosis

31 • Spitz's Nevus

Criteria for diagnosis of this Spitz's nevus (junctional type)

This is a nevus because:

1. The neoplasm is symmetric.
2. It is well-circumscribed.
3. Nests of melanocytes are discrete.
4. Nests of melanocytes are relatively uniform in size and shape.
5. Nuclei of melanocytes are relatively monomorphous.

This is a Spitz's nevus because:

1. Some melanocytes have largish nuclei, abundant cytoplasm, and oval, spindle, and polygonal shapes.
2. Some nests of melanocytes are elongated.
3. Some nests of melanocytes are separated from adjacent keratinocytes by clefts.
4. There are subtle hyperkeratosis, hypergranulosis, and hyperplasia of spinous cells.
5. Globules within the spinous zone are seen to be dull pink in sections stained by hematoxylin and eosin.

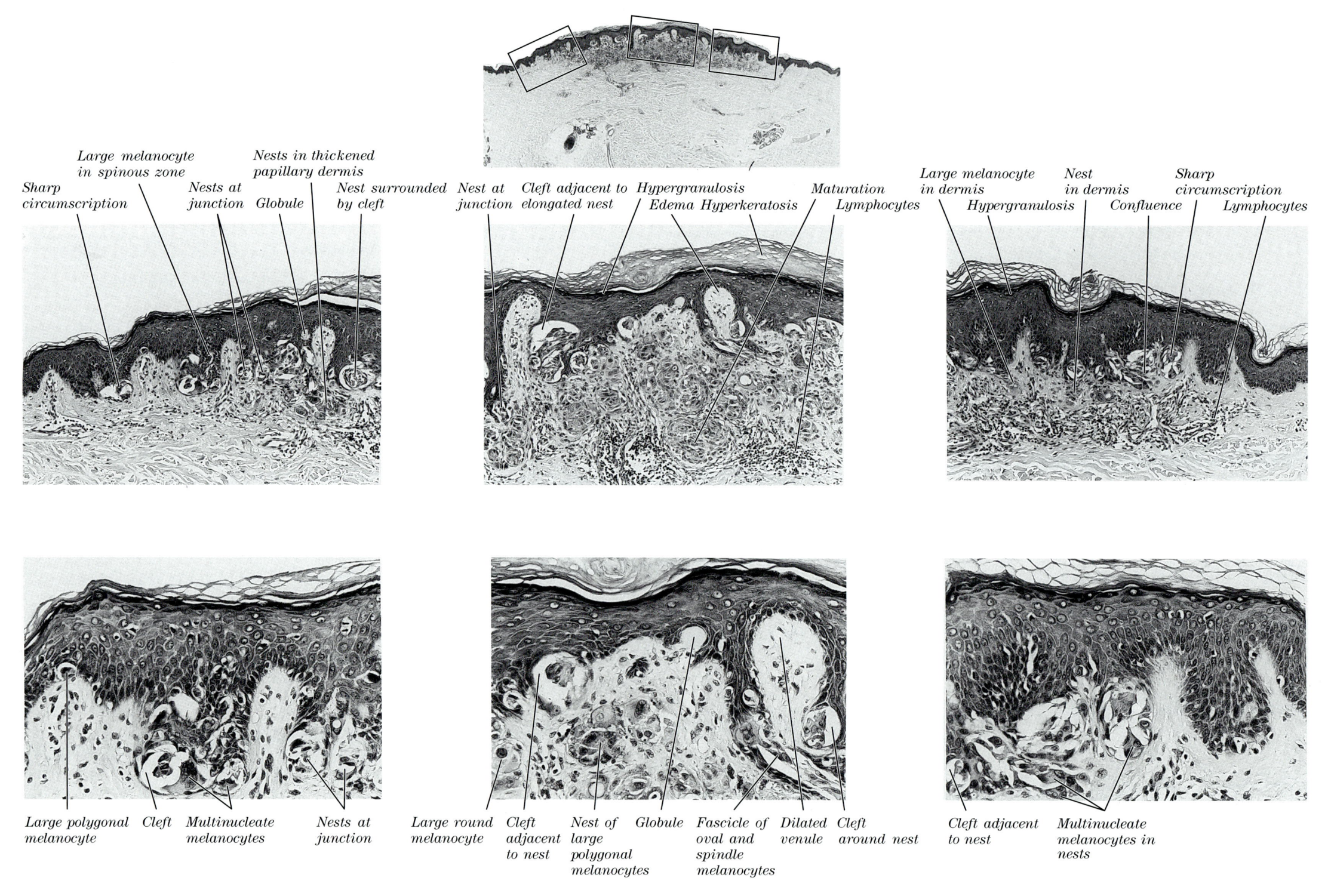

32 • Spitz's Nevus

Criteria for diagnosis of this Spitz's nevus (compound type)

This neoplasm is benign because:

1. It is relatively symmetric.
2. It is well-circumscribed.
3. Most melanocytes within the epidermis are disposed in nests, rather than as solitary units.
4. Most nests within the epidermis are situated at the dermo-epidermal junction, not above it.
5. Melanocytes mature.

This is a Spitz's nevus because:

1. Many melanocytes have large nuclei, abundant cytoplasm, and round, oval, spindle, and polygonal shapes.
2. There are hyperkeratosis, hypergranulosis, and irregular spinous-cell hyperplasia.
3. Prominent clefts separate many nests of melanocytes from adjacent keratinocytes.

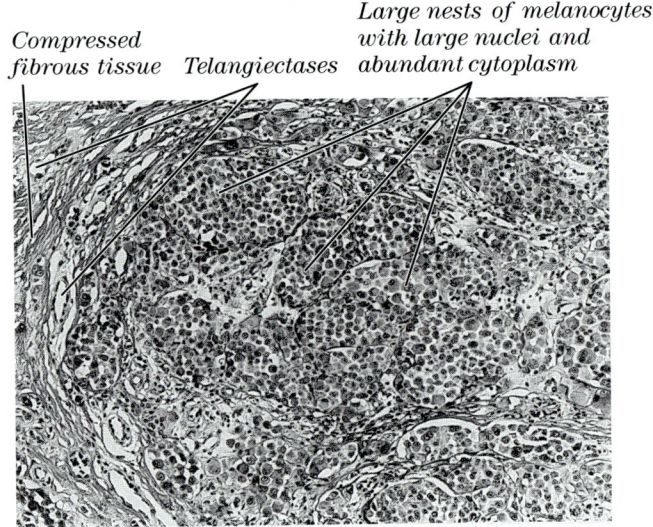

Compressed fibrous tissue — *Telangiectases* — *Large nests of melanocytes with large nuclei and abundant cytoplasm* — *Melanocytes with large nuclei* — *Maturation* — *Clefts in the stroma* — *Multinucleate melanocytes with large nuclei* — *Mononuclear, binucleate, and multinucleate melanocytes with large nuclei* — *Multinucleate melanocytes with large nuclei* — *Cluster of bi- and multinucleate melanocytes* — *Dilated venules*

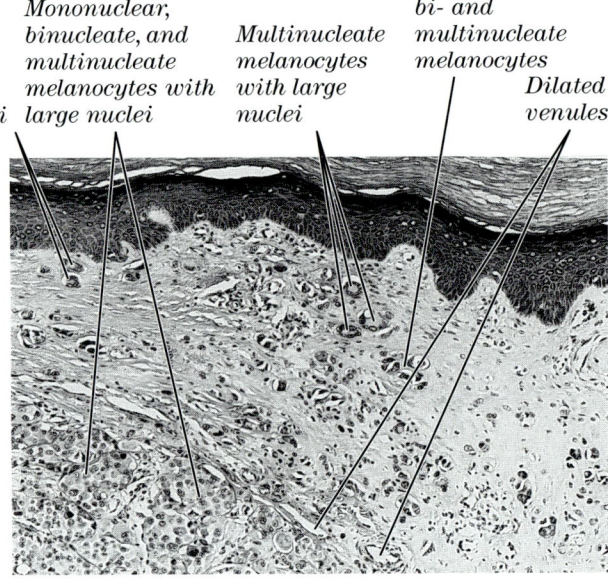

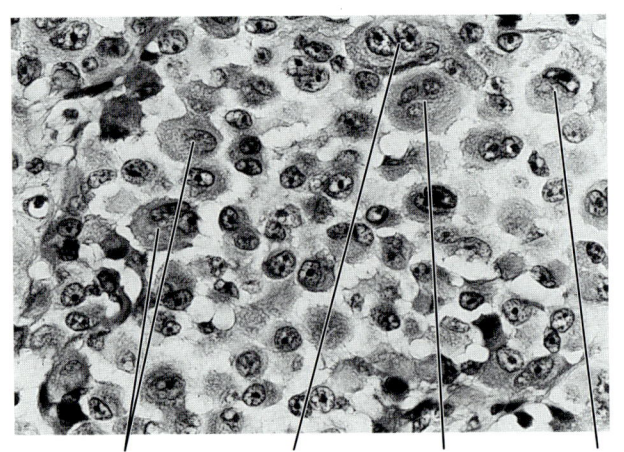

Melanocytes with large nuclei and abundant cytoplasm — *Binucleate melanocyte with large nuclei* — *Trinucleate melanocyte with large nuclei* — *Mononuclear melanocyte with large nucleus*

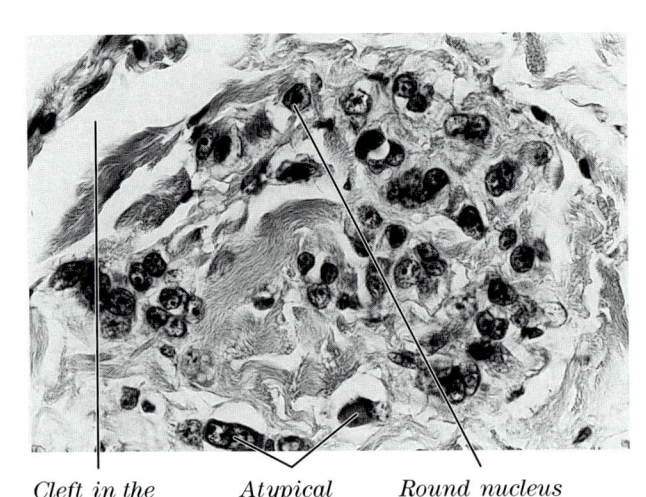

Cleft in the stroma — *Atypical oval nuclei* — *Round nucleus*

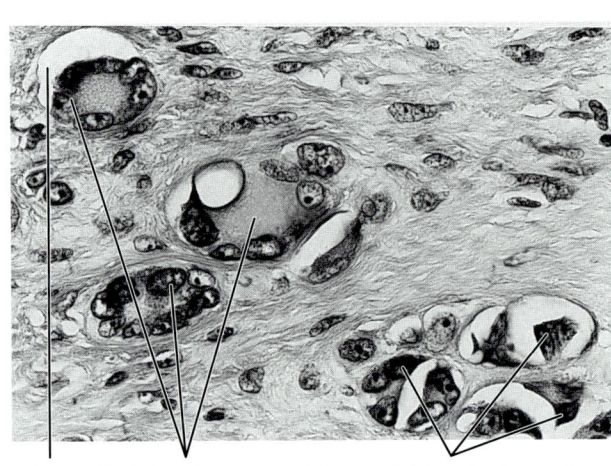

Cleft — *Multinucleate melanocytes with large nuclei* — *Nests of binucleate and multinucleate melanocytes with large polygonal nuclei*

33 • Spitz's Nevus

Criteria for diagnosis of this
Spitz's nevus (intradermal type)

This is a nevus because the neoplasm is:

1. Tiny, i.e., less than 3.0 mm in greatest diameter.
2. Symmetric.
3. Well-circumscribed, in part by a collarette of adnexal epithelium.
4. Wedge-shaped.

This is a Spitz's nevus because:

1. Some nuclei of melanocytes are atypical.
2. The shapes of melanocytes are round, oval, and polygonal.
3. The cytoplasm of melanocytes is abundant and amphophilic.
4. There are numerous multinucleate melanocytes.

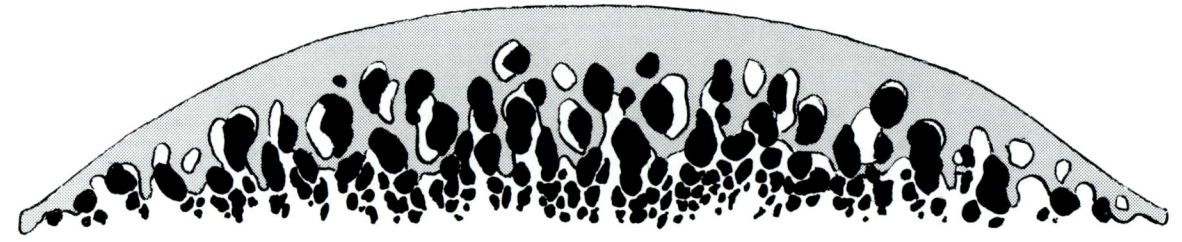

Fig. 34. Spitz's nevus. The neoplasm is benign because it is symmetric, well-circumscribed, and characterized by maturation of melanocytes with progressive descent into the dermis, that is, individual melanocytes become smaller as they go deeper into the dermis. From silhouette alone, the neoplasm can be diagnosed as a Spitz's nevus because there are epidermal hyperplasia, clefts between elongated nests of melanocytes and adjacent keratinocytes, and scatter of nests above the dermo-epidermal junction. In short, this constellation of findings, recognizable by architectural pattern alone, is diagnostic of a compound type of Spitz's nevus.

A common type of Spitz's nevus, termed "pigmented spindle-cell tumor" by those who do not consider it to be a Spitz's nevus, is a brown, gently domed-shaped papule clinically and a neoplasm confined to either the epidermis alone or to the epidermis and papillary dermis histopathologically. In the epidermis, melanocytes are oval (Fig. 37) and, uncommonly, spindle-shaped (Fig. 38), and are arranged in fascicles oriented mostly perpendicular to the surface of the skin. The nuclei are but slightly large and the cytoplasm is scant. Dendrites of neoplastic melanocytes may be prominent within the epidermis (Fig. 39). Such lesions have nearly all of the other features of Spitz's nevi already enumerated, including dull pink globules sometimes, except that the nuclei are not very large and the cytoplasm is not very abundant. In brief, the term "pigmented spindle-cell tumor" is misleading because it implies a specific distinctive nevus when, in our view, it really is nothing more than one of many morphologic expressions of Spitz's nevus.

Dull pink globules within the epidermis of a proliferation of melanocytes are a highly suggestive evidence of Spitz's nevus (Figs. 34, 37). They are PAS-positive, diastase-resistant, and trichrome-positive. Practically never are those globules found in Unna's, Miescher's, or Clark's nevi, and only rarely do they appear in melanomas. The globules consist of components of necrotic melanocytes and keratinocytes, and of fibronectin. They are situated mostly at the periphery of intra-epidermal nests of melanocytes and above suprapapillary plates. Because melanocytes within the epidermis of Spitz's nevus replicate rapidly, necrotic melanocytes constitute an important component of the globules. The globules are positioned in the epidermis only, not in the dermis.

Another common variant of Spitz's nevus is papillated, often pink, and comprised mostly of large polygonal melanocytes with either large monomorphous or pleomorphic nuclei and abundant amphophilic cytoplasm (Fig. 40). The polygonal melanocytes tend to be separated from one another by narrow spaces, giving them the appearance of "acantholytic" cells. A pink color is imparted to the lesions by a combination of numerous widely dilated venules and near absence of melanin.

Sometimes, at scanning magnification, a particular Spitz's nevus may be thought to be an example of granulomatous dermatitis, so closely do the melanocytes resemble histiocytes (Figs. 41, 42). That is the reason why the most popular title for this nevus prior to nearly universal acceptance of the designation "Spitz's nevus" was some variation on a theme of "spindle-cell and epithelioid cell nevus." Not only do individual neoplastic melanocytes resemble epithelioid histiocytes (both have oval nuclei and pink cytoplasm in sections stained by hematoxylin and eosin), but also collections of melanocytes simulate granulomas (in both the neoplastic and inflammatory process, oval cells seem to touch one another like components of an epithelium). When, therefore, a histopathologist encounters a melanocytic neoplasm that at first glance is thought to be granulomatous inflammation, serious consideration must be given to the possibility of a Spitz's nevus.

Numerous other variants of Spitz's nevus are identified by topographic features, distribution of melanocytes, cytologic features of melanocytes, and presence or absence of nuclear atypia. If criteria for histopathologic diagnosis of a nevus in general are employed strictly, and if the least common denominators for diagnosis of Spitz's nevus are sought carefully, then diagnosis of Spitz's nevus may be made with confidence in lesions that have been excised completely, despite the many histopathologic features that some Spitz's nevi share with melanoma. All too often, however, biopsy specimens of Spitz's nevi are inadequate, removed as they are by superficial shave or by narrow punch technique. In such instances, it may be impossible to differentiate a Spitz's nevus from a melanoma (see Table 7). As a consequence of such paltry biopsy specimens, errors in histopathologic diagnosis may be made. The implications of these errors are serious when more surgery than necessary is performed for a Spitz's nevus that was diagnosed incorrectly as a melanoma, but they may result in death when a melanoma is misread as a Spitz's nevus. The three criteria crucial for differentiation of Spitz's nevus from melanoma—symmetry, sharp circumscription, and maturation (Fig. 43)—cannot be assessed adequately in many biopsy specimens taken by shave technique. Whenever possible, biopsy of a melanocytic neoplasm suspected of being a Spitz's nevus or a melanoma should be by excision in toto.

No benign proliferation of melanocytes in skin poses greater problems in histopathologic differentiation from melanoma than does that in some Spitz's nevi. The reason for this vexing situation is that the two proliferations of melanocytes of wholly different biologic natures often have more histopathologic features in common than they have differences between them. The shared features are an increased number of melanocytes arranged as solitary units and in nests within the epidermis, not only at the dermo-epidermal junction but also above it and sometimes throughout the entire thickness of the epidermis, including the granular zone and cornified

Text continues on page 86

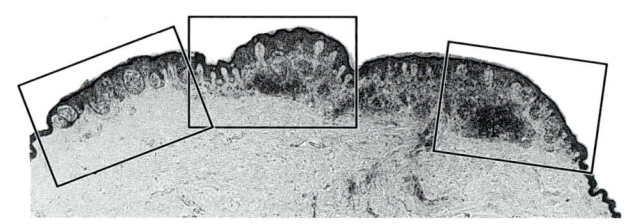

Sharp circumscription · *Cleft* · *Hyperkeratosis* · *Hypergranulosis* · *Discrete nests* · *Elongated nest perpendicular to surface*

Nests vary · *Globules* · *Nests partially obscured by lymphocytes* · *Confluence* · *Hypergranulosis* · *Hyperkeratosis* · *Scatter*

Globule Scatter · *Nest at junction* · *Nest in spinous zone* · *Confluence* · *Sharp circumscription* · *Globules*

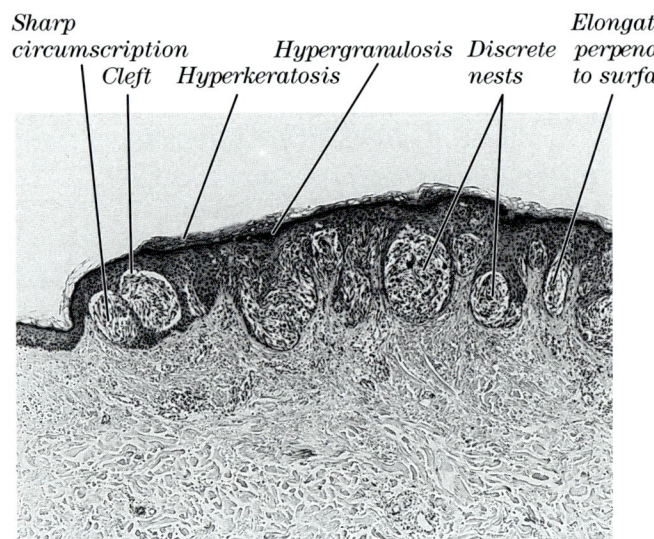 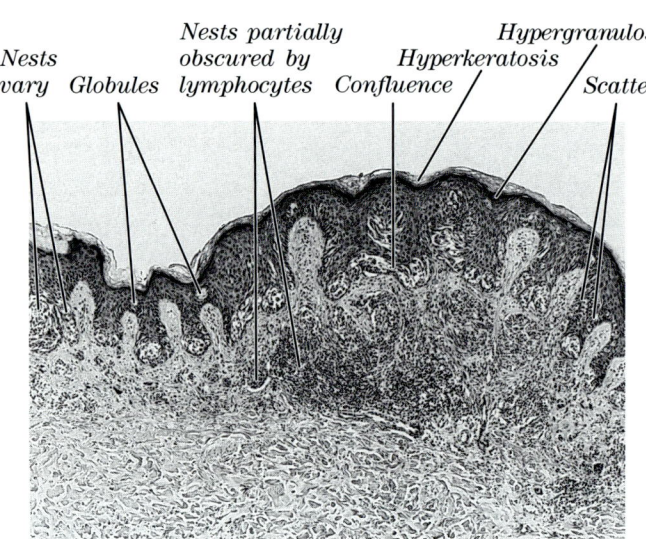 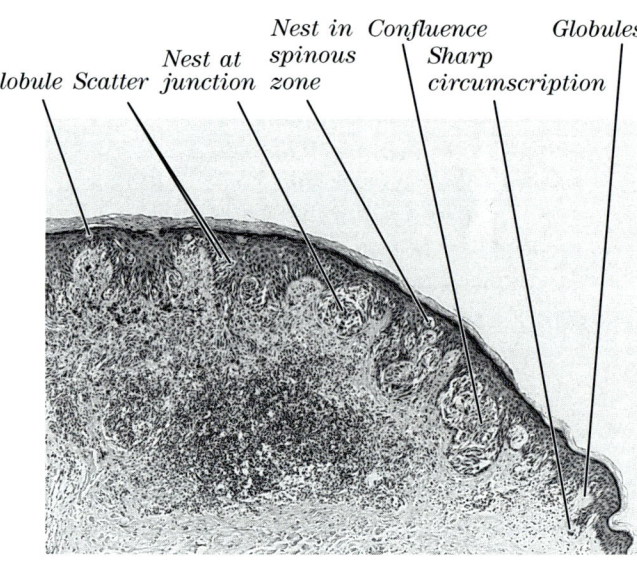

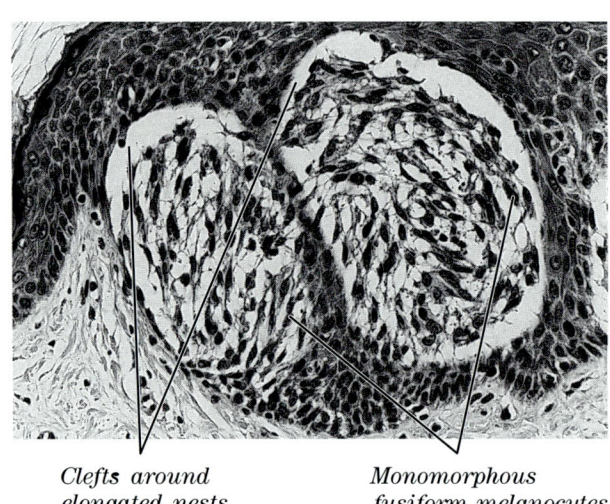 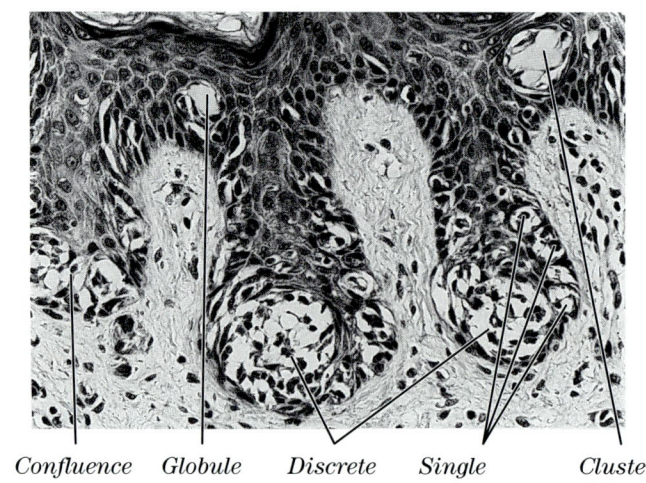 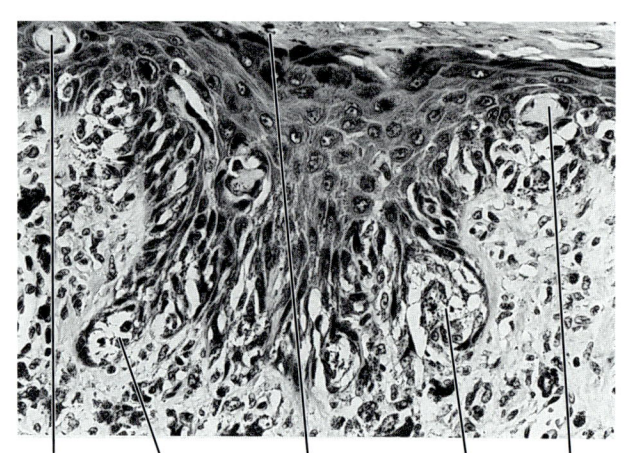

Clefts around elongated nests · *Monomorphous fusiform melanocytes*

Confluence · *Globule* · *Discrete nests* · *Single melanocytes* · *Cluster of globules*

Globule · *Nest at junction* · *Melanocyte in cornified layer* · *Nest at junction* · *Globule*

35 • Spitz's Nevus

Criteria for diagnosis of this Spitz's nevus (compound type)

This neoplasm is benign because:

1. The neoplasm is well-circumscribed.
2. Nests of melanocytes within the epidermis predominate over melanocytes arranged as solitary units.
3. Nests of melanocytes within the epidermis are discrete.
4. Melanocytes mature.
5. Nuclei of melanocytes are oval and monomorphous.

This is a Spitz's nevus because:

1. Many melanocytes have largish nuclei, abundant cytoplasm, and oval shape.
2. There are hyperkeratosis, hypergranulosis, and hyperplasia of spinous cells.
3. Clefts are present between some elongated nests of melanocytes and adjacent keratinocytes.
4. Some nests of melanocytes are oriented perpendicularly to the skin surface.
5. Homogeneous globules are present in clusters within the epidermis.

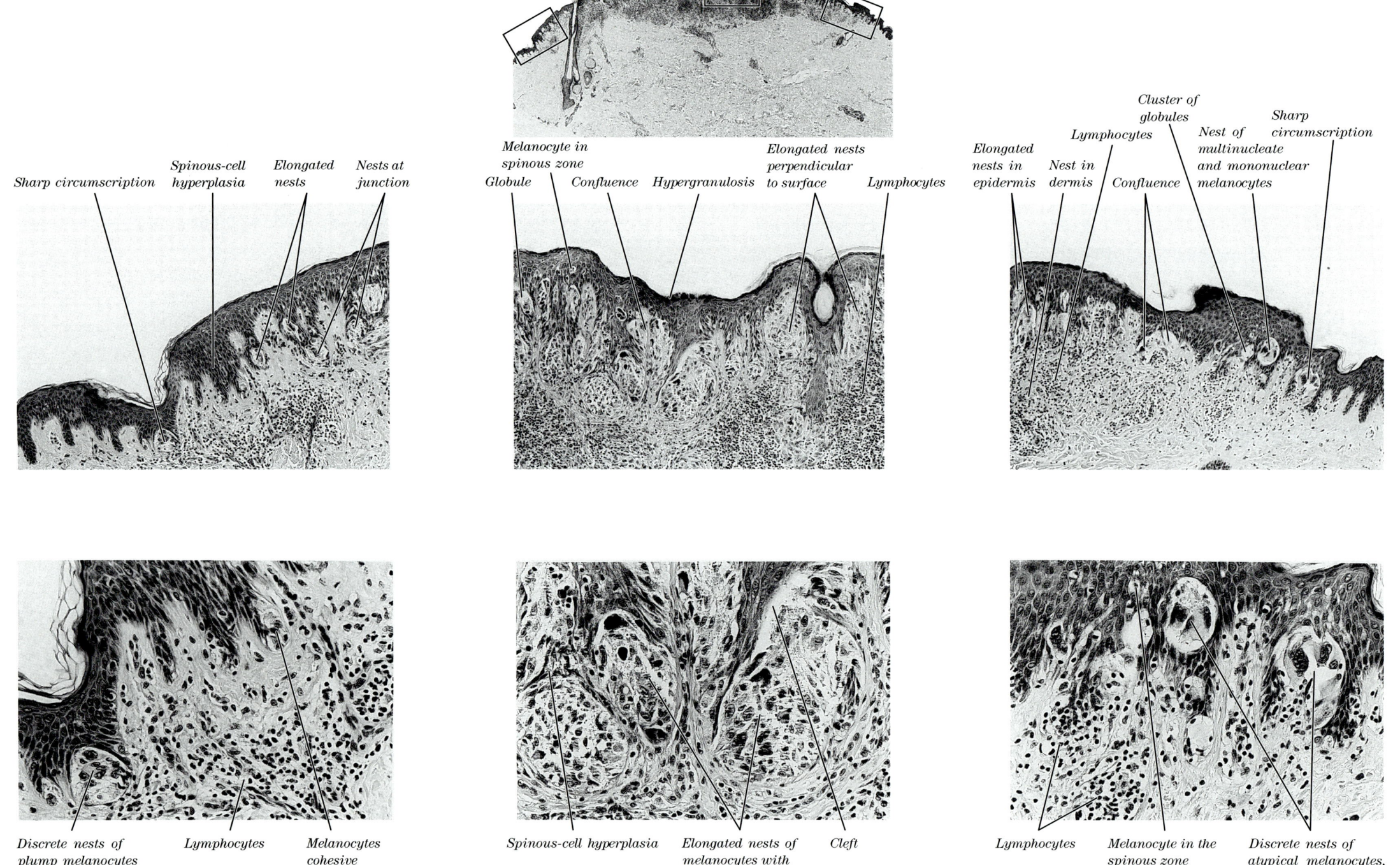

36 · Spitz's Nevus

Criteria for diagnosis of this Spitz's nevus (compound type)

This is a nevus because:

1. The neoplasm is symmetric.
2. It is well-circumscribed.
3. Melanocytes within the epidermis are arranged mostly in nests, rather than as solitary units.
4. Most nests of melanocytes are present at the dermo-epidermal junction, rather than above it.
5. Nests of melanocytes within the epidermis are relatively equidistant from one another.

This is a Spitz's nevus because:

1. Many melanocytes have large pleomorphic nuclei, abundant cytoplasm, and oval, round, spindle, and polygonal shapes.
2. Many melanocytes are multinucleate.
3. There are hyperkeratosis, hypergranulosis, and hyperplasia of spinous cells.
4. Some melanocytes arranged as solitary units and in nests are present above the dermo-epidermal junction.
5. Many nests are oriented perpendicular to the skin surface.
6. Clefts separate some nests of melanocytes from adjacent keratinocytes.
7. A patchy lymphocytic infiltrate is present around blood vessels throughout the neoplasm.

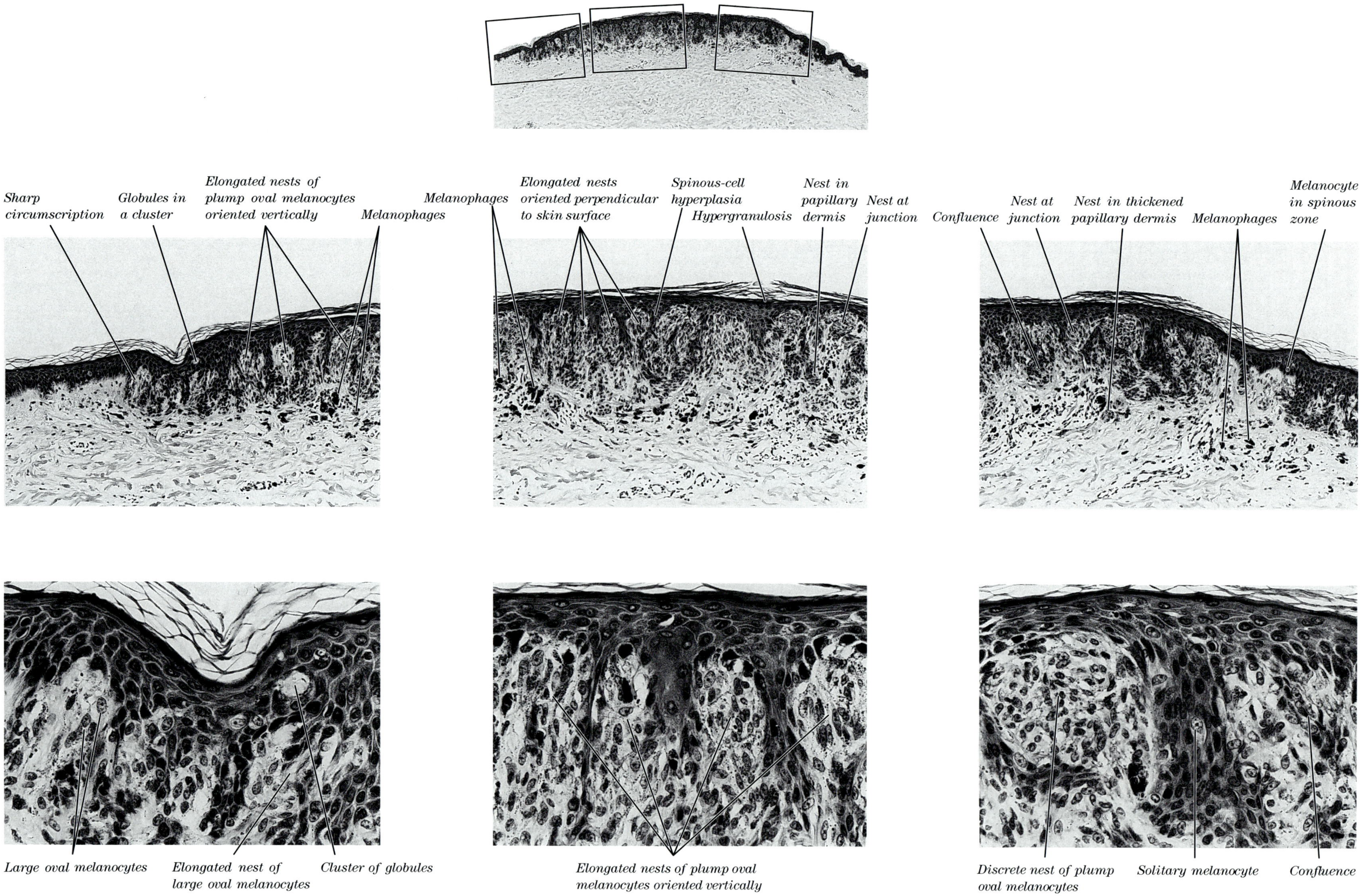

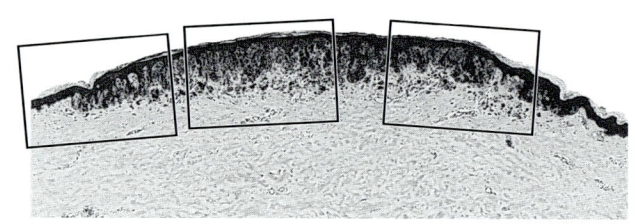

37 • Spitz's Nevus *("pigmented spindle-cell" type)*

Criteria for diagnosis of this Spitz's nevus ("pigmented spindle-cell" type)

This is a nevus because:

1. The neoplasm is symmetric.
2. It is well-circumscribed.
3. Melanocytes within the epidermis are arrayed mostly in nests, rather than as solitary units.
4. Nests of melanocytes within the epidermis are situated at the dermo-epidermal junction and not above it.
5. Nests of melanocytes within the epidermis are relatively equidistant from one another.
6. Nuclei of melanocytes are relatively monomorphous.
7. Melanin is distributed throughout the neoplasm in relatively uniform fashion.

This is a Spitz's nevus because:

1. The melanocytes have slightly largish nuclei, abundant cytoplasm, and plump oval shape.
2. Many nests of melanocytes are oriented vertically to the skin surface.
3. Globules within the spinous zone are stained dull pink by hematoxylin and eosin.
4. There are slight hyperkeratosis, hypergranulosis, and irregular hyperplasia of spinous cells.

This is a "pigmented spindle-cell" variant of Spitz's nevus because:

1. Most melanocytes are oval.
2. The neoplasm is pigmented heavily by melanin, both melanocytes and macrophages.
3. The neoplasm is superficial, i.e., confined to the epidermis and papillary dermis.

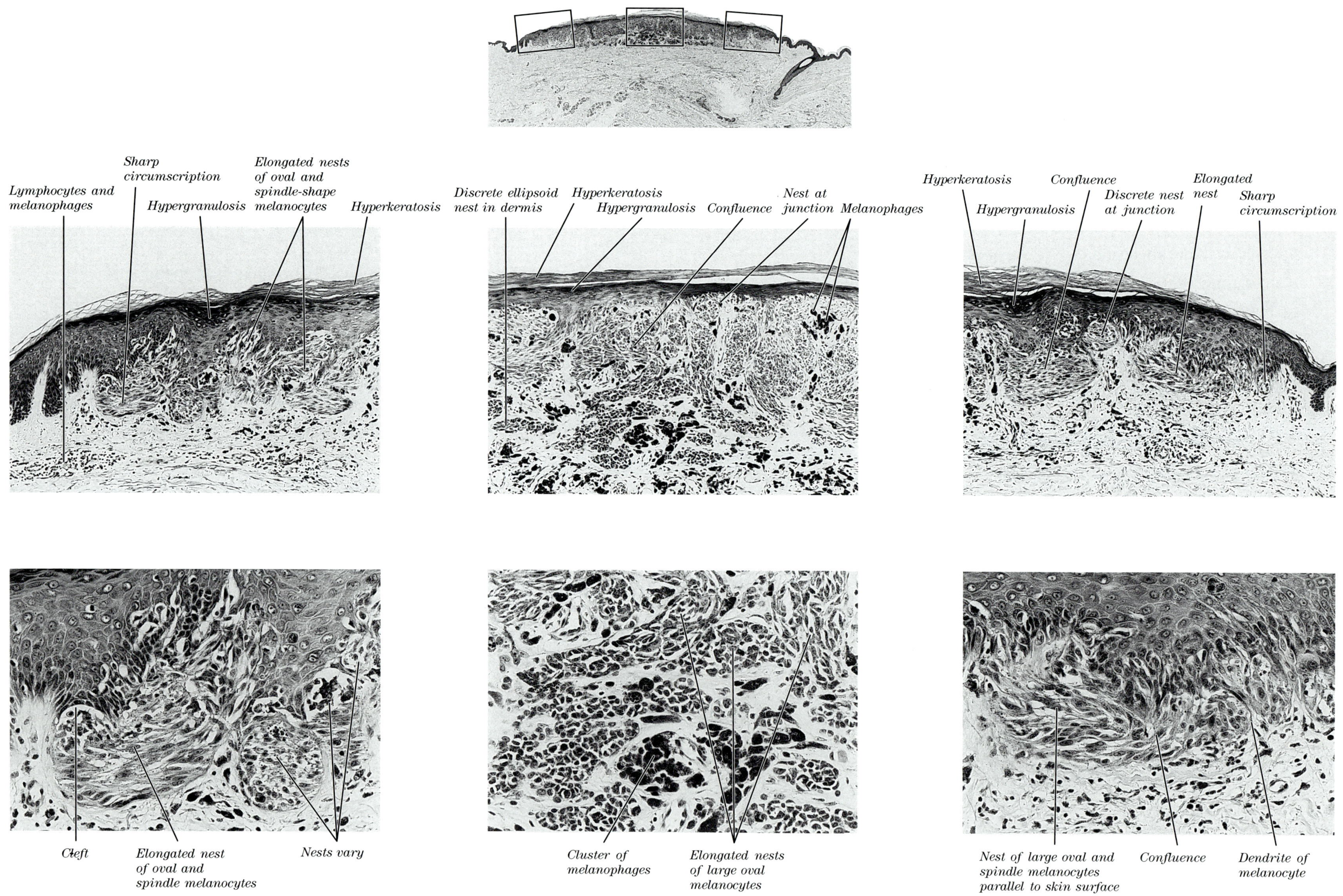

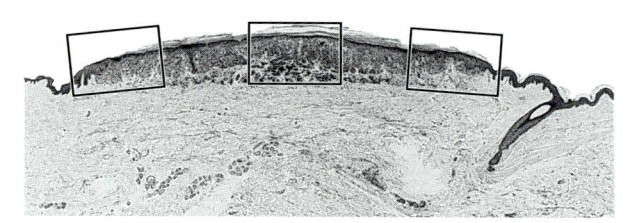

38 • Spitz's Nevus *("pigmented spindle-cell" type)*

Criteria for diagnosis of this Spitz's nevus ("pigmented spindle-cell" type)

This lesion is benign because:

1. It is symmetric.
2. It is well-circumscribed.
3. It has a flat bottom.
4. Melanocytes mature.
5. Nests of melanocytes within the epidermis predominate over melanocytes arranged as solitary units.
6. Nests of melanocytes are situated mostly at the dermo-epidermal junction.
7. Melanin is distributed in relatively uniform fashion throughout the neoplasm.

This is a Spitz's nevus because:

1. The nuclei of many melanocytes are largish, oval-spindle, and monomorphous.
2. There are hyperkeratosis, hypergranulosis, and hyperplasia of spinous cells.
3. Some nests of melanocytes are elongated and oriented perpendicularly to the skin surface.
4. Some melanocytes arrayed as solitary units are scattered above the dermo-epidermal junction.

In contrast to other variants of Spitz's nevus, the pigmented spindle-cell type is marked by both relatively small size and absence of pleomorphism of nuclei. Almost always, the lesion is but gently domed and confined to the dermo-epidermal junction and thickened papillary dermis. That it is truly a Spitz's nevus can be concluded from the aforementioned criteria and by the fact that this lesion often is accompanied by numerous dull pink globules within the epidermis.

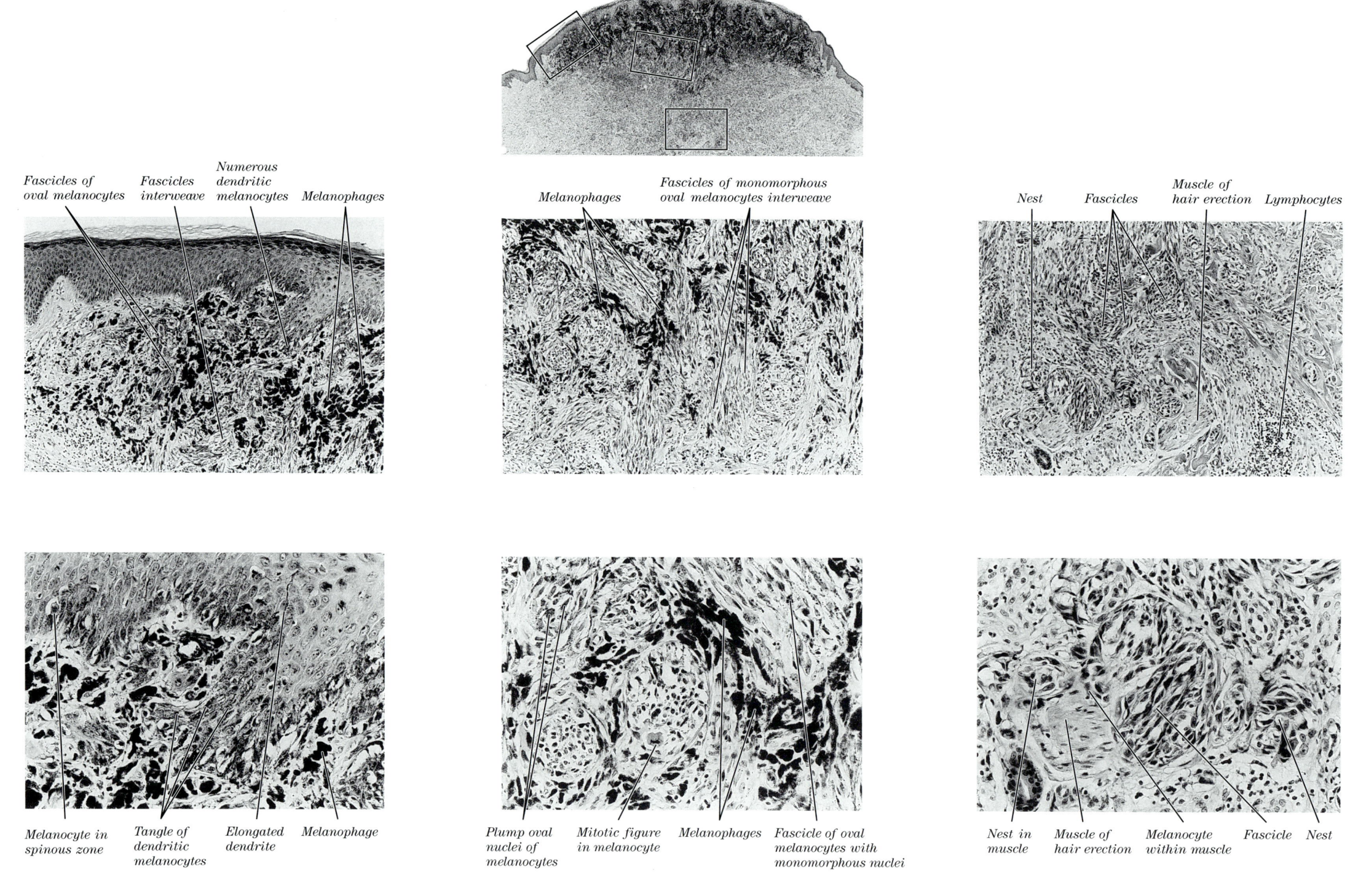

39 • Spitz's Nevus *("pigmented spindle-cell" type)*

Criteria for diagnosis of this Spitz's nevus ("pigmented spindle-cell type")

This is a nevus because:

1. The neoplasm is symmetric.
2. The neoplasm is wedge-shaped.
3. It is well-circumscribed.
4. Melanocytes within the epidermis are situated mostly at the dermo-epidermal junction, not above it.
5. There is maturation of melanocytes.
6. Nuclei of melanocytes are monomorphous.

This is a Spitz's nevus because:

1. Some melanocytes in the upper part of the neoplasm have largish nuclei, abundant cytoplasm, and oval and dendritic shapes.
2. There are hyperkeratosis, hypergranulosis, and spinous-cell hyperplasia.
3. Melanocytes within the dermis are arranged in elongated fascicles.
4. Some mitotic figures are present within the dermal component of the neoplasm.

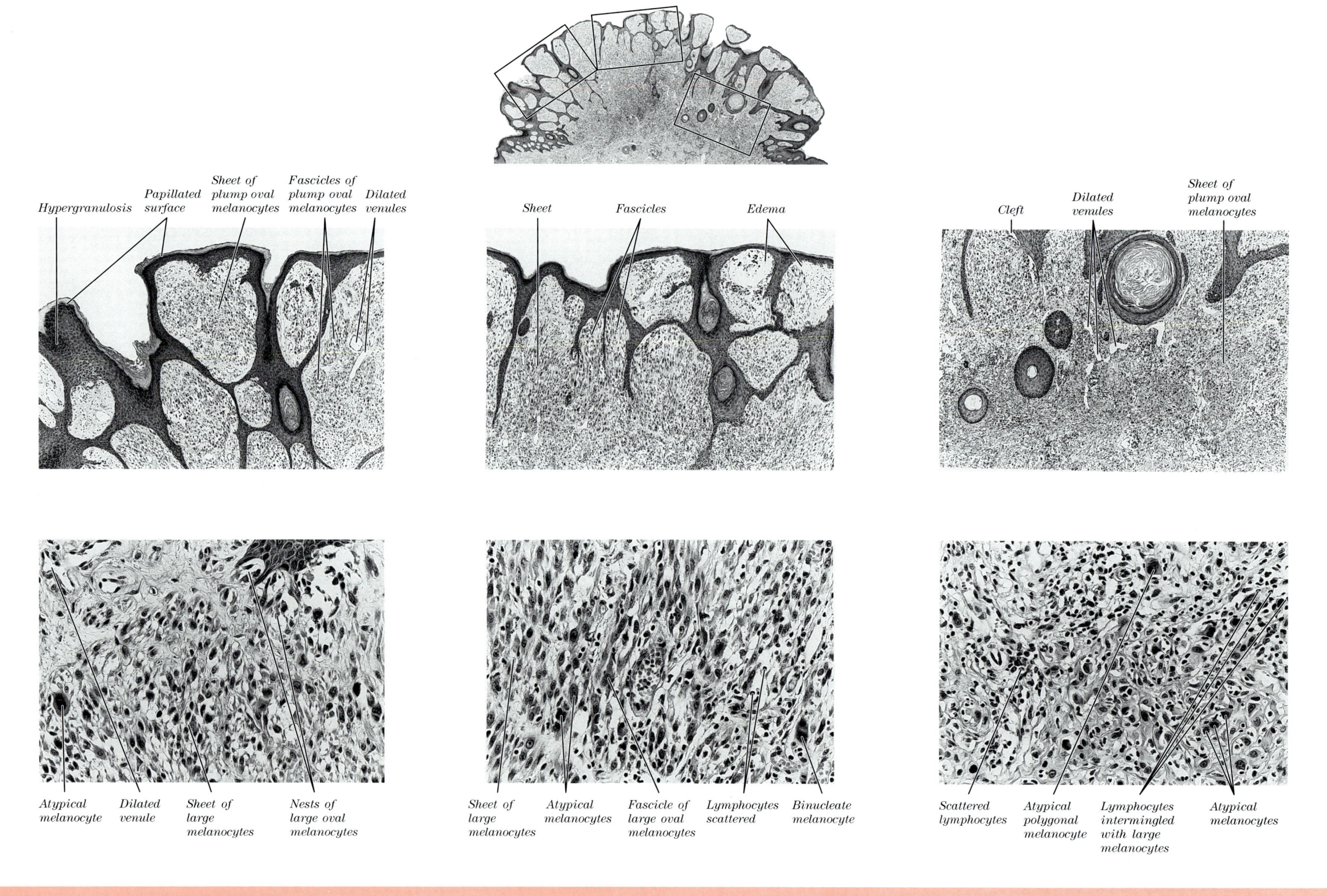

40 • Spitz's Nevus

Criteria for diagnosis of this Spitz's nevus (compound type)

This is a nevus because:

1. The neoplasm is symmetric.
2. It is well-circumscribed.
3. Melanocytes mature.
4. Melanocytes arranged both as solitary units and in nests are situated at the dermo-epidermal junction, not above it.
5. Epithelial structures of adnexa are preserved.

This is a Spitz's nevus because:

1. Numerous neoplastic melanocytes have large pleomorphic nuclei, abundant cytoplasm, and plump oval, spindle, and polygonal shapes; many are binucleate and multinucleate.
2. There are edema of the papillary dermis, an increased number of widely dilated blood vessels, and a sprinkling of lymphocytes throughout the neoplasm.
3. Hyperkeratosis, hypergranulosis, and both epidermal and adnexal epithelial hyperplasia are apparent.

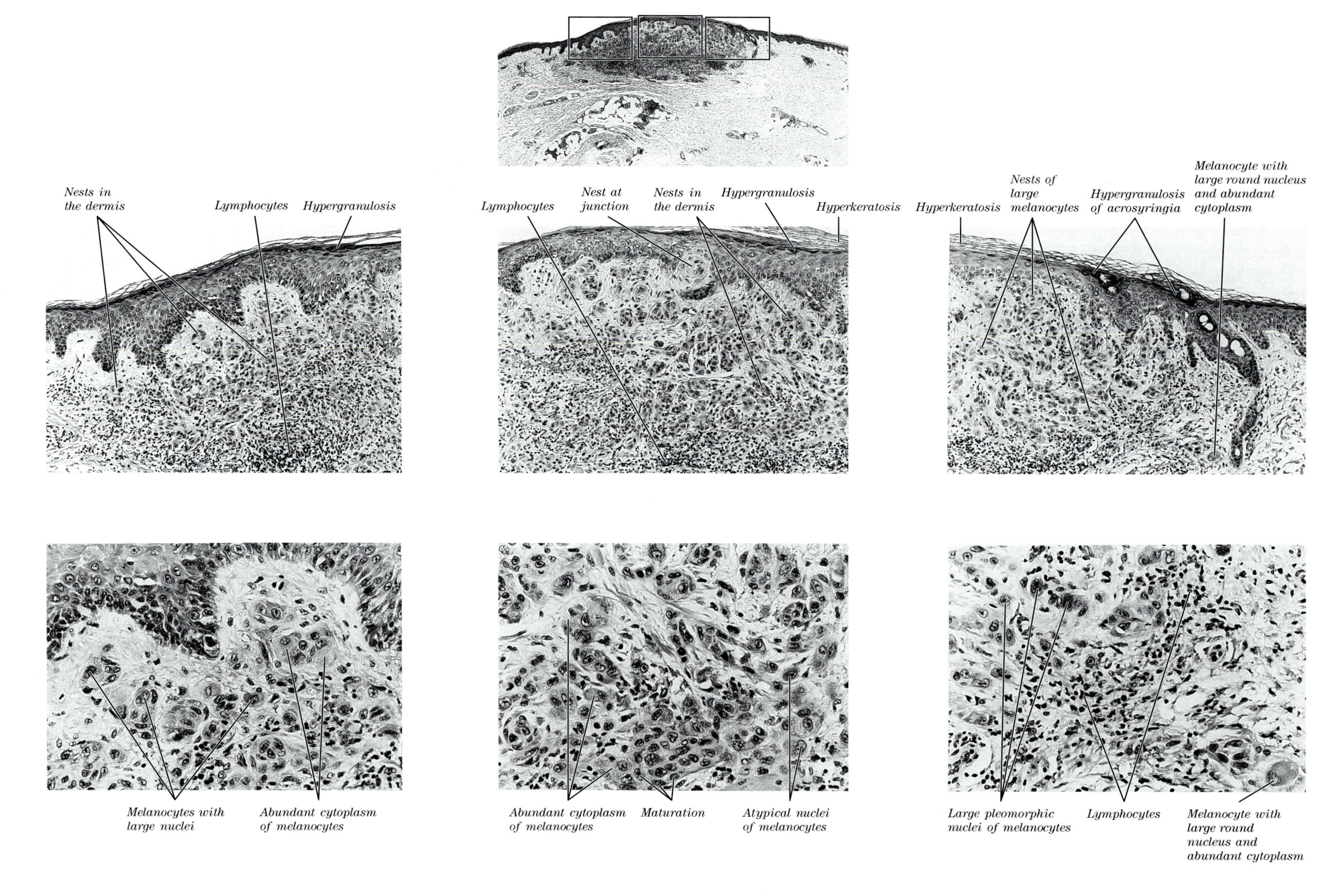

41 • Spitz's Nevus

Criteria for diagnosis of this Spitz's nevus (compound type)

This neoplasm is benign because:

1. It is small, yet it extends into the upper part of the reticular dermis.
2. It is symmetric.
3. It is well-circumscribed.
4. There is maturation of melanocytes.

This is a Spitz's nevus because:

Most of the melanocytes have large nuclei, abundant cytoplasm, and oval and round shapes.

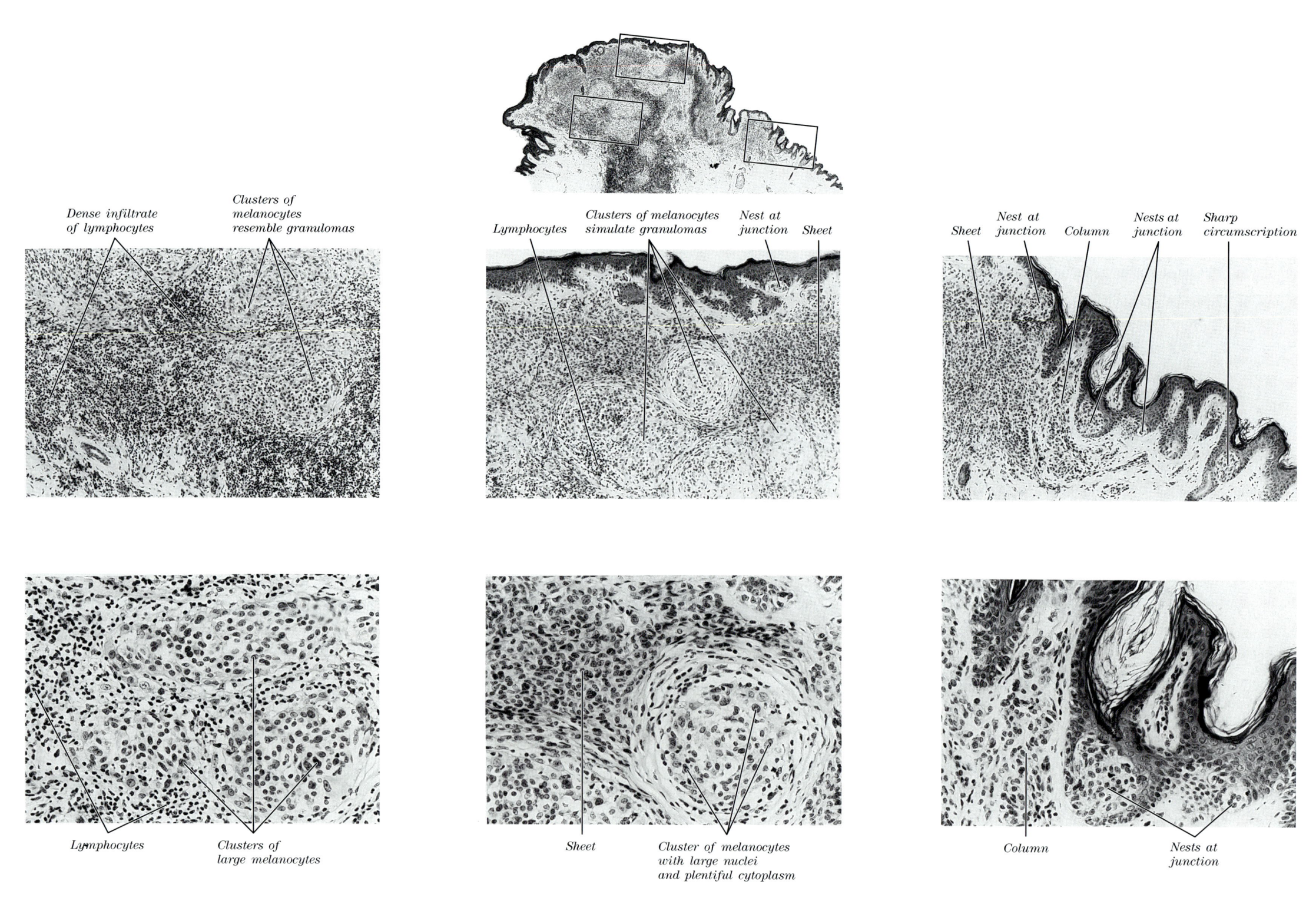

42 • Combined Nevus (Clark's and Spitz's)

Criteria for diagnosis of this combined nevus (Clark's and Spitz's with "granulomatous" features)

This neoplasm is benign because:

1. It is oriented vertically.
2. It is wedge-shaped.
3. It is well-circumscribed.
4. Nests of melanocytes in the epidermis are situated at the dermo-epidermal junction.

This is a combined nevus because:

1. There are two types of acquired nevi in these sections: a Clark's nevus on the right and beneath the epidermis, and a Spitz's nevus in the reticular dermis.
2. The Clark's nevus is seen best on the right of the neoplasm where there are discrete nests of melanocytes at the dermo-epidermal junction and nests, cords, and strands of melanocytes in a thickened papillary dermis.
3. The Spitz's nevus is seen best in the center of the neoplasm where large oval and round melanocytes possess abundant cytoplasm.

The nests of "epithelioid" melanocytes in Spitz's nevus resemble closely collections of epithelioid histiocytes in granulomatous inflammation.

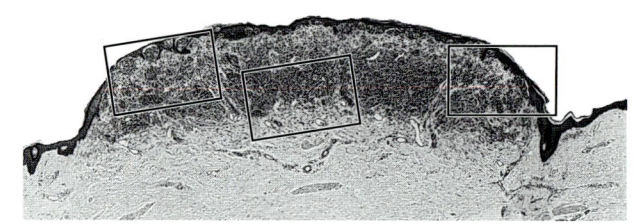

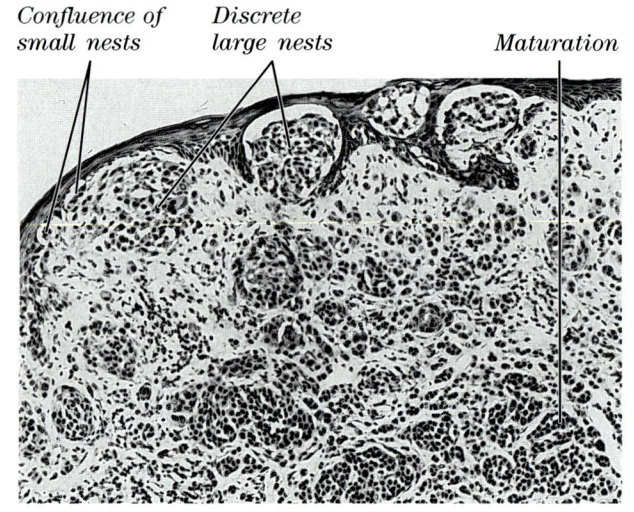

Confluence of small nests | Discrete large nests | Maturation

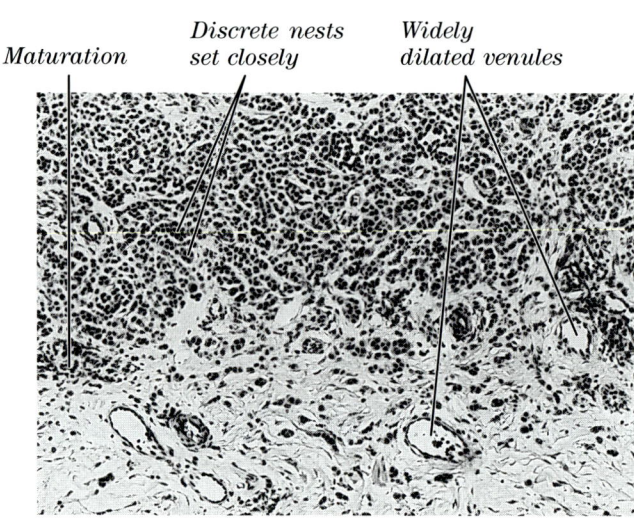

Maturation | Discrete nests set closely | Widely dilated venules

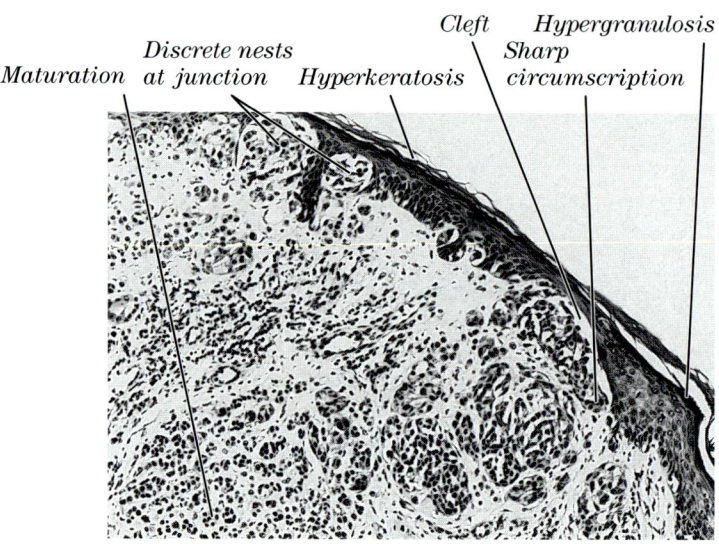

Maturation | Discrete nests at junction | Hyperkeratosis | Cleft | Hypergranulosis | Sharp circumscription

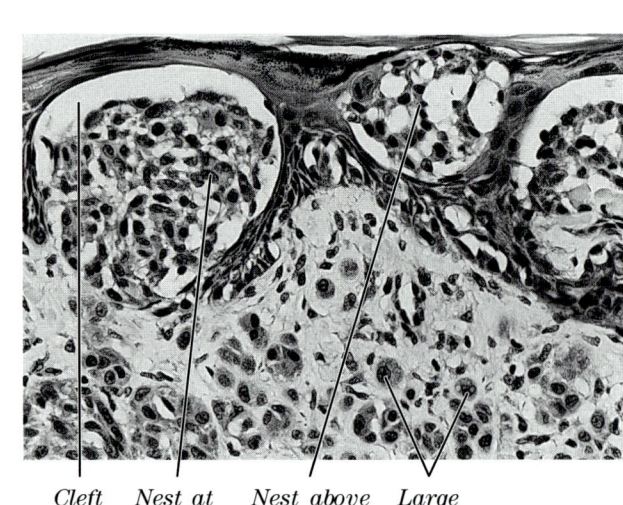

Cleft | Nest at junction | Nest above junction | Large melanocytes

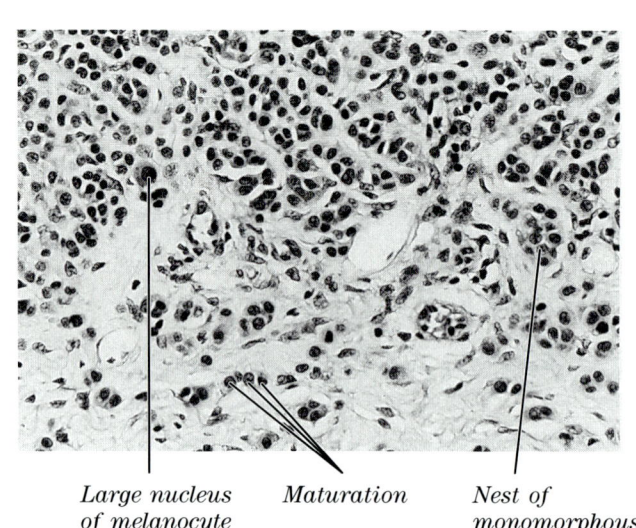

Large nucleus of melanocyte | Maturation | Nest of monomorphous melanocytes

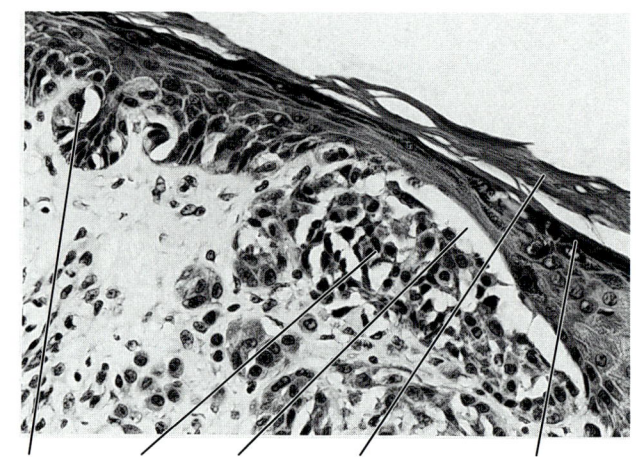

Atypical melanocyte | Elongated nest | Cleft | Hyperkeratosis | Hypergranulosis

43 • Spitz's Nevus

Criteria for diagnosis of this Spitz's nevus (compound type)

This neoplasm is benign because:

1. It is symmetric.
2. It is well-circumscribed.
3. Its base is flattish.
4. Melanocytes mature.
5. Nests of melanocytes within the epidermis predominate over melanocytes disposed as solitary units there.

This is a Spitz's nevus because:

1. Many of the melanocytes, both within the epidermis and the dermis, have large nuclei, abundant cytoplasm, and round and oval shapes.
2. There are hyperkeratosis, hypergranulosis, and spinous-cell hyperplasia.
3. Clefts are present between some nests of melanocytes and adjacent keratinocytes.
4. The neoplasm is richly vascularized.

layer, nests of melanocytes that are not equidistant from one another, nests that vary in size and shape, confluence of some nests, extension of melanocytes far down epithelial structures of adnexa, melanocytes with atypical nuclei, melanocytes in mitosis, some of which even may be abnormal, necrotic melanocytes, and dense lymphocytic infiltrates. Despite these features in common, Spitz's nevus can be recognized as the wholly benign nevus that it is by its symmetry, sharp circumscription, and maturation of melanocytes with progressive descent into the dermis; in short, by its silhouette.

4. Clark's nevus. Clark's nevus known currently, but confusingly, as the dysplastic nevus or atypical mole, is the commonest acquired nevus in our experience. It is named for Wallace H. Clark, Jr., who, in 1978, drew attention to it originally as the B-K mole, studied it intensively, popularized it, and magnetized the interest of colleagues to it.

Clinically, Clark's nevus is flat at the outset and slightly elevated with a smooth or gently mamillated surface later. A tan or pink, usually narrow, rim often surrounds the slightly elevated darker center, which commonly is brown. Colors range widely, however, and include pink, fawn, dark brown, and, rarely, black. An overwhelming majority of Clark's nevi are diagnosed with facility as nevi clinically because the neoplasms fulfill all the criteria for benignancy: relative symmetry, sharp circumscription, smooth borders, and uniform color. Uncommonly, however, a Clark's nevus may be asymmetric, poorly circumscribed with notched borders, and variegated in shades of brown admixed with pink and black. Such a lesion may be indistinguishable, seemingly, from melanoma, and unequivocal diagnosis must await histopathologic examination and interpretation, which, nearly always, resolves the issue because the two neoplasms are diametric. Study of pigmented lesions that may, episodically, simulate melanoma clinically, such as some Clark's nevi, some seborrheic keratoses, some thrombosed capillary aneurysms, and some pigmented basal-cell carcinomas, by epiluminescent methods (dermoscopy) often enhances the possibility of resolving the diagnostic dilemma prior to biopsy. In brief, the overwhelming majority of Clark's nevi do not resemble melanoma at all, either clinically or histopathologically. That is not surprising because they are nevi.

Clark's nevi are found mostly in skin that has been exposed to sunlight, especially the trunk and extremities, but they may be seen also on the buttocks and other covered parts, e.g., the suprapubic parts and genitalia.

TABLE 3. Criteria for Histopathologic Diagnosis of Clark's Nevus

Architectural
1. Symmetric
2. Sharply circumscribed
3. Melanocytes mature
4. Melanocytes arranged as solitary units and in nests situated at the dermo-epidermal junction, not above it
5. Nests of melanocytes are relatively uniform in size and shape
6. Melanocytes in nests are cohesive
7. Nests of melanocytes throughout the epidermis predominate over melanocytes arranged as solitary units
8. Melanocytes arranged as solitary units within the epidermis are relatively equidistant from one another
9. Changes within epithelial structures of adnexa are just like those in the epidermis

Cytologic
1. Melanocytes are monomorphous
2. No melanocytes are in mitosis
3. No melanocytes are necrotic

The nevus, when compound, is slightly elevated, and nests of melanocytes are confined to the dermo-epidermal junction and papillary dermis.

More than 90% of Clark's nevi are less than 5.0 mm in greatest diameter. But some surely are broader, i.e., sometimes more than 1.0 cm in diameter (one patient whom we have examined clinically and whose sections we have studied histopathologically has some Clark's nevi that are more than 5.0 cm in diameter). The fundamental histopathologic findings in Clark's nevi, irrespective of size, color, and topographic features, are repeatable, especially symmetry topographically, sharp circumscription, and maturation of melanocytes.

By the time most biopsies of Clark's nevus are taken, the neoplasm already has become compound, i.e., it is present in both the epidermis and the papillary dermis (Table 3). What makes a compound type of Clark's nevus distinctive is the combination of slight elevation of the center of the lesion with confinement of melanocytes to the dermo-epidermal junction and papillary dermis. If the reticular dermis is involved at all, as it is very uncommonly, only a few melanocytes are present focally and then in the uppermost part where they are splayed between bundles of collagen in the manner of superficial congenital nevi, which, conceivably, they could be.

When viewed with scanning magnification of a conventional microscope, a compound type of Clark's nevus is slightly elevated in its center (by nests of melanocytes situated at the dermo-epidermal junction and in the papillary dermis) and flat at its periphery (because nests of melanocytes are positioned at the junction only) (Figs. 44, 45), findings that reflect changes seen clinically (Table 3). The central, larger, slightly elevated portion is either smooth-surfaced or gently papillated. In this central portion, melanocytes in increased numbers are situated at the dermo-epidermal junction and arranged there as solitary units and, as a rule, in small nests. The subjacent papillary dermis houses melanocytes in nests and sometimes in cords and strands, and as individual units. The intradermal melanocytic component varies from scant to profuse, and the latter circumstance causes the papillary dermis to thicken markedly (Fig. 46). A junctional component of the nevus extends as "shoulders" beyond the intradermal component of the nevus for a distance of from but a single rete ridge to more than twenty-five of them (Fig. 47). The peripheral extent of the junctional component of Clark's nevus parallels precisely the extent of the tannish or pink rim seen clinically. The melanocytes arranged as solitary units and in nests within the epidermis across the central front of the nevus and at the "shoulders" possess small, oval, monomorphous nuclei and, often, abundant pale cytoplasm that may appear to be dusted by melanin. There is no nuclear atypia. The epidermis itself may be hyperplastic and slightly hyperkeratotic. Immediately beneath some nests of melanocytes situated at the dermo-epidermal junction there may be alterations of collagen bundles that have been described as (a) "concentric fibroplasia" in which wiry bundles of collagen follow the undulating course formed by epidermal rete ridges and dermal papillae, and (b) "lamellar fibroplasia" in which bundles of collagen are stacked in parallel immediately beneath nests of melanocytes at bases of rete ridges (Fig. 45). So-called concentric and lamellar fibroplasia seem to be variations on a single theme that reflects their position anatomically and the orientation of histopathologic sections. Furthermore, so-called concentric and lamellar fibroplasia are not specific for any single melanocytic neoplasm, being found in such disparate conditions as simple lentigo and melanoma. "Concentric" and "lamellar" fibroplasia may be found wherever melanocytes, typical or atypical, proliferate at the dermo-epidermal junction. In addition to alterations in melanocytes and changes in collagen bundles, the papillary dermis of a compound type of Clark's nevi also contains melanophages in variable numbers, an infiltrate of lymphocytes of variable density, and dilated venules.

In some examples of Clark's nevi, the lymphocytic infiltrate may be so dense that the neoplastic melanocytes are obscured partially or entirely by it (Fig. 48). Such a lesion usually is devoid of a halo clinically, but it is identical histopathologically to an authentic halo nevus. In actuality, a true halo nevus nearly always is simply one variant of Clark's nevus in which a dense infiltrate of lymphocytes destroys all the melanocytes in the nevus, both in the dermis and in the epidermis. The sine qua non for indubitable diagnosis of halo nevus is not histopathologic findings, however, but the clinical sign of a macular white "halo" around a nevus.

A junctional type of Clark's nevus has all the features just described in the intra-epidermal component of a compound type of Clark's nevus (Fig. 49), and an intradermal type of Clark's nevus is like the intradermal component of a compound type of Clark's nevus (Fig. 50). A junctional type is flattish, and an intradermal type is elevated in proportion to the number of melanocytes situated in the papillary dermis. A simple lentigo, which consists of an increased number of melanocytes arranged as solitary units of elongated, hyperpigmented rete ridges, is a stage in the evolution of a junctional nevus, most often a Clark's nevus (Fig. 51). A simple lentigo differs from a reticulated lentigo which is a cutaneous analogue of oral labial lentigo (which is the mucus membrane equivalent of melanosis of the genitalia). If a papillary dermis is packed with melanocytes, an intradermal type of Clark's nevus may be elevated noticeably. At compound and intradermal stages, a Clark's nevus is differentiated easily by silhouette, clinically and histopathologically, from Unna's nevus, Miescher's nevus, and Spitz's nevus; at the junctional stage, however, it is not possible to differentiate among Clark's, Unna's, and Miescher's nevi because, in the beginning, all three have nests of melanocytes only at the dermo-epidermal junction. A histopathologist is not likely to encounter a junctional type of Unna's or Miescher's nevus. When fully formed and compound, though, a Clark's nevus, in contrast to a Unna's nevus and a Miescher's nevus, is slightly elevated in its center, and melanocytes that constitute it are restricted to the dermo-epidermal junction and papillary dermis. Although an occasional melanocyte may be detected focally above the junction in the spinous zone, the granular zone, and even in the cornified layer, especially in a junctional or compound type of Clark's nevus on a palm or sole, melanocytes practi-

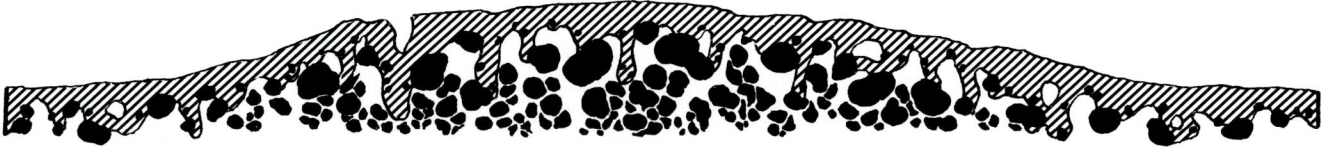

Fig. 44. Clark's nevus. This compound type of melanocytic nevus is gently domed and confined to the dermo-epidermal junction and papillary dermis. Invariably, nests of melanocytes within the epidermis extend for variable distances beyond the intradermal component of the nevus. In short, the silhouette of the nevus pictured here is diagnostic of what currently and enigmatically is termed a "dysplastic nevus" or an "atypical mole." The concept of dysplastic nevus is supposed to hinge on the presence of atypical nuclei in some melanocytes, but we are unable to recognize any nuclear atypia in these nevi. Furthermore, the fact that a neoplasm such as this one can be diagnosed for what it is by silhouette alone, without heed to nuclear detail, indicates that the term "dysplastic nevus" is a misnomer and that the nevus in point is better named eponymically for Clark.

cally never are scattered in the upper part of the epidermis across the entire front of a Clark's nevus (Fig. 52). If those changes are spotted in the absence of signs of trauma, e.g., erosion or crust, they represent melanoma in situ in association with a pre-existing Clark's nevus (or a part of a neoplasm that is melanoma entirely). The histopathologic findings of lymphocytes, melanophages, fibroplasia, and telangiectases are not differentiating, individually or collectively, from other types of nevi or from melanoma; they, like "concentric" and "lamellar" fibroplasia, are non-specific.

A Clark's nevus may be combined with Unna's, Miescher's, or Spitz's nevus, and even with more than one of them in a single biopsy specimen (Fig. 42). Furthermore, a Clark's nevus may house a combination of two or more cytologic types of melanocytes (Fig. 53).

About 20 to 25% of all melanomas in Caucasians begin in association with pre-existing acquired nevi and, for practical purposes, nearly all of those nevi are Clark's type. The melanomas that arise in Clark's nevi are situated mainly on the trunk and proximal parts of the extremities. Virtually all melanomas on the head and neck, including the face, and on the distal parts of the extremities, including palms, soles, and nail units, begin de novo, i.e., not in association with a nevus of any kind. More than 99.9% of all Clark's nevi never eventuate in melanomas. Nearly all melanomas in Africans and Asians arise de novo, i.e., unassociated with a pre-existing nevus.

We do not use the terms "dysplasia," "dysplastic cells," "dysplastic nevi," and "dysplastic nevus syndrome" because there is no unanimity among pathologists, dermatologists, surgeons, and other physicians and basic scientists about what those terms mean. No author seems to have been able to define "dysplasia" in the same way from article to article, or even sometimes in the same article. For that reason, we eschew those terms and all other terms that contribute to pathobabel, i.e., a tower of Babel in pathology. The chaos that surrounds the so-called dysplastic nevus (and the syndrome predicated upon it) is like the confusion more than 40 years ago that swirled around the nevus named today for Spitz, and almost 40 years ago that enveloped the lesion Allen called "active junctional nevus." In 1948, Spitz titled her paper in *The American Journal of Pathology* "Melanomas in Childhood" because, as she stated definitively then, she considered them to be malignant melanomas in children, indistinguishable histopathologically from malignant melanomas in adults ("The term 'melanoma' in this paper, as in common usage, has been applied only as an abbreviation for malignant melanoma."). Within a few years, it became apparent to Spitz, and others, that the lesion was not a malignant melanoma at all, but a melanocytic nevus. The name was then changed to "juvenile melanoma," but physicians, especially surgeons, continued to confuse those nevi with malignant melanomas as a result of the flawed nomenclature. Therefore, the name of the nevus was changed again, this time to "benign juvenile melanoma," but as long as the word "melanoma" was retained, confusion about it persisted. Not until the neoplasm described by Spitz was renamed "Spitz's nevus" and that designation adopted almost universally, did the wholly benign nature of the lesion come to be appreciated universally. Only when physicians were made to understand that the lesion was merely a nevus and not a melanoma were patients, many of them children, spared mutilating surgery that was routine practice for melanomas as recently as a few decades ago.

In 1953, Allen, in the journal *Cancer*, introduced the notion of an "active junctional nevus." Although he termed the lesion a nevus, his photomicrograph of it showed all of the findings of melanoma in situ, and Allen acknowledged in his legend that he considered the neoplasm to be a "melanocarcinoma in situ." Designating a melanoma a nevus was bound to lead to chaos, and that, in fact, was the result. So-called active junctional nevi and nevi with junctional activity were removed wholesale by surgeons, ostensibly to prevent them from eventuating in melanoma. The entire exercise was unnecessary and might have been prevented had Allen diagnosed what he acknowledged was melanoma as "melanoma."

The situation today vis-a-vis "dysplastic nevi" is analogous to that which obtained for "melanomas in childhood" and "active junctional nevi."

No two pathologists, dermatologists, or surgeons seem to be able to define "dysplastic nevus" in the same way clinically, histopathologically, and biologically. There is no agreement about what the lesion is, what the criteria for diagnosis of it are, and what to do about it, let alone concurrence about criteria for diagnosis of a "syndrome" based upon identification of that nevus, namely, a "dysplastic nevus syndrome" (some authors claim that a single "dysplastic nevus" constitutes that syndrome and thereby places patients at markedly increased risk, i.e., 500 times, for development of melanoma, whereas other authors aver that hundreds of these nevi are required for diagnosis of the purported syndrome). For these reasons, we advocate designating the nevus under discussion here "Clark's nevus," in the same spirit as melanomas in childhood and juvenile melanomas were renamed Spitz's nevus with excellent practical results, to wit, colleagues were less confused and patients were better served.

Last, Clark's nevus, as we employ it, is *not* a synonym for dysplastic nevus. Clark and co-workers describe dysplastic nevi clinically as "lesions that have a macular component, have irregular and indistinct borders, vary in color (including tan, brown, dark brown, and pink), are frequently larger than 4 to 5 mm . . ." A Clark's nevus, clinically, usually is small (often tiny), symmetric, well-circumscribed, and relatively uniform in color. Very rarely does it simulate a melanoma clinically. Clark and associates describe a dysplastic nevus histopathologically as having "basilar melanocytic hyperplasia of large epithelioid melanocytes, concentric eosinophilic fibroplasia, and lamellar fibroplasia. For Clark and co-workers, the sine qua non for diagnosis of dysplastic nevus is the presence of atypical nuclei in melanocytes. A Clark's nevus histopathologically, when compound, is slightly elevated in the center, and nests composed of small melanocytes are confined to the dermo-epidermal junction and papillary dermis. There is no nuclear atypia of melanocytes.

The term "atypical mole" is devoid of meaning because no definition has yet been proferred for a "typical mole." All moles, i.e., melanocytic nevi, are atypical in the sense that they are expressions of a pathologic process. Although some authors have propounded the notion of a "normal mole," the concept lacks legitimacy because all moles are abnormal, as should be obvious from the fact that they are discussed in textbooks of histopathology, not in ones devoted to histology. In brief, impenetrable terms like "dysplastic nevi," "atypical moles", and "normal moles" should be eschewed and we do that throughout this book.

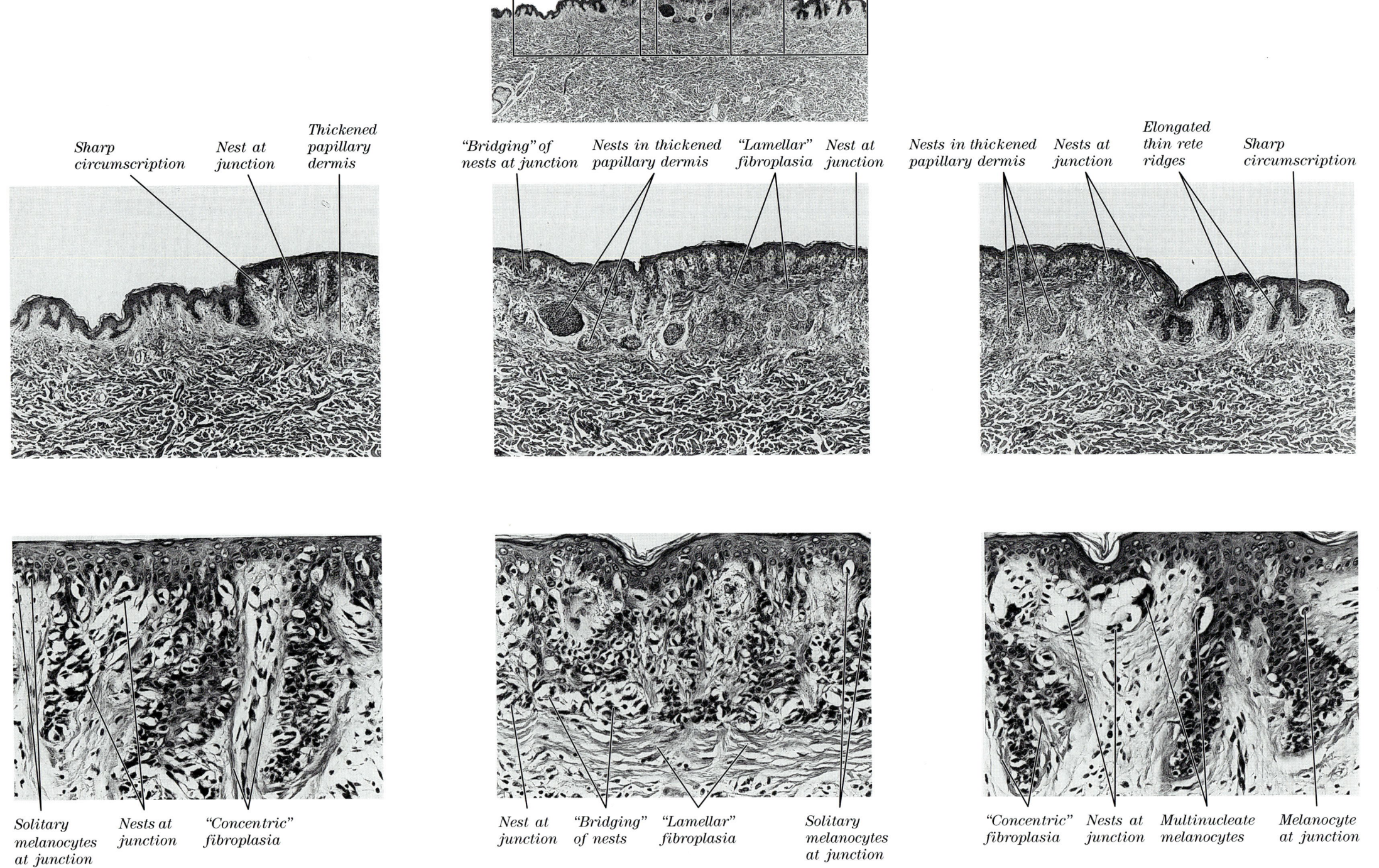

45 · Clark's Nevus

Criteria for diagnosis of this Clark's nevus (compound type)

This is a nevus because:

1. The neoplasm is symmetric.

2. It is well-circumscribed.

3. Melanocytes mature.

4. Most melanocytes, both those arranged as solitary units and those in nests, are situated at the dermo-epidermal junction.

5. Nuclei of melanocytes are relatively monomorphous.

This is a Clark's nevus because:

1. The neoplasm is but slightly elevated in its center.

2. Melanocytes arranged as solitary units and in nests are confined to the dermo-epidermal junction and thickened papillary dermis.

Other ancillary findings are:

1. The junctional component of the nevus extends beyond the intradermal component.

2. "Lamellar" and "concentric" fibroplasia are present in the papillary dermis.

3. Nests of melanocytes at bases of elongated rete ridges show evidences of "bridging."

4. In foci, the junctional component of the lesion resembles a simple lentigo.

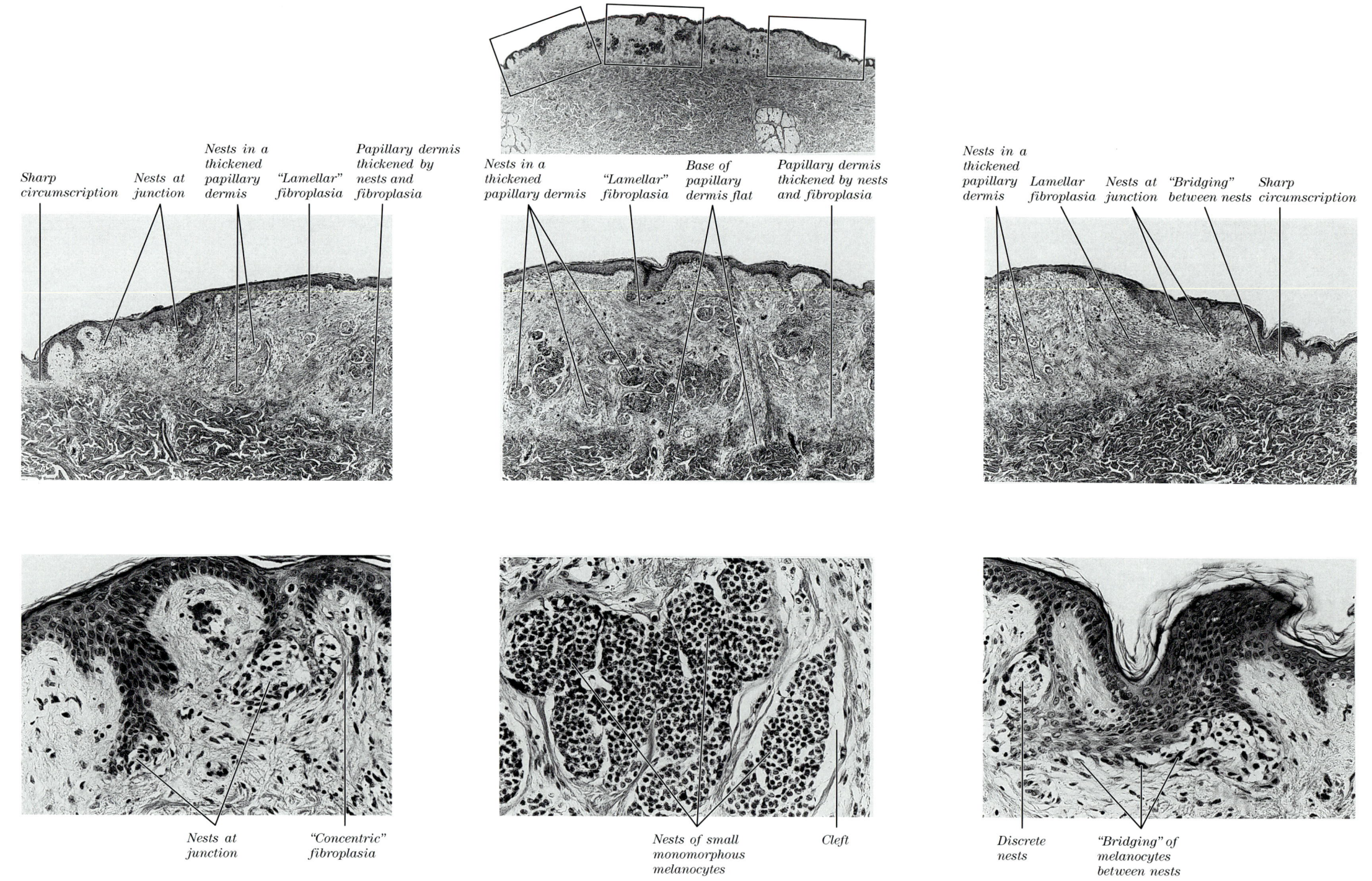

46 • Clark's Nevus

Criteria for diagnosis of this Clark's nevus (compound type)

This is a nevus because:

1. The neoplasm is symmetric.
2. It is well-circumscribed.
3. The thickened papillary dermis has a flat bottom.
4. Melanocytes mature in the thickened papillary dermis.
5. Melanocytes have small, oval, monomorphous nuclei.

This is a Clark's nevus because:

1. The neoplasm is slightly domed.
2. It is gently mammillated.
3. Nests of melanocytes are confined to the dermo-epidermal junction and markedly thickened papillary dermis.

Other ancillary findings are:

1. The junctional component extends beyond the intradermal component.
2. There is "bridging" of melanocytes at bases of rete ridges.
3. "Lamellar" and "concentric" fibroplasia are present just beneath the proliferation of melanocytes.

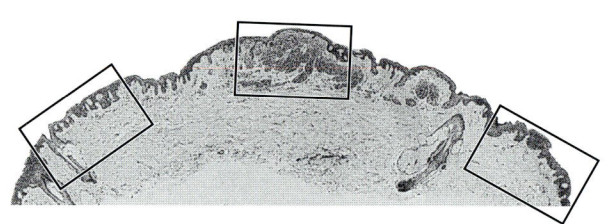

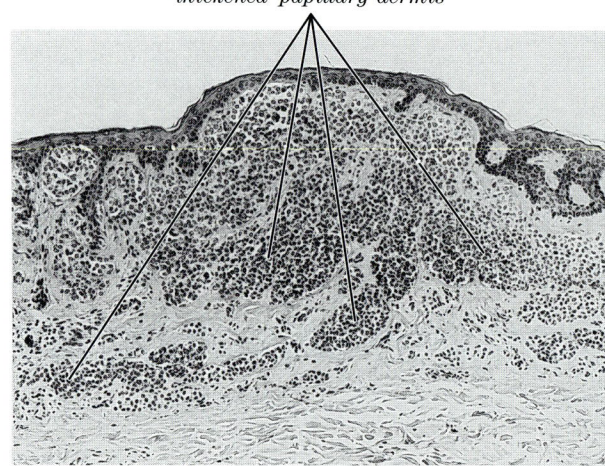

Cluster of melanocytes at margin | Single melanocytes at junction | Melanocyte with small nucleus and abundant pale cytoplasm | Tiny nest at junction

Small oval monomorphous melanocytes in markedly thickened papillary dermis

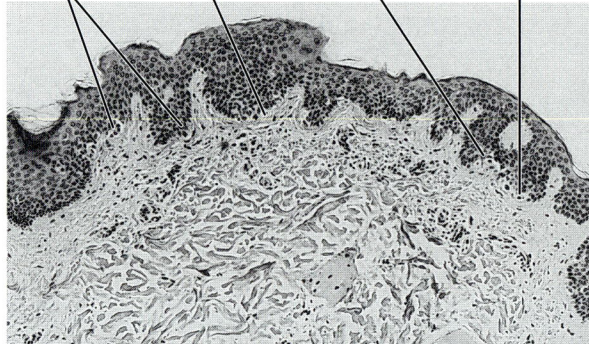

Tiny nests at junction | "Concentric" fibroplasia | Discrete nest at junction | Sharp circumscription

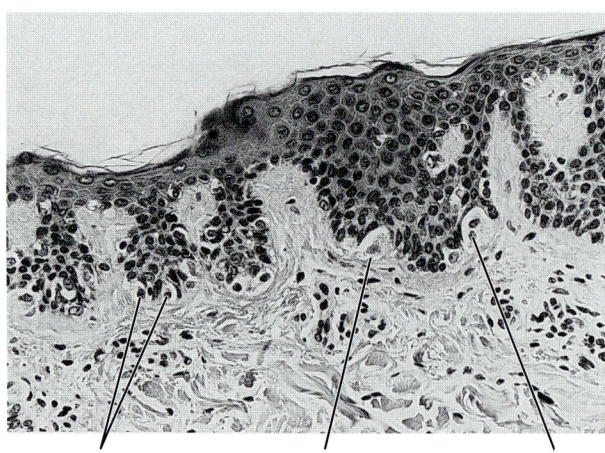

Single melanocytes at junction | Melanocyte with small nucleus and abundant pale cytoplasm | Tiny nest of small oval monomorphous melanocytes with abundant pale cytoplasm

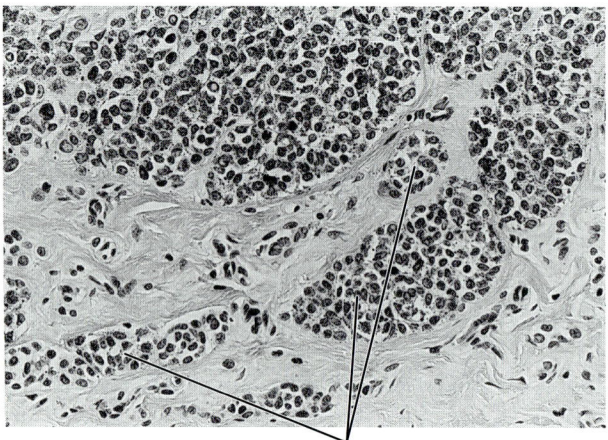

Small oval monomorphous melanocytes in a thickened papillary dermis

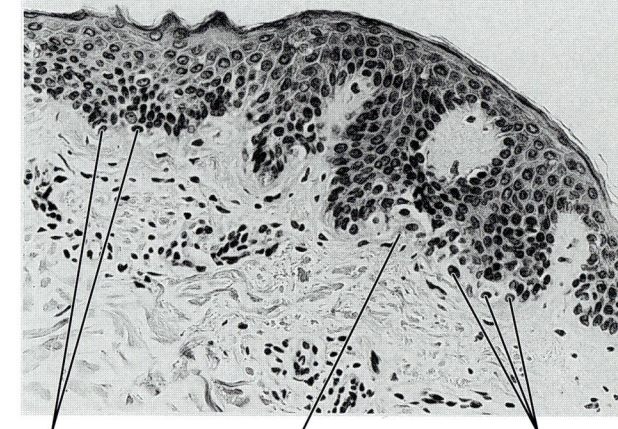

Single melanocytes at junction | Small nest of monomorphous melanocytes with abundant pale cytoplasm at junction | Small oval monomorphous melanocytes at junction

47 • Clark's Nevus

Criteria for diagnosis of this Clark's nevus (compound type)

This neoplasm is benign because:

1. It is symmetric.
2. It is well-circumscribed.
3. Melanocytes within the epidermis, both those arranged as solitary units and those in nests, are situated at the dermo-epidermal junction, not above it.
4. Melanocytes mature.
5. Melanocytes within the epidermis and the dermis have small, oval, monomorphous nuclei.

This is a compound nevus because:

Nests of melanocytes are present within the epidermis and the dermis.

This is a Clark's nevus because:

1. The neoplasm is slightly elevated.
2. Melanocytes that constitute the neoplasm are confined to the dermo-epidermal junction and thickened papillary dermis.
3. Nuclei of melanocytes are small, oval, and monomorphous.

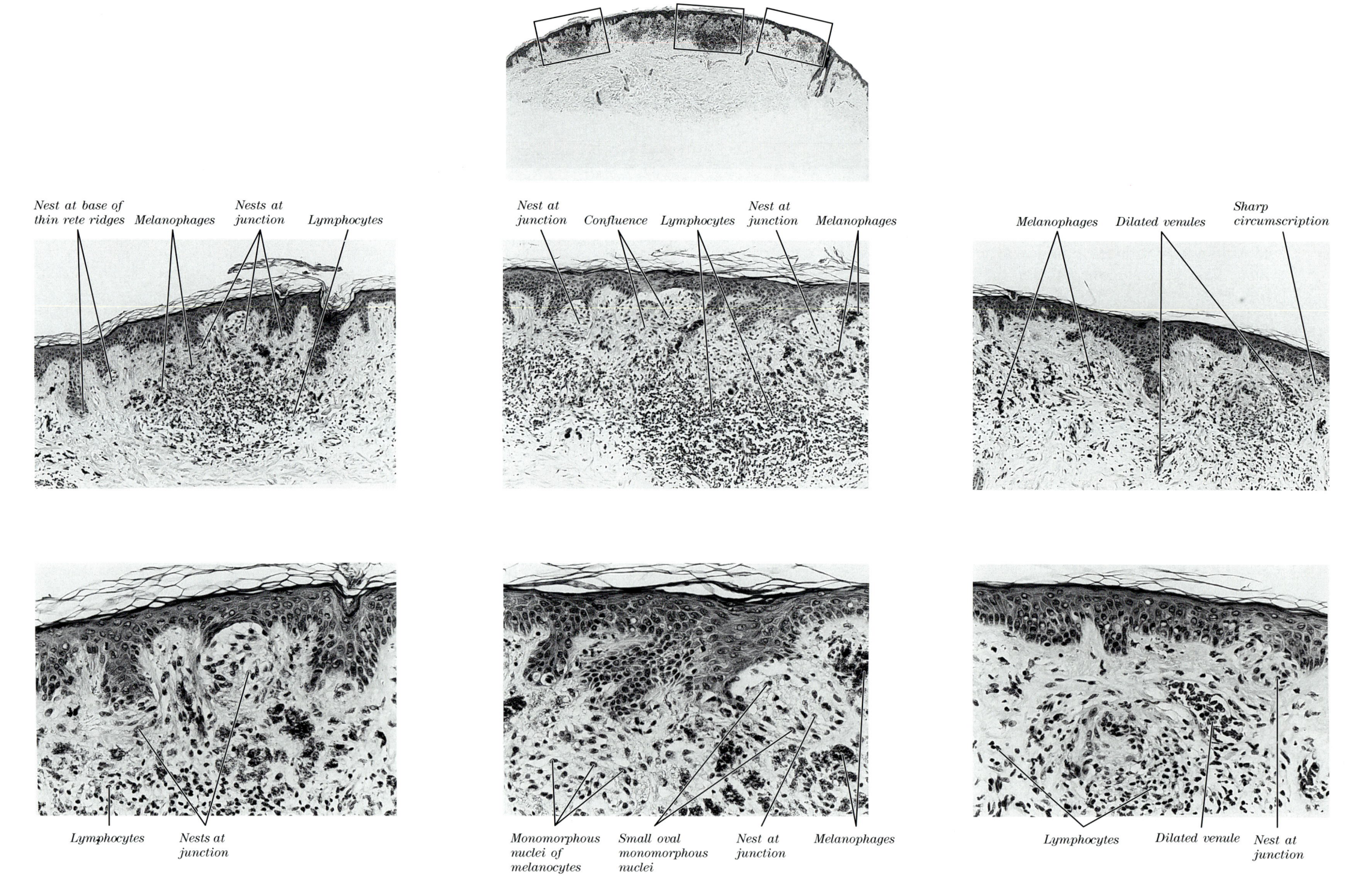

48 • Clark's Nevus

Criteria for diagnosis of this Clark's nevus (compound type)

This neoplasm is benign because:

1. The lesion is relatively symmetric.
2. It is well-circumscribed.
3. Melanocytes arrayed as solitary units and in nests are situated at the dermo-epidermal junction, not above it.
4. There is maturation of melanocytes.
5. The melanocytes themselves have small, oval, monomorphous nuclei.

This is a Clark's nevus because:

The lesion is slightly elevated and domed, and nests of melanocytes are confined to the dermo-epidermal junction and thickened papillary dermis.

Ancillary findings are:

1. "Concentric" and "lamellar" fibroplasia are present in a thickened papillary dermis.
2. A patchy lichenoid infiltrate of lymphocytes, an expected finding in many nevi of this type, is present in the thickened papillary dermis where there also are numerous melanophages.

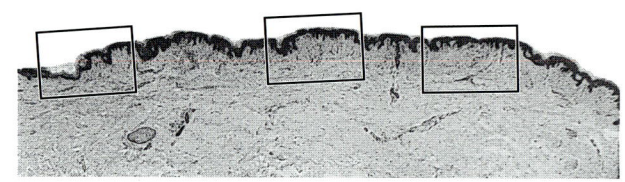

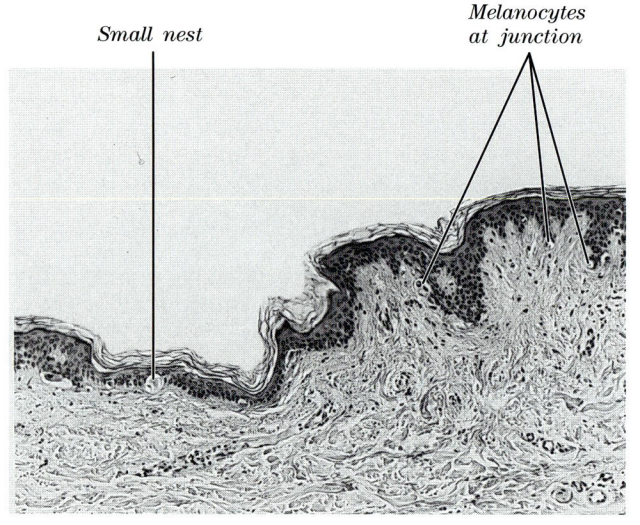
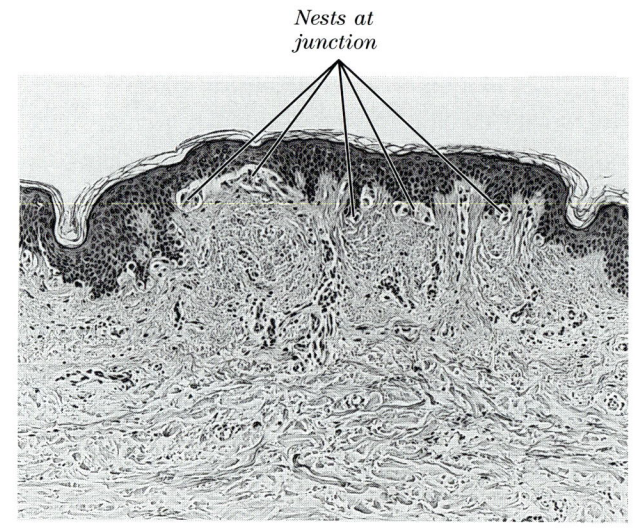
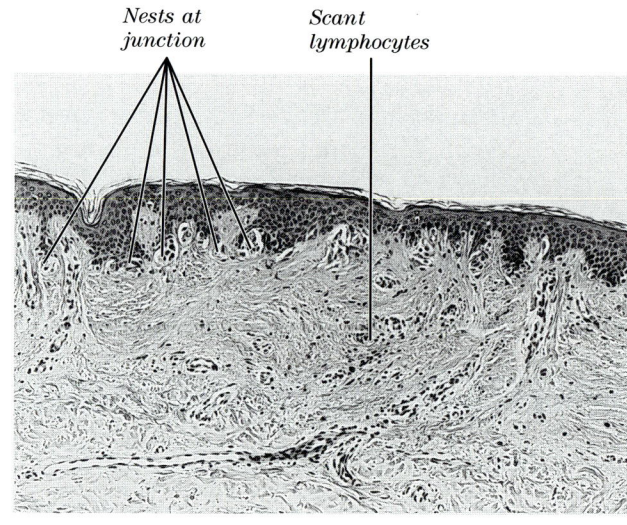

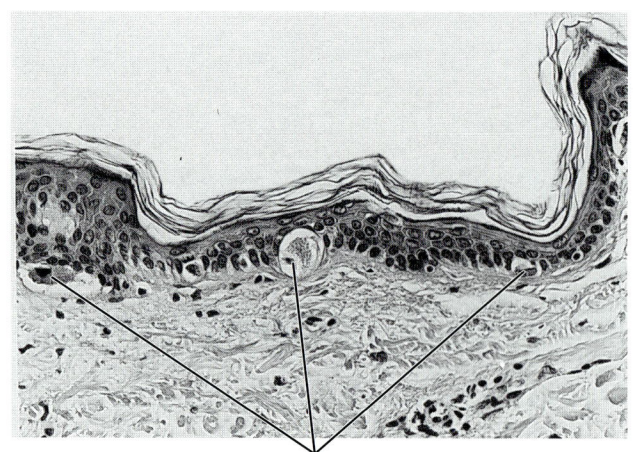
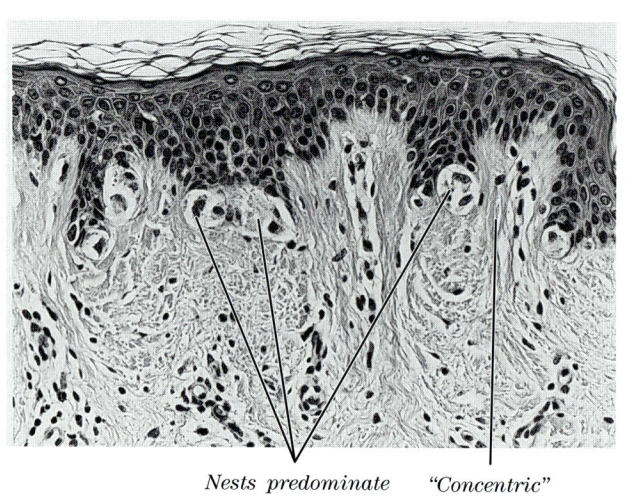
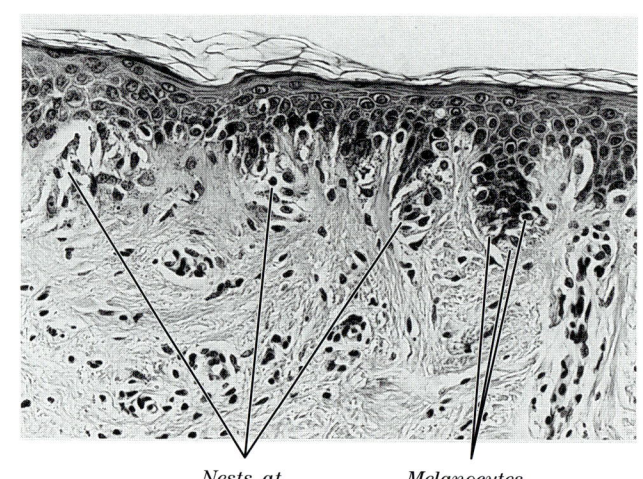

49 • Clark's Nevus

Criteria for diagnosis of this Clark's nevus (junctional type)

This neoplasm is benign because:

1. The lesion is relatively symmetric.
2. Melanocytes are arranged mostly in nests, rather than as solitary units.
3. The nests of melanocytes are positioned at the dermo-epidermal junction.
4. The melanocytes have relatively monomorphous nuclei.

This is a Clark's nevus because:

1. Nests of melanocytes are small.
2. The melanocytes themselves are small, oval, and monomorphous, and the cytoplasm is abundant and pale.
3. There are many melanocytes disposed as solitary units, as well as in nests, and all of them are situated at the dermo-epidermal junction.
4. There are distinctive types of fibroplasia (so-called concentric and lamellar) in the papillary dermis.
5. A sparse perivascular lymphocytic infiltrate is present in the thickened papillary dermis.
6. There are numerous telangiectases.

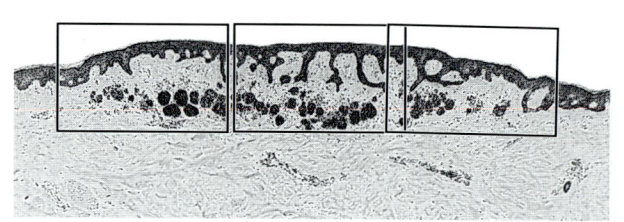

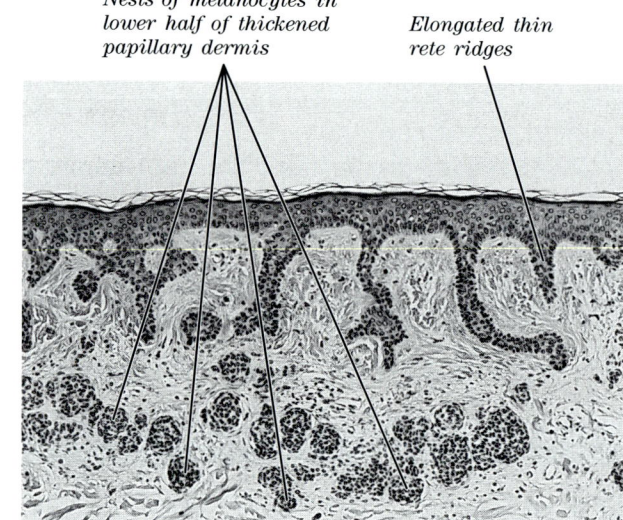
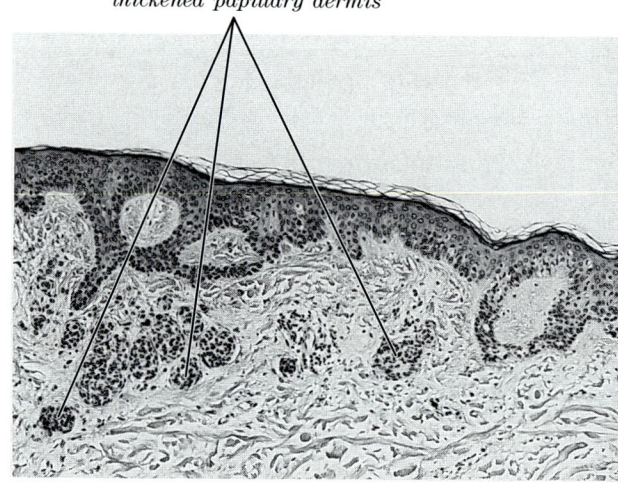

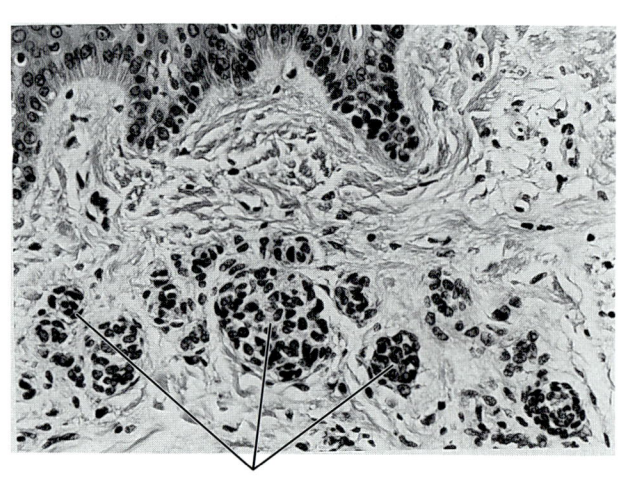
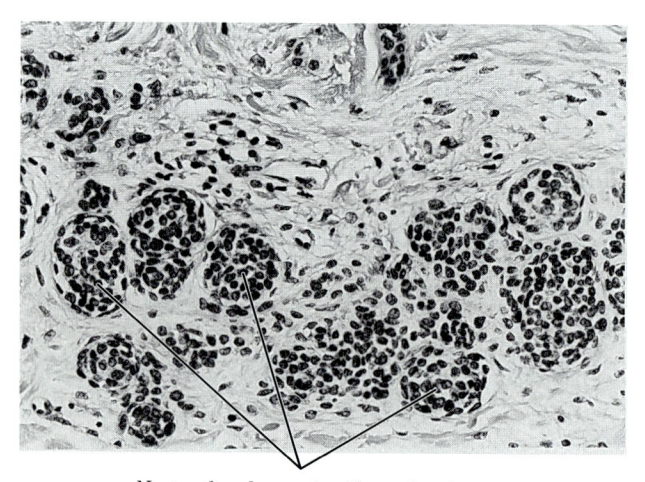
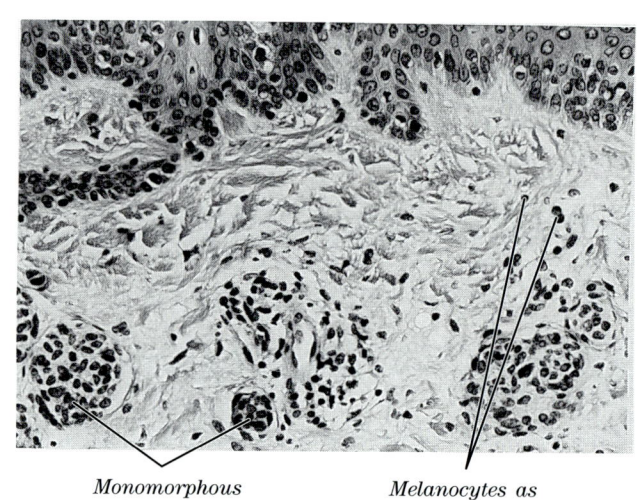

50 • Clark's Nevus

Criteria for diagnosis of this
Clark's nevus (intradermal type)

This neoplasm is benign because:

1. It is symmetric.
2. It is well-circumscribed.
3. Its base is flattish.
4. Nests within the dermis are relatively uniform in size and shape.
5. Nuclei of melanocytes are plump oval and monomorphous.

This is an intradermal Clark's nevus because:

Nests of melanocytes are confined to a thickened papillary dermis, but one not nearly as thick as in Unna's nevus.

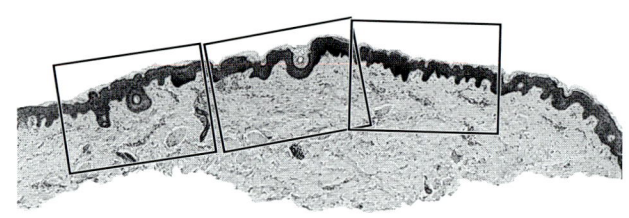

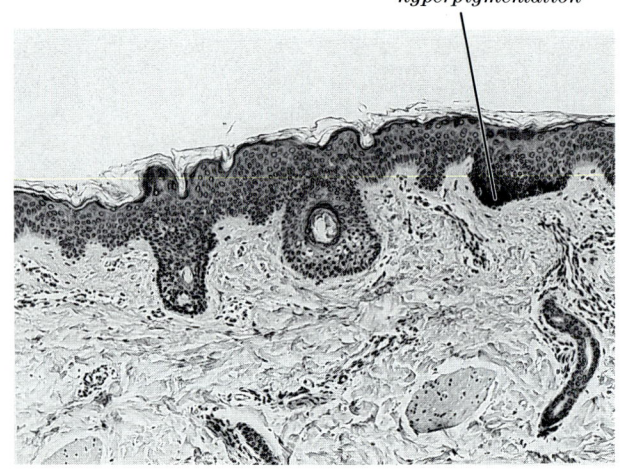
Epidermal hyperpigmentation

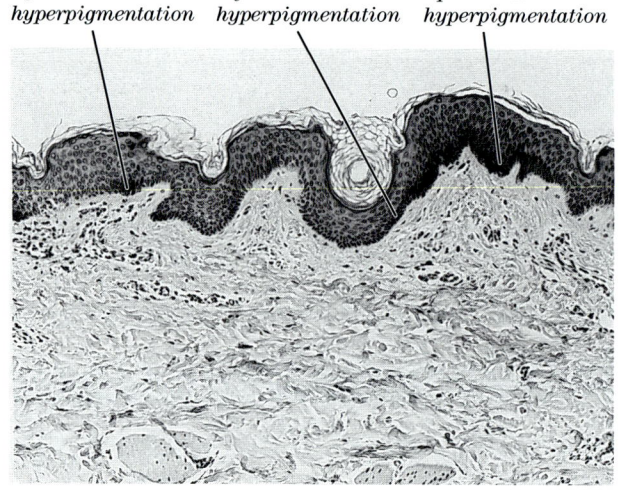
Epidermal hyperpigmentation *Infundibular hyperpigmentation* *Epidermal hyperpigmentation*

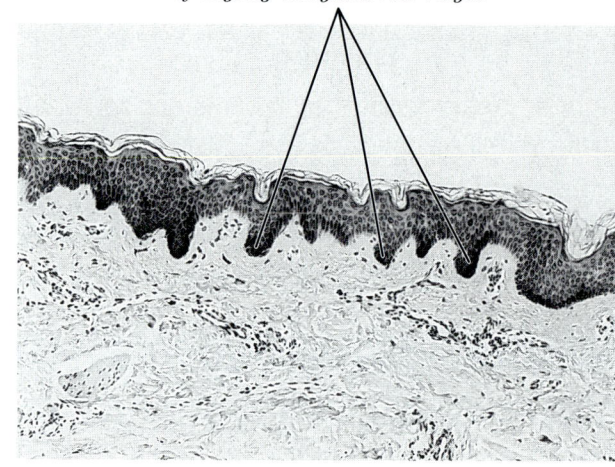
Prominent hyperpigmentation of slightly elongated rete ridges

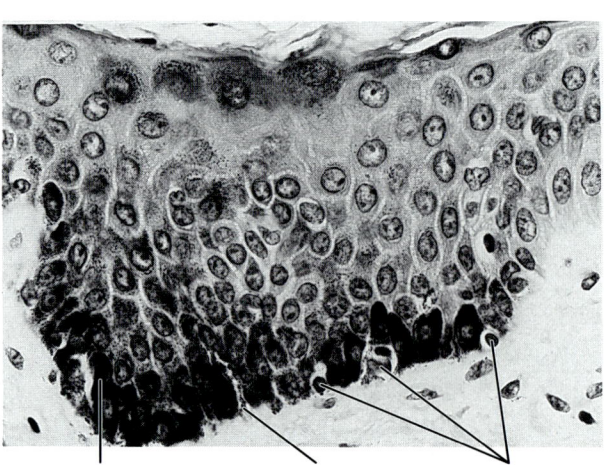
Hyperpigmentation of lower part of epidermis *Dendrite of melanocyte* *Slightly increased number of solitary melanocytes*

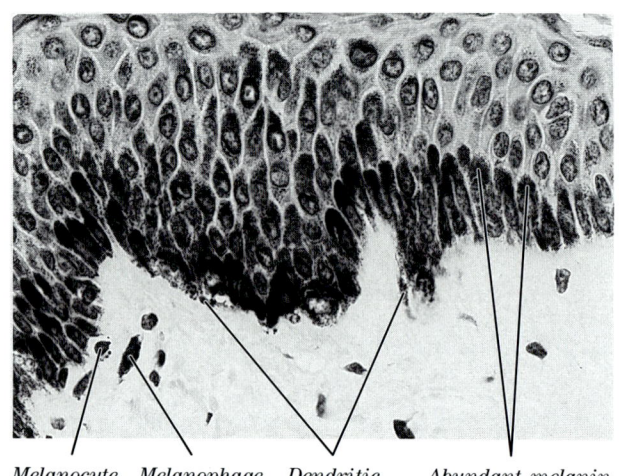
Melanocyte *Melanophage* *Dendritic melanocytes* *Abundant melanin in basal keratinocytes*

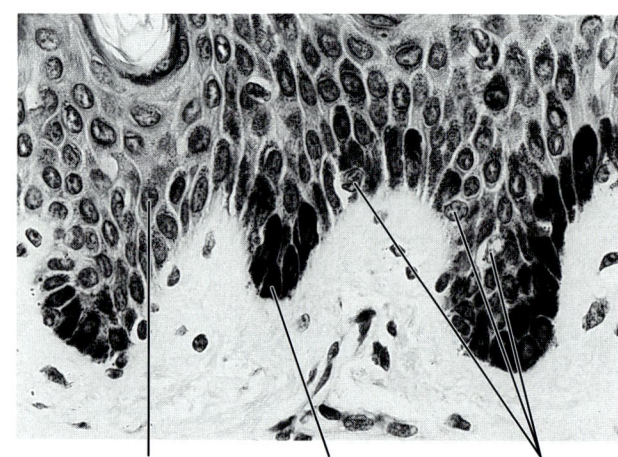
Increased melanin in spinous keratinocyte *Pigment in basal keratinocytes markedly increased* *Melanocytes*

51 · Simple Lentigo

Criteria for diagnosis of this simple lentigo

This lesion is benign because:

1. It is small.
2. Neoplastic melanocytes, increased in number, are situated at the dermo-epidermal junction only.
3. The melanocytes have uniform nuclei.

This is a simple lentigo because:

1. Melanocytes appear wholly as solitary units at the dermo-epidermal junction.
2. Hyperpigmentation of the epidermis is uniform.
3. Melanin is distributed mostly at bases of rete ridges, rather than in suprapapillary plates.
4. Dendrites of melanocytes are noticeable.
5. Melanin, increased in amount throughout the entire thickness of the epidermis, is most apparent in the basal layer.

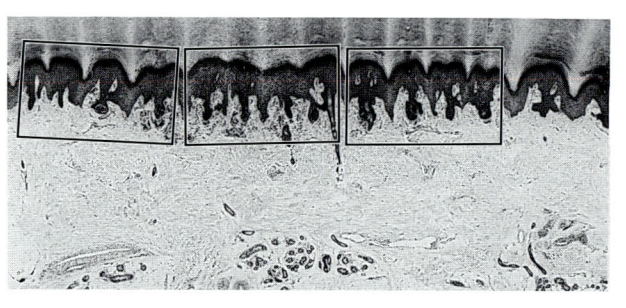

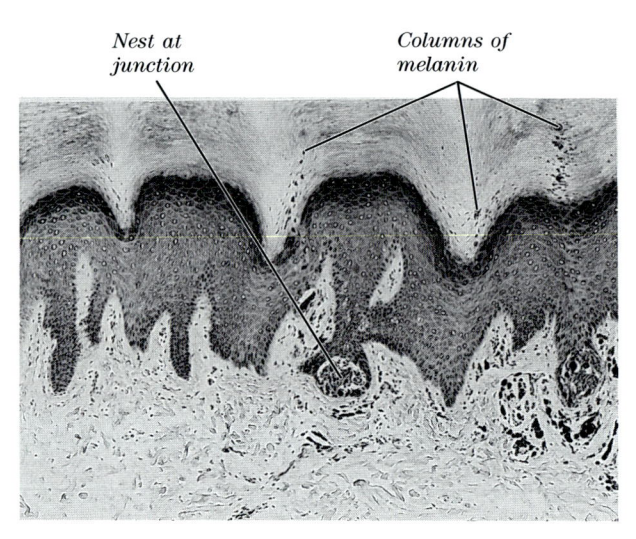

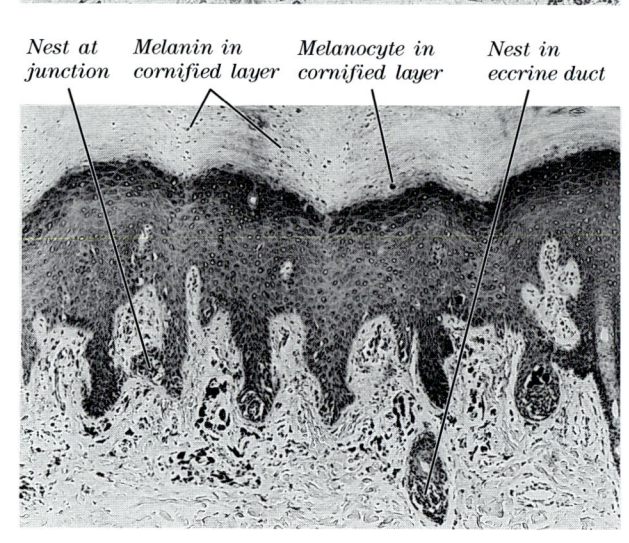

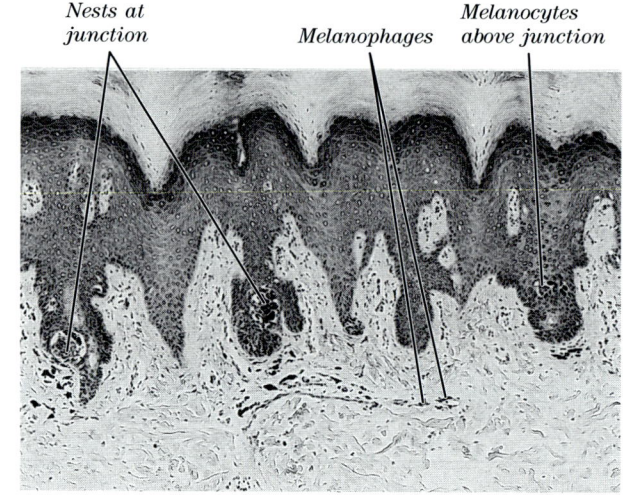

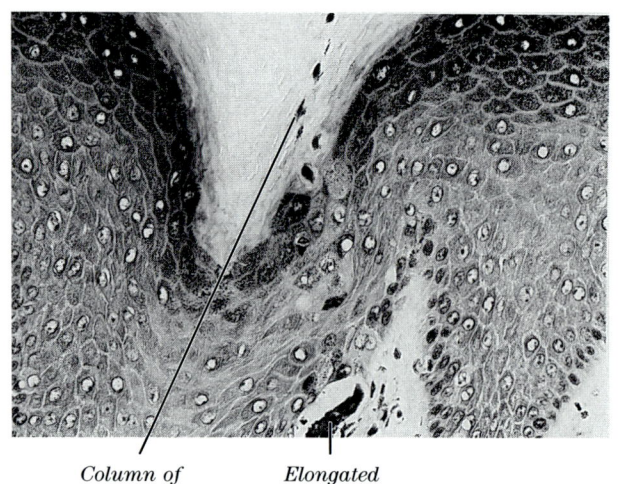

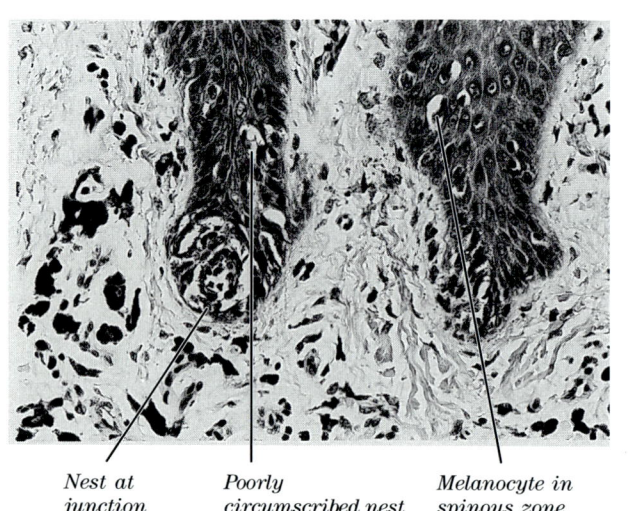

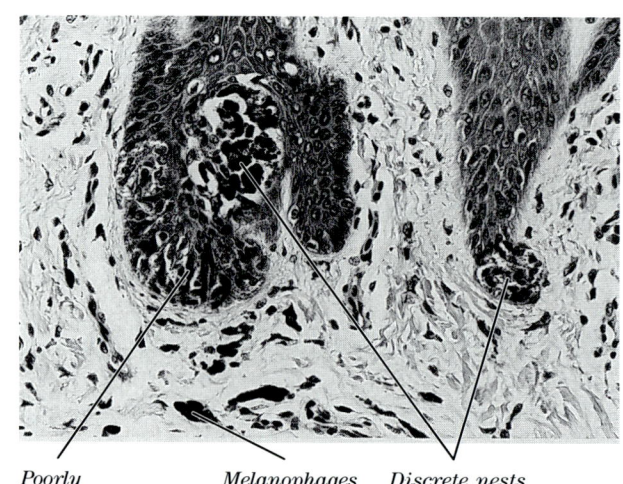

52 • Clark's Nevus

Criteria for diagnosis of this Clark's nevus (junctional type) on volar skin

This neoplasm is benign because:

1. The lesion is symmetric.
2. It is well-circumscribed.
3. Nests of melanocytes are numerous in this lesion that is less than 4.0 mm in greatest diameter.
4. Nests of melanocytes are discrete.
5. Nests of melanocytes are relatively uniform in size and shape.
6. Melanin is distributed in relatively uniform fashion across the lesion.
7. Discrete columns of melanin are present in the cornified layer above nests stationed at bases of rete ridges.
8. Nuclei of melanocytes are monomorphous.

This is a Clark's nevus because:

1. The lesion is gently mammillated, and the nests of melanocytes are located at the dermo-epidermal junction.
2. Nests of melanocytes are small.
3. The nuclei of melanocytes are small, oval, and monomorphous.

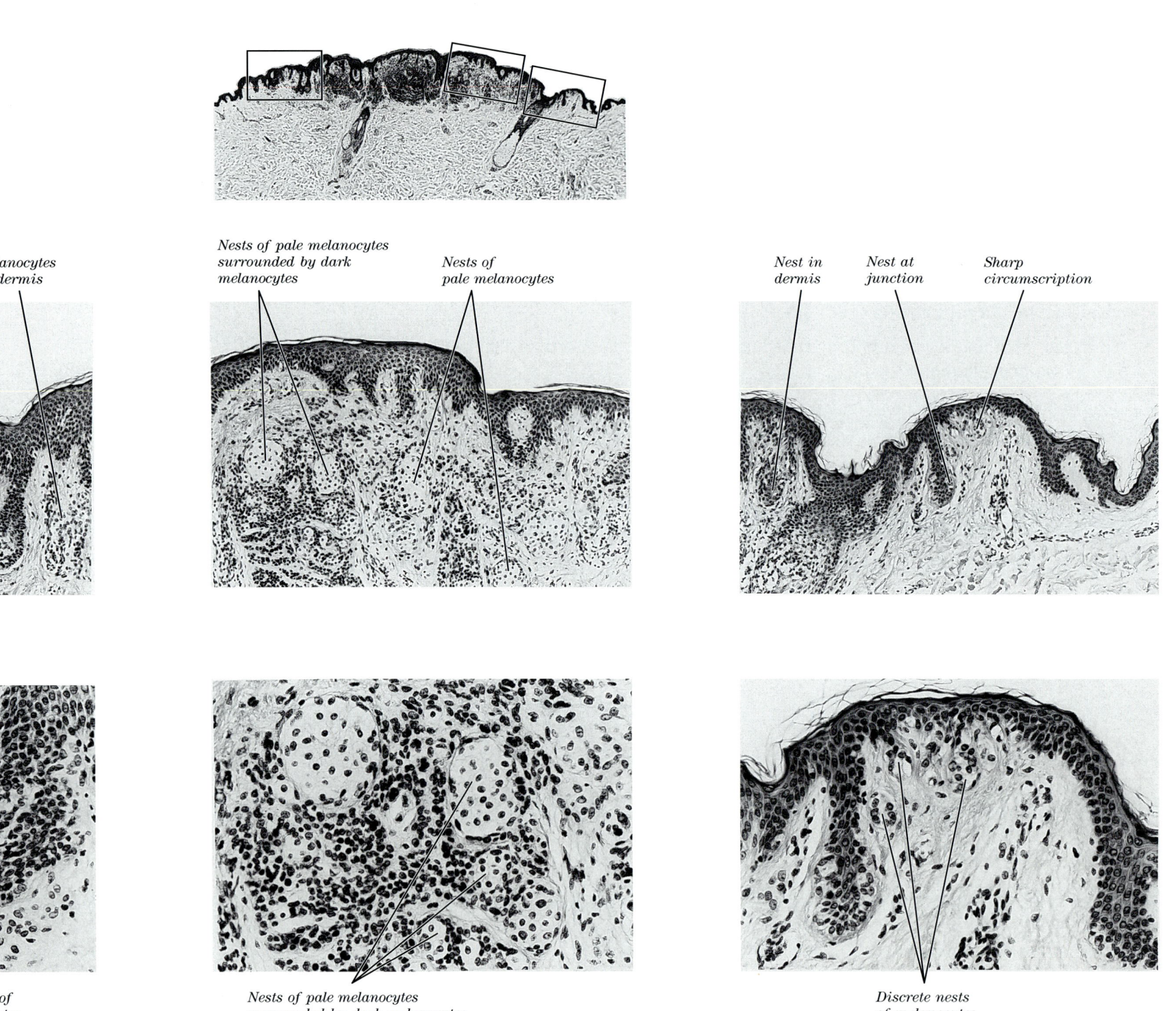

53 • Clark's Nevus *(combined type)*

Criteria for diagnosis of this Clark's nevus
(with several populations of melanocytes)

This neoplasm is benign because:

1. It is symmetric.
2. It is well-circumscribed.
3. Nests of melanocytes and solitary melanocytes are positioned at the dermo-epidermal junction and not above it.
4. There is maturation of melanocytes.
5. Nuclei of melanocytes are monomorphous.

This is a Clark's nevus because:

1. The neoplasm is slightly elevated and gently mammillated.
2. Melanocytes that constitute it are confined to the dermo-epidermal junction and thickened papillary dermis.

The combination of neoplastic melanocytes in this Clark's nevus includes the following types:

1. Small oval with scant cytoplasm (dark cells).
2. Round with abundant pale cytoplasm, i.e., pagetoid melanocytes (pale cells).

III. Melanomas

A. Definition

A melanoma is a malignant neoplasm of melanocytes that may cause death as a consequence of the effects of metastases.

B. Principles

Clinically, histopathologically, and biologically, melanomas are diametric to nevi. Clinically, melanomas, like acquired nevi, begin small, but unlike nevi, continue to grow in unrestrained fashion and, with time, become progressively larger, more asymmetric, and outlined more dramatically by notched, scalloped, and jagged borders. Instead of being a relatively uniform brown, as nevi generally are, colors of melanomas range in brown from fawn to deep chocolate and include other colors such as pink, blue, and black. The surface of a melanoma often fails to preserve the normal dermatoglyphic pattern and, instead, may be uneven, e.g., smooth in some parts, scaly in others, flat focally, and elevated elsewhere. Whereas an acquired nevus begins as a macule that tends to become a papule, a melanoma starts as a macule that may become a papule, then a nodule, and finally even a tumor, or a patch upon which a papule, a nodule, or a tumor may develop, or a patch that eventuates in a plaque that eventually may be surmounted by one or more nodules or tumors. Not uncommonly, a nodule or tumor of melanoma ulcerates. Virtually all cutaneous melanomas originate as macules, including those that begin in association with acquired nevi.

Histopathologically, melanomas also are polar to acquired nevi (see Table 4) (Fig. 54). Despite that fact, melanocytes that constitute melanomas have the same shapes and components as nevi (see Table 5): small round, large round, pagetoid, balloon, polygonal, oval, spindle, dendritic, wavy, and multinucleate. The ten types of melanocytes may appear in a melanoma on any anatomic site, in either sex, and at any age. In Asians and Africans, melanomas commonly comprise, at least in part, markedly pigmented, strikingly dendritic melanocytes, especially within the epidermis and epithelial structures of adnexa. A melanoma begins tiny, like all acquired lesions in skin, and until it is about 2.0 mm in diameter or more by the time a specimen is submitted to a pathology laboratory, it cannot be diagnosed with confidence histopathologically. In such a tiny melanoma confined to the epidermis and adnexal epithelium, nests of melanocytes will not predominate over melanocytes disposed as solitary units across the entire front of the flat neoplasm. In fact, at a very early stage in the evolution of virtually every melanoma, all of the neoplastic melanocytes are disposed as solitary units at the dermo-epidermal junction. Once a melanoma reaches a diameter of approximately 3.0 mm, however, nests of melanocytes may predominate over melanocytes arranged as solitary units within the epidermis. A stereotypic melanoma, irrespective of size, tends to be asymmetric, poorly circumscribed, i.e., atypical melanocytes arranged as solitary units are present at or above the dermo-epidermal junction beyond the last recognizable nest of melanocytes within the epidermis,* and characterized

TABLE 4. Criteria for Histopathologic Diagnosis of Malignant Melanoma

Architectural pattern
1. Asymmetric
2. Poorly circumscribed
3. No maturation of melanocytes with progressive descent into the dermis
4. Nests of melanocytes within the epidermis are not equidistant from one another
5. Nests of melanocytes vary markedly in sizes and shapes
6. Some nests of melanocytes become confluent
7. Melanocytes in some "nests" are not cohesive
8. Scatter of melanocytes above the dermo-epidermal junction
9. Melanocytes arranged as solitary units predominate over nests of melanocytes in some high-power fields
10. Melanocytes arranged as solitary units are not equidistant from one another
11. Melanocytes extend far down epithelial structures of adnexa in the same pattern as they are arrayed within the epidermis
12. Melanin is not distributed symmetrically within the epidermis, adnexa, and dermis

Cytologic features
1. Melanocytes may be atypical
2. Melanocytes in mitosis
3. Melanocytes may be necrotic

---

*It is inevitable that melanocytes in evolving nevi, especially Spitz's nevi, may extend as solitary units for a very short distance, e.g., the breadth of about one rete ridge, beyond the last nest of melanocytes. That is not considered to be poor circumscription.

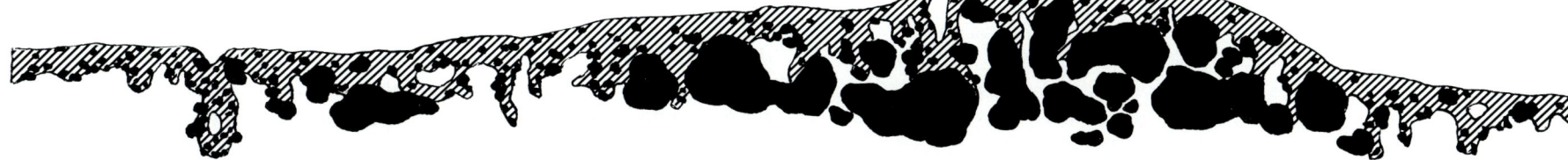

Fig. 54. Melanoma. The silhouette of the neoplasm illustrated here is that of a melanoma because it is asymmetric, poorly circumscribed by melanocytes arranged as solitary units above the dermo-epidermal junction beyond the last nest of melanocytes at the periphery of the neoplasm, and characterized by nests of melanocytes within the epidermis that are not equidistant from one another, vary in size and shape, and have become confluent. Melanocytes arranged as solitary units and in small nests are present above the dermo-epidermal junction, even in the upper reaches of the epidermis. Similar changes are present within epithelial structures of adnexa. Nests of melanocytes within the dermis also vary markedly in size and shape and some have become confluent. For all these reasons, this neoplasm is a melanoma, and that judgment can be made on the basis of silhouette alone.

TABLE 5. Criteria for Differentiation of Melanocytes of Unna's, Miescher's, and Clark's Nevi from Small Melanocytes of Melanomas

Melanocytes of Nevi	Small Melanocytes of Melanomas
MAJOR CRITERIA	
1. Monomorphic nuclei	1. Pleomorphic nuclei
2. No or inconspicuous nucleoli	2. Prominent nucleoli
3. Nuclei 7 to 10 microns in greatest diameter	3. Nuclei sometimes more than 10 microns in greatest diameter
4. No mitotic figures	4. Mitotic figures common
5. No necrotic cells	5. Necrotic cells sometimes
6. No plasma cells at bases of lesions	6. Plasma cells at bases of some thick lesions
7. No continuity with overlying melanoma cells	7. Continuity with overlying melanoma cells
8. Nests at bases of lesions small with smooth borders	8. Nests at bases of lesions occasionally large with irregular borders
MINOR CRITERIA	
1. No pigment in quantity at bases of lesions as a rule	1. Abundant pigment at bases of lesions as a rule, at least in foci
2. Cells in the reticular dermis often arranged as solitary units	2. Cells in discrete nests in the reticular dermis rather than as solitary units mostly
3. Little discernible cytoplasm in cells at bases of lesions	3. Discernible cytoplasm in some cells at bases of lesions
4. Delicate fibrillary collagen between individual cells	4. No delicate fibrillary collagen between individual cells

Modified after Maize, J., and Ackerman, A.B.: *Pigmented Lesions of the Skin.* Philadelphia, Lea & Febiger, 1987, pp. 183–4.

both by neoplastic melanocytes that fail to mature with progressive descent into the dermis and by nests that do not consistently become smaller as they go deeper. Furthermore, within the epidermis, nests of melanocytes of melanoma are not equidistant from one another, nests vary markedly in size and shape, often nests are not discrete but tend to confluence, melanocytes in some "nests" are not cohesive, and melanocytes arranged as solitary units commonly predominate over melanocytes arranged as nests in one or more high-power fields (Table 4). The changes just enumerated within the epidermis of melanomas tend to be present also within epithelial structures of adnexa, i.e., folliculo-sebaceous units and eccrine ducts.

C. Melanoma in situ

All primary melanomas in skin, with the exception of some of those that begin in deep congenital nevi, originate at the dermo-epidermal junction (Fig. 55). A tiny pigmented macule that may be too small to identify as a melanoma clinically may consist only of a proliferation of typical melanocytes arranged as solitary units at the dermo-epidermal junction. Such a proliferation cannot be diagnosed with conviction as melanoma in situ because the changes simply are too subtle. If, however, the individual melanocytes are not at all equidistant from one another and if melanin is not distributed evenly within the epidermis, or if melanocytes are not disposed symmetrically, then a diagnosis of an early stage of melanoma in situ may be suggested to the managing physician. In time, as the macule expands, nuclei of some melanocytes become atypical and, later, some individual melanocytes appear above the dermo-epidermal junction, mostly in the lower part of the spinous zone (Fig. 56). At this still macular stage, a diagnosis of melanoma in situ can be made definitively in most instances (the major simulator of it being a very early junctional Spitz's nevus). As the small flat lesion of melanoma continues to enlarge asymmetrically, tiny nests of melanocytes come into being at the dermo-epidermal junction (Fig. 57), and in the course of years, as more and more melanocytes appear within the epidermis, both as solitary units and in nests, the lesion becomes slightly elevated (Fig. 58). Melanocytes arranged as solitary units and in nests come to be lodged not only at the dermo-epidermal junction and immediately above it, but far above the junction in the upper reaches of the epidermis, including the granular zone and the cornified layer, and also within the upper portion of epithelial structures of adnexa (Fig. 59). These changes, in concert, in a macule or patch of melanoma, represent the fullest histopathologic expression of melanoma in situ. "In situ" means "in place," and the epidermis and upper portion of epithelial structures of adnexa are the places where melanocytes reside normally in the skin.

The term "melanoma in situ" is preferable to "intra-epidermal melanoma" (which does not incorporate the reality of neoplastic melanocytes within folliculo-sebaceous and eccrine units), to "intra-epithelial melanoma" (which fails to specify which epithelium is affected, i.e., epidermal,

Text continues on page 120

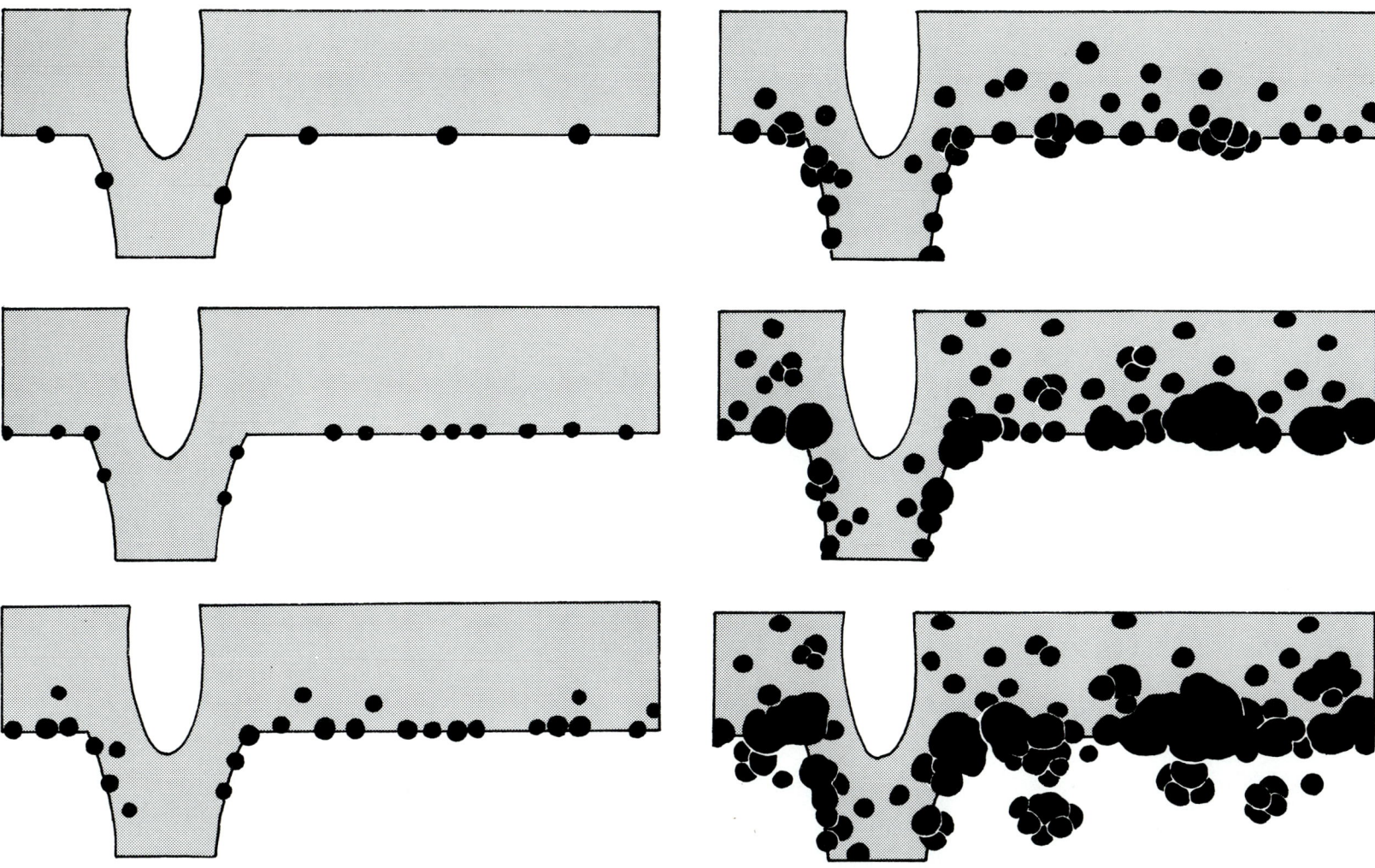

Fig. 55. Chronologic sequence in the evolution of melanoma. *(Top left)* Normal melanocytes in normal epidermis are situated at the dermo-epidermal junction mostly and are positioned nearly equidistant from one another. Primary de novo cutaneous melanoma begins with proliferation of relatively typical melanocytes arranged as solitary units at the dermo-epidermal junction. Those melanocytes are not equidistant from one another. In time, nuclei of some of the melanocytes become atypical and some of those melanocytes come to be disposed above the dermo-epidermal junction and within epithelial structures of adnexa: infundibula and eccrine ducts *(Top right)*. Still later, nests of atypical melanocytes form at the dermo-epidermal junction. The nests vary in size and shape. Concurrent with these changes, more and more melanocytes come to be present above the dermo-epidermal junction and at progressively higher levels of the epidermis. As the process continues, nests of melanocytes often become confluent, and some of those nests also appear above the dermo-epidermal junction. Similar changes occur within epithelial structures of adnexa. From the outset until this time, all of the neoplastic melanocytes have been confined to the epidermis and epithelial structures of adnexa, that is, the melanoma has been in situ. As long as the melanoma is confined to epithelium, it is benign biologically. Only when neoplastic melanocytes descend into the dermis is a person at any risk for metastasis, and then only after the neoplasm has reached a thickness of more than about 0.7 mm. After nests of melanocytes have formed at the dermo-epidermal junction and have become sufficiently large, neoplastic melanocytes may descend from the epidermis into the dermis. When even a single atypical melanocyte is detected within the dermis, the diagnosis no longer is melanoma in situ, but melanoma unmodified.

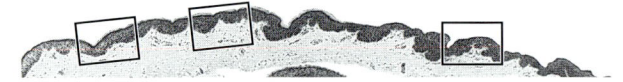

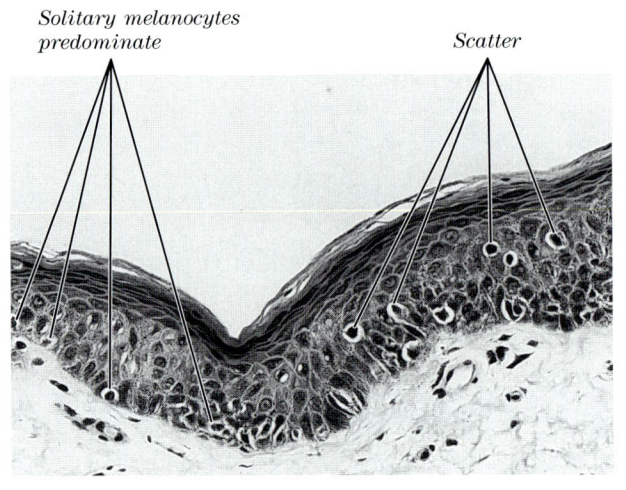

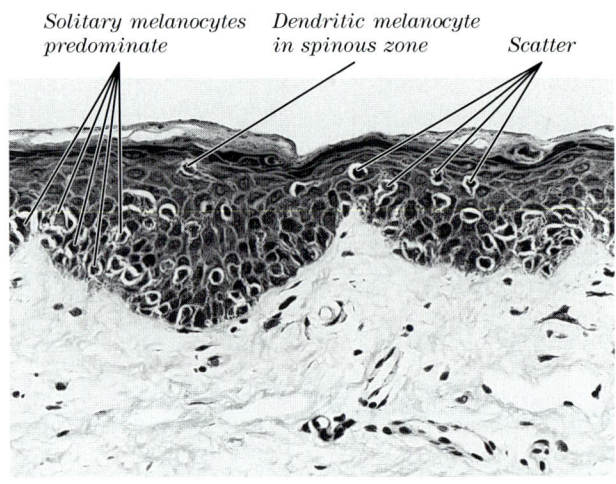

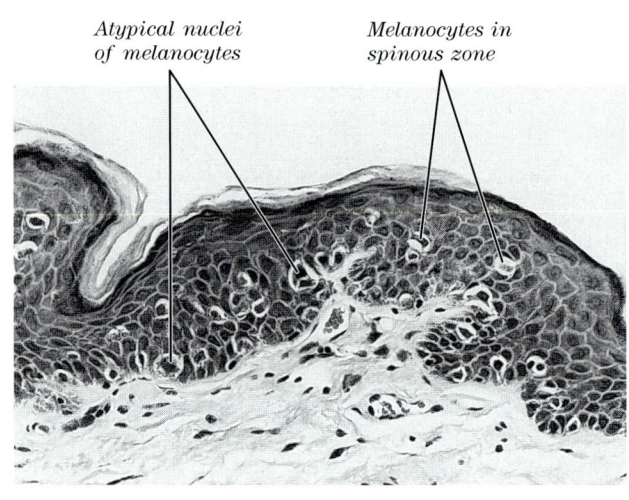

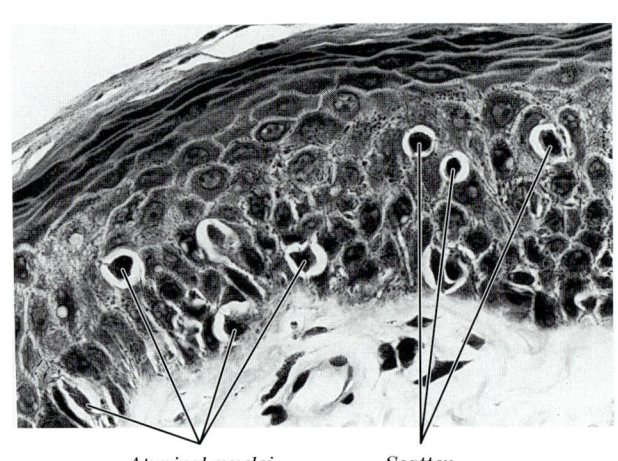

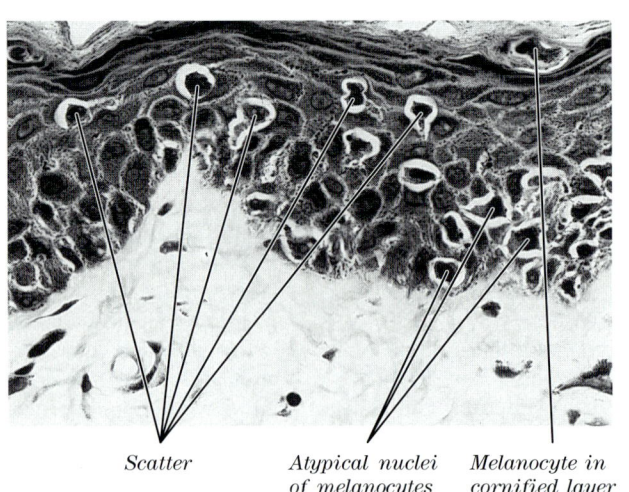

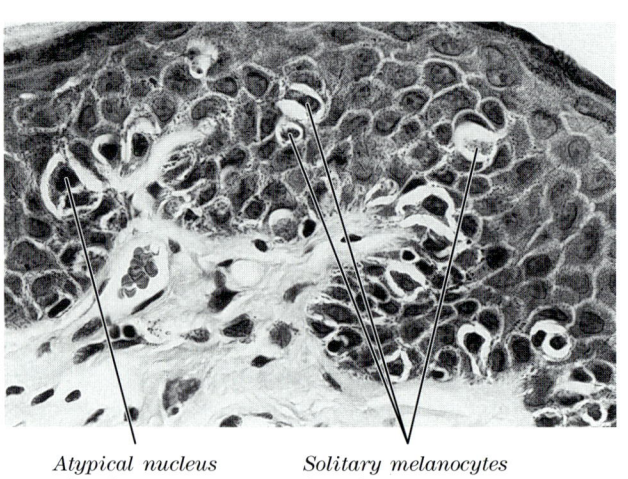

56 • Melanoma in situ

Criteria for diagnosis of this melanoma in situ

This is a melanoma in situ because:

1. Atypical melanocytes arranged almost entirely as solitary units are present not only at the dermo-epidermal junction, but also above it.

2. Although most of the melanocytes are positioned in the lower half of the epidermis, some are apparent in the cornified layer.

3. Melanocytes arrayed as solitary units are not equidistant from one another.

4. Nuclei of melanocytes are pleomorphic.

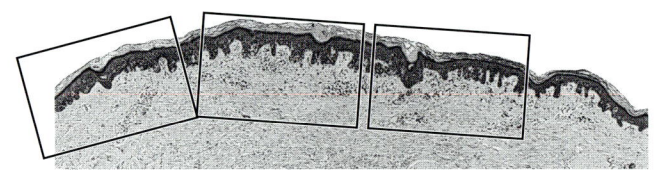

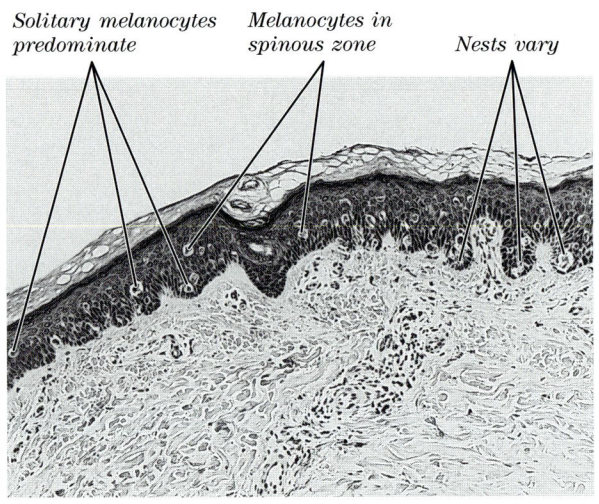
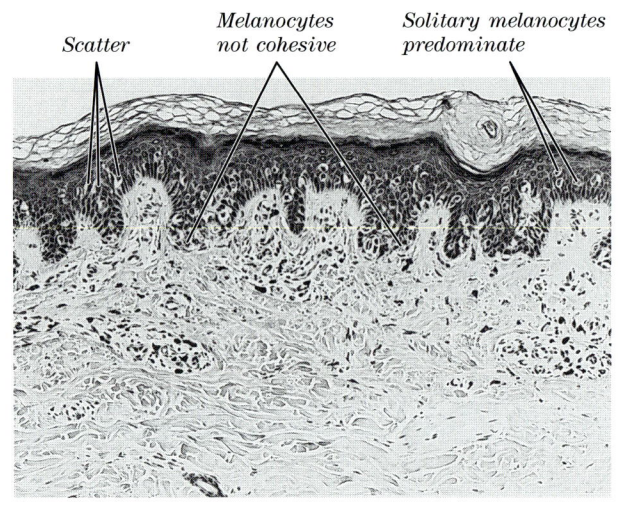
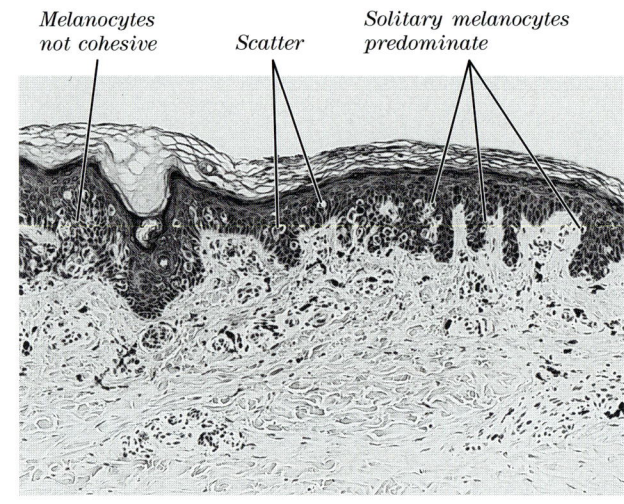

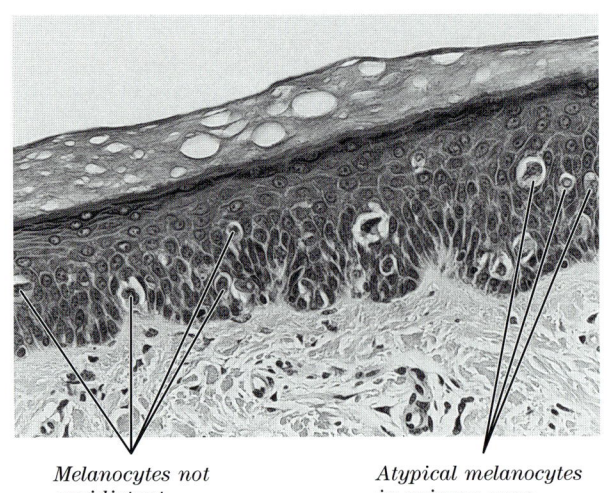
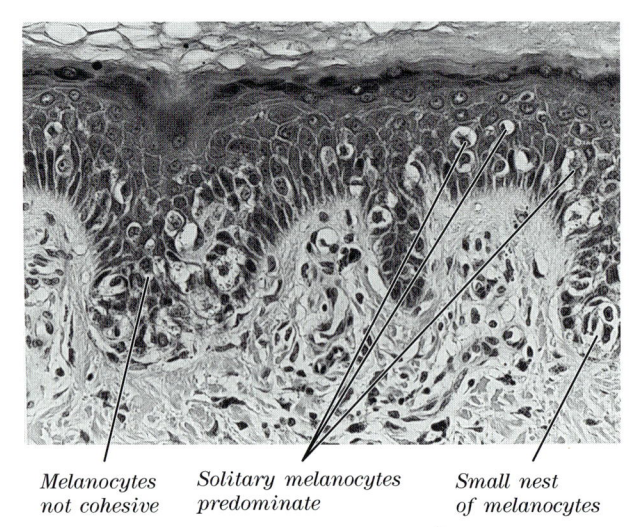
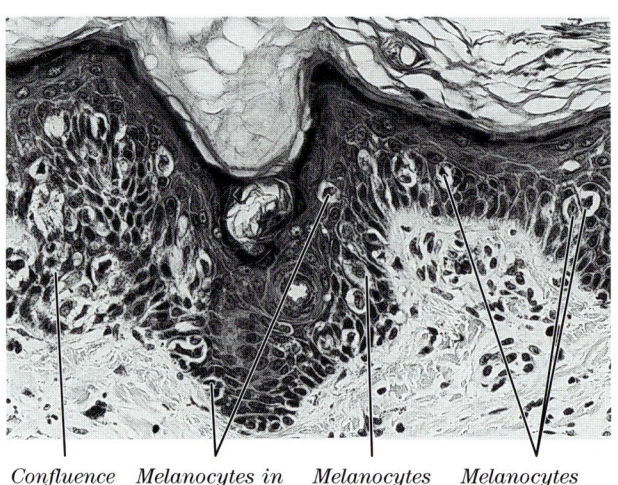

57 • Melanoma in situ

Criteria for diagnosis of this melanoma in situ

This is a melanoma in situ because:

1. The neoplasm is poorly circumscribed.

2. Nests of melanocytes within the epidermis are not equidistant from one another.

3. Some nests of melanocytes are not discrete, and melanocytes within them are not cohesive.

4. Some nests have become confluent.

5. Melanocytes disposed as solitary units predominate over nests of them in many high-power fields.

6. Melanocytes arrayed as solitary units are scattered far above the dermo-epidermal junction.

7. Changes like those in the epidermis are present within an eccrine duct.

8. Many neoplastic cells have atypical nuclei.

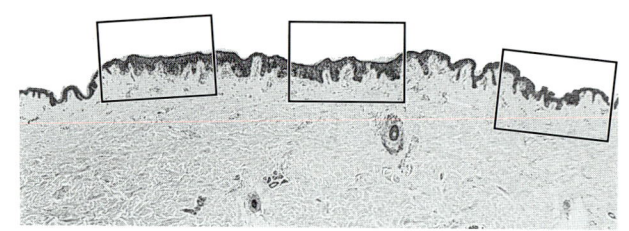

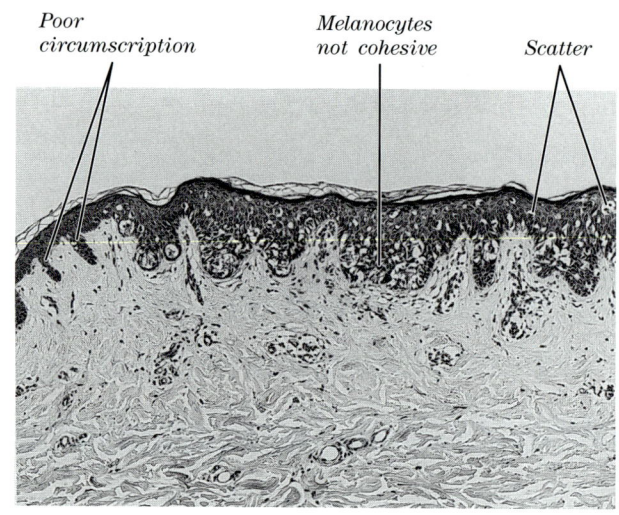

Poor circumscription | Melanocytes not cohesive | Scatter

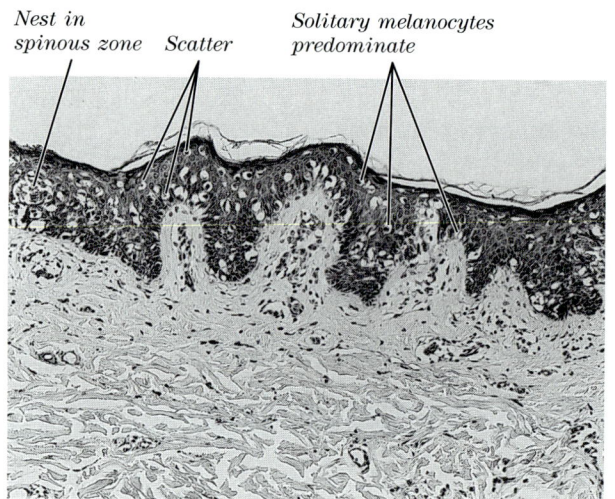

Nest in spinous zone | Scatter | Solitary melanocytes predominate

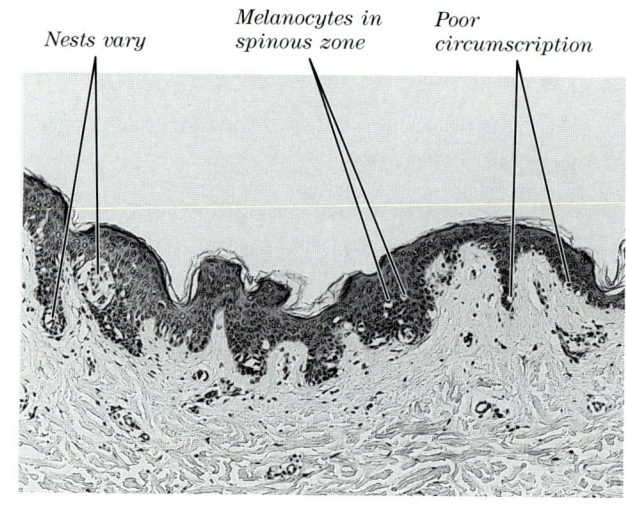

Nests vary | Melanocytes in spinous zone | Poor circumscription

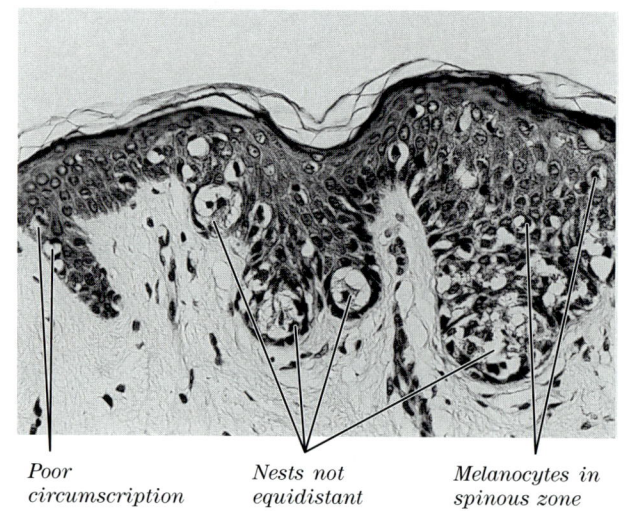

Poor circumscription | Nests not equidistant and vary | Melanocytes in spinous zone

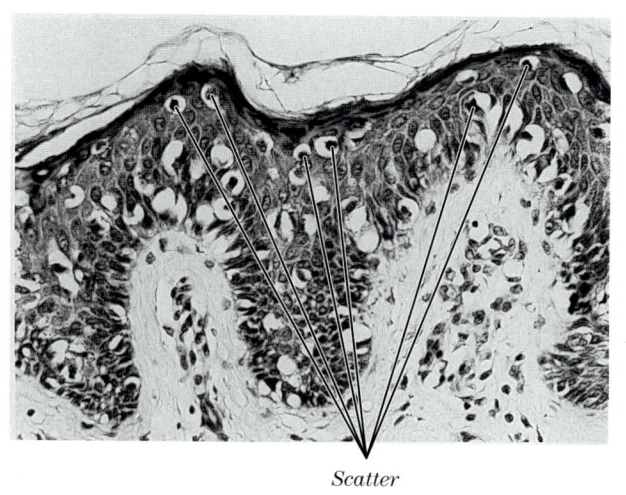

Scatter

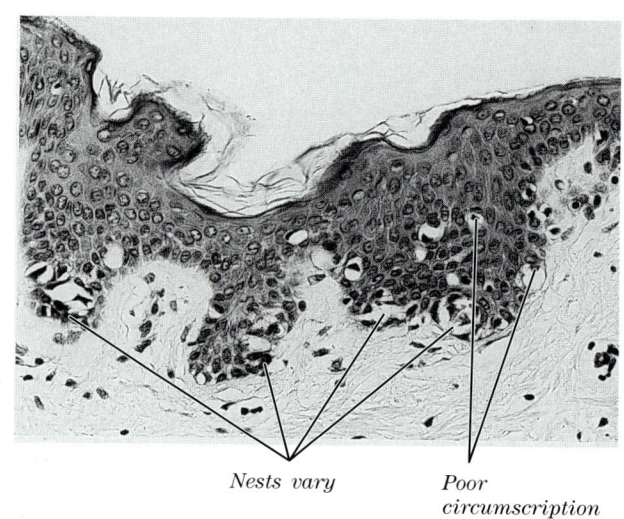

Nests vary | Poor circumscription

58 • Melanoma in situ

Criteria for diagnosis of this melanoma in situ

This is a melanoma in situ because:

1. The neoplasm is asymmetric, e.g., there are many more melanocytes on the left than on the right of it.
2. The lesion is poorly circumscribed.
3. Nests of melanocytes are not equidistant from one another.
4. Nests of melanocytes vary in size and shape.
5. Some nests of melanocytes have become confluent.
6. Melanocytes arranged as solitary units predominate over nests in many high-power fields.
7. Melanocytes arrayed both as solitary units and in nests are scattered at all levels of the epidermis.
8. Melanocytes disposed as solitary units are not equidistant from one another.
9. Nuclei of melanocytes are atypical.

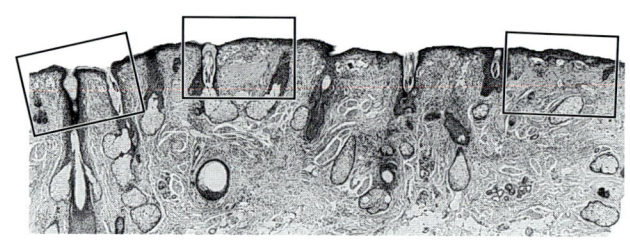

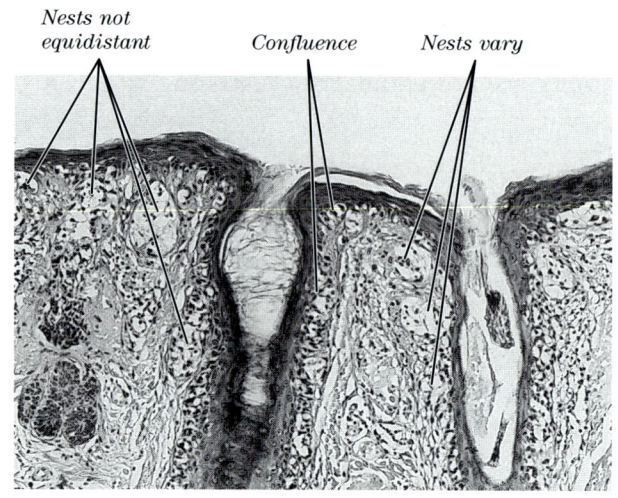

Nests not equidistant | Confluence | Nests vary

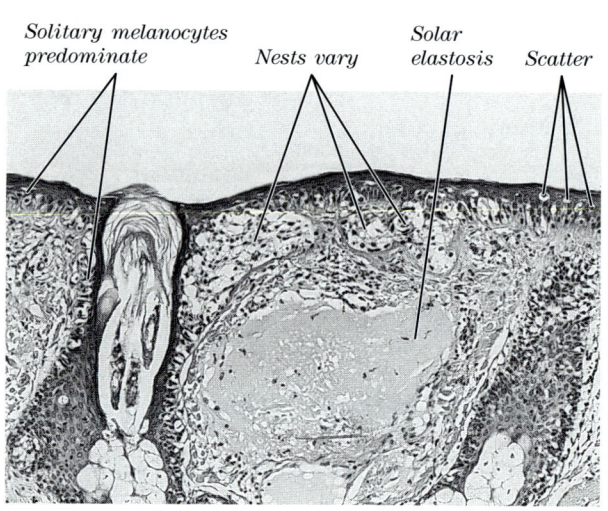

Solitary melanocytes predominate | Nests vary | Solar elastosis | Scatter

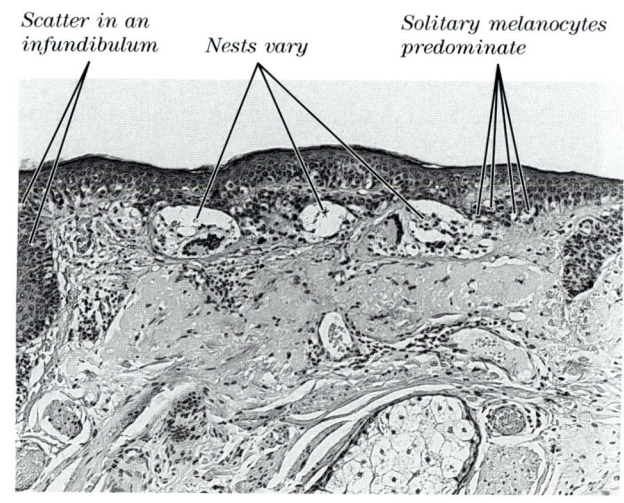

Scatter in an infundibulum | Nests vary | Solitary melanocytes predominate

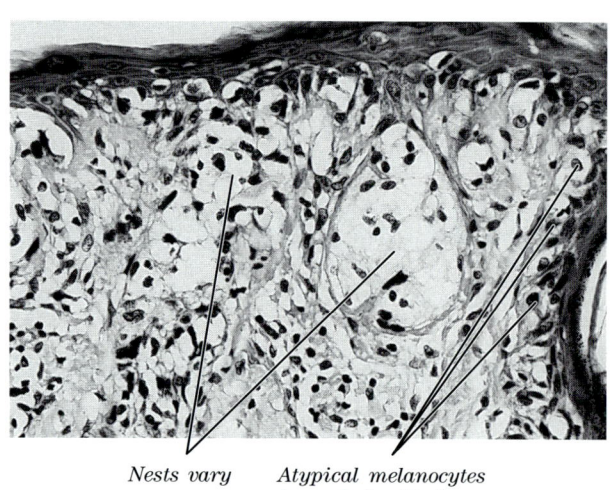

Nests vary | Atypical melanocytes in an infundibulum

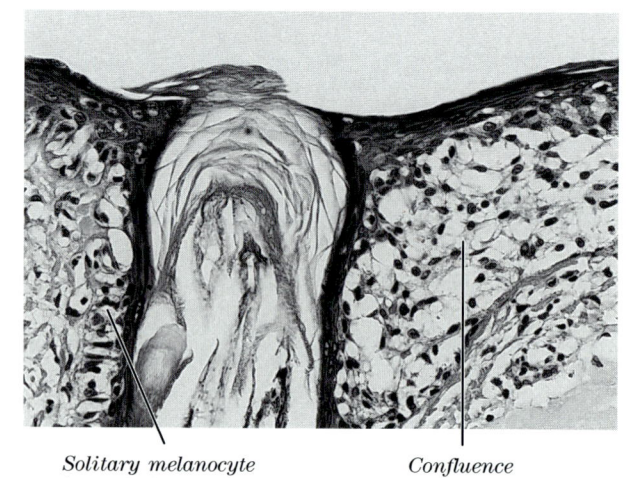

Solitary melanocyte in an infundibulum | Confluence

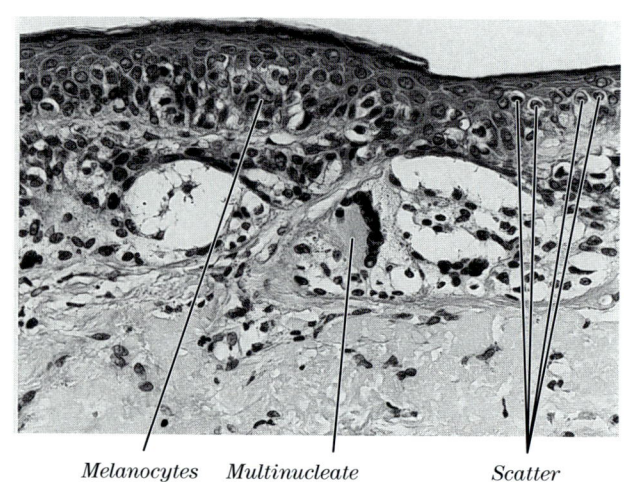

Melanocytes not cohesive | Multinucleate atypical melanocyte | Scatter

59 • Melanoma in situ

Criteria for diagnosis of this melanoma in situ

This is a melanoma in situ because:

1. The melanocytic proliferation on skin of a face damaged severely by sunlight is broad, i.e., more than 1.0 cm in greatest diameter.

2. Melanocytes are present not only at the dermo-epidermal junction, but well above it and far down infundibula to the level of sebaceous units.

3. Nests of melanocytes vary in size and shape.

4. Nests of melanocytes have become confluent.

5. Nests of melanocytes are not equidistant from one another.

6. Melanocytes arranged as solitary units predominate over nests of melanocytes in some high-power fields within the epidermis and epithelial structures of adnexa.

7. Nuclei of melanocytes are pleomorphic.

It is difficult sometimes to determine whether nests of melanocytes are positioned entirely at the dermo-epidermal junction or whether they are separated from the junction by a thin zone of dermis. That conundrum is illustrated in the photomicrograph in the lower right, i.e., is this melanoma in situ or not? In our opinion, the melanoma is in situ and the appearance of nests in the dermis is a consequence of the section having been cut at a slight tangent.

adnexal, mucosal), and to a variety of inaccurate descriptions that are not diagnoses at all, such as "lentigo maligna," "precancerous circumscribed melanosis," "atypical melanocytic dysplasia," "severe melanocytic dysplasia," "basilar melanocytic hyperplasia, slightly atypical," and "pagetoid melanocytic proliferation." In January 1992, the panel of an NIH Consensus Conference concurred with the view set forth here when it stated: "Melanoma in situ is a specific diagnosis for flat or elevated lesions with histologic features identical to those described for melanoma but confined to the full thickness of the epidermis and adnexal epithelium." We demur only in regard to "full thickness;" the diagnosis of melanoma in situ sometimes can be made when no melanocytes are present above the basal layer.

The concept of melanoma in situ is analogous to that of squamous-cell carcinoma in situ (Bowen's disease and bowenoid papulosis) and to adenocarcinoma in situ (extramammary Paget's disease) in which neoplastic cells are confined to the epidermis and to adnexal epithelial structures. In short, a diagnosis of melanoma in situ should not be rendered when only an increased number of *typical* melanocytes is stationed at the dermo-epidermal junction. A diagnosis of melanoma in situ should be entertained seriously, however, when an increased number of *atypical* melanocytes arranged as solitary units, not equidistant from one another, is observed at the junction between epidermis and dermis, between infundibula and dermis, and sometimes between the uppermost part of eccrine ducts and dermis. When atypical melanocytes arranged as solitary units are present above the dermo-epidermal junction of a lesion that is symmetric and poorly circumscribed, a diagnosis of melanoma in situ usually can be made with near surety, especially when that proliferation of melanocytes is situated on skin that shows signs of having been damaged badly by sunlight. The criteria for histopathologic (and clinical) diagnosis of melanoma in situ are the same for all anatomic sites (Figs. 58, 59, 60). Last, it must be stressed that cytologic atypia is *not* a sine qua non for diagnosis of melanoma in situ; architectural pattern is.

In sum, melanomas in skin nearly always begin at the dermo-epidermal junction. When they are confined to epithelium (epidermal and adnexal), they may be considered melanomas in situ. The same criteria used to make a diagnosis of melanoma that involves both the epidermis and the dermis are utilized for making a diagnosis of melanoma in the epidermis alone, minus criteria that pertain to the dermis, to wit, failure of maturation of melanocytes with progressive descent into the dermis, marked variation in size and shape of nests of melanocytes within the dermis, confluence of nests of melanocytes to form sheets of cells within the dermis, and presence of mitotic figures in the dermal portion of the neoplasm (Fig. 61). In short, most of the criteria for diagnosis of melanoma, unqualified, obtain also for diagnosis of melanoma in situ, even when one or more foci of regression are noted in the papillary dermis (Fig. 62). Parenthetically and for practical purposes, a diagnosis of primary cutaneous melanoma, no matter how small the lesion (Fig. 63), should not be made unless there is indubitable evidence of melanoma in situ. The criteria, as enumerated and illustrated here, enable diagnosis of melanoma in situ to be made at an early stage, e.g., when melanocytes within the epidermis and adnexal epithelia are arranged only as solitary units and not at all in nests. Of course, it is incumbent upon histopathologists not to overdiagnose melanomas and particularly melanomas in situ, but when changes such as those just described are observed histopathologically, criteria for melanoma are fulfilled. If clinicians are able to diagnose small flat lesions of melanoma, so, too, should histopathologists. If all small flat lesions of melanoma could be diagnosed and removed, no one would ever die of cutaneous melanoma.

D. Desmoplastic Melanoma, Neurotropic Melanoma, and Melanoma with Neural Differentiation

A distinctive, but uncommon variant of melanoma is typified by extensive fibroplasia and a tendency, though not invariable, to neurotropism (Figs. 64, 65). This desmoplastic, neurotropic expression of melanoma develops mostly on the face, exhibits little, if any, pigment clinically, and demonstrates scant proliferation of melanocytes within the epidermis in most specimens. In desmoplastic melanoma, crucial clues to diagnosis are found in the dermis and subcutaneous fat especially. One clue is moderately dense infiltrates of lymphocytes around venules throughout the dermis, especially the lower half of it, and in the upper part of the subcutaneous fat. Another clue is perineural fibroplasia in the form of fibrillary or wiry bundles of collagen displayed concentrically. A third clue is the presence of neoplastic cells within nerve fascicles. The definitive diagnostic findings, however, are the asymmetry of the neoplasm in concert with signs of melanoma in situ, no matter how subtle. The neoplastic cells in the dermis and subcutaneous fat have thin oval, spindle, and wavy nuclei and scant cytoplasm. A smidgen of brown granular (melanin) pigment may be present in the cytoplasm of some neoplastic cells and in macrophages, but some neoplasms are amelanotic. The proclivity of neoplastic melanocytes in this type of melanoma for nerve fascicles within the dermis and in the subcutis accounts for the designation "desmoplastic, neurotropic melanoma." It must be emphasized, however, that melanomas may be neurotropic and not desmoplastic. Neurotropic melanoma must be distinguished from melanoma with neural differentiation in which wavy neoplastic melanocytes form structures that resemble caricatures of authentic nerve fascicles, in contrast to hyperplasia of pre-existing nerve fascicles by neoplastic melanocytes in neurotropic melanoma (Fig. 65). Both patterns may appear together in the same section, i.e., fascicles of melanocytes with neural differentiation and neurotropism of melanocytes.

In desmoplastic melanoma, discrete nests of melanocytes are few or absent; mitotic figures are scant; the stroma is abundant and constituted of delicate, fibrillary bundles of collagen, and mucin may be prominent within the stroma (Fig. 66). The triad of wavy nuclei, fibrillary bundles of collagen, and mucin suggest neural differentiation in general and, in the absence of signs of melanoma in situ or of melanin, a desmoplastic melanoma may be misinterpreted as a benign neoplasm with neural differentiation. Subtle signs of melanoma in situ may be detected if enough sections are cut and scrutinized, but not always. Immunoperoxidase stains for S-100 protein and HMB-45 are positive for the neoplastic melanocytes within the dermis and may unmask neoplastic melanocytes within the epidermis, epithelial structures of adnexa, and nerve fascicles, thereby confirming a diagnosis of melanoma. When spindle-shaped melanocytes monopolize a dermoplastic melanoma, stain for S-100 protein may be negative.

Desmoplastic melanoma poses diagnostic problems clinically and histopathologically. Clinically, it is confused easily with a fibroma because of lack of pigment and the sensation of hardness. Histopathologically, it is misinterpreted easily as a benign neural or other non-epithelial neoplasm because changes of melanoma in situ so often are hardly noticeable, no melanin may be detectable, no nests of melanocytes may be apparent, and lack of striking nuclear atypia is the rule. The remarkable proclivity of neoplastic cells for nerve fascicles explains why neoplastic melanocytes in desmoplastic melanoma situated on a face follow nerves in the skin backward through foramina in the skull into the brain. Desmoplastic melanoma also has the capability for metastasis, so that patients afflicted with it sometimes die agonizing deaths as a consequence both of direct effects of extension of neoplastic melanocytes into the brain and of metastases there and elsewhere.

Desmoplastic melanoma is not the only type of primary melanoma that may be non-pigmented. Episodically, a pink macule or patch on a face thought to be Bowen's disease, a superficial basal-cell carcinoma, or even a lichen planus-like keratosis, may be discovered on histopathologic examination to be melanoma in situ or a thin, non-dermoplastic melanoma.

In summary, it is our practice to make a diagnosis of melanoma, unmodified, except for extraordinary examples such as those of the desmoplastic, neurotropic variety that has a distinctive appearance and behavior. We do not qualify melanomas as lentigo maligna, borderline, minimal deviation, without capability for metastasis, etc., because we do not consider those designations accurate, valid, or beneficial to patients.

Another distinctive morphologic variant of melanoma, and a rare one, is characterized by large quantities of mucin in the immediate vicinity of neoplastic melanocytes (Fig. 67). The abundance of mucin is disconcerting, but the underlying neoplasm still can be determined to be a melanoma on the basis of the same criteria employed histopathologically to identify all primary cutaneous melanomas, irrespective of nuance or variation.

In conclusion, it cannot be emphasized too strongly that a diagnosis of melanoma or of a benign simulator of it, such as Spitz's nevus, should not be made on the basis of a single morphologic criterion, but predicated on a constellation of criteria. Rarely, mitotic figures may be noted at the base of a Spitz's nevus and dull pink globules within the epidermis of melanoma. In those exceptional instances, scrutiny of all the histopathologic findings, especially those that pertain to silhouette, will enable a correct diagnosis to be reached in the vast majority of cases. Truistic though it be, there are exceptions to every statement that can be made about nevi and melanomas. Therefore, just as criteria (rules) for diagnosis and clues (hints) to diagnosis of those neoplasms must be known well, so, too, must exceptions to them.

E. Thickness as a Measure of Prognosis

All cutaneous malignant neoplasms confined to epithelium, including melanoma, are biologically benign because all of the neoplastic cells are restricted to an avascular compartment. When neoplastic melanocytes of melanoma descend, however, as they do so often and without premonitory

Text continues on page 131

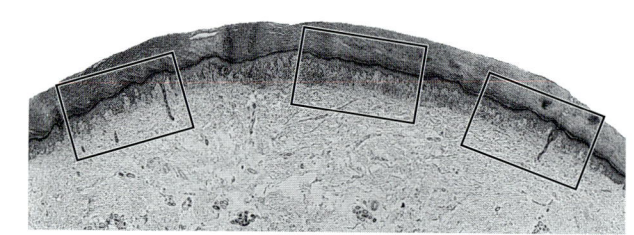

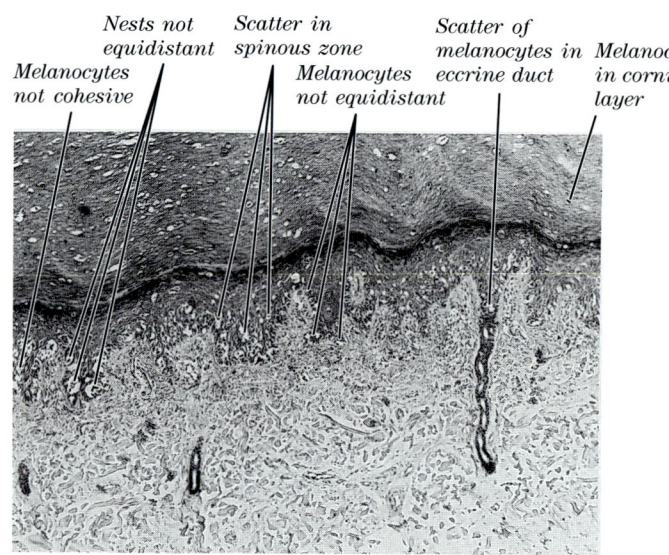

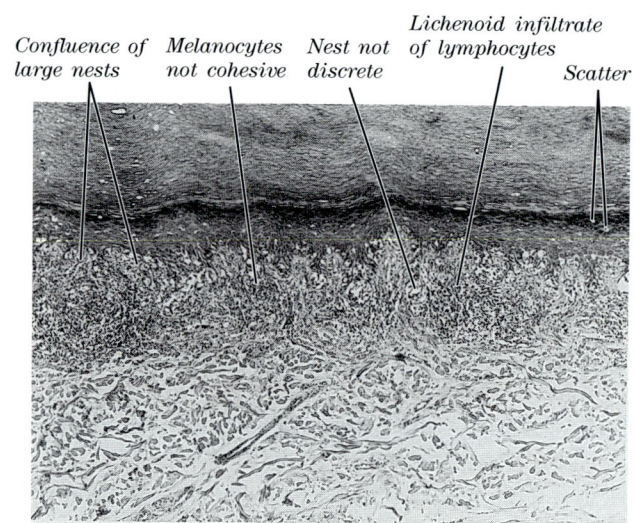

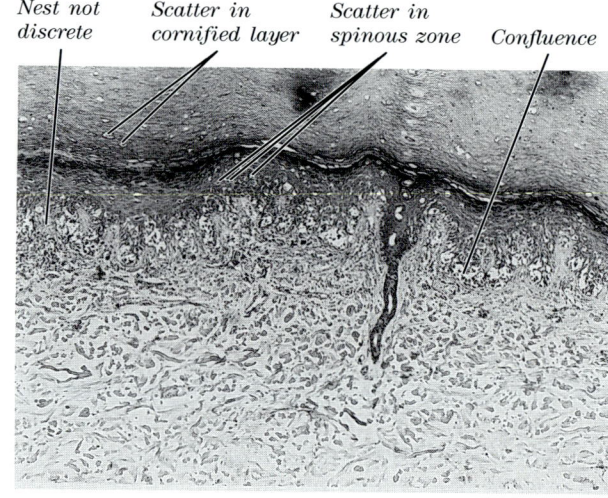

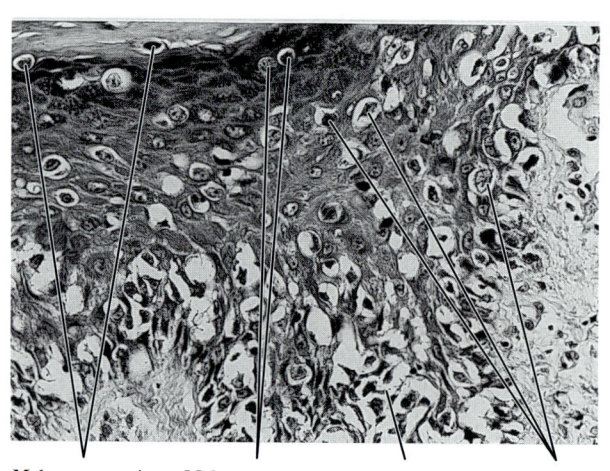

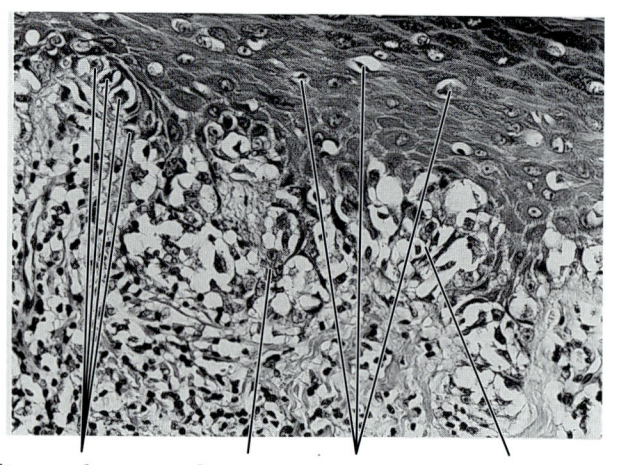

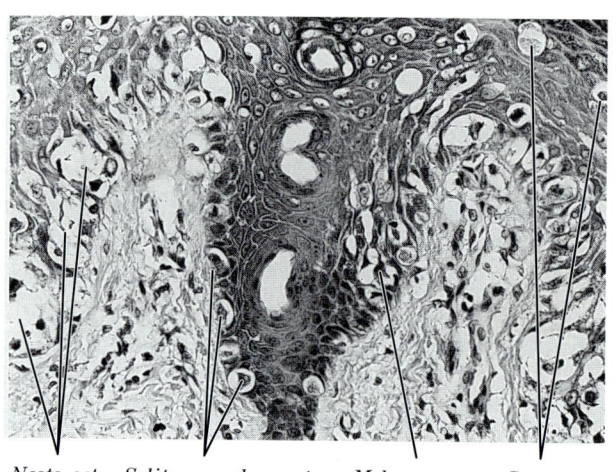

60 · Melanoma in situ

Criteria for diagnosis of this melanoma in situ (on volar skin)

This is a melanoma in situ because:

1. Atypical melanocytes are disposed both as solitary units and in nests at all levels of the epidermis, including the cornified layer, and far down eccrine ducts.

2. Melanocytes arranged as solitary units predominate over melanocytes in nests.

3. There are many more melanocytes per unit area of epidermis than is found in any kind of junctional nevus.

4. Nests of melanocytes are not equidistant from one another.

5. Nests of melanocytes vary in size and shape.

6. Some nests of melanocytes have become confluent.

7. Some nests of melanocytes have peculiar shapes, i.e., they are neither round nor oval.

8. Nuclei of melanocytes are strikingly atypical.

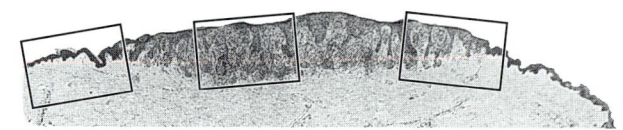

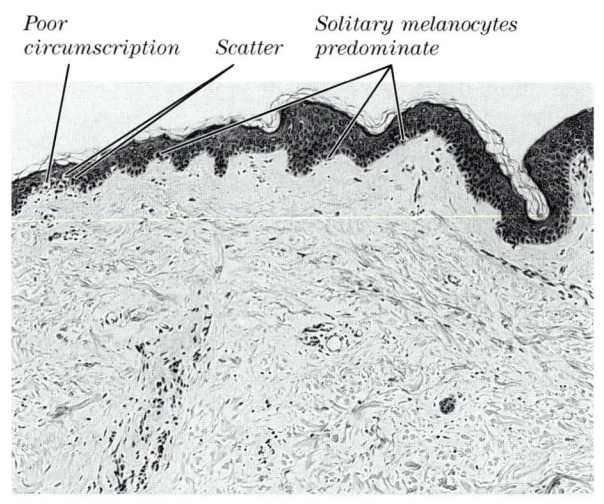
Poor circumscription | Scatter | Solitary melanocytes predominate

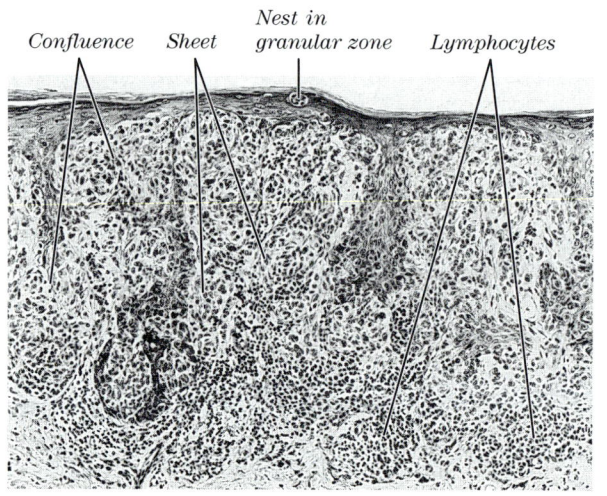
Confluence | Sheet | Nest in granular zone | Lymphocytes

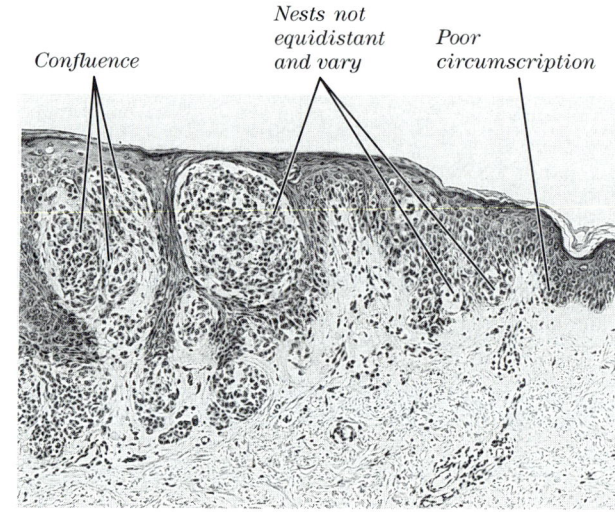
Confluence | Nests not equidistant and vary | Poor circumscription

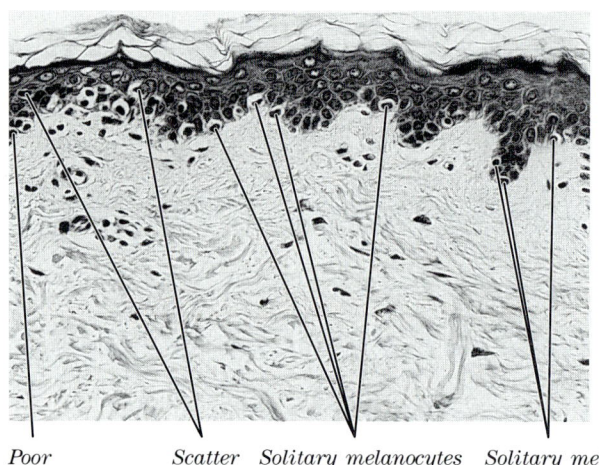
Poor circumscription | Scatter | Solitary melanocytes predominate | Solitary melanocytes not equidistant

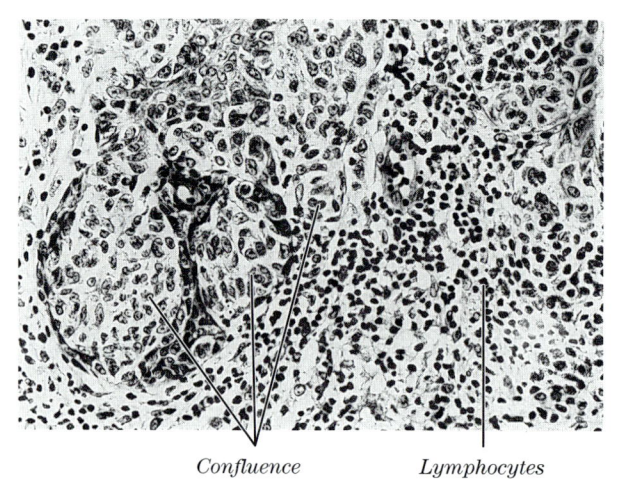
Confluence | Lymphocytes

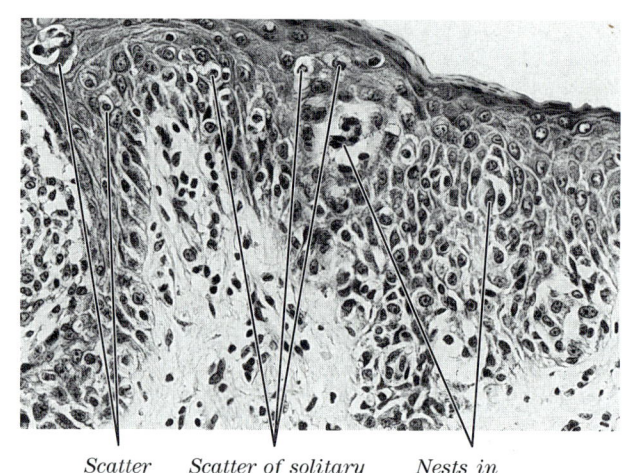
Scatter | Scatter of solitary melanocytes | Nests in spinous zone

61 • Melanoma

Criteria for diagnosis of this melanoma

This is a melanoma because:

1. The neoplasm is asymmetric.
2. It is poorly circumscribed.
3. Nests of melanocytes within the epidermis are not equidistant from one another.
4. Nests of melanocytes within the epidermis vary in size and shape.
5. Nests of melanocytes within the epidermis and the dermis have become confluent.
6. Atypical melanocytes are present within epithelial structures of adnexa.
7. Pagetoid melanocytes are arrayed in pagetoid pattern.
8. Melanocytes do not mature.
9. Nuclear atypia is striking.

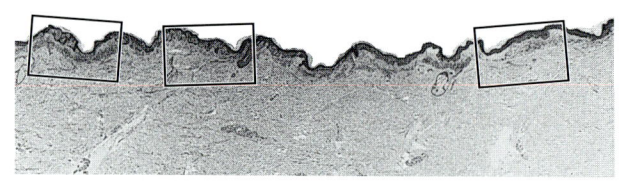

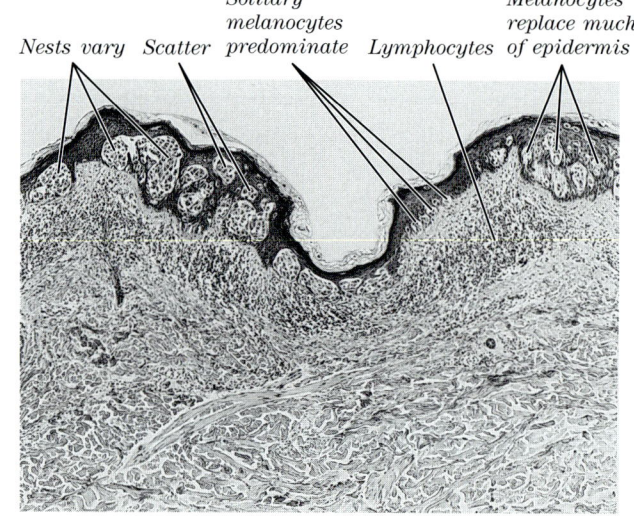
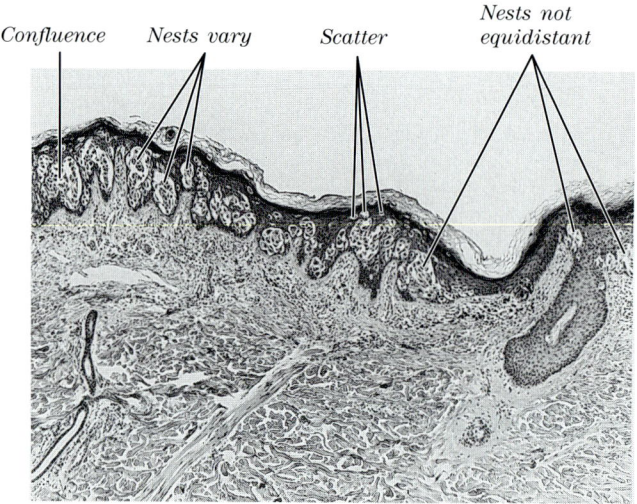
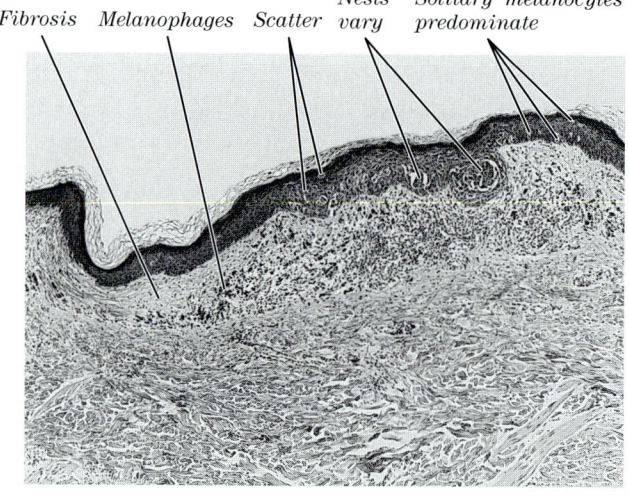

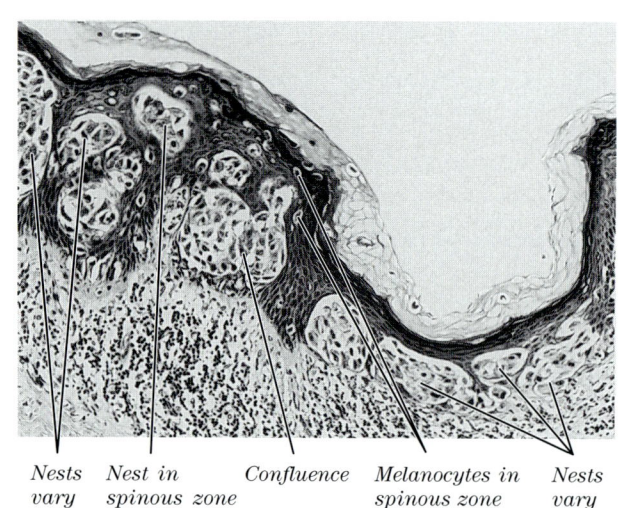
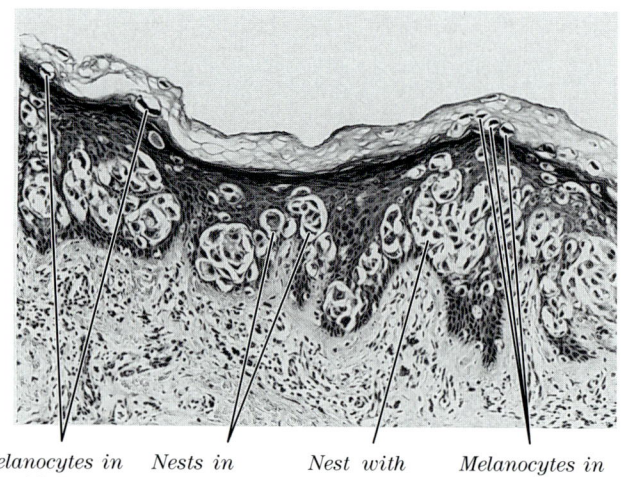
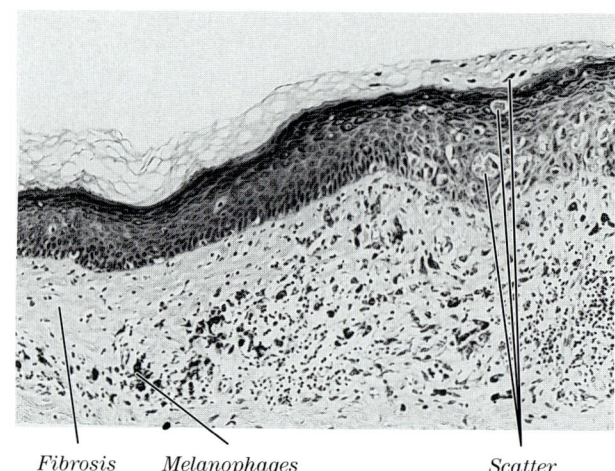

126   **62 • Melanoma in situ**

Criteria for diagnosis of this melanoma in situ

This is a melanoma in situ because:

1. The proliferation of melanocytes is broad, i.e., considerably more than 1.0 cm in greatest diameter.

2. Melanocytes organized as solitary units and in nests are present throughout the entire thickness of the epidermis, including the granular zone and cornified layer.

3. Nests of melanocytes are not equidistant from one another.

4. Nests of melanocytes vary in size and shape.

5. Some nests of melanocytes have bizarre shapes, i.e., they are neither round nor oval.

6. Melanocytes arrayed as solitary units predominate over nests in some high-power fields.

7. The pattern of distribution of melanocytes within the epidermis is present also within epithelial structures of adnexa.

8. Nuclei of melanocytes are atypical.

9. Focal regression of the neoplasm is apparent in the form of a papillary dermis thickened by fibrosis, numerous melanophages, and a patchy lichenoid infiltrate of lymphocytes.

    This neoplasm must be diagnosed as melanoma in situ on the basis of morphologic criteria, but the presence of regression seems to indicate that some neoplastic melanocytes of melanoma had entered the papillary dermis where they were destroyed by the effects of lymphocytes.

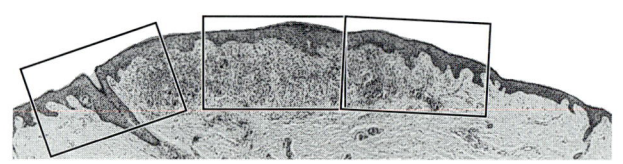

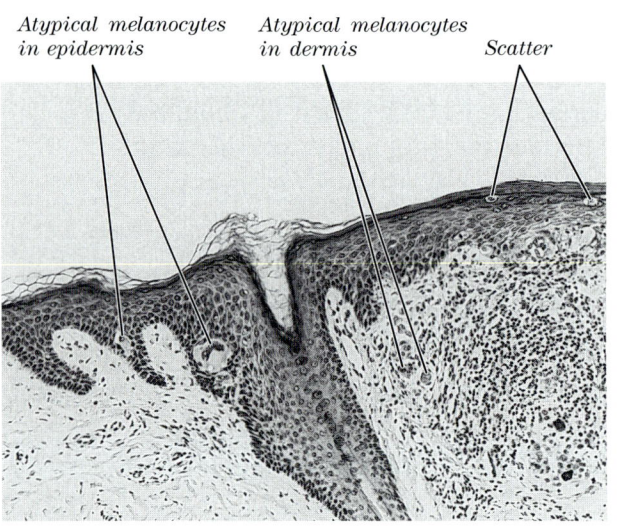

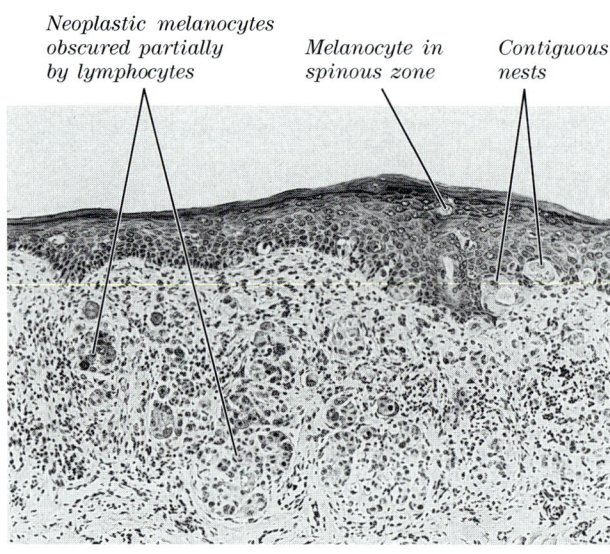

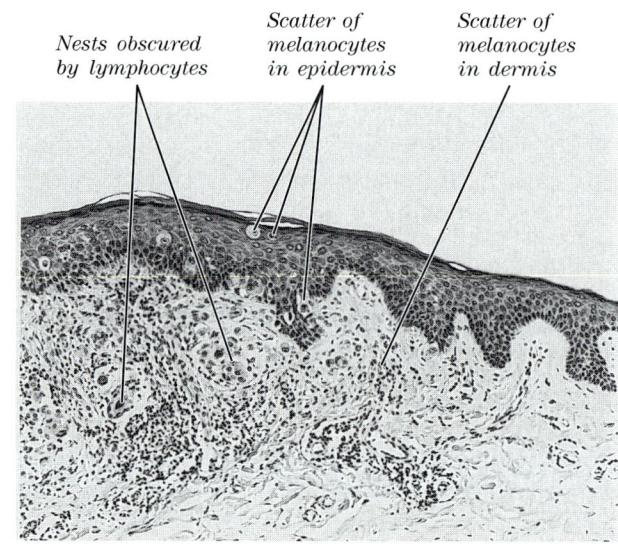

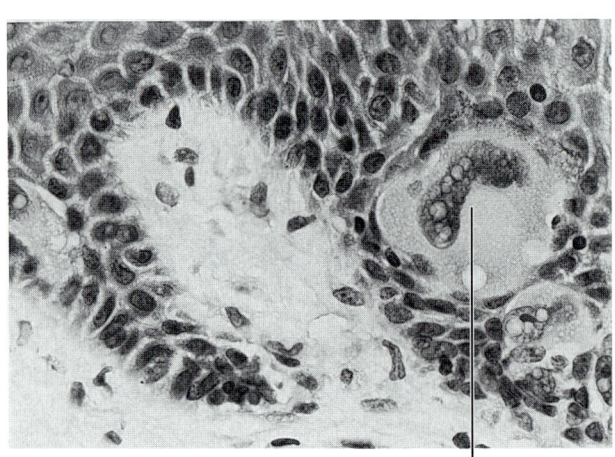

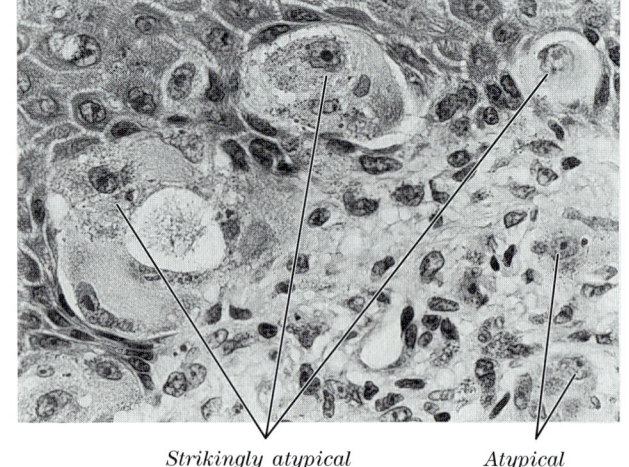

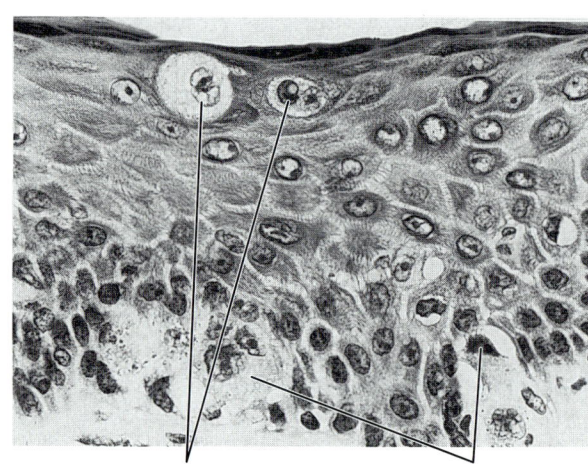

63 • Melanoma

Criteria for diagnosis of this melanoma

This is a melanoma because:

1. The neoplasm is slightly asymmetric, i.e., it has a snub nose on the left and a pointed nose on the right.
2. It is poorly circumscribed.
3. Nests of melanocytes are few and are not equidistant from one another.
4. Nests of melanocytes within the epidermis vary in size and shape.
5. Atypical melanocytes disposed as solitary units are not equidistant from one another.
6. Melanocytes are scattered at all levels of the epidermis and throughout epithelial structures of adnexa.
7. Melanocytes do not mature.
8. Melanocytes arranged as solitary units predominate over nests throughout the epidermis.
9. Nests of melanocytes within the dermis have become confluent.
10. Melanin is not distributed uniformly either within the nests themselves or from nest to nest.
11. Nuclear atypia is striking, and nucleoli are prominent.

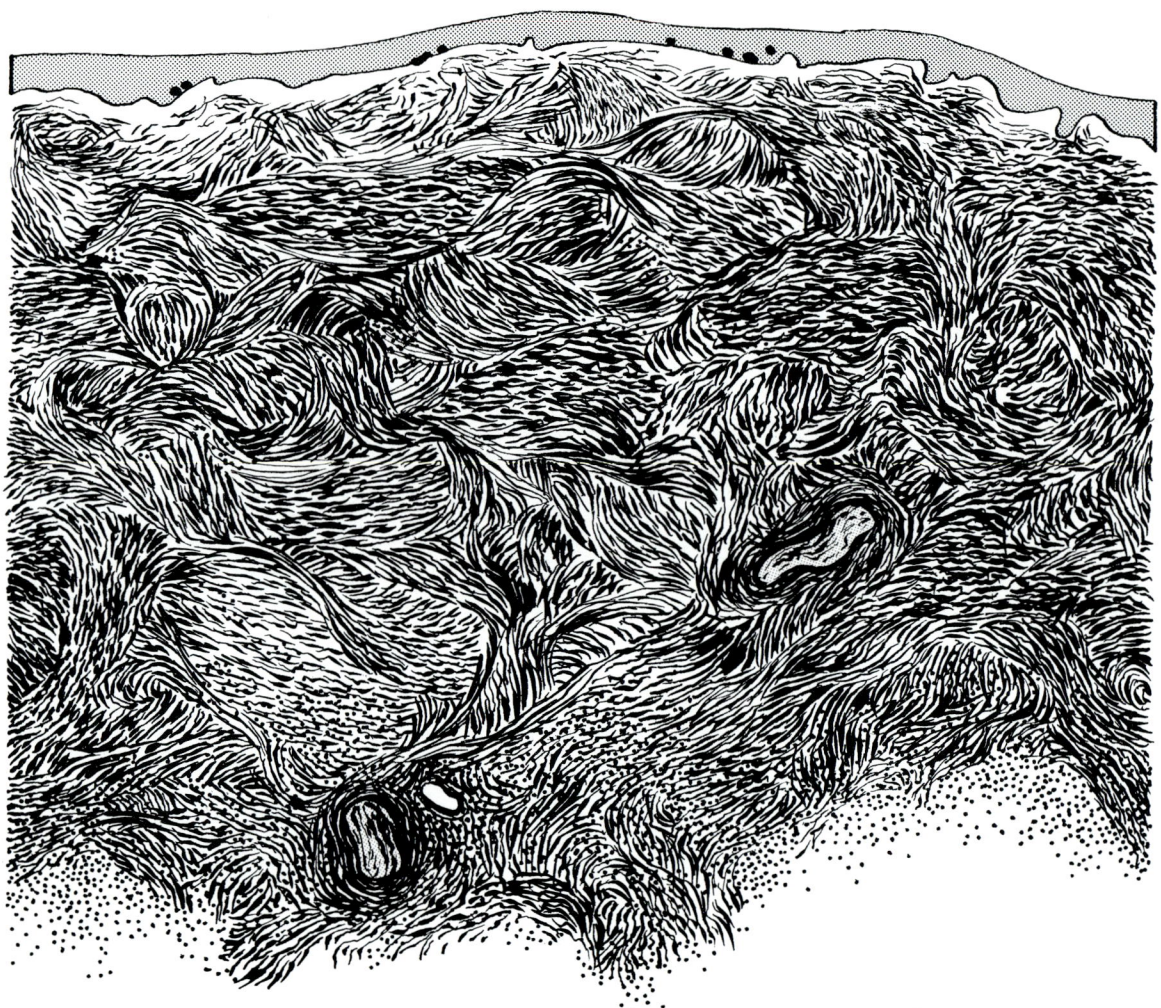

Fig. 64. Desmoplastic melanoma. With scanning magnification, the neoplasm could be misinterpreted as a benign neoplasm with neural differentiation or a dermatofibrosarcoma protuberans. In truth, it is a malignant melanoma with striking desmoplasia and neurotropism, i.e., a desmoplastic melanoma. Note the subtle proliferation focally of melanocytes arranged as solitary units and in small nests at the dermo-epidermal junction and slightly above it, evidences of melanoma in situ. Within the lower half of the reticular dermis, neoplastic cells are present within nerve fascicles. The storiform pattern within the dermis consists of striking, delicate fibroplasia, in concert with a proliferation of oval, thin, and wavy nuclei of melanocytes.

signs, into the papillary dermis and beyond it, a person who bears such a lesion is at risk, theoretically, for metastasis because numerous blood and lymph vessels are housed there. Curiously, though, metastasis of melanocytes from a melanoma situated in a papillary dermis occurs uncommonly. Most metastases of melanoma take place through vessels located in the reticular dermis. Therefore, most "thin" melanomas, those that measure less than 1.0 mm in thickness (as determined by a micrometer placed within an ocular of a microscope and measured from the top of the granular zone of the epidermis to the base of the neoplasm) are benign biologically, i.e., they did not metastasize before the melanoma was excised (Fig. 68). In general, the thicker a melanoma, the worse the prognosis. Melanomas whose neoplastic melanocytes have extended from the epidermis through the entire dermis and near or into the subcutaneous fat have the worst prognosis (Fig. 69). The late Alexander Breslow, who conceived of measuring thickness of melanomas in order to predict prognosis, thought that thickness of a melanoma was a rough estimate of the volume of melanocytes in a neoplasm, and that volume was the most important guide to prognosis. Measurement of thickness of melanomas, as advocated by Breslow, is a more reliable gauge of prognosis than assessment of "levels of invasion" of melanomas advocated by Clark. No method, however, is able to indicate precisely how a person with a melanoma will fare because there are so many factors at play, e.g., age (young persons do worse), sex (men do worse), site (scalp is worst), mitotic figures (many is worse), necrosis (en masse is worse), and, furthermore, the most important determinants have yet to be established. Some persons with thin melanomas die of metastatic disease; yet others with very thick melanomas survive. In brief, just as "levels of invasion" have become passe for predicting prognosis of melanoma, so, too, it is inevitable that the same will be true for thickness as a reliable gauge of prognosis. Most important, thickness of a melanoma should not guide a surgeon's hand in the decision about how wide and deep margins of excision should be. They should not be wider for thicker melanomas, nor should they be deeper. The precept that should underlie surgical extirpation of melanoma, irrespective of thickness, is complete removal as judged by a surgeon's keen clinical assessment and a histopathologist's critical appraisal of margins of excision. There is not a jot of evidence in support of the contention that extraction of centimeters of normal skin and subcutaneous fat in the immediate vicinity of a melanoma, no matter how thick the melanoma, enhances prognosis a whit.

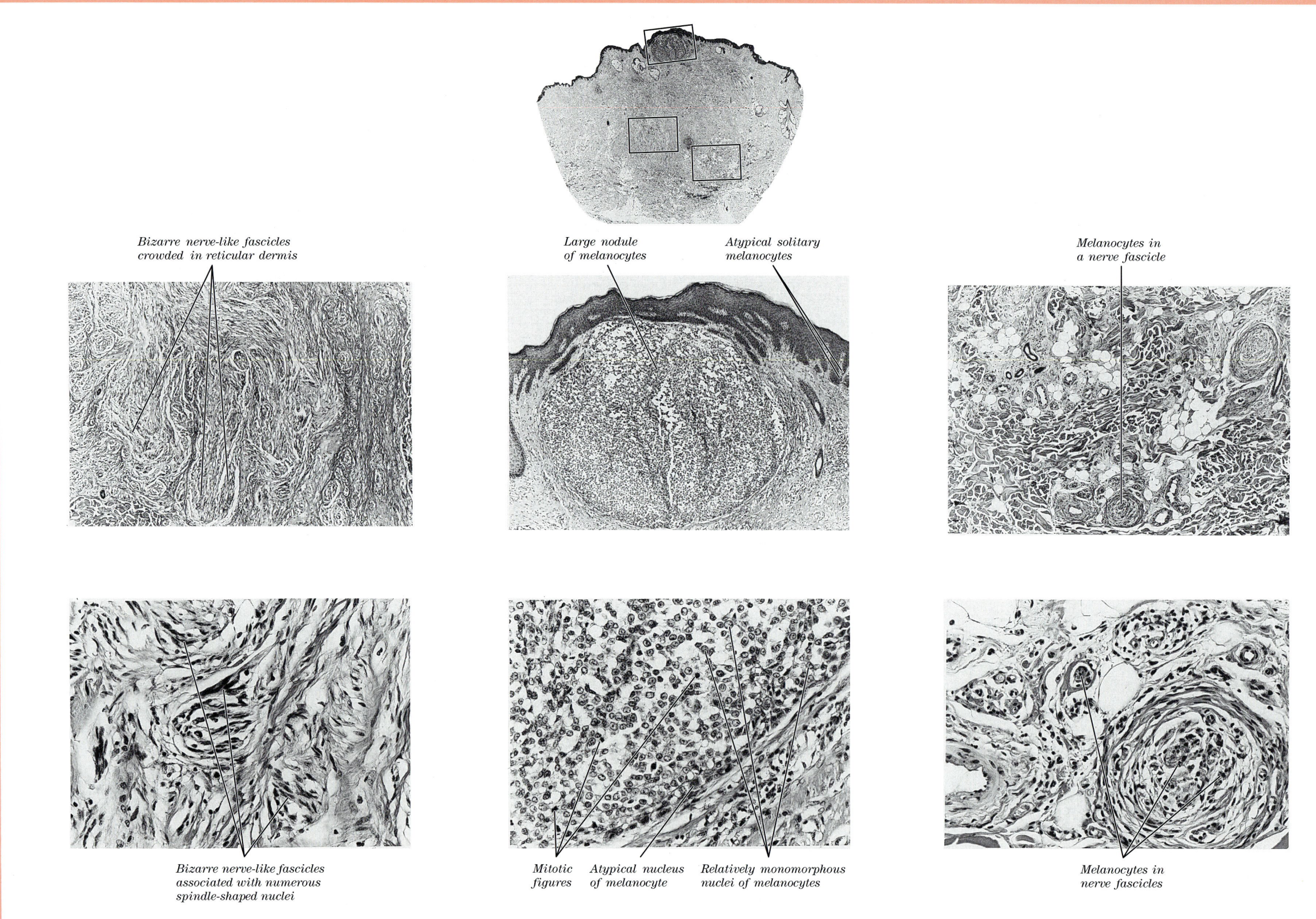

132 65 · Melanoma *(with neurotropism and neural differentiation)*

Criteria for diagnosis of this melanoma

This is a melanoma because:

1. The neoplasm is asymmetric.
2. Neoplastic melanocytes are arranged in sheets.
3. Neoplastic melanocytes have pleomorphic nuclei.

This melanoma exhibits neurotropism (seen on the right) because:

1. Neoplastic melanocytes, arranged as solitary units and in nests, are present within the substance of nerve fascicles.

This melanoma shows neural differentiation (seen on the left) because:

1. Numerous elongated structures that resemble caricatures of nerve fascicles are seen to interweave in haphazard fashion.
2. The bizarre simulators of fascicles consist, in large measure, of cells with thin wavy nuclei.
3. Some of the nuclei are atypical.

This melanoma demonstrates the difference between neurotropism of neoplastic melanocytes and neural differentiation of neoplastic melanocytes. Melanomas have the capability to do both: to extend into pre-existing nerve fascicles and to differentiate in the direction of nerve fascicles. The architectural and cytologic differences are demonstrated well in this section. Parenthetically, indubitable signs of melanoma in situ also are present in this specimen.

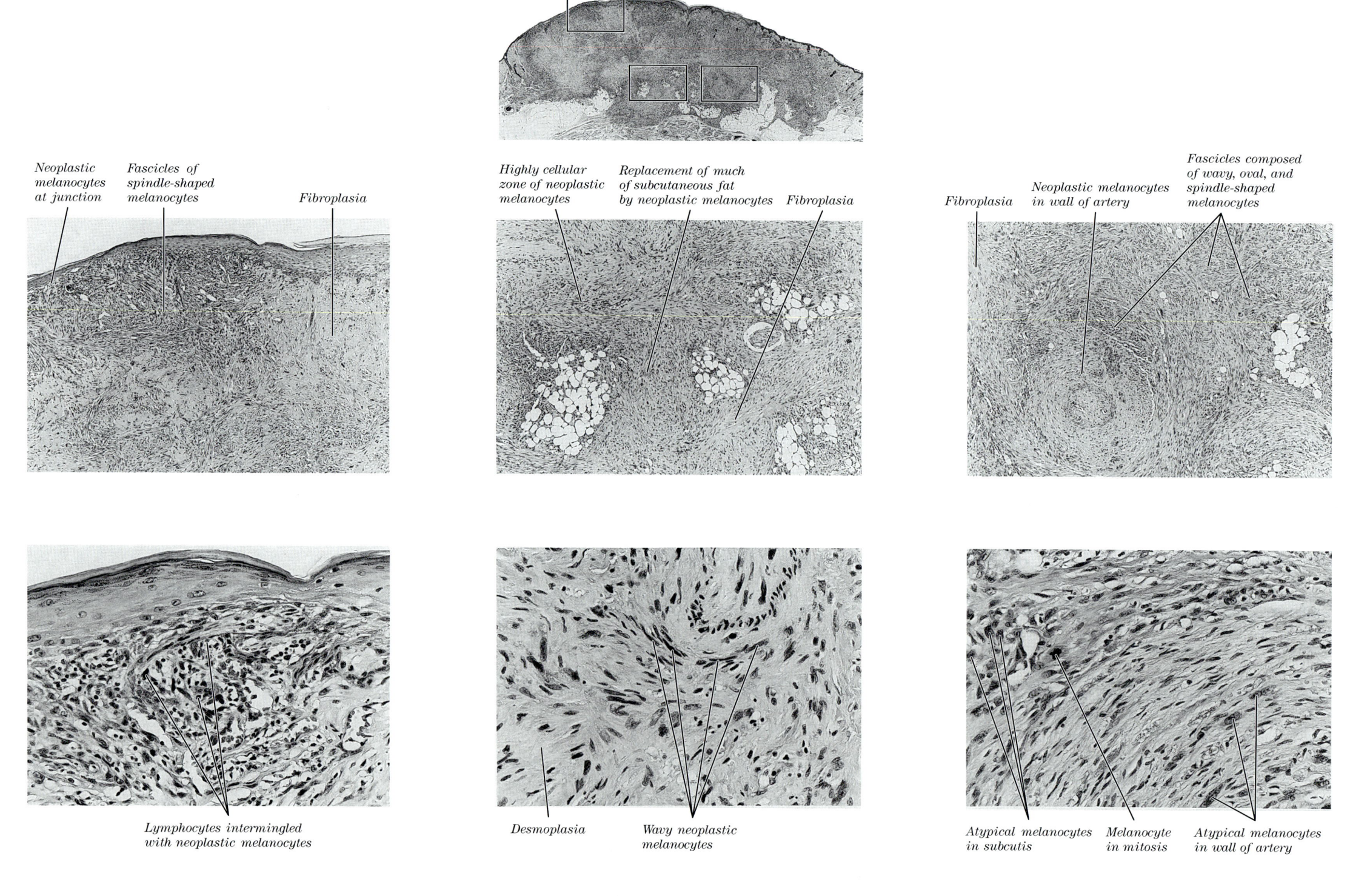

66 • Melanoma *(desmoplastic type)*

Criteria for diagnosis of this melanoma (desmoplastic type)

This is a melanoma because:

1. The neoplasm is asymmetric.
2. Nests of melanocytes within the epidermis are not equidistant from one another.
3. Nests of melanocytes within the epidermis vary in size and shape.
4. Nests of melanocytes within the epidermis have become confluent.
5. A few melanocytes arrayed as solitary units are present just above the dermo-epidermal junction.
6. Neoplastic cells throughout the dermis and the subcutaneous fat are arranged in sheets.
7. Nuclei of melanocytes are atypical.
8. Some neoplastic melanocytes in the dermis and the subcutaneous fat are in mitosis.

This is a desmoplastic melanoma because:

1. Prominent fibroplasia accompanies the proliferation of atypical melanocytes in the dermis and the subcutaneous fat.
2. Nuclei of some fibrocytes are impossible to distinguish from those of neoplastic melanocytes, but the latter are often wavy and atypical.
3. Neoplastic melanocytes within the dermis and the subcutaneous fat are organized mostly as solitary units, rather than mostly in nests.

This is a melanoma with neurotropism because:

1. Atypical neoplastic melanocytes are present within nerve fascicles in the dermis and the subcutaneous fat.
2. There is extensive perineural fibroplasia displayed as whorls.

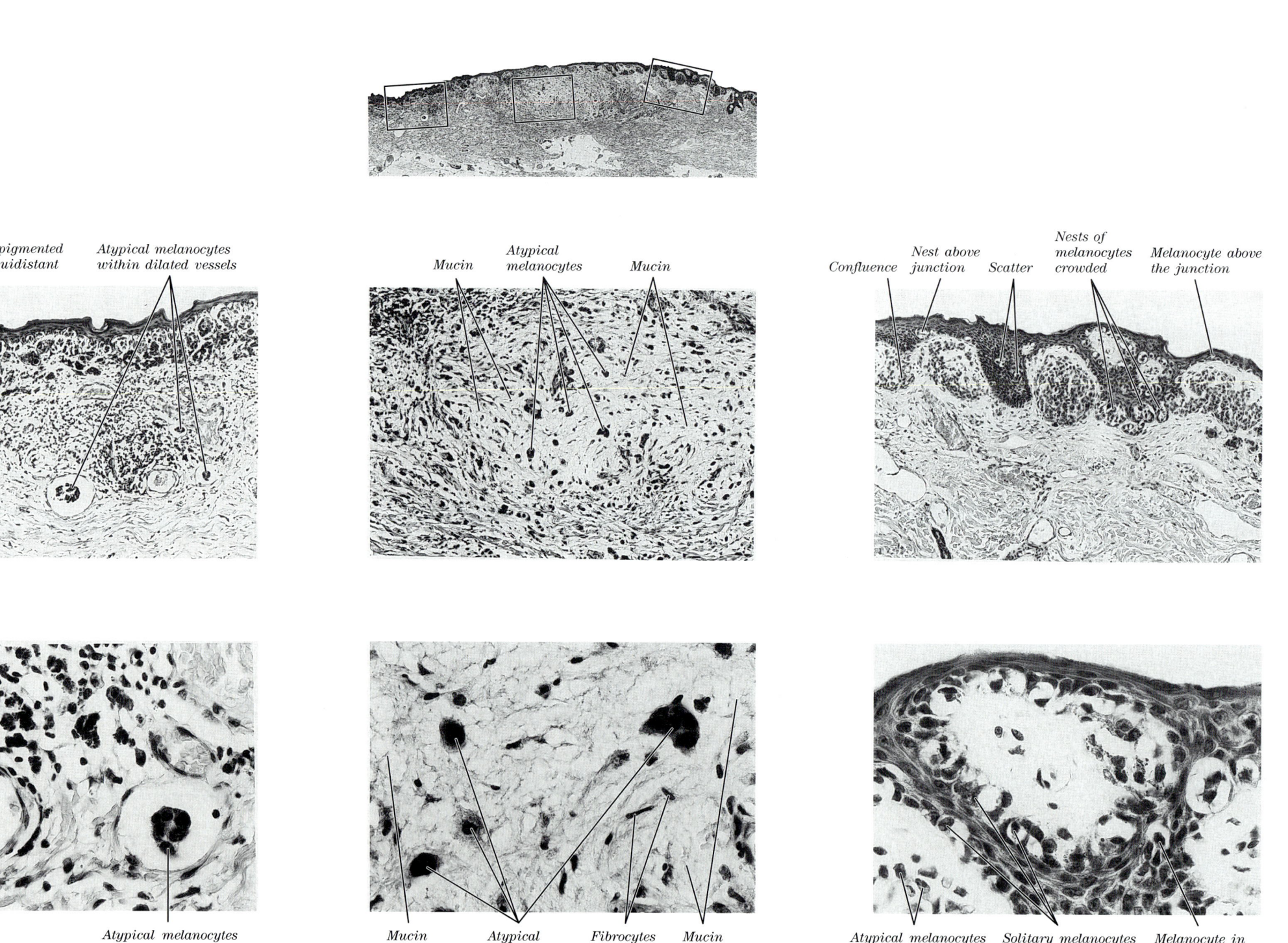

67 • Melanoma *(with abundant mucin)*

Criteria for diagnosis of this melanoma (associated with abundant mucin)

This is a melanoma associated with abundant mucin because:

1. Atypical melanocytes disposed as solitary units and in nests are present at all levels of the epidermis.

2. Nests of melanocytes within the epidermis are not equidistant from one another.

3. Nests of melanocytes vary in size and shape.

4. Some nests of melanocytes have become confluent.

5. There is no maturation of melanocytes.

6. Atypical melanocytes within the dermis are scattered throughout zones of abundant mucin.

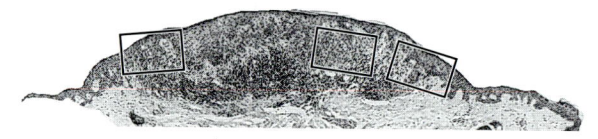

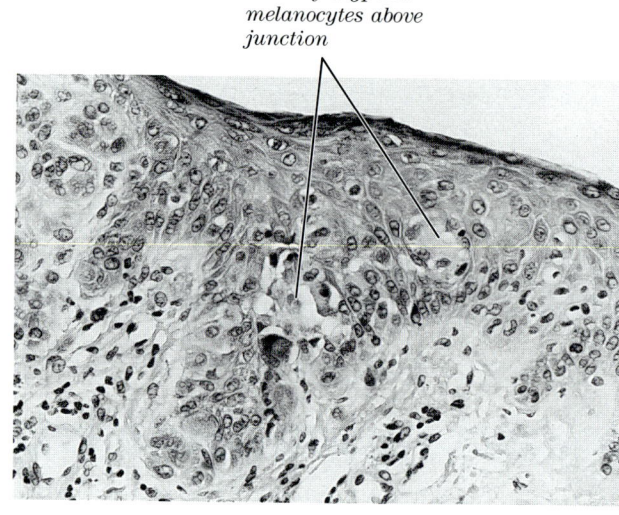

Poor circumscription of nests of atypical melanocytes

Confluence

Nests of atypical melanocytes above junction

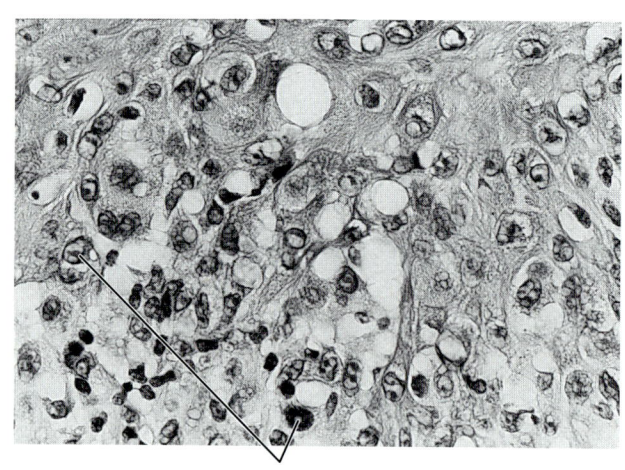

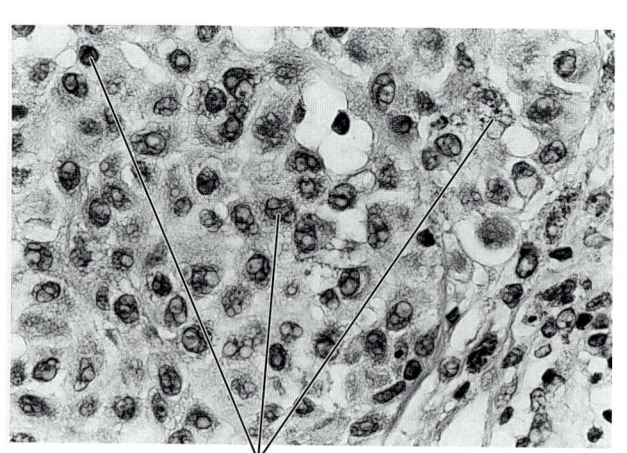

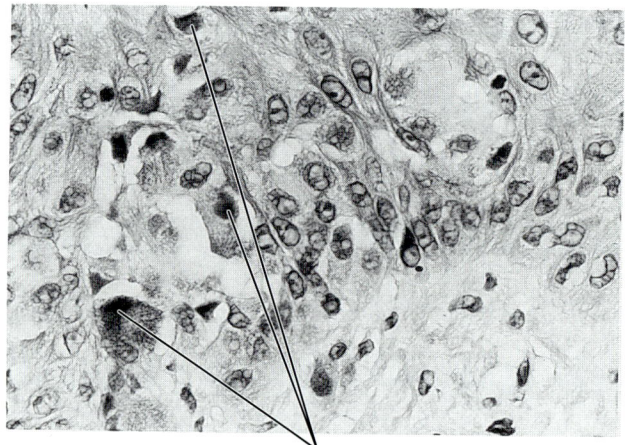

Atypical nuclei of melanocytes

Variation in staining of pleomorphic nuclei

Pleomorphic nuclei of melanocytes

68 • Melanoma

Criteria for diagnosis of this melanoma

This is a melanoma because:

1. The neoplasm is asymmetric, i.e., many more lymphocytes are present on the left of it.
2. Nests of melanocytes within the epidermis are not equidistant from one another.
3. Nests of melanocytes within the epidermis and the dermis have become confluent.
4. Confluence of nests of melanocytes within the upper part of the dermis has resulted in sheets of them.
5. Atypical nuclei are discernible.
6. Nuclear staining of melanocytes varies in intensity.

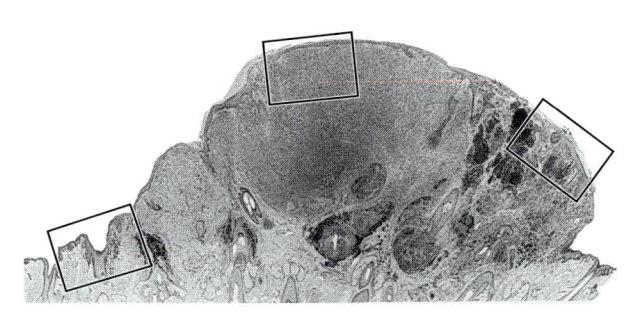

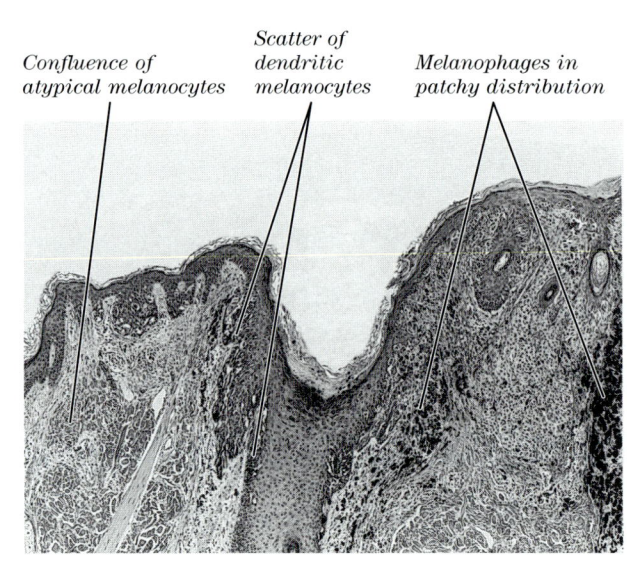
Confluence of atypical melanocytes — Scatter of dendritic melanocytes — Melanophages in patchy distribution

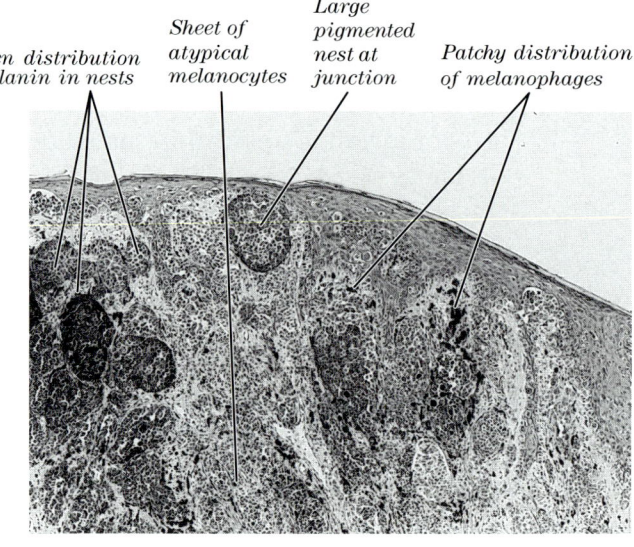
Sheet of atypical melanocytes

Uneven distribution of melanin in nests — Sheet of atypical melanocytes — Large pigmented nest at junction — Patchy distribution of melanophages

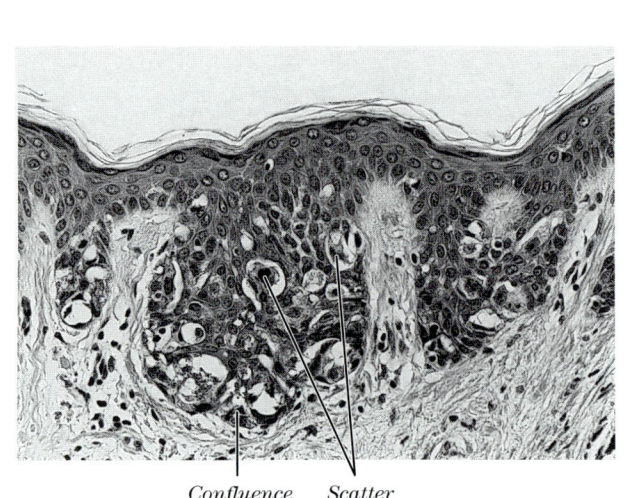
Confluence   Scatter

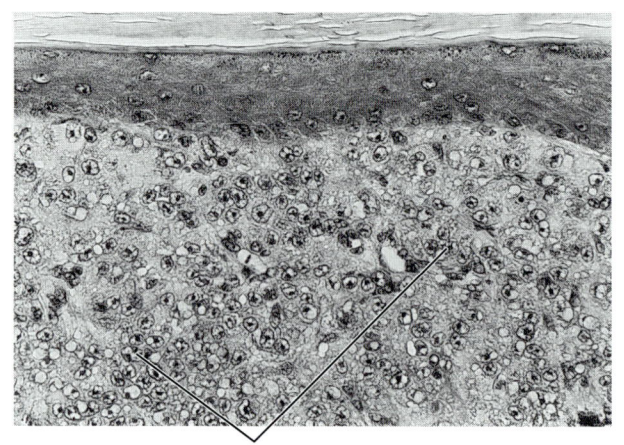
Sheet of atypical melanocytes

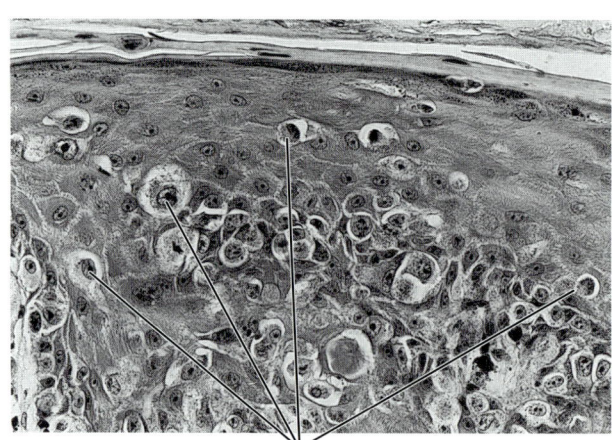
Scatter of atypical melanocytes

69 • Melanoma

Criteria for diagnosis of this melanoma

This is a melanoma because:

1. There is striking asymmetry.
2. The neoplasm is poorly circumscribed.
3. Melanin is not distributed in uniform fashion throughout the neoplasm.
4. Melanocytes do not mature.
5. Nests of melanocytes within the epidermis are not equidistant from one another.
6. Nests of melanocytes within the epidermis and the dermis vary in size and shape.
7. Nests of melanocytes within the epidermis and the dermis have become confluent and, in the dermis, have formed sheets.
8. Melanocytes arranged as solitary units and in nests are present at all levels of the epidermis and, in the same pattern, far down epithelial structures of adnexa.
9. Pagetoid melanocytes are disposed in pagetoid pattern.
10. There is striking nuclear atypia.
11. Many melanocytes are in mitosis.

IV. Melanoma in Association with a Nevus

It is difficult at times for a clinician to detect a melanoma in association with a nevus, and there are several reasons for that. By the time a patient has sought consultation for a melanoma that is a plaque, a nodule, or a tumor, it is likely that the melanomatous component of the neoplasm has overrun any pre-existing nevus and thereby either obscured the nevus or obliterated it. For another, melanomas often are variegate in their surface characteristics, outlines, and color, and a nevus caught up in such a melanoma would be mistaken clinically for part of the melanoma. Yet another reason for the difficulty experienced by clinicians in spotting a nevus in association with a melanoma is that the nevus usually is so small, only a few millimeters in diameter, in contrast to the melanoma which usually is considerably larger, and simply is dwarfed by the melanoma. A related pitfall in diagnosis is that a nevus, especially a tiny one, is banal morphologically, e.g., uniform in color and undramatic in other aspects, whereas a melanoma tends to be eye-catching because of its striking variegation in all respects. Last, with naked-eye examination alone, a rare Clark's nevus may be indistinguishable clinically from a melanoma, and when a melanoma is continuous with such a nevus, no clinical criteria are available currently that allow those two neoplasms to be differentiated from one another. Only in a meager minority of instances is a nevus in association with a melanoma recognized clinically prior to biopsy.

Less than 1.0% of nevi in which melanomas develop are congenital nevi, the vast majority of those being superficial (Fig. 70). A tiny fraction of 1.0% are deep congenital nevi (Fig. 71). Rare, too, is development of a melanoma in a pre-existing blue nevus. Except for an occasional Unna's or Miescher's nevus, the remainder of acquired nevi in which melanomas originate in Caucasians are Clark's nevi, most of which are compound (Fig. 72) or intradermal (Fig. 73), and only a few of which are junctional. Whether a melanoma arises de novo, in association with a pre-existing superficial congenital nevus, or in company with an acquired nevus, the sequential steps of melanoma are traced clinically and histopathologically in repeatable fashion, beginning with a tiny pigmented macule marked by proliferation of small melanocytes disposed as solitary units at the dermo-epidermal junction.

For a clinician to identify a Clark's nevus in continuity with a melanoma, criteria for diagnosis of both the benign and malignant neoplasms, and differentiation of them from one another, must be understood well. In short, Clark's nevi, the commonest type of nevus in man in our experience, are usually small, symmetric, well-circumscribed, relatively uniform in a shade of brown, flat or slightly elevated in their centers, and smooth-surfaced or gently mammillated. A tannish rim of variable breadth often surrounds the slightly elevated, darker central component. Uncommonly, Clark's nevi are mostly pink or black, and very uncommonly they are broad, i.e., greater than 1.0 cm in diameter and, exceedingly rarely, as great as several centimeters in diameter. When a flattish melanoma is juxtaposed to a conventional Clark's nevus, a diagnosis of melanoma in association with a nevus can be made clinically because the two neoplasms are so different. Distinction between the benign and malignant neoplasm cannot be accomplished, however, if a melanoma has destroyed a pre-existing nevus.

Problems posed by histopathologic diagnosis of a melanoma in company with a nevus are several. The most obvious arises when such a lesion is removed by shave or punch technique, and either the melanoma or, more often, the nevus has not been delivered in the biopsy specimen. An analogous pitfall in diagnosis occurs when, as a consequence of technical imprecision, a nevus is present in a biopsy specimen that consists mostly of melanoma, but sections cut from that specimen fail to include the melanoma. Another trap that a histopathologist must avoid in interpreting correctly a tiny nevus (particularly a Clark's nevus (Fig. 74), but also a small superficial congenital one) (Fig. 75) in association with a melanoma is failure to detect a few melanocytes of the nevus among the innumerable neoplastic melanocytes of the melanoma, especially a melanoma whose nuclei are small like those in the cells of the nevus. When a nevus is continuous with a melanoma, the transition between them may be so smooth that cytologic differences in the two neoplasms may not be recognizable (Table 5). Melanocytes of a melanoma may be misinterpreted histopathologically as those of a nevus in the uncommon circumstance where a melanoma demonstrates maturation of its melanocytes with progressive descent into the dermis. The melanocytes of the melanoma become smaller the further they descend and at the base of the neoplasm may resemble melanocytes of a nevus (Fig. 76). Sometimes a nevus is situated immediately beneath a melanoma, usually in a markedly thickened papillary dermis, and at the interface between the two neoplasms of melanocytes, melanocytes of the melanoma merge almost imperceptibly with those of the nevus. When that occurs, the nevus may be misread as melanoma that matured. Despite these caveats, in most instances a histopathologist should be able to differentiate cells of a nevus from cells of a melanoma if the criteria set forth here are utilized.

There is no compelling evidence that melanomas that arise in association with a nevus have a better prognosis than melanomas that originate de novo.

The association between nevi and melanomas is not fortuitous; the two neoplasms of melanocytes, one benign and the other malignant, are related to one another intimately in more than 20% of all melanomas that develop in Caucasians (but hardly every are they joined in melanomas that occur in Africans and Asians). Such is not the case with a variety of other incidental associations that involve nevi and melanomas, with the exception of follicular cysts that develop frequently in Miescher's nevi. These cysts tend to rupture with consequent suppurative, granulomatous, and fibrosing inflammation. Incidental inflammatory, neoplastic, hamartomatous, and "degenerative" diseases may be seen in sections from the same biopsy specimen as a nevus, a melanoma, or a melanoma in association with a nevus. A melanoma on skin injured severely by sunlight may be accompanied, in the same histopathologic section, by another neoplasm induced by sunlight such as a thin squamous-cell carcinoma like solar keratosis and Bowen's disease, a thicker squamous-cell carcinoma, including a keratoacanthomatous squamous-cell carcinoma, a basal-cell carcinoma, or a malignant fibrous histiocytoma. In brief, for practical purposes, the only repeatable association with melanoma is a nevus (and that linkage is observed in a decided minority of melanomas and a minuscule minority of nevi), but a host of coincidental pathologic processes appear episodically in specimens that harbor a nevus or a melanoma.

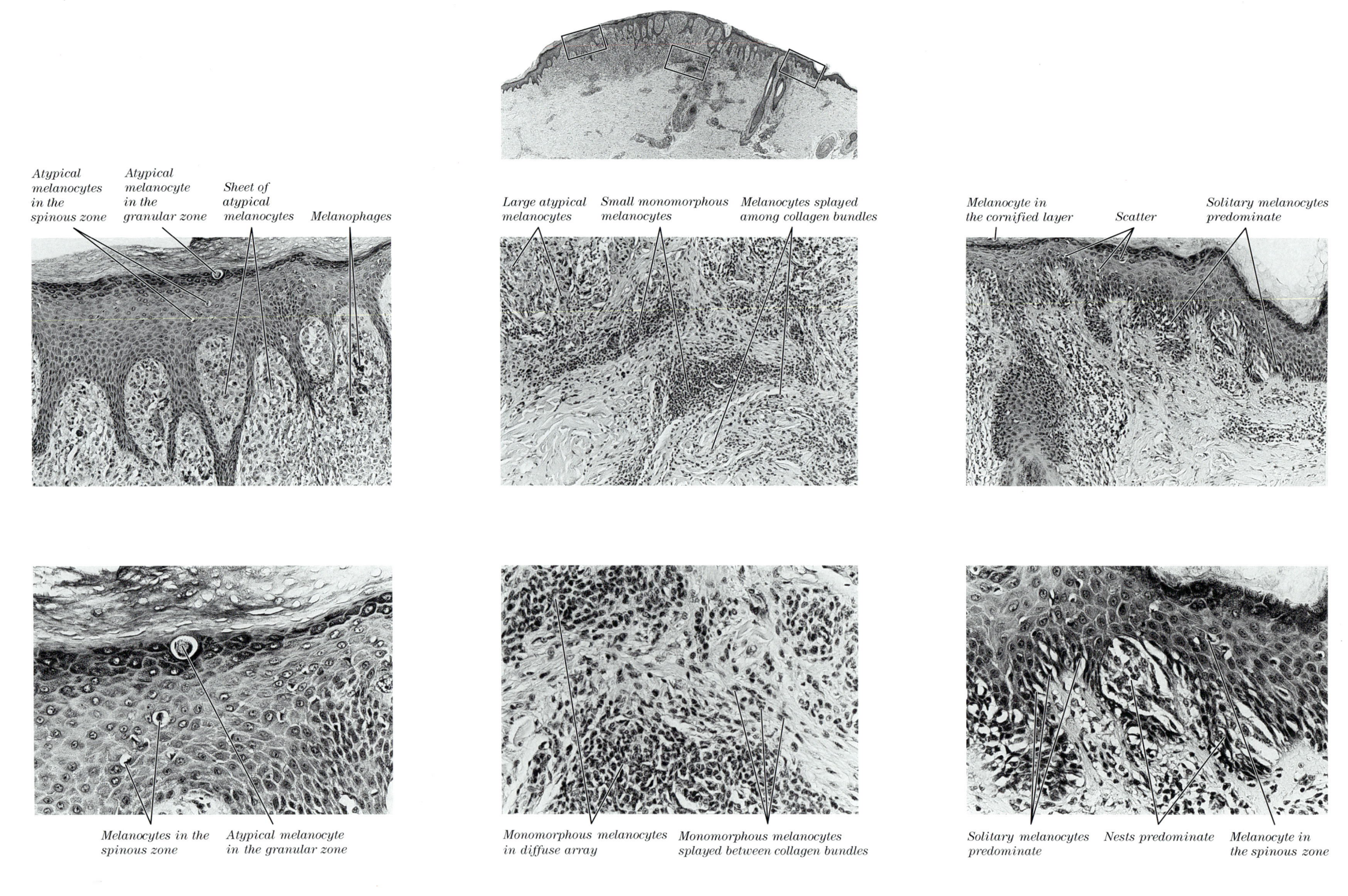

70 · **Melanoma and Congenital Nevus** *(superficial type)*

Criteria for diagnosis of this melanoma that began in association with a non-blue congenital nevus (superficial type)

The neoplasm that extends across the entire upper portion of this lesion is a melanoma because:

1. It is asymmetric.
2. It is poorly circumscribed.
3. Nests of melanocytes within the epidermis are not equidistant from one another.
4. Melanocytes arranged as solitary units predominate over nests of melanocytes within the epidermis in some high-power fields.
5. Melanocytes within epithelial structures of adnexa are disposed in the same pattern as within the epidermis.
6. Melanocytes are scattered at all levels of the epidermis, including the granular zone and the cornified layer.
7. Melanocytes within the dermis have become confluent and thereby formed sheets.
8. There is no maturation of melanocytes.
9. Nuclei of melanocytes are atypical.

The remainder of the lesion is an intradermal nevus because:

1. Melanocytes within the dermis have small, plump oval, monomorphous nuclei.
2. Melanocytes do not exhibit nuclear atypia.

The nevus is a superficial congenital one because:

1. Nearly all of the melanocytes of the nevus are present above the mid-reticular dermis.
2. Melanocytes are splayed between collagen bundles in foci within the reticular dermis.
3. The apparent linearity of melanocytes within the reticular dermis is a consequence of angiocentricity and eccrocentricity.

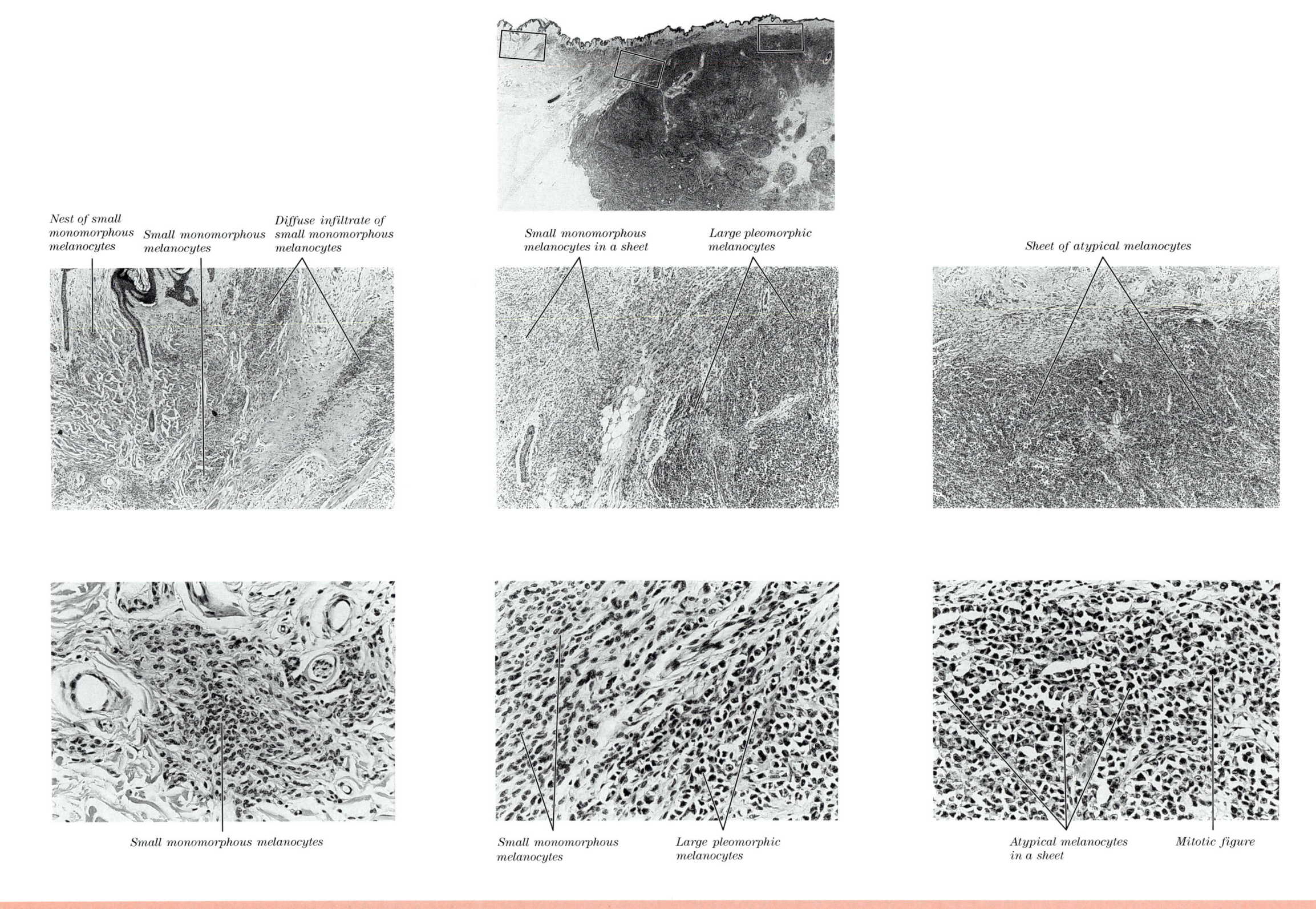

71 • Melanoma and Congenital Nevus (deep type)

Criteria for diagnosis of this melanoma that arose in a pre-existing non-blue congenital nevus (deep type)

This is a melanoma in the center and on the right because:

1. Nodules of different sizes and shapes are present throughout the dermis and far into the subcutaneous fat.
2. The nodules consist of atypical melanocytes that are in striking contrast to the melanocytes of the congenital nevus on the left.
3. Many melanocytes are in mitosis and some of them are abnormal.

This is a pre-existing deep congenital nevus because:

Throughout the reticular dermis and far into septa of the subcutaneous fat are monomorphous melanocytes distributed diffusely.

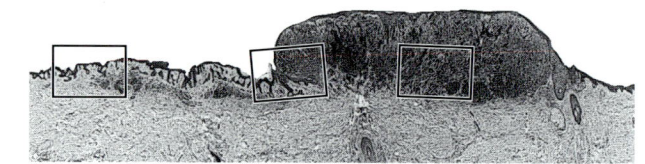

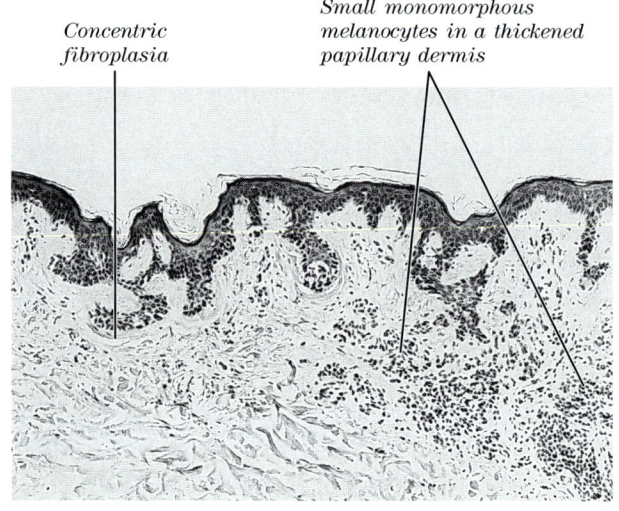

Concentric fibroplasia · Small monomorphous melanocytes in a thickened papillary dermis

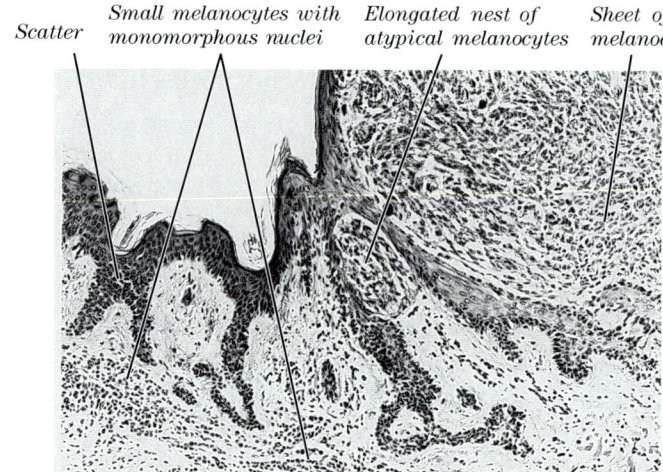

Scatter · Small melanocytes with monomorphous nuclei · Elongated nest of atypical melanocytes · Sheet of atypical melanocytes

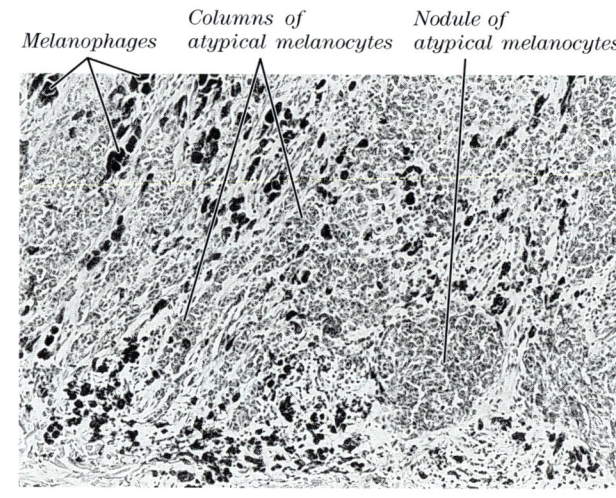

Melanophages · Columns of atypical melanocytes · Nodule of atypical melanocytes

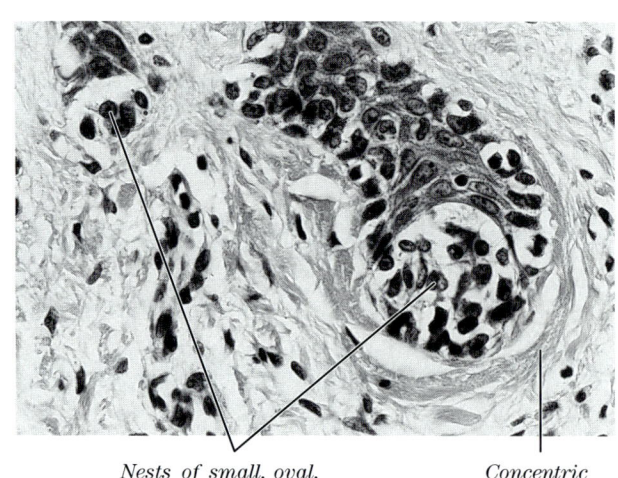

Nests of small, oval, monomorphous melanocytes · Concentric fibroplasia

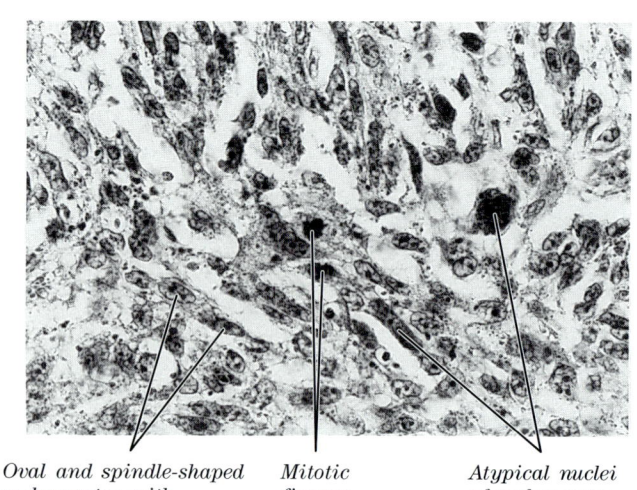

Oval and spindle-shaped melanocytes with pleomorphic nuclei · Mitotic figures · Atypical nuclei of melanocytes

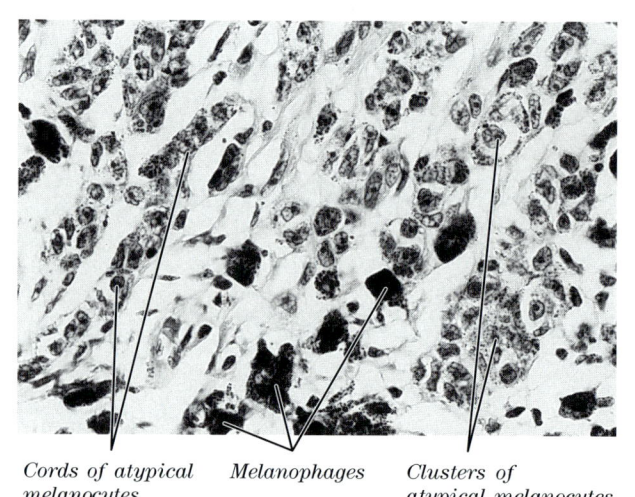

Cords of atypical melanocytes · Melanophages · Clusters of atypical melanocytes

72 · Melanoma and Clark's Nevus

Criteria for diagnosis of this melanoma in association with a Clark's nevus (compound type)

On the right side is a melanoma because:

1. It is asymmetric.
2. It is poorly circumscribed.
3. Melanocytes are scattered as solitary units within the epidermis.
4. Neoplastic cells are arranged in sheets.
5. The base of the neoplasm is not flat.
6. Melanocytes do not mature.
7. Melanocytes have atypical nuclei.
8. Many melanocytes are in mitosis.

On the left side is a Clark's nevus because:

1. It is slightly elevated and gently mammillated.
2. The melanocytic component is confined to the dermo-epidermal junction and papillary dermis.
3. The melanocytes are small, oval, and monomorphous.
4. There are no mitotic figures.

   The different patterns of the melanoma and the nevus are apparent at scanning magnification. One important difference between them is the distribution of melanin: it is abundant in the melanoma and scant in the nevus.

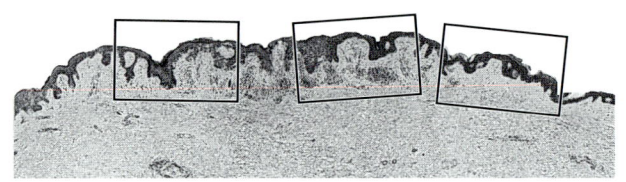

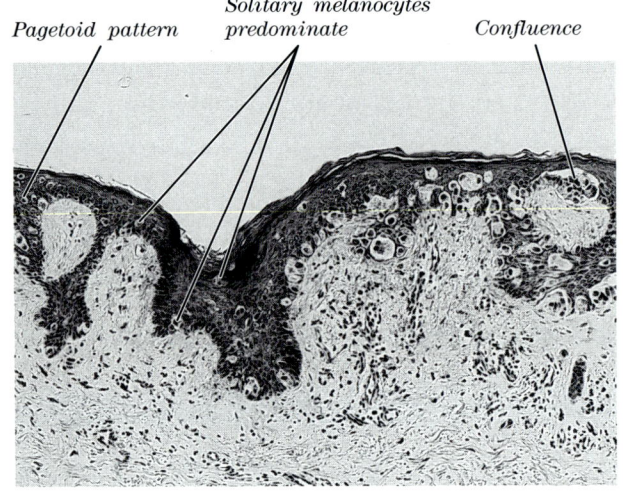

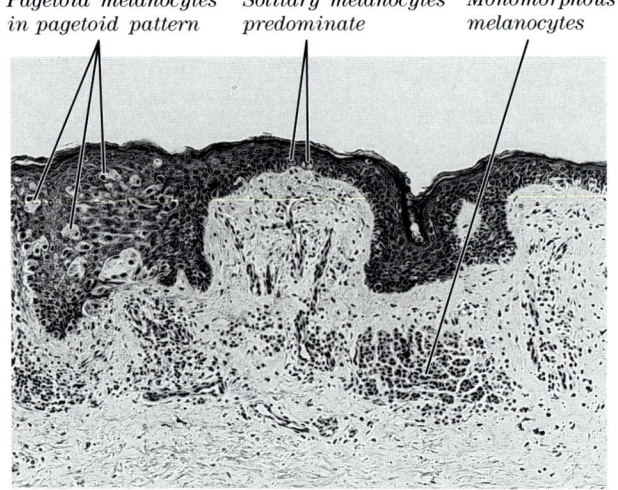

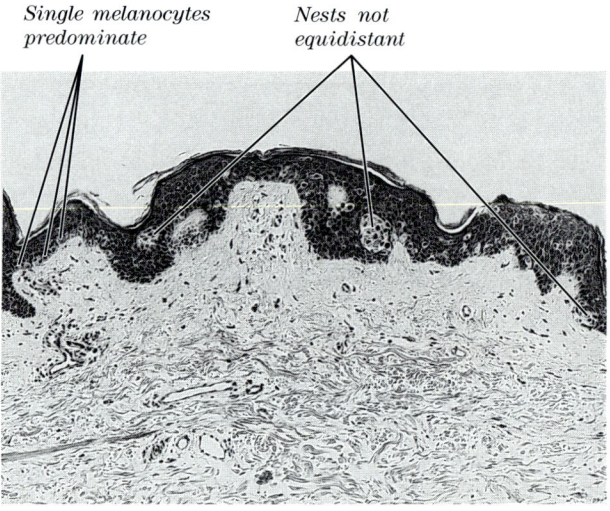

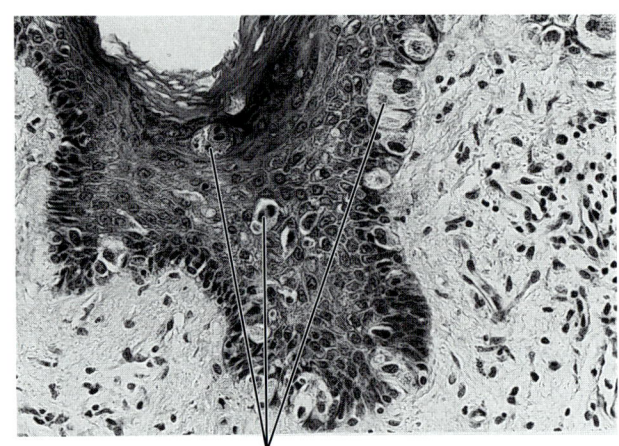

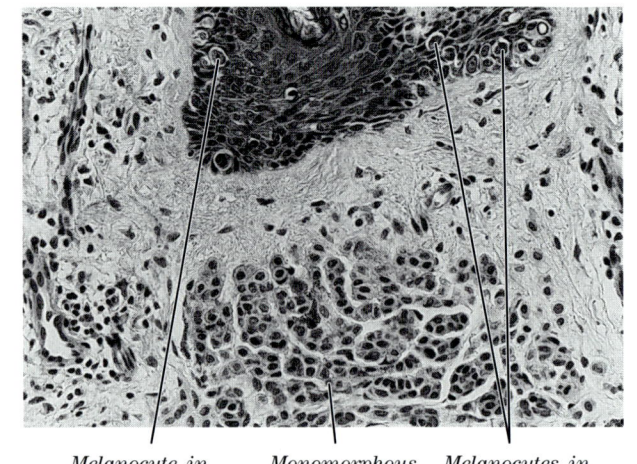

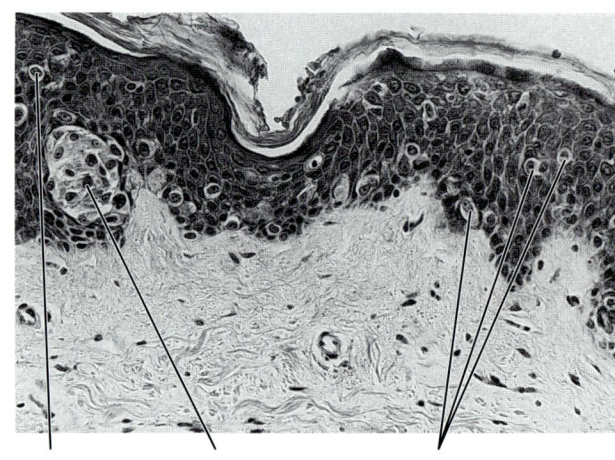

73 • Melanoma and Clark's Nevus

Criteria for diagnosis of this melanoma in association with a Clark's nevus (intradermal type)

This is a melanoma because:

1. The neoplasm is poorly circumscribed.

2. Atypical pagetoid melanocytes in pagetoid pattern are present within the surface and adnexal epithelia.

3. Melanocytes within the epidermis arranged as solitary units predominate over nests of melanocytes in some high-power fields.

4. Nests of melanocytes are not equidistant from one another.

5. Nests of melanocytes vary in size and shape.

6. Epithelial structures of adnexa are involved by the proliferation of melanocytes in the same fashion as is the epidermis.

7. Nuclei of melanocytes are atypical.

The intradermal nevus is of Clark's type because:

The melanocytes of the nevus are confined to a thickened papillary dermis, but one that is much less exophytic than an Unna's nevus.

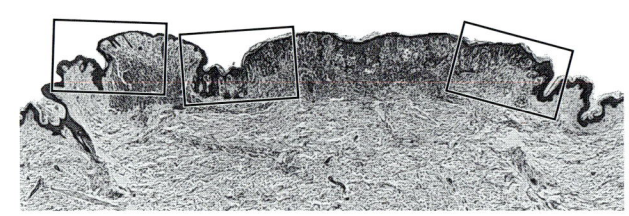

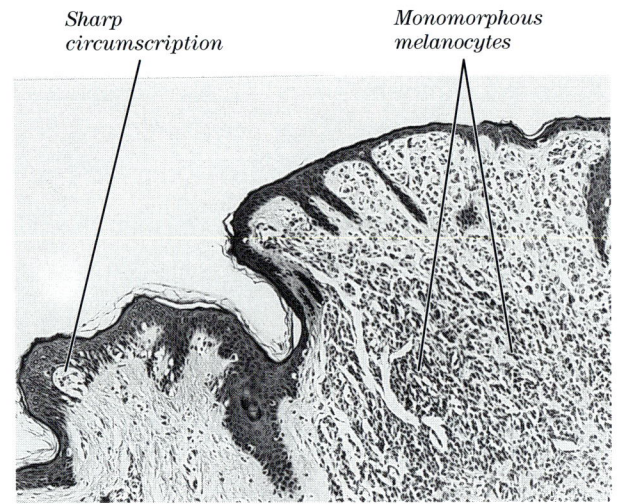
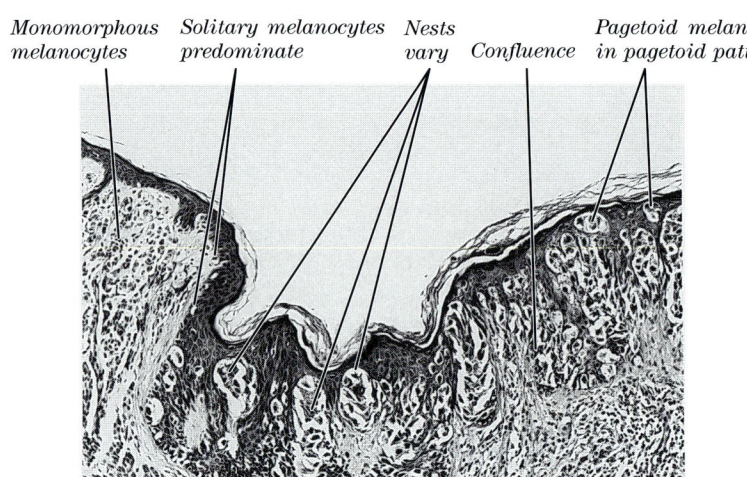
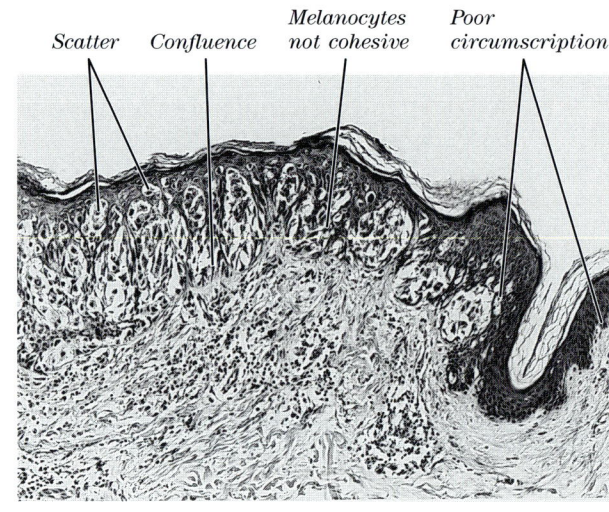

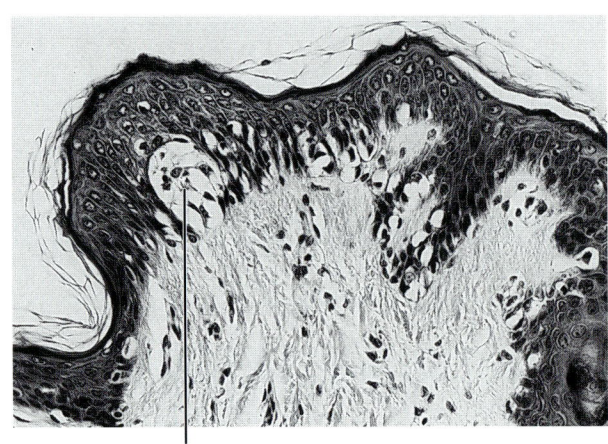
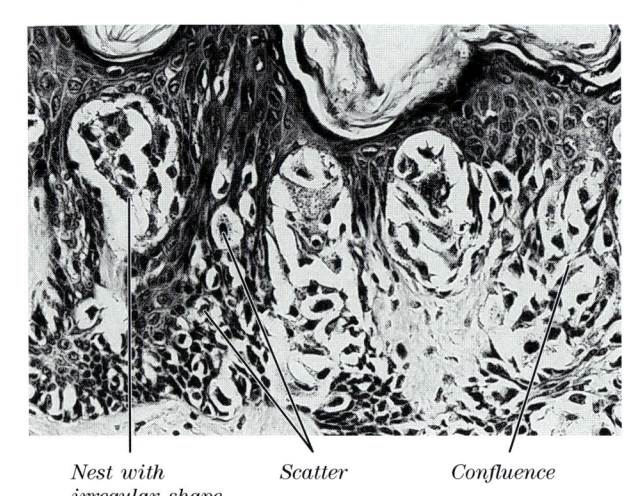
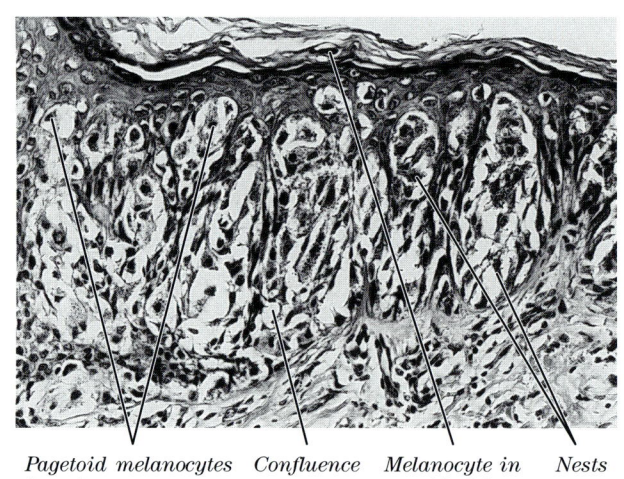

74 • Melanoma and Clark's Nevus

Criteria for diagnosis of this melanoma in situ in association with a Clark's nevus (compound type)

The lesion in the center and on the right is a melanoma in situ because:

1. Atypical melanocytes, arranged as solitary units and in nests, are scattered at all levels of the epidermis.
2. Nests of melanocytes are not equidistant from one another.
3. Nests of melanocytes have become confluent.
4. Some aggregations of melanocytes have jagged peripheries.
5. Many melanocytes are pagetoid and arrayed in pagetoid pattern.

The lesion on the left is a Clark's nevus because:

1. Melanocytes are confined almost entirely to the dermo-epidermal junction and thickened papillary dermis.
2. The surface of the lesion is mammillated.
3. The junctional component of the nevus extends beyond the intradermal component.
4. Nuclei are small, oval, and monomorphous.

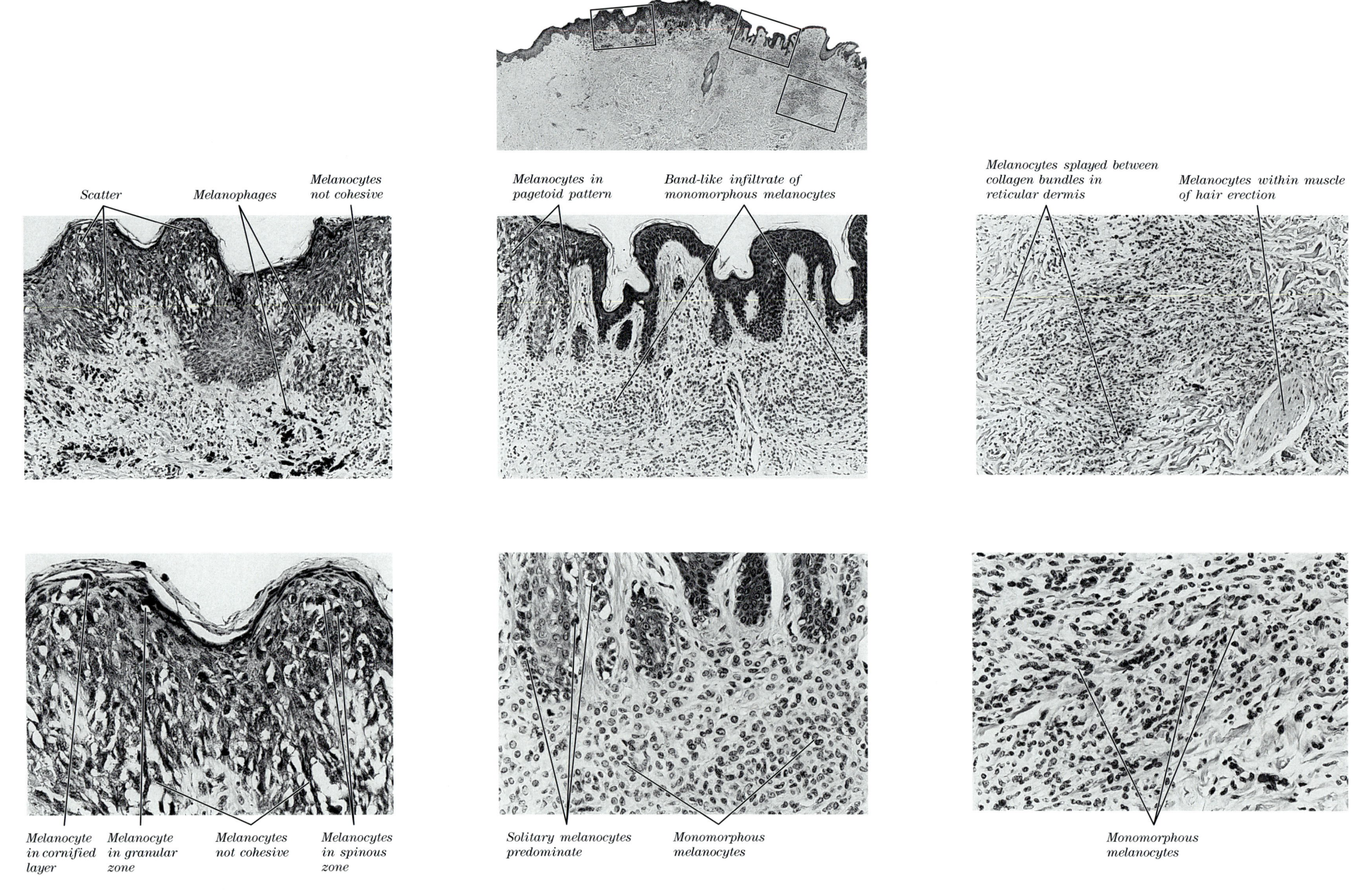

75 • Melanoma and Congenital Nevus *(superficial type)*

Criteria for diagnosis of this melanoma in situ in association with a non-blue congenital nevus (superficial type)

This is a melanoma in situ because:

1. Melanocytes arranged as solitary units, many of them dendritic, are scattered far above the dermo-epidermal junction, including the granular zone and cornified layer.

2. Melanin is not distributed in uniform fashion within the epidermal neoplasm or in melanophages within the dermis.

3. Nests of melanocytes within the epidermis are not equidistant from one another.

This is a superficial congenital nevus because:

1. Melanocytes are arranged in band-like fashion in the upper part of the dermis.

2. Melanocytes are arrayed in angiocentric and adnexocentric fashion in the upper part of the reticular dermis.

3. Melanocytes are splayed between collagen bundles in foci in the upper half of the reticular dermis.

4. Some melanocytes are present within smooth muscles of hair erection.

5. Melanocytes within the epidermis are disposed as solitary units and in nests at the dermo-epidermal junction only, and not above it.

  In addition to the criteria for differentiation of the melanoma and the nevus already mentioned, the two neoplasms that are housed in this section can be distinguished by the distribution of melanin: the melanoma is pigmented strikingly; the nevus is not.

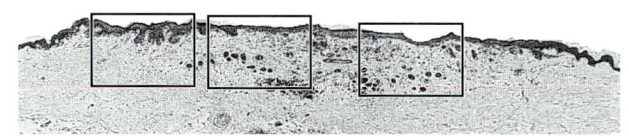

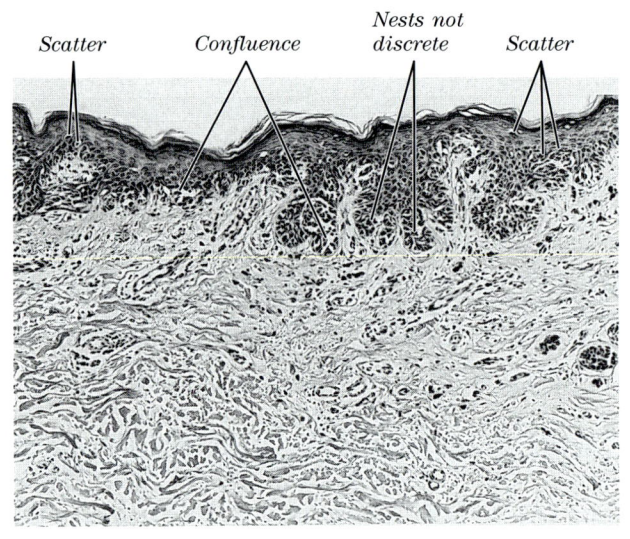

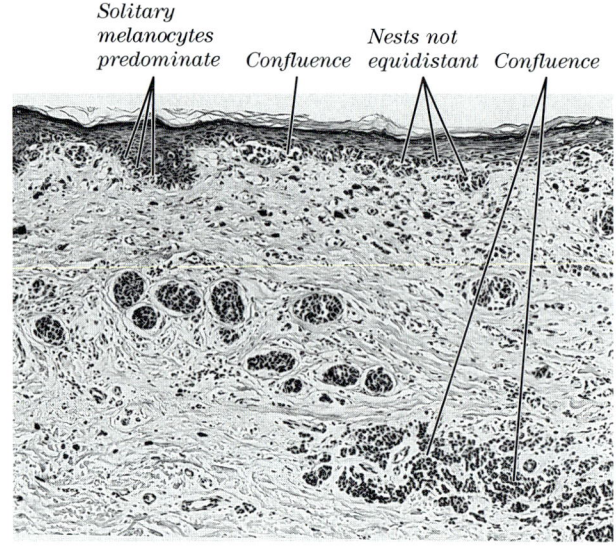

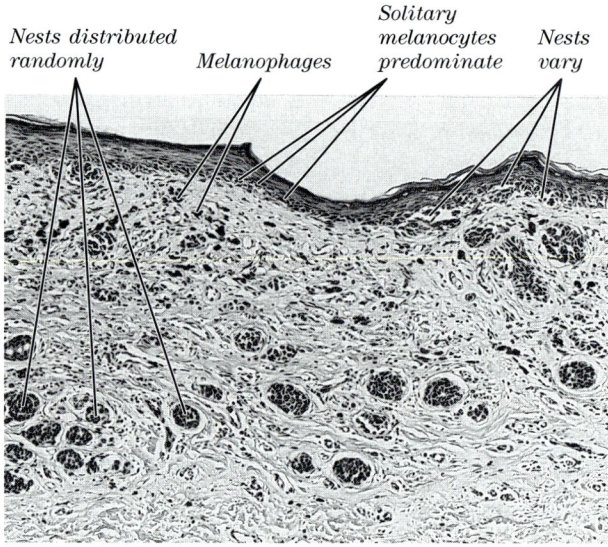

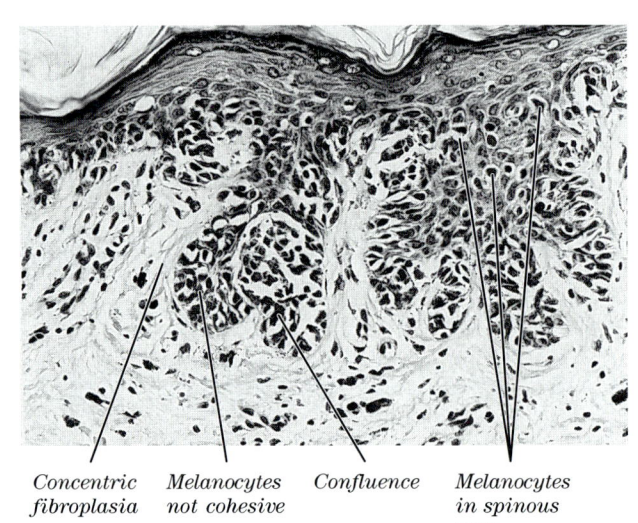

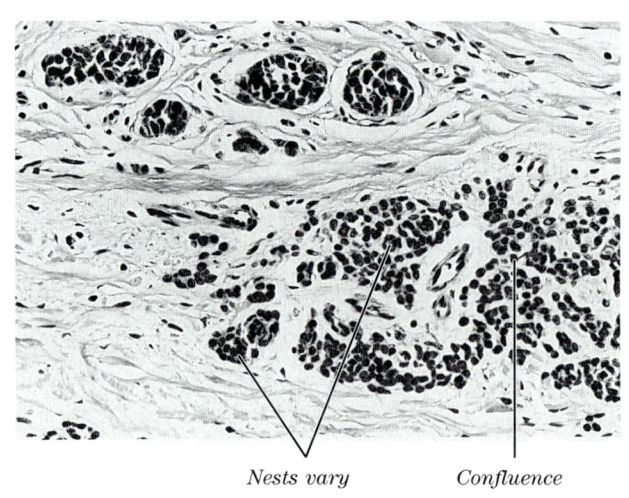

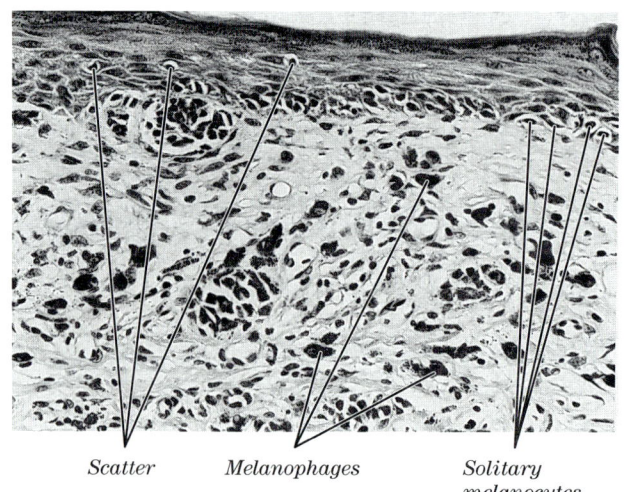

76 • Melanoma

Criteria for diagnosis of this melanoma

This is a melanoma because:

1. The neoplasm is asymmetric.
2. It is poorly circumscribed.
3. Nests of melanocytes within the epidermis are not equidistant from one another.
4. Nests of melanocytes vary in size and shape.
5. Some nests of melanocytes within the epidermis have become confluent.
6. Melanocytes within the epidermis arranged as solitary units predominate over nests of melanocytes in some high-power fields.
7. Melanocytes arrayed as solitary units and in small nests are scattered far above the dermo-epidermal junction.
8. Nests of melanocytes at the base of the neoplasm have irregular shapes and have become confluent.
9. Nuclei of some neoplastic melanocytes are atypical.

V. Regression of Melanoma

Regression of primary melanoma is a phenomenon that involves the superficial vascular plexus, a thickened papillary dermis, and the epidermis. Requirements for induction of regression are (1) neoplastic melanocytes of melanoma in the epidermis and papillary dermis, and (2) lymphocytic infiltrates around the vessels of the superficial plexus, in lichenoid array within the melanomatous component of the papillary dermis, and scattered among neoplastic melanocytes of melanoma within the epidermis (Fig. 77). In brief, cytotoxic products of lymphocytes kill neoplastic cells of melanoma situated in the papillary dermis and epidermis. Rarely, all of the cells of the melanoma in the epidermis are destroyed by the effects of lymphocytes, a condition termed "complete regression" of melanoma (Fig. 78). Often, all of the neoplastic melanocytes of melanoma in a discrete focus of the papillary dermis and epidermis are obliterated by the action of lymphocytes, a circumstance designated "focal regression" of melanoma (Fig. 79). Episodically, neoplastic cells of a melanoma are eliminated partially in the papillary dermis and in the epidermis or entirely in the papillary dermis and not at all in the epidermis, a phenomenon known as "partial regression" (Fig. 80).

Morphologically, the effects of the battle between lymphocytes and neoplastic melanocytes of melanoma express themselves in three fashions: fibrosis, melanosis, and a combination of fibrosis and melanosis. These descriptive terms, i.e., fibrosis and melanosis, apply to residual changes of complete and focal regression of primary melanoma in a thickened papillary dermis beneath an epidermis whose normal undulations have been muted or effaced. Fibrosis refers to fibroplasia, usually of delicate fibrillary bundles of collagen, in a thickened papillary dermis. Sometimes the papillary dermis may be more than five times its normal thickness and measures more than 1.0 mm as a consequence of formation of new collagen by fibrocytes. Fibrosis often is accompanied by diffuse deposits of mucin, sparse lymphocytic infiltrates, variable numbers of melanophages, i.e., from practically none to many, and telangiectases. In contrast, melanosis denotes a dense band of melanophages in a papillary dermis that may be as thickened by macrophages as it may be by fibroplasia (Fig. 81). The epidermis above a zone of melanosis also shows diminution in the normal pattern of rete ridges and dermal papillae. In some specimens, sections exhibit features of both fibrosis and melanosis in the same thickened papillary dermis. In those cases, fibrosis tends to be present in the upper part of the expanded papillary dermis and melanosis in the lower part. When melanosis is noted, a diagnosis of regression of melanoma may be issued without equivocation. The findings of melanosis are specific. That is not the case for fibrosis in regression of melanoma. Changes indistinguishable from it may be found in regression of lichen planus-like keratosis, a solar lentigo-reticulated seborrheic keratosis that attracts lichenoid infiltrates of lymphocytes to it and is subsequently destroyed by them. Even the numerous necrotic keratinocytes so often observed in the epidermis and papillary dermis of a regressing lichen planus-like keratosis may be noted in some lesions of melanoma undergoing regression by fibrosis. Regression of "halo" nevus as a result of the effects of lymphocytes on melanocytes also takes the form of fibroplasia, but never of melanosis. A "halo" nevus that has regressed completely can be distinguished, usually, at scanning magnification from a melanoma that has regressed completely by fibrosis: the two have different silhouettes. In most instances, a regressed "halo" nevus has the silhouette of a Clark's nevus, i.e., it is small, symmetric, and slightly domed, whereas a melanoma usually is broader, asymmetric, and flattish.

What is the significance of regression of primary melanoma? Complete regression of melanoma, in our experience, is synonymous with the existence of metastases from that primary melanoma. As we conceive it, prior metastasis to a regional lymph node is mandatory for occurrence of complete regression of primary melanoma. Sensitized lymphocytes return from the involved node to the skin where they "home in" on the melanoma and destroy it. Different authors have different interpretations concerning the significance of focal regression of primary melanoma. Some aver that it is a good prognostic sign, whereas others claim that it has no prognostic significance. We are not certain of the meaning of focal regression of primary melanoma, biologically, but we infer that if complete regression signifies a grave prognosis, focal regression probably does not herald a good one.

Last, there is the subject of regression of metastasis of melanoma to skin. That phenomenon is seen rarely, but when it is encountered, the setting tends to be a satellite metastasis in the same histopathologic section as a primary melanoma. When melanophages in discrete collections marked by jagged outlines are discerned in foci within the reticular dermis and even within the subcutaneous fat, the diagnosis is melanosis as a consequence of regression of a metastasis of melanoma.

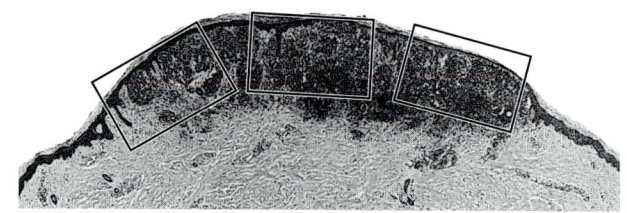

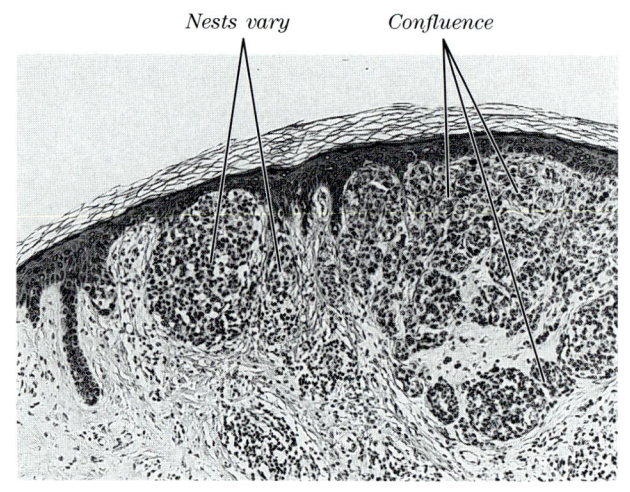
Nests vary   *Confluence*

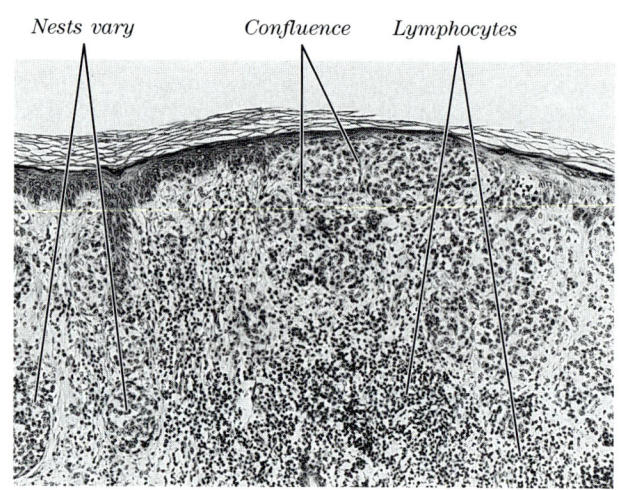
Nests vary   *Confluence*   *Lymphocytes*

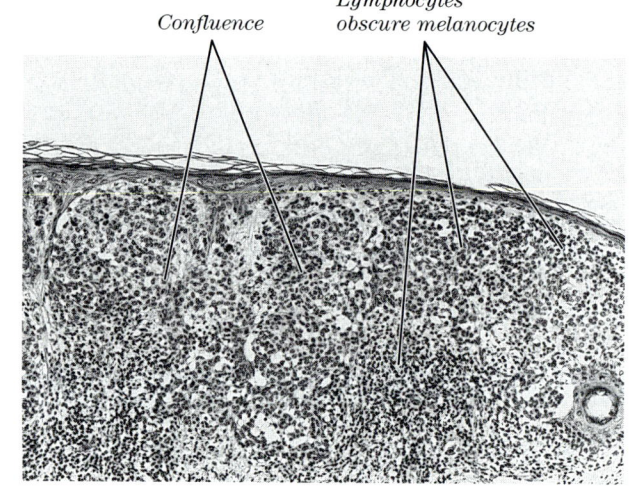
Confluence   *Lymphocytes obscure melanocytes*

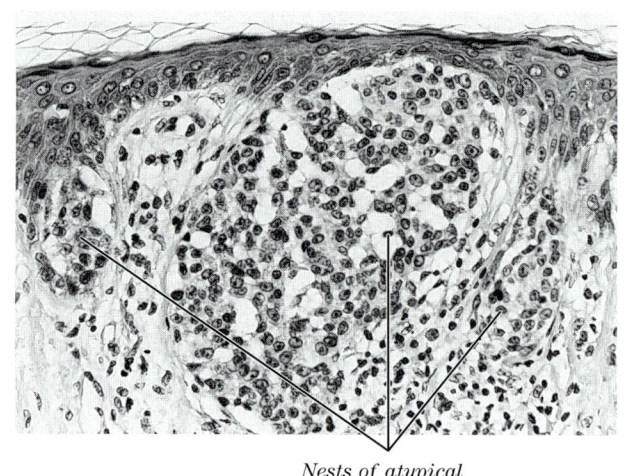
Nests of atypical melanocytes vary

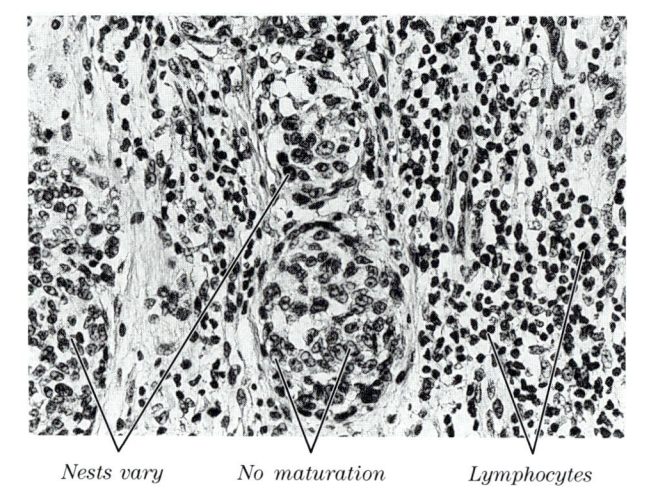
Nests vary   *No maturation*   *Lymphocytes*

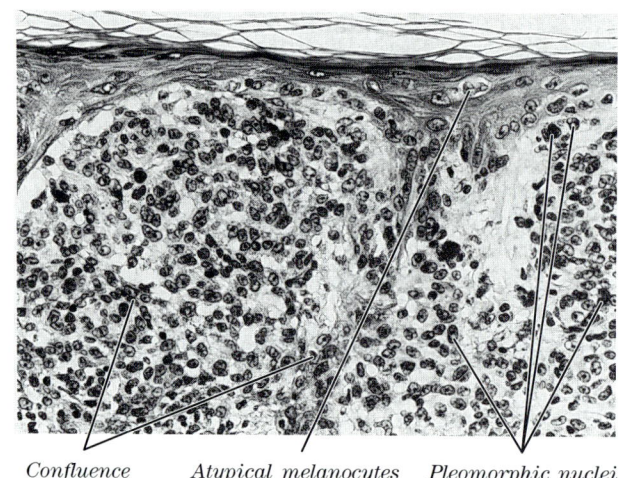
Confluence   *Atypical melanocytes above junction*   *Pleomorphic nuclei of melanocytes*

77 • Melanoma

Criteria for diagnosis of this melanoma

This is a melanoma because:

1. It is asymmetric.

2. Nests of melanocytes within the epidermis are not equidistant from one another.

3. Nests of melanocytes within the epidermis and the dermis vary in size and shape.

4. Nests of melanocytes within the epidermis and the dermis have become confluent.

5. Some melanocytes within the epidermis are present far above the dermo-epidermal junction.

6. Melanocytes do not mature.

7. Lymphocytes are not distributed in symmetric fashion, i.e., they are much more numerous on the right side of the neoplasm than on the left.

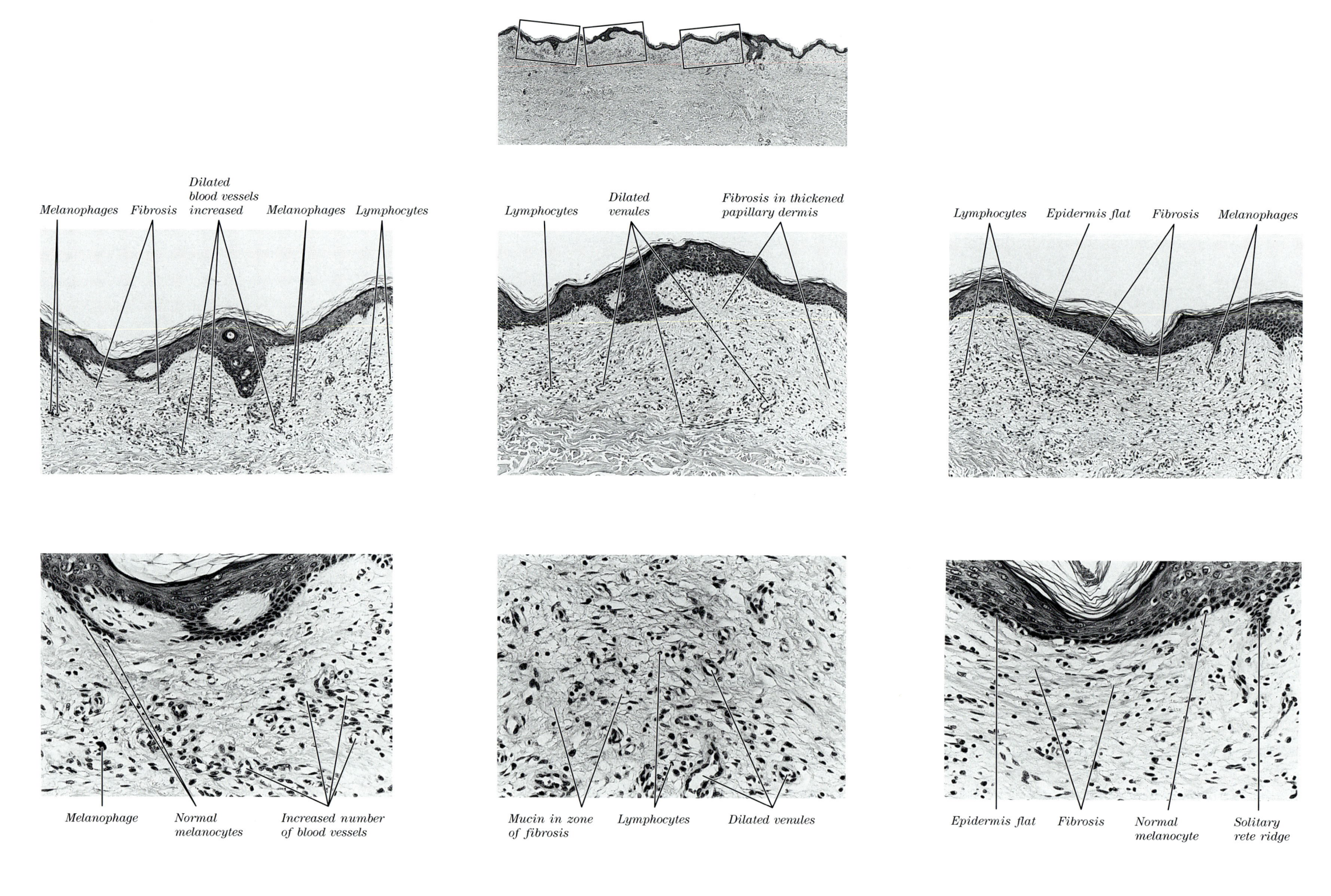

78 • Melanoma *(with complete regression by fibrosis)*

Criteria for diagnosis of complete regression of this melanoma

Signs of complete regression of melanoma at this site are:

1. Across the entire section, the papillary dermis is thickened extensively by fibroplasia in concert with telangiectases, a sprinkling of lymphocytes, and a few melanophages.

2. The normal pattern of undulations between rete ridges and dermal papillae is altered; rete ridges in many foci have been obliterated.

3. The only melanocytes that remain within the epidermis are normal melanocytes situated at the dermo-epidermal junction.

4. The reticular dermis is unaffected.

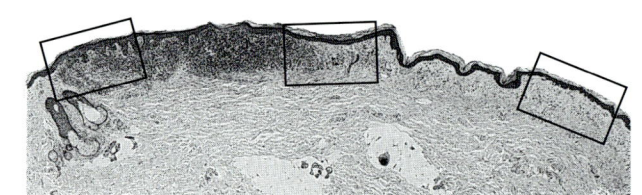

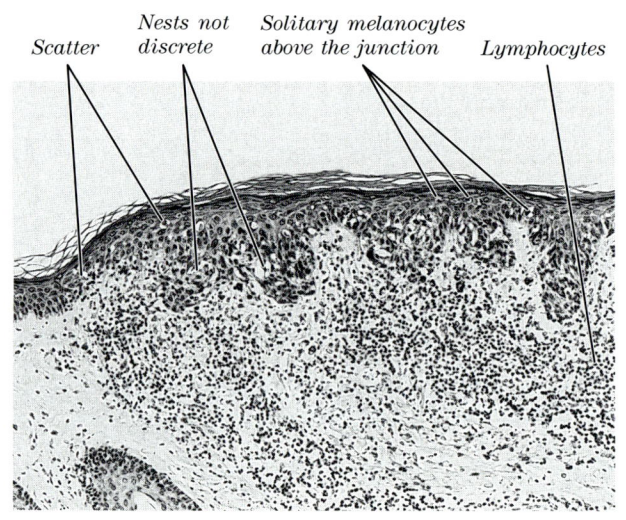

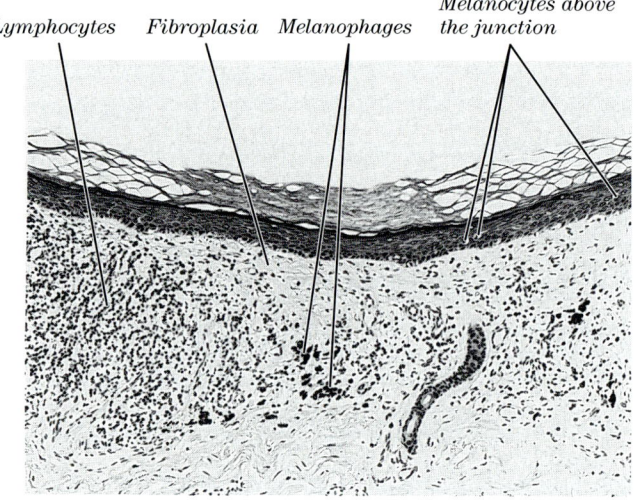

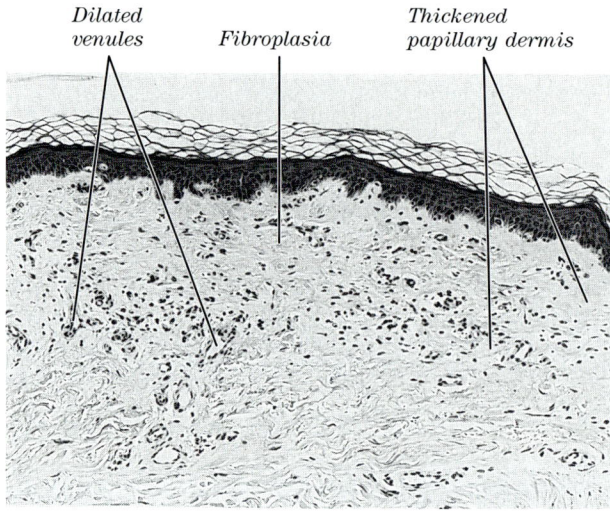

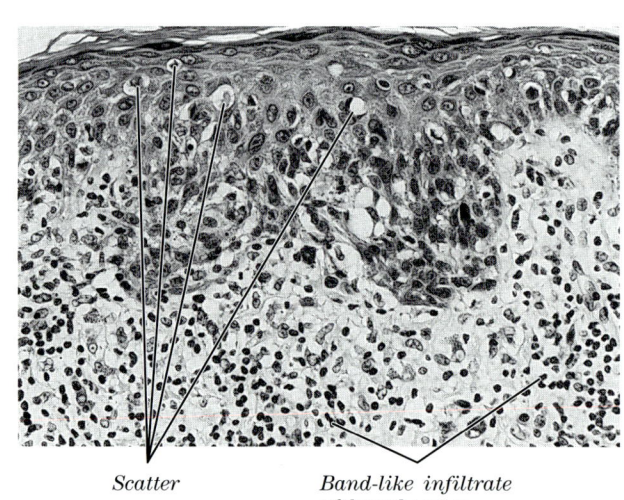

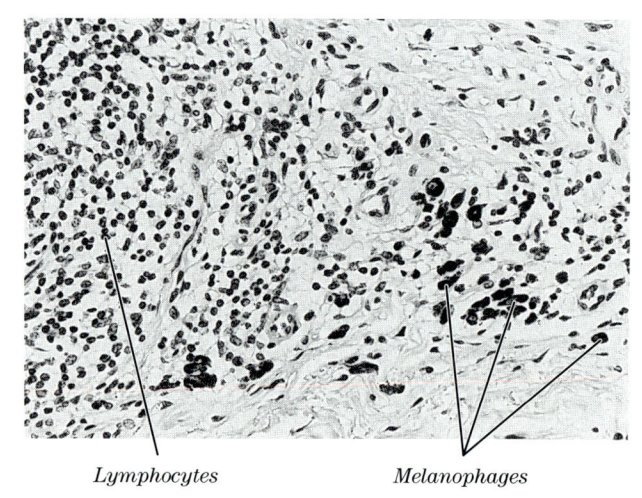

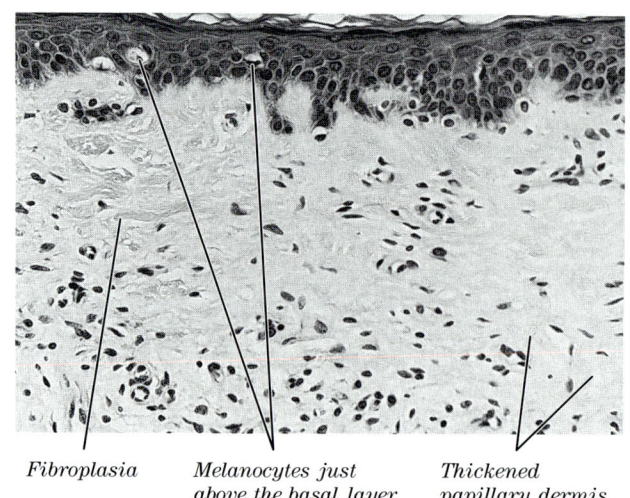

79 • Melanoma *(with focal regression by fibrosis)*

Criteria for diagnosis of focal regression of this melanoma

This is a melanoma because:

1. Nests of melanocytes within the epidermis are not equidistant from one another.
2. Nests of melanocytes vary in size and shape.
3. Some nests of melanocytes within the epidermis are not discrete.
4. Some melanocytes arranged as solitary units are present within the spinous zone.
5. Some nuclei of melanocytes within the epidermis are atypical.
6. A few atypical melanocytes may be present in the patchy lichenoid infiltrate of lymphocytes.

This is focal regression of melanoma because:

1. The papillary dermis, in foci, is thickened markedly by fibroplasia; the fibroplasia does not extend across the entire front of the lesion.
2. Within the thickened fibrotic papillary dermis there are telangiectases, melanophages, and a sprinkling of lymphocytes.
3. The epidermis above the zone of fibrosis is thinned and devoid of the usual undulating pattern between rete ridges and dermal papillae.
4. No nests of melanocytes are found within the epidermis, and only a few individual melanocytes are present above the dermo-epidermal junction, and they are not diagnostic of melanoma in situ.

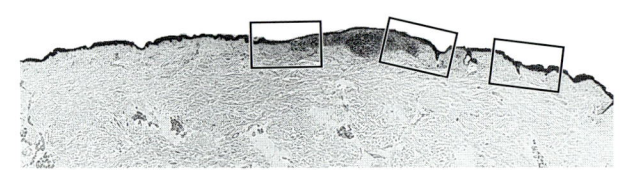

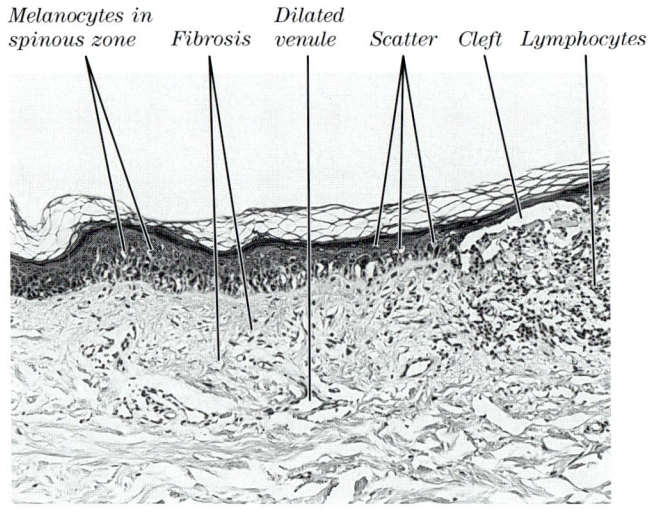

Melanocytes in spinous zone | Fibrosis | Dilated venule | Scatter | Cleft | Lymphocytes

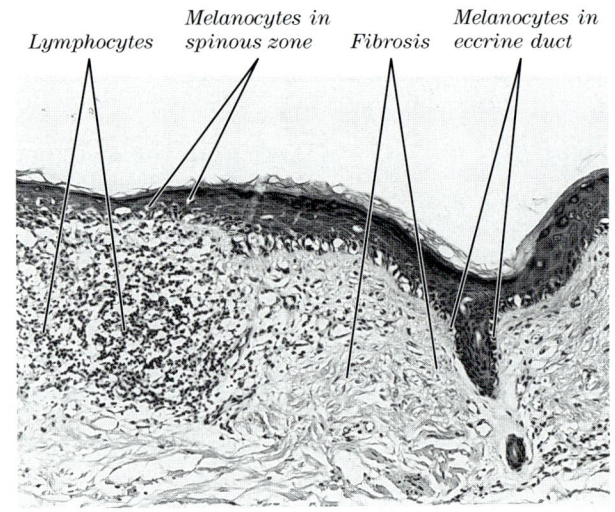

Lymphocytes | Melanocytes in spinous zone | Fibrosis | Melanocytes in eccrine duct

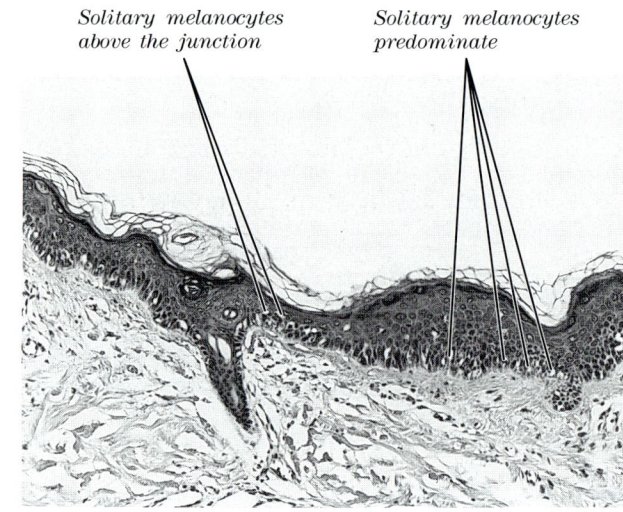

Solitary melanocytes above the junction | Solitary melanocytes predominate

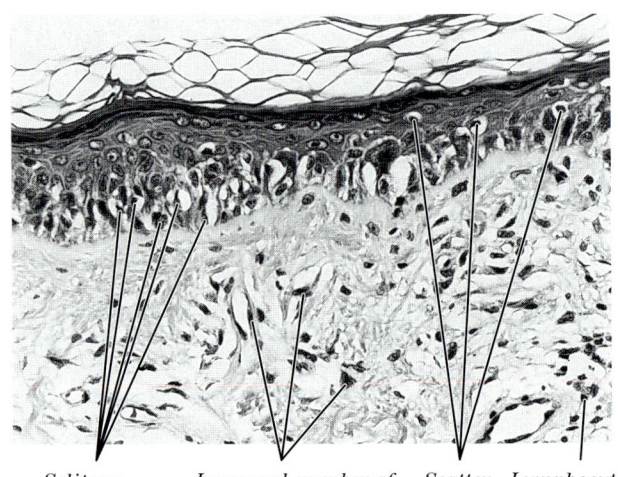

Solitary melanocytes predominate | Increased number of fibrocytes in zone of fibroplasia | Scatter | Lymphocytes

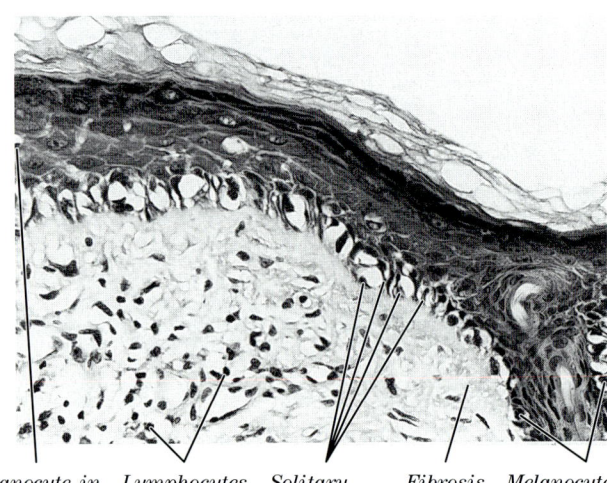

Melanocyte in spinous zone | Lymphocytes | Solitary melanocytes predominate | Fibrosis | Melanocytes along acrosyringium

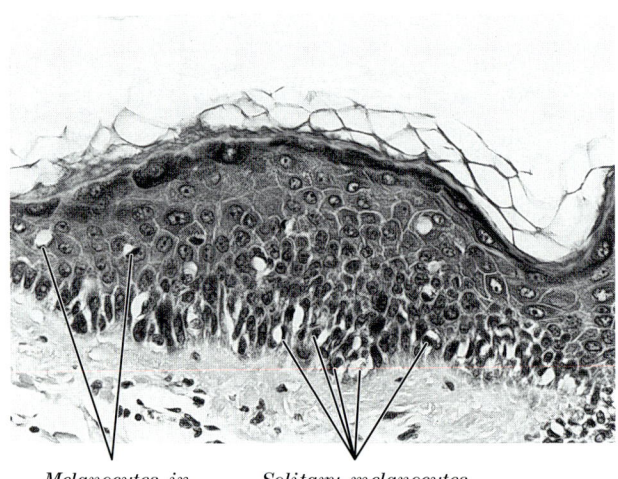

Melanocytes in spinous zone | Solitary melanocytes predominate

80 • Melanoma in situ *(with partial regression by fibrosis)*

Criteria for diagnosis of partial regression of this melanoma in situ

This is a melanoma in situ because:

1. The neoplasm is not symmetric.
2. The neoplasm is poorly circumscribed.
3. Melanocytes arranged as solitary units predominate over melanocytes arranged in nests in many high-power fields.
4. Melanocytes disposed as solitary units are not equidistant from one another.
5. Many melanocytes arrayed as solitary units are present far above the dermo-epidermal junction.
6. Nests of melanocytes are not equidistant from one another.
7. Nests of melanocytes vary in size and shape.
8. Melanocytes organized as solitary units extend far down epithelial structures of adnexa.
9. Nuclei of melanocytes are atypical.

The signs of partial regression in this melanoma are:

1. The papillary dermis, in some foci, is thickened markedly by fibroplasia, in association with telangiectases, melanophages, and a patchy lymphocytic infiltrate.
2. Signs of melanoma in situ are apparent above the zone of fibroplasia.

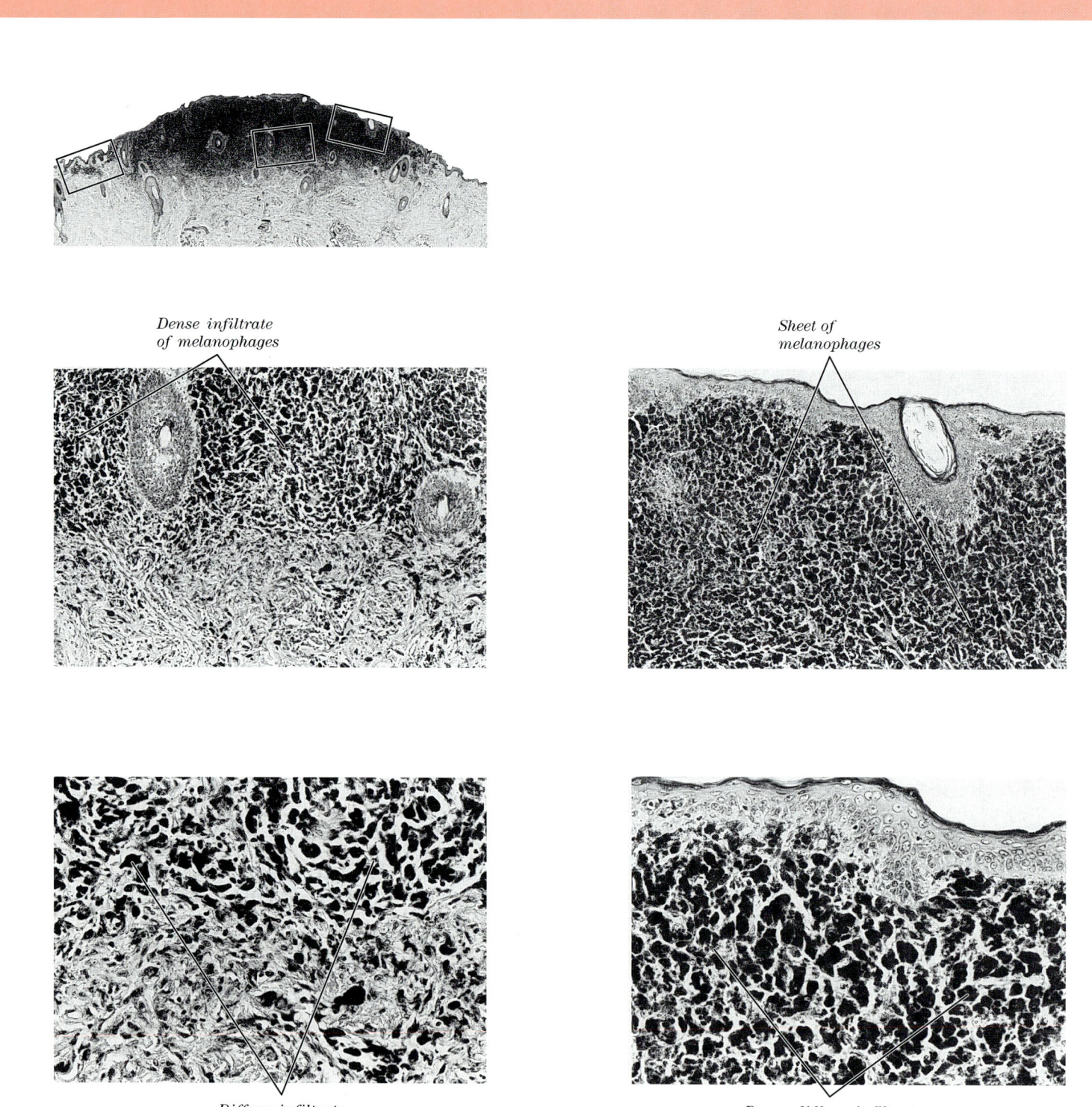

81 • Melanoma *(with complete regression by melanosis)*

Criteria for diagnosis of complete regression of this melanoma

This melanoma has regressed completely because:

1. There is a broad, band-like zone of melanophages in a dome-shaped, markedly thickened papillary dermis (and in the uppermost part of the reticular dermis), i.e., melanosis.

2. There are no signs of melanoma in situ in the form of atypical melanocytes arranged as solitary units and/or in nests within the neoplasm.

VI. Metastases of Melanoma to Skin

In a particular histopathologic section, a metastasis of melanoma to the skin may comprise a single focus of neoplastic melanocytes or of numerous foci of them, be confined to the dermis immediately beneath the epidermis (Fig. 82) or to the subcutaneous fat, or be present at both sites (Fig. 83) and be positioned in the upper part of the dermis and the epidermis (epidermotropically metastatic melanoma). It may be pigmented by melanin in variable amounts or be devoid entirely of melanin, associated with striking nuclear atypia or little atypia, marked by many mitotic figures, some of which may be abnormal, or stamped by few mitotic figures, constituted of a constellation of cytologic types of melanocytes or of a single cytologic type, and joined by neoplastic melanocytes within vascular lumina or lack intravascular involvement by neoplastic cells. A metastasis of melanoma to the skin may be no challenge diagnostically, or it may pose formidable problems in diagnosis because of simulation of numerous conditions that include inflammatory diseases like sarcoidosis, benign neoplasms like Spitz's nevus, and primary malignant neoplasms like angiosarcoma and especially primary melanoma (Table 6). When lymphatics in the upper part of the reticular dermis of a melanoma are stuffed with neoplastic melanocytes, that melanoma must be metastatic to skin (Fig. 84). Histopathologic denominators in common for all types of metastases of melanoma to the skin are asymmetry of the neoplasm, some nuclear atypia, and some mitotic figures. A sign that a metastasis is one of melanoma is melanin within the cytoplasm of neoplastic cells (or melanin within macrophages contiguous with neoplastic cells). If a metastasis is amelanotic, clues to its melanomatous nature are neoplastic cells arranged in nests and protrusions of cytoplasm into nuclei of neoplastic cells where they often appear as large pink inclusions. If the common denominator, specific signs, and clues are heeded, metastatic melanoma to skin can be diagnosed in most instances in sections stained only by hematoxylin and eosin. When doubt persists about the identity of a neoplasm in question, a positive response to an immunoperoxidase stain for S-100 protein and HMB-45 should resolve the issue.

Several patterns of metastasis of melanoma to skin are so characteristic that they deserve mention. One is a large nodule of neoplastic cells within a vein in the subcutaneous fat. Another is a starburst appearance of neoplastic melanocytes within the dermis, a consequence of centrifugal migration of cells that have emerged from a central blood vessel that brought them to the skin. Yet another pattern resembles that of inflammatory carcinoma of the breast in which widely dilated lymphatics throughout the dermis house aggregations of neoplastic melanocytes.

Of all the patterns of metastatic melanoma to skin, one of the most intriguing and baffling diagnostically is epidermotropically metastatic melanoma (Fig. 85). That neoplasm may simulate a small primary melanoma so closely that the two simply cannot be distinguished from one another by conventional microscopy (Table 6). Both the primary and the metastatic melanoma may be small and well-circumscribed, involve both the epidermis and the upper part of the dermis only, consist of atypical melanocytes that often are pagetoid and arranged in pagetoid pattern within the epidermis and epithelial structures of adnexa, have nests of melanocytes that are not equidistant from one another, vary markedly in size and shape, have become confluent, and are accompanied by an infiltrate of lymphocytes. Despite these similarities, the two expressions of cutaneous melanoma usually can be distinguished from one another at scanning magnification by noting in some lesions of epidermotropically metastatic melanoma that: neoplastic melanocytes are present within vascular spaces beneath a "thin" melanoma, the intradermal component of the melanoma extends beyond the intra-epidermal component rather than vice versa, few nests and soli-

TABLE 6. Criteria for Histopathologic Differentiation of Epidermotropically Metastatic Melanoma From Primary Melanoma

1. Dome-shaped with symmetric topography
2. Rather sharp circumscription
3. Nests in both the epidermis and dermis, yet the lesion usually is small, e.g., less than 3.0 mm
4. No proliferation of atypical melanocytes arranged as solitary units at the dermo-epidermal junction
5. Some nests in the uppermost part of the dermis often are larger than nests in the epidermis
6. Intradermal portion of the neoplasm sometimes extends beyond the intra-epidermal component
7. Neoplastic melanocytes may be present within vascular lumina in a "thin" lesion

tary units of melanocytes within the epidermis are seated precisely at the dermo-epidermal junction, but most are scattered randomly above and below it, neoplastic melanocytes arranged as solitary units do not predominate over nests of melanocytes in any high-power field, and the small neoplasm may be almost as deep as it is broad. Patients with many tiny metastases that range in color from pink to black may have some lesions that are epidermotropic and others that show similar findings, except for absence, of epidermal involvement. Curiously, some of the metastases seem to be epidermotropic entirely, no neoplastic melanocytes being detectable in the dermis. No explanation for that enigmatic phenomenon is satisfying.

Metastases of melanoma are categorized conventionally as satellite (Fig. 86), in-transit, regional, and distant. Traditionally, satellite metastases are those within 5.0-cm radices of a primary melanoma, in-transit metastases are those more than 5.0 cm from the primary neoplasm but short of regional lymph nodes, regional metastases are within regional lymph nodes, and distant metastases are those that have spread beyond the nodes. Like all classifications, this one is artificial, but it also is misleading because it implies that prognosis is progressively worse as metastases express themselves in satellite, in-transit, regional, and distant fashion. In our judgment, a metastasis of melanoma is a metastasis, irrespective of modifier, and implies systemic involvement with a grave prognosis. A "satellite" metastasis presages the same grim end as does a "distant" one. Neoplastic melanocytes are not carried by vessels for just 4.9 cm; they are transported by the blood stream throughout the body. It is not surprising, therefore, that the histopathologic findings in the skin of a satellite metastasis (sometimes present at a short distance from the primary melanoma and in the same biopsy specimen) are no different than those in in-transit and distant metastases to skin. Furthermore, sustained management of patients with satellite metastases reveals an inordinate tendency for death from distant metastases even when the primary melanoma with the "satellites" has been excised.

The presence of a metastasis of melanoma does not necessarily denote imminent death. Although most patients with metastases of melanoma die within a few years as a consequence of the effects of those deposits of neoplastic cells, some survive for decades without therapy. We know of patients who have lived with metastases of melanoma for more than 30 years.

Text continues on page 182

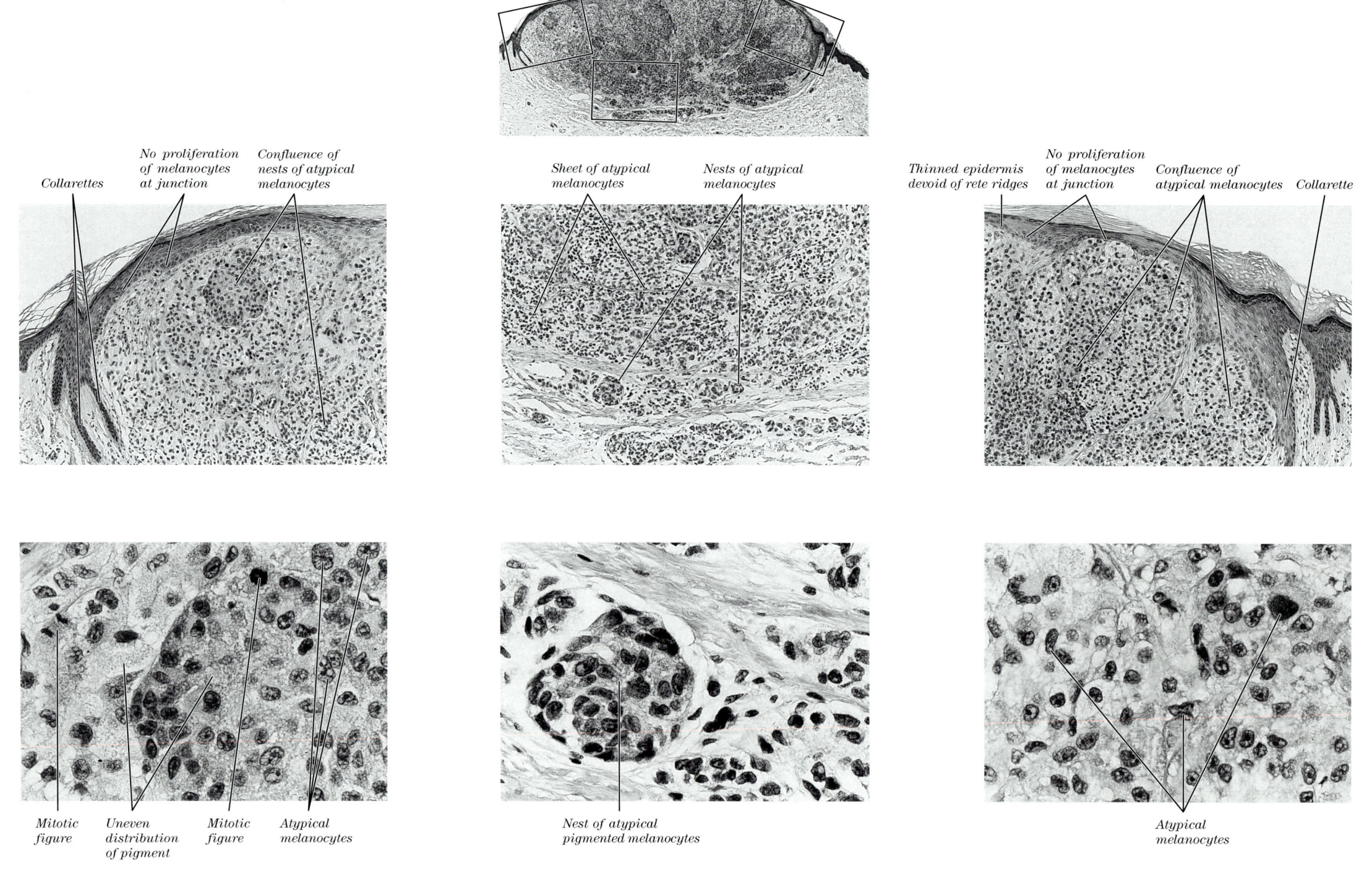

82 • Metastasis of Melanoma

Criteria for diagnosis of this metastasis of melanoma

This neoplasm is malignant because:

1. It is asymmetric.
2. Melanin is not distributed in uniform fashion throughout it.
3. Nests of melanocytes vary in size and shape.
4. Nests of melanocytes have become confluent, forming sheets.
5. Melanocytes do not mature.
6. Nuclei of melanocytes are strikingly atypical.
7. Some neoplastic melanocytes are in mitosis.

This is a metastasis of melanoma, rather than a primary melanoma, because:

There is no proliferation of neoplastic melanocytes at the dermo-epidermal junction. Without signs of melanoma in situ, a diagnosis of primary melanoma cannot be made. This melanoma, therefore, must be a metastasis.

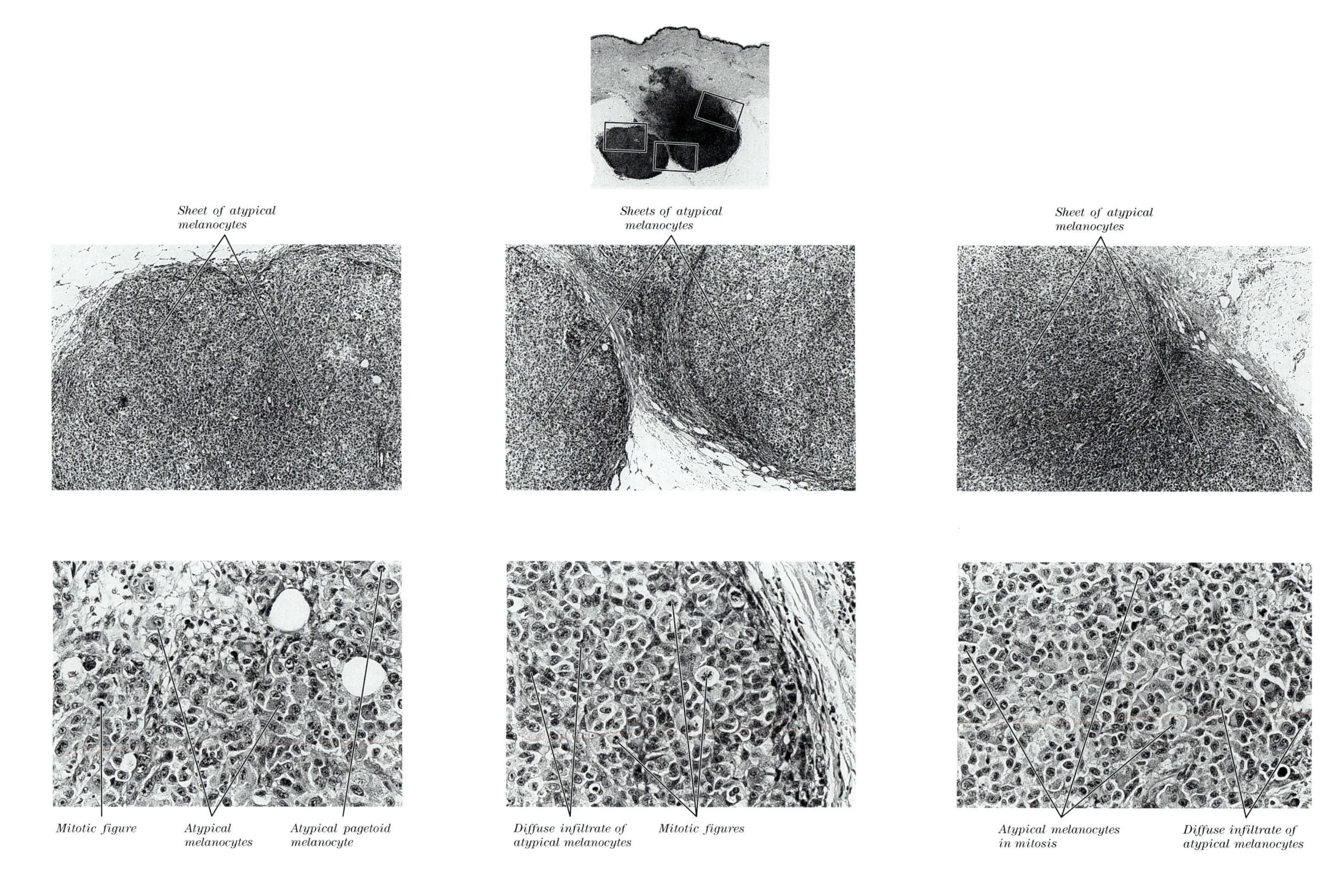

83 • Metastasis of Melanoma

Criteria for diagnosis of this metastasis of melanoma

This is a metastasis of melanoma because:

1. The neoplasm is asymmetric.

2. It is positioned in the lower half of the reticular dermis and the subcutaneous fat.

3. The upper portion of the larger aggregation has a jagged periphery.

4. Neoplastic cells are arranged in sheets.

5. The neoplastic cells have strikingly atypical nuclei.

6. Many neoplastic cells are in mitosis, and some of them are abnormal.

7. There is no evidence of melanoma in situ.

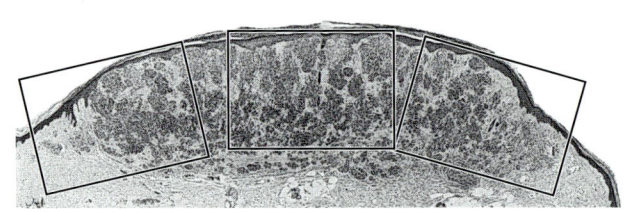

84 • Metastasis of Melanoma

Criteria for diagnosis of this metastasis of melanoma

This is a metastasis of melanoma because:

1. At the sides of the neoplasm, rather than at the base of it, aggregations of neoplastic melanocytes are present within endothelium-lined spaces.

2. No neoplastic melanocytes are present at the dermo-epidermal junction, i.e., there are no atypical melanocytes arranged as solitary units or in nests at that junction (melanoma in situ).

3. The neoplasm is "bottom-heavy," i.e., the base is broader than the surface.

4. Practically no infiltrate of lymphocytes is present at the base of the neoplasm.

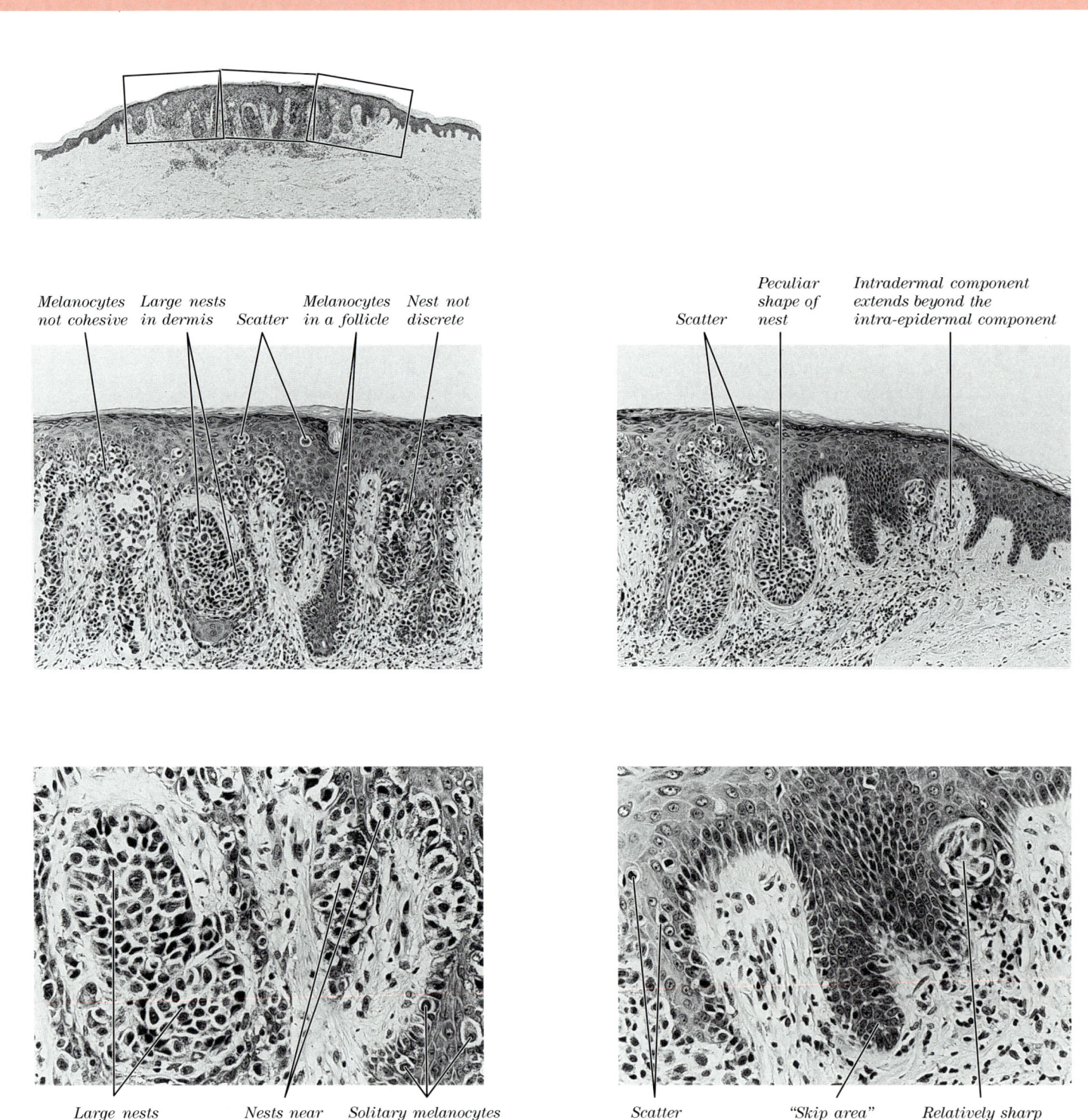

85 • Metastasis of Melanoma *(epidermotropic)*

Criteria for diagnosis of this metastasis of melanoma (epidermotropic)

This is an epidermotropically metastatic melanoma because:

1. It is tiny, i.e., less than 2.0 mm in diameter, yet comprised of many large nests of atypical melanocytes in the epidermis.

2. Large nests of atypical melanocytes, some larger than those in the epidermis, are situated in the uppermost part of the dermis.

3. There are "skip areas" devoid of atypical melanocytes at the dermo-epidermal junction.

4. In some foci, more melanocytes are disposed as solitary units and in nests above the dermo-epidermal junction than at the junction.

5. The intra-epidermal component extends only a little beyond the intradermal component on one side; on the other side, the intradermal component extends beyond the intra-epidermal one.

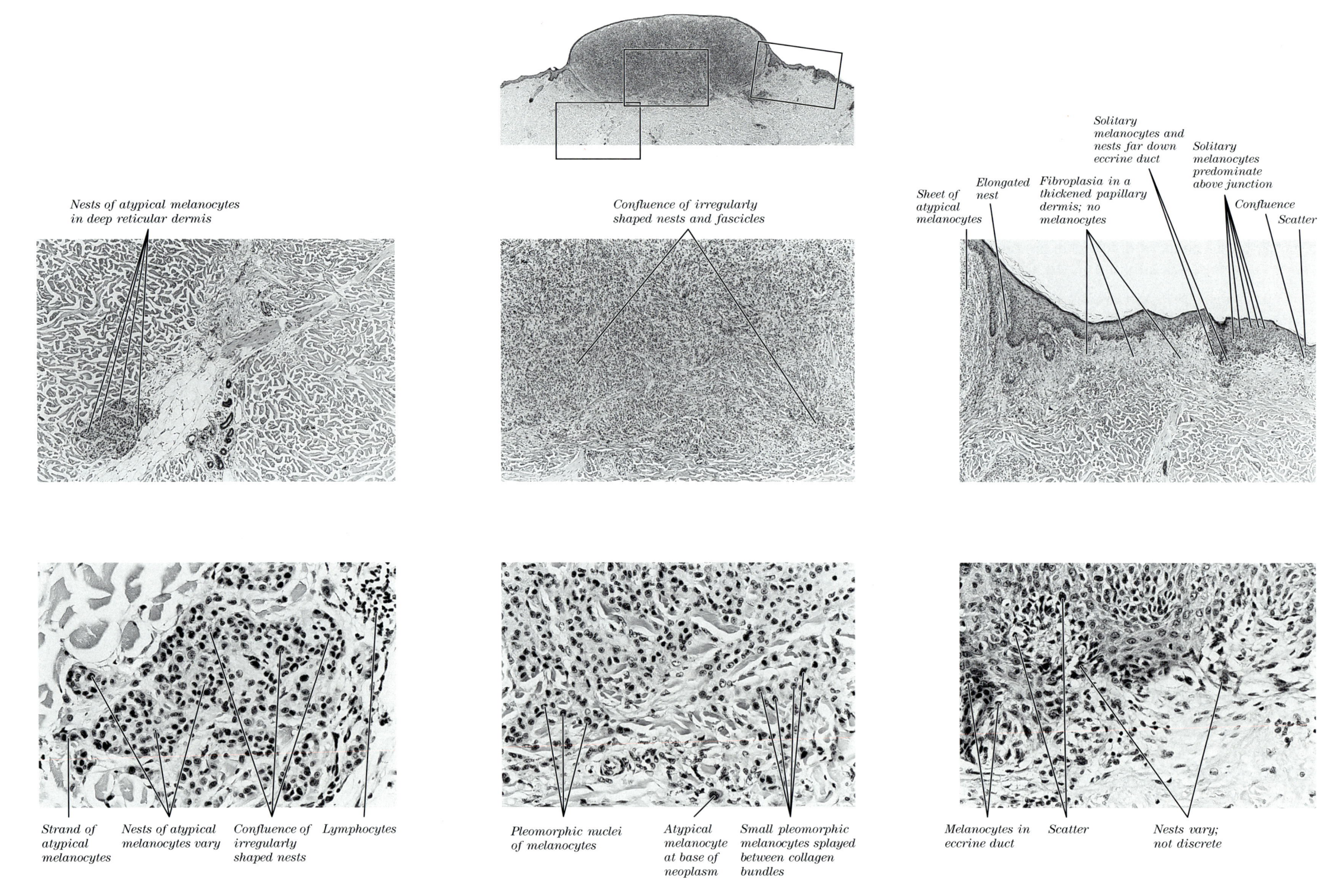

86 • Melanoma with Satellite Metastasis

Criteria for diagnosis of this primary melanoma with satellite metastasis

This is a primary melanoma because:

1. The neoplasm is asymmetric.

2. It is poorly circumscribed.

3. Some melanocytes within the epidermis have become confluent.

4. Some melanocytes disposed as solitary units are present far above the dermo-epidermal junction.

5. Melanocytes within the dermis are arrayed in a sheet.

6. Not all melanocytes mature with progressive descent, i.e., some melanocytes at the base are larger than those above it.

7. Numerous mitotic figures are present within the dermal component and some of those are near the base of the neoplasm.

8. There is a zone of regression of melanoma characterized by fibrosis in the thickened papillary dermis.

There is also a satellite metastasis of melanoma because:

1. In the deep reticular dermis, in a well-circumscribed focus far from the primary melanoma, there are aggregations of atypical melanocytes that vary in size and shape, and have become confluent.

2. Cytologic features of neoplastic cells at a distance from the primary neoplasm are the same as those within the primary melanoma.

VII. Benign Simulators of Melanoma*

A. Melanocytic Simulators

Some proliferations of melanocytes may simulate melanoma by virtue of shared architectural attributes, others by shared cytologic features, and still others by both shared architectural and cytologic findings. The following are melanocytic proliferations that may resemble primary melanoma closely.

1. Spitz's nevi
2. Combined nevi
3. Persistent (recurrent) nevi
4. Halo nevi
5. Ancient Miescher's and Unna's nevi
6. Congenital nevi in newborns and infants
7. Nevi on genitalia of young adults
8. Nevi on palms and soles
9. Nevi in association with lichen sclerosus et atrophicus in the anogenital region
10. Junctional nevi above a band of melanophages
11. Melanosis of the genitalia
12. Melanocytic proliferation in the epidermis above some intradermal Miescher's nevi
13. Melanocytic proliferation in the epidermis above some fibrous papules of the face
14. Melanocytic proliferation in the epidermis of skin damaged severely by sunlight, especially on the face
15. Melanocytic proliferation within some solar lentigines
16. Melanocytic proliferation in the epidermis of some normal eyelids

---

*Much of this section comes from a chapter by A. Bernard Ackerman in *Pathobiology and Recognition of Malignant Melanomas*, edited by Martin C. Mihm, Jr., George F. Murphy, and Nathan Kaufman, published by Williams & Wilkins, Baltimore, 1988.

TABLE 7. Histopathologic Features in Common Between Spitz's Nevi and Melanomas

Architectural
1. Scatter of melanocytes above the dermo-epidermal junction
2. Nests of melanocytes vary in size and shape
3. Some nests of melanocytes have become confluent
4. Extension of melanocytes far down epithelial structures of adnexa
5. Nests of melanocytes not necessarily equidistant from one another
6. Lymphocytic infiltrates within the dermis
7. Base of neoplasm neither flat nor wedge-shaped

Cytologic
1. Atypical melanocytes
2. Melanocytes in mitosis
3. Necrotic melanocytes sometimes

Spitz's Nevi. As has been emphasized previously, Spitz's nevi are wholly benign neoplasms that differ histopathologically from melanomas by being symmetric and sharply circumscribed, and by showing maturation of melanocytes with progressive descent into the dermis. These three features indicate that Spitz's nevi are benign. But Spitz's nevi may have many architectural and cytologic features in common with melanoma: nests of melanocytes within the epidermis that vary in size and shape, nests with shapes other than round or oval, tendency of nests to become confluent, scatter of melanocytes arranged as solitary units and in nests above the basal layer (sometimes within the granular zone and cornified layer), extension of melanocytes far down epithelial structures of adnexa, nuclear atypia that may be striking (Fig. 87), melanocytes in mitosis (some of them even abnormal), and necrotic melanocytes (Table 7). Despite the numerous features that Spitz's nevi may share with melanoma, they can be recognized for what they are by the findings, in addition to symmetry, sharp circumscription, and maturation, of compact orthokeratosis, hypergranulosis, irregular spinous-cell hyperplasia, clefts between elongated nests of melanocytes and adjacent keratinocytes, dull pink globules in the epidermis of junctional and compound types, and melanocytes with large nuclei, abundant cytoplasm, and oval, spindle, round, and polygonal shapes. Multinucleate melanocytes may be numerous and even may predominate. Dendritic melanocytes are seen commonly in Spitz's nevi in Asians and in Africans, in whom they occur rarely.

Combined Nevi. Combined nevi result from (1) any combination of the four morphologic expressions of acquired nevi (Unna, Miescher, Spitz, and Clark) or congenital nevi (blue and non-blue), and from (2) any combination of cytologic types of melanocytes other than small/large round and multinucleate (e.g., small round and pagetoid, small round and balloon). A combined nevus usually is a manifestation of a congenital nevus. In short, combinations of nevi may develop as a result of the appearance in the same lesion of more than one type of nevus, e.g., Unna's and Spitz's (Fig. 88), or as a consequence of more than one cytologic type of melanocyte, e.g., a congenital analogue of Miescher's nevus (dendritic with abundant cytoplasm and non-dendritic with scant cytoplasm) (Figs. 89, 90).

A common combined nevus is one that combines Spitz's nevus with architectural elements of another type of nevus. A Spitz's nevus may be combined with an Unna's, Miescher's, or Clark's nevus. The large melanocytes of Spitz's nevus may be situated above, below, or at the side of small melanocytes of those other types of nevi, or they may be intermingled with them. Unlike typical Spitz's nevi, which are patently symmetric, combined Spitz's nevi usually are asymmetric because two basic types of nevi are wedded and at least two types of melanocytes are distributed peculiarly. Combined nevi with a component of Spitz's nevus are well circumscribed and show maturation of melanocytes with progressive descent into the dermis, signs that confirm their benignancy. Nonetheless, these nevi, which frequently occur in youngsters and adolescents, are misdiagnosed often as melanomas.

Less common than combined nevi with a component of Spitz's nevus are combinations of the other three basic types of acquired nevi such as those of Clark and Unna. A very common combination joins small melanocytes and pagetoid melanocytes in the reticular dermis of a distinctive congenital nevus. They are recognizable readily as benign because they are small and well-circumscribed. As a rule, these nevi are compound in type, and the pagetoid melanocytes are positioned wholly in the intradermal component, usually in the lower half of it, and often in angiocentric and adnexocentric fashion with some pagetoid melanocytes splayed between bundles of collagen. The majority of the melanocytes in a combined nevus with pagetoid cells tend to be small round ones. Pagetoid melanocytes with small round (or oval) nuclei and abundant pale cytoplasm filled with dusty melanin nearly always are surrounded by numerous melanophages. These striking changes are apparent at scanning magnification, the clue to the diagnosis being a melanocytic nevus with asymmetric, patchy distribution of melanophages in the reticular dermis. Combined nevi with pagetoid melanocytes have two features in common with pagetoid melanoma: pagetoid cells and asymmetric distribution of those cells and of melanophages. In melanoma, pagetoid cells tend to be found within the epidermis as well as within the dermis, and their nuclei are atypical; in contrast, pagetoid cells in a combined nevus are situated completely within the dermis and their nuclei are small and monomorphous.

What has just been written about combined nevi with pagetoid melanocytes applies in large measure to combined nevi with balloon melanocytes. They, too, display most of the architectural features of nevi, are usually compound in type, exhibit nuclear characteristics typical of melanocytes of a nevus, and consist of at least some melanocytes whose cytoplasm is ballooned (Fig. 91). The number of cells of a nevus that are ballooned ranges from few to many, the remainder of the melanocytes being small and round. The two types of melanocytes are distributed asymmetrically. The architectural and cytologic features of a balloon-cell nevus may cause problems in histopathologic differentiation from melanoma. In balloon-cell melanomas, neoplastic melanocytes within the epidermis fulfill criteria for melanoma in situ, whereas neoplastic melanocytes within the epidermis of combined nevi with balloon cells are arranged mostly in nests that are situated at the dermo-epidermal junction. Balloon melanocytes of melanomas have atypical nuclei, some of which may be in mitosis, whereas balloon melanocytes of nevi are typical and not in mitosis.

Other combinations of cytologic types of melanocytes in acquired nevi may present problems, on occasion, in differentiation from melanoma, but combined nevi with pagetoid melanocytes and combined nevi with balloon melanocytes are among the most formidable challenges to a histopathologist.

Combinations of architectural patterns of nevi on the one hand and of cytologic types of melanocytes on the other (and both together) are found in acquired nevi as well as in congenital ones. In fact, most combined nevi seem to be congenital. The same principles for differentiation of combined congenital nevi from melanomas obtain for distinguishing combined acquired congenital nevi from melanomas.

Text continues on page 194

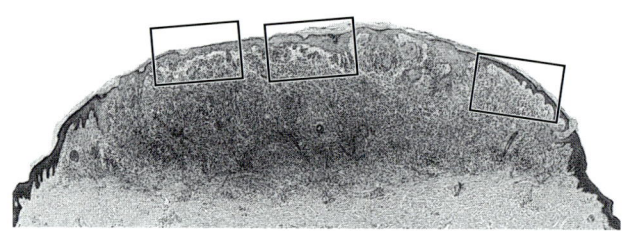

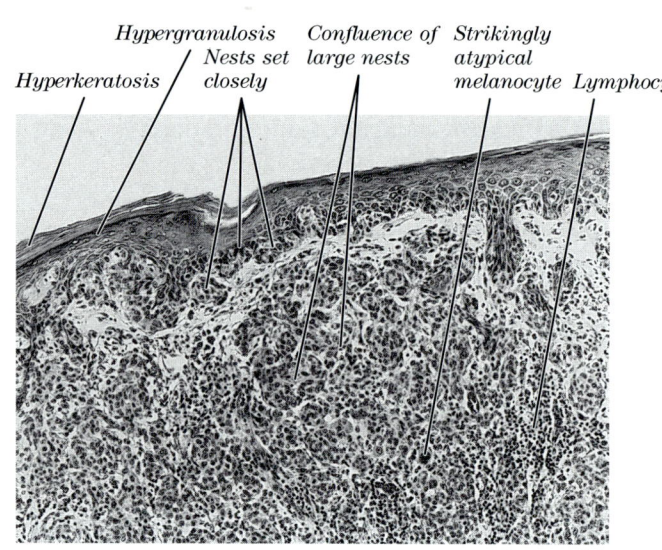
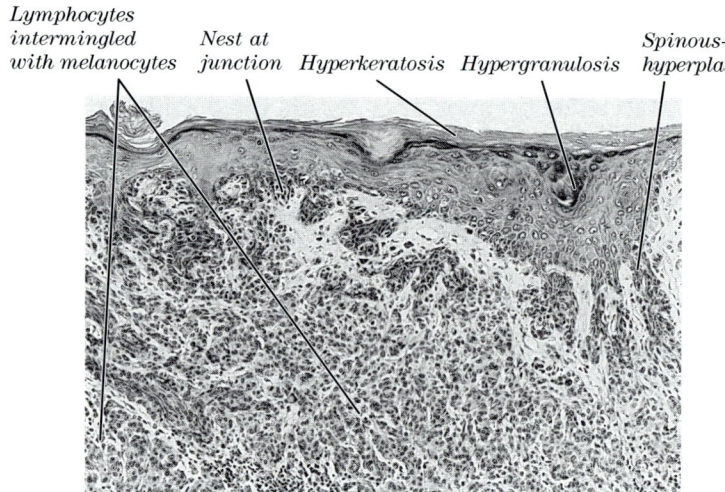
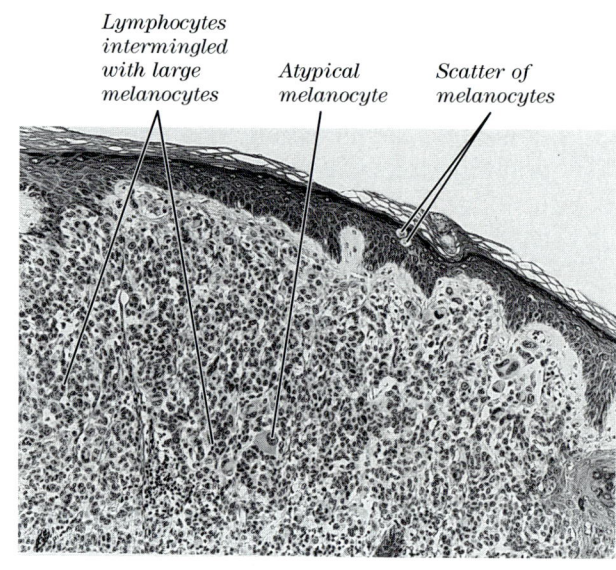

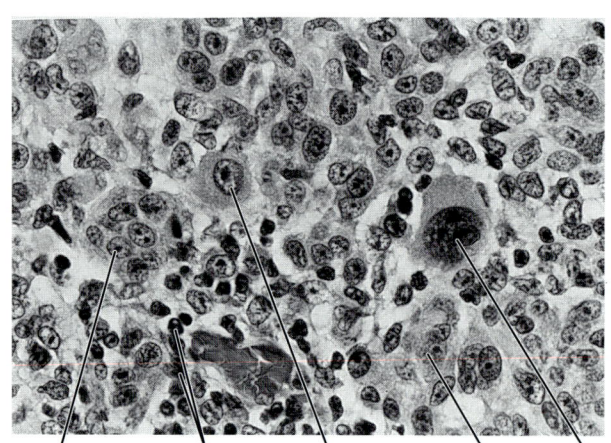
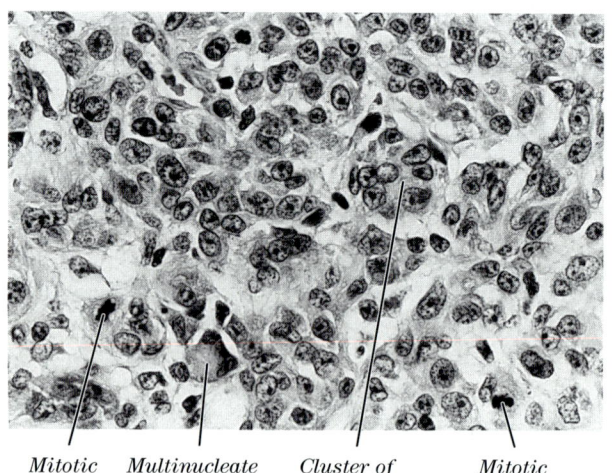
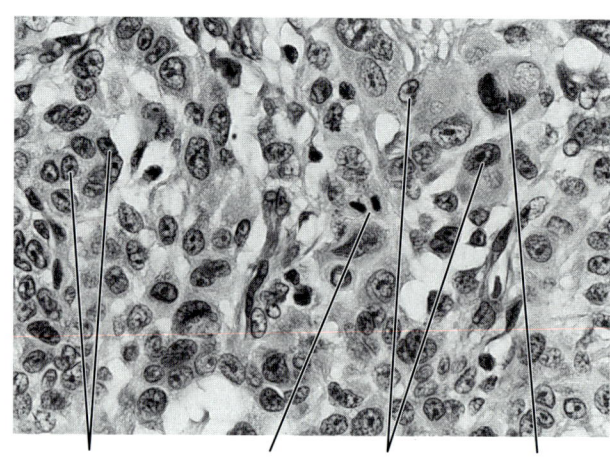

87 • Spitz's Nevus

Criteria for diagnosis of this Spitz's nevus

This neoplasm is benign because it is:

1. Symmetric.
2. Well-circumscribed.
3. Flat at its base.
4. Associated with maturation of melanocytes.

This is a Spitz's nevus because:

1. Many melanocytes have large nuclei, abundant cytoplasm, and round and oval shapes.
2. There are slight hyperkeratosis, hypergranulosis, and epidermal hyperplasia.
3. A perivascular infiltrate of lymphocytes is present throughout the neoplasm.

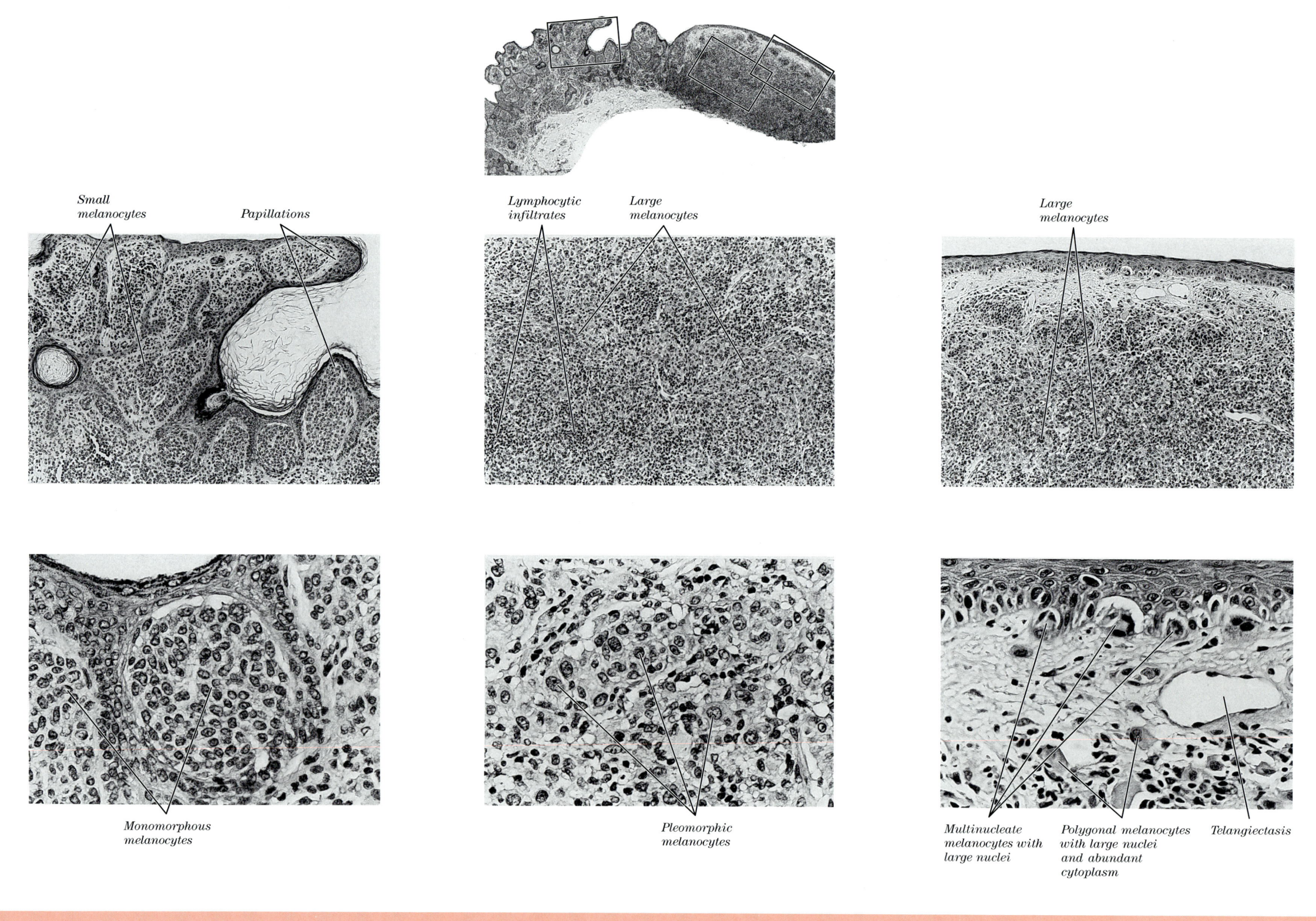

88 • Combined Nevus *(Unna's and Spitz's)*

Criteria for diagnosis of this combined nevus (Unna's and Spitz's)

This is a combined nevus because:

Two different types of melanocytic nevi are represented in this specimen: a Unna's nevus on the left and a Spitz's nevus on the right.

This is a Unna's nevus on the left because:

1. The lesion is both exo- and endophytic, but mostly exophytic.
2. The surface is papillated.
3. The process is confined to a thickened papillary dermis.
4. The melanocytes have oval nuclei and scant cytoplasm.

This is a Spitz's nevus on the right because:

1. Many of the melanocytes have large nuclei, abundant cytoplasm, and round, oval, and polygonal shapes.
2. Many of the melanocytes are multinucleated.
3. A dense, mostly perivascular infiltrate of lymphocytes is present throughout the neoplasm.
4. Many widely dilated blood vessels are present within the neoplasm.

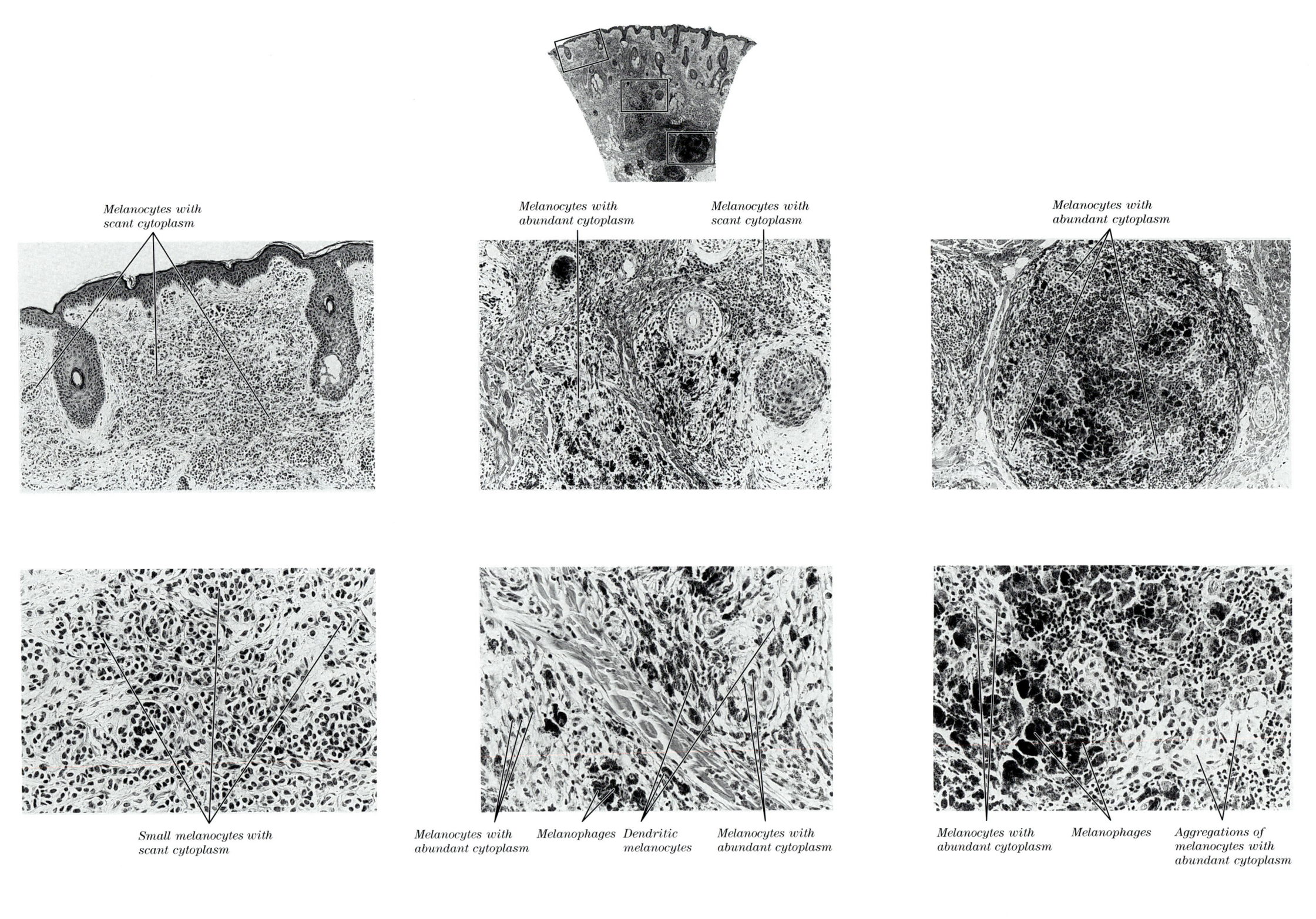

89 • Miescher's Nevus *(combined type)*

Criteria for diagnosis of this combined nevus

This is a nevus because:

1. Melanocytes mature.
2. Epithelial structures of adnexa are preserved.
3. Nuclei of melanocytes are typical.
4. Nuclei of melanocytes are monomorphous throughout the lesion.

This is a Miescher's nevus because:

The nevus is slightly domed, entirely endophytic in a wedge shape, and on the face.

This is a combined nevus because:

There is more than one population of melanocytes: those on the left with scant cytoplasm and those on the right with abundant cytoplasm (associated with which are numerous melanophages) and dendrites.

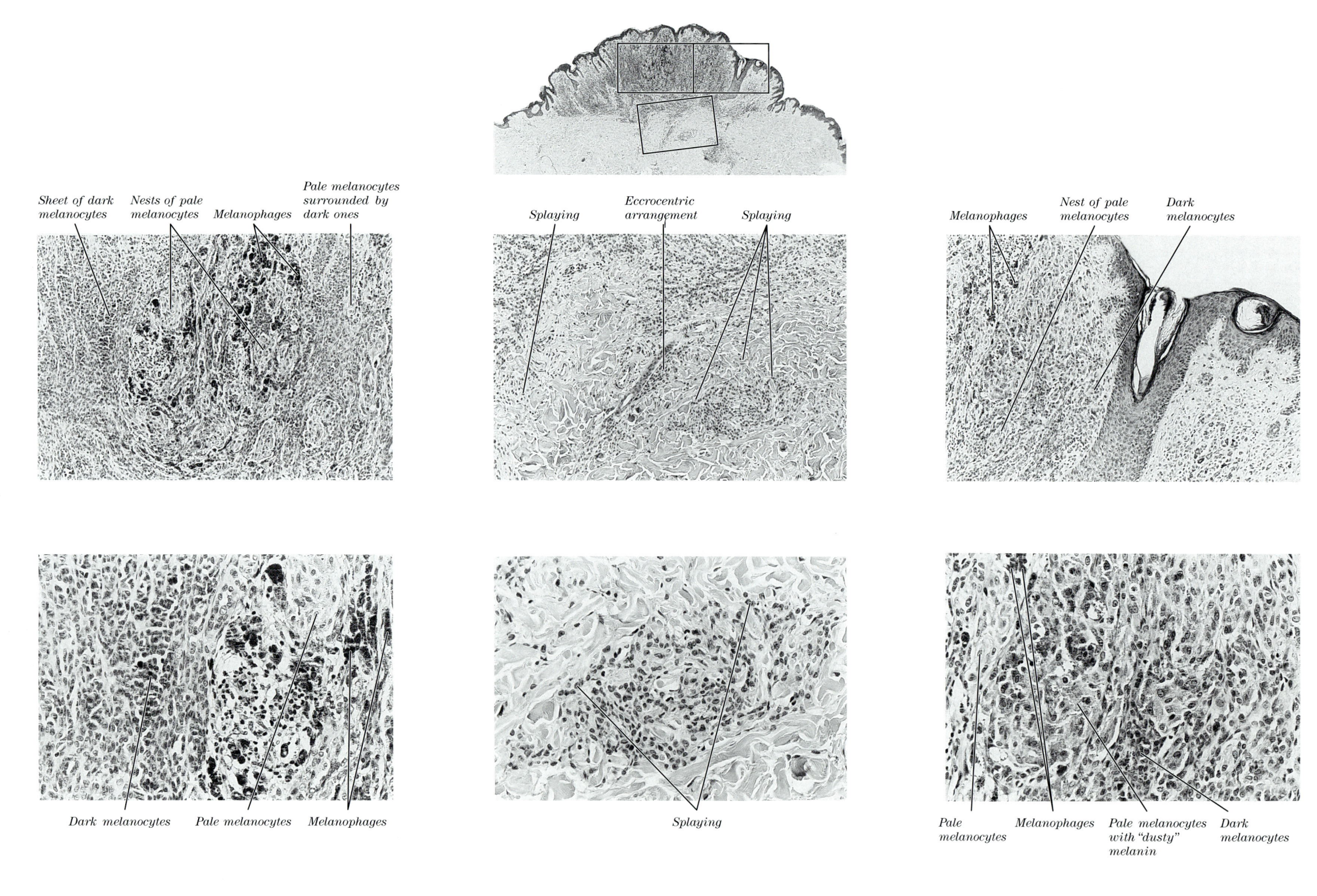

90 • Congenital Nevus *(superficial type, combined)*

Criteria for diagnosis of this non-blue congenital nevus (superficial type, combined)

This is a congenital nevus because:

1. Melanocytes are splayed between collagen bundles in the reticular dermis.
2. Melanocytes are distributed in angiocentric and adnexocentric fashion.

This is a combined nevus because:

1. There are two different populations of melanocytes within the intradermal portion of the nevus: cells with small oval nuclei and scant cytoplasm, and cells with small oval nuclei and abundant pale cytoplasm that houses dusty melanin.
2. Melanophages are particularly numerous in zones where there are melanocytes with abundant pale cytoplasm and dusty melanin.

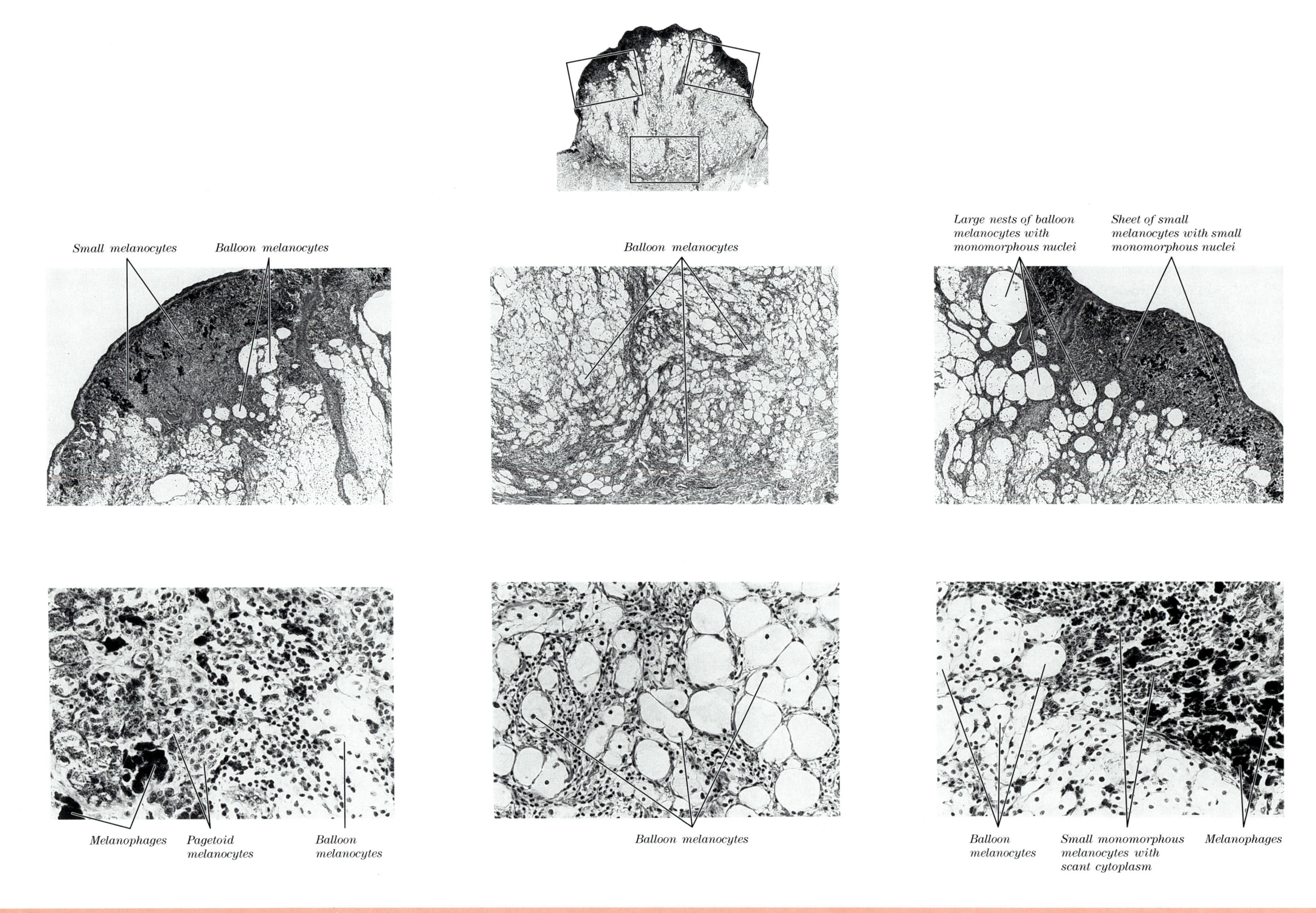

91 • Miescher's Nevus *(with balloon cells)*

Criteria for diagnosis of this Miescher's nevus (combined type, with balloon cells)

This lesion is benign because:

1. It is symmetric.
2. It is vertically oriented.
3. It is sharply circumscribed.
4. Melanocytes mature with progressive descent into the dermis.
5. Nuclei of melanocytes are small and relatively monomorphous.

This is a Miescher's nevus because:

1. It is dome-shaped.
2. It is mostly endophytic.
3. The shape is vaguely like that of a wedge.

This is a combined nevus because:

Three different populations of melanocytes constitute the neoplasm: those with small roundish and oval nuclei surrounded by scant cytoplasm (like those that usually constitute a Miescher's nevus), small round nuclei and abundant pale cytoplasm that contains "dusty" melanin (pagetoid melanocytes), and cells with small roundish nuclei and extraordinarily abundant cytoplasm (balloon cells). A nevus such as this one is known colloquially as "balloon-cell nevus."

Persistent (Recurrent) Melanocytic Nevi. When compound or intradermal types of nevi, usually those situated on the upper half of the body of young adults, are removed by superficial shave technique and sometimes subjected then to light electrodesiccation, the melanocytes of the nevi may not be removed completely and, therefore, may persist and proliferate at the local site, only to reappear in several weeks. Clinically, "recurrent" nevi may resemble flat melanomas by being asymmetric, poorly circumscribed, and variegate in shades of brown.

Histopathologically, these lesions usually show some features in the epidermis and epithelial structures of adnexa that resemble melanoma (Figs. 92, 93). At times, there also may be findings like those of melanoma in the upper part of the dermis. Fibrosis is apparent beneath the proliferation of melanocytes and represents a sign of one or more previous destructive procedures at the site. Beneath the scar may reside monomorphous melanocytes of the original nevus. Intra-epidermal features of persistent melanocytic nevi may be misinterpreted as those of melanoma in situ because nests of melanocytes are not equidistant from one another, they vary in size and shape, and they may have irregular shapes. Furthermore, nests of melanocytes often become confluent, melanocytes arranged as solitary units predominate over nests of melanocytes in some high-power fields, and some melanocytes may be found above the dermo-epidermal junction, sometimes far above it. Similar changes may be seen within epithelial structures of adnexa.

Whenever a histopathologist suspects a proliferation of melanocytes to be that of a recurrent nevus, sections from the original biopsy specimen taken by shave technique should be examined to ascertain whether they show a nevus or a melanoma that was misinterpreted as a nevus. Review of the original sections is particularly important for recurrent melanocytic lesions in which indubitable melanocytes of a nevus, a clue to the wholly benign nature of the lesion, are not present in the dermis beneath the scar.

Histopathologic clues to the benign character of recurrent nevi are their sharp circumscription, failure of the intra-epidermal proliferation of melanocytes to extend beyond the scar, presence of nests of melanocytes mostly at the dermo-epidermal junction, absence of striking nuclear atypia, and typical melanocytes of a nevus beneath the scar, when they are present.

Re-excision of a persistent nevus usually is performed within weeks or a few months after the original procedure. Sometimes, however, the persistent nevus is removed years after the shave excision has been obtained. Even after years, changes that simulate melanoma may be observed in the epidermis and in the upper part of the dermis.

Halo Nevi. Halo nevi are sometimes confused with melanomas by histopathologists who consider a dense lymphocytic infiltrate throughout a melanocytic neoplasm to be a sign of malignancy. In actuality, the significance for differential diagnosis of a lymphocytic infiltrate within melanocytic neoplasms turns completely upon the distribution of the lymphocytes, rather than the density of them. Symmetric distribution of lymphocytes usually signifies a nevus, whereas asymmetric distribution tends to indicate melanoma. Infiltrates of lymphocytes in Spitz's nevi and Clark's nevi are arranged symmetrically. Halo nevus, in most instances, is merely a compound type of Clark's nevus in which the infiltrate of lymphocytes destroys the nevus and leaves a vitiliginous macule as residuum (Figs. 94, 95). Halo nevi may be recognized as benign at scanning magnification, because they usually are small, slightly dome-shaped, mostly symmetric, well-circumscribed, and characterized by a flat bottom that rests upon the reticular dermis. With higher magnification, nests of melanocytes are seen to be positioned at the dermo-epidermal junction and in the papillary dermis, nests of melanocytes predominate over melanocytes arranged as solitary units in the epidermis and within epithelial structures of adnexa, and melanocytes mature with progressive descent. The only other features, besides lymphocytic infiltrates, that halo nevi have in common with melanoma are nuclear atypia of some melanocytes, especially those that are surrounded by the densest infiltrates of lymphocytes, and some tendency to confluence of nests of melanocytes within the epidermis. Those latter two findings are not seen with repeatability in halo nevi.

Regression of halo nevus has several features in common with manifestations of regression of melanoma in which fibroplasia predominates: fibrosis, telangiectases, patchy lymphocytic infiltrates, and some melanophages in a thickened papillary dermis are found in both. A regressed halo nevus, in contrast to a regressed melanoma, usually is small, domed, and associated with fewer melanophages. There never are signs of melanosis in regression of a halo nevus (Fig. 96).

Last, it is important to know that "halo nevus" is a clinical diagnosis, not a histopathologic one. The same histopathologic findings seen in indubitable halo nevi (in which a white "halo" surrounds a nevus) may be noted

Text continues on page 199

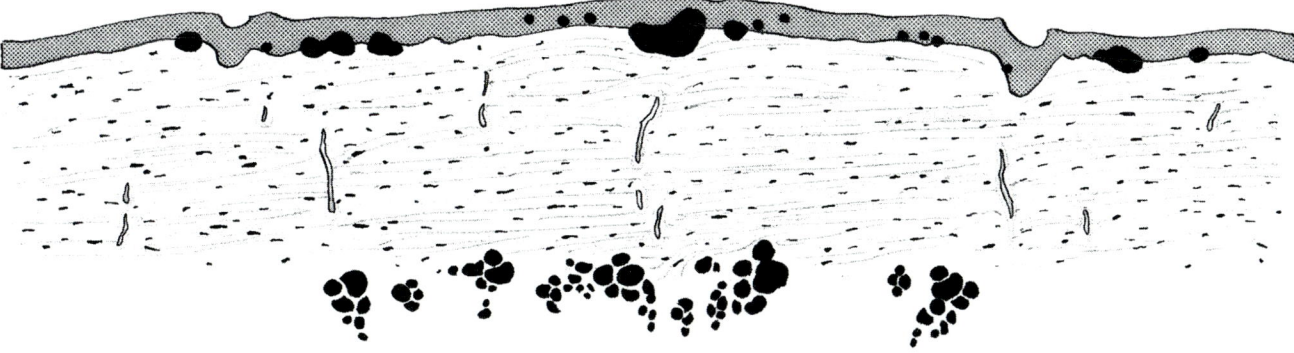

Fig. 92. Persistent (recurrent) nevus. If attention is paid solely to changes within the epidermis, a neoplasm such as this one easily could be misinterpreted as a melanoma in situ. Nests of melanocytes within the epidermis are not equidistant from one another, they vary in size and shape, some have become confluent, and melanocytes arranged as solitary units are present above the dermo-epidermal junction. The findings just enumerated, however, are not those of a melanoma, but are expected ones in a melanocytic nevus that previously has been removed partially by shave technique. As a consequence of that procedure, a scar develops in the upper part of the dermis, as is seen here in the form of collagen bundles and thin fibrocytes oriented parallel to the skin surface, and dilated blood vessels oriented perpendicular to it. Beneath the scar, the residuum of the original melanocytic nevus is seen as nests, cords, and strands of melanocytes. The changes within the epidermis represent recurrence of the melanocytic nevus at that site. Sometimes, the scar may be subtle, and there may be no residual nests of melanocytes of a nevus beneath it. In those circumstances, histopathologists and surgeons must be alert to the danger of overdiagnosing a proliferation of melanocytes such as this one as melanoma.

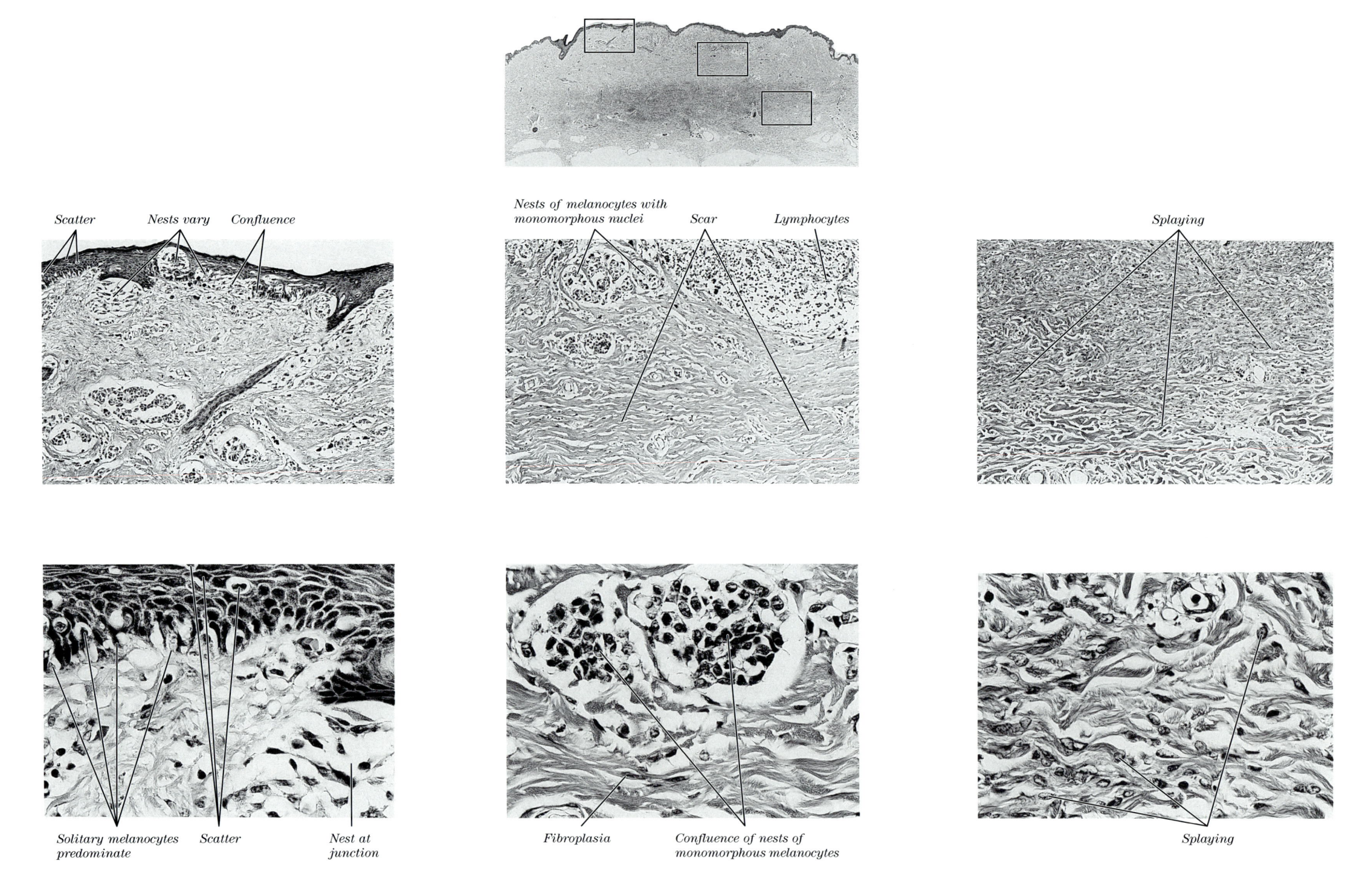

93 • Congenital Nevus *(superficial type, persistent)*

Criteria for diagnosis of this congenital nevus (superficial type, persistent)

This is a nevus because:

1. The neoplasm seems to be symmetric.
2. It appears to be well-circumscribed.
3. Melanocytes within the epidermis and the dermis have relatively monomorphous nuclei.
4. Melanocytes mature.

This is a superficial congenital nevus because:

1. Most of the melanocytes are confined to the upper half of the dermis.
2. Melanocytes of the nevus are splayed focally between collagen bundles in the reticular dermis.
3. Some melanocytes of the nevus are present around adnexal structures within the reticular dermis.

This is a recurrent nevus because:

1. A scar, a consequence of a previous surgical procedure, is apparent in the upper half of the dermis.
2. Above the scar, neoplastic melanocytes within the epidermis are present not only at the dermo-epidermal junction, but also above it.
3. Above the scar, in some high-power fields, some melanocytes within the epidermis are arrayed as solitary units and predominate over nests of melanocytes.

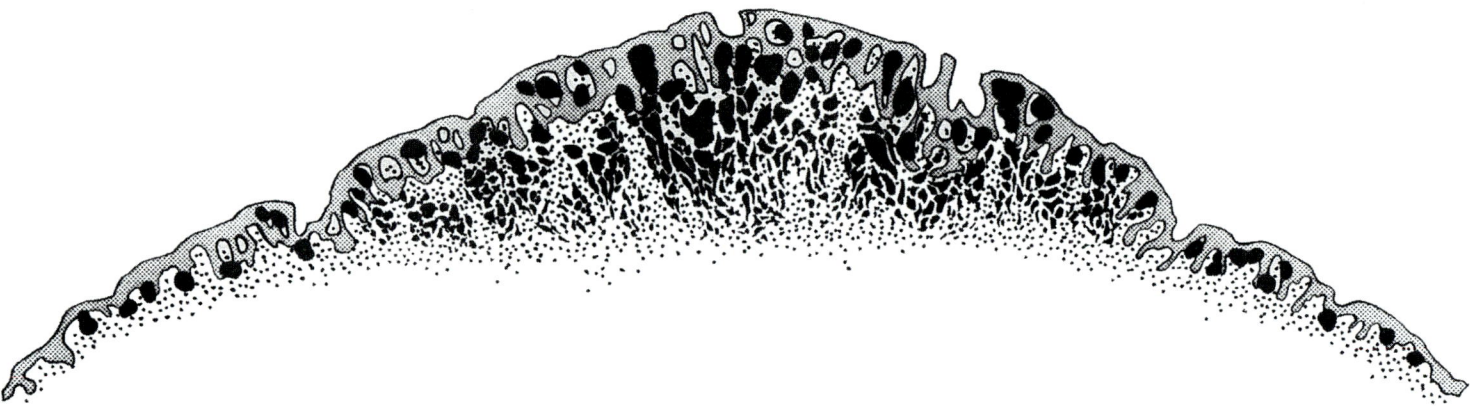

Fig. 94. Halo nevus. At scanning magnification, the silhouette indicates that this neoplasm is benign. It is symmetric, well-circumscribed, and characterized by nests of melanocytes positioned at the dermo-epidermal junction and not above it. Furthermore, there is maturation of melanocytes with progressive descent into the dermis. The base of the neoplasm is flat, another sign of benignancy. The nevus is Clark's type because it is slightly elevated and gently mammillated, and nests of melanocytes are confined to the dermo-epidermal junction and the papillary dermis. This is a halo nevus because a dense infiltrate of lymphocytes partially obscures the Clark's nevus. Eventually, that infiltrate will destroy the nevus.

in Clark's nevi that were not accompanied by a "halo" clinically. Without that clinical sign, a definitive diagnosis of halo nevus cannot and should not be made.

Ancient Miescher's and Unna's Nevi. Episodically, sections from a biopsy specimen of a Miescher's nevus removed from a face, especially a cheek or ear, but also rarely from another site such as the trunk of an older person, one who is more than 60 years of age as a rule, shows distinctive histopathologic changes that may be misread as those of melanoma. As is generally the situation in Miescher's nevi, the neoplasm is domed, mostly endophytic, nearly or entirely intradermal, and often wedge-shaped. Furthermore, the topographic attributes of the neoplasm are symmetry as a rule and sharp circumscription. Clefts may separate the compressed fibrous tissue that surrounds the lesion from the adjacent normal skin and subcutaneous fat. Maturation of melanocytes is striking. All of these features mark the neoplasm as benign. In some instances, however, the nevus is asymmetric because of the distribution of nests of melanocytes, some of which are very large.

Two populations of melanocytes constitute an ancient Miescher's nevus: those with large round, sometimes atypical nuclei and abundant cytoplasm that form an umbrella-like zone across the upper part of the reticular dermis, and those with smaller round nuclei and scant cytoplasm that make up the remaining bulk of it. Both types of melanocytes exhibit prominent nucleoli. Scattered throughout the neoplasm are mitotic figures. All of the features just described may be found also in Unna's nevus (Fig. 97).

This specific manifestation of Miescher's or Unna's nevus is designated "ancient" because it occurs in older persons of both sexes and shares numerous features of a well-recognized benign neoplasm with neural differentiation named "ancient schwannoma." Within and in between the large aggregations of neoplastic melanocytes of an ancient Miescher's or Unna's nevus there tend to be many widely dilated venules, thrombi, patchy zones of hemorrhage and resultant siderophages, clotted blood, rims of sclerosis around dilated venules, delicate fibrillary bundles of collagen, and an edematous and mucinous stroma, all of which are findings integral to an ancient schwannoma, too.

If heed is paid to the overall architectural pattern of an ancient Miescher's or Unna's nevus, the benign nature of it should be apparent. If too close attention is directed to cytologic features, however, risk of misdiagnosis as melanoma is courted.

Congenital Nevi in Newborns and Infants. When a biopsy of a congenital nevus is performed in infants, especially in the first few days after parturition but even for many months thereafter, the histopathologic changes in the dermis and subcutaneous fat may be like those expected in congenital nevi, but the intra-epidermal component of a superficial or deep, non-blue type of congenital nevus may show features that are misread easily as those of melanoma in situ. For example, there may be pagetoid melanocytes disposed as solitary units and nests, not only at the dermo-epidermal junction but also far above it (some pagetoid melanocytes even being present in the granular zone and cornified layer). Nests of melanocytes within the epidermis tend to vary in size and shape, and some nests may become confluent (Fig. 98). Those changes pose a vexing problem in differentiation from melanoma in situ. If a congenital nevus is wholly junctional, i.e., without any intradermal component, or if it involves the epidermis and dermis but has been removed by superficial shave technique that fails to deliver melanocytes in the dermis, differentiation from melanoma in situ may not be possible. Even if the intradermal component of a congenital nevus, where the characteristic and specific features reside, is not available for study, an important sign for differentiation is present in the epidermis. Pagetoid melanocytes within the epidermis of a congenital nevus in a biopsy specimen taken shortly after birth do not have atypical nuclei. Usually, the nuclei are small, but even if they are large, they are monomorphous, not pleomorphic.

Another pitfall in diagnosis of a deep congenital nevus in a biopsy specimen extracted shortly after birth concerns the dermis, where there may be one or several small nodules of melanocytes surrounded by typical melanocytes of the nevus. In such a nodule, the melanocytes have large nuclei and scant cytoplasm, many of them may be in mitosis, and many may be necrotic (Figs. 99, 100). Such a nodule could be misinterpreted as one of melanoma that resides in the intradermal component of a deep congenital nevus of a newborn. If, however, a nodule (or nodules) is situated mostly in the upper half of the nevus, is symmetric and rather well-circumscribed, and if the large melanocytes that constitute it are monomorphous, almost certainly it is a part of the nevus, not a melanoma. Rarely, such a nodule is not small and cannot be extirpated completely. Even in those circumstances, no metastases appear and infants who bear the lesions develop in normal fashion.

Text continues on page 212

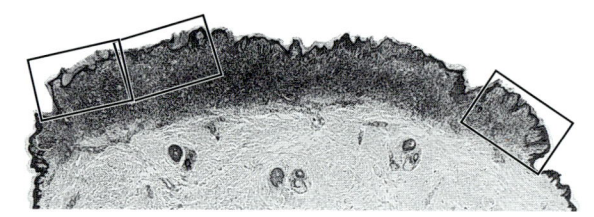

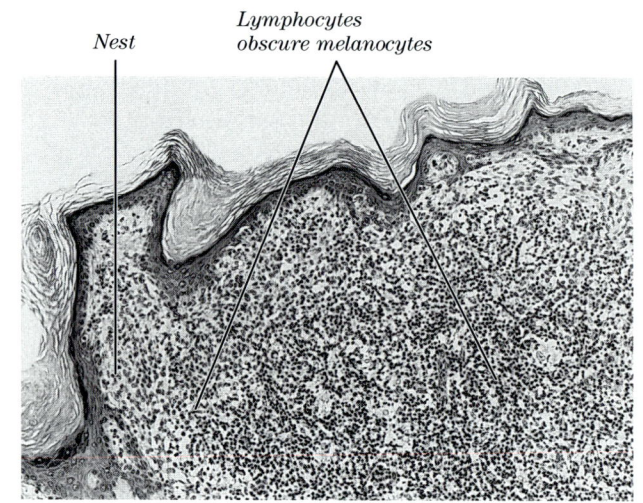
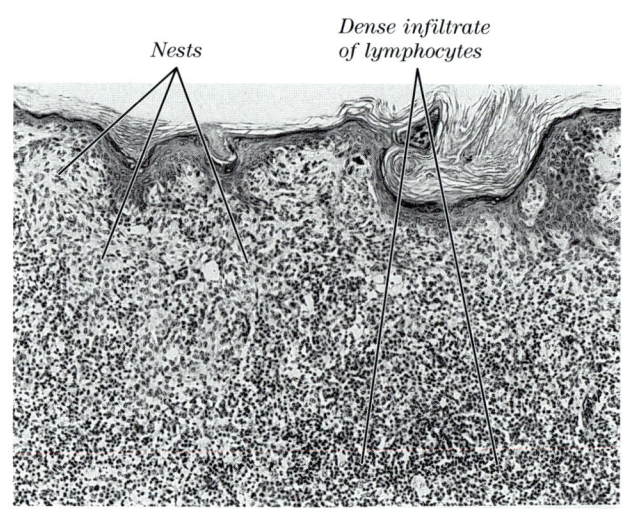
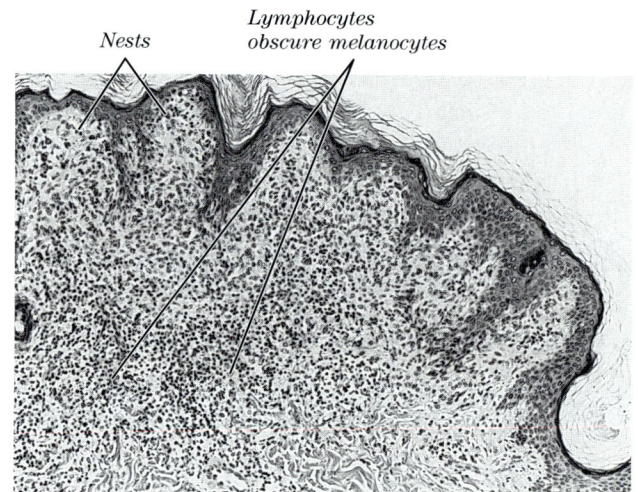

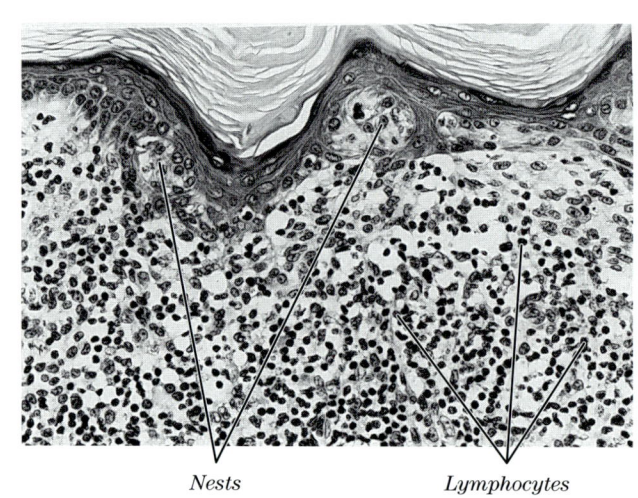
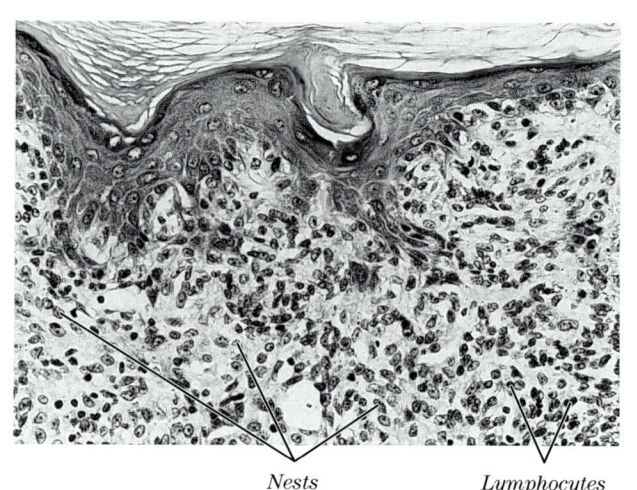
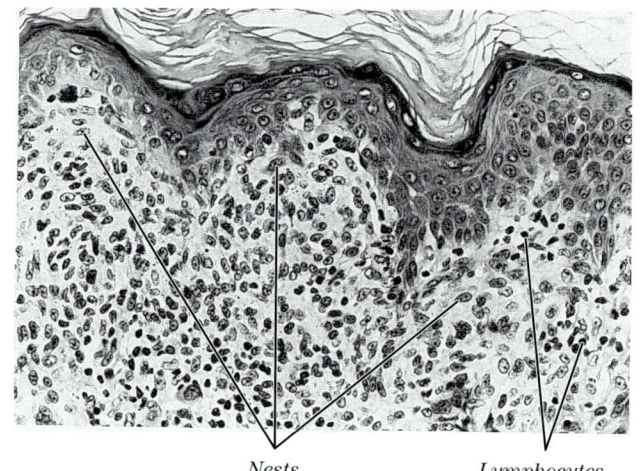

95 • Clark's Nevus *(halo type)*

Criteria for diagnosis of this Clark's nevus (halo type)

This neoplasm is benign because:

1. It is relatively symmetric.

2. It is very well-circumscribed.

3. Its bottom is flat.

4. Melanocytes within the epidermis, both those arranged as solitary units and those in nests, are situated at the dermo-epidermal junction, not above it.

5. There is maturation of melanocytes.

This is a compound nevus because:

The lesion is slightly elevated and mammillated, and nests of melanocytes are confined to the dermo-epidermal junction and thickened papillary dermis. In short, this is a Clark's nevus.

This is a halo nevus because:

There is a dense, patchy, diffuse infiltrate of lymphocytes throughout the intradermal and intraepidermal portions of the neoplasm.

A halo nevus usually is a Clark's nevus in which dense infiltrates of lymphocytes are present throughout the neoplasm. However, not all nevi with this histopathologic appearance are associated with a "halo" clinically.

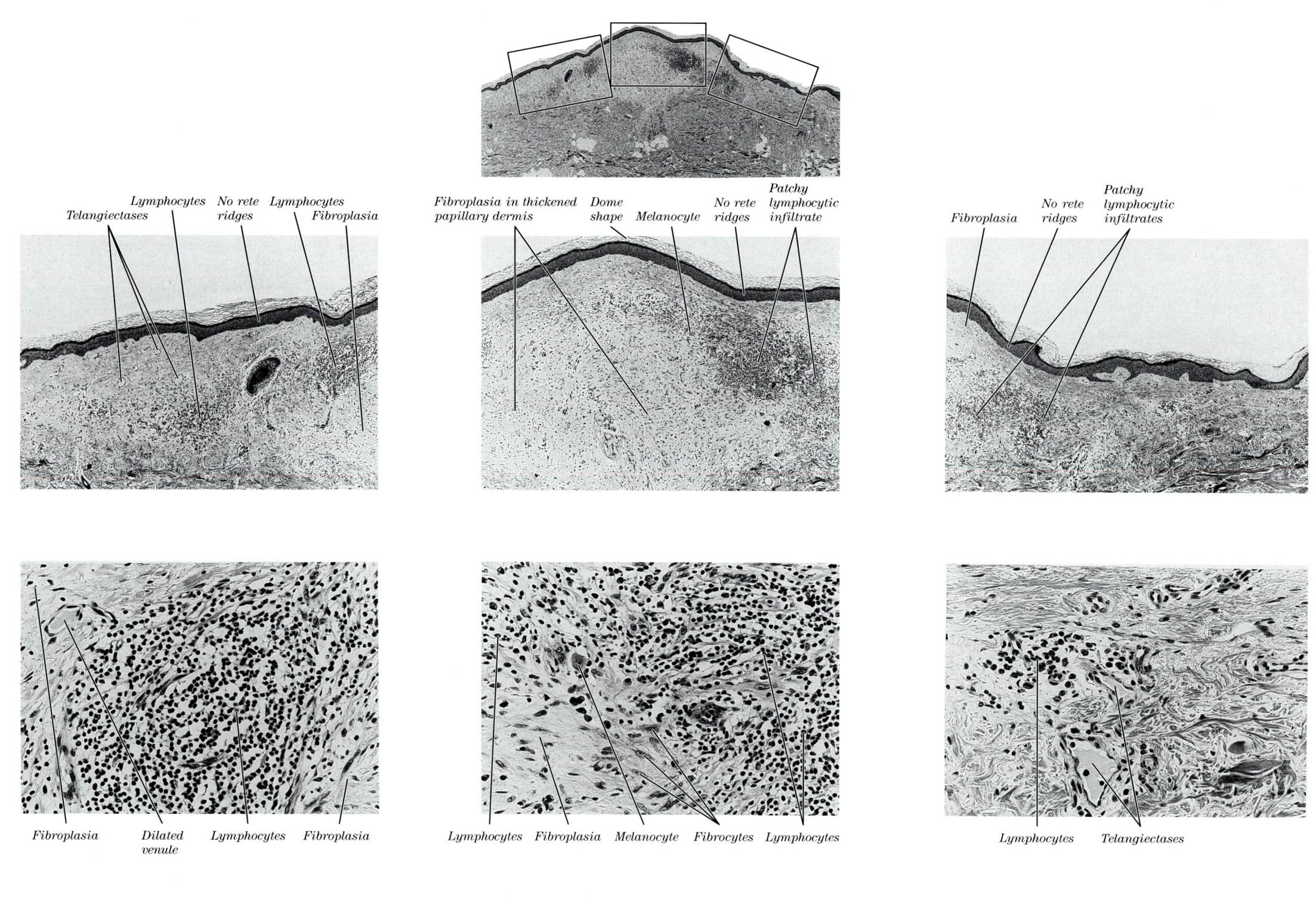

96 • Clark's Nevus *(halo type, with nearly complete regression)*

Criteria for diagnosis of this Clark's nevus (halo type) that has undergone near total regression

This is a nevus because:

1. A few melanocytes still can be identified in the markedly thickened papillary dermis.
2. The shape of the lesion and the confinement of its cells to a markedly thickened papillary dermis are consonant with the shape and distribution of melanocytes in a Clark's nevus.

This is a nearly regressed halo nevus because:

1. A moderately dense, patchy lymphocytic infiltrate is present within a thickened papillary dermis.
2. The papillary dermis is thickened mostly by fibrosis.
3. The epidermis is devoid of the undulating pattern formed normally by rete ridges and dermal papillae.
4. The number of melanocytes and the amount of melanin within the epidermis at the sides of the dome-shaped component of the lesion are both decreased.
5. Most of the melanocytes that formerly constituted this lesion have been destroyed, leaving only a few melanocytes as residuum.

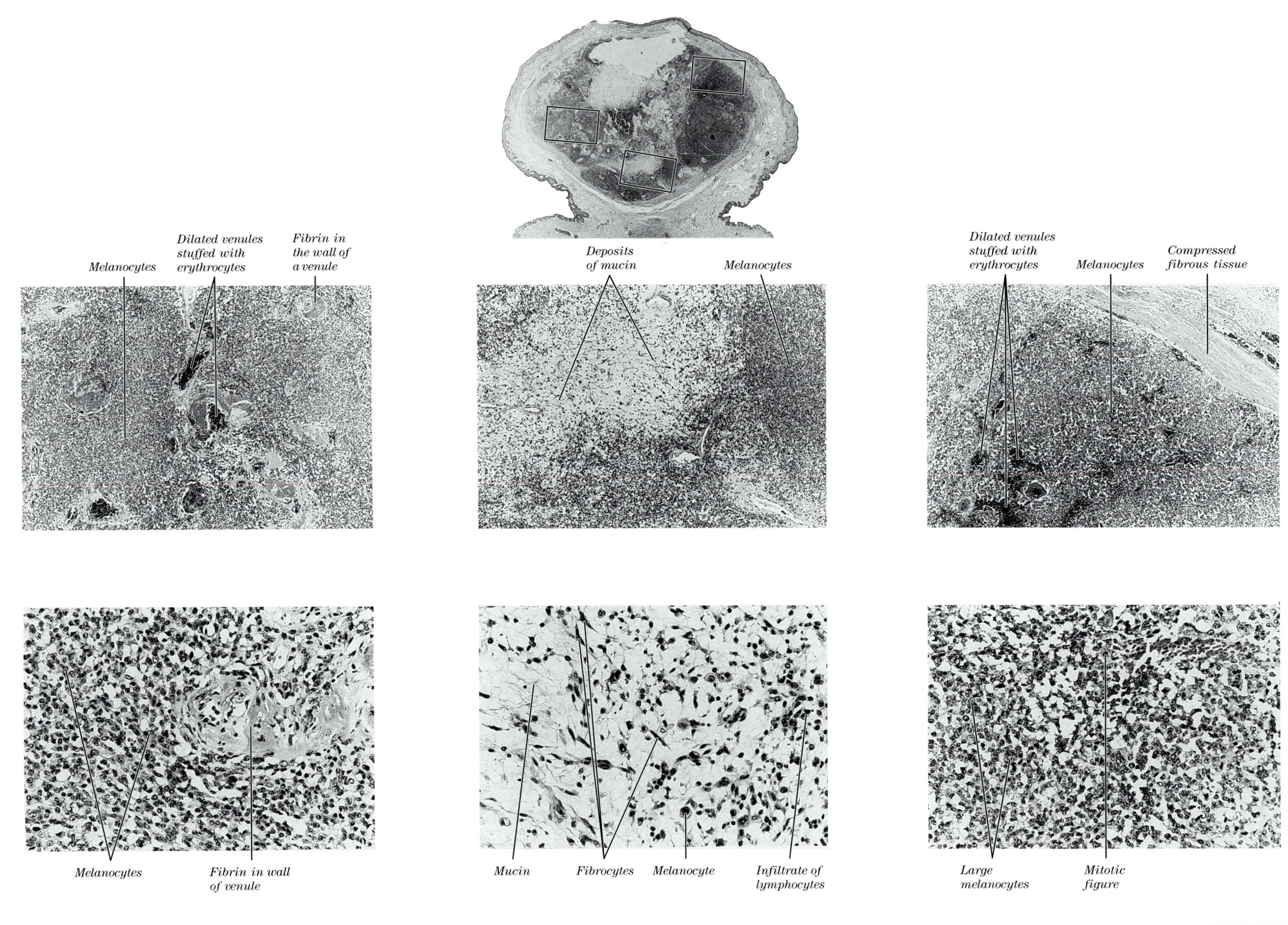

97 • Unna's Nevus *(ancient)*

Criteria for diagnosis of this ancient Unna's nevus

This neoplasm is benign because:

1. It is relatively symmetric.
2. It is well-circumscribed.
3. Clefts are present between compressed fibrous tissue that surrounds the neoplasm and the adjacent normal skin.
4. There is maturation of melanocytes.

This is an Unna's nevus because:

1. The neoplasm is polypoid.
2. The melanocytes are confined to a markedly thickened papillary dermis.

This is an ancient type of Unna's nevus because:

1. Abundant fibrin is present in the walls of numerous venules.
2. Thrombi are lodged within lumina of venules.
3. Numerous erythrocytes are extravasated in the vicinity of altered blood vessels.
4. Abundant mucin is deposited focally.
5. Many melanocytes have atypical nuclei.
6. Some melanocytes are in mitosis.

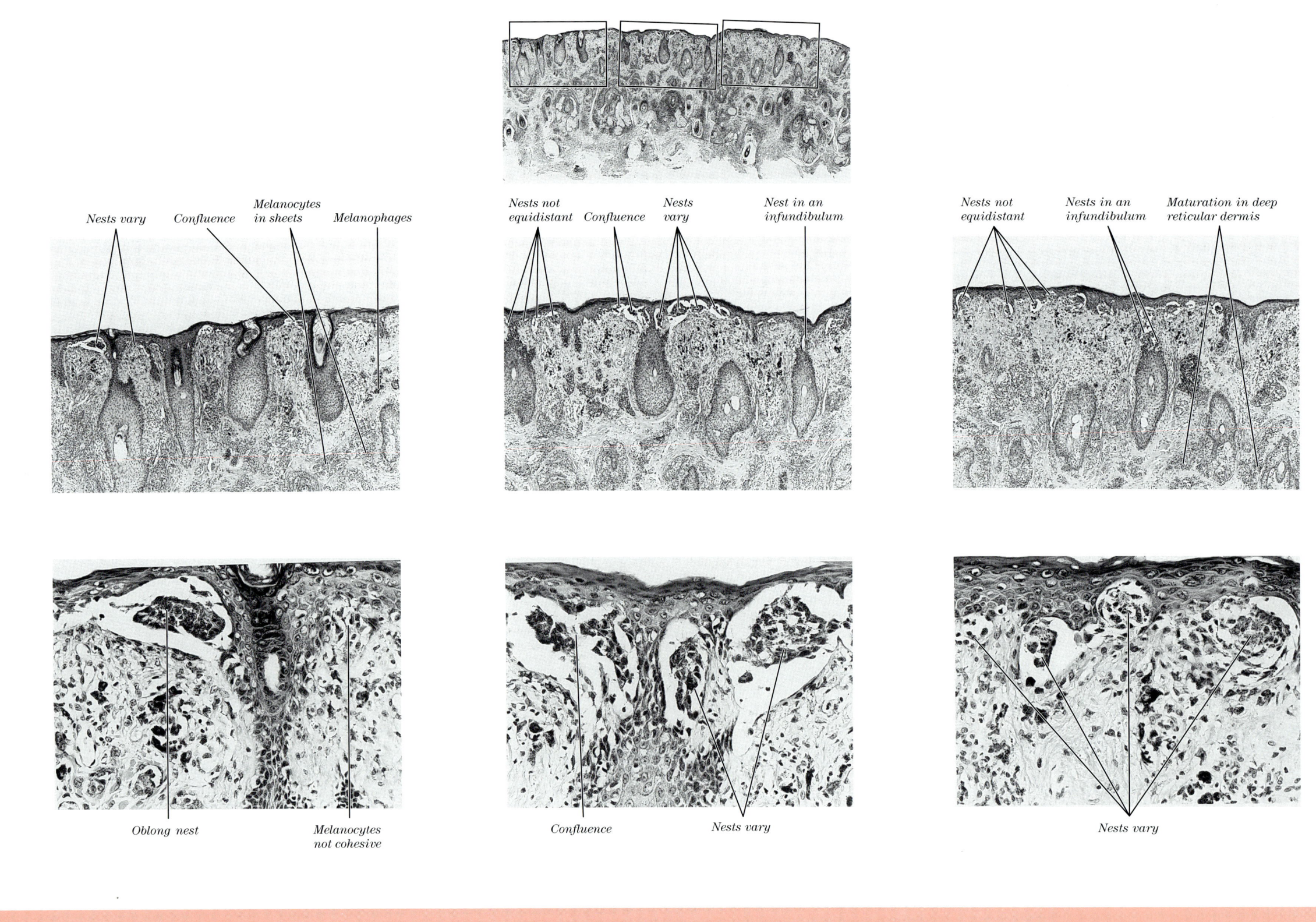

98 • Congenital Nevus *(deep type)*

Criteria for diagnosis of this non-blue congenital nevus (deep type)

This is a nevus because:

1. Nests of melanocytes within the epidermis are situated at the dermo-epidermal junction, not above it.
2. Nests of melanocytes within the epidermis are relatively equidistant from one another.
3. Nests of melanocytes within the epidermis are relatively uniform in size and shape.
4. Melanocytes mature.

This is a congenital non-blue nevus because:

1. Melanocytes are splayed between bundles of collagen throughout the reticular dermis.
2. Some melanocytes exhibit a tendency to angiocentricity and adnexocentricity.
3. The nevus is broad, i.e., greater than 2.0 cm in diameter.
4. Some melanocytes extend to the base of the reticular dermis and into septa of the subcutaneous fat.

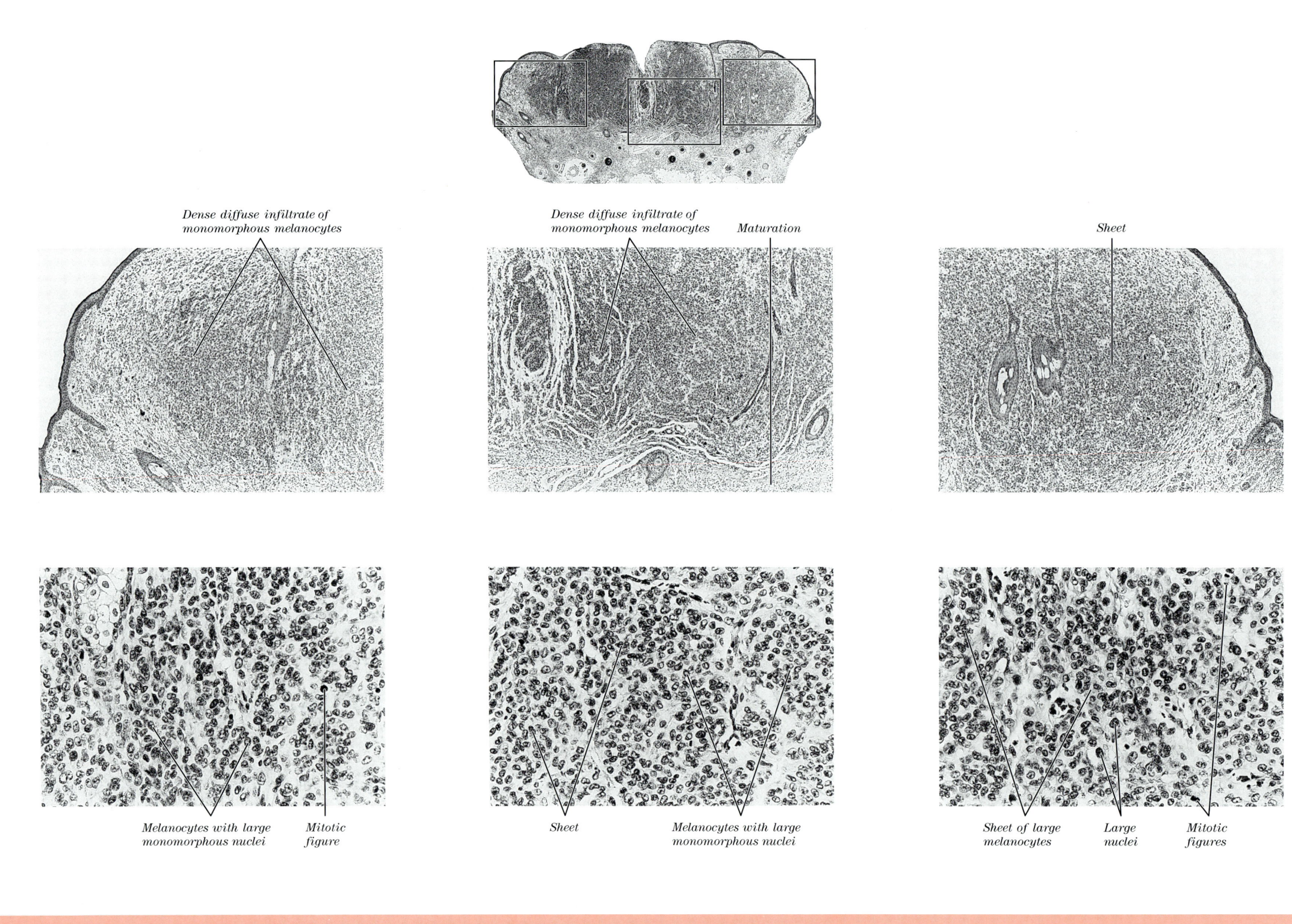

99 • Congenital Nevus *(deep type)* Biopsied Shortly After Birth

Criteria for diagnosis of this non-blue congenital nevus (deep type) biopsied shortly after birth

This is a deep non-blue congenital nevus because:

1. Throughout the entire dermis and within septa of the subcutaneous fat, to the base of the specimen, is a dense diffuse infiltrate of melanocytes.
2. The infiltrate of melanocytes is mostly monomorphous.
3. Epithelial structures of adnexa are preserved throughout.

This is a non-blue congenital nevus biopsied shortly after birth because:

1. In some nodular foci, some melanocytes have atypical nuclei.
2. There is a markedly increased number of melanocytes in mitosis within the nodules.
3. Terminal hair follicles are puny, an indication of skin of a newborn.

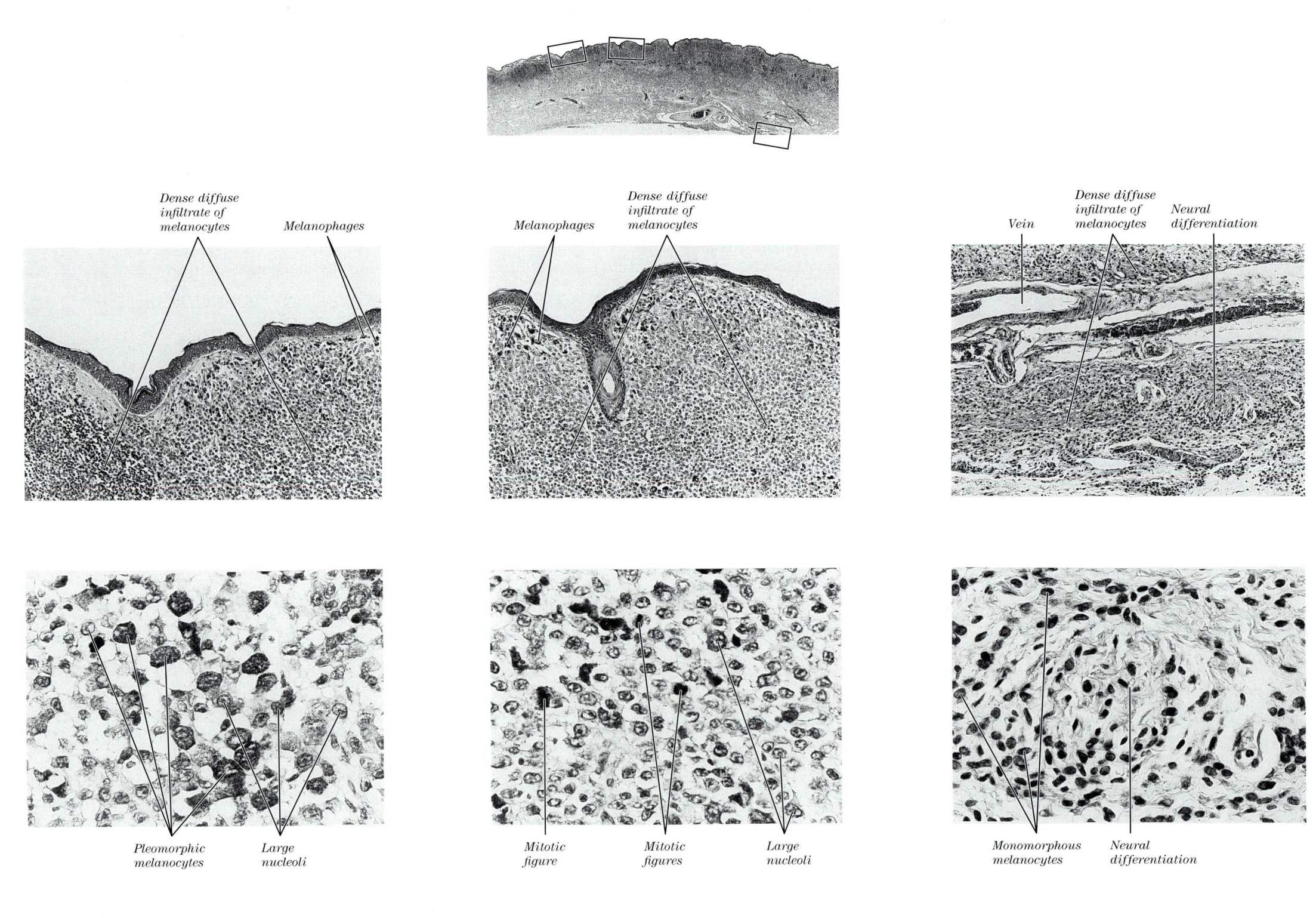

100 • Congenital Nevus *(deep type)* Biopsied Shortly After Birth

Criteria for diagnosis of this non-blue congenital nevus (deep type) biopsied shortly after birth

This is a deep non-blue congenital nevus because:

1. At scanning magnification, the infiltrate of melanocytes seems to be monomorphous.

2. At higher magnification, the melanocytes are relatively monomorphous, although their nuclei are large.

3. There is maturation of melanocytes.

4. The dermis is of uniform thickness across the entire lesion.

5. Melanophages are distributed in relatively uniform fashion in the upper part of the dermis.

Numerous mitotic figures in melanocytes is an expected finding in a section of a biopsy specimen removed from a deep congenital nevus shortly after birth.

Nevi on Genitalia of Young Adults. Melanocytic nevi on genitalia that pose the greatest problem in differentiation from melanoma are situated on the vulva, and, to a lesser extent, on the shaft of the penis. Like acquired nevi in general, those on the genitalia are symmetric, well-circumscribed, and show maturation of melanocytes with progressive descent into the dermis. Within the dermis, typical melanocytes are arranged in nests and cords. The intradermal melanocytes are located in the upper part of the dermis, and the intra-epidermal melanocytic component extends beyond the intradermal component, two features found repeatably in Clark's nevi. The changes that simulate those of melanoma are confined to the epidermis: nests of melanocytes within the epidermis that are not equidistant from one another, nests that vary in size and shape, some nests that have jagged shapes, some nests that have become confluent, and some melanocytes disposed as solitary units and/or nests may be situated above the dermo-epidermal junction (Fig. 101). The melanocytes themselves have large nuclei (although not decidedly pleomorphic or hyperchromatic ones) and abundant pale cytoplasm. This combination of findings causes nevi on the genitalia of young adults to resemble pagetoid melanoma in situ. In melanocytic nevi on the genitalia, however, few, if any, melanocytes are scattered in the upper reaches of the epidermis, and nests of melanocytes within the epidermis predominate over melanocytes arranged as solitary units across the whole front of the neoplasm. Last, the unusual changes within the epidermis are sharply circumscribed and extend across the entire intradermal portion of the nevus, that latter portion being stereotypic of a nevus.

In sum, nevi on the genitalia may be recognized for what they are by their symmetry, sharp circumscription, and maturation of melanocytes. Furthermore, within the epidermis, nests of melanocytes predominate overwhelmingly over melanocytes arranged as solitary units, and the nests are situated mostly at the dermo-epidermal junction. Last, the nuclei of melanocytes within the epidermis, although large, are monomorphous.

All of the aforementioned statements apply equally to junctional and compound nevi found on an areola of a breast, on an umbilicus, or on perianal skin.

Nevi on Palms and Soles. Melanocytic nevi situated on volar skin have all of the features of acquired nevi save one, some melanocytes arranged as solitary units and in small nests may be present in the spinous and granular zones and even in the cornified layer (Fig. 102), a finding also seen in many melanomas. In contrast to the situation in melanomas, however, melanocytes in the upper reaches of the epidermis of nevi on palms and soles have typical, rather than atypical, nuclei. The vast majority of nests are present at the dermo-epidermal junction, and nests of melanocytes predominate dramatically over melanocytes arranged as solitary units. Last, an additional clue to diagnosis of a junctional or compound nevus on a palm or sole is discrete columns of pigment in the cornified layer. When that sign, which appears above nests seated at the dermo-epidermal junction, is noted, the diagnosis is nevus, not melanoma, on volar skin.

Scatter of melanocytes above the epidermal basal layer in nevi on volar skin may be a consequence of trauma, but it is a common finding irrespective of cause, and must not lead to overdiagnosis as melanoma. Melanocytes in the cornified layer are separated from corneocytes by clefts, whereas corneocytes pigmented by melanin are cohesive and unassociated with clefts.

Nevi in Association with Lichen Sclerosus et Atrophicus in Anogenital Region. Although this association is uncommon, it may be a thorny dilemma for histopathologists seeking to diagnose a proliferation of melanocytes in the anogenital region of children and adolescents who have lichen sclerosus et atrophicus. The nevi are either junctional or compound, and the intra-epidermal changes in them may be confused with those of melanoma in situ. In the epidermis, melanocytes are arranged mostly in nests that vary in size and shape, nests have irregular shapes, and nests tend strikingly to confluence (Fig. 103). Despite these features, a proliferation of melanocytes within the epidermis above lichen sclerosus et atrophicus may be identified as those of a junctional nevus, rather than of a melanoma in situ, because virtually all of the melanocytes are arranged in nests, the nests are seated at the dermo-epidermal junction and not above it, there is no nuclear atypia, and an intradermal component, if present, consists of characteristic nests of typical melanocytes of a nevus.

Junctional Nevi above Band of Melanophages. Regression of melanoma in the form of melanosis may be simulated by a benign proliferation of melanocytes, namely, a junctional nevus with a band of melanophages across a thickened papillary dermis (Fig. 104). The melanophages are not a consequence of the effects of infiltrates of inflammatory cells on neoplastic melanocytes, but of the extraordinary synthesizing capability of melanocytes arranged in nests at the dermo-epidermal junction. When nests are spotted there, the diagnosis becomes junctional nevus, and regression of melanoma in the form of melanosis, which it simulates, no longer is a consideration. A pitfall in diagnosis is the striking band of heavily pigmented melanophages that distract a histopathologist from the often hardly noticeable nests of melanocytes at the junction.

Melanosis of the Genitalia. This condition, an analogue of oral labial lentigo, occurs mostly on the vulva of young women and less often on the penis of young men. Clinically, the lesions are flat and may be indistinguishable from those of melanoma in situ, being asymmetric, poorly circumscribed with notched, scalloped, or crenulated borders, and variegated in hues of brown. Some zones may be black. "Skip areas" of normal skin are common. A lesion of melanosis may be less than 1.0 cm or more than 5.0 cm in greatest diameter.

Histopathologically, melanosis of the genitalia is characterized by a slight increase in the number of slightly dendritic melanocytes seated at the dermo-epidermal junction (Fig. 105). The dendrites are revealed to be more elongated when they are colored by the Fontana-Masson silver stain. Nuclei of the melanocytes are small and monomorphous. There is no atypia. Early lesions of melanoma in situ on genital skin and on mucous membranes also are typified by a proliferation of dendritic melanocytes, but the dendrites are strikingly elongated, some of them extending to near the surface of those epithelia. The melanocytes in those intra-epithelial melanomas, in contrast to those in melanosis of the genitalia, may have atypical nuclei, are not equidistant from one another, may be situated above the dermo-epidermal junction, and may be nested subtly. None of these findings, including nests of melanocytes, are ever seen in melanosis of the genitalia.

Melanocytic Proliferation in the Epidermis above Some Intradermal Miescher's Nevi. Sometimes above typical intradermal nevi, especially of Miescher, but also of Unna, there may be a proliferation of melanocytes with large nuclei at the dermo-epidermal junction and just above the junction, and at the junction of epithelial structures of adnexa and the dermis and just above it. In addition to possessing large, roundish, monomorphous nuclei, the melanocytes sometimes have abundant cytoplasm. Most of the melanocytes, however, are situated at those junctions and not above them. Furthermore, they are all arranged as solitary units there, not in nests, and the individual units are relatively equidistant from one another.

A proliferation of large monomorphous melanocytes arranged as solitary units at the dermo-epidermal junction above some intradermal Miescher's nevi is an expected finding and should not be misconstrued as an early melanoma in situ.

Melanocytic Proliferation in the Epidermis above Some Fibrous Papules of the Face. Fibrous papule of the face, known also as perifollicular fibroma, has the same histopathologic features as do lesions of adenoma sebaceum in patients with tuberous sclerosis. In contrast, fibrous papule usually is a solitary lesion situated on the nose. The condition is fundamentally a hamartoma with pecular follicular, perifollicular, and angiomatous features. It is small, symmetric, and well-circumscribed. Numerous stellate and multinucleated fibrocytes are scattered throughout the dermis, in concert with perifollicular fibroplasia and telangiectases. Follicles often are malformed and are oriented peculiarly. In a minority of instances, proliferation of large melanocytes is seen at the dermo-epidermal junction and sometimes at the junction of epithelial structures of adnexa and dermis (Fig. 106). These changes are similar to those described in the epidermis above intradermal nevi of Miescher and of Unna, i.e., the melanocytes, although increased in number and large, are monomorphous and equidistant from one another. They, too, are expected findings and pose a problem in diagnosis only when a fibrous papule has been removed by shave biopsy technique performed so superficially that the specimen consists almost entirely of epidermis. Sections from such thin specimens have, on occasion, been misinterpreted as "lentigo maligna," a euphemism for melanoma in situ.

Melanocytic Proliferation in the Epidermis of Severely Sun-Damaged Skin, Especially of a Face. Biopsy specimens from skin badly injured by ultraviolet light, especially of the face, often reveal an increased number of melanocytes, some of them atypical, at the dermo-epidermal junction only, not above it (Fig. 107). An increased number of such melanocytes also may be present in the upper portions of epithelial structures of adnexa. It may be impossible to differentiate those findings from the earliest stage of melanoma in situ. The ultimate judgment about such changes must be the responsibility of the clinician; a histopathologist is unable to render a deci-

Text continues on page 228

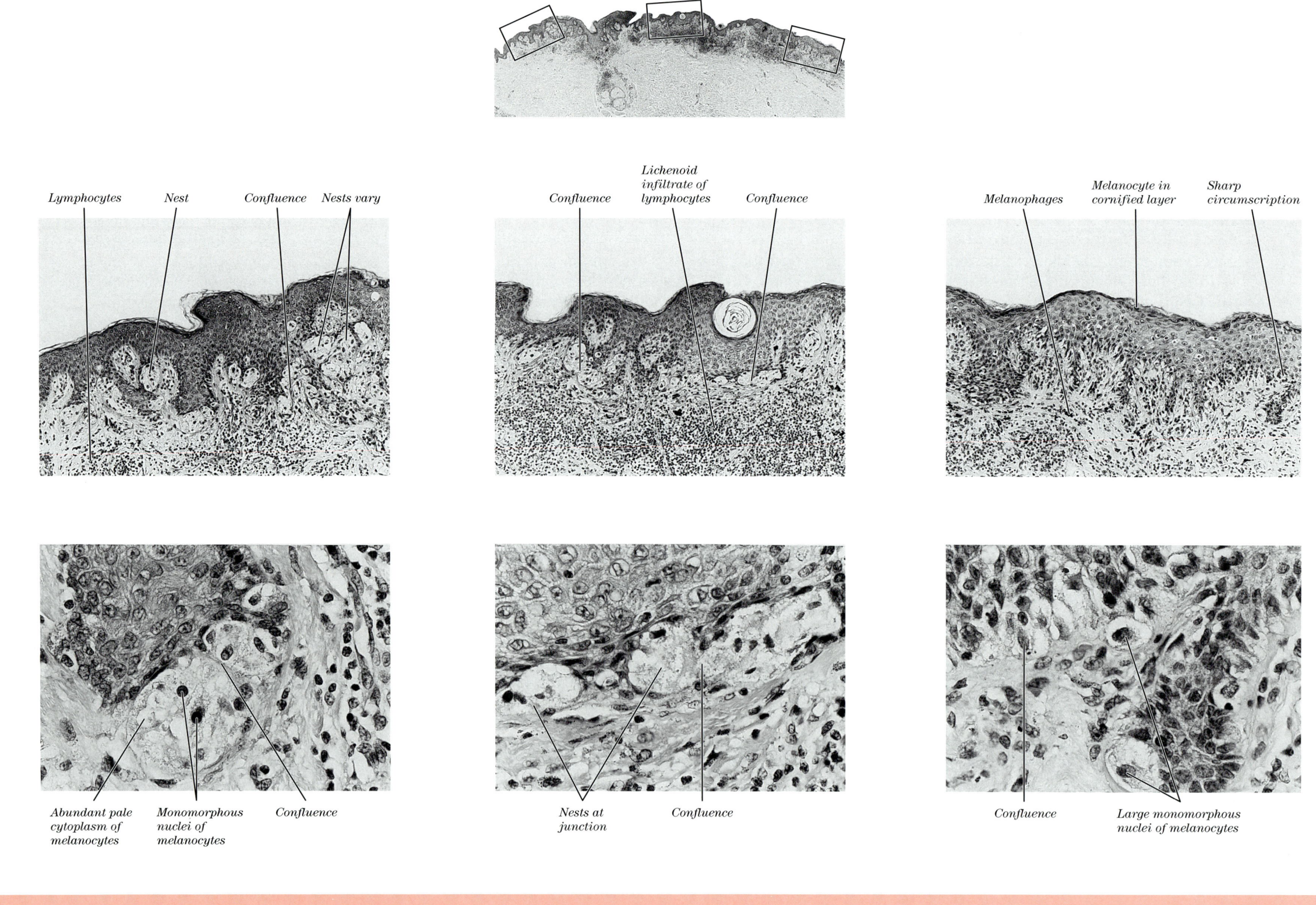

214 101 • Clark's Nevus *(on genital skin)*

Criteria for diagnosis of this Clark's nevus (compound type) on genital skin

This is a nevus because:

1. The lesion is well-circumscribed.
2. Melanocytes arranged in nests within the epidermis predominate overwhelmingly over melanocytes arrayed as solitary units there.
3. Nests of melanocytes within the epidermis are seated wholly at the dermo-epidermal junction; none are above it.
4. Most melanocytes within the epidermis have relatively monomorphous nuclei.

This is a Clark's nevus because:

1. The lesion is slightly elevated and gently mammillated.
2. Nests of melanocytes are confined to the epidermis and the equivalent of a thickened papillary dermis.

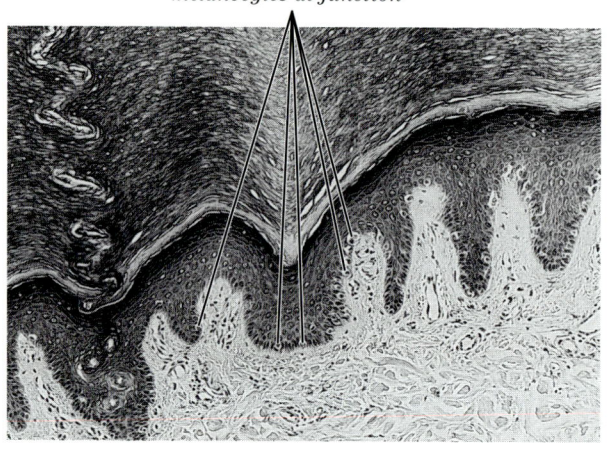
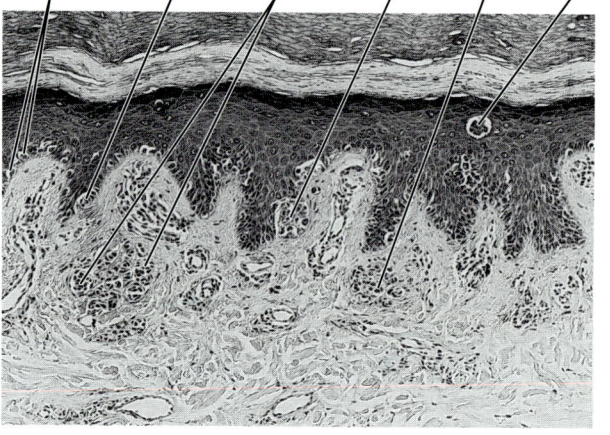
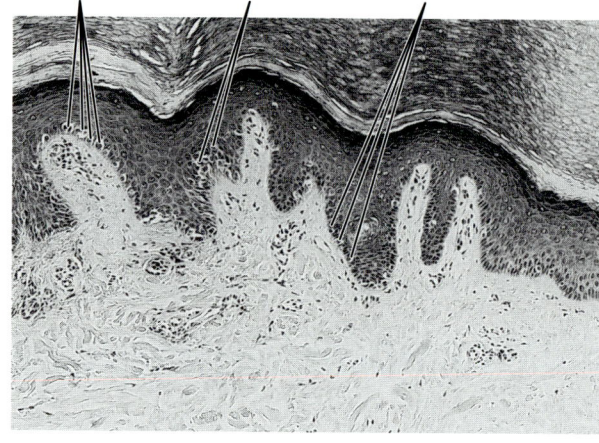
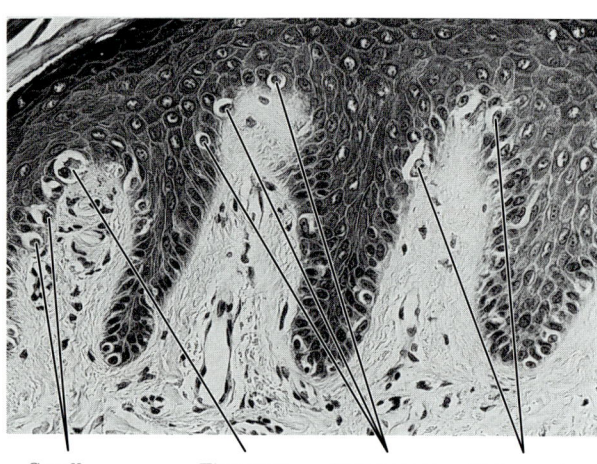
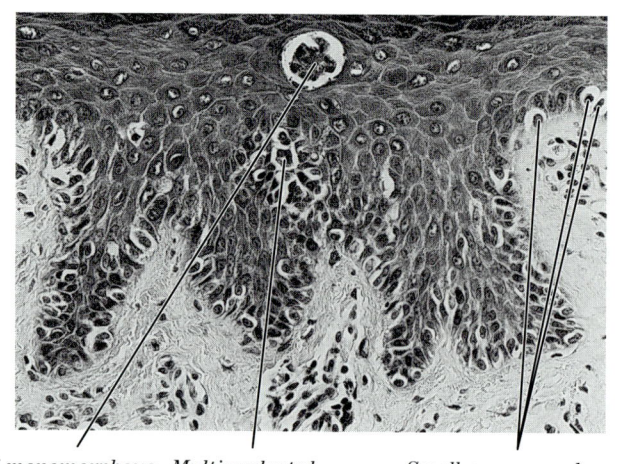
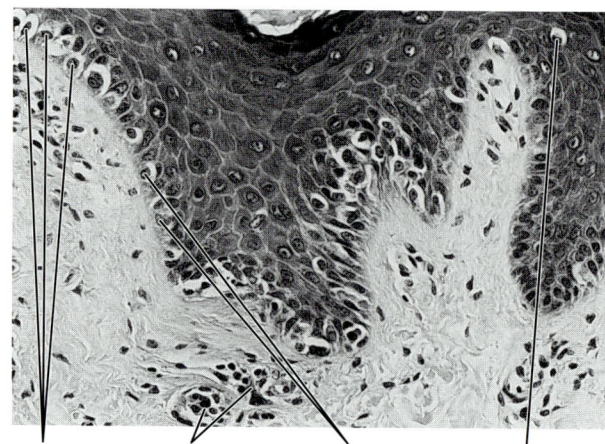

102 • Clark's Nevus

Criteria for diagnosis of this Clark's nevus (compound type) on volar skin

This is a nevus because:

1. The lesion is symmetric.
2. Melanocytes mature.
3. Melanocytes within the epidermis have relatively monomorphous nuclei.
4. Most melanocytes within the epidermis are situated at the dermo-epidermal junction.

This is a Clark's nevus because:

The slightly elevated nevus is confined to the epidermis and thickened papillary dermis.

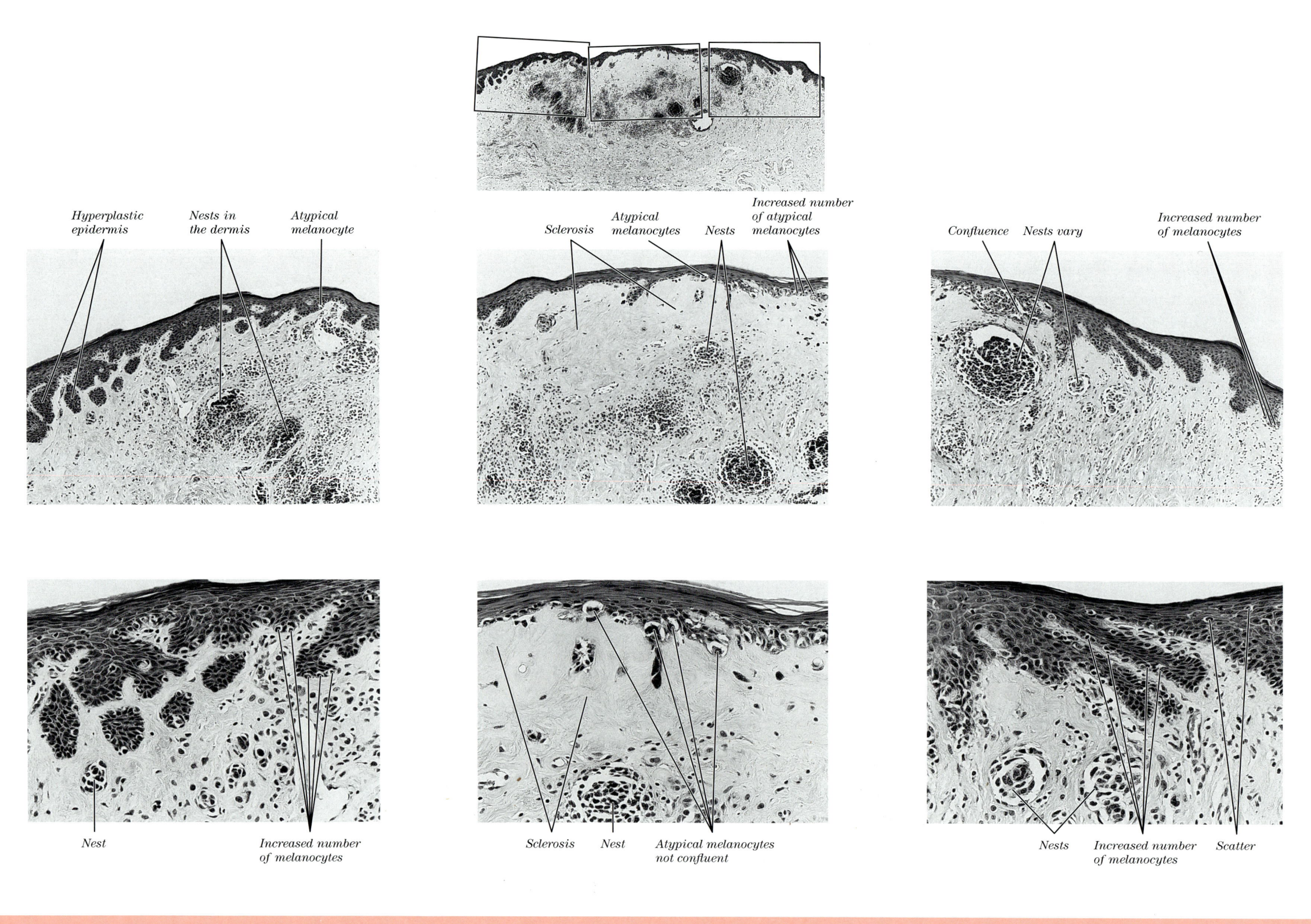

103 • Clark's Nevus and Lichen Sclerosus et Atrophicus

Criteria for diagnosis of this Clark's nevus (compound type) in association with lichen sclerosus et atrophicus

This is lichen sclerosus et atrophicus because:

A zone of sclerosis is present across a front of thickened papillary dermis.

This is a compound nevus because:

There are nests of melanocytes within the epidermis and in the upper part of the dermis.

This is a Clark's nevus because:

Nests of melanocytes are confined to the epidermis and thickened papillary dermis of the slightly elevated lesion.

The proliferation of melanocytes within the epidermis above the zone of lichen sclerosis et atrophicus could be misinterpreted as that of melanoma in situ because melanocytes arranged as solitary units predominate over nests in some high-power fields, the nests of melanocytes are not equidistant from one another, some nests of melanocytes have become confluent, melanocytes in some "nests" are not cohesive, and the nuclei of some melanocytes are atypical. Despite these findings, the overall architectural pattern of the melanocytic neoplasm, that is, its relative symmetry, sharp circumscription, and maturation of melanocytes, all indicate that this lesion is a nevus and not a melanoma.

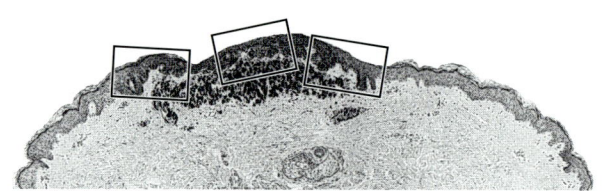

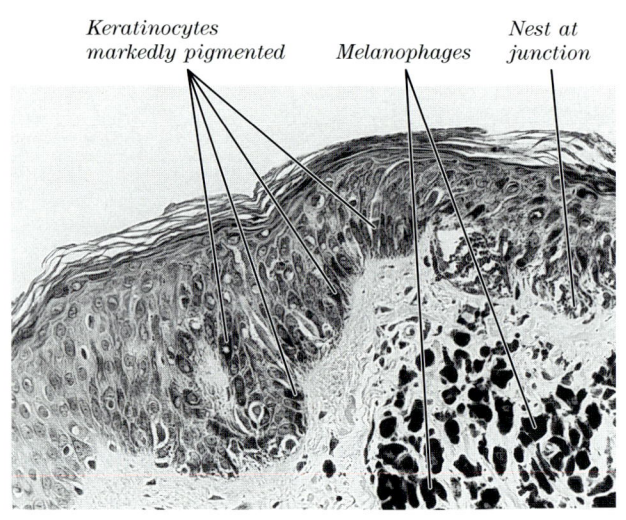

Keratinocytes markedly pigmented | Melanophages | Nest at junction

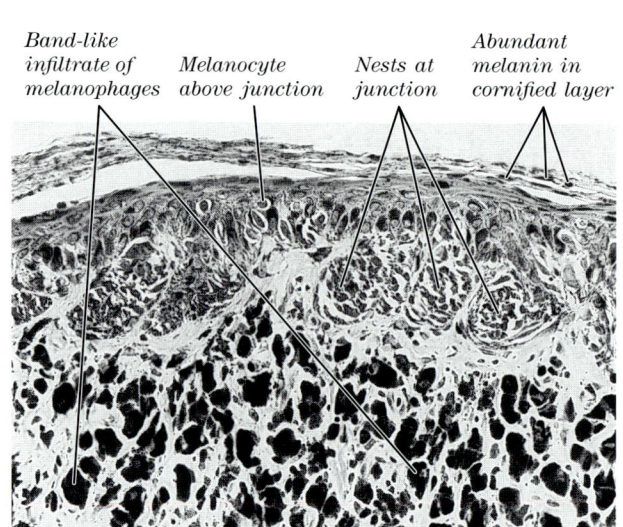

Band-like infiltrate of melanophages | Melanocyte above junction | Nests at junction | Abundant melanin in cornified layer

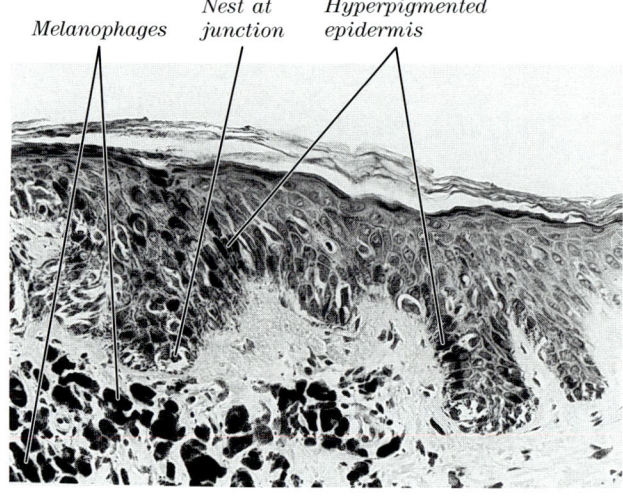

Melanophages | Nest at junction | Hyperpigmented epidermis

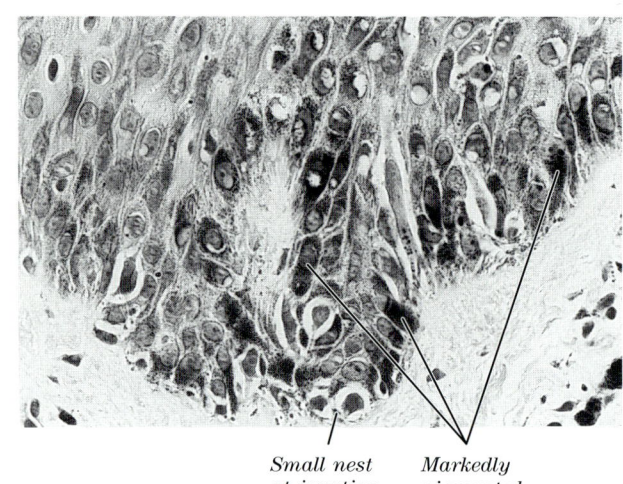

Small nest at junction | Markedly pigmented keratinocytes

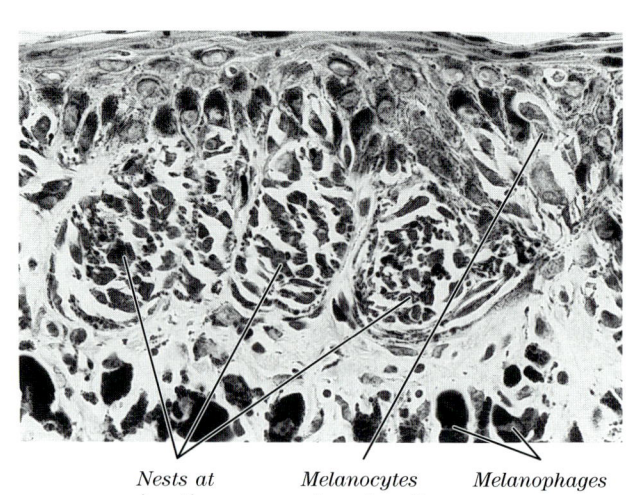

Nests at junction | Melanocytes above junction | Melanophages

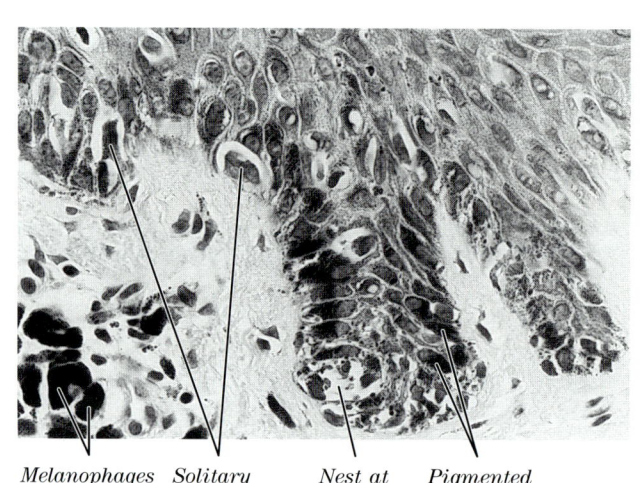

Melanophages | Solitary melanocytes at junction | Nest at junction | Pigmented keratinocytes

104 • Clark's Nevus

Criteria for diagnosis of this Clark's nevus (junctional type) above a band of melanophages

This is a junctional nevus because:

1. The neoplasm is very small.
2. The neoplasm is well-circumscribed.
3. Melanocytes within the epidermis are arranged mostly in nests rather than as solitary units.
4. Nests of melanocytes are situated at the dermo-epidermal junction, not above it.
5. Nuclei of melanocytes are relatively monomorphous.
6. A few melanocytes arrayed as solitary units are dendritic and present above the dermo-epidermal junction, but all of them are situated in the lower part of the epidermis.

The epidermis is markedly pigmented as a consequence of the proliferation of melanocytes. Pigmentation is seen particularly well in the cornified layer where abundant melanin is apparent. The band of melanophages in the thickened papillary dermis could be confused with melanosis, one sign of regression of melanoma. The fact that the band is present beneath a junctional nevus, however, indicates that it is related to the nevus and not to regression of a melanoma.

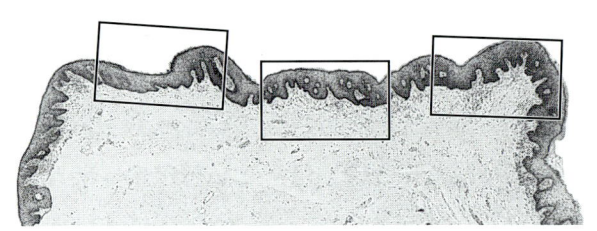

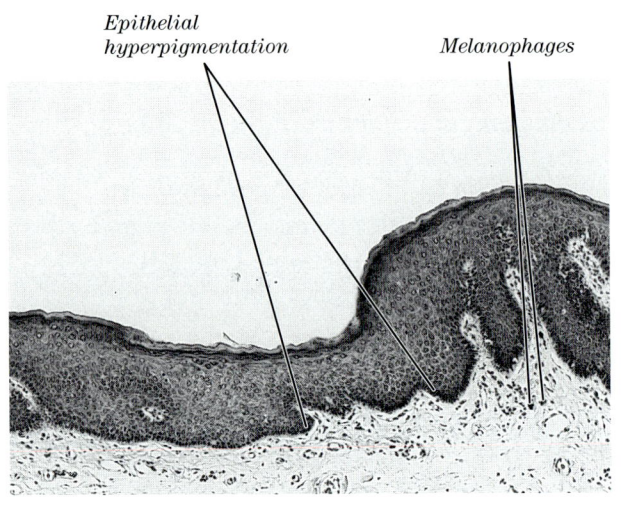
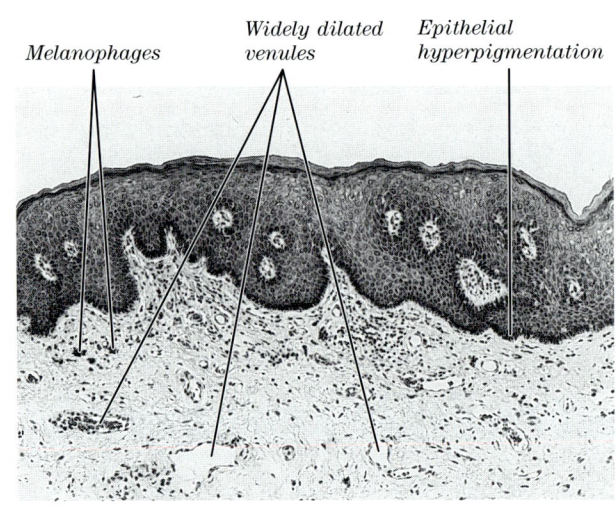
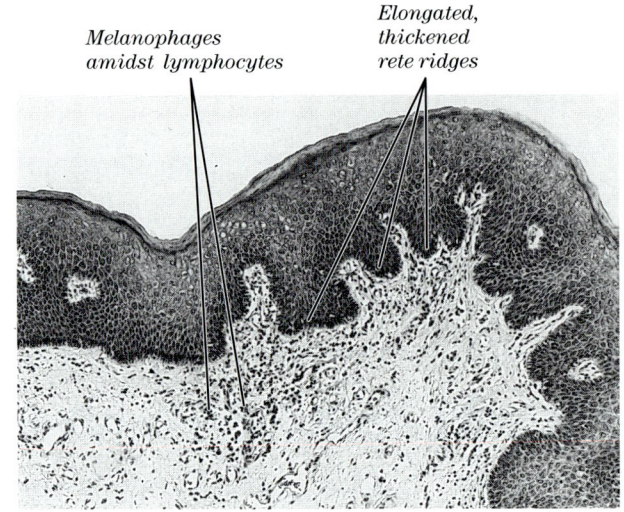

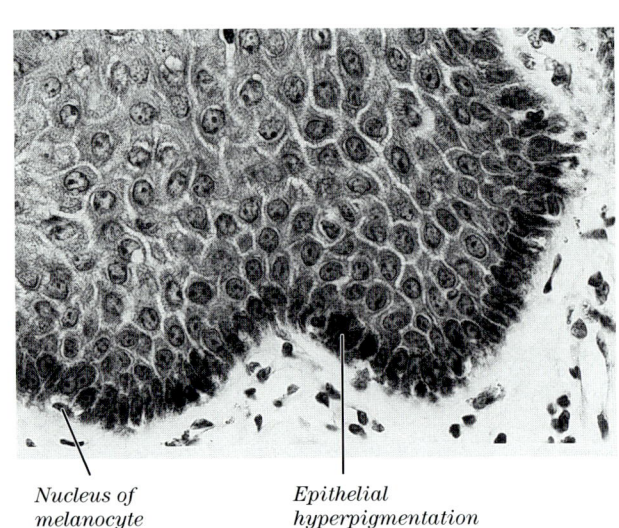
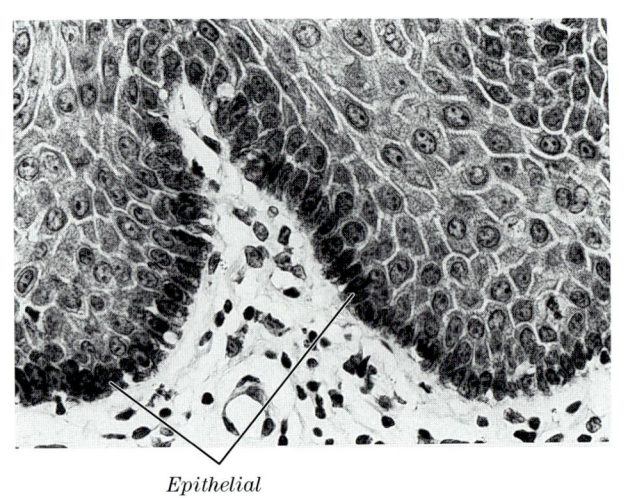
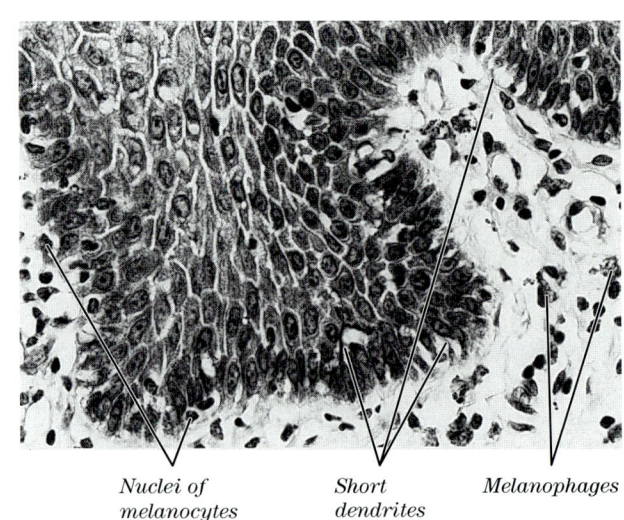

105 • Melanosis of the Genitalia

Criteria for diagnosis of melanosis of the genitalia

This is melanosis of the genitalia because:

1. Across a broad front, there is a slight increase in the number of typical melanocytes arranged as solitary units at the dermo-epidermal junction, and some of those melanocytes have stubby, but discernible, dendrites.

2. An increased amount of melanin is distributed in rather uniform fashion across the entire lesion.

3. The lesion is situated on genital skin.

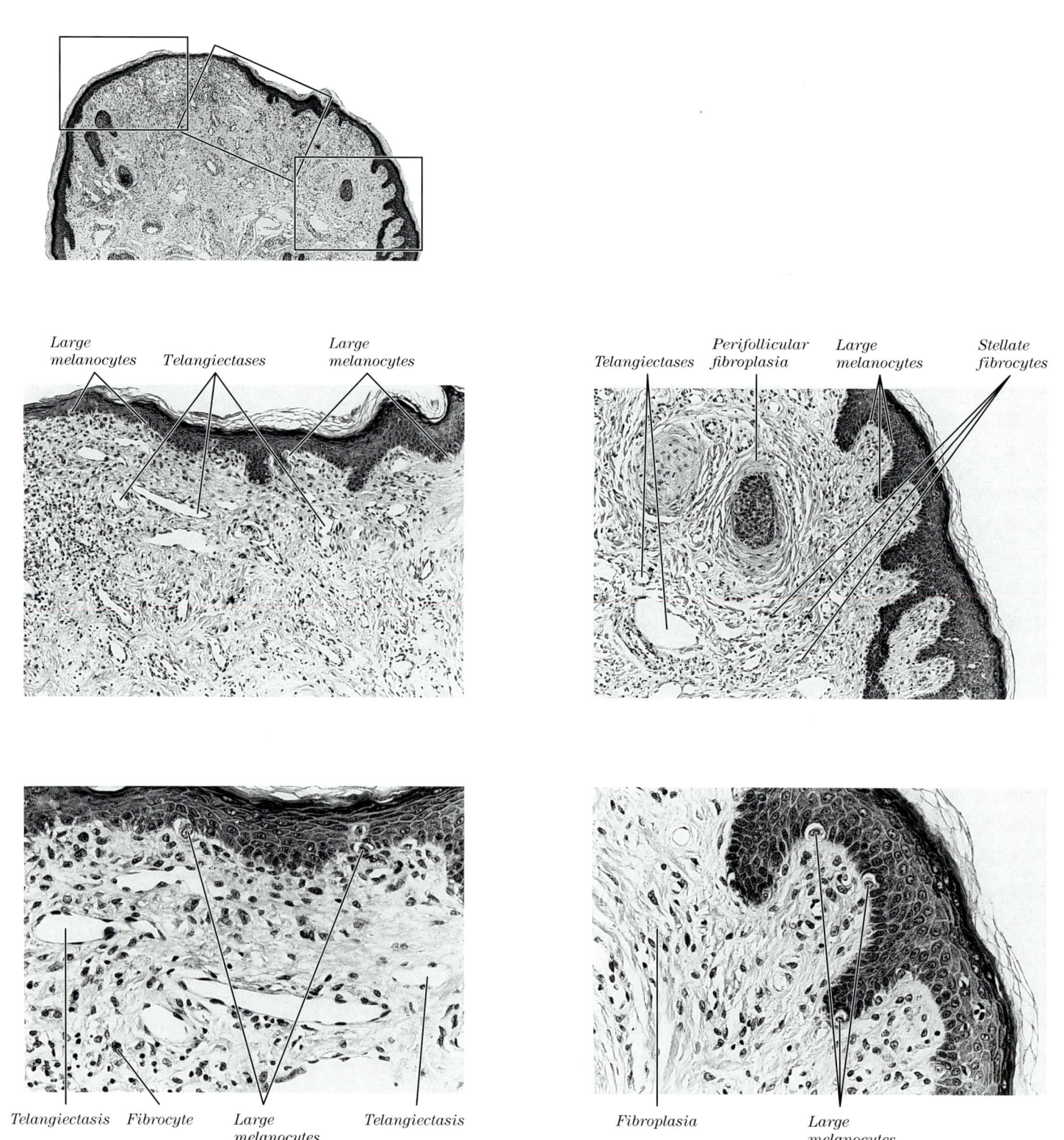

224

106 • Fibrous Papule of the Face

Criteria for diagnosis of this fibrous papule of the face

This is a fibrous papule because:

1. The lesion is small, well-circumscribed, and domed.
2. Hair follicles are not distributed in uniform fashion.
3. There is striking perifollicular fibroplasia.
4. Angiofibromatous features are prominent.
5. An increased number of large melanocytes with slightly pleomorphic nuclei are situated at the dermo-epidermal junction.

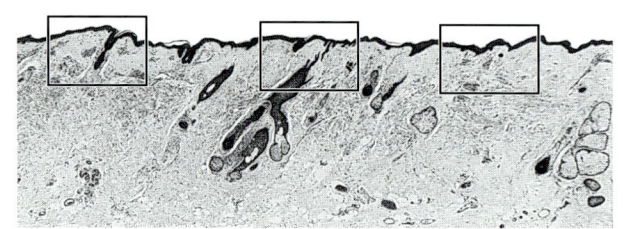

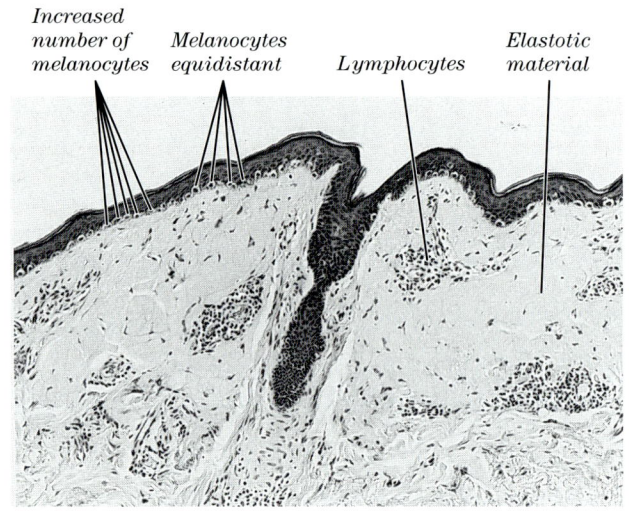

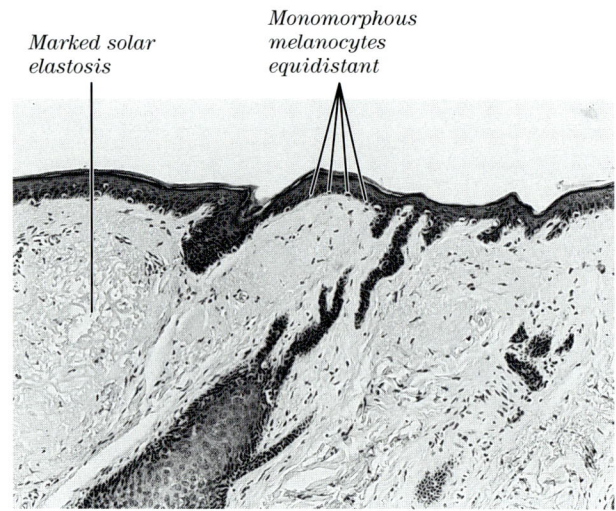

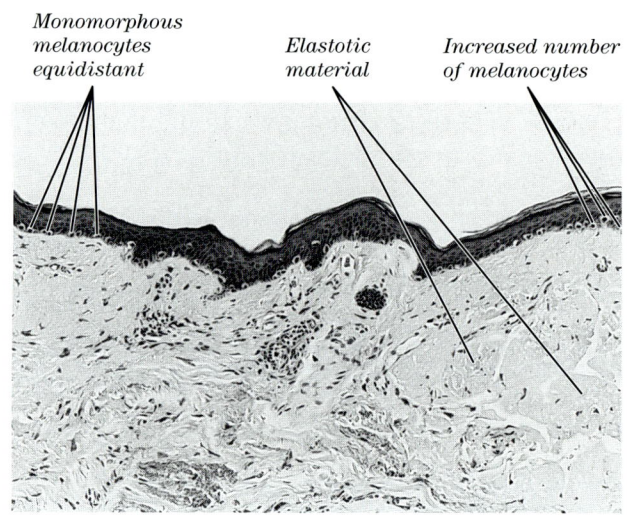

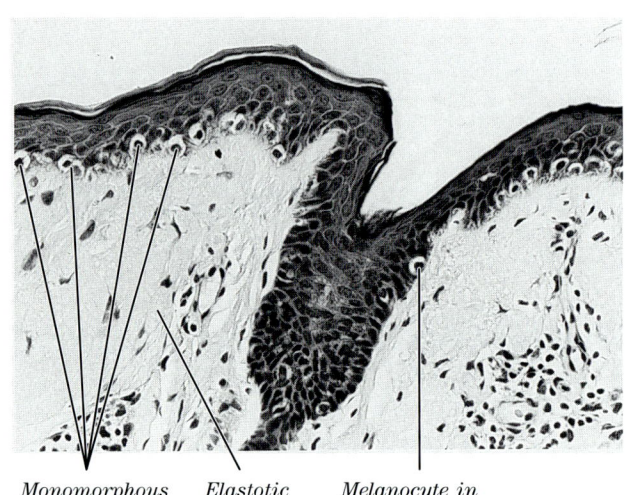

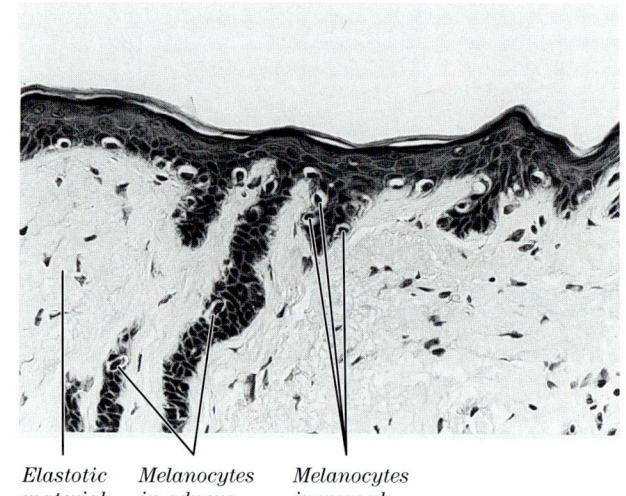

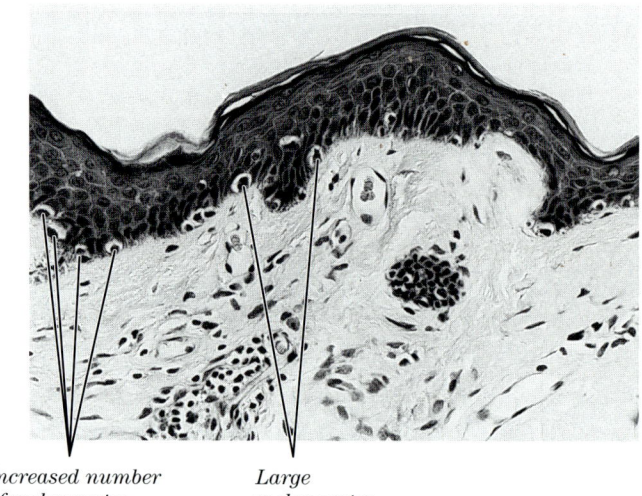

107 · Melanocytes on Sun-Damaged Skin

Criteria for diagnosis of this benign proliferation of melanocytes at the dermo-epidermal junction above a dermis that is badly damaged by ultraviolet light

This is a benign proliferation of melanocytes at the dermo-epidermal junction above sun-damaged dermis because:

1. Virtually all the melanocytes are situated at the dermo-epidermal junction or in the basal layer.//

2. The melanocytes are approximately equidistant from one another.

3. The nuclei of melanocytes are monomorphous, i.e., they are smallish, oval, and devoid of nucleoli.

4. Only a few melanocytes are present in the upper part of epithelial structures of adnexa.

5. Extensive solar elastosis is apparent throughout the reticular dermis.

sion about them with surety. Together at a microscope, clinician and histopathologist can come to a decision that is in the best interest of the patient.

A difficult and related problem for a histopathologist is assessment of margins of melanomas in situ on severely sun-damaged skin of the face. Even if a surgeon removes several centimeters of apparently normal skin around such a melanoma, there may be an increased number of melanocytes at the dermo-epidermal junction in the margins. Some nuclei of those melanocytes may be atypical. Has the neoplasm in question been removed completely or is more surgery necessary? Again, a histopathologist may not be able to answer that question with certainty. The decision must be the surgeon's based upon clinical observations and practical considerations, e.g., whether there is any evidence of a residual pigmented lesion, whether the patient is sufficiently responsible and reliable that meticulous follow-up can be assured in order to discover signs of persistence of the pigmented lesion should it recur, and whether it is feasible to excise more skin at that particular anatomic site.

Melanocytic Proliferation in the Epidermis of Solar Lentigines. Solar lentigines are proliferations of keratinocytes on skin that has been exposed chronically to the damaging effects of ultraviolet light. In contrast, simple lentigines are proliferations of melanocytes disposed as solitary units in the basal layer of an epidermis in skin that has not been injured by sunlight. Solar lentigines eventuate in reticulated seborrheic keratoses, whereas simple lentigines in time become junctional nevi. Although solar lentigines are hyperpigmented as a consequence of an increased amount of melanin within keratinocytes, they generally are not accompanied by a strikingly increased number of melanocytes. Sometimes, however, there is a definite increase in number of large melanocytes in the row of basal cells in solar lentigines (Fig. 108). This feature may be misinterpreted as an early stage in the development of melanoma in situ. The dilemma is particularly trying when the diagnosis of the clinician is "solar lentigo rule out lentigo maligna." That the finding is merely an integral component of some solar lentigines and unrelated to melanoma may be deduced from the facts that the melanocytes are seated entirely in the basal layer of the epidermis, not above it, are equidistant from one another, and are unassociated with nests of melanocytes, even tiny ones. Furthermore, the nuclei of the large melanocytes are monomorphous.

Melanocytic Proliferation in the Epidermis of Normal Skin of an Eyelid. For reasons not yet explicable, sections from biopsy specimens removed from ostensibly normal eyelids of adults often show what seem to be an increased number of large melanocytes at the dermo-epidermal junction (Fig. 109). Sometimes, the changes are accompanied by solar elastosis in variable quantities, but in most instances the dermis is normal. In either circumstance, the proliferation of large melanocytes within the epidermis can be confused for a very early lesion of melanoma in situ. The wholly benign nature of the findings on an eyelid is confirmed by noting their positions equidistant from one another, their location entirely at the dermo-epidermal junction, their expression as solitary units only, never in nests, and their monomorphous quality.

B. Non-Melanocytic Simulators

A variety of conditions devoid of any proliferation of melanocytes may simulate melanoma histopathologically. They include changes within the epidermis that resemble melanoma in situ, e.g., "clear cell" artifacts in keratinocytes induced during the processing of specimens, extramammary Paget's disease, mammary Paget's disease, pagetoid Bowen's disease, and pagetoid reticulosis (Woringer-Kolopp disease, mycosis fungoides); alterations within the dermis that can be confused with a metastasis of melanoma, e.g., carbon tattoo and histiocytoma-dermatofibroma laden with siderophages, and changes that resemble regression of primary melanoma, e.g., regression of lichen planus-like keratosis and caricatures of postinflammatory pigmentary alteration.

In brief, clefts that result from shrinkage of cytoplasm of keratinocytes in the process of preparing tissues for sectioning form immediately around nuclei, whereas artefacts of similar cause in melanocytes surround narrow rims of cytoplasm (Fig. 110). In extramammary Paget's disease, a primary apocrine adenocarcinoma that originates within the epidermis, there is no proliferation of neoplastic cells at the dermo-epidermal junction, only in the basal layer and above it (Fig. 111). The neoplastic cells contain abundant acid mucosubstances that cause them to resemble signet rings. In mammary Paget's disease, an adenocarcinoma that begins in lactiferous ducts and extends by continuity into the epidermis, and that represents an entirely different pathologic process from extramammary Paget's disease, there also are no neoplastic cells at the dermo-epidermal junction, only in the basal layer and above it. The absence of neoplastic cells arranged as solitary units or in nests at the dermo-epidermal junction precludes the possibility of melanoma. Pagetoid Bowen's disease, an expression of squamous-cell carcinoma in situ, shows evidences of cornification in the form of dyskeratosis and either orthokeratosis or parakeratosis, findings that are not usual in melanoma. Furthermore, neoplastic cells are not positioned at the dermo-epidermal junction, only above it (Fig. 112). Pagetoid reticulosis, a euphemism for one manifestation of mycosis fungoides, differs from other pagetoid simulators of melanoma by absence of abundant pale cytoplasm. Because the neoplastic cells are lymphocytes, they possess scant cytoplasm. Moreover, the lymphocytes are not seated at the dermo-epidermal junction, but are scattered randomly on either side of it, being aligned often as solitary units within the basal layer of the epidermis itself (Fig. 113).

Carbon in tattoos is scattered mostly extracellularly, never in neoplastic cells, but sometimes in macrophages. In addition, the jet black pigment is darker than melanin and is distributed in clumps that have jagged outlines (Fig. 114). The many siderophages in some histiocytomas-dermatofibromas may be misinterpreted as melanophages of a metastasis of melanoma, but they can be recognized for what they are by the yellowish hue and refractile quality of hemosiderin. Confirmation of the iron-containing nature of those macrophages can be accomplished by exposing them to Perls' stain, which colors them aquamarine.

Lichen planus-like keratosis is a solar lentigo or seborrheic keratosis, usually reticulated, that attracts a dense, band-like infiltrate of lymphocytes to it and, in the process, is destroyed by the products of those lymphocytes (Fig. 115). En route to regression, when lichen planus-like keratosis is fully developed, it may be confused with the lichenoid lymphocytic stage in regression of melanoma. When the keratosis regresses, it leaves residua that are nearly indistinguishable from those of regression of melanoma, to wit, a papillary dermis thickened by fibroplasia, patchy lymphocytic infiltrates, scattered melanophages, and telangiectases (Fig. 116). Furthermore, the presence of numerous necrotic keratinocytes (colloid bodies, Civatte bodies, apoptotic bodies) in the papillary dermis of lichen planus-like keratosis is not differentiating from melanoma. The same structures may be noted in a zone of regression of melanoma.

In short, it may be impossible at times to distinguish between regression of a lichen planus-like keratosis and regression of melanoma. If a remnant of a solar lentigo or reticulated seborrheic keratosis can be identified contiguous with a zone of regression, it is presumptive evidence of a lichen planus-like keratosis that has undergone regression.

In dark-skinned persons, especially in Africans or those of African descent, the aftermath of inflammatory processes that affect the dermo-epidermal junction may be changes that resemble, to variable extent, those of regression of melanoma. Those changes, in brief, are melanophages, a patchy lymphocytic infiltrate, and telangiectases in a thickened papillary dermis. The findings that follow inflammatory reactions that injure basal keratinocytes, but also melanocytes at the dermo-epidermal junction, differ from those in the most common expression (fibrosis) of regression of melanoma by absence of prominent fibroplasia in the altered papillary dermis and from those in the less uncommon expression (melanosis) of melanoma by exhibiting far fewer melanophages. Furthermore, the melanophages in post-inflammatory pigmentary changes tend to be in perivascular, rather than in lichenoid, array. Despite its similarities to regression of melanoma, post-inflammatory pigmentary alteration differs from it in several respects.

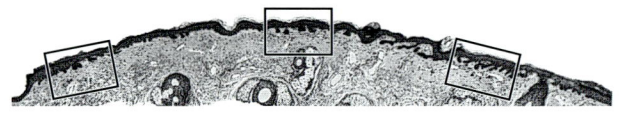

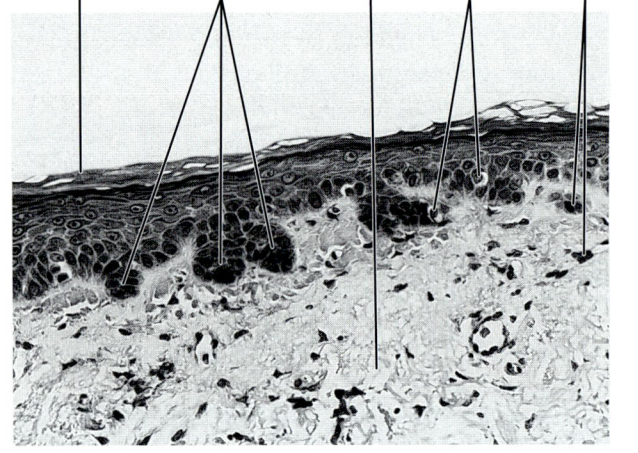

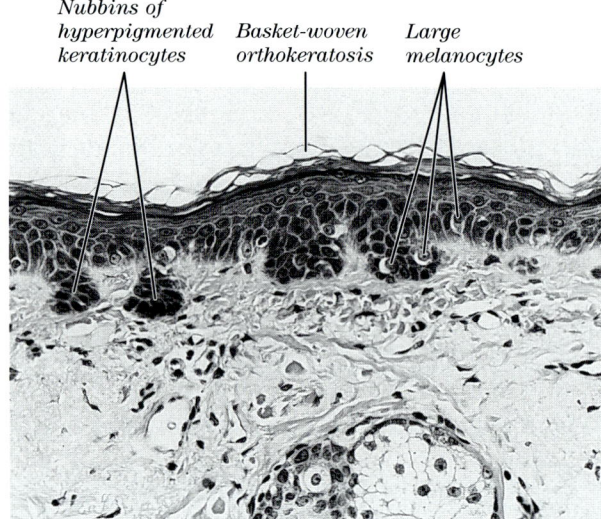

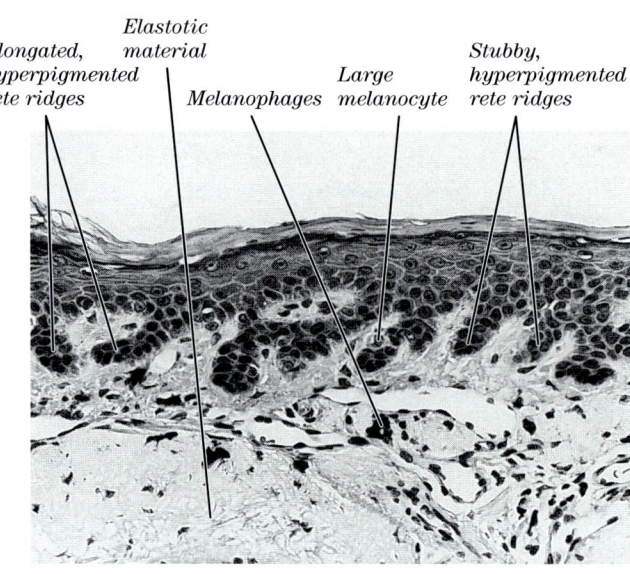

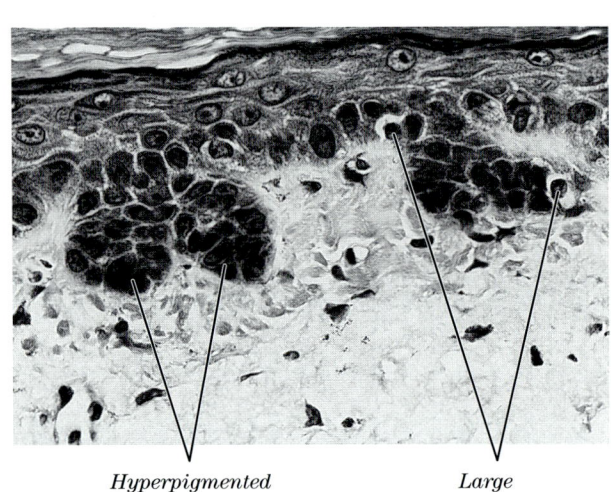

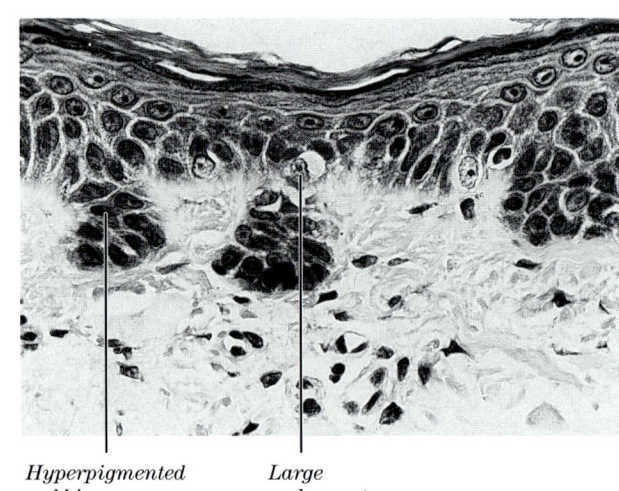

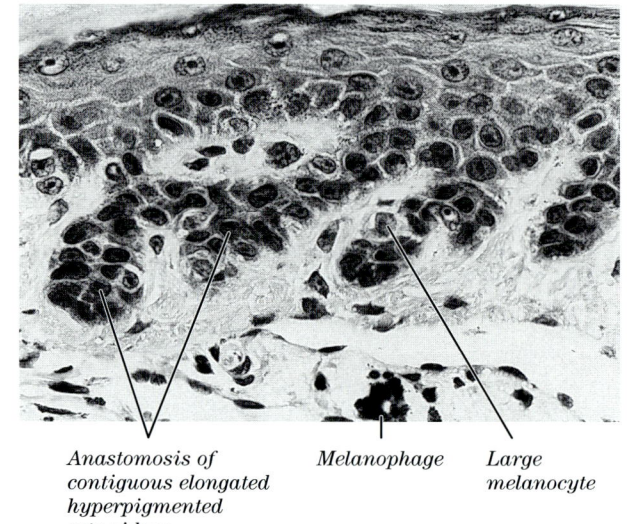

108 • Solar Lentigo

Criteria for diagnosis of this solar lentigo

This is a solar lentigo because:

1. Nubbins, cords, and columns of hyperpigmented keratinocytes are all confined to the papillary dermis.

2. Abundant elastotic material (solar elastosis) is present in the upper part of the dermis.

3. An increased number of large melanocytes are disposed as solitary units in the basal layer, and those melanocytes are monomorphous and equidistant from one another.

4. The cornified layer is thickened in compact, laminated, and basket-weave configuration.

5. Melanin is distributed in uniform fashion throughout the lesion.

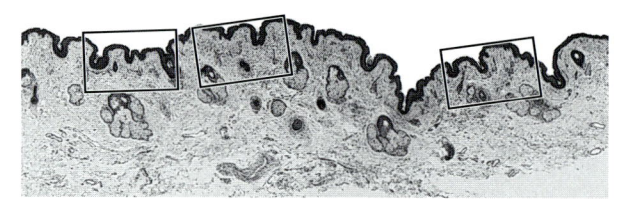

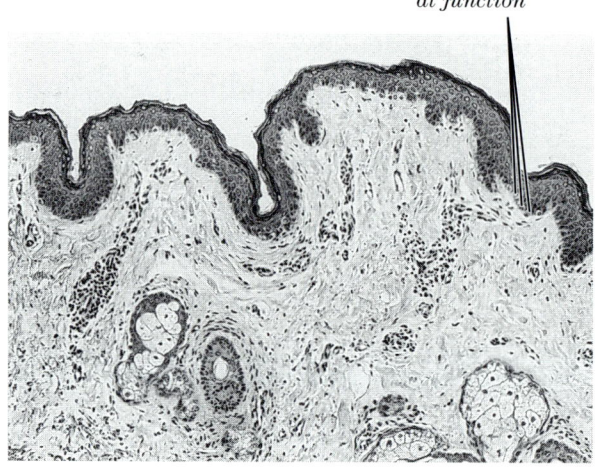
Increased number of melanocytes at junction

Large melanocytes

Increased number of melanocytes

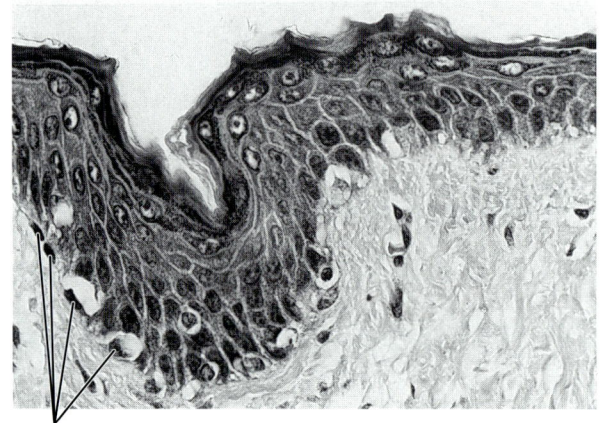
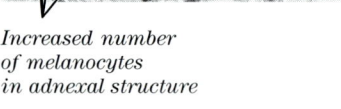
Increased number of melanocytes in adnexal structure

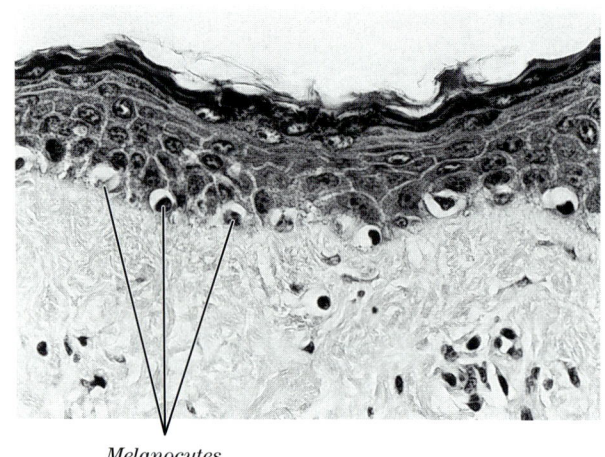
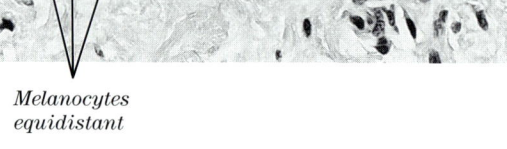
Melanocytes equidistant

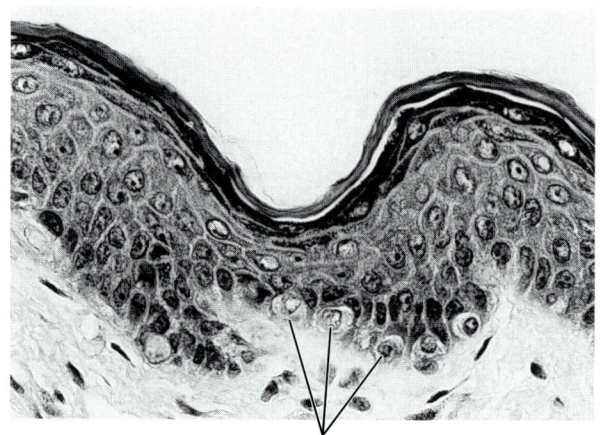
Large melanocytes

109 • Melanocytes on Eyelid Skin

Criteria for diagnosis of this example of normal skin of an eyelid

1. Although melanocytes situated at the dermo-epidermal junction seem to be increased in number, they are equidistant from one another.

2. All of the melanocytes in this section are positioned at the dermo-epidermal junction and not above it.

3. Nuclei of melanocytes are monomorphous.

4. All the melanocytes are arranged as solitary units; none are in nests.

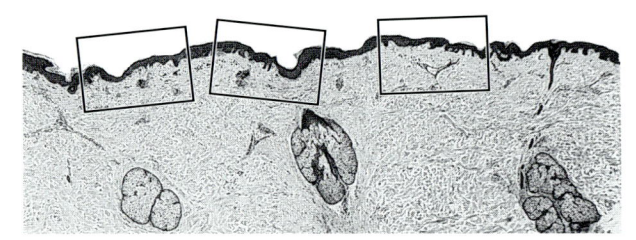

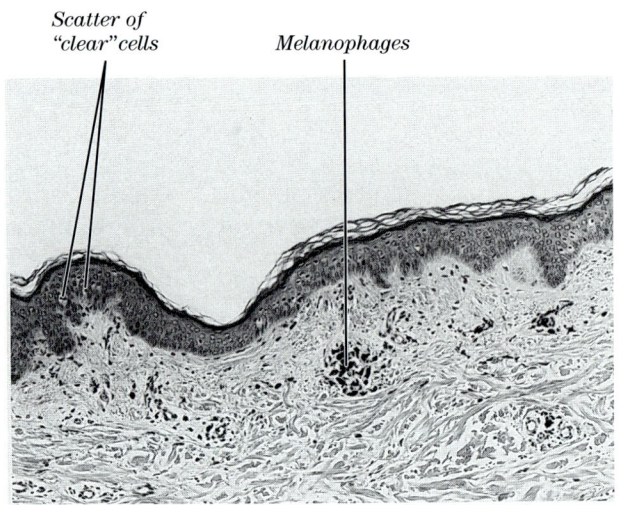

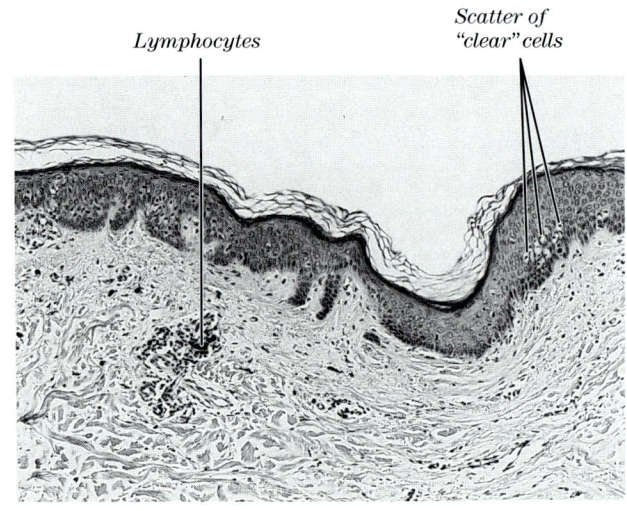

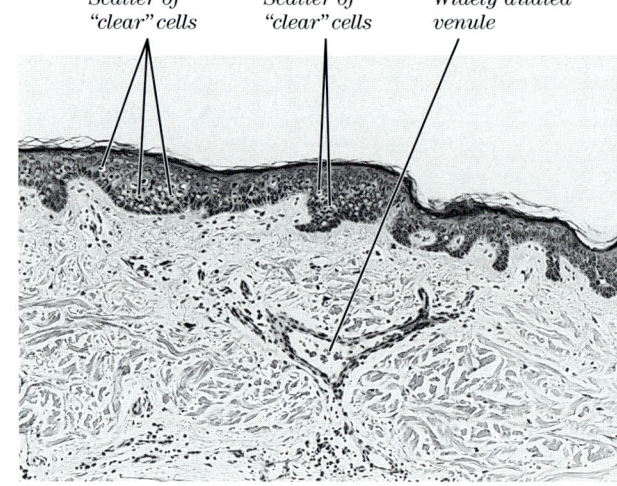

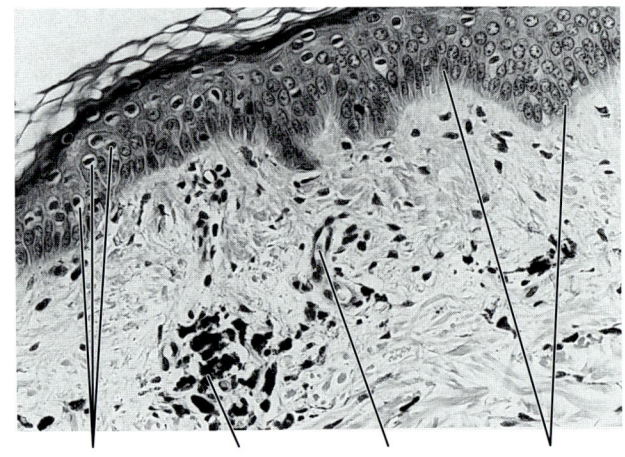

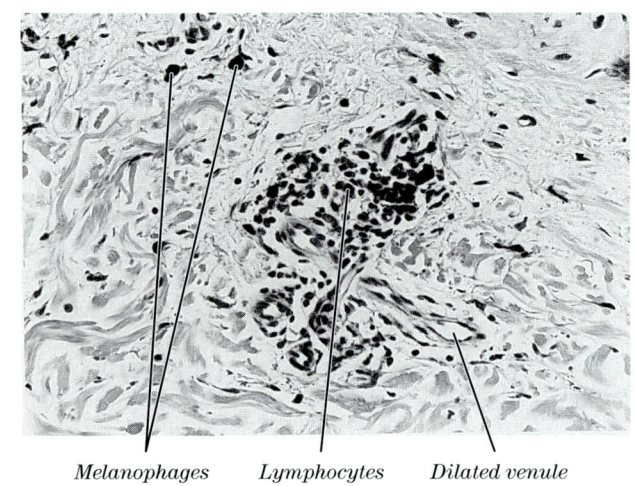

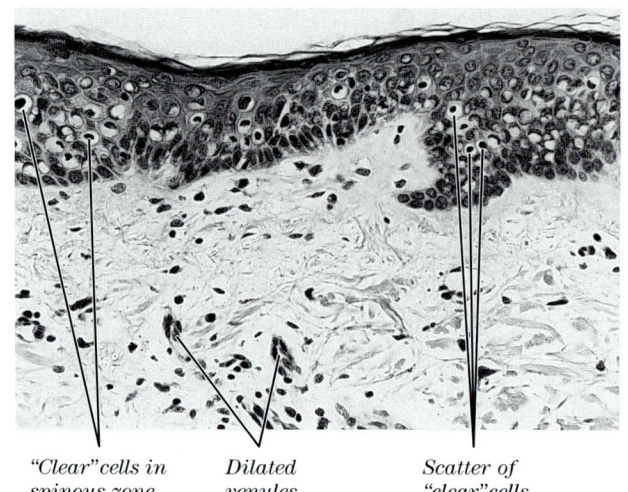

110 • Artifactual Changes Around Keratinocytes

Criteria for diagnosis of this artifact around keratinocytes

This is an artifact because:

1. Halos are present around nuclei of keratinocytes in the spinous and granular zones, in contrast to halos around melanocytes in melanoma in situ that appear around cytoplasm, rather than around the nuclei themselves.

2. There are no "clear" cells at the dermo-epidermal junction or in the basal layer, unlike the situation in melanoma in situ where there always are some melanocytes ("clear" cells) at the junction or in the basal layer.

3. Numerous melanophages are present in the papillary dermis and around the vessels of the superficial plexus in the absence of a proliferation of melanocytes, either as solitary units or in nests, at the dermo-epidermal junction.

In short, these are the changes of post-inflammatory pigmentary alteration in concert with an artifact of keratinocytes within the epidermis, and not those of melanoma in situ.

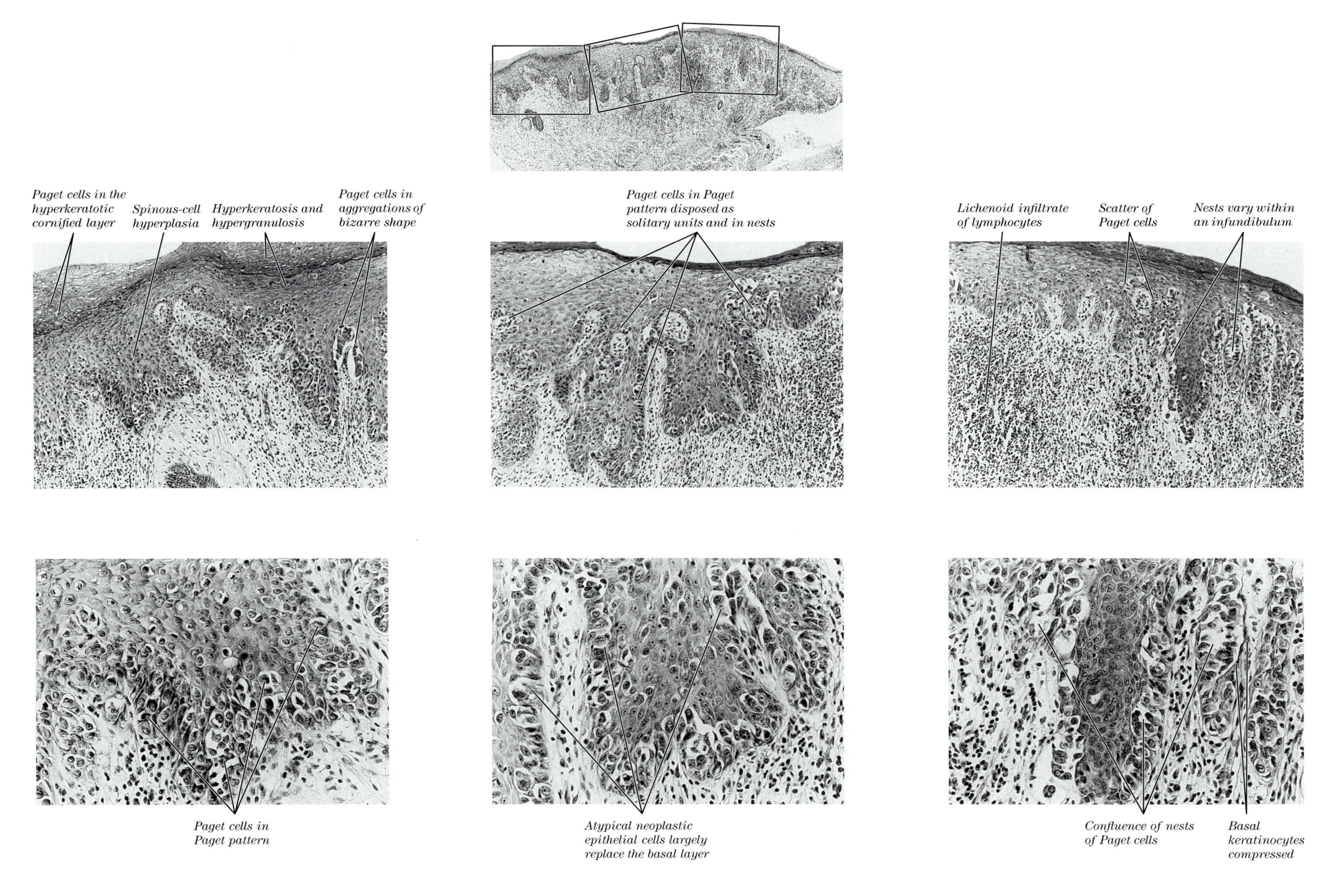

111 • Extramammary Paget's Disease

Criteria for diagnosis of this lesion of extramammary Paget's disease

This is extramammary Paget's disease because:

1. Atypical epithelial cells, both those arranged as solitary units and those in nests, are situated within the basal layer and above it, but hardly at all at the dermo-epidermal junction.

2. Nuclei of some neoplastic cells are eccentric (signet-ring cells).

3. Basal keratinocytes in some foci are compressed by aggregations of neoplastic cells.

Lichen simplex chronicus in the form of marked compact orthokeratosis, hypergranulosis, and spinous-cell hyperplasia is observed episodically in association with extramammary Paget's disease, but not at all in concert with melanoma. It is particularly common to see lichen simplex chronicus superimposed upon extramammary Paget's disease of the vulva.

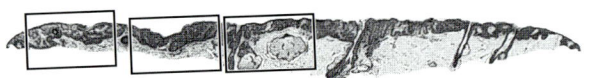

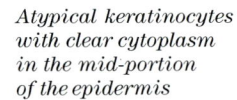
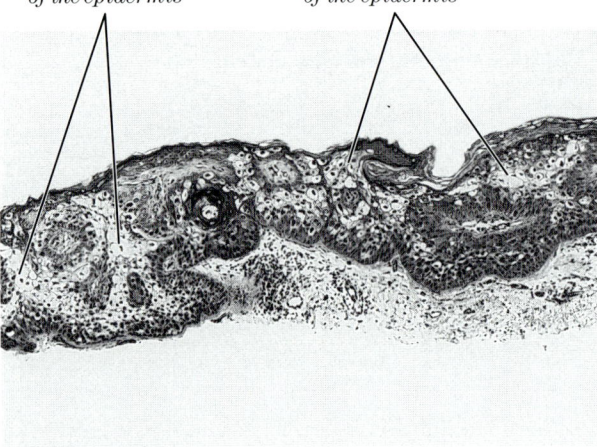
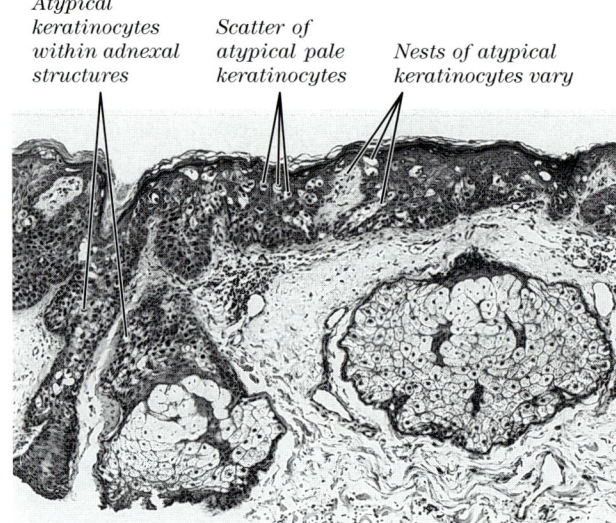
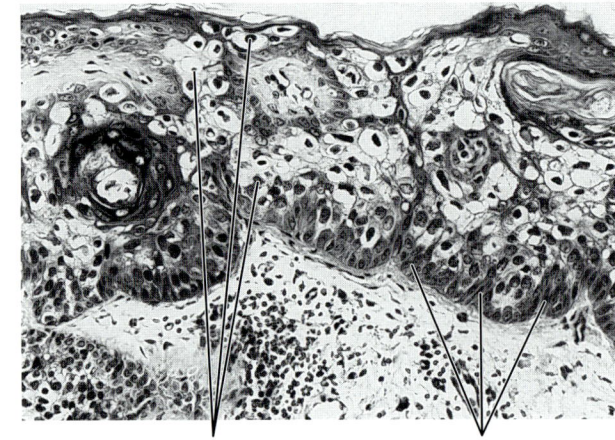
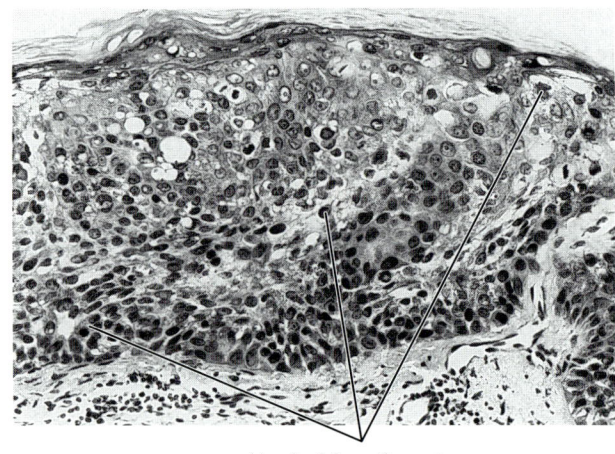
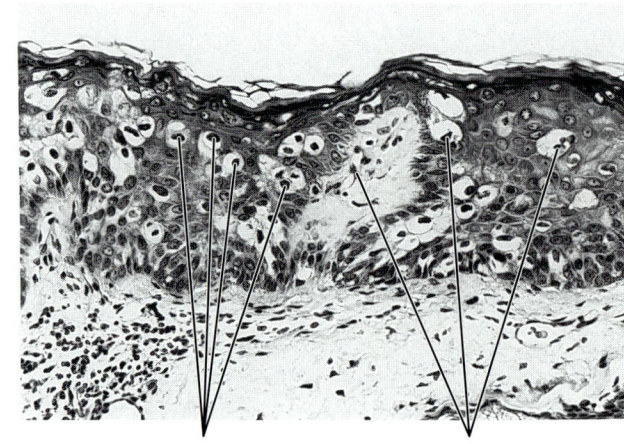

112 • Bowen's Disease *(pagetoid type)*

Criteria for diagnosis of this example of Bowen's disease (pagetoid type)

This is a squamous-cell carcinoma in situ of Bowen's type because:

1. Atypical keratinocytes are present throughout the entire thickness of the thickened epidermis.
2. Atypical keratinocytes also extend far down epithelial structures of adnexa.

This is a pagetoid expression of Bowen's disease because:

Atypical keratinocytes with abundant pale and clear cytoplasm are present as solitary units, nests, and sheets within a thickened epidermis and within epithelial structures of adnexa.

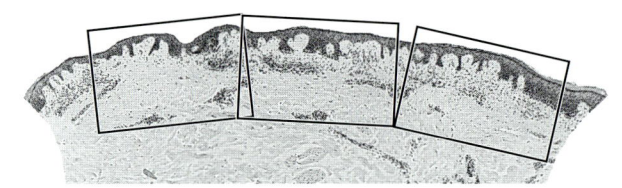

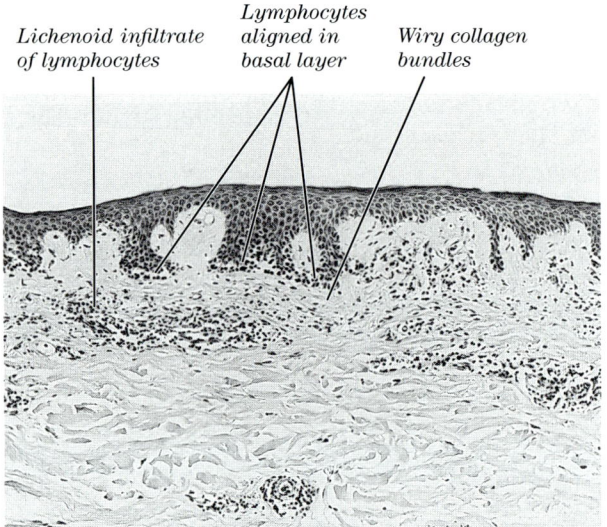

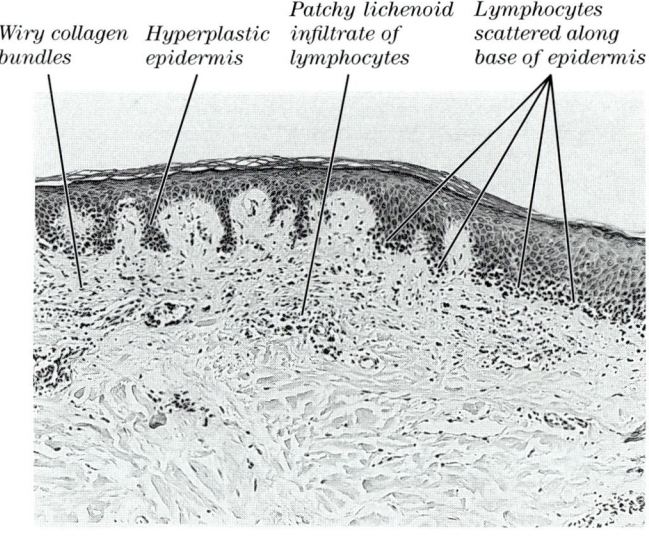

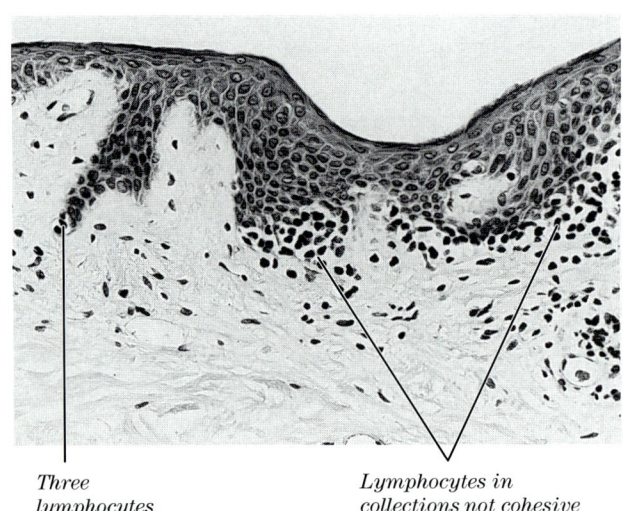

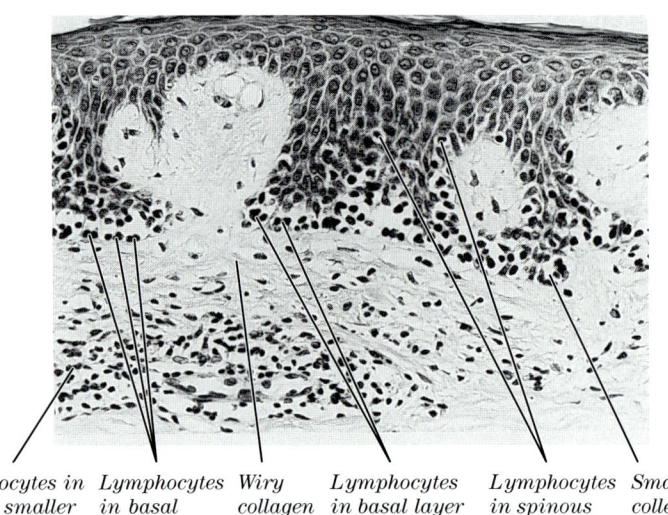

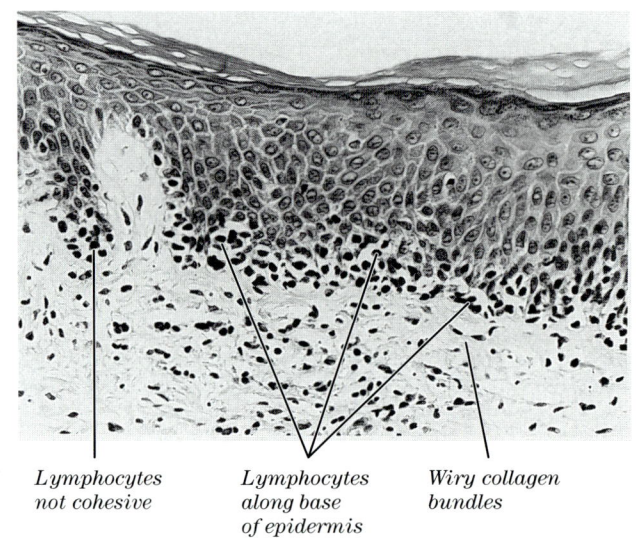

113 • Mycosis Fungoides

Criteria for diagnosis of this plaque of mycosis fungoides

This is a plaque of mycosis fungoides because:

1. Mononuclear cells consist almost entirely of a nucleus, with practically no cytoplasm, i.e., like lymphocytes that they are.

2. Lymphocytes are sprinkled along the dermo-epidermal junction, above it, and immediately beneath it, but not precisely at the junction.

3. Lymphocytes are aligned as solitary units in the basal layer in many foci.

4. No nests of cells are present at the junction.

5. There are no discrete nests in which cells are cohesive.

6. Many lymphocytes in the epidermis are larger than those in the dermis.

7. The papillary dermis is thickened by wiry bundles of collagen in haphazard array; no bundles of collagen are arrayed in lamellar or "concentric" fashion.

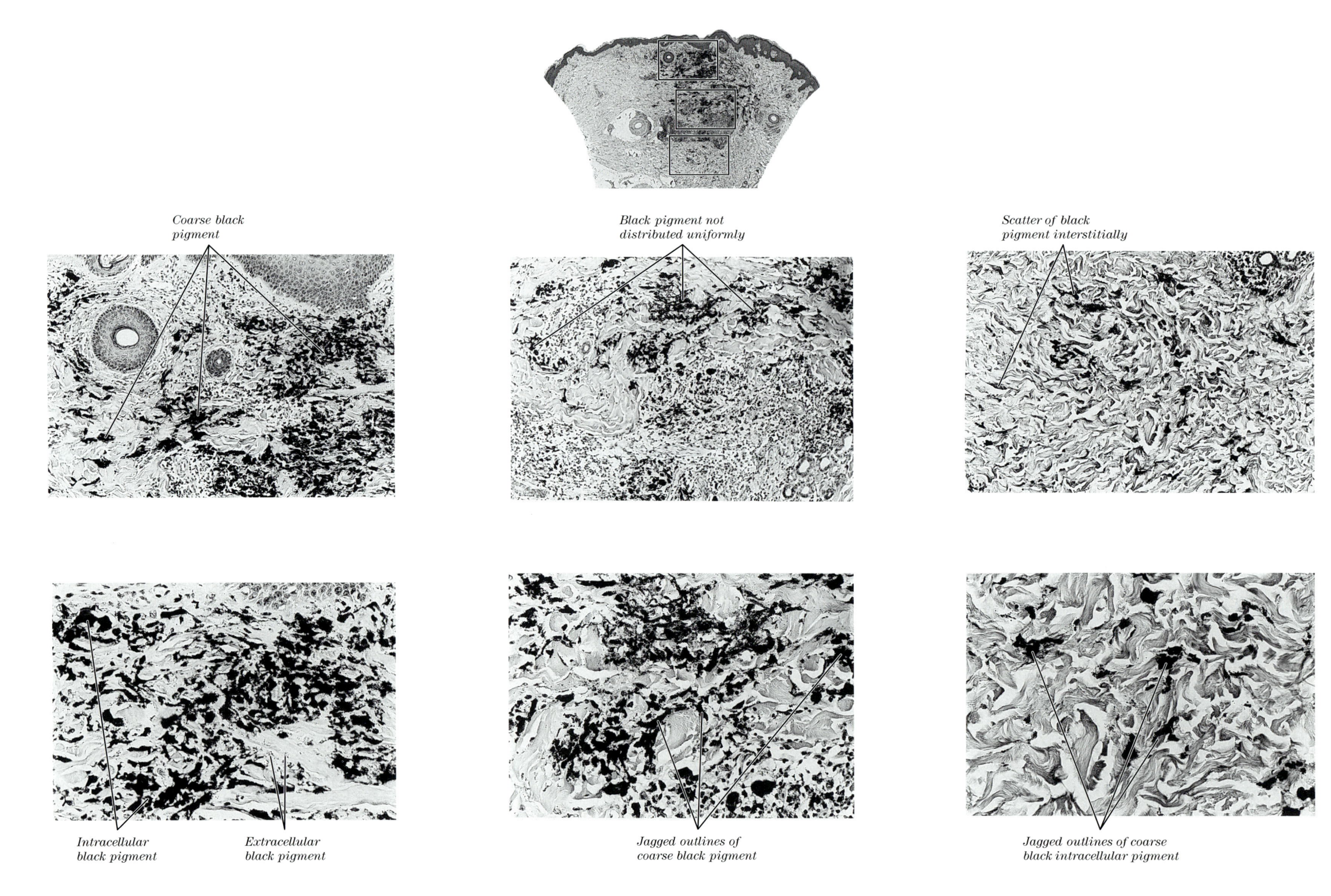

114 • Tattoo by Carbon

Criteria for diagnosis of this tattoo by carbon

This is a tattoo because:

1. Much of the pigment is extracellular.
2. The pigment is arranged in irregularly shaped clumps.
3. The number of melanocytes in the epidermis above the abundant pigment is not increased.
4. The pigment is black, not dark brown like melanin, in sections stained by hematoxylin and eosin.

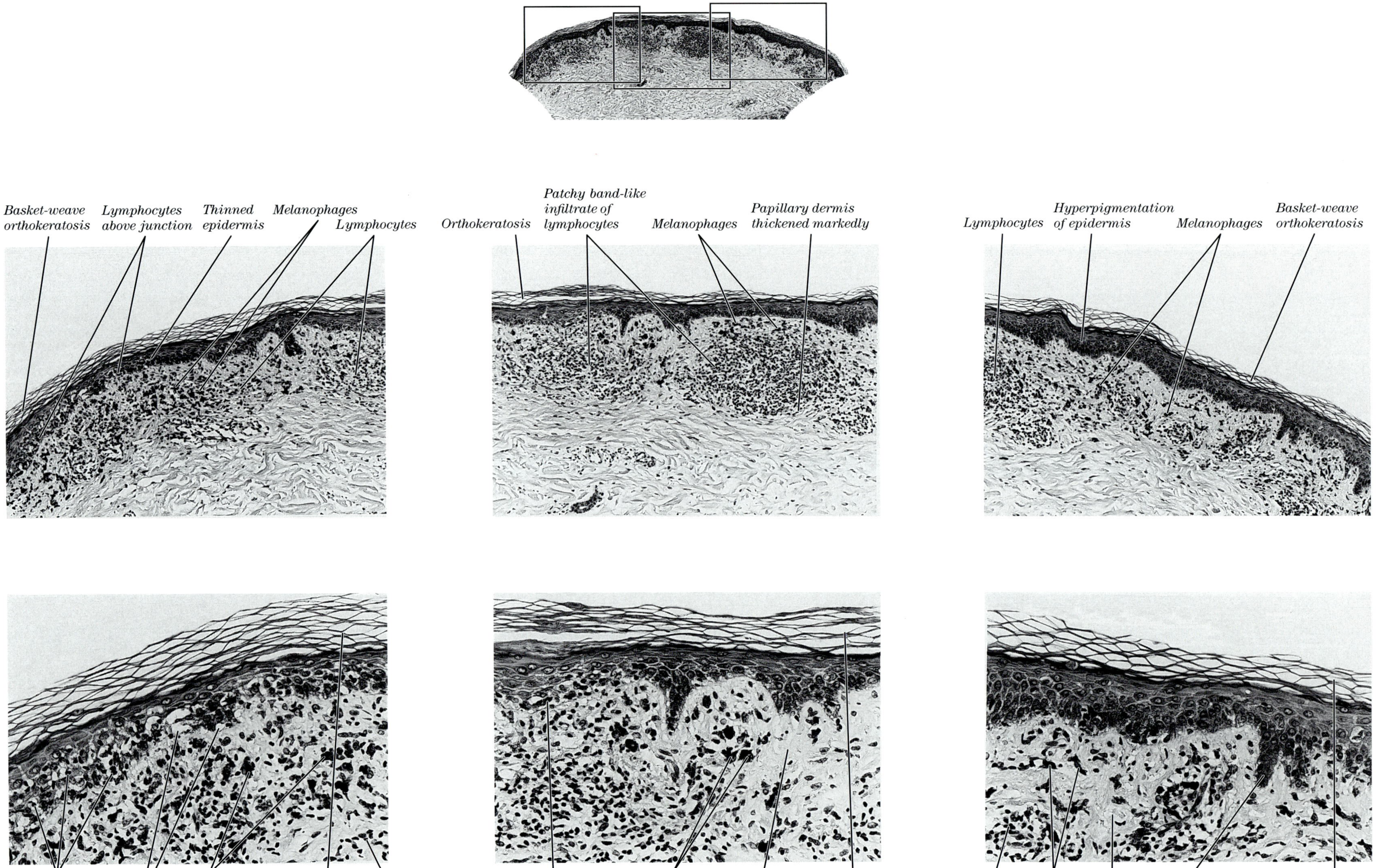

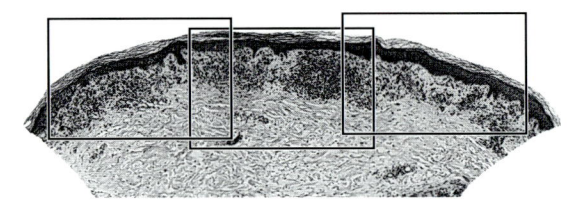

115 • Lichen Planus-Like Keratosis *(with partial regression)*

Criteria for diagnosis of this partially regressed lichen planus-like keratosis

This is a partially regressed lichen planus-like keratosis because:

1. A patchy lichenoid infiltrate consisting mostly of lymphocytes is still present in a thickened papillary dermis.

2. Numerous melanophages are present within the thickened papillary dermis.

3. Fibroplasia accompanies the lichenoid infiltrate of lymphocytes and melanophages in the thickened papillary dermis.

4. The epidermis is thinned focally and devoid, in those zones, of prominent rete ridges.

5. The cornified layer has been restored to basket-weave configuration, but remains hyperkeratotic.

6. The dermo-epidermal junction is obscured, focally, by lymphocytes and vacuolar alteration.

7. There is focal spongiosis.

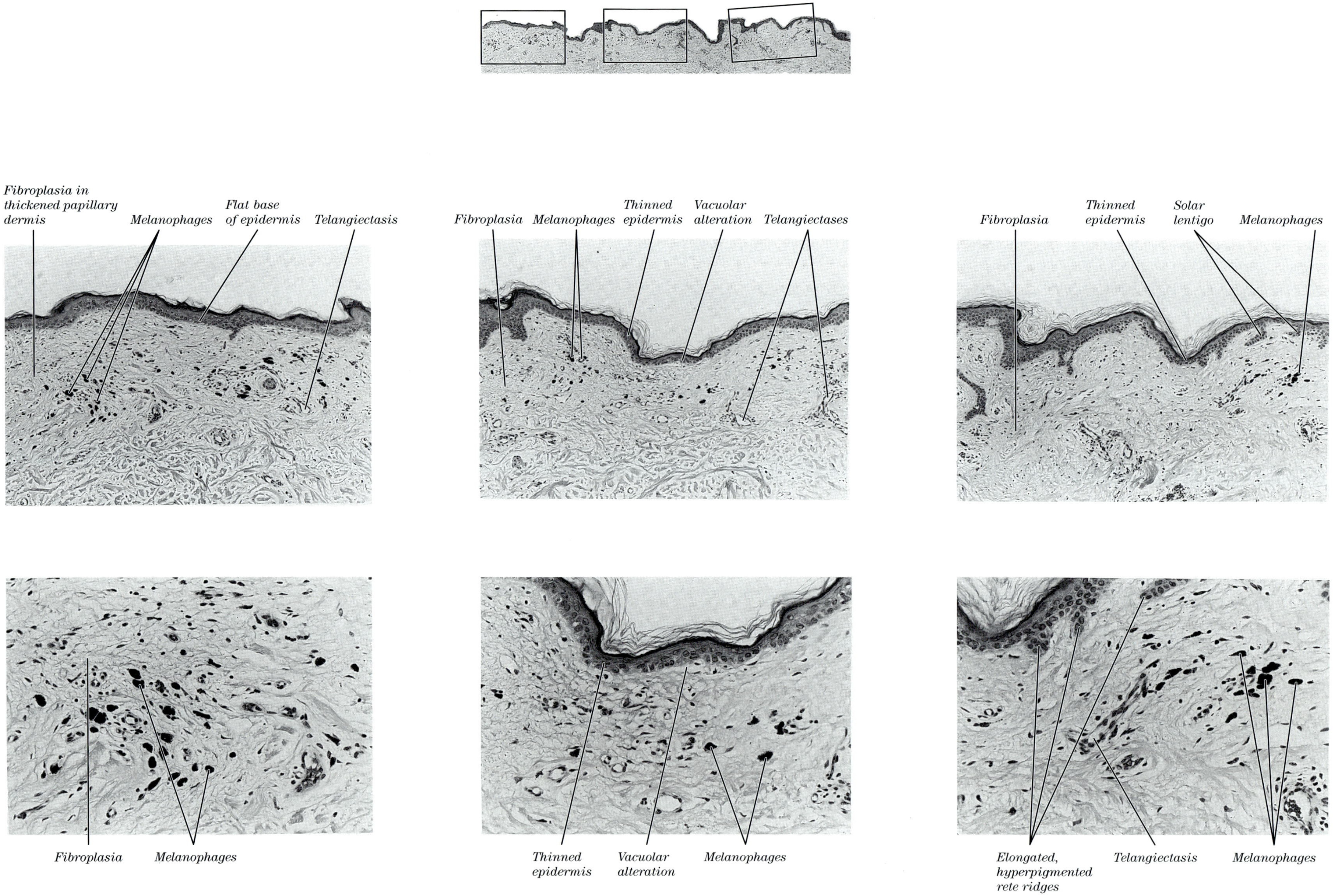

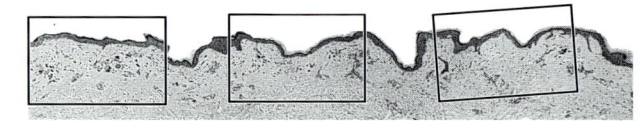

116 • Complete Regression of Lichen Planus-Like Keratosis

Criteria for diagnosis of regression of lichen planus-like keratosis

This is regression of a pigmented lesion consequent to an infiltrate of inflammatory cells because:

1. The papillary dermis is thickened markedly by fibroplasia, melanophages, a sprinkling of lymphocytes, and telangiectases.
2. The epidermis is thinned and nearly devoid of normal rete ridges.
3. Slight vacuolar alteration is present at the dermo-epidermal junction.

This is most likely a lichen planus-like keratosis that underwent regression because:

At the periphery of the lesion are signs of a solar lentigo in the form of elongated and hockey-stick shaped hyperpigmented rete ridges above elastotic material.

VIII. Confusing Concepts

Histopathologists routinely describe neoplastic cells as being benign or malignant, but "benign" and "malignant" are biologic concepts, not cytologic ones. Nuclei may be described properly as "typical" or "atypical," but not as "benign" or "malignant." Cytologic atypia, no matter how startling, is not synonymous with biologic malignancy. Because Spitz's nevi often have more strikingly atypical nuclei than have many melanomas (as well as more mitotic figures, some of them even abnormal), it is not uncommon for histopathologists to misinterpret some Spitz's nevi as melanomas. That can be avoided if criteria for histopathologic diagnosis and differential diagnosis are heeded fastidiously, if scanning magnification is used scrupulously to assess silhouette, and if fanciful terms like "invasion," "invasive," and "invading" for neoplasms, and "wicked," "vicious," and "worrisome" for neoplastic cells are avoided punctiliously.

The terms "invasion," "invasive," and "invading" have no place in description of melanocytic neoplasms, or any neoplasms for that matter. A histopathologist who views a Spitz's nevus or a melanoma through a conventional microscope cannot assess movement of melanocytes, because those cells are immobile. Words like "invasion," "invasive," and "invading" (and "infiltrating," "penetrating," and "pushing") are animistic because they attribute vitality to elements that no longer are alive. This is not merely a semantic quibble; it has profound implications for patients. When histopathologists use the terms "invasion," "invasive," and "invading," they mean that the neoplasm under study is malignant, just as they do when they describe nuclei as being suspicious, ugly, evil, monstrous, and frightening. Histopathologists never use those terms to describe benign neoplasms. In reality, Spitz's nevus frequently is more "invasive" biologically, i.e., in vivo, than any melanoma because it often grows much more rapidly and descends much more quickly from the epidermis into the dermis. In vivo, neoplastic melanocytes of a Spitz's nevus, just like those of a melanoma, move from the epidermis into the dermis and, in this sense, both the benign and the malignant neoplasm are invasive. Histopathologists can and should make specific diagnoses in the language of clinical dermatology, e.g., nevus, melanoma, dermatofibroma, verruca vulgaris, seborrheic keratosis, based upon repeatable criteria, without resort to animistic allusions and illusions such as "invasion."

The notion of "invasive melanoma without competence for metastasis" is a speculation biologically and an oxymoron linguistically. All melanomas in situ (in the absence of signs of regression) are benign because all of the neoplastic melanocytes are confined to the epidermis and epithelial structures of adnexa, from whence they cannot and do not metastasize. Once neoplastic melanocytes of melanoma enter the dermis rich in vascular channels, however, a person who bears that melanoma is at risk for metastasis. It is extremely rare for thin melanomas to metastasize, but that phenomenon may occur and does. Therefore, a histopathologist can advise a surgeon managing a patient with a thin melanoma that the prognosis for that patient is excellent, but a histopathologist is well-advised to refrain from ex cathedra pronouncements about capability for metastasis in regard to melanomas in the dermis. Too much still is unknown about this subject to issue dogmatic statements about prognoses based upon thickness and upon "levels of invasion" that are neither repeatable nor reliable. In general, it is true that thin melanomas have a favorable prognosis and thick melanomas an unfavorable one, but there are exceptions to these generalities, and the broad zone between thin and thick is gray. Episodically, some thin melanomas metastasize and some very thick melanomas have not metastasized by the time that neoplasm is removed surgically. Levels of invasion (Clark) and measurements of thickness (Breslow) are only rough estimates of prognosis, not precise determinants of it. Surgeons should not alter their procedures based upon these gauges of prognosis. The treatment of melanoma is the same regardless of thickness. An excision should be designed to remove the entire melanoma and little more than that for good measure, and if that goal has been accomplished, a surgeon should do no more.

The concepts of a "radial growth phase" and a "vertical growth phase" of melanoma are interesting theories, but only theories; they lack value in practice. First, "radial" and "vertical" are not contrasting. Vertical is a component of radial. Second, what is called the "radial growth phase" involves the epidermis and the papillary dermis, an indication that that phase, too, has a vertical dimension (some neoplastic cells, in their movement in vivo from the epidermis into the dermis, must have taken a vertical route). Third, for many years no criteria were given that could enable histopathologists to recognize a "radial" and a "vertical" growth phase of melanoma and to differentiate them from one another. Recently, criteria for that differentiation have been put forth, but they are recondite, highly subjective, and not applicable with repeatability. One criterion for recognition of the so-called vertical growth phase is detection of an "expansile nodule" in the dermis. Both the words "expansile" and "nodule" are flawed in this setting. The "nodule" referred to is a tiny collection of neoplastic melanocytes in the papillary dermis. Nodules, clinically and histopathologically, are large structures, yet the "nodules" of the supposed "vertical growth phase" are minuscule. When viewed through a conventional microscope, aggregations of neoplastic cells, whether nodules or not, are not expansile. In histopathologic sections, nothing is expansile; "nodules" cannot swell in vitro. "Expansile nodules" in a "vertical growth phase" of melanoma are illustrative of the phenomenon of pathobabel, the tower of Babel in the language of pathology in general and of dermatopathology in particular. In brief, they are incomprehensible. Last, concepts of "radial" and "vertical" growth phases are not relevant, either to diagnosis of melanoma or to its management. Clinical and histopathologic diagnosis of melanoma are based on morphologic criteria and do not require knowledge of "growth phases," and neither does proper treatment of melanoma, i.e., complete surgical excision of it.

The just mentioned criticism of terms like "invading," "infiltration," and "expanding" as they are employed in morphologic description is equally applicable to the active verb "penetrating," particularly as it is used in the appellation "deep penetrating nevus" (Fig. 117). That benign neoplasm is distinctive, having the silhouette and dendritic melanocytes of a blue nevus, but being compound, in some specimens, unlike a blue nevus. In addition, some nuclei are large and pleomorphic, and some of them may be in mitosis, features that are seen often in Spitz's nevi. By the time that a biopsy specimen of a "deep penetrating nevus" (plexiform spindle-cell nevus) has been taken, the proliferation of melanocytes frequently has involved most, if not all, of the reticular dermis, and sometimes the upper part of the subcutaneous fat, yet "deep penetrating nevus" begins superficial. Even the deep distribution of melanocytes in a nevus, however, is not peculiar to "deep penetrating nevus." All deep forms of congenital nevi (and deep penetrating nevi seem to be congenital) involve the deep reticular dermis and usually the subcutaneous fat. So, too, do Masson's blue neuro-nevi and other expressions of bulbous blue nevi. Some examples of Spitz's nevi also involve the subcutaneous fat (Fig. 118). In short, although a histopathologist can judge whether a nevus is superficial or deep, a realistic determination cannot be made through a microscope about whether that nevus is "penetrating" or not.

Some pathologists have written of "malignant Spitz's nevi" and "metastasizing Spitz's nevi." Surely those neoplasms are not Spitz's nevi, but melanomas that simulate Spitz's nevi because they consist of oval, spindle, or polygonal melanocytes that harbor large nuclei. Spitz's nevus, as the name denotes, is a nevus, and a nevus does not metastasize. If a neoplasm diagnosed histopathologically as a Spitz's nevus metastasizes, it behooves a pathologist to acknowledge error rather than to retreat behind a transparent diagnosis of "metastasizing Spitz's nevus." Of course, Spitz's nevi may simulate melanomas closely histopathologically (and vice versa), and, therefore, errors in differentiation of the benign from the malignant neoplasm are inevitable. No person in the Western world has ever practiced dermatopathology or general pathology for long and not misinterpreted at least one Spitz's nevus as a melanoma and one melanoma as a Spitz's nevus. Most have erred far more often than that. In order to prevent such misinterpretations in the future, lessons must be learned from those painful mistakes in the past. That cannot be accomplished by covering them up with phrases like "metastasizing Spitz's nevus."

As already has been stated, the concept of "malignant blue nevus" is as illogical as that of "metastasizing Spitz's nevus." A nevus, by definition, cannot be malignant, but a melanoma can arise in association with any type of melanocytic nevus, including blue nevus. When that happens, as it does extremely rarely, the malignant neoplasm should be designated "melanoma" and not "malignant blue nevus." More frequent than the circumstance of melanoma originating in a blue nevus is the phenomenon of metastatic melanoma in which strikingly elongated pigmented melanocytes simulate those of a blue nevus, thereby prompting misinterpretation of the metastasis as a "malignant blue nevus" (Fig. 119).

The terms "minimal deviation melanoma" and "borderline melanoma" are merely hedges against commitment by a histopathologist to a straight-forward diagnosis of melanoma (or nevus). No melanomas can be diagnosed with repeatability as "minimal deviation" (deviation from what?) or "borderline" (straddling what border?). Surely it is fitting and proper to acknowledge uncertainty in regard to diagnosis of some melanocytic neoplasms, because some of them are incredibly irksome diagnostically. The more honest, instructive, and beneficial response in those circumstances is "I don't know," rather than posturing behind non-diagnoses like "minimal deviation melanoma" and "borderline melanoma." All diagnoses in dermatopathology, including those that pertain to melanocytic neoplasms, should

Text continues on page 256

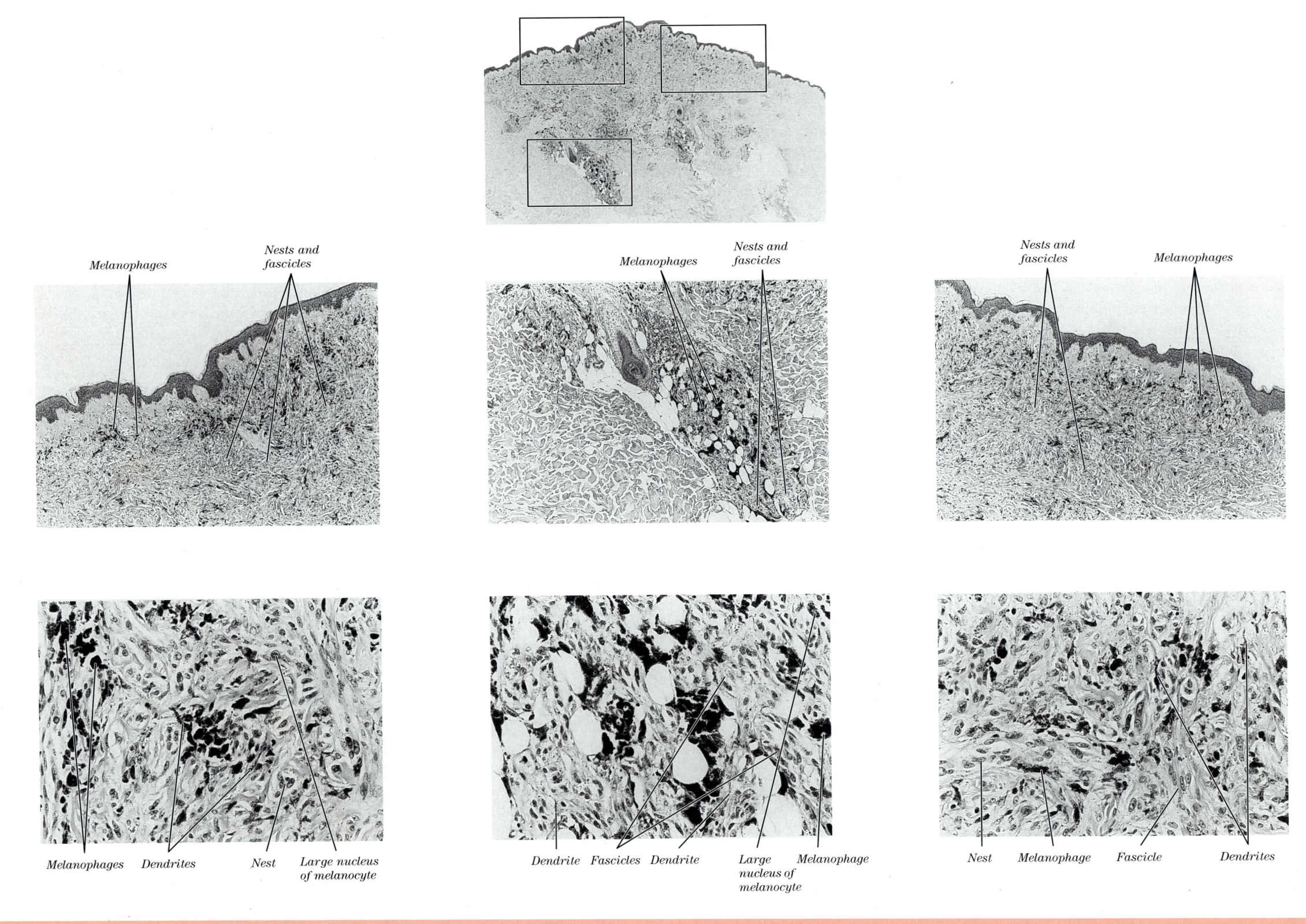

117 • "Deep Penetrating Nevus"

Criteria for diagnosis of this "deep penetrating nevus"

This neoplasm is benign because:

1. It is relatively symmetric.
2. It is wedge-shaped.
3. There is maturation of melanocytes.
4. There are no signs of melanoma in situ.

This is a so-called deep penetrating nevus because:

1. The neoplastic melanocytes tend to involve the deep reticular dermis and the subcutaneous fat.
2. The nuclei of some melanocytes are large and their cytoplasm abundant, like those of Spitz's nevi.
3. There are numerous markedly pigmented dendritic melanocytes, like those of blue nevi.
4. The cytoplasm of many melanocytes is pale and contains dusty melanin.

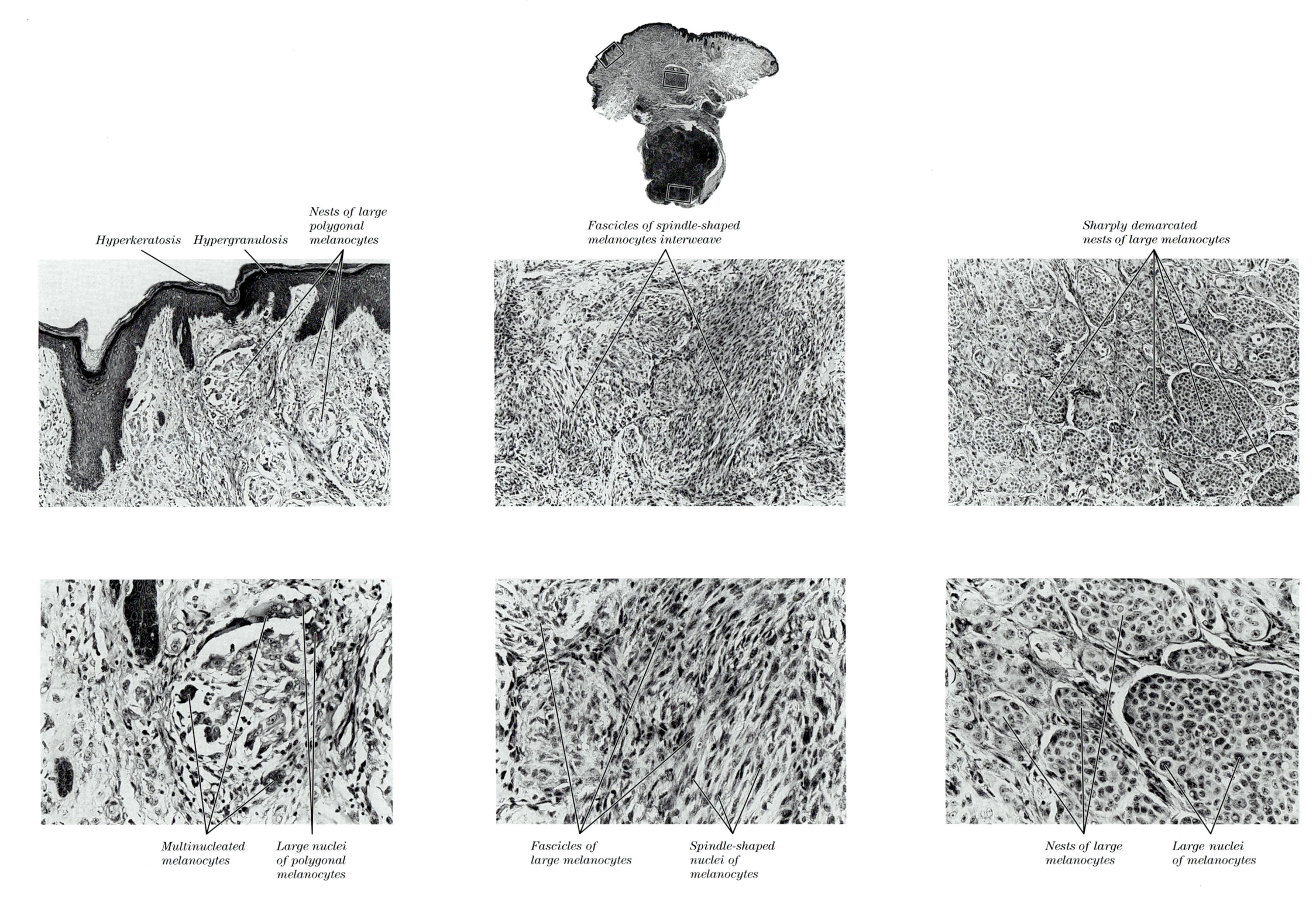

118 • Spitz's Nevus

Criteria for diagnosis of this Spitz's nevus

This neoplasm is benign because:

1. It is oriented vertically.
2. It is well-circumscribed.
3. Melanocytes mature.
4. Clefts separate a rim of compressed connective tissue around nodules of melanocytes from the "normal" dermis and subcutaneous fat.

This is a Spitz's nevus because:

Many of the melanocytes have large nuclei, abundant cytoplasm, and round, oval, and spindle shapes.

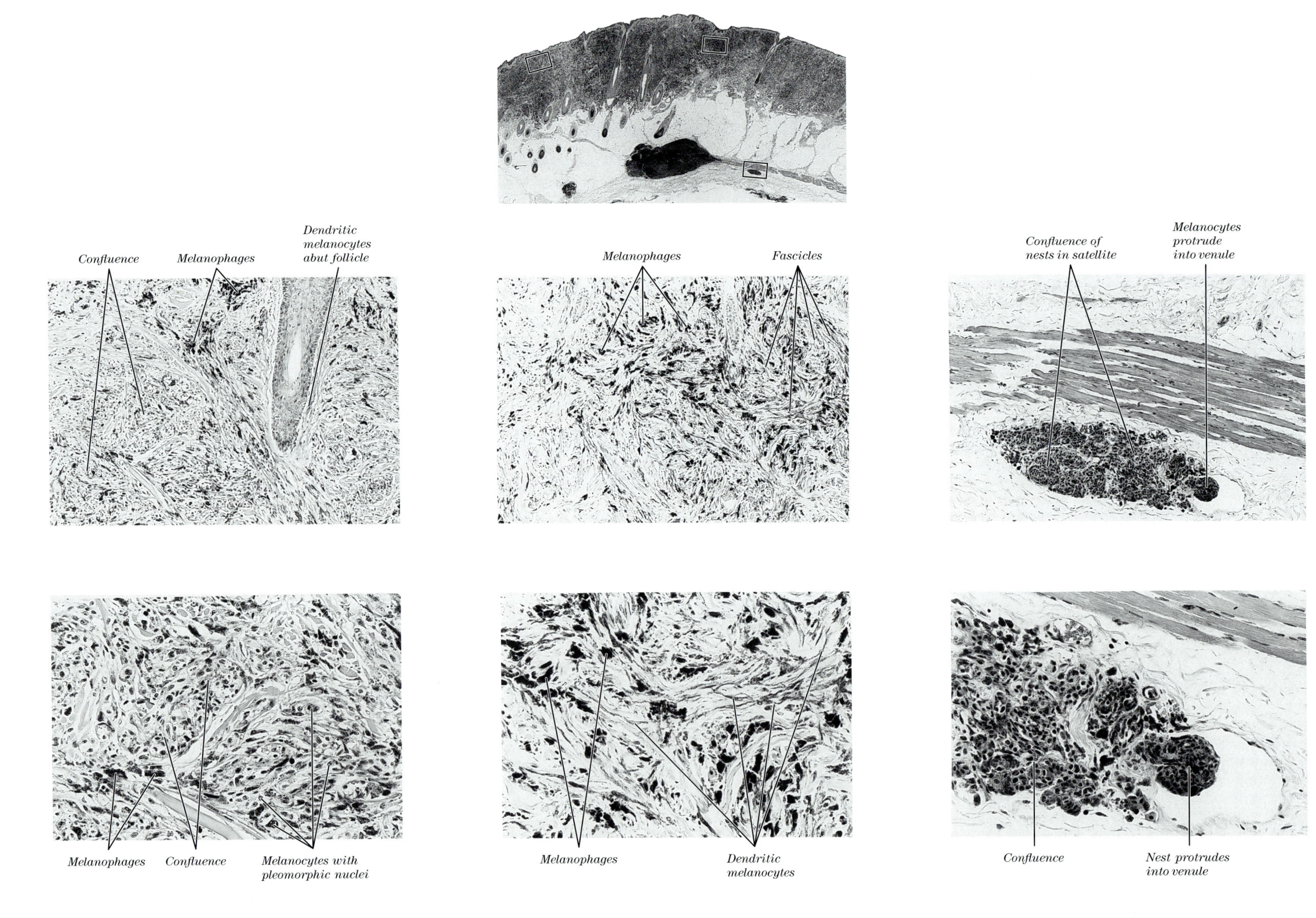

119 • Melanoma with Satellite Metastases

Criteria for diagnosis of this primary melanoma with satellite metastases

This is a melanoma because:

1. Sheets of atypical melanocytes extend throughout the entire dermis and into the upper part of the subcutaneous fat.

2. At some distance from the primary neoplasm, aggregations of neoplastic cells (satellite metastases) are present in the deep subcutaneous fat, fascia, and skeletal muscle.

3. Beneath skeletal muscle, some aggregations of atypical neoplastic cells protrude into vascular lumina.

Step sections through the specimen failed to reveal any sign of melanoma in situ, which militates against this being a conventional primary cutaneous melanoma. The entire neoplasm is a melanoma; there is no evidence of a pre-existing blue nevus. The fact that the neoplasm was present for many years, but surely was not present at birth, favors an exceedingly rare example of a primary melanoma that arose in the dermis and gave rise to satellite metastases. The history is not consonant with metastatic melanoma as an explanation for the entire neoplasm.

be couched in the language of clinical dermatology. Dermatologists never make diagnoses of "minimal deviation melanoma" and "borderline melanoma." In the realm of melanocytic neoplasia, dermatologists make only three diagnoses: nevus, melanoma, or melanoma in association with a nevus. Those are the very diagnoses that histopathologists should make.

The terms "dysplasia," "dysplastic cells," "dysplastic nevi," and "dysplastic nevus syndrome" should be eschewed because they lack meaning, i.e., they have not been defined in a repeatable, comprehensible way, and, therefore, they are confusing to physicians in general, to dermatologists and pathologists in particular, and to patients. Just as the erroneous implication of "juvenile melanoma" was rectified by naming the nevus in debate eponymically for Spitz, who called attention to and helped clarify it, so, too, "dysplastic nevus" can be demystified by naming it for Clark, who popularized it.

A panel at a Consensus Conference that convened at the National Institutes of Health between January 27 and 29, 1992, in Bethesda, Maryland, advised that the "term 'dysplastic nevus' has been used in significantly different ways by different investigators, generating a great deal of controversy and has outlived its usefulness. . . . Because of the controversy surrounding use of the term 'dysplastic nevus,' it seems appropriate to discontinue use of that diagnosis. . . " Unfortunately, the NIH panel proposed that "the clinical lesions should be described as 'atypical moles'" and histopathologically as "'nevus with architectural disorder' with a statement as to the presence and degree of melanocytic atypia." Because no definitions of "architectural order" and of "typical moles" are extant, the proposal of the NIH panel in this regard lacks validity. The "atypical mole" doubtlessly will come to the same sorry end as the "dysplastic nevus."

Although we deny the legitimacy of a "dysplastic nevus syndrome," we acknowledge the authenticity of familial melanoma in patients who also have Clark's nevi, sometimes many of them and some of them large. Whether these persons have a "dysplastic nevus syndrome" cannot be determined because that syndrome has not been defined lucidly. Some authors insist that it may consist of but a single "dysplastic nevus," whereas others contend that there must be scores or even hundreds of them. Some aver that the nevi may be small, i.e., less than 4.0 mm; others are adamant that nothing less than 8.0 mm suffices. Unquestionably, there are families with strong histories of melanoma, i.e., familial melanoma, but that rare genetic aberration is not synonymous with a yet to be clearly defined "dysplastic nevus syndrome." It should be stated, parenthetically, that familial melanoma may occur in the absence of nevi of any kind.

The terms "familial" and "sporadic" for types of "dysplastic nevi" reputed to develop in persons with a personal or family history of melanoma and in persons without such a history, respectively, also are confusing. The nevi in both "familial" and "sporadic" types are indistinguishable clinically, histopathologically, and biologically. Much of the confusion that swirls around the subject of these nevi might be dissipated if all of them, familial and sporadic, were referred to simply as "Clark's nevi." Parenthetically, "familial" and "sporadic" are not contrasting. The opposite of "familial" is "non-familial," and of "sporadic" is "persistent."

The purported histopathologic types of "dysplastic" nevi are "lentiginous" and "epithelioid." This terminology is confusing because these terms, too, are not contrasting. "Lentiginous" refers to an increased *number* of melanocytes disposed as solitary units within elongated rete ridges, and "epithelioid" describes the *cytologic features* of those melanocytes, to wit, oval and cohesive like epithelial cells.

It has been stated repeatedly that "dysplastic nevi" are the commonest precursors of melanomas. They are not. "Normal" melanocytes situated at the dermo-epidermal junction and unassociated with a nevus of any kind are the commonest precursors of melanoma. In our experience, 75 to 80% of all melanomas in Caucasians arise de novo; 20 to 25% begin in association with pre-existing nevi, most of them Clark's nevi. Other students of this subject aver that 50% or more of all melanomas arise in pre-existing nevi. Not only is this figure twice our own, but it does not take into account that virtually all melanomas in Africans and Asians do not originate in association with nevi; they develop de novo. If the worldwide incidence of the association of melanomas and nevi were surveyed, it is likely that less than 10% of all melanomas would be found to be continuous with a nevus.

Clark and co-workers long have asserted that primary melanomas could be classified as lentigo maligna, superficial spreading, acrolentiginous, and nodular types. In our view, this schema is not valid clinically, histopathologically, and biologically. In brief, virtually all melanomas on all cutaneous sites are characterized clinically by asymmetry, poor circumscription, and variegation in shades of brown. Nearly all melanomas, irrespective of anatomic site, are typified histopathologically by asymmetry, poor circumscription, failure of maturation of melanocytes, predominance of single melanocytes over nests of melanocytes in some high-power fields within the epidermis, nests of melanocytes within the epidermis that are not equidistant from one another, nests that vary markedly in size and shape, and nests that have become confluent, scatter of melanocytes above the dermo-epidermal junction, cytologic atypia, melanocytes in mitosis, and necrotic melanocytes. Melanomas on all anatomic sites are notable biologically for relatively similar behavior at similar thicknesses, a truth that was expressed succinctly about melanomas at sites of severe sun damage in the title of an article by proponents of Clark's classification: "Lentigo-maligna melanoma has no better prognosis than other forms of melanoma."

The idea that "lentigo maligna melanoma," "superficial spreading melanoma," "acrolentiginous melanoma," and "nodular melanoma" are distinctive types of melanoma, clinically, histopathologically, and biologically, lacks authenticity. They are simply different names for melanomas on different anatomic sites. The advocates of this classification have yet to present compelling reasons for its legitimacy. Not only do these supposed types of melanoma look fundamentally the same, clinically and histopathologically, but also they behave in a similar fashion, thickness for thickness.

BANS areas are not sites in which melanomas, thickness for thickness, behave in a more lethal way. BANS is an acronym for *b*ack, *a*rms, *n*eck, and *s*houlders. Like so much that has been stated and written about melanomas in the past 35 years, the concept of BANS had a short life span, i.e., less than 5 years, from about 1980 to 1985. During that period, BANS was the rage as a vehicle for identifying sites purported to be ones that spawned melanomas with the most aggressive behavior. BANS is never mentioned now, except as an historical relic.

Partial regression is said by some authors to be a favorable prognostic sign for melanoma, but it probably is not. The worst prognostic sign of melanoma, clinically and histopathologically, is complete regression of the neoplasm in the absence of therapy for it (the regression is not "spontaneous" because nothing is spontaneous; neoplastic melanocytes of melanoma are destroyed by products of dense infiltrates of lymphocytes). Nearly all patients whose primary melanoma has undergone regression completely, die of metastatic melanoma (possibly because the melanoma metastasized to a lymph node *prior* to the onset of regression, which probably was mediated by sensitized lymphocytes). If total regression is a poor prognostic sign, it is unlikely that partial regression can be a good one.

The amount of melanin in a melanoma has no influence on prognosis of the neoplasm, conflicting statements to the contrary. Even "amelanotic" melanomas possess melanosomes when they are viewed through an electron microscope. In that sense, they are not truly "amelanotic." In brief, so-called amelanotic melanomas do not have a worse prognosis than melanotic melanomas. The amount of melanin in a melanoma is irrelevant to its behavior.

It is untrue that nearly 11.0% of all melanomas arise in small congenital nevi as some colleagues have claimed. In our experience, far fewer than 10% of all melanomas begin in congenital nevi, irrespective of breadth or depth of them.

The terms "nevus" and "lentigo" confound all too many students of melanocytic proliferations. The word "nevus" means a spot, particularly one that is present at birth, such as a congenital melanocytic nevus (which is a hamartoma). Yet the name "nevus" has come to be applied to pigmented hamartomas that are not associated with proliferations of melanocytes such as Becker's nevus, benign neoplasms of melanoctyes such as the acquired nevi of Unna, Miescher, Spitz, and Clark, and to cells that constitute those nevi, namely, "nevus cells" that, in fact, are melanocytes. In addition, the designation "nevus" is given to a variety of hamartomas such as nevus flammeus, nevus lipomatosus, elastic tissue nevus, nevus sebaceus, and hair follicle nevus. If sense is to be made of this potpourri of uses for the word "nevus," it seems reasonable to avoid calling melanocytes of a melanocytic nevus "nevus cells," "nevocytes," and "nevo-melanocytes" when they are really melanocytes. For the other well-established conditions named "nevi," the appellation "nevus" should always be modified to insure precision and clarity.

The term "lentigo" comes from lentil and is used for a slew of unrelated conditions such as simple lentigo (a stage in the evolution of junctional nevus), solar lentigo (a stage in the evolution of reticulated seborrheic keratosis), and labial lentigo (a distinctive proliferation of melanocytes arranged as solitary units on mucous membranes and muco-cutaneous junctions; it is not related to simple lentigo because it never eventuates in a junctional nevus or to melanoma of the genitalia because it remains small and well-circumscribed and has short rather than long dendrites) (Fig. 120). Furthermore, there is lentigo maligna (a melanoma in situ in skin damaged severely by sunlight) and acrolentiginous melanoma (melanoma on palms, soles, and nail units that is not different fundamentally from melanoma on any other anatomic site). Confusion can be reduced if lentigo maligna is diagnosed for what it is as melanoma in situ, if acrolentiginous melanoma is

Text continues on page 262

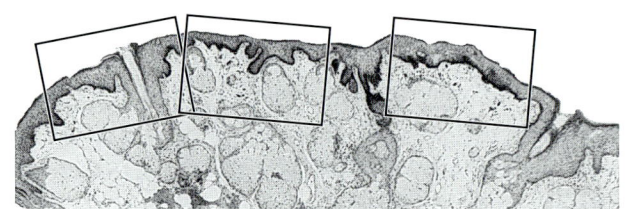

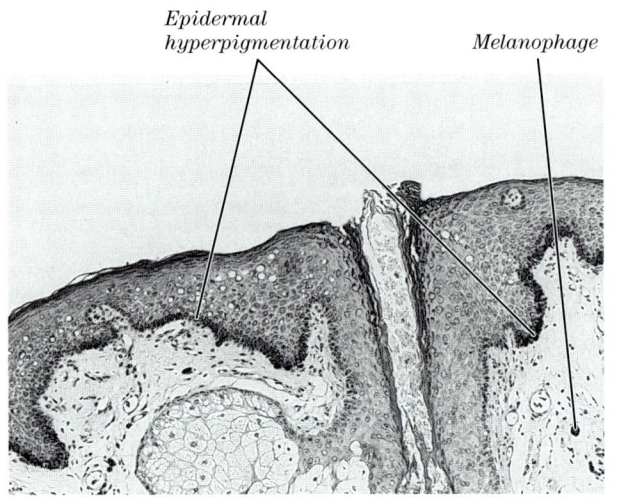
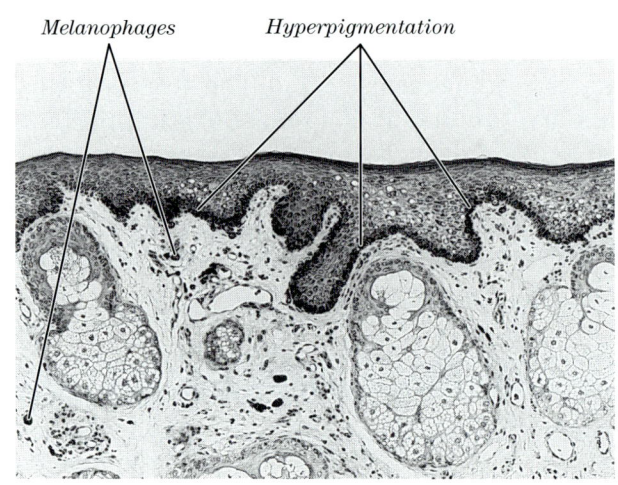
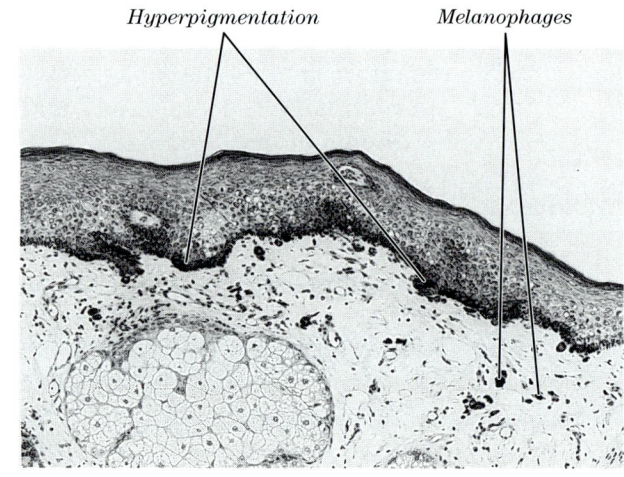

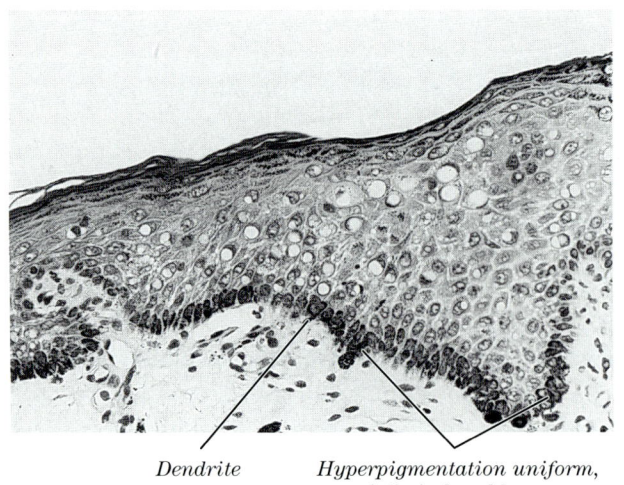
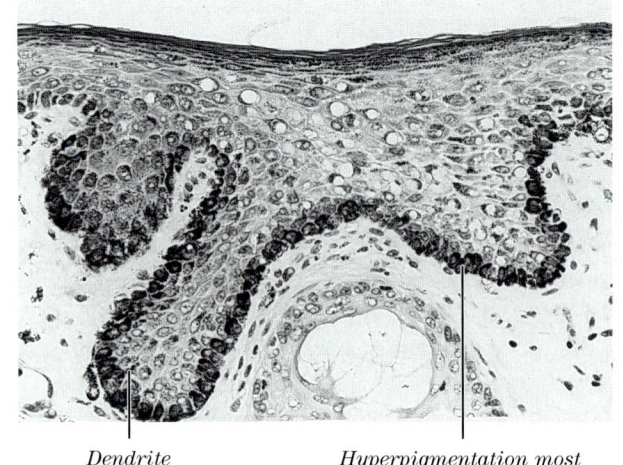
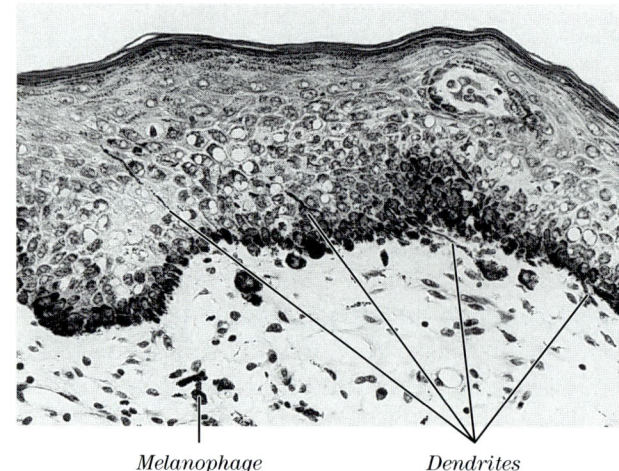

120 • Labial Lentigo

Criteria for diagnosis of this labial lentigo

This is a labial lentigo because:

1. The lesion is situated on a labium, in this instance, a labium majus.

2. Markedly pigmented dendritic melanocytes are disposed as solitary units at the dermo-epidermal junction.

3. The epidermis is hyperpigmented, and melanin is distributed in uniform fashion across the breadth of the lesion, particularly noticeable in the basal layer.

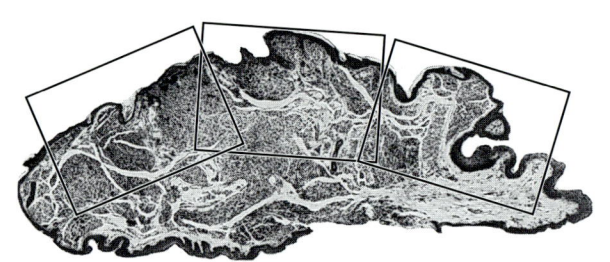

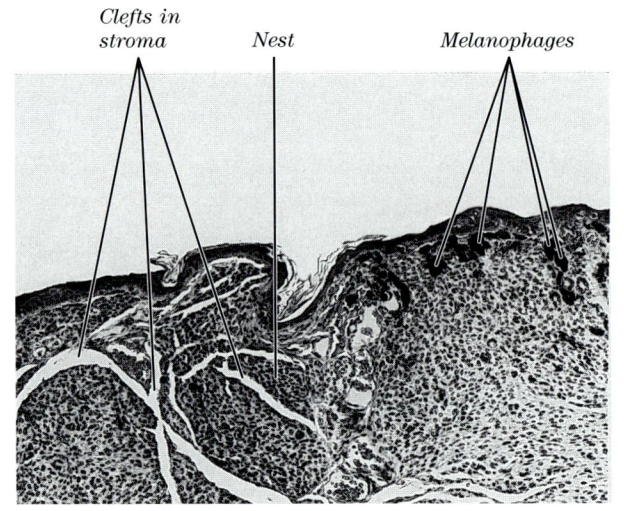
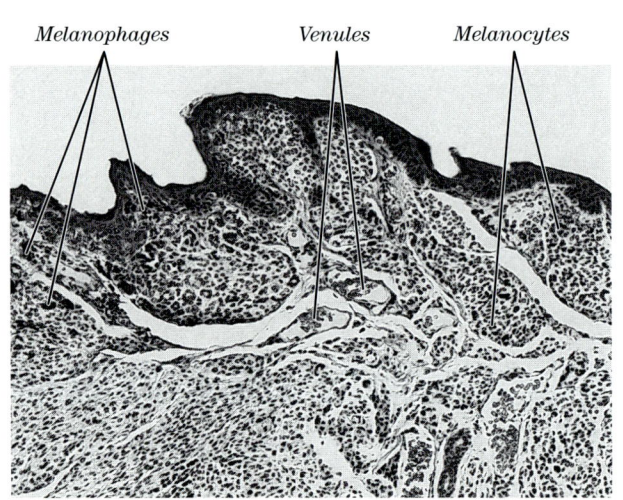
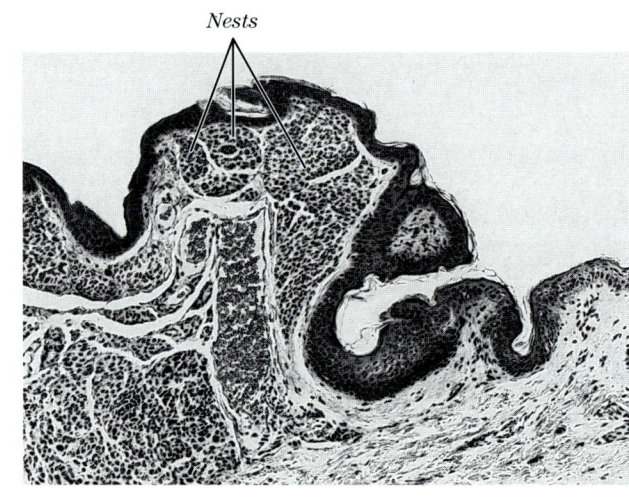

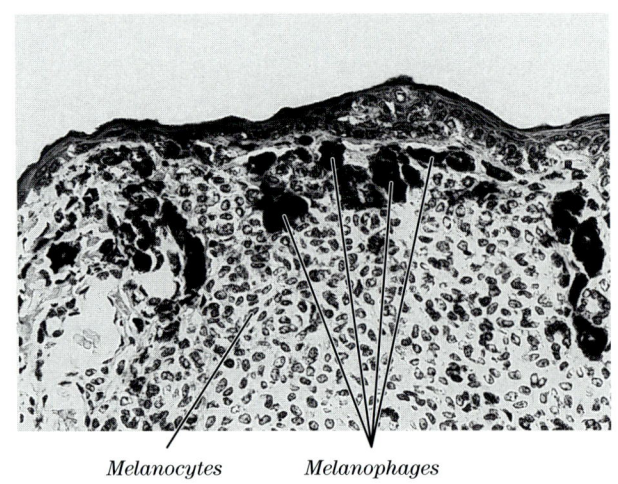
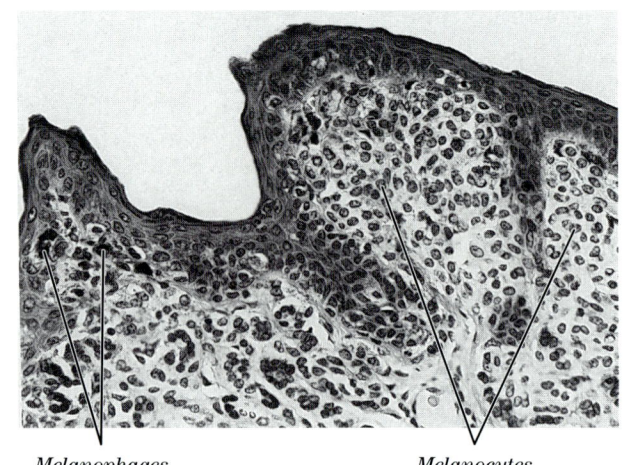
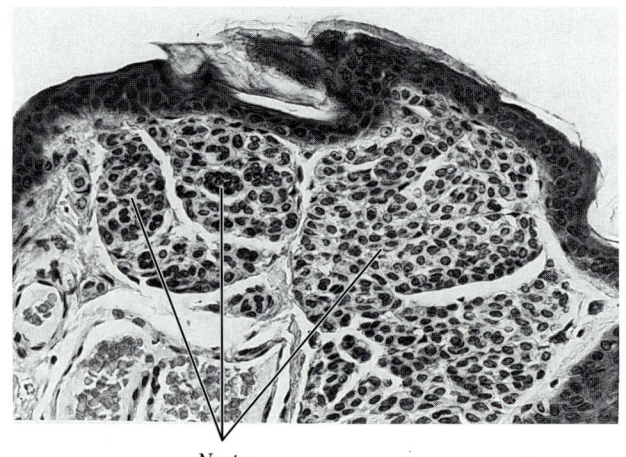

121 • Unna's Nevus *(excised during pregnancy)*

Criteria for diagnosis of this Unna's nevus (removed during pregnancy)

This is a nevus because:

There are nests, cords, and strands of small, oval, monomorphous melanocytes within the dermis in concert with a few tiny nests of melanocytes at the dermo-epidermal junction.

This is an Unna's nevus because:

The silhouette of the lesion is indistinguishable from that of an acrochordon: it is mostly exophytic and papillated, and melanocytes fill the markedly thickened papillary dermis.

This is a nevus removed during pregnancy because:

The history was that of a nevus removed during pregnancy. In short, a histopathologist cannot identify a nevus removed from someone pregnant by using any single morphologic criterion or any constellation of criteria. There are numerous melanophages in the upper part of the dermis of this lesion, and they could be responsible for the darkening said to occur in nevi during pregnancy.

diagnosed simply as melanoma, and if the very different conditions designated "lentigo" are modified by "simple," "solar," and "labial."

There is no evidence that pregnancy induces nevi to resemble melanoma or to convert to melanoma (Fig. 121). During pregnancy, nevi may become darker as a consequence of the play of adrenocorticotropic hormone (ACTH) and melanocyte-stimulating hormone (MSH) on them, but nevi are not transformed into melanoma as a consequence of hormones or any other effects of pregnancy. Nevi in those who are pregnant have all the clinical and histopathologic signs of a benign proliferation of melanocytes, i.e., a nevus of Unna, Miescher, Spitz, or Clark. Of course, a melanoma may develop in someone who is pregnant, just as a melanoma may originate in a child or in an octogenarian, but there is no evidence that pregnancy causes nevi to eventuate in melanoma. A melanoma in a woman who is pregnant has the same features as it does in any other person.

Last, a few lines should be devoted to the myth of an "epidemic" of melanoma. That reputed epidemic is in large measure a reflection of markedly enhanced capability for diagnosis of melanoma, clinically and histopathologically, when the lesion is small and flat. A mere 30 years ago, medical students were taught that melanoma is a large, fungating, black tumor that killed almost always. Melanoma in those days practically never was diagnosed when it was confined to epidermal and adnexal epithelium. Now, competent clinicians are able to diagnose melanoma when it is but a few millimeters in diameter and flat, and able histopathologists can make a diagnosis of melanoma in situ with facility, even when the melanocytes are disposed as solitary units only. Virtually all melanomas begin in situ and if dermatologists can diagnose that neoplasm when flat as melanoma, so, too, should histopathologists be able to do that, aided as they are by lenses of various magnifications. Furthermore, the diagnosis of melanoma in situ, which is made so commonly today, was guised in a variety of euphemisms in the past, among them activated junctional nevus, atypical melanocytic hyperplasia, severe melanocytic dysplasia, and pagetoid melanocytic proliferation. The increasing use of the word "melanoma" in diagnosis, rather than evasions from it, also contributes to the seemingly increased incidence of melanoma. In conclusion, there may have been a slight increase in the prevalence of melanoma during the past several decades, but surely nothing that resembles an epidemic. The situation for melanoma is not equivalent to that of Kaposi's sarcoma in acquired immunodeficiency syndrome (AIDS).

It cannot be stressed too emphatically that there are exceptions to every "rule" in morphologic diagnosis. Nowhere does that obtain more poignantly than in matters of melanoma and simulators of it.

This book is not a treatise about theoretic and philosophic aspects of melanomas. It is intended to be thoroughly practical in pursuit of its purpose to teach histopathologists to avoid pitfalls in diagnosis of melanoma by having firm, dependable, repeatable criteria for diagnosis predicated mostly upon silhouette. Being exquisitely alert to pitfalls in diagnosis is achieved best by what is learned as a consequence of having fallen into pits. What follows is an opportunity to profit immeasurably from that uncomfortable experience.

Bibliography

Ackerman, A.B.: Malignant melanoma: A unifying concept. Hum. Pathol. 11:591–597, 1980.

Ackerman, A.B.: Clinical diagnosis of malignant melanoma in situ. *In* Pathology of Malignant Melanoma, edited by A.B. Ackerman. New York, Masson USA, 1981, pp. 57–58.

Ackerman, A.B.: Classification of malignant melanomas: A view of the current controversy. Am. J. Dermatopathol. 4:447–452, 1982.

Ackerman, A.B.: Conventional microscopy: Signs that stamp pigmented melanocytic nevi as benign. Am. J. Dermatopathol. 4:461–466, 1982.

Ackerman, A.B.: Disagreements with the current classification of malignant melanomas. Am. J. Surg. Pathol. 6:733–743, 1982.

Ackerman, A.B.: Macular and patch lesions of malignant melanoma: Malignant melanoma in situ. J. Dermatol. Surg. Oncol. 9:615–618, 1983.

Ackerman, A.B., and Scheiner, A.M.: How wide and deep is wide and deep enough? A critique of surgical practice in excisions of primary cutaneous malignant melanoma. Hum. Pathol. 14:743–744, 1983.

Ackerman, A.B.: From the Editor. More than conventional microscopy is now required for study of moles and malignant melanomas. Am. J. Dermatopathol. 6:10–12 (Suppl.), 1984.

Ackerman, A.B., and Godomski, J.: Neurotropic malignant melanoma and other neurotropic neoplasms in the skin. Am. J. Dermatopathol. 6:63–80 (Suppl.), 1984.

Ackerman, A.B.: Controversies in Dermatopathology. Histopathologists can diagnose malignant melanoma in situ correctly and consistently. Am. J. Dermatopathol. 6:103–108 (Suppl.), 1984.

Ackerman, A.B., and Scheiner, A.M.: A critique of surgical practice in excisions of primary cutaneous malignant melanoma. Am. J. Dermatopathol. 6:109–112 (Suppl.), 1984.

Ackerman, A.B.: Critical commentary on statements in "Precursors to malignant melanoma." Am. J. Dermatopathol. 6:181–183 (Suppl.), 1984.

Ackerman, A.B.: Editorial. No one should die of malignant melanoma. J. Am. Acad. Dermatol. 12:115–116, 1985.

Ackerman, A.B., and Mihara, I.: Dysplasia, dysplastic melanocytes, dysplastic nevi, the dysplastic nevus syndrome, and the relation between dysplastic nevi and malignant melanomas. Hum. Pathol. 16:87–91, 1985.

Ackerman, A.B.: Malignant melanoma in situ. Pathology. 17:298–300, 1985.

Ackerman, A.B., and Elder, D.E.: An exchange of ideas about dysplastic nevi and malignant melanoma. Am. J. Dermatopathol. 7:99–105 (Suppl.), 1985.

Ackerman, A.B.: Das maligne Melanom in situ. Hautarzt 36:317–319, 1985.

Ackerman, A.B., and David, K.M.: A unifying concept of malignant melanoma. Biologic aspects. Hum. Pathol. 17:438–440, 1986.

Ackerman, A.B.: The concept of malignant melanoma in situ. *In* Pathobiology of Malignant Melanoma, edited by D.E. Elder. Basel, Karger, 1987, pp. 205–210.

Ackerman, A.B.: What naevus is dysplastic, a syndrome and the commonest precursor of malignant melanoma? A riddle and an answer. Histopathology 13:241–256, 1988.

Ackerman, A.B., and Magana-Garcia, M.: Naming acquired melanocytic nevi: Unna's, Miescher's, Spitz's, Clark's. Am. J. Dermatopathol. 12:193–209, 1990.

Ackerman, A.B., and Borghi, S.: "Pagetoid melanocytic proliferation" is the latest evasion from a diagnosis of "melanoma in situ." Am. J. Dermatopathol. 13:583–604, 1991.

Ackerman, A.B., Sood, R., and Koenig, M.: Primary acquired melanosis of the conjunctiva is melanoma in situ. Mod. Pathol. 4:253–263, 1991.

Ackerman, A.B., and Milde, P.: Naming Acquired Melanocytic Nevi: Common and Dysplastic, Normal and Atypical, or Unna, Miescher, Spitz, and Clark. Am. J. of Dermatopathol. 14:447–453, 1992.

Ackerman, A.B.: A Critique of an NIH Consensus Development Conference about "Early Melanoma." Am. J. of Dermatopathol. 15, 1993.

Ackerman, A.B.: Critique of definitions about melanocytic proliferations formulated by an N.I.H. panel. Am. J. of Dermatopathol. 14:238–244, 1992.

Albert, L.S., Rhodes, A.R., and Sober, A.J.: Dysplastic melanocytic nevi and cutaneous melanoma: Markers of increased melanoma risk for affected persons and blood relatives. J. Am. Acad. Dermatol. 22:69–75, 1990.

Allen, A.C.: Juvenile melanomas. Ann. N.Y. Acad. Sci. 100:29–48, 1963.

Aloi, F.G., Coverlizza, S., and Pippione, M.: Balloon cell melanoma: A report of two cases. J. Cutan. Pathol. 15:230–233, 1988

Balch, C.M., et al.: Cutaneous melanoma, Philadelphia, J.B. Lippincott, 1992.

Bale, S.J., et al.: Mapping the gene for hereditary cutaneous malignant melanoma—dysplastic nevus to chromosome 1p. N. Engl. J. Med. 320:1367–1372, 1989.

Barnhill, R.L., and Mihm, Jr., M.C.: Pigmented spindle cell naevus and its variants: distinction from melanoma. Br. J. Dermatol. 121:717–726, 1989.

Barnhill, R.L. and Roush, G.C.: Histopathologic spectrum of clinically atypical melanocytic nevi. Arch. Dermatol. 126:1315–1318, 1990.

Barnhill, R.L., et al.: Genital lentiginosis: A clinical and histopathologic study. J. Am. Acad. Dermatol. 22:453–460, 1990.

Barnhill, R.L., Roush, G.C., and Duray, P.H.: Correlation of histologic architectural and cytoplasmic features with nuclear atypia in atypical (dysplastic) nevomelanocytic nevi. Hum. Pathol. 21:51–58, 1990.

Barnhill, R.L.: Current status of the dysplastic melanocytic nevus. J. Cutan. Pathol. 18:147–159, 1991.

Barnhill, R.L., Barnhill, M.A., Berwick, M., and Mihm, Jr., M.C.: The histologic spectrum of pigmented spindle cell nevus: A review of 120 cases with emphasis on atypical variants. Hum. Pathol. 22:52–58, 1991.

Barnhill, R.L., Mihm, Jr., M.C., and Magro, C.M.: Plexiform spindle cell naevus: a distinctive variant of plexiform melanocytic naevus. Histopathology 18:243–247, 1991.

Barr, R.J., Morales, R.V., and Graham, J.H.: Desmoplastic nevus: a distinct histologic variant of mixed spindle cell and epithelioid cell nevus. Cancer 46:557–564, 1980.

Bergman, W., Ruiter, D.J., Scheffer, E., and van Vloten, W.A.: Melanocytic atypia in dysplastic nevi. Cancer 61:1660–1666, 1988.

Bhuta, S., Mirra, J.M., and Cochran, A.J.: Myxoid malignant melanoma: A previously undescribed histologic pattern noted in metastatic lesions and a report of four cases. Am. J. Surg. Pathol. 10:203–211, 1986.

Black, W.C., and Hunt, W.C.: Histologic correlations with the clinical diagnosis of dysplastic nevus. Am. J. Surg. Pathol. 14:44–52, 1990.

Breslow, A.: Thickness, cross-sectional areas and depth of invasion in the prognosis of cutaneous melanoma. Ann. Surg. 172:902–908, 1970.

Breslow, A.: Prognostic factors in the treatment of cutaneous melanoma. J. Cutan. Pathol. 6:208–212, 1979.

Bronson, D.M., and Ackerman, A.B.: Clefts as clues to melanocytes in the stratum corneum. Am. J. Dermatopathol. 6:161–162 (Suppl.), 1984.

Christensen, W.N., Friedman, K.J., Woodruff, J.D., and Hood, A.F.: Histologic characteristics of vulvar nevocellular nevi. J. Cutan. Pathol. 14:87–91, 1987.

Clark, Jr., W.H., From, L., Bernardino, E.A., and Mihm, M.C.: The histogenesis and biologic behavior of primary human malignant melanomas of the skin. Cancer Res. 29:705–727, 1969.

Clark, Jr., W.H., et al.: Origin of familial malignant melanomas from heritable melanocytic lesions: "The B-K mole syndrome". Arch. Dermatol. 114:732–738, 1978.

Clark, Jr., W.H., et al.: A study of tumor progression: The precursor lesions of superficial spreading and nodular melanoma. Hum. Pathol. 15:1147–1165, 1984.

Clark, Jr., W.H., Elder, D.E., and van Horn, M.: The biologic forms of malignant melanoma. Hum. Pathol. 17:443–450, 1986.

Clark, Jr., W.H., and Ackerman, A.B.: An exchange of views regarding the dysplastic nevus controversy. Semin. Dermatol. 8:229–250, 1989.

Clark, Jr., W.H., et al.: Model predicting survival in stage I melanoma based on tumor progression. J. Natl. Cancer Inst. 81:1893–1904, 1989.

Clemente, C., et al.: Histopathologic diagnosis of dysplastic nevi: Concordance among pathologists convened by the World Health Organization melanoma programme. Hum. Pathol. 22:313–319, 1991.

Clemmensen, O.J., and Kroon, S.: The histology of "congenital features" in early acquired melanocytic nevi. J. Am. Acad. Dermatol. 19:742–746, 1988.

Conley, J., Lattes, R., and Orr, W.: Desmoplastic malignant melanoma (a rare variant of spindle cell melanoma). Cancer 28:914–936, 1971.

Cook, M.G., and Fallowfield, M.E.: Dysplastic naevi—an alternative view. Histopathology 16:29–35, 1990.

Cooper, P.H.: Deep penetrating (plexiform spindle cell) nevus. J. Cutan. Pathol. 19:172–180, 1992.

Duray, P.H., and Ernstoff, M.S.: Dysplastic nevus in histologic contiguity with acquired nonfamilial melanoma. Arch. Dermatol. 123:80–84, 1987.

Egbert, B., Kempson, R., and Sagebiel, R.: Desmoplastic malignant melanoma. Cancer 62:2033–2041, 1988.

Elder, D.E., et al.: Dysplastic nevus syndrome: A phenotypic association of sporadic cutaneous melanoma. Cancer 46:1787–1794, 1980.

Elder, D.E., et al.: The dysplastic nevus syndrome. Am. J. Dermatopathol. 4:455–460, 1982.

Elder, D.E., and Murphy, G.F.: Atlas of tumor pathology. Melanocytic tumors of the skin. Washington, D.C., Armed Forces Institute of Pathology, 1991.

Feibleman, C.E., Stoll, H., and Maize, J.C.: Melanomas of the palm, sole, and nailbed: A clinicopathologic study. Cancer 46:2492–2504, 1980.

Fletcher, V., and Sagebiel, R.W.: The combined nevus: Mixed patterns of benign melanocytic lesions must be differentiated from malignant melanomas. *In* Pathology of Malignant Melanoma, edited by A.B. Ackerman. New York, Masson USA, 1981, pp. 273–283.

Friedman, R.J., and Ackerman, A.B.: Difficulties in the histologic diagnosis of melanocytic nevi on the vulvae of premenopausal women. *In* Pathology of Malignant Melanoma, edited by A.B. Ackerman. New York, Masson USA, 1981, pp. 119–127.

From, L., et al.: Origin of the desmoplasia in desmoplastic malignant melanoma. Hum. Pathol. 14:1072–1080, 1983.

Gartmann, H.: Der pigmentierte Spindelzelltumor (PSCT). Z. Hautkr. 56:862–876, 1981.

Gartmann, H., and Ganser, M.: Der Spitz-Naevus. Z. Hautkr. 60:22–28, 1985.

Gottlieb, G.J., and Ackerman, A.B.: Mitotic figures may be seen in cells of banal melanocytic nevi. Am. J. Dermatopathol. 7:87–91 (Suppl.), 1985.

Greene, M.H., et al.: Acquired precursors of cutaneous malignant melanoma. N. Engl. J. Med. 312:91–97, 1985.

Hastrup, N., Osterlind, A., Drzewiecki, K.T., and Hou-Jensen, K.: The presence of dysplastic nevus remnants in malignant melanomas. Am. J. Dermatopathol. 13:378–385, 1991.

Hendrickson, M.R., and Ross, J.C.: Neoplasms arising in congenital giant nevi. Am. J. Surg. Pathol. 5:109–135, 1981.

Illig, L., et al.: Congenital nevi <10 cm as precursors to melanoma. Arch. Dermatol. 121:1274–1281, 1985.

Jain, S. and Allen, P.W.: Desmoplastic malignant melanoma and its variants: A study of 45 cases. Am. J. Surg. Pathol. 13:358–373, 1989.

Jones, Jr., R.E., Cash, M.E., and Ackerman, A.B.: Malignant melanomas mistaken histologically for junctional nevi. *In* Pathology of Malignant Melanoma, edited by A.B. Ackerman. New York, Masson USA, 1981, pp. 93–106.

Kamino, H., and Ackerman, A.B.: Malignant melanoma in situ: The evolution of malignant melanoma within the epidermis. *In* Pathology of Malignant Melanoma, edited by A.B. Ackerman. New York, Masson USA, 1981, pp. 59–91.

Kamino, H., and Ackerman, A.B.: The problems of interpreting the meanings of atypical melanocytes and unusual patterns of melanocytes within the epidermis. *In* Pathology of Malignant Melanoma, edited by A.B. Ackerman. New York, Masson USA, 1981, pp. 129–157.

Kamino, H., and Tam, S.T.: Compound blue nevus: A variant of blue nevus with an additional junctional dendritic component. Arch. Dermatol. 126:1330–1333, 1990.

Kamino, H., Kiryu, H., and Ratech, H.: Small malignant melanomas: Clinicopathologic correlation and DNA ploidy analysis. J. Am. Acad. Dermatol. 22:1032–1038, 1990.

Kaye, V.N., and Dehner, L.P.: Spindle and epithelioid cell nevus (Spitz nevus). Arch. Dermatol. 126:1581–1583, 1990.

Kerl, H., Hoedl, S., and Stettner, H.: Acral lentiginous melanoma. *In* Pathology of Malignant Melanoma, edited by A.B. Ackerman. New York, Masson USA, 1981, pp. 217–242.

Kerl, H., Hoedl, S., Kresbach, H., and Stettner, H.: Diagnosis and prognosis of the early stages of cutaneous malignant melanoma. Clin. Oncol. 1:433–453, 1982.

Kerl, H., Trau, H., and Ackerman, A.B.: Differentiation of melanocytic nevi from malignant melanomas in palms, soles, and nail beds solely by signs in the cornified layer of the epidermis. Am. J. Dermatopathol. 6:159–160 (Suppl.), 1984.

Kerl, H., Smolle, J., Hoedl, S., and Soyer, H.P.: Kongenitales Pseudomelanom. Z. Hautkr. 64:564–568, 1989.

Kernan, J.A., and Ackerman, L.V.: Spindle cell nevi and epithelioid cell nevi (so-called juvenile melanomas) in children and adults. Cancer 13:612–625, 1960.

Klein, L.J., and Barr, R.J.: Histologic atypia in clinically benign nevi. J. Am. Acad. Dermatol. 22:275–282, 1990.

Kopf, A.W., Bart, R.S., and Hennessey, P.: Congenital nevocytic nevi and malignant melanomas. J. Am. Acad. Dermatol. 1:123–130, 1979.

Kopf, A.W., Bart, R.S., Rodriguez-Sains, R., and Ackerman, A.B.: Malignant Melanoma. New York, Masson USA, 1979.

Kopf, A.W., Friedman, R.J., and Rigel, D.S.: Atypical mole syndrome. J. Am. Acad. Dermatol. 22:117–118, 1990.

Kornberg, R., and Ackerman, A.B.: Pseudomelanoma. Arch. Dermatol. 111:1588–1590, 1975.

Kornberg, R., Harris, M., and Ackerman, A.B.: Epidermotropically metastatic malignant melanoma. Arch. Dermatol. 114:67–69, 1978.

Kuehnl-Petzoldt, C., et al.: Histology of congenital nevi during the first year of life. Am. J. Dermatopathol. 6:81–88 (Suppl.), 1984.

Lynch, H.T., et al.: A review of hereditary malignant melanoma including biomarkers in familial atypical multiple mole melanoma syndrome. Cancer Genet. Cytogenet. 8:325–358, 1983.

Macy-Roberts, E., and Ackerman, A.B.: A critique of techniques for biopsy of clinically suspected malignant melanomas. Am. J. Dermatopathol. 4:391–398, 1982.

Maize, J., and Ackerman, A.B.: Pigmented Lesions of the Skin. Philadelphia, Lea & Febiger, 1987.

Mark, G.J., et al.: Congenital melanocytic nevi of the small and garment type. Hum. Pathol. 4:395–418, 1973.

McGovern, V.J., Shaw, H.M., and Milton, G.W.: Prognosis in patients with thin malignant melanoma: Influence of regression. Histopathology 7:673–680, 1983.

Mehregan, A.H.: Dysplastic nevi: A histopathological investigation. J. Cutan. Pathol. 15:276–281, 1988.

Michalik, E.E., Fitzpatrick, T.B., and Sober, A.J.: Rapid progression of lentigo maligna to deeply invasive lentigo maligna melanoma. Arch. Dermatol. 119:831–835, 1983.

Miescher, G., and von Albertini, A.: Histologie de 100 cas de naevi pigmentaires d'apres les methodes de Masson. Bull. Soc. Fr. Dermatol. Syph. 42:1265–1273, 1935.

Mihm, Jr., M.C., Murphy, G.F., and Kaufman, N., (eds.): Pathobiology and Recognition of Malignant Melanoma. Baltimore, Williams & Wilkins, 1988.

Mihm, Jr., M.C., and Googe, P.B.: Problematic Pigmented Lesions. Philadelphia, Lea & Febiger, 1990.

Murphy, G.F., and Halpern, A.: Dysplastic melanocytic nevi. Arch. Dermatol. 126:519–521, 1990.

NIH Consensus Conference 1983: Precursors to malignant melanoma. J. Am. Acad. Dermatol. 10:683–688, 1984.

NIH Consensus Conference 1991: Early melanoma—Histologic terms. Am. J. Dermatopathol. 13:579–582, 1991.

Nix, M., and Ackerman, A.B.: Differentiation of "melanocytic angiofibromas" (fibrous papules of the face) from early evolving malignant melanomas in situ in specimens removed by superficial shave technique. Am. J. Dermatopathol. 6:163–168 (Suppl.), 1984.

Paniago-Pereira, C., Maize, J.C., and Ackerman, A.B.: Nevus of large spindle and/or epithelioid cells (Spitz's nevus). Arch. Dermatol. 114:1811–1823, 1978.

Park, H.K., Leonard, D.D., Arrington III, J.H., and Lund, H.Z.: Recurrent melanocytic nevi: Clinical and histologic review of 175 cases. J. Am. Acad. Dermatol. 17:285–292, 1987.

Patterson, R.H., and Helwig, E.B.: Subungual malignant melanoma: A clinical-pathologic study. Cancer 46:2074–2087, 1980.

Peters, M.S., and Goellner, J.R.: Spitz naevi and malignant melanomas of childhood and adolescence. Histopathology 10:1289–1302, 1986.

Piepkorn, M., et al.: The dysplastic melanocytic nevus: A prevalent lesion that correlates poorly with clinical phenotype. J. Am. Acad. Dermatol. 20:407–415, 1989.

Piepkorn, M.: A hypothesis incorporating the histologic characteristics of dysplastic nevi into the normal biological development of melanocytic nevi. Arch. Dermatol. 126:514–518, 1990.

Plotnick, H., Rachmaninoff, N., and Van den Berg, Jr., H.J.: Polypoid melanoma: A virulent variant of nodular melanoma. J. Am. Acad. Dermatol. 23:880–884, 1990.

Price, N.M., Rywlin, A.M., and Ackerman, A.B.: Histologic criteria for the diagnosis of superficial spreading malignant melanoma: Formulated on the basis of proven metastatic lesions. Cancer 38:2434–2441, 1976.

Reed, R.J., and Leonard, D.D.: Neurotropic melanoma. Am. J. Surg. Pathol. 3:301–311, 1979.

Reed, R.J.: A classification of melanocytic dysplasias and malignant melanomas. Am. J. Dermatopathol. 6:195–206 (Suppl.), 1984.

Reed, R.J.: Minimal deviation melanoma. Hum. Pathol. 21:1206–1211, 1990.

Reed, R.J., Webb, S.V., and Clark, Jr., W.H.: Minimal deviation melanoma (halo nevus variant). Am. J. Surg. Pathol. 14:53–68, 1990.

Requena, L., and Sanchez Yus, E.: Pigmented spindle cell naevus. Br. J. Dermatol. 123:757–763, 1990.

Requena, L., et al.: Malignant combined nevus. Am. J. Dermatopathol. 13:169–173, 1991.

Rhodes, A.R., et al.: The malignant potential of small congenital nevocellular nevi. An estimate of association based on a histologic study of 234 primary cutaneous melanomas. J. Am. Acad. Dermatol. 6:230–241, 1982.

Rhodes, A.R., et al.: Dysplastic melanocytic nevi in histologic association with 234 primary cutaneous melanomas. J. Am. Acad. Dermatol. 9:563–574, 1983.

Rhodes, A.R., et al.: Increased intraepidermal melanocyte frequency and size in dysplastic melanocytic nevi and cutaneous melanoma. A comparative quantitative study of dysplastic melanocytic nevi, superficial spreading melanoma, nevocellular nevi, and solar lentigines. J. Invest. Dermatol. 80:452–459, 1983.

Rhodes, A.R., Silverman, R.A., Harrist, T.J., and Melski, J.W.: A histologic comparison of congenital and acquired nevo-melanocytic nevi. Arch. Dermatol. 121:1266–1273, 1985.

Rhodes, A.R., Mihm, Jr., M.C., and Weinstock, M.A.: Dysplastic melanocytic nevi: A reproducible histologic definition emphasizing cellular morphology. Mod. Pathol. 2:306–319, 1989.

Rigel, D.S., et al.: Dysplastic nevi. Cancer 63:386–389, 1989.

Rivers, J.K., Cockerell, C.J., McBride, A., and Kopf, A.W.: Quantification of histologic features of dysplastic nevi. Am. J. Dermatopathol. 12:42–50, 1990.

Rogers, G.S., Advani, H., and Ackerman, A.B.: A combined variant of Spitz's nevi: How to differentiate them from malignant melanomas. Am. J. Dermatopathol. 7:61–78 (Suppl.), 1985.

Roses, D.F., et al.: Assessment of biopsy techniques and histopathologic interpretations of primary cutaneous malignant melanoma. Ann. Surg. 189:294–297, 1979.

Roses, D., Harris, M., and Ackerman, A.B. (eds.): Diagnosis and Management of Cutaneous Malignant Melanoma. Philadelphia, W.B. Saunders, 1983.

Roth, M.E., et al.: Melanoma in children. J. Am. Acad. Dermatol. 22:265–274, 1990.

Roth, M.E., et al.: The histopathology of dysplastic nevi. Am. J. Dermatopathol. 13:38–51, 1991.

Sagebiel, R.W., Chinn, E.K., and Egbert, B.M.: Pigmented spindle cell nevus. Am. J. Surg. Pathol. 8:645–653, 1984.

Sagebiel, R.W., Banda, P.W., Schneider, J.S., and Crutcher, W.A.: Age distribution and histologic patterns of dysplastic nevi. J. Am. Acad. Dermatol. 13:975–982, 1985.

Sagebiel, R.W.: The dysplastic melanocytic nevus. J. Am. Acad. Dermatol. 20:496–501, 1989.

Saida, T., and Yoshida, N.: Guidelines for histopathologic diagnosis of plantar malignant melanoma. Dermatologica 181:112–116, 1990.

Schmoeckel, C., and Braun-Falco, O.: Prognostic index in malignant melanoma. Arch. Dermatol. 114:871–873, 1978.

Schmoeckel, C., Castro, C.E., and Braun-Falco, O.: Nevoid malignant melanoma. Arch. Dermatol. Res. 277:362–369, 1985.

Seab, Jr., J.A., Graham, J.H., and Helwig, E.B.: Deep penetrating nevus. Am. J. Surg. Pathol. 13:39–44, 1989.

Shapiro, L., and Ackerman, A.B.: Solitary lichen planus-like keratosis. Dermatologica 132:386–392, 1966.

Sheibani, K., and Battifora, H.: Signet-ring cell melanoma. Am. J. Surg. Pathol. 12:28–34, 1988.

Silvers, D.N., and Helwig, E.B.: Melanocytic nevi in neonates. J. Am. Acad. Dermatol. 4:166–175, 1981.

Sison-Torre, E.Q., and Ackerman, A.B.: Melanosis of the vulva: A clinical simulator of malignant melanoma. Am. J. Dermatopathol. 7:51–60 (Suppl.), 1985.

Smith, K.J., et al.: Spindle cell and epithelioid cell nevi with atypia and metastasis (malignant Spitz's nevus). Am. J. Surg. Pathol. 13:931–939, 1989.

Smith, N.P.: The pigmented spindle cell tumor of Reed: An underdiagnosed lesion. Semin. Diagn. Pathol. 4:75–87, 1987.

Spitz, S.: Melanomas of childhood. Am. J. Pathol. 24:591–609, 1948.

Steijlen, P.M., et al.: The efficacy of histopathological criteria required for diagnosing dysplastic naevi. Histopathology 12:289–300, 1988.

Stolz, W., Schmoeckel, C., Landthaler, M., and Braun-Falco, O.: Association of early malignant melanoma with nevocytic nevi. Cancer 63:550–555, 1989.

Tièche, M.: Ueber benigne Melanome ("Chromatophorome") der Haut—"blaue Naevi". Virchows Arch. Pathol. Anat. 186:212–229, 1906.

Trau, H., et al.: Regression in malignant melanoma. J. Am. Acad. Dermatol. 8:363–368, 1983.

Unna, P.G.: The Histopathology of the Diseases of the Skin. New York, Macmillan & Co., 1896.

Urso, C., Giannotti, B., and Bondi, R.: Myxoid melanoma of the skin. Arch. Pathol. Lab. Med. 144:527–528, 1990.

Weedon, D.: Unusual features of nevocellular nevi. J. Cutan. Pathol. 9:284–292, 1982.

IX. Pitfalls   Figures 1–101

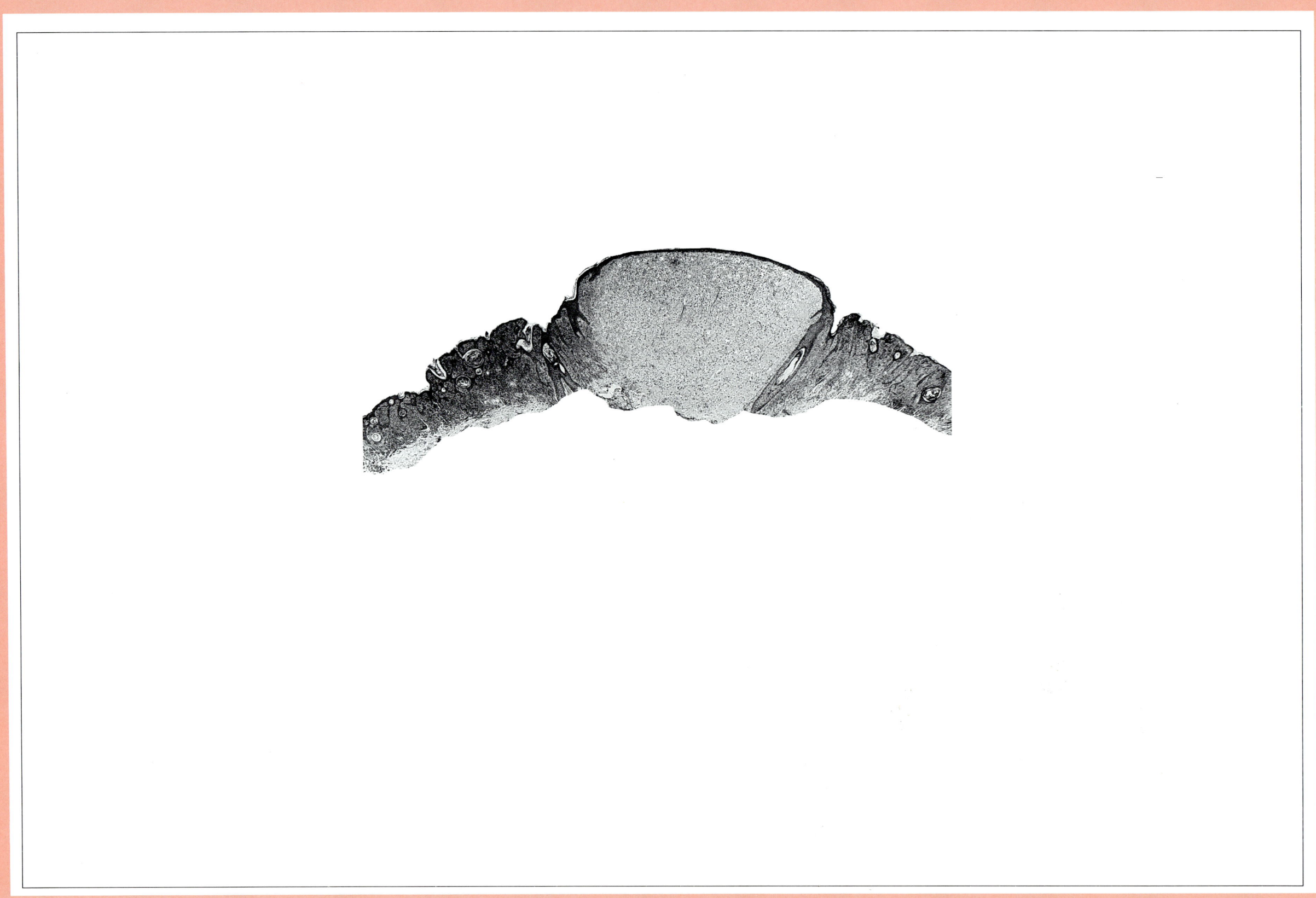

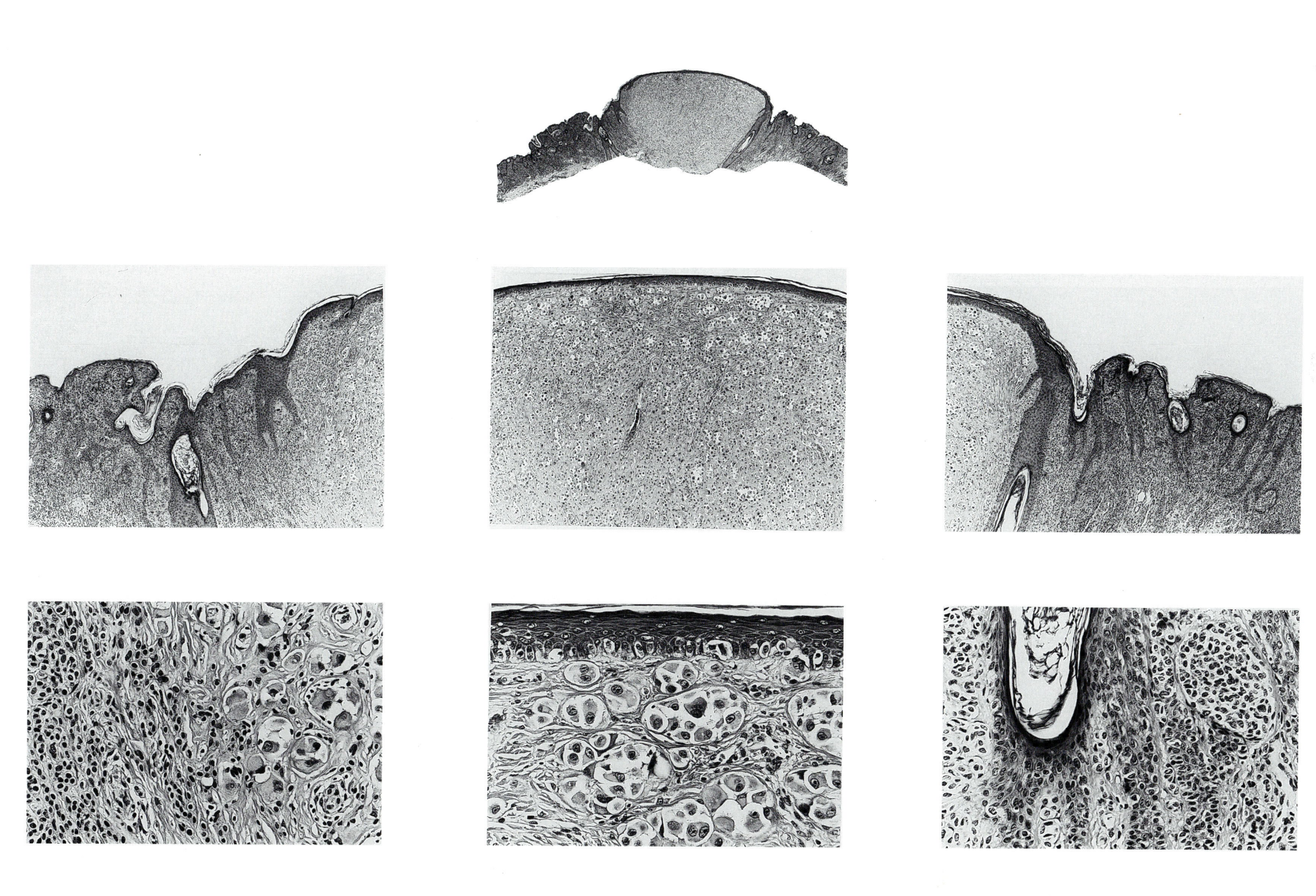

1. What is your diagnosis?

A sharply circumscribed lesion of uniform color on the back of a 15-year-old boy. Clinical diagnosis: nevus. Patient is in good health after 5 years.

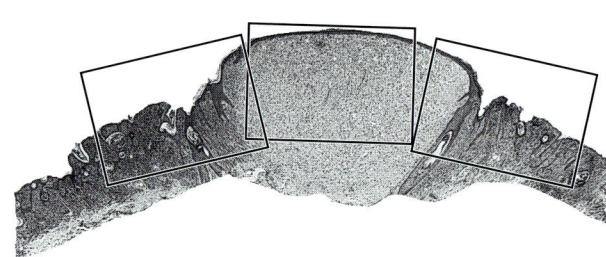

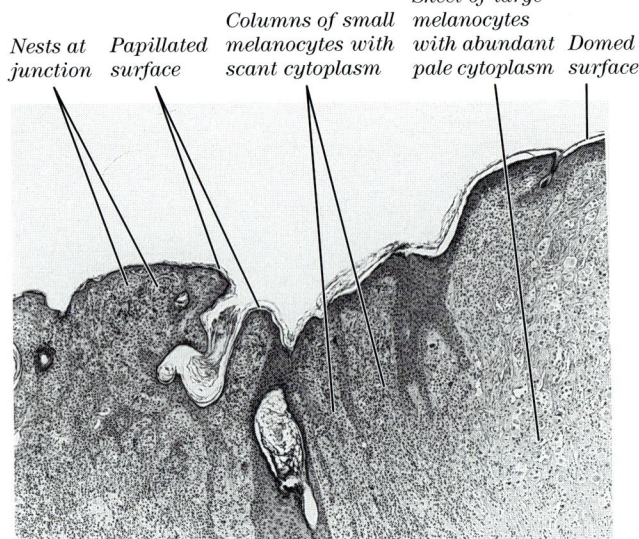

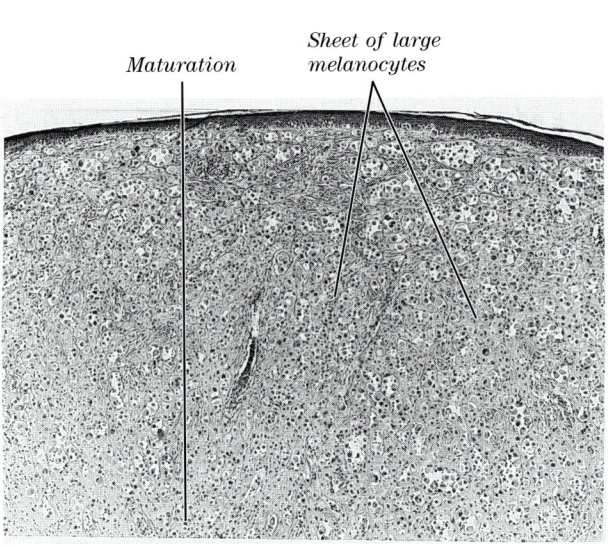

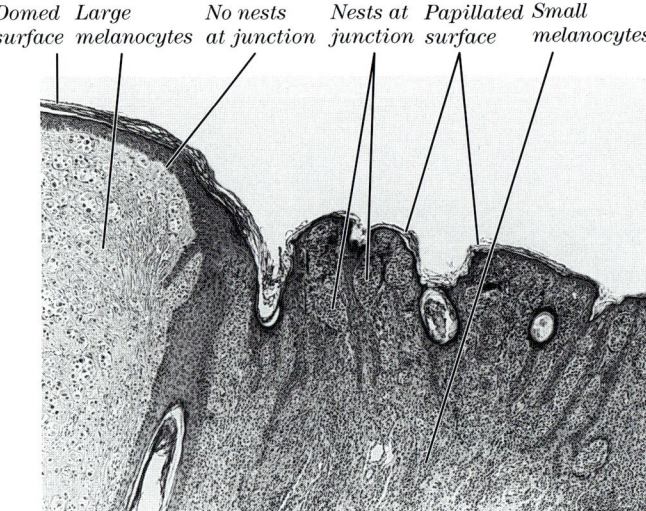

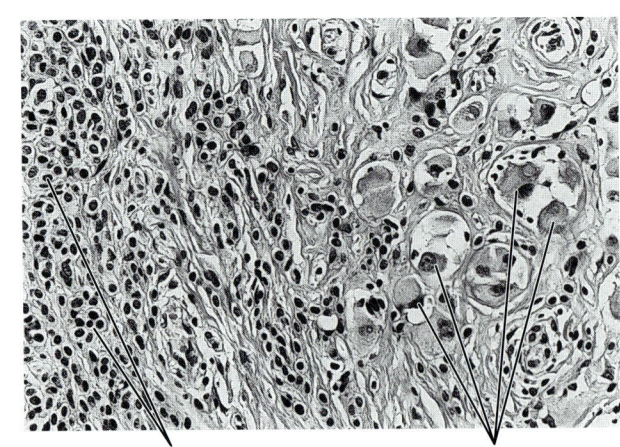

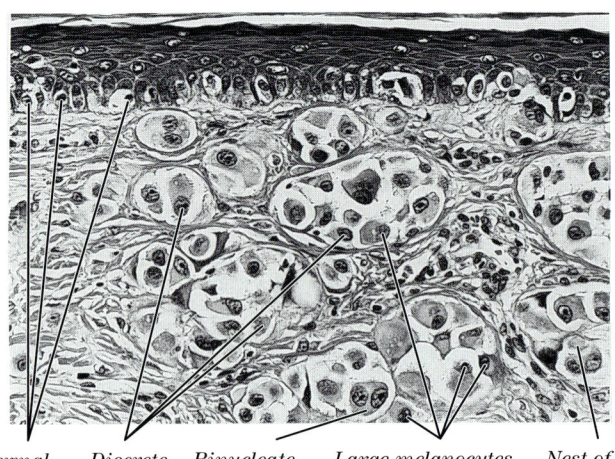

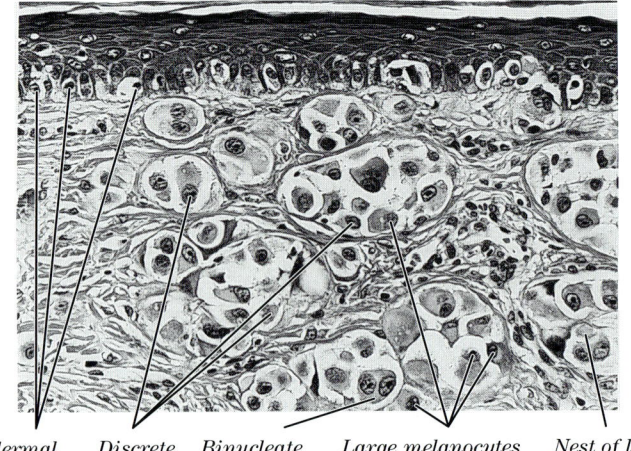

Nests at junction · *Papillated surface* · *Columns of small melanocytes with scant cytoplasm* · *Sheet of large melanocytes with abundant pale cytoplasm* · *Domed surface*

Maturation · *Sheet of large melanocytes*

Domed surface · *Large melanocytes* · *No nests at junction* · *Nests at junction* · *Papillated surface* · *Small melanocytes*

Small melanocytes with oval nuclei and scant cytoplasm · *Large polygonal melanocytes with atypical nuclei and abundant cytoplasm*

Intraepidermal proliferation of melanocytes with pleomorphic nuclei · *Discrete nests* · *Binucleate melanocyte* · *Large melanocytes with pleomorphic nuclei and abundant cytoplasm* · *Nest of large polygonal melanocytes*

Nests of melanocytes with small oval nuclei and scant cytoplasm

1 • Combined Nevus *(Clark's and Spitz's)*

Criteria for diagnosis of this combined nevus (Spitz's and Clark's)

This neoplasm is benign because:

1. The central papule is oriented vertically.
2. Melanocytes within the central papule exhibit maturation with progressive descent into the dermis.
3. There are no mitotic figures.
4. Changes at the sides of the central papule are those of a compound Clark's nevus.

This is a combined nevus because:

1. Two types of acquired melanocytic nevus are presented in this section: a central Spitz's nevus and a peripheral Clark's nevus.

Pitfall in diagnosis

This combined (Spitz's and Clark's) nevus could be misinterpreted as a melanoma because:

1. Two distinct populations of melanocytes constitute this neoplasm.
2. Atypical nuclei of many melanocytes are seen in the central papule.
3. Within the epidermis of the central papule are atypical melanocytes disposed as solitary units at the dermo-epidermal junction and above it.
4. Neoplastic melanocytes within the papule are arranged in sheets.

At scanning magnification, the clue to benignancy of the central papular component of this neoplasm is its tiny size (little more than 2.0 mm in greatest diameter), vertical orientation, and partial embrace by adnexal epithelium. Because the melanocytes that constitute the papule have strikingly atypical nuclei in no way alters the reality of the neoplasm being benign. It is a combined nevus because the architectural pattern of each of the two components is that of a benign neoplasm.

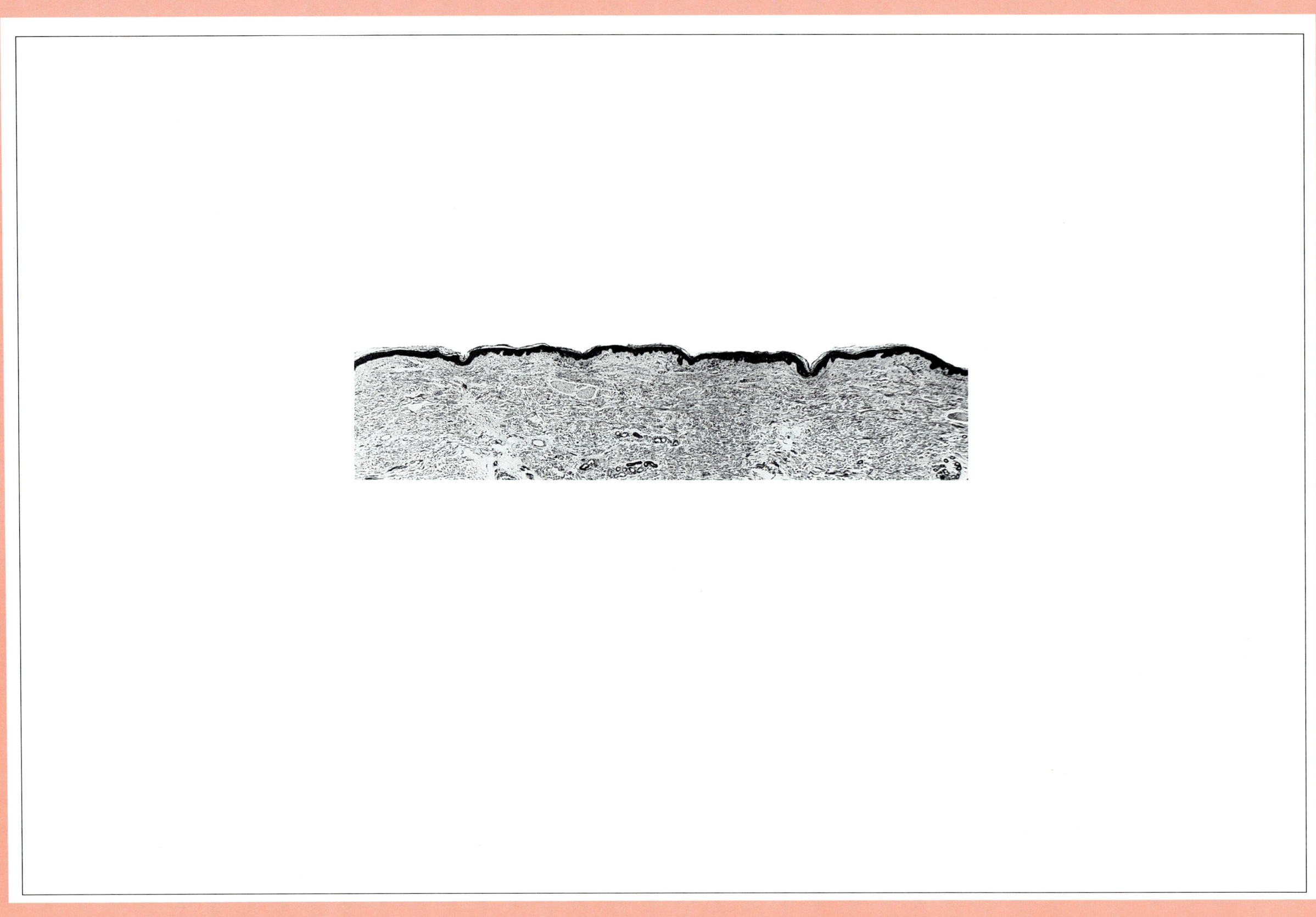

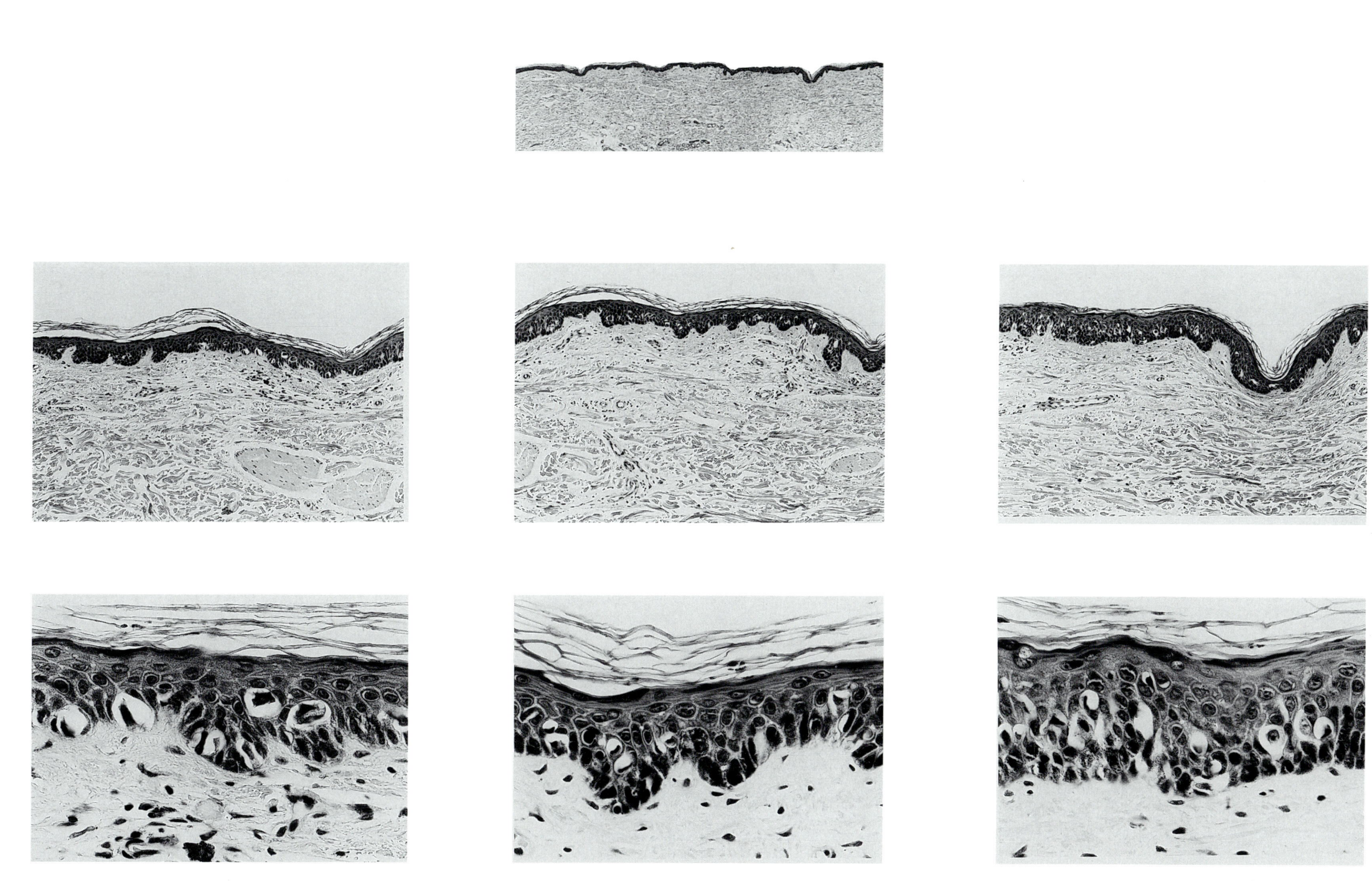

2. What is your diagnosis?

Pigmented lesion from the left calf of a 58-year-old man with a history of melanoma. Clinical diagnosis: melanocytic nevus. No follow-up information is available.

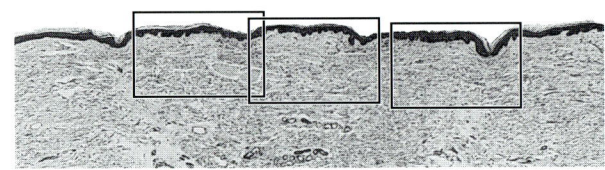

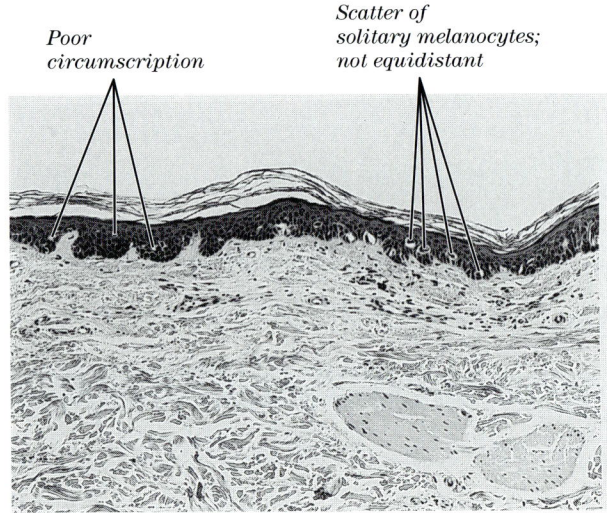

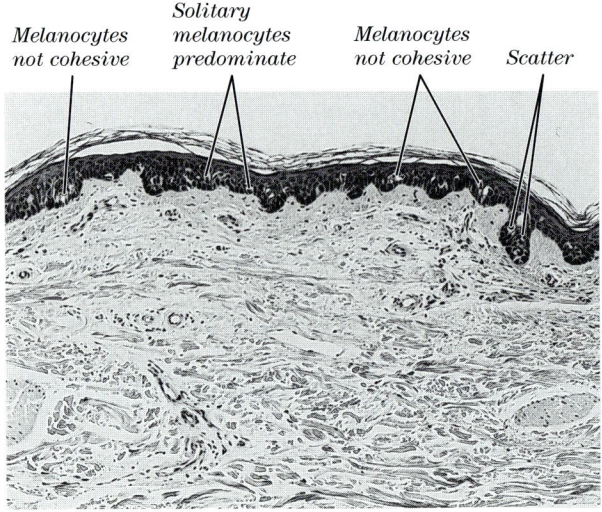

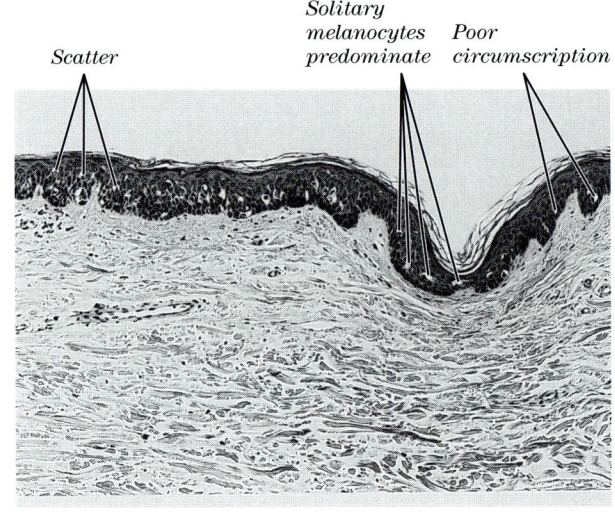

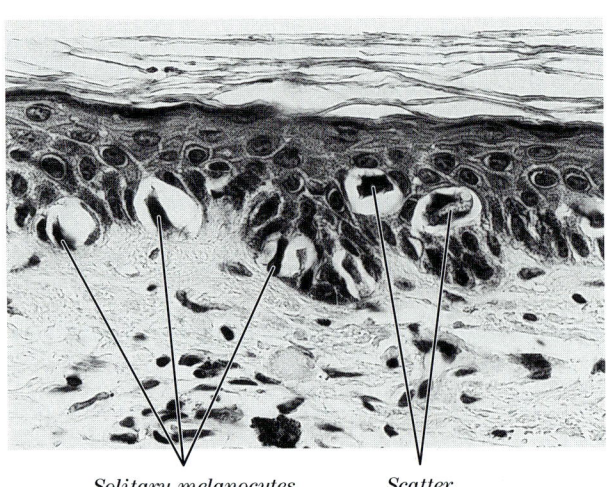

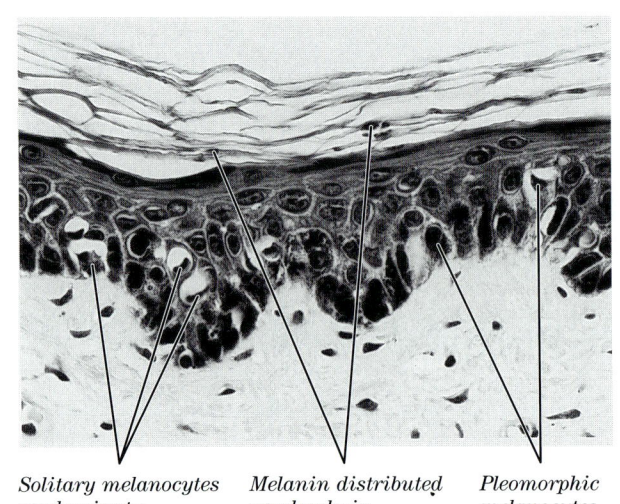

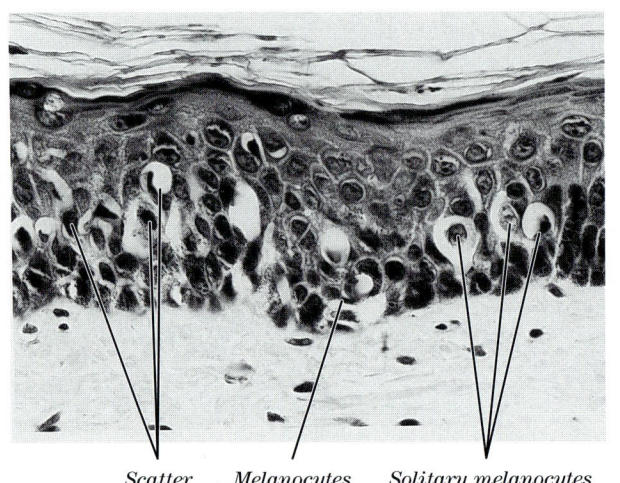

2 • Melanoma in situ

Criteria for diagnosis of this melanoma in situ

This is a melanoma in situ because:

1. Melanocytes within the epidermis are not seated wholly at the dermo-epidermal junction, but are scattered above it.

2. More melanocytes are present above the dermo-epidermal junction than at it.

3. Melanocytes arranged as solitary units are not equidistant from one another.

4. Some melanocytes have atypical nuclei.

5. Melanin is not distributed in uniform fashion within the epidermis, a finding reflected best in the cornified layer.

Pitfall in diagnosis

This melanoma in situ could be misinterpreted as an early junctional Spitz's nevus because:

1. The vast majority of melanocytes within the epidermis are disposed as solitary units.

2. Melanocytes are positioned mostly in the lower half of the epidermis.

3. There is little, if any, nuclear atypia in many melanocytes.

The reason for the variegate colors in melanomas in situ as they present themselves clinically is uneven distribution of melanin within the epidermis and papillary dermis. That phenomenon is illustrated well in this section. Melanin is not distributed uniformly across the entire epidermis, and melanophages are scattered haphazardly in the papillary dermis. In short, attention to distribution of melanin within melanocytic neoplasms may be as important to specific diagnosis as scrutiny of melanocytes themselves.

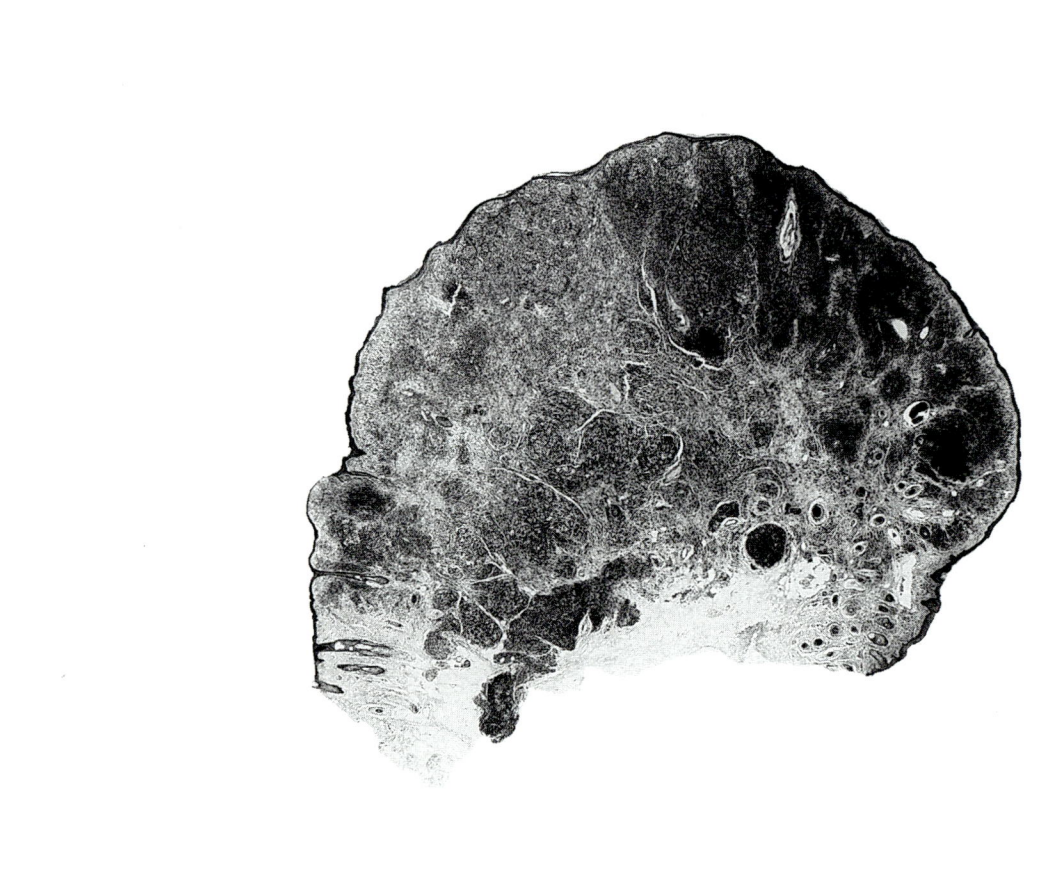

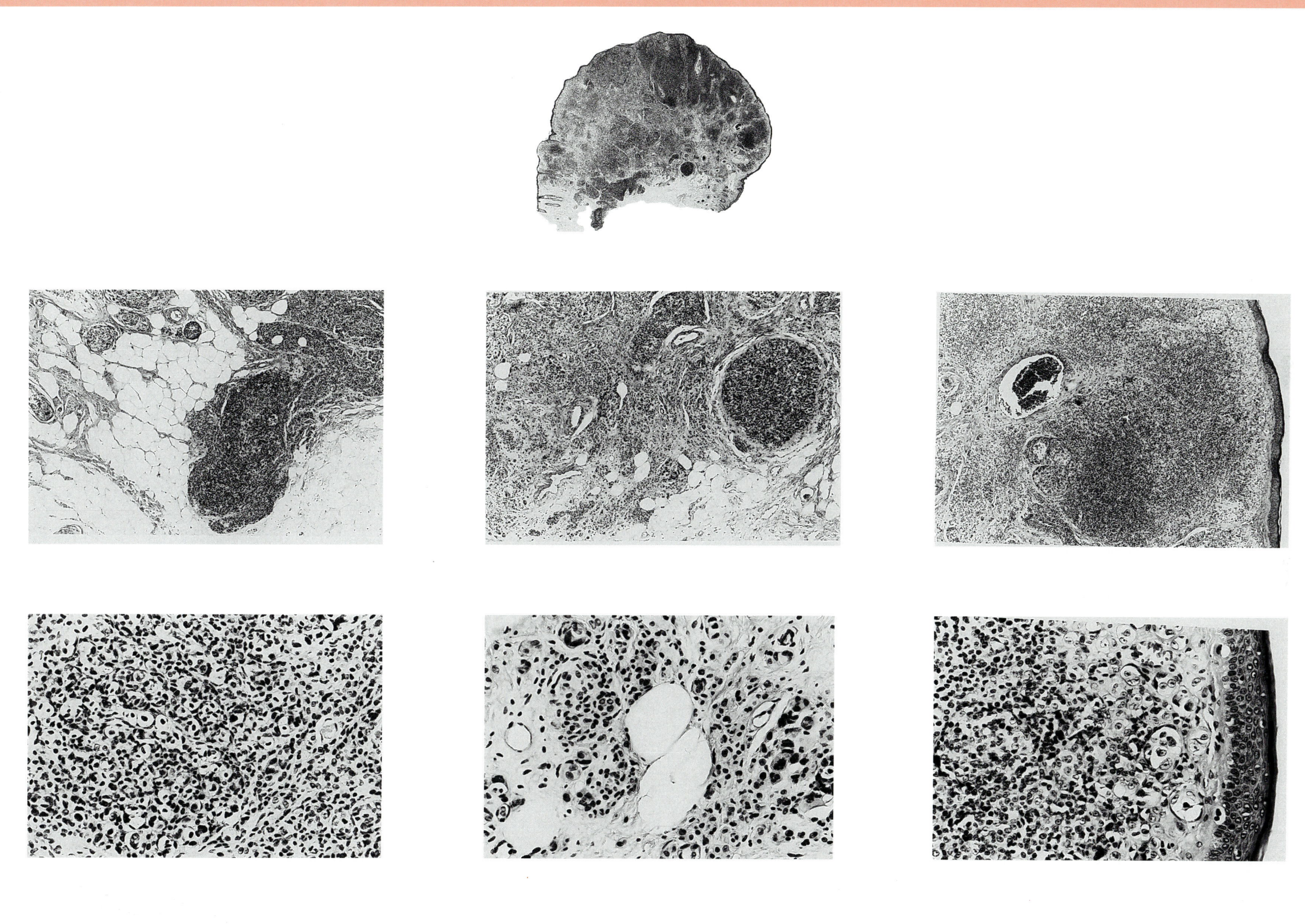

3. What is your diagnosis?

Reddish-brown lesion on the left auricle of a 60-year-old woman. The lesion was excised completely. Patient was free of disease after 1 year.

Small aggregations of small melanocytes *Large aggregation of large melanocytes*

Small melanocytes *Cleft* *Large melanocytes* *Aggregations of large melanocytes*

Small melanocytes *Widely dilated venule* *Sheet of large melanocytes* *Dilated venule*

Confluence of nests of large melanocytes

Large melanocytes *Nests of small melanocytes* *Mitosis* *Atypical melanocyte*

Small melanocytes *Large melanocytes*

3 • Miescher's Nevus *(ancient)*

Criteria for diagnosis of this Miescher's nevus (ancient)

This is a nevus because:

1. The neoplasm is well-circumscribed.
2. There is maturation of melanocytes.
3. The process is wholly intradermal, i.e., there is no sign of melanoma in situ.

This is a Miescher's nevus because:

1. The neoplasm is dome-shaped.
2. It is exo-endophytic.
3. The process is vaguely wedge-shaped.
4. Neoplastic melanocytes extend throughout the reticular dermis and into the subcutaneous fat.

This is an ancient Miescher's nevus because:

1. There are two populations of melanocytes within the dermis and subcutaneous fat: small and large.
2. Some of the neoplastic melanocytes are atypical, i.e., in addition to being large, they are pleomorphic and hyperchromatic.
3. Some neoplastic melanocytes are in mitosis.
4. Nests of melanocytes within the reticular dermis and the subcutaneous fat are both very large and very small.
5. There are exceptionally dilated vessels filled with erythrocytes.

Pitfall in diagnosis

This ancient Miescher's nevus could be misread as a melanoma because:

1. The neoplasm is strikingly asymmetric.
2. Neoplastic cells extend throughout the reticular dermis and into the subcutaneous fat.
3. Epithelial structures of adnexa, especially vellus follicles, are preserved much better on the right of the lesion than on the left of it.
4. Some neoplastic melanocytes have atypical nuclei.
5. Some neoplastic melanocytes near the base of the neoplasm are in mitosis.

Neoplastic cells in this neoplasm are confined to the dermis and subcutaneous fat. For practical purposes, a diagnosis of primary cutaneous melanoma cannot be made in the absence of signs of melanoma in situ. Surely this is not a metastasis of melanoma because typical melanocytes of a nevus are present in many foci throughout the neoplasm, and there are signs of maturation of melanocytes with progressive descent into the dermis and subcutaneous fat. If this melanocytic neoplasm is neither a primary nor a metastatic melanoma, it must be a nevus. The lesion fulfills criteria for Miescher's nevus, the "ancient" expression of which, illustrated here, may be confused histopathologically with melanoma.

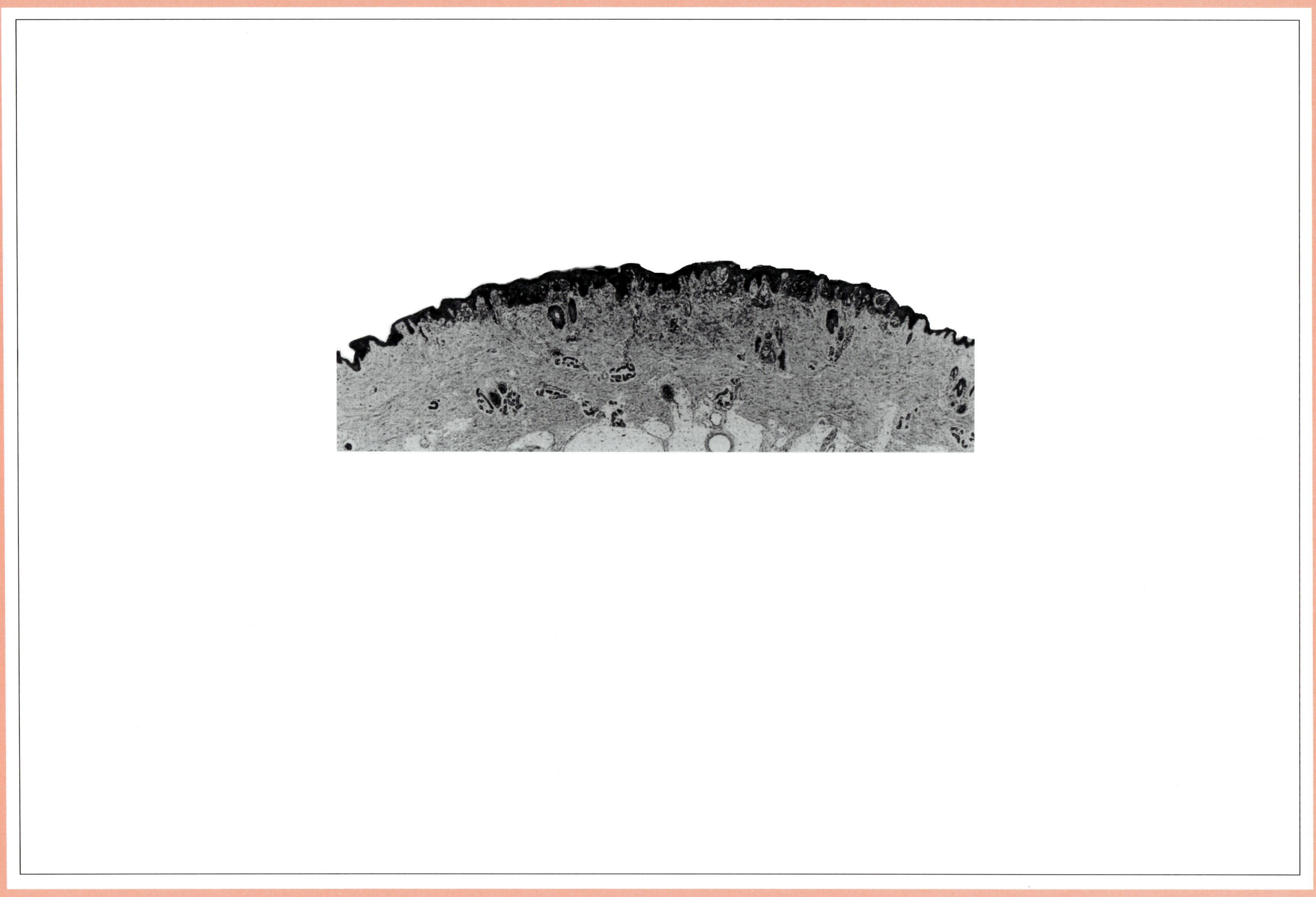

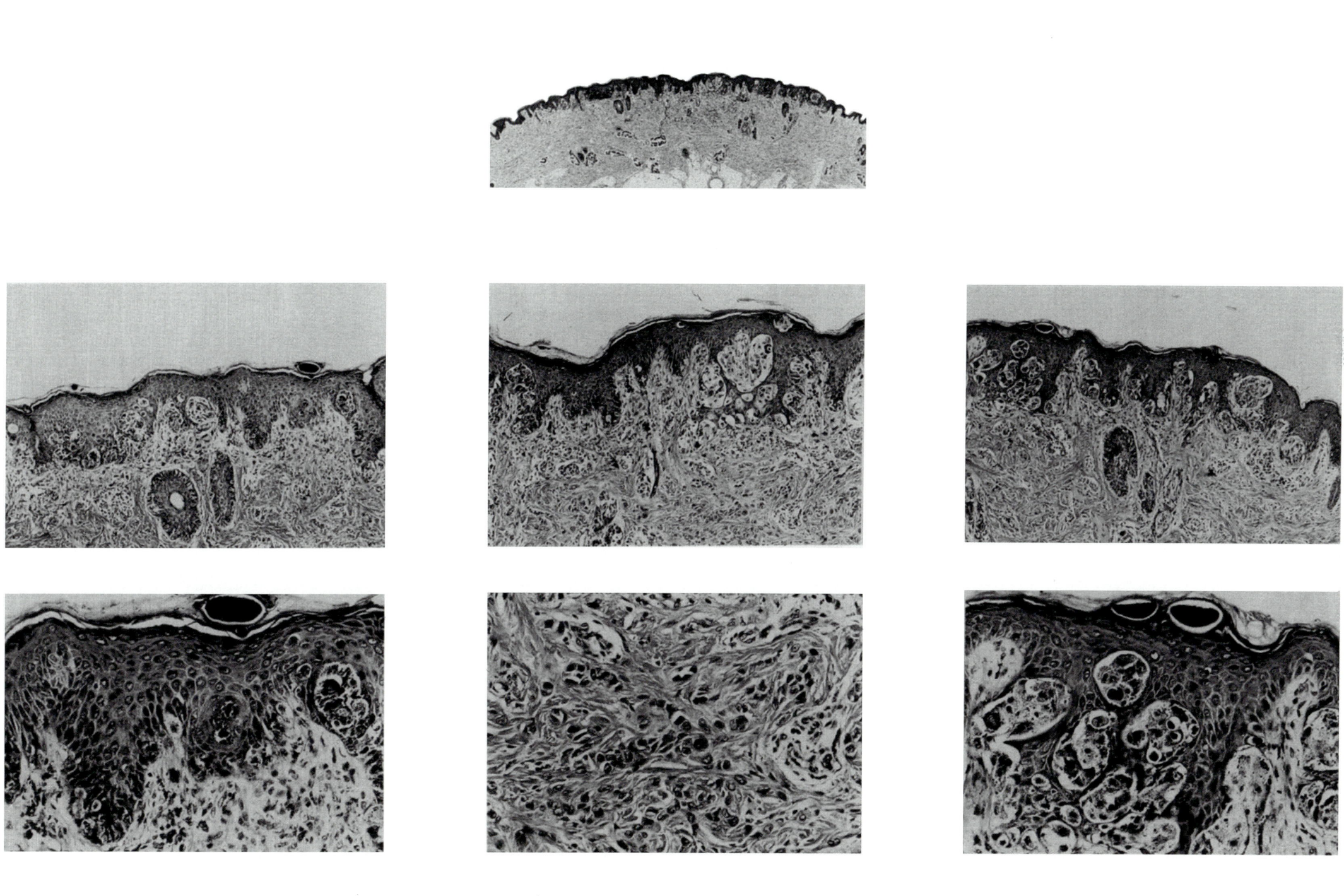

4. What is your diagnosis?

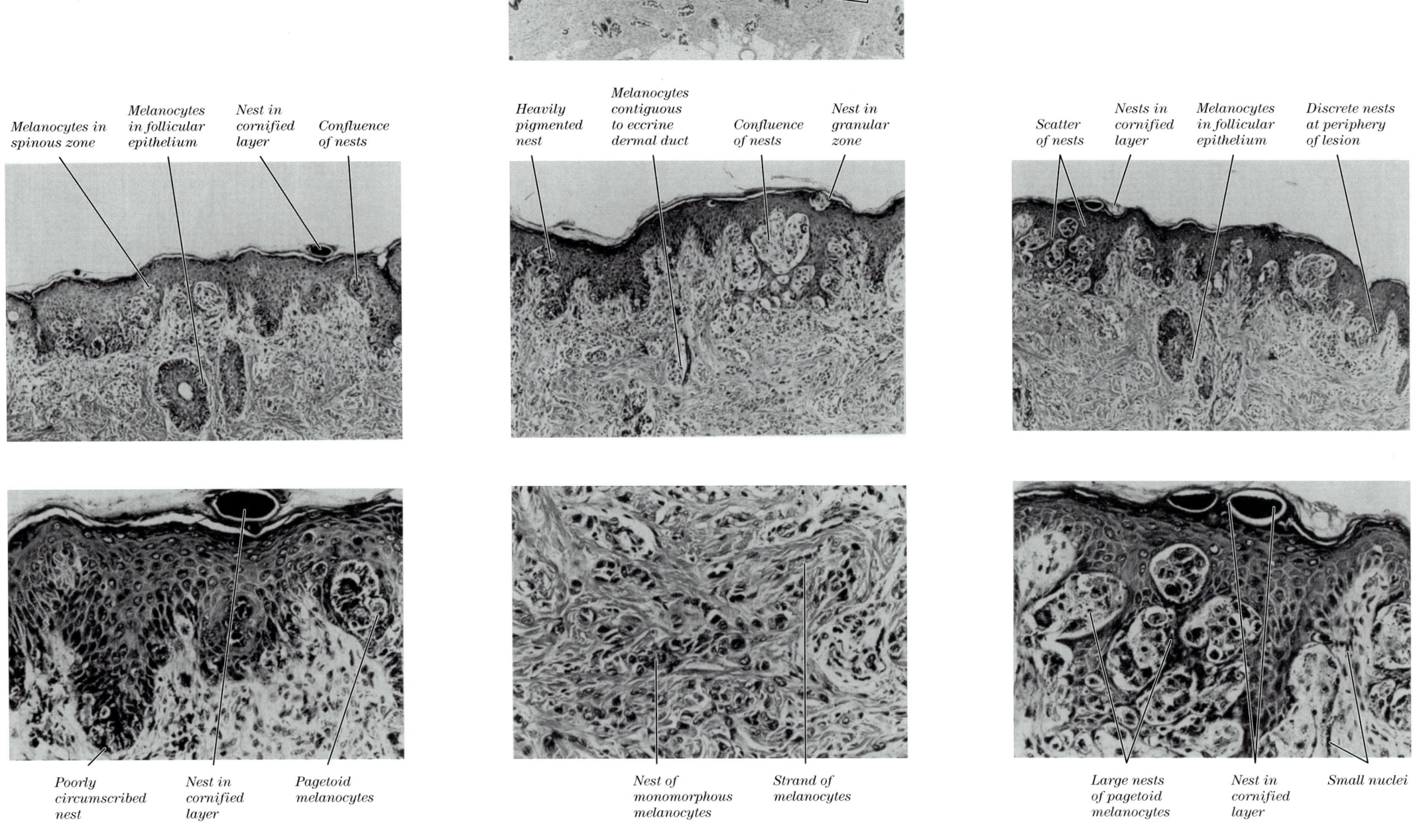

4 • Congenital Nevus *(superficial type)* Biopsied Shortly After Birth

Criteria for diagnosis of this congenital melanocytic nevus biopsied shortly after birth

This is a nevus because:

1. The lesion is symmetric.
2. It is very well-circumscribed.
3. There is maturation of melanocytes with progressive descent into the dermis.
4. Melanocytes arrayed in nests within the epidermis predominate over melanocytes arranged as solitary units there.
5. Nuclei of pagetoid melanocytes are small.

This is a congenital nevus because:

1. There is splaying of melanocytes between collagen bundles in the reticular dermis.
2. Melanocytes are present around epithelial structures of adnexa within the reticular dermis.

Pitfall in diagnosis

This congenital melanocytic nevus could be misread as a melanoma because:

1. Pagetoid melanocytes are in pagetoid pattern within the epidermis and epithelial structures of adnexa.
2. Nests of melanocytes are not equidistant from one another.
3. Nests of melanocytes vary markedly in size and shape.
4. Some nests of melanocytes have become confluent.
5. Melanin is not distributed evenly within intra-epidermal melanocytes.

Congenital nevi biopsied shortly after birth or even in the first month of life display findings that simulate melanoma much more often than they exhibit signs of authentic melanoma. Histopathologists should be wary of making an unequivocal diagnosis of primary melanoma in a congenital nevus of a newborn unless the much more common simulation of melanoma has been excluded definitively.

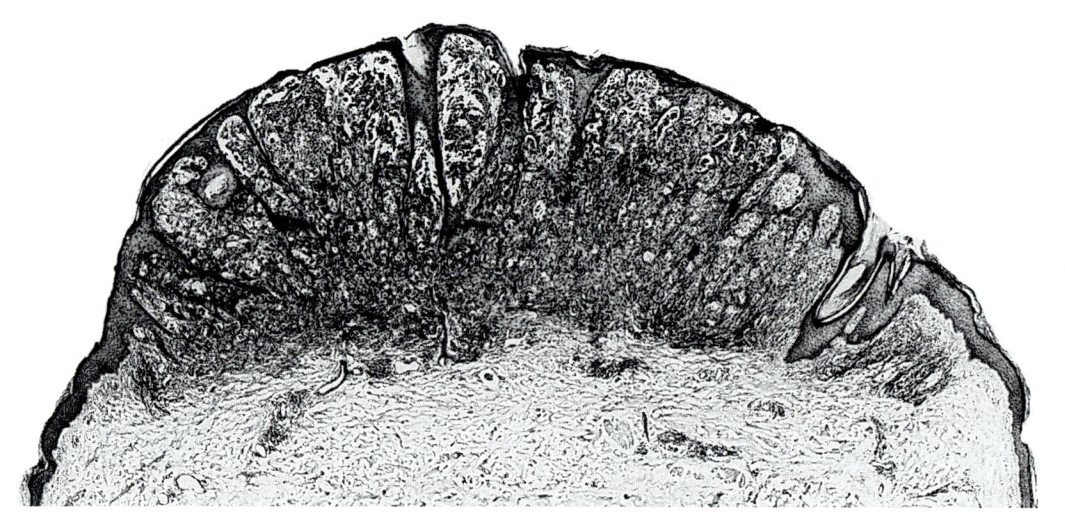

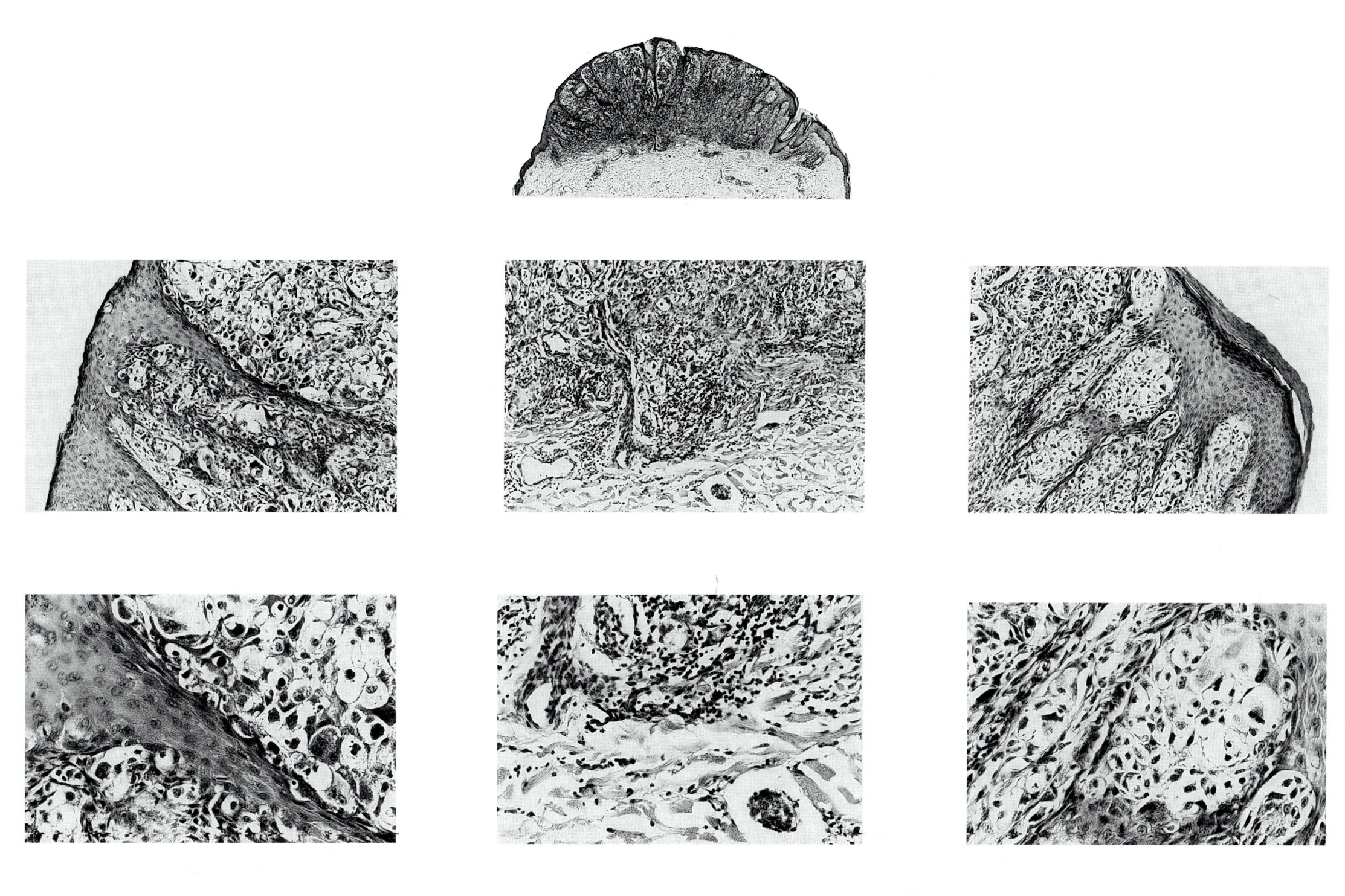

5. What is your diagnosis?

Pigmented lesion on the right calf of a 39-year-old woman that grew rapidly over a period of 7 months. Clinical diagnosis: dermatofibroma or seborrheic keratosis. Lesion was excised completely. No signs of persistence locally or metastasis were noted after 1 year.

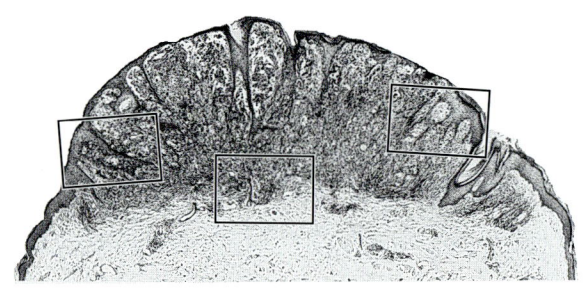

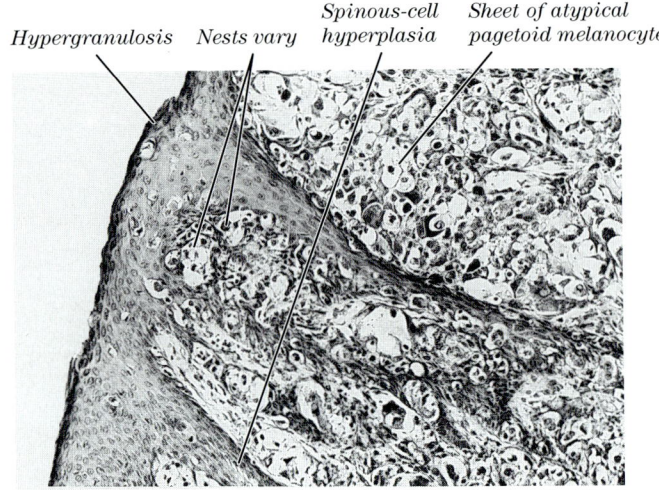

Hypergranulosis — Nests vary — Spinous-cell hyperplasia — Sheet of atypical pagetoid melanocytes

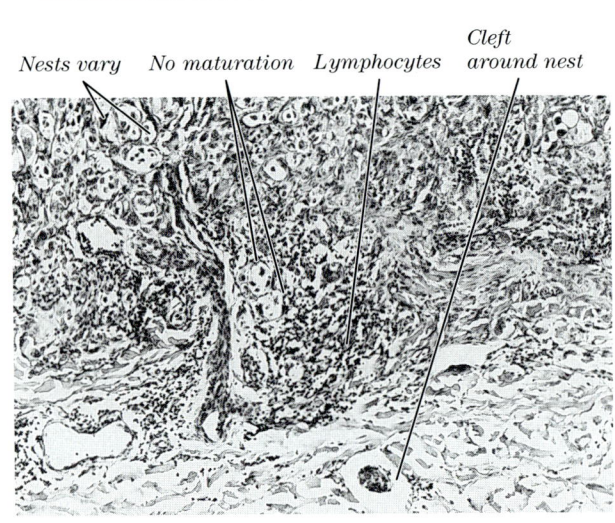

Nests vary — No maturation — Lymphocytes — Cleft around nest

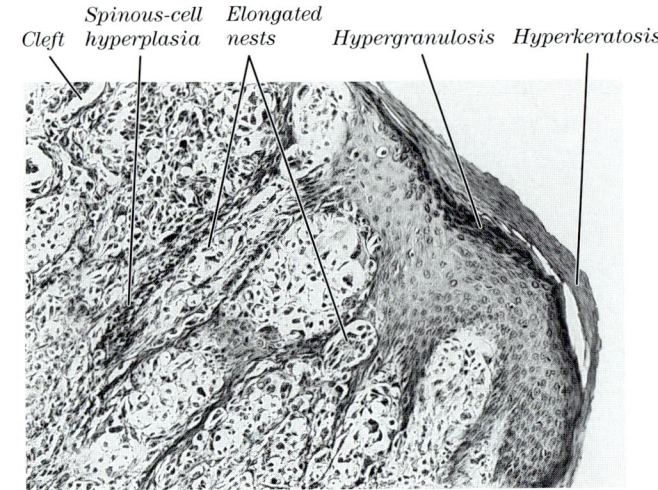

Cleft — Spinous-cell hyperplasia — Elongated nests — Hypergranulosis — Hyperkeratosis

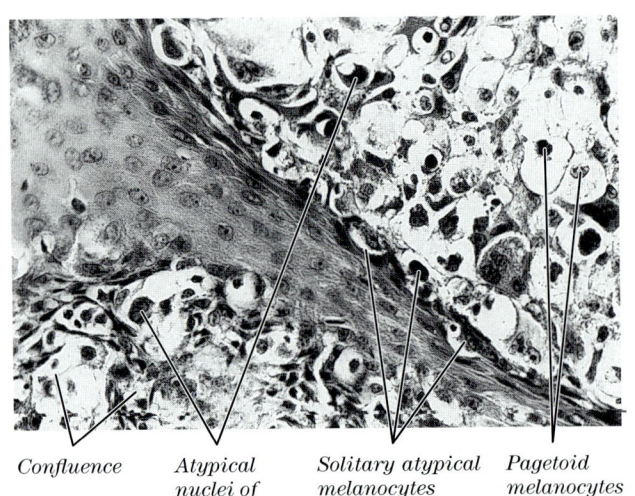

Confluence — Atypical nuclei of melanocytes — Solitary atypical melanocytes predominate — Pagetoid melanocytes

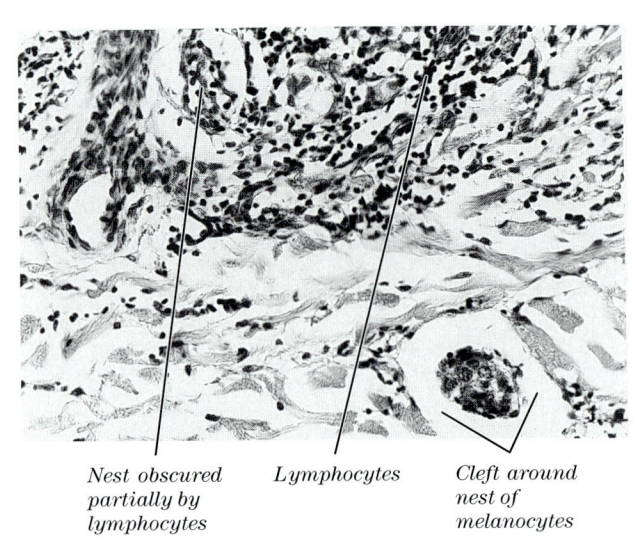

Nest obscured partially by lymphocytes — Lymphocytes — Cleft around nest of melanocytes

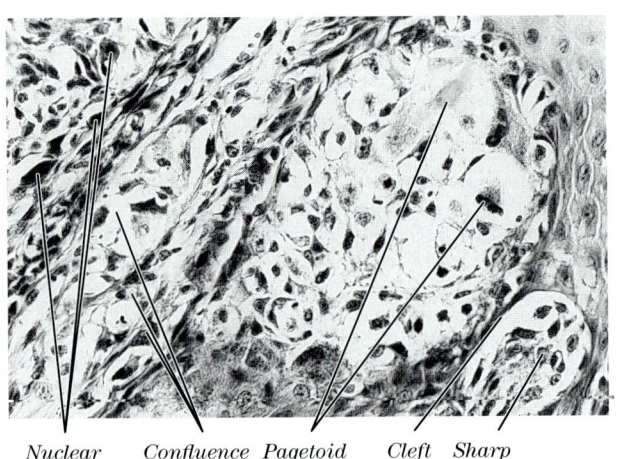

Nuclear atypia of melanocytes — Confluence — Pagetoid melanocytes — Cleft — Sharp circumscription by nest of oval melanocytes

5 • Melanoma

Criteria for diagnosis of this melanoma

This is a melanoma because:

1. The neoplasm is asymmetric (atypical melanocytes are present within the epidermis and epithelial structures of adnexa on the left, but not on the right).
2. Melanocytes disposed as solitary units predominate over nests within some epithelial structures of adnexa on the left.
3. Nests of melanocytes within the epidermis are not equidistant from one another.
4. Nests of melanocytes within the epidermis vary in size and shape.
5. Some nests of melanocytes have become confluent.
6. Pagetoid melanocytes within the epidermis are arranged in pagetoid pattern.
7. Nests of melanocytes within the dermis vary in size and shape and some have become confluent.

Pitfall in diagnosis

This melanoma could be misinterpreted as a Spitz's nevus because:

1. The neoplasm is well-circumscribed.
2. There are hyperkeratosis, hypergranulosis, and uneven epidermal hyperplasia.
3. Clefts are present between some elongated nests of melanocytes and adjacent epidermal keratinocytes.
4. A nest of melanocytes at the base of the neoplasm seems to be present within a lymphatic, but the space actually is an artifactual cleft.
5. A perivascular lymphocytic infiltrate is present throughout the neoplasm.
6. At scanning magnification, the base of the neoplasm is relatively flat.

At first glance with scanning magnification, the neoplasm could be misconstrued as a compound Spitz's nevus. More careful scrutiny, however, even at that low magnification, reveals striking asymmetry. The right half of the neoplasm surely is not a mirror image of the left half. The finding of asymmetry should alert a histopathologist to the likelihood of melanoma.

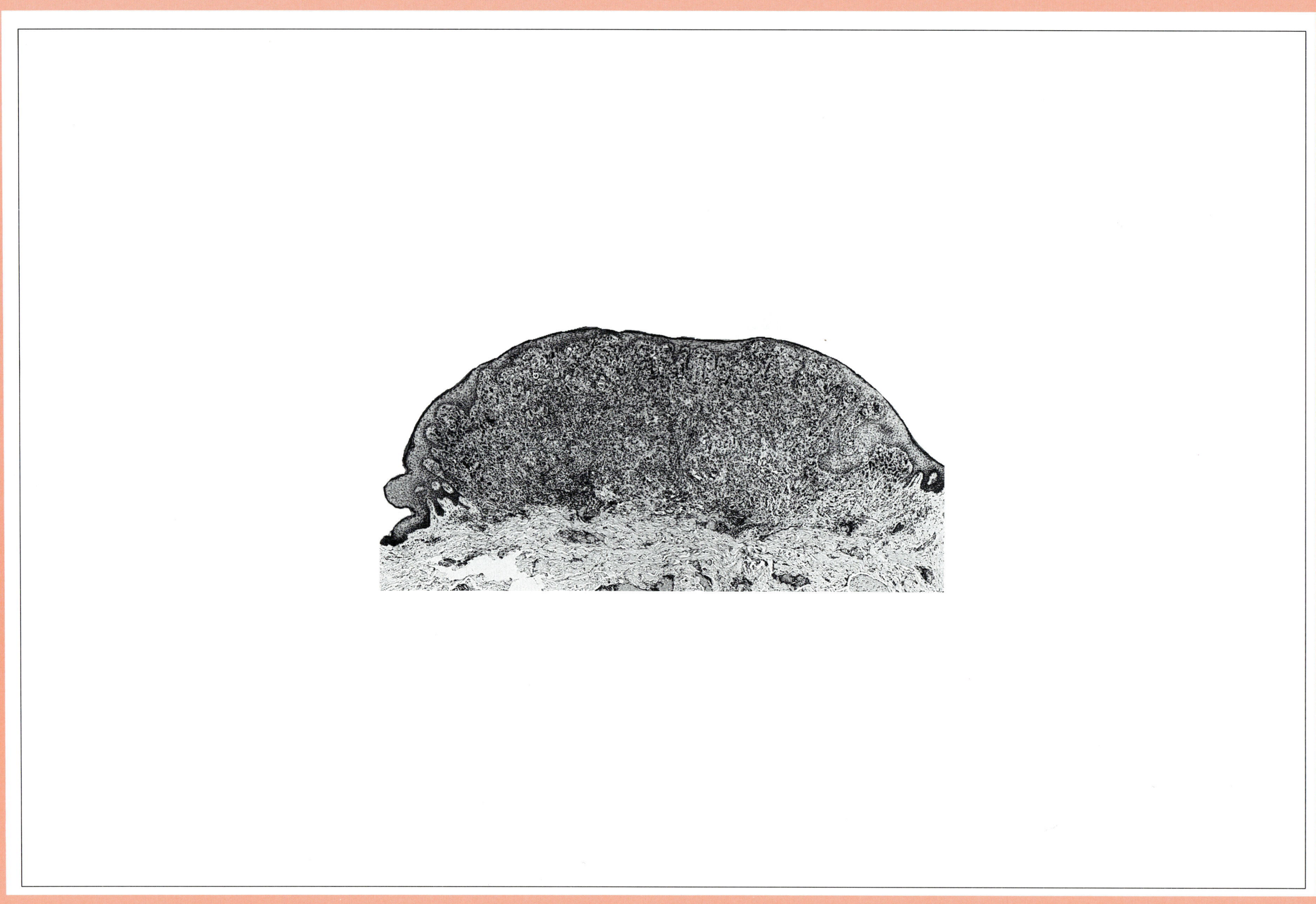

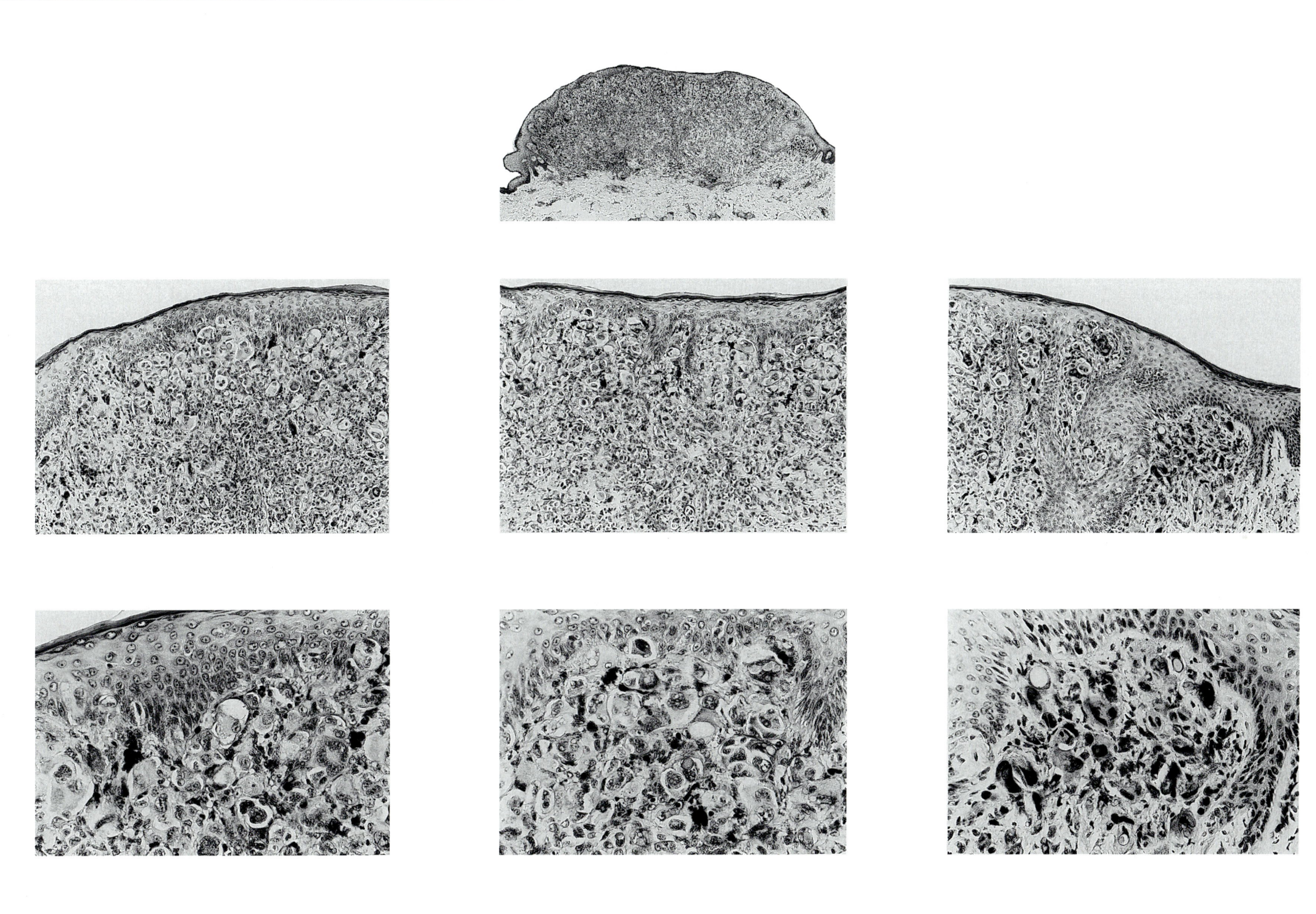

6. What is your diagnosis?

Pigmented lesion in the right nasolabial fold of a 29-year-old woman. Clinical diagnosis: nevus. Patient was free of disease after 1 year.

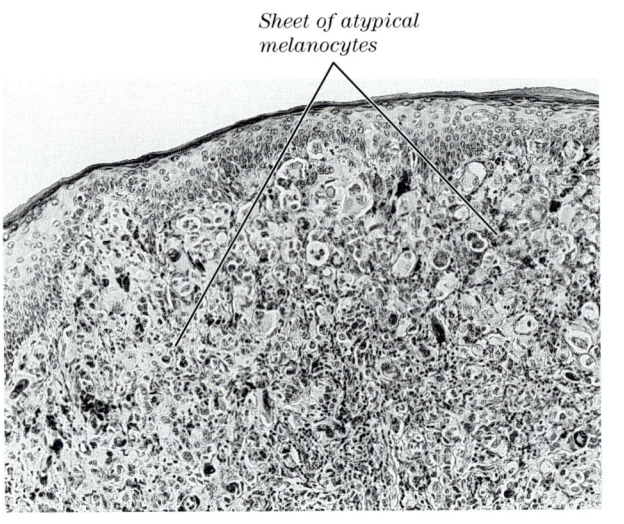
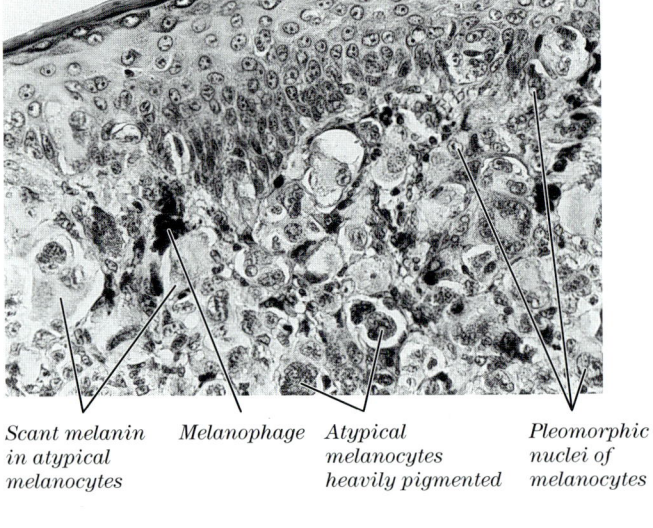
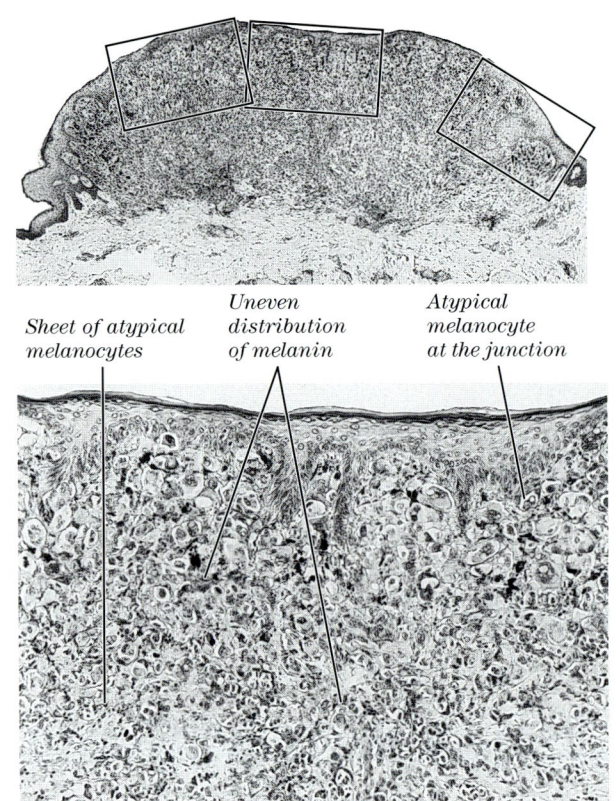
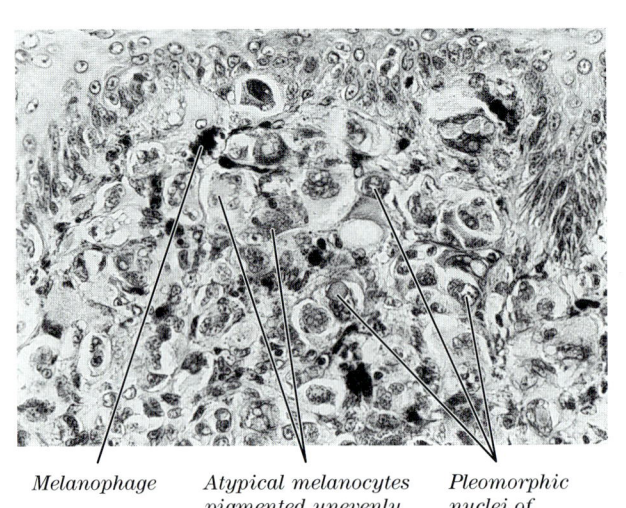
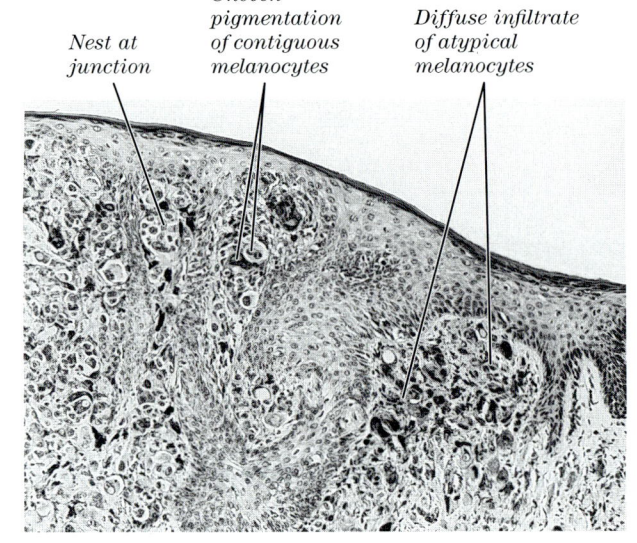
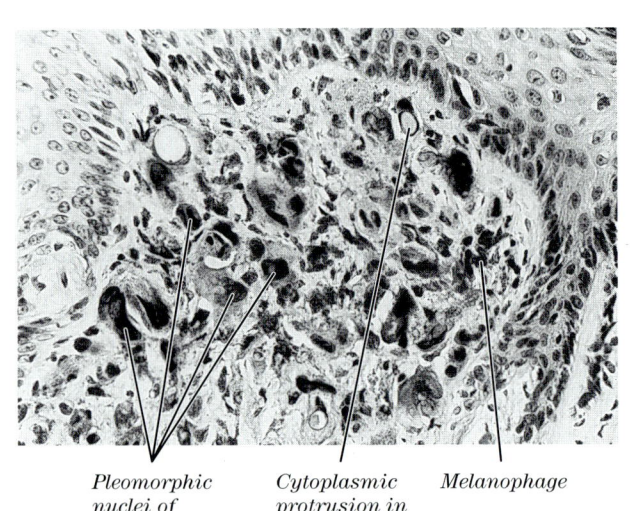

6 • Melanoma

Criteria for diagnosis of this melanoma

This is a melanoma because:

1. The neoplasm is asymmetric.

2. Its base is neither flat nor wedge-shaped.

3. Nests of melanocytes within the dermis have become confluent and formed sheets.

4. Most of the melanocytes are pagetoid, i.e., consisting of large roundish nuclei and abundant pale cytoplasm that contains "dusty" melanin.

5. Melanin is not distributed in uniform fashion throughout the neoplasm.

Pitfall in diagnosis

This melanoma could be misinterpreted as a Spitz's nevus because:

1. The neoplasm is symmetric topographically.

2. The neoplasm is well-circumscribed.

3. There is some maturation of melanocytes with progressive descent into the dermis.

4. Nuclei of melanocytes are atypical.

5. Cytoplasm of melanocytes is abundant.

6. There are hyperkeratosis, hypergranulosis, and irregular spinous-cell hyperplasia.

7. A perivascular lymphocytic infiltrate is present throughout the neoplasm.

8. Many of the neoplastic melanocytes are multinucleate.

Although this neoplasm is symmetric topographically, it is asymmetric in distribution of melanin (melanin is much more abundant on the left side than on the right side). Furthermore, many of the neoplastic cells are pagetoid, and nests of them have become confluent with formation of sheets of melanocytes. These findings, in toto, are diagnostic of melanoma.

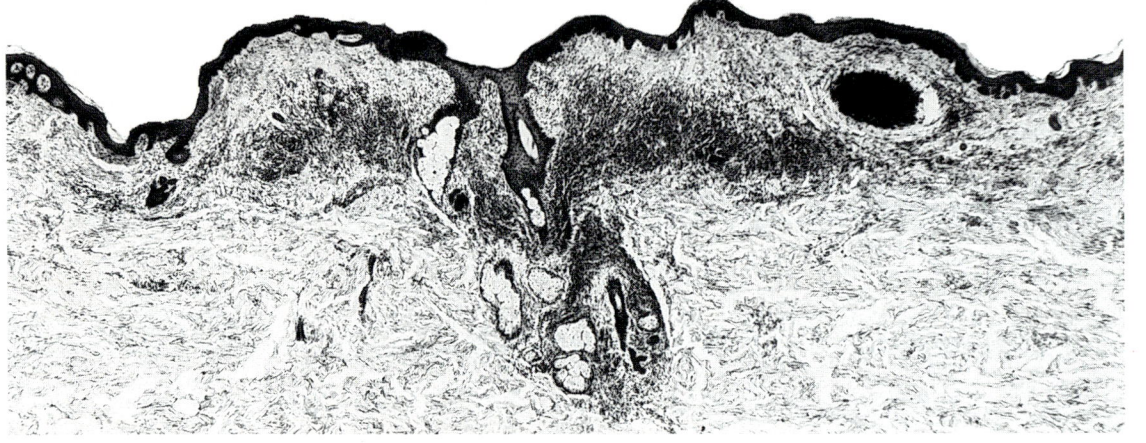

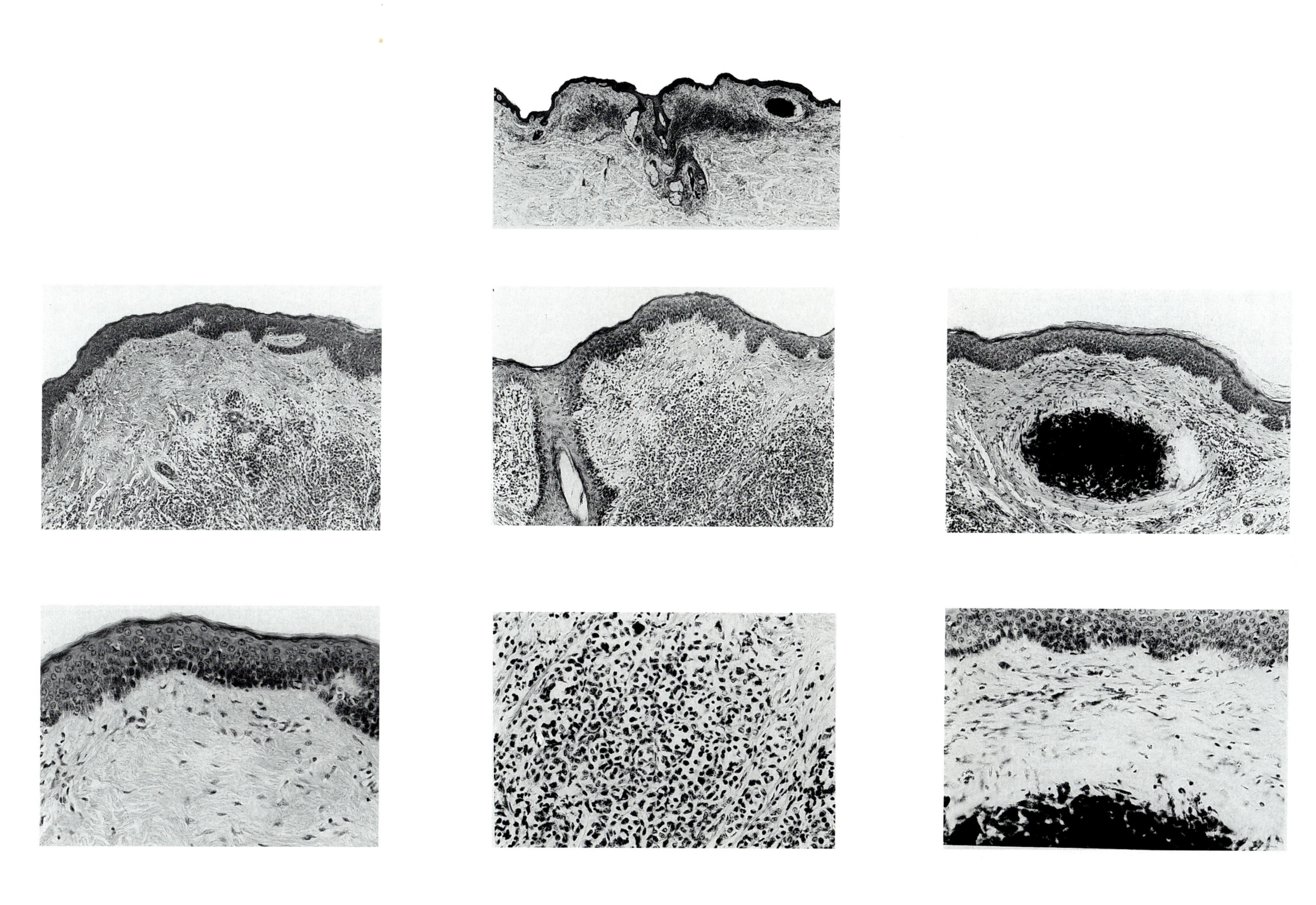

7. What is your diagnosis?

Pigmented lesion on the midback of a 35-year-old woman. The lesion was excised completely. One lymph node in the right axilla contained metastases of melanoma. The patient was alive and well after 4 years.

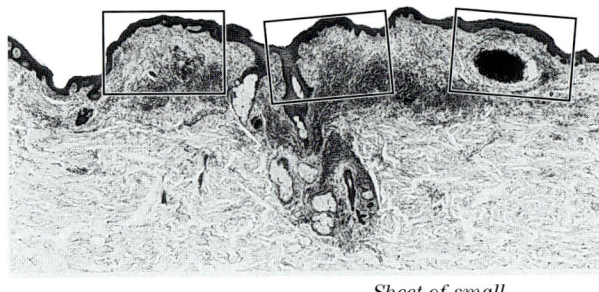

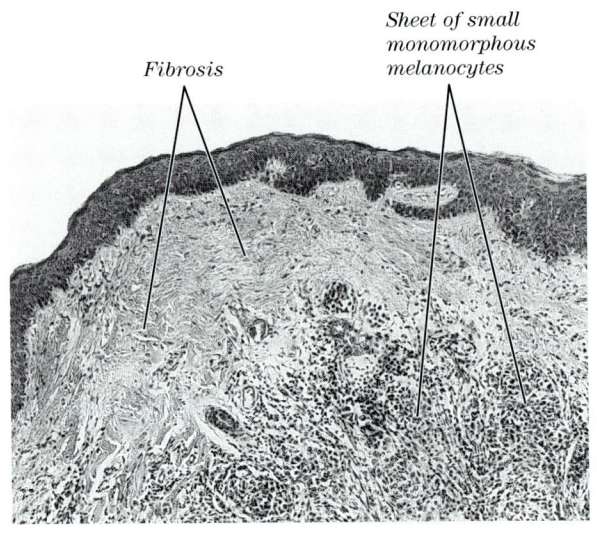

Fibrosis — *Sheet of small monomorphous melanocytes*

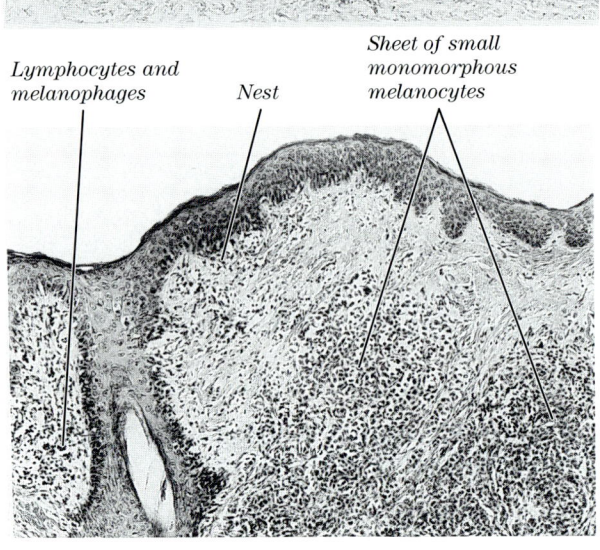

Lymphocytes and melanophages — *Nest* — *Sheet of small monomorphous melanocytes*

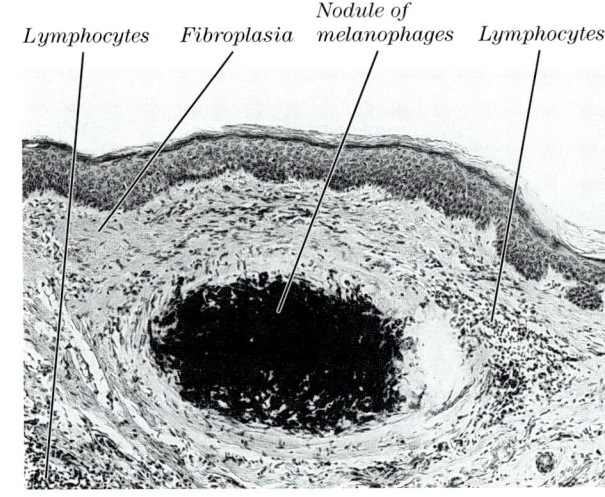

Lymphocytes — *Fibroplasia* — *Nodule of melanophages* — *Lymphocytes*

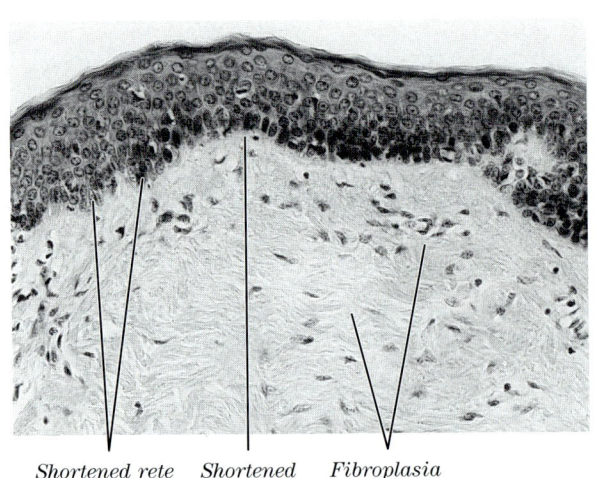

Shortened rete ridges — *Shortened papilla* — *Fibroplasia*

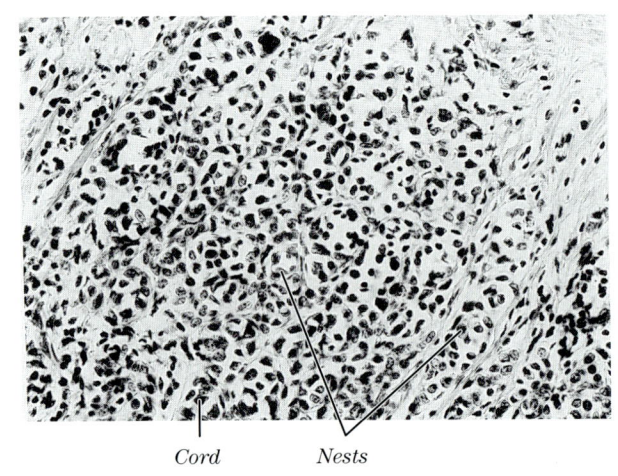

Cord — *Nests*

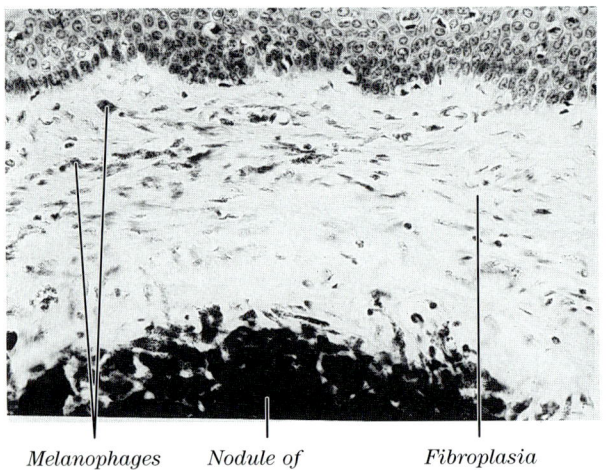

Melanophages — *Nodule of melanophages* — *Fibroplasia*

7 • Melanoma *(with regression)* and Clark's Nevus

Criteria for diagnosis of this melanoma (with regression) in association with a Clark's nevus

This is regression of melanoma because:

1. On the right, the papillary dermis is thickened markedly by fibroplasia, a sprinkling of lymphocytes, and a large ovoid collection of melanophages.

2. On the left, the papillary dermis also is thickened by fibrosis within which there are dilated venules and a sprinkling of lymphocytes and melanophages.

This is a compound Clark's nevus because:

1. The neoplasm is gently domed.

2. The melanocytic process is confined to the dermo-epidermal junction and markedly thickened papillary dermis.

3. Nests of melanocytes within the epidermis are situated at the dermo-epidermal junction and not above it.

4. There are orderly nests, cords, and strands of monomorphous melanocytes in the thickened papillary dermis.

Pitfall in diagnosis

This regressed melanoma in association with a pre-existing Clark's nevus could be misinterpreted as a halo nevus because:

1. The predominant melanocytic process is a compound Clark's nevus.

2. Lymphocytes are scattered within the intradermal portion of the nevus.

3. Fibroplasia is present in the thickened papillary dermis.

4. Melanophages are present within the thickened papillary dermis.

Two entirely different patterns can be observed in this lesion. One is an indubitable Clark's nevus and the other a large cluster of melanophages surrounded by fibroplasia and a lymphocytic infiltrate. The latter changes are those of regression of melanoma, the two major signs of which are fibroplasia and melanosis, and both of them are shown. That this interpretation is correct is fortified by the knowledge that the patient developed a metastasis of melanoma to a regional lymph node.

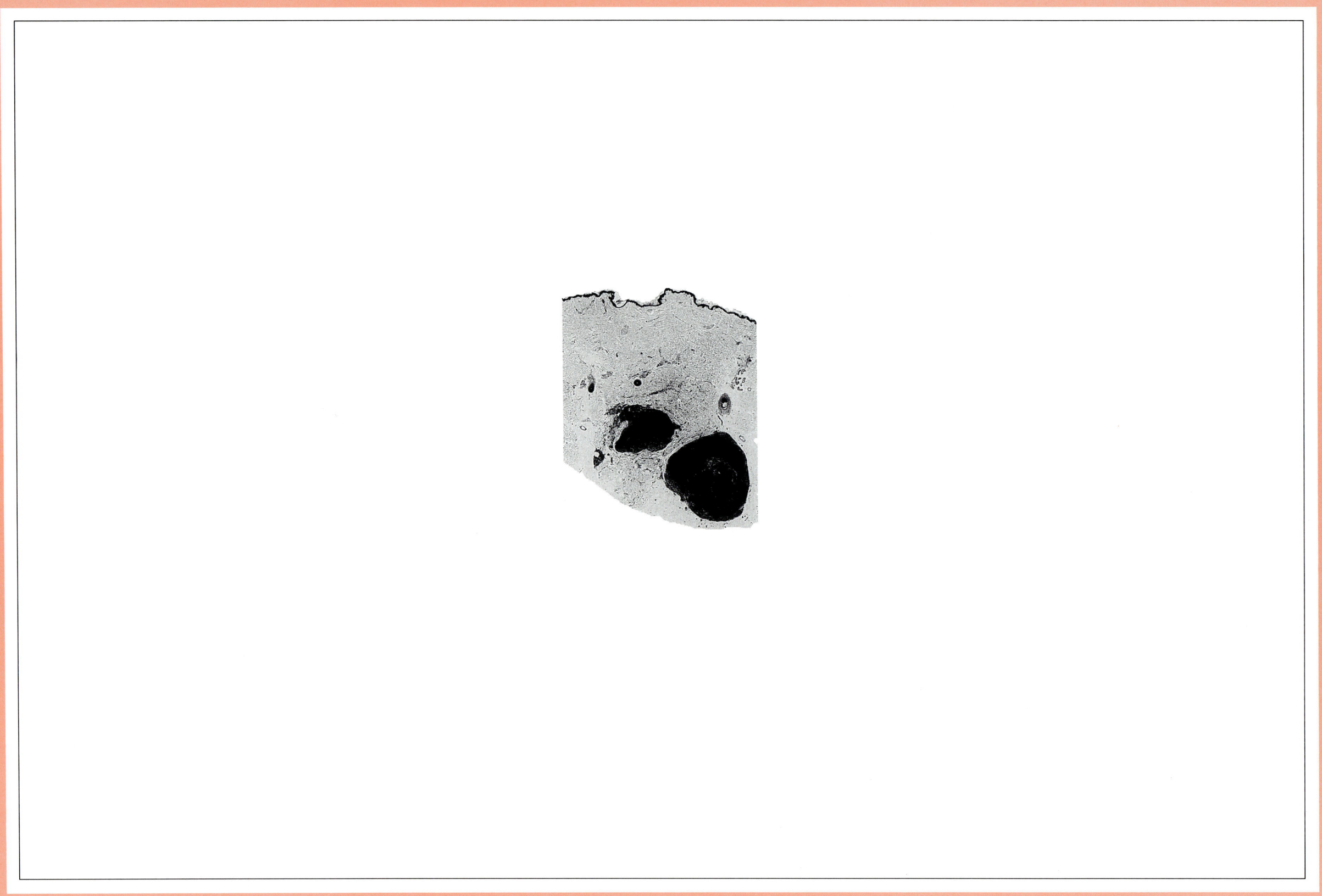

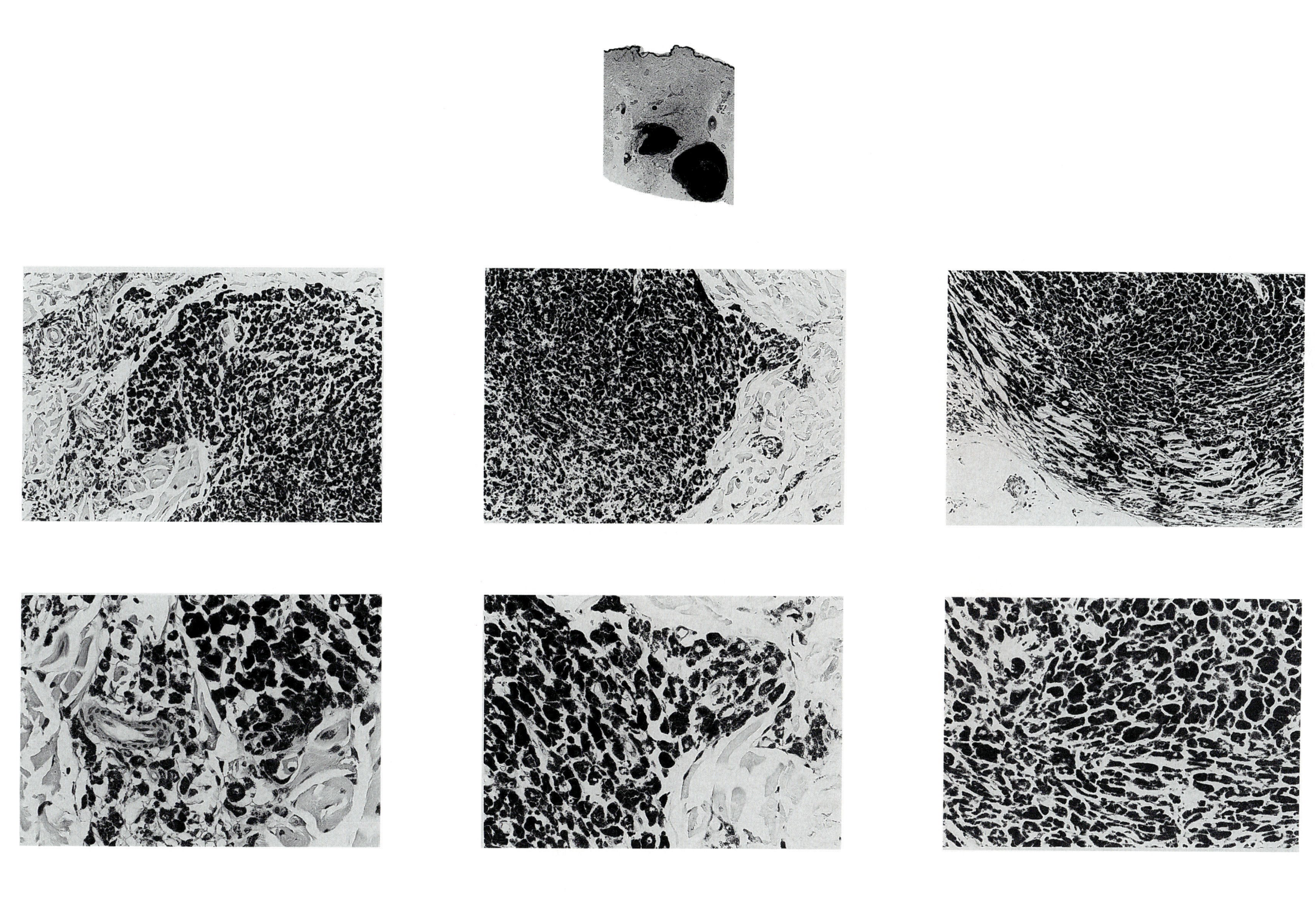

8. What is your diagnosis?

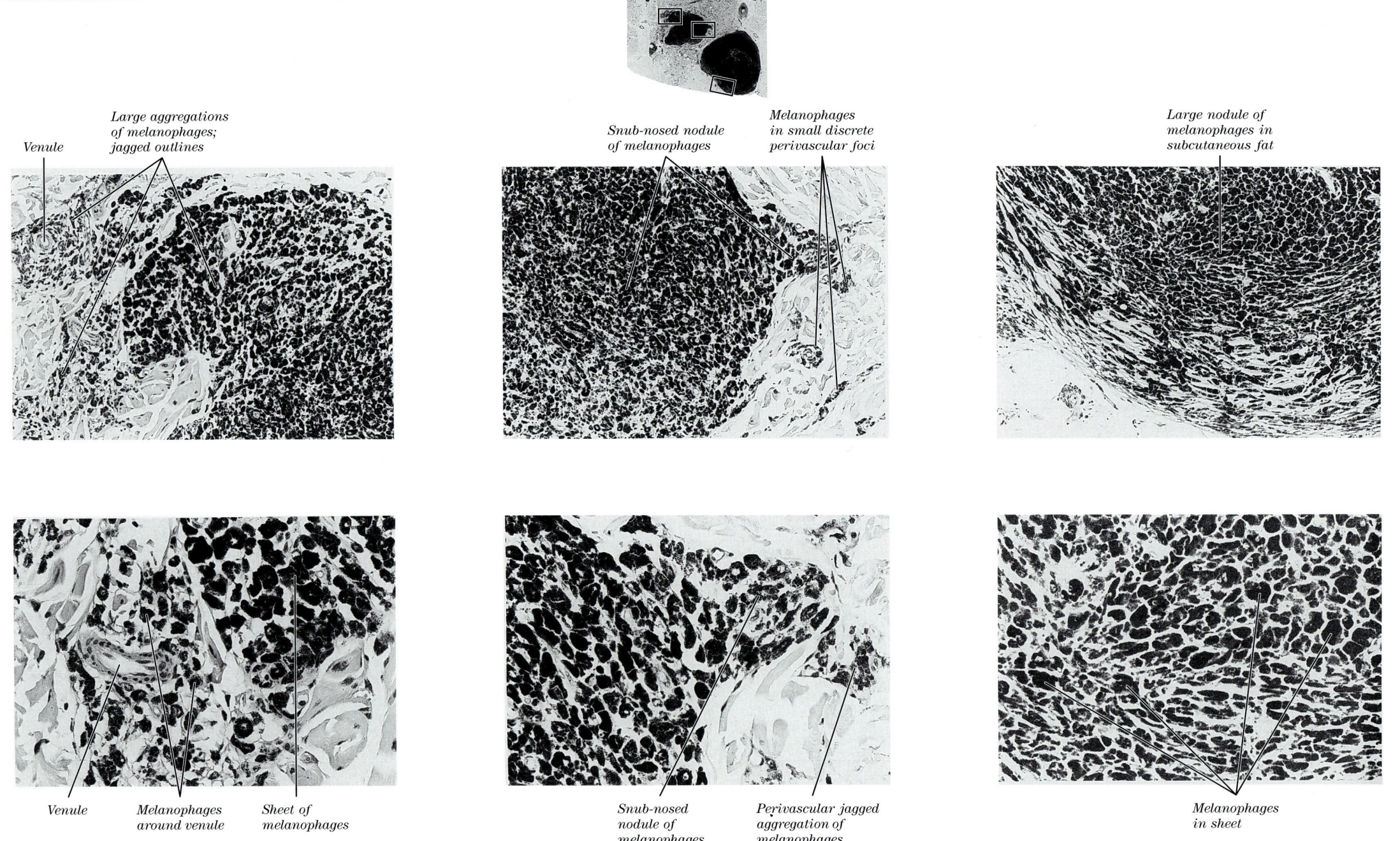

8 • Metastases of Melanoma (completely regressed)

Criteria for diagnosis of these metastases of melanoma (completely regressed)

These are metastases of melanoma because of:

1. Asymmetric distribution of pigmented cells.
2. Aggregations composed entirely of melanophages; no neoplastic melanocytes.
3. Aggregations of pigmented cells are positioned in two large foci in the deep reticular dermis and the subcutaneous fat; none are present in the rest of the dermis.

Pitfall in diagnosis

These regressed metastases of melanoma could be misconstrued as components of a blue nevus because:

1. Aggregations of pigmented cells are discrete.
2. Aggregations are pigmented markedly by melanin.
3. Many melanophages are present.

Even though, at scanning magnification, this lesion could be judged to be a blue nevus, that notion should be dispelled at higher magnifications where all of the cells can be observed to be melanophages. There are no neoplastic melanocytes. These changes, therefore, represent complete regression of a metastasis of melanoma, analogous to melanosis in the papillary dermis, which signifies regression of a primary melanoma.

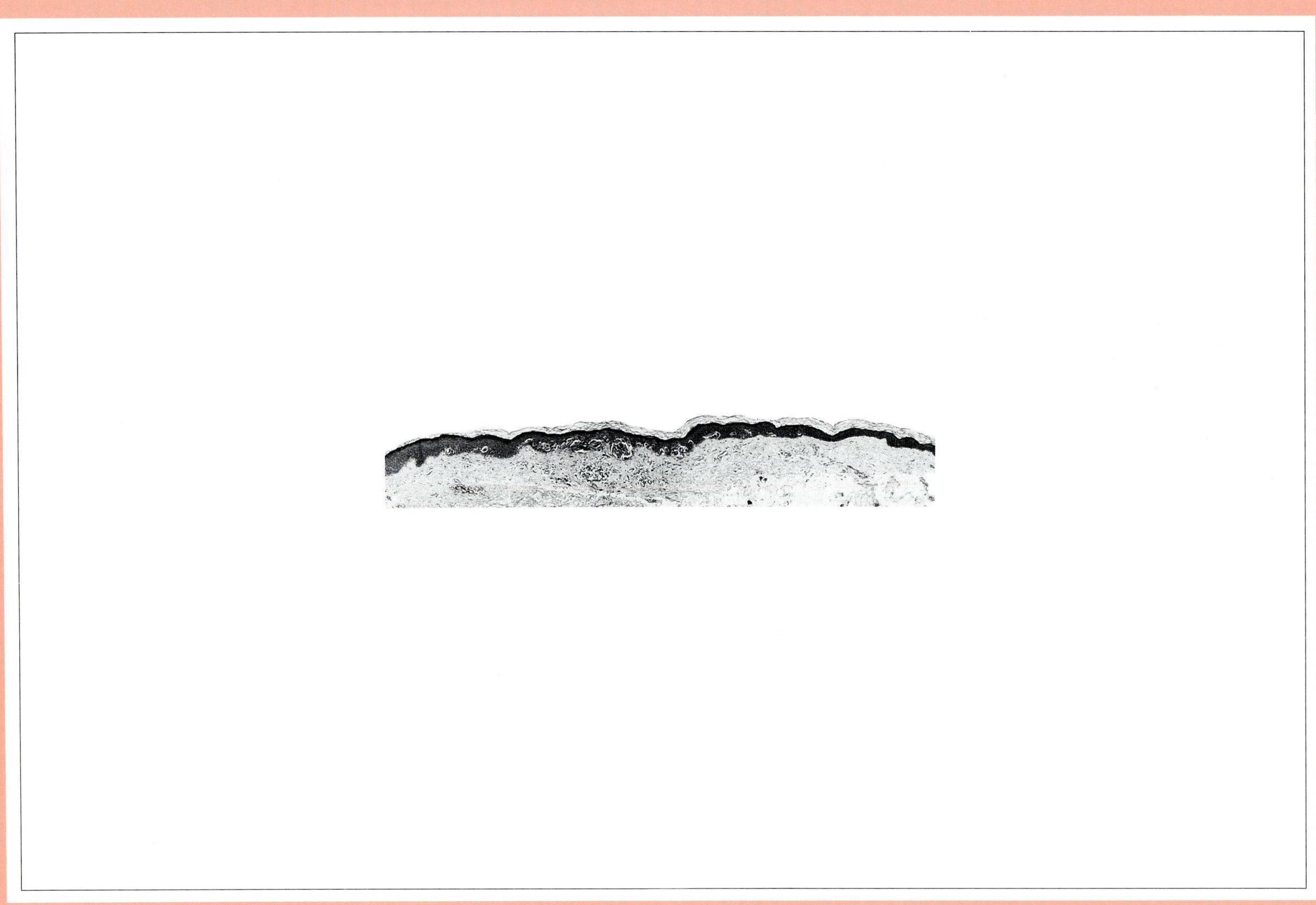

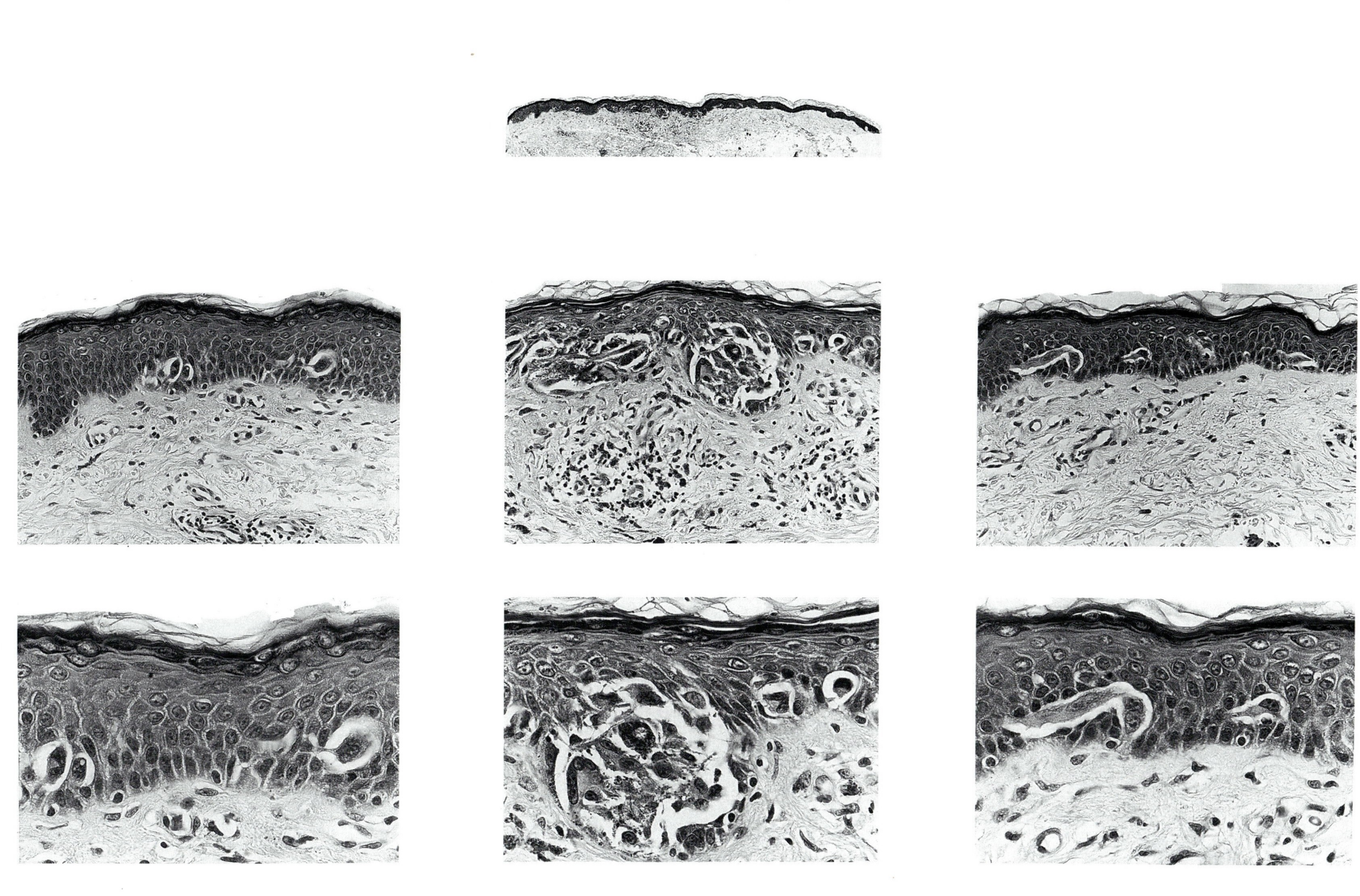

9. What is your diagnosis?

Slightly elevated brown papule on the right thigh of a 27-year-old woman. Clinical diagnosis: nevus.

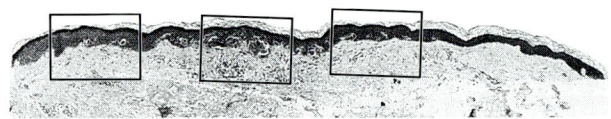

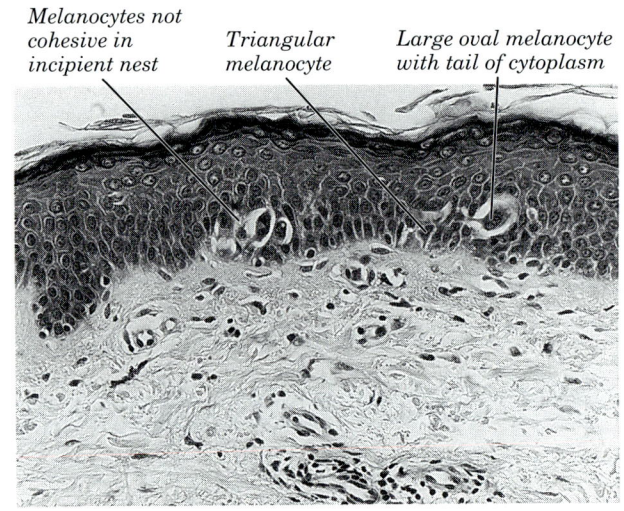

Melanocytes not cohesive in incipient nest — *Triangular melanocyte* — *Large oval melanocyte with tail of cytoplasm*

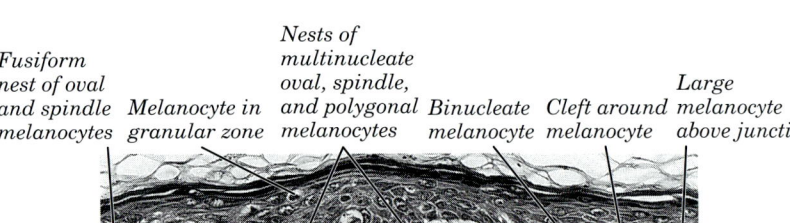

Fusiform nest of oval and spindle melanocytes — *Melanocyte in granular zone* — *Nests of multinucleate oval, spindle, and polygonal melanocytes* — *Binucleate melanocyte* — *Cleft around melanocyte* — *Large melanocyte above junction*

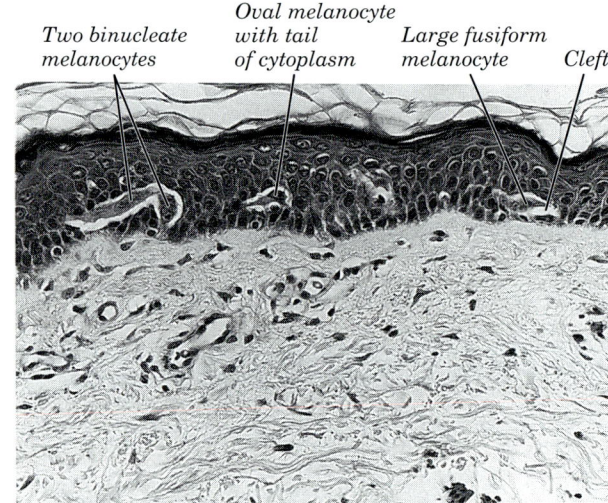

Two binucleate melanocytes — *Oval melanocyte with tail of cytoplasm* — *Large fusiform melanocyte* — *Cleft*

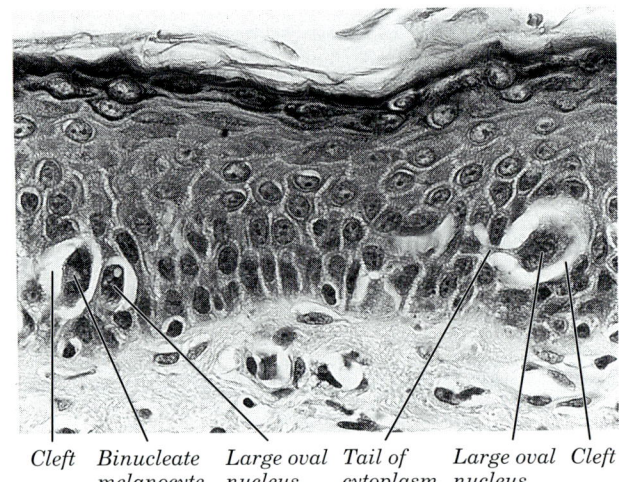

Cleft *Binucleate melanocyte* *Large oval nucleus* *Tail of cytoplasm* *Large oval nucleus* *Cleft*

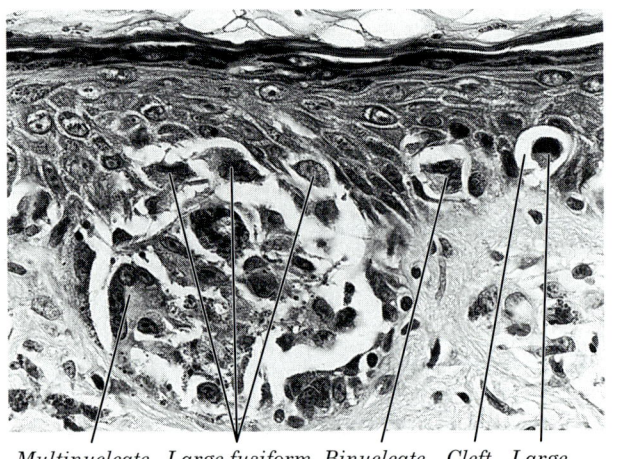

Multinucleate melanocyte *Large fusiform melanocytes* *Binucleate melanocyte* *Cleft* *Large melanocyte*

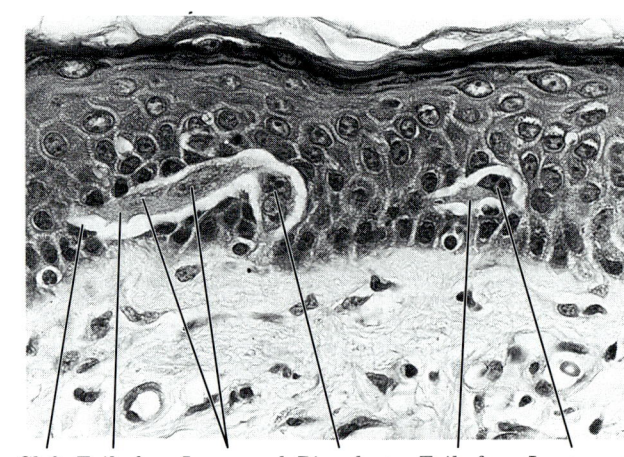

Cleft *Tail of cytoplasm* *Large oval nuclei* *Binucleate melanocyte* *Tail of cytoplasm* *Large oval nucleus*

9 • Spitz's Nevus

Criteria for diagnosis of this Spitz's nevus (junctional type)

This is a nevus because:

1. It is relatively symmetric.
2. Melanocytes arranged in nests are situated at the dermo-epidermal junction, not above it.
3. Nuclei of melanocytes, both those disposed as solitary units and those in nests, are relatively monomorphous.

This is a Spitz's nevus because:

1. Melanocytes have large nuclei, abundant cytoplasm, and plump oval, polygonal, round, and sometimes dendritic shapes.
2. Many neoplastic melanocytes are binucleate and multinucleate.
3. Prominent clefts exist between individual melanocytes and adjacent keratinocytes and between nests of melanocytes and adjacent keratinocytes.

Pitfall in diagnosis

This junctional Spitz's nevus could be misread as a melanoma in situ because:

1. Nests of melanocytes within the epidermis are not equidistant from one another.
2. Throughout most of the neoplasm, melanocytes arranged as solitary units predominate over nests.
3. Many melanocytes arrayed as solitary units are present above the dermo-epidermal junction.
4. Melanocytes disposed as solitary units are not equidistant from one another.

This Spitz's nevus has many features in common with melanoma in situ, but can be differentiated from it by the relative symmetry (nests of melanocytes mostly in the center and melanocytes arranged as solitary units at the periphery), position of nests of melanocytes at the dermo-epidermal junction, and monomorphous quality of nuclei of melanocytes.

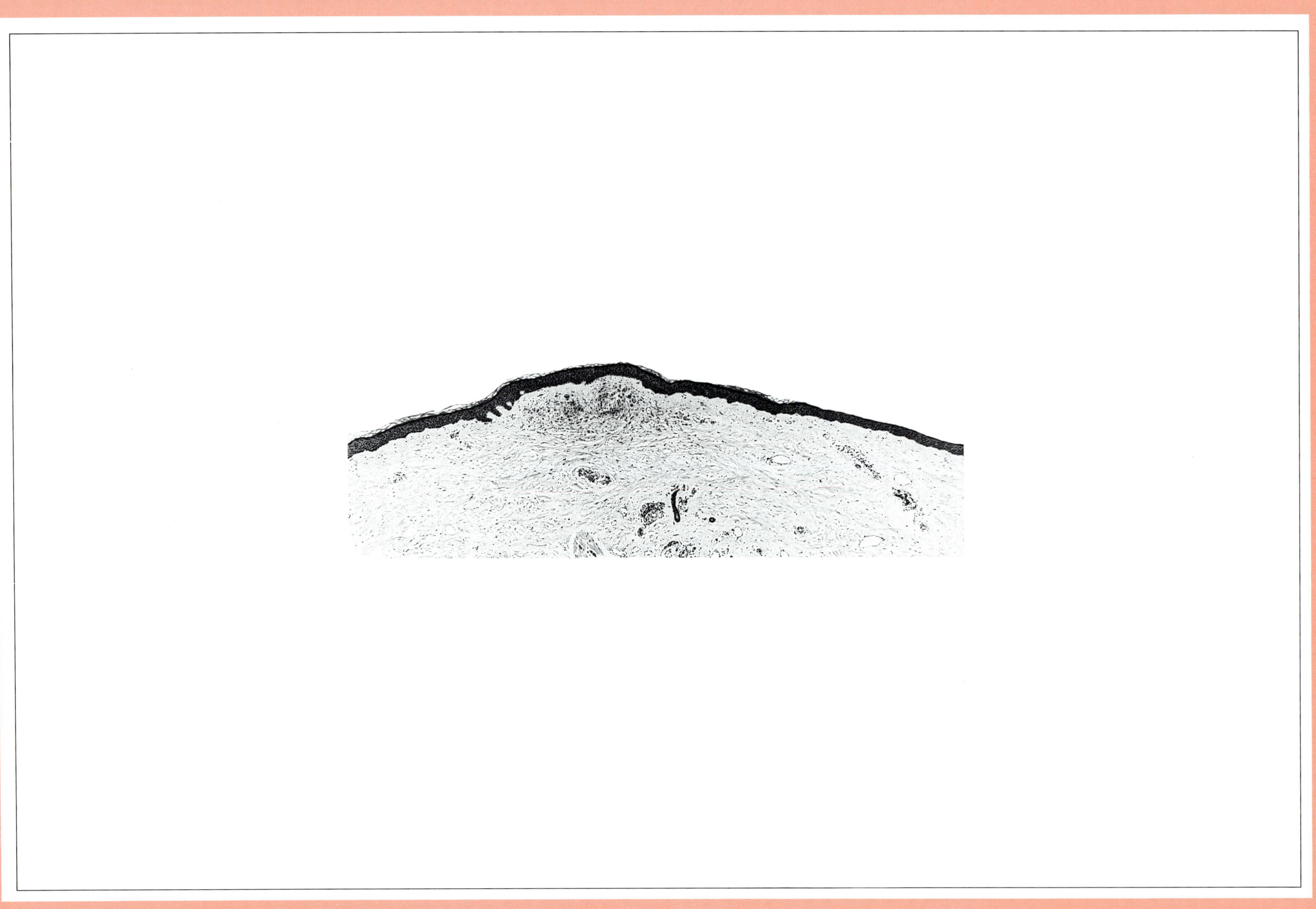

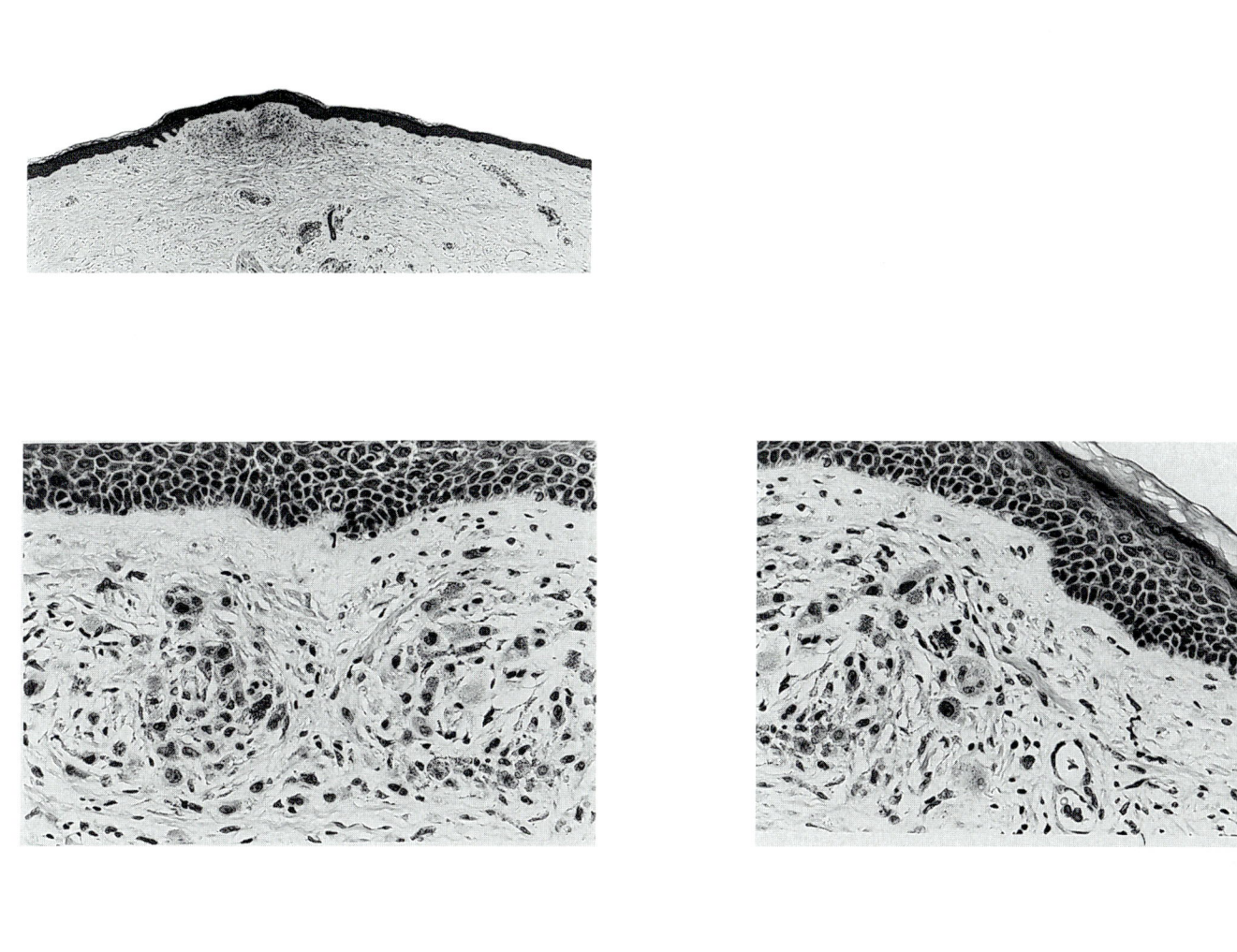

10. What is your diagnosis?

Pigmented lesion of 3 months duration on the right leg of a 65-year-old woman. Patient had a history of melanoma with satellite metastases. Clinical diagnosis: metastatic melanoma. The patient was alive after 1 year.

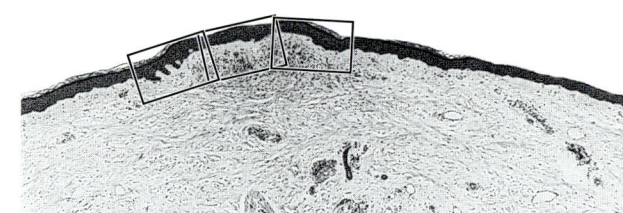

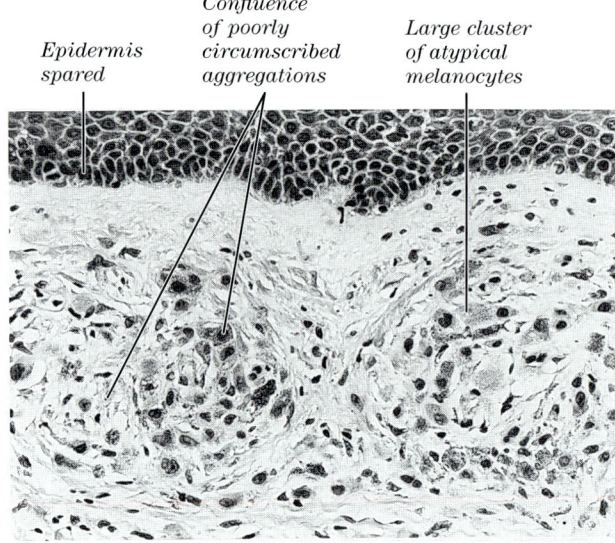

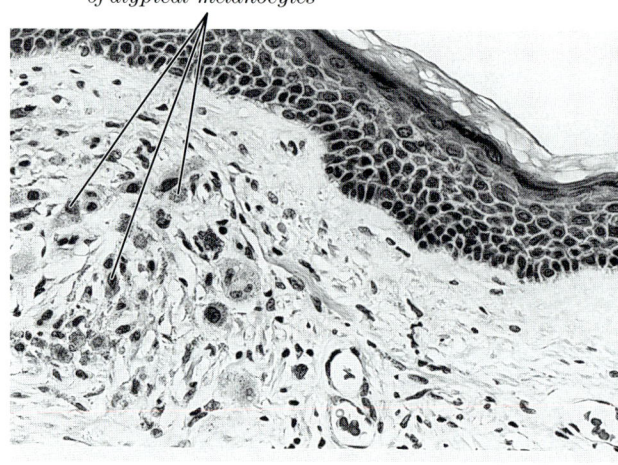

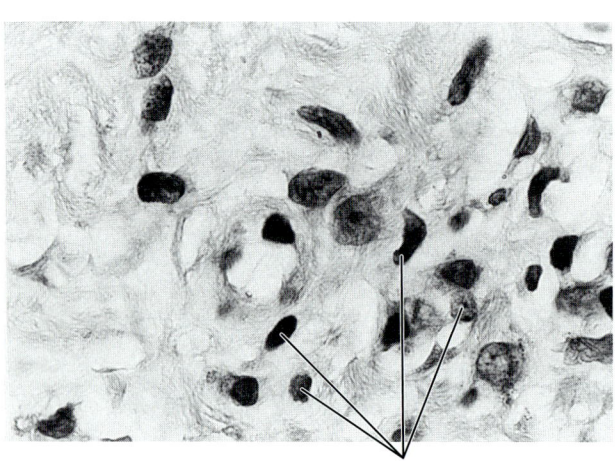

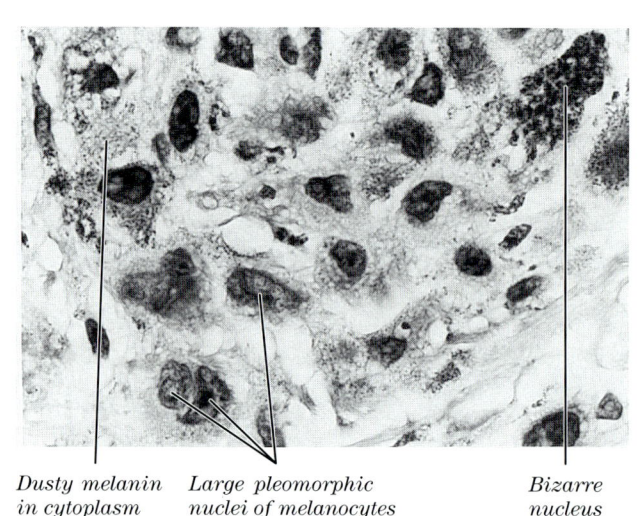

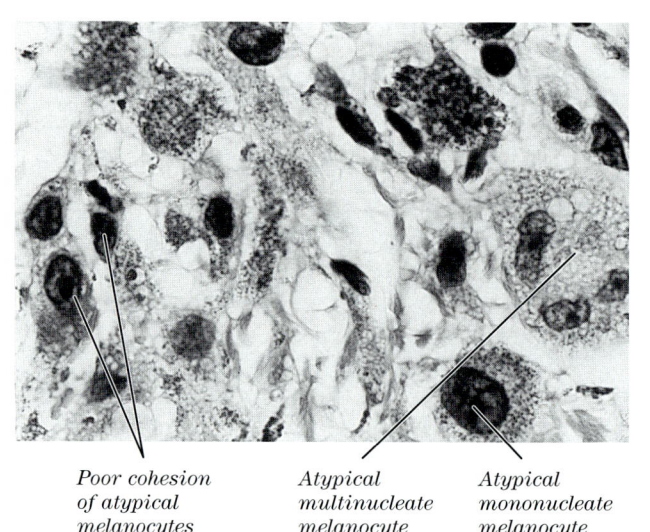

10 • Metastasis of Melanoma

Criteria for diagnosis of this metastasis of melanoma

This is a metastasis of melanoma because:

1. The neoplasm is asymmetric.

2. Melanocytes within the dermis are not arranged in discrete nests but in vague aggregations, some of which have become confluent.

3. Some nuclei of melanocytes are not simply round, oval, or polygonal, but have arciform and other geometric shapes.

4. There is striking pleomorphism of nuclei of melanocytes that are contiguous with one another.

5. Many neoplastic melanocytes, some of them multinucleate, have abundant pale cytoplasm within which is "dusty" melanin.

6. Some neoplastic melanocytes are present within vascular spaces in the upper part of the dermis.

7. The quantity of cytoplasm of neoplastic melanocytes varies markedly from cell to cell.

Pitfall in diagnosis

This metastasis of melanoma could be misinterpreted as an intradermal Spitz's nevus because:

1. The neoplasm is small.

2. The neoplasm is relatively well-circumscribed.

3. The neoplasm is confined to the upper part of the dermis.

4. Nuclei of melanocytes are large, cytoplasm is abundant, and shapes are round, oval, and polygonal.

5. Several neoplastic melanocytes are multinucleate.

6. Mitotic figures are relatively few.

Just as atypical pagetoid melanocytes in pagetoid pattern enable differentiation of many melanomas from Spitz's nevi, so, too, presence of pagetoid melanocytes within the dermis helps in distinguishing primary and metastatic melanoma from Spitz's nevus. In general, pagetoid melanocytes are not found in Spitz's nevi. Other findings that permit this metastasis of melanoma to be distinguished from an intradermal Spitz's nevus are asymmetry, uneven distribution of melanin within neoplastic cells and macrophages, and poor circumscription of aggregations of neoplastic cells.

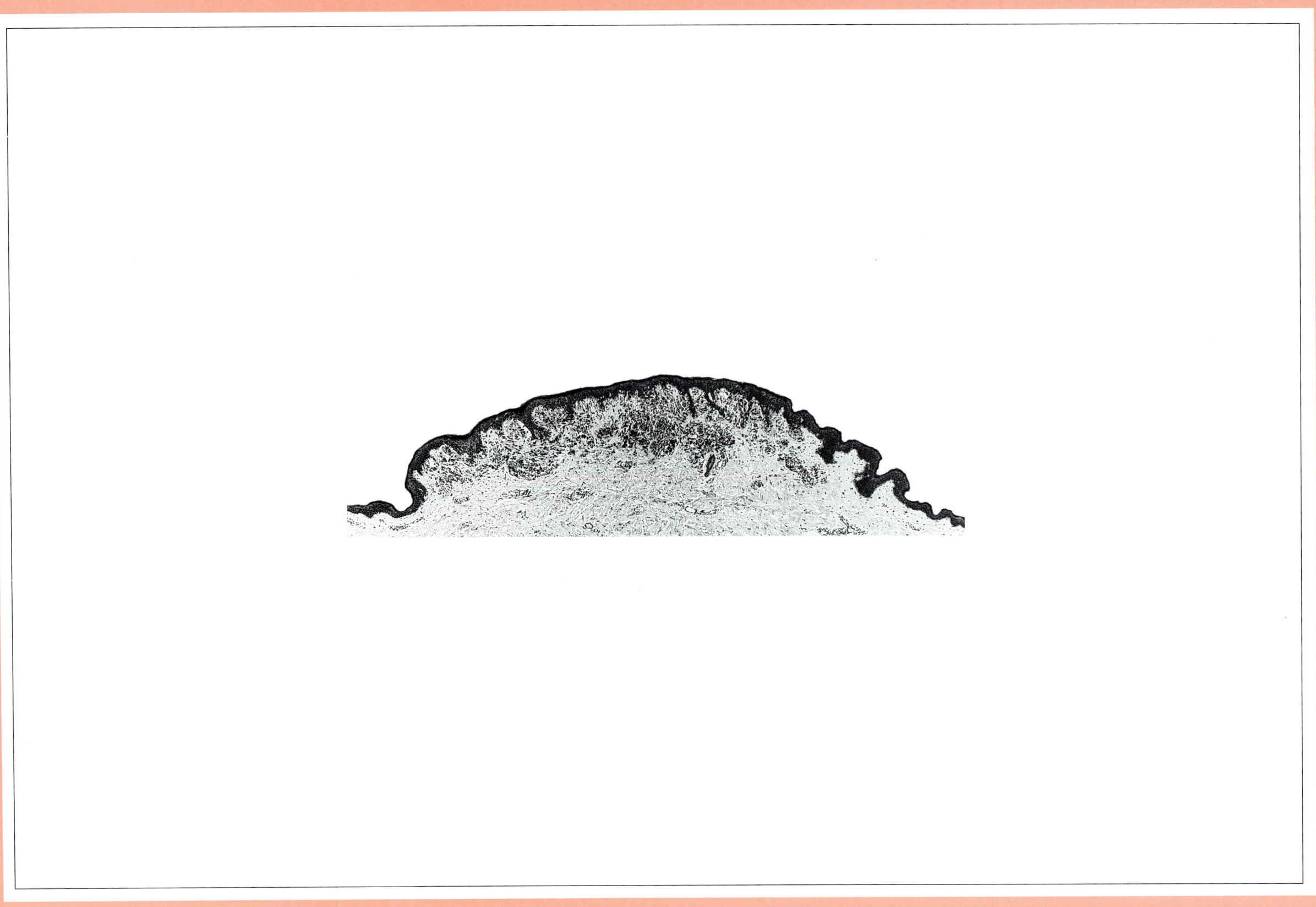

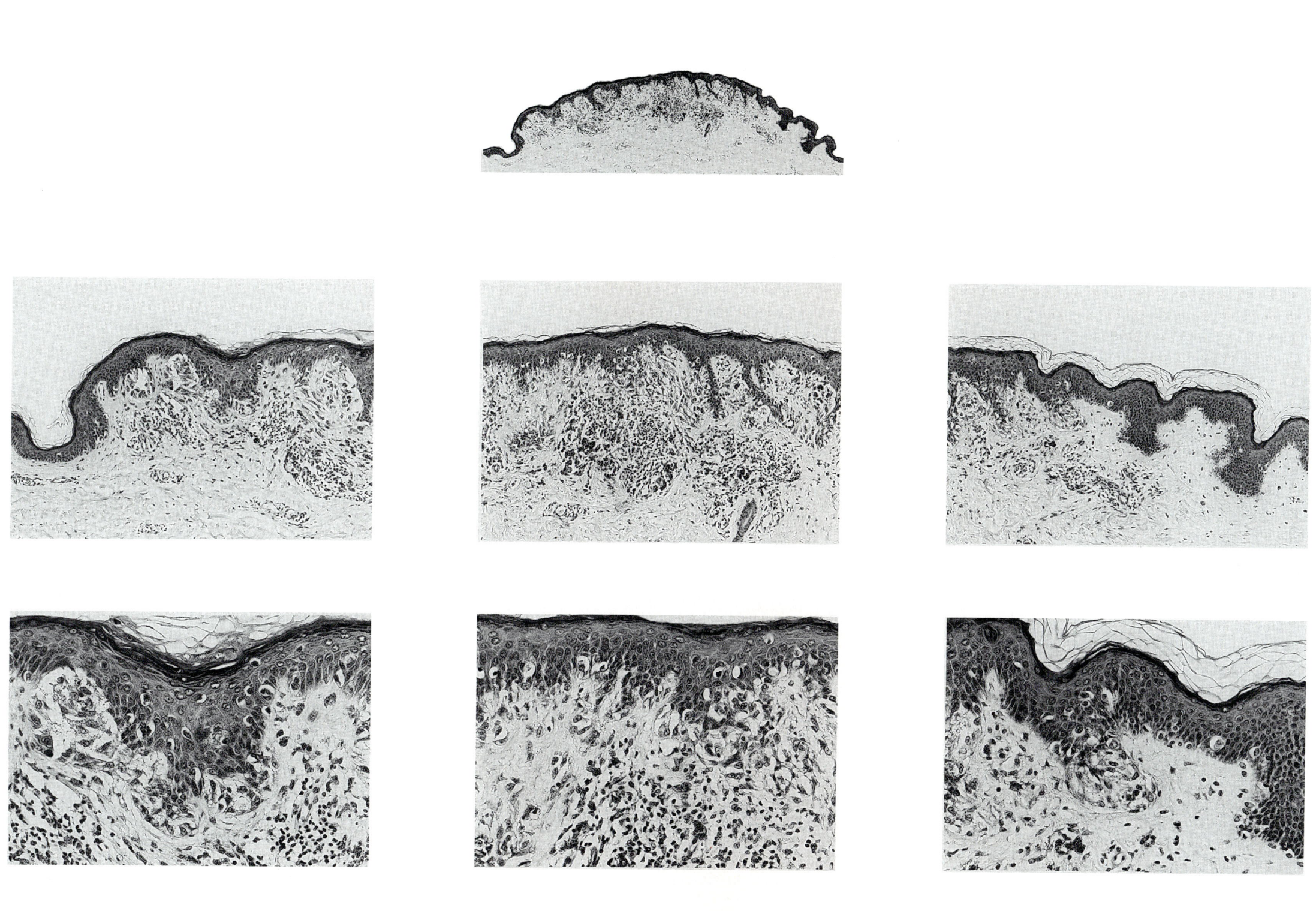

11. What is your diagnosis?

Small, pigmented, slightly raised, sharply delineated lesion on a leg of a 40-year-old woman. Clinical diagnosis: nevus. A wide excision of the site was performed and no evidence of residual neoplasm was found in the specimen. Patient was well after 3 years.

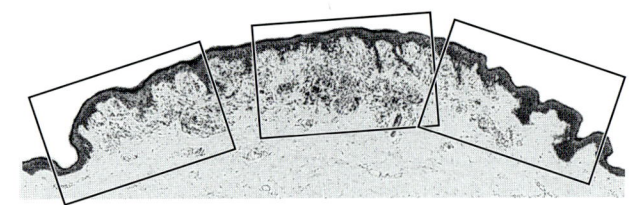

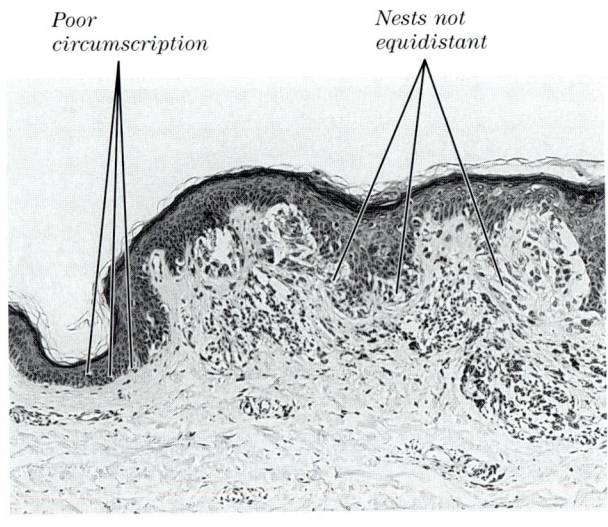

Poor circumscription   *Nests not equidistant*

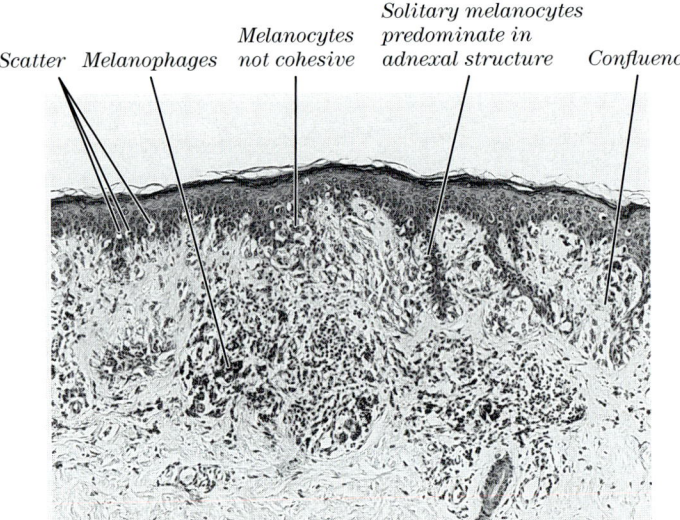

Scatter   *Melanophages*   *Melanocytes not cohesive*   *Solitary melanocytes predominate in adnexal structure*   *Confluence*

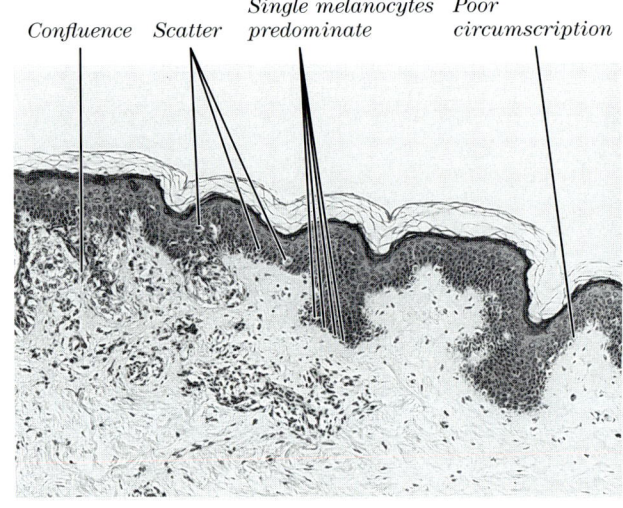

Confluence   *Scatter*   *Single melanocytes predominate*   *Poor circumscription*

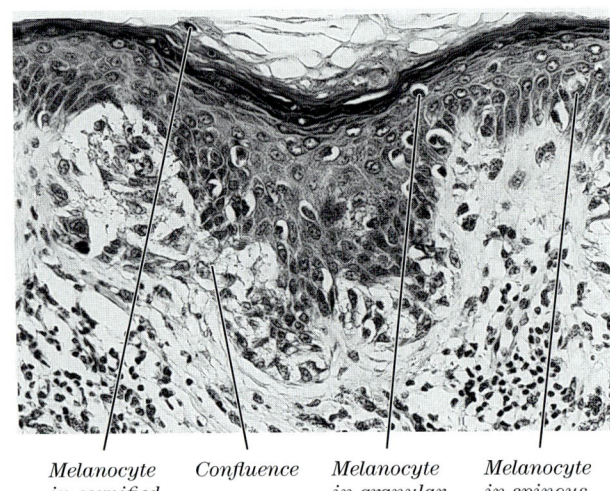

Melanocyte in cornified layer   *Confluence*   *Melanocyte in granular zone*   *Melanocyte in spinous zone*

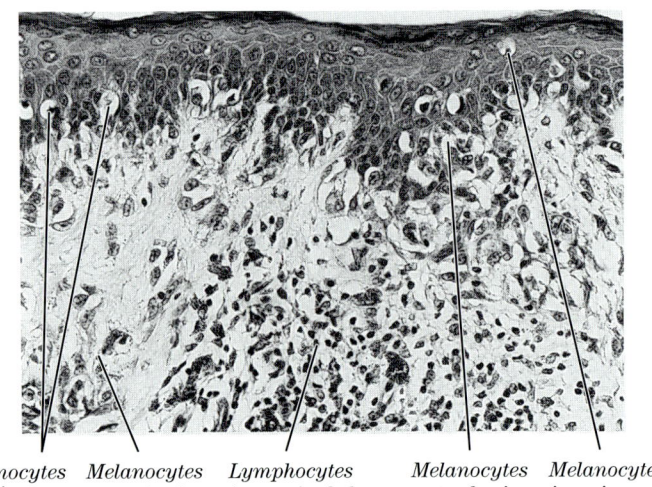

Melanocytes in spinous zone   *Melanocytes not cohesive*   *Lymphocytes intermingled with melanocytes*   *Melanocytes not cohesive*   *Melanocyte in spinous zone*

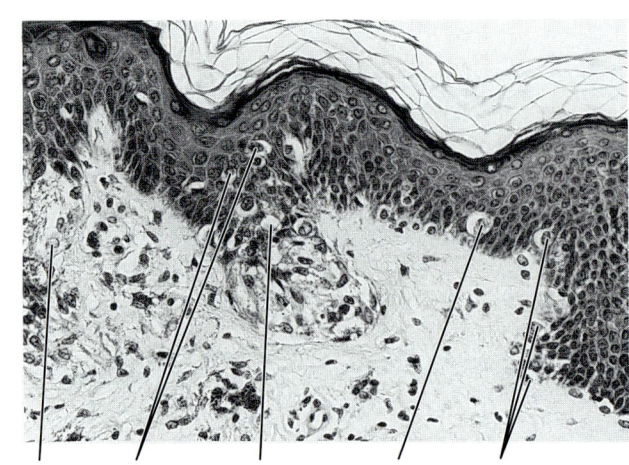

Confluence   *Melanocytes in spinous zone*   *Melanocytes not cohesive*   *Melanocyte in spinous zone*   *Poor circumscription*

11 • Melanoma

Criteria for diagnosis of this small melanoma

This is a melanoma because:

1. The neoplasm is asymmetric.
2. The neoplasm is poorly circumscribed.
3. Nests of melanocytes within the epidermis are not equidistant from one another.
4. Nests of melanocytes vary in size and shape.
5. Some nests of melanocytes have become confluent.
6. Melanocytes disposed as solitary units within the epidermis predominate over nests of melanocytes in some high-power fields.
7. Melanocytes disposed as solitary units are scattered throughout the entire thickness of the epidermis.
8. Melanin is not distributed in uniform fashion throughout the neoplasm.

Pitfall in diagnosis

This small melanoma could be misinterpreted as a compound Clark's nevus because:

1. It is small.
2. Nests of melanocytes are situated mostly at the dermo-epidermal junction.
3. The neoplasm is confined to the epidermis and papillary dermis.
4. Perivascular lymphocytic infiltrates are accompanied by melanophages.
5. The junctional component of the neoplasm extends beyond the intradermal component of it.

Despite whatever similarities this small melanoma may have in common with a Clark's nevus, it cannot be a Clark's nevus because of the scatter of melanocytes arrayed as solitary units in the spinous, granular, and cornified layers. Furthermore, those findings do not represent "dysplasia"; they are features of melanoma.

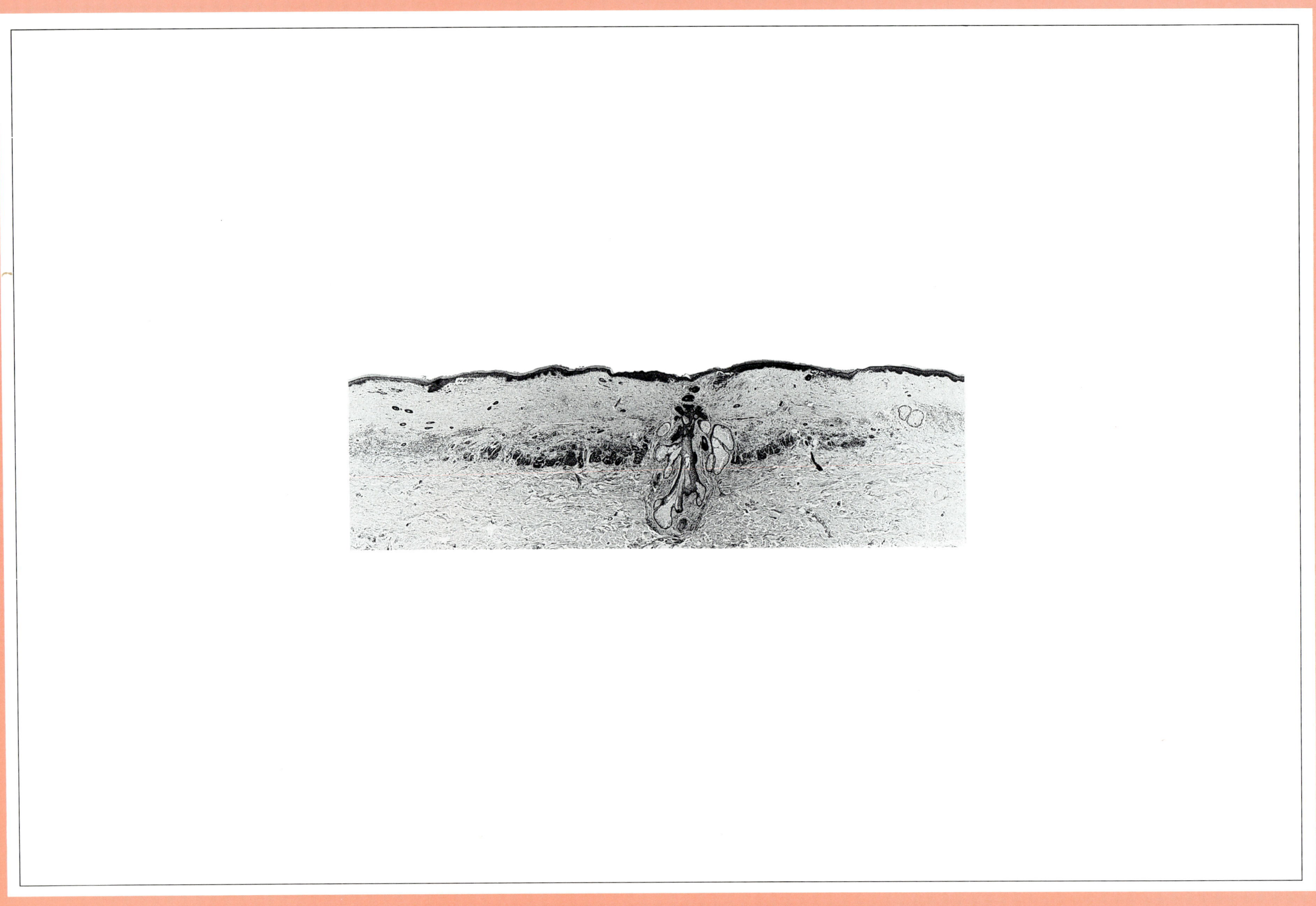

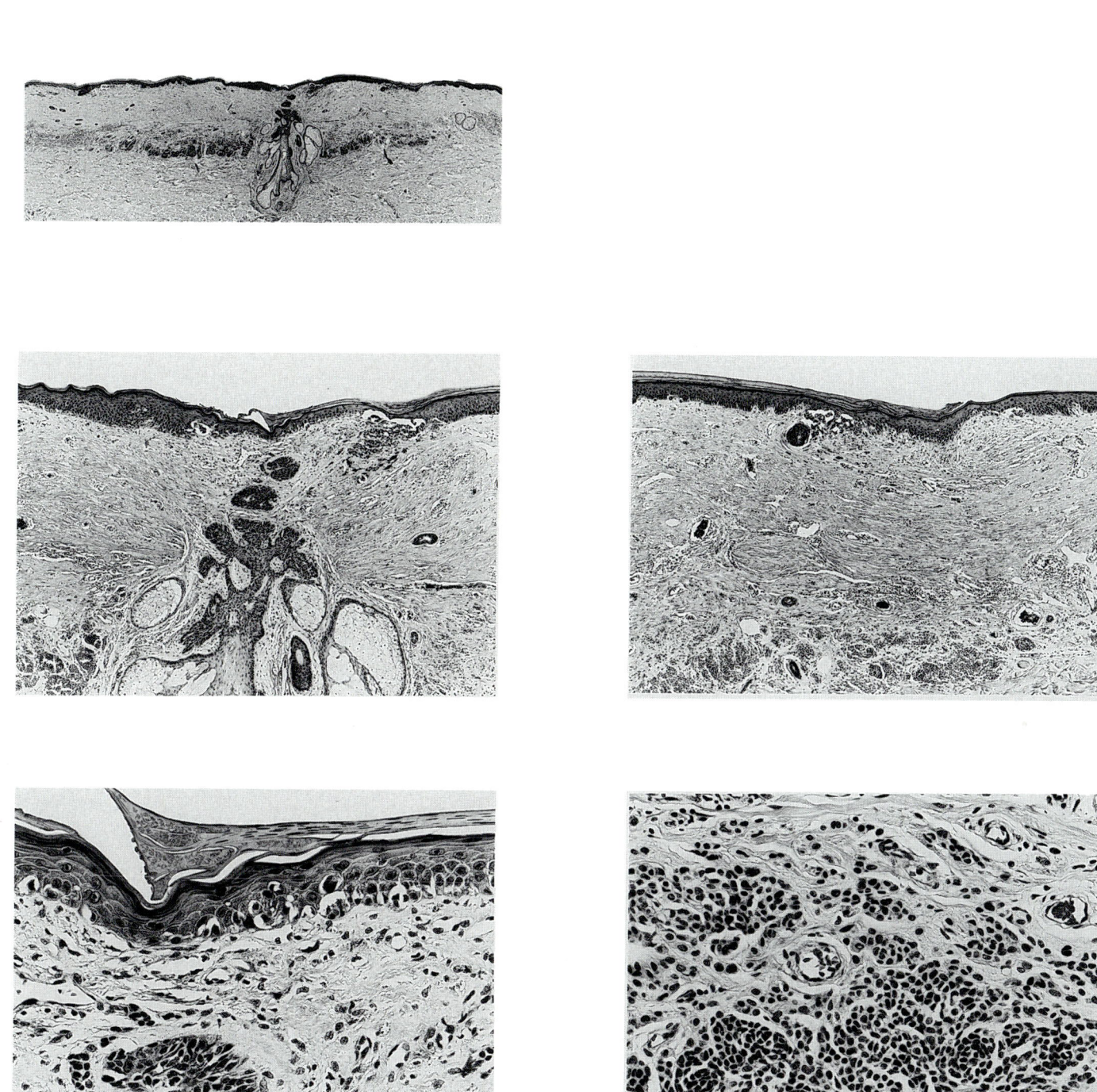

12. What is your diagnosis?

Lesion on the upper part of the back of a 64-year-old man. Clinical diagnosis: dysplastic nevus, rule out basal-cell carcinoma and malignant melanoma. No follow-up data are available.

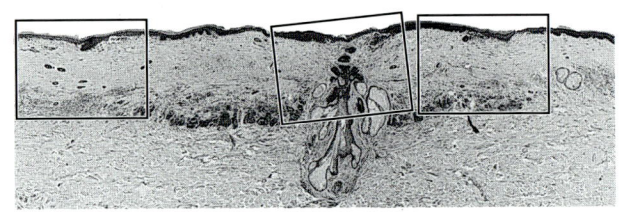

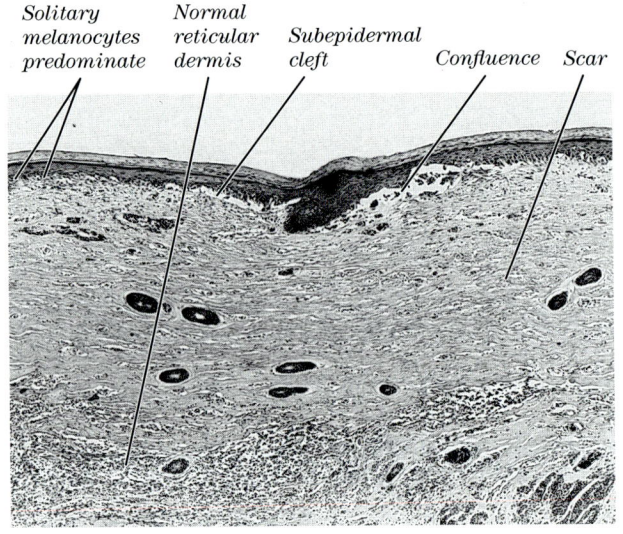

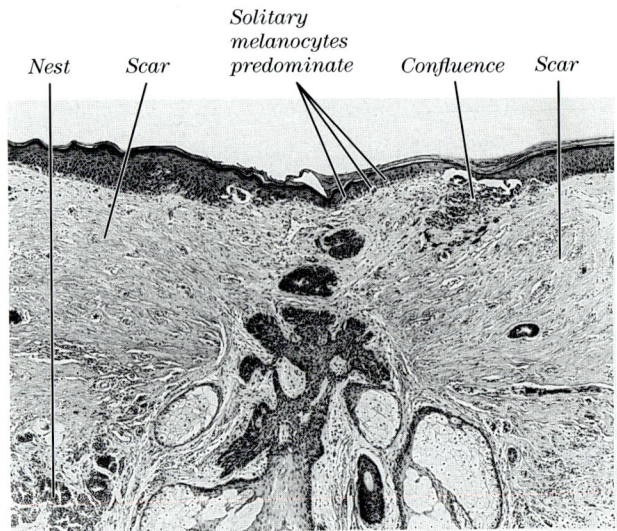

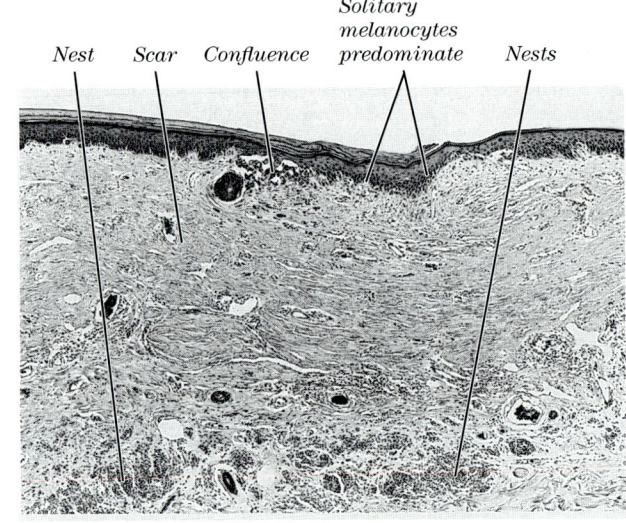

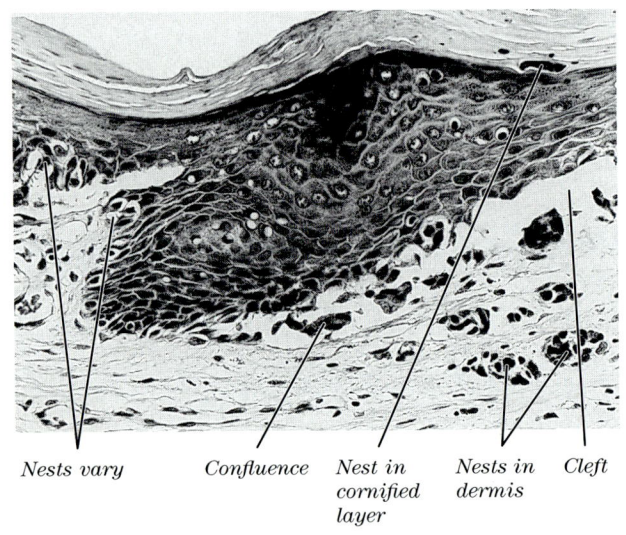

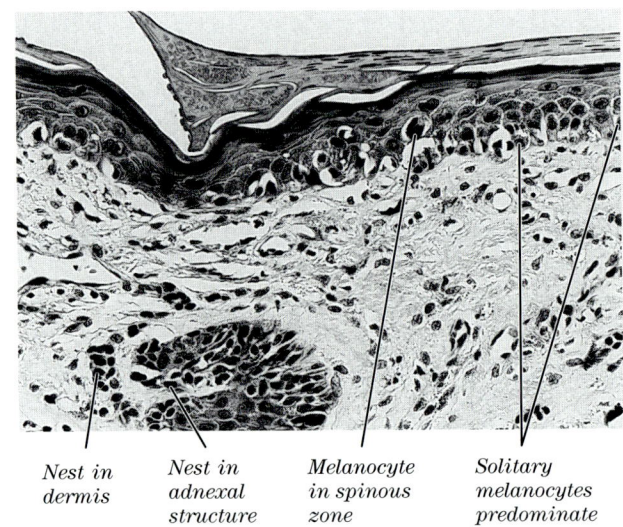

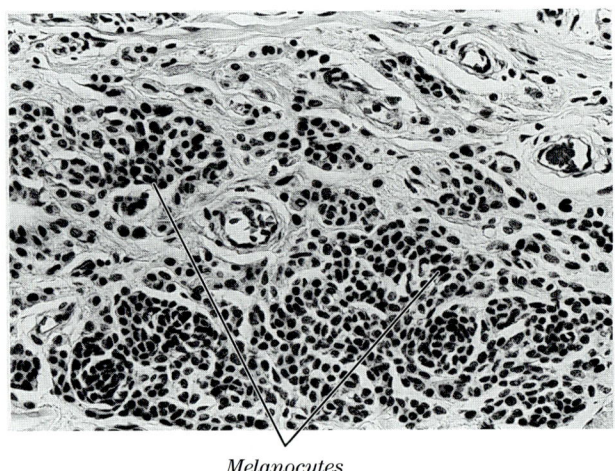

12 • Congenital Nevus *(superficial, persistent)*

Criteria for diagnosis of this congenital nevus (superficial type, persistent).

This is a superficial type of congenital nevus because:

1. The lesion is relatively symmetric.

2. An indubitable small congenital nevus is present beneath a scar that represents the site of previous surgical excision by shave technique.

3. Nuclei in melanocytes of the nevus beneath the scar are smaller than those within the epidermis and the uppermost part of the fibrotic dermis.

4. Most of the nuclei within the epidermis and the upper part of the fibrotic dermis are small, round, and monomorphous.

Pitfall in diagnosis

This persistent superficial congenital nevus could be misdiagnosed as a melanoma in association with a nevus because:

1. An unquestionable nevus is present in the upper half of the dermis.

2. Proliferation of melanocytes is apparent at all levels of the epidermis, including the cornified layer.

3. Proliferation of melanocytes within epithelial structures of adnexa, especially infundibula, is in a pattern like that within the epidermis.

4. Nests of melanocytes within the epidermis are not equidistant from one another.

5. Nests of melanocytes within the epidermis vary in size and shape.

6. Some nests of melanocytes within the epidermis have peculiar shapes, i.e., they are neither round nor oval.

7. Some nests of melanocytes within the epidermis have become confluent.

8. Melanocytes disposed as solitary units within the epidermis predominate over nests of melanocytes there in some high-power fields.

Were only the findings in the epidermis of this section examined, this neoplasm could be misdiagnosed as a melanoma in situ. In fact, more features in the epidermis favor melanoma in situ than they do a nevus. Beneath the scar in the upper part of the dermis, however, are indubitable signs of a nevus. That informs a microscopist that the changes in the epidermis (and within the scar) almost certainly are those of a persistent nevus. In every instance in which the diagnosis of persistent nevus or persistent melanoma is in doubt, sections from the original biopsy specimen must be obtained and scrutinized.

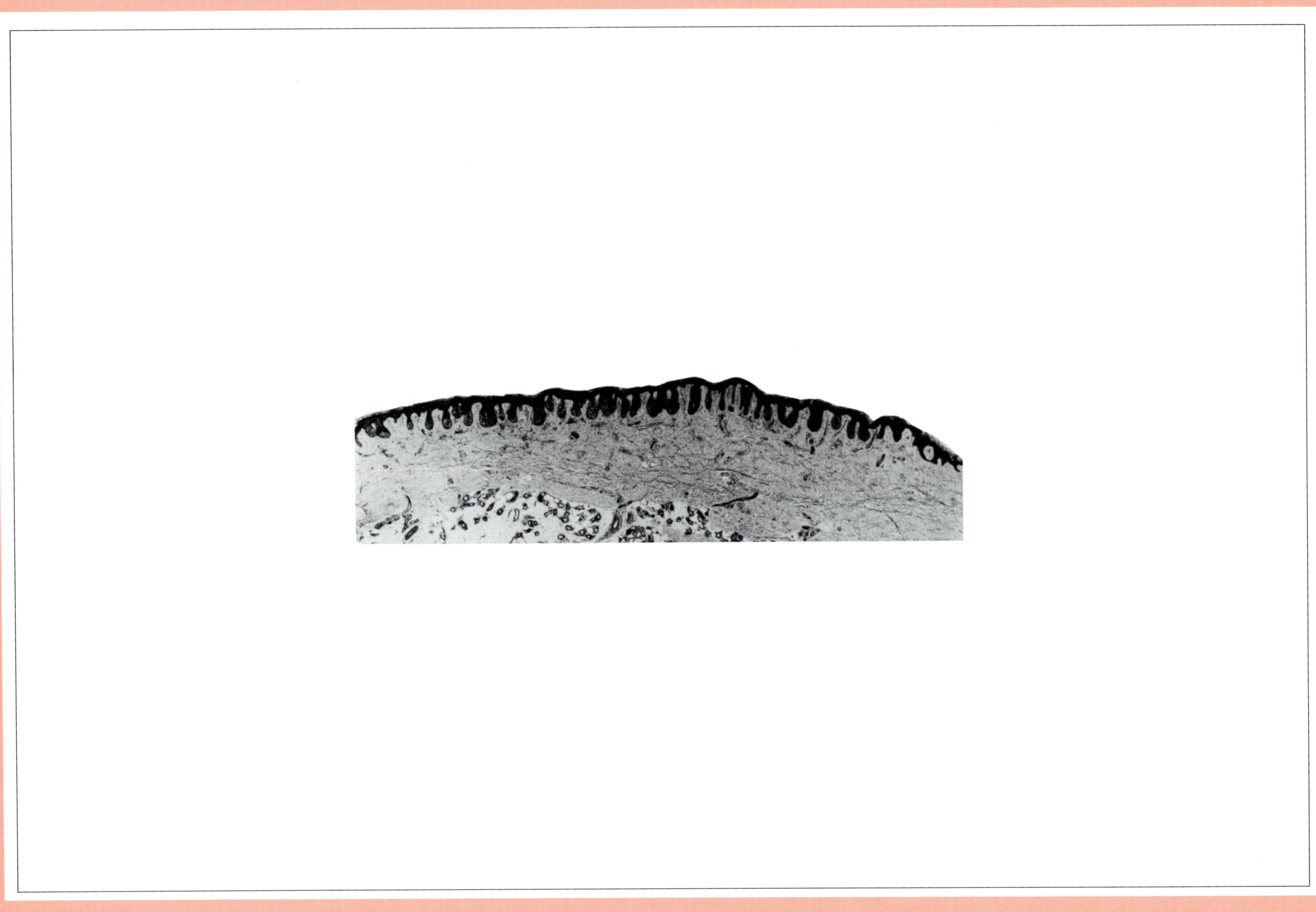

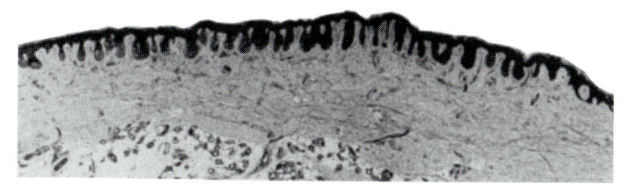

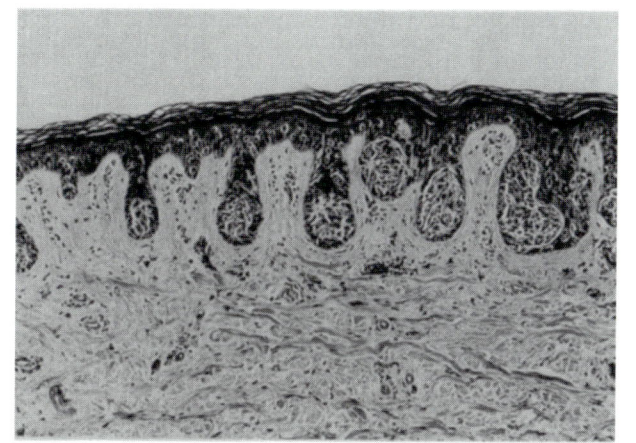
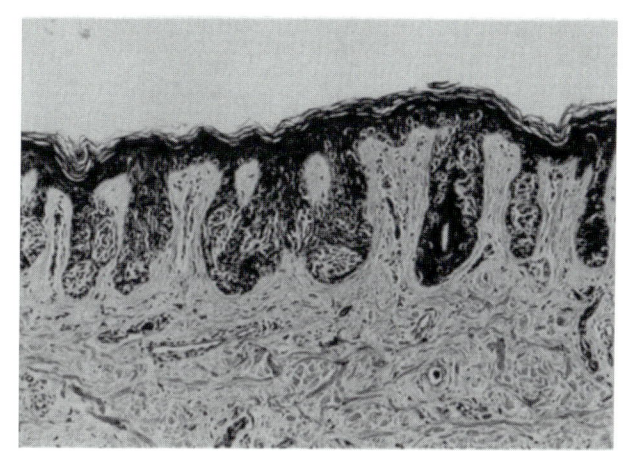
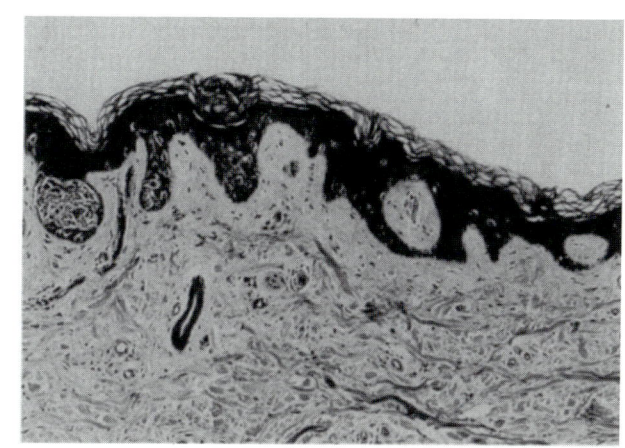
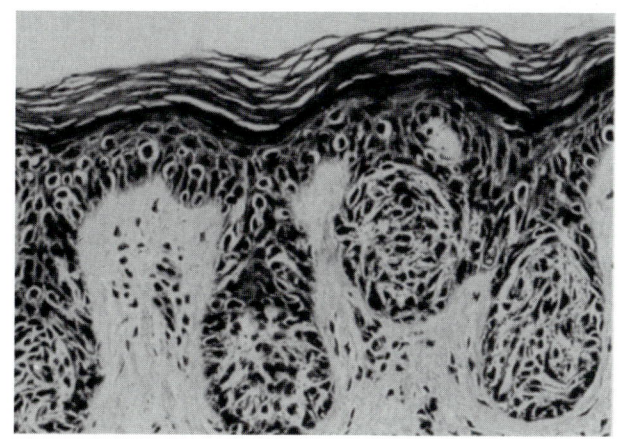
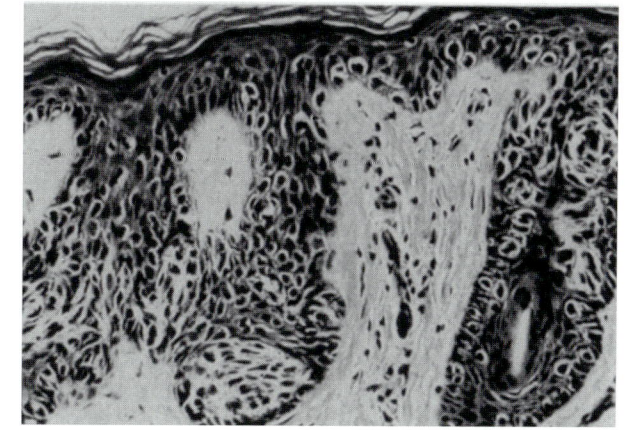
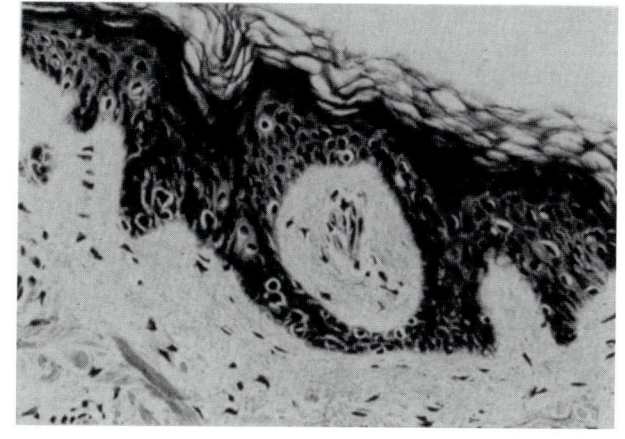

13. What is your diagnosis?

Pigmented lesion on the third toe of the left foot of a 72-year-old man. No clinical diagnosis or follow-up was available.

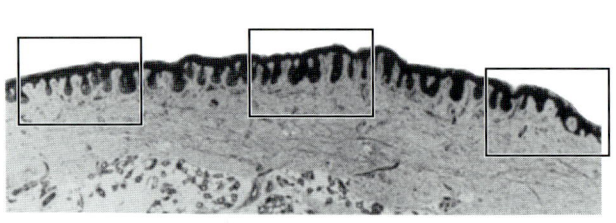

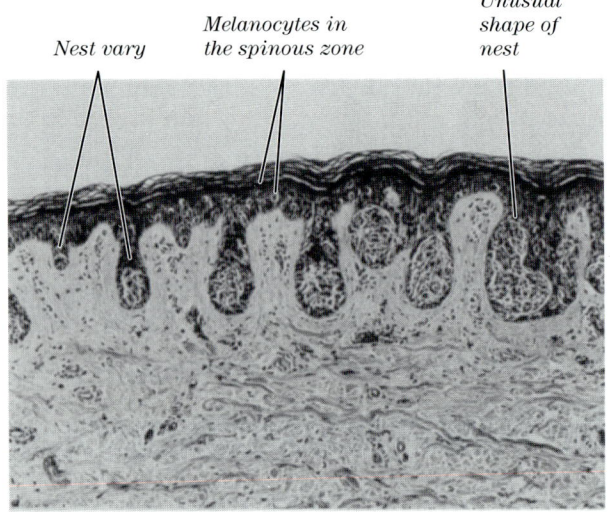

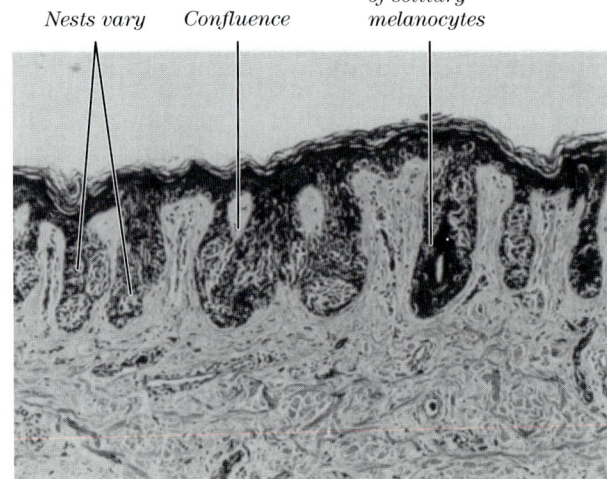

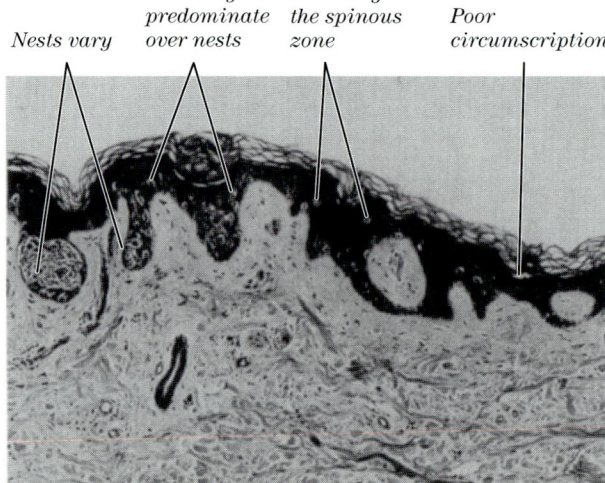

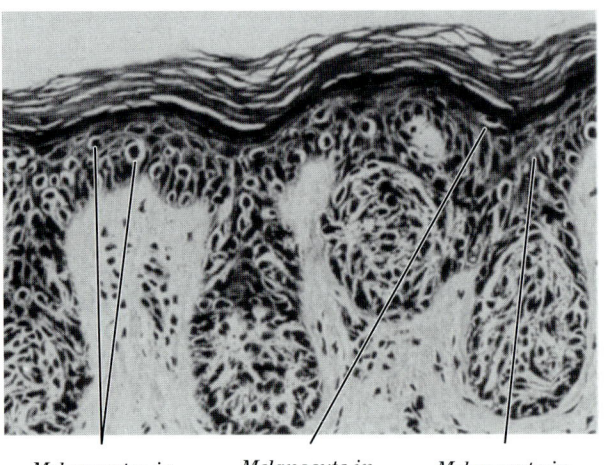

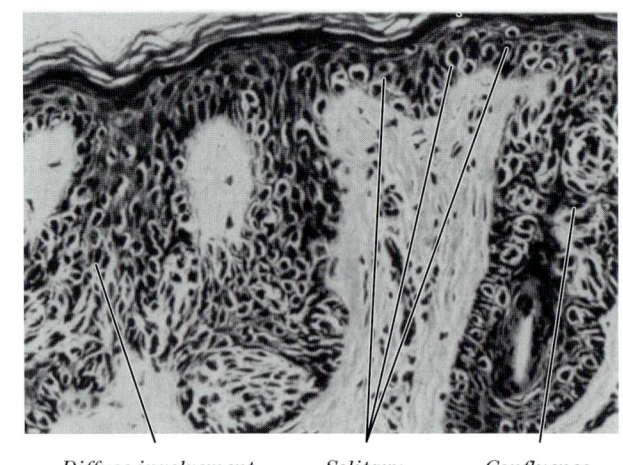

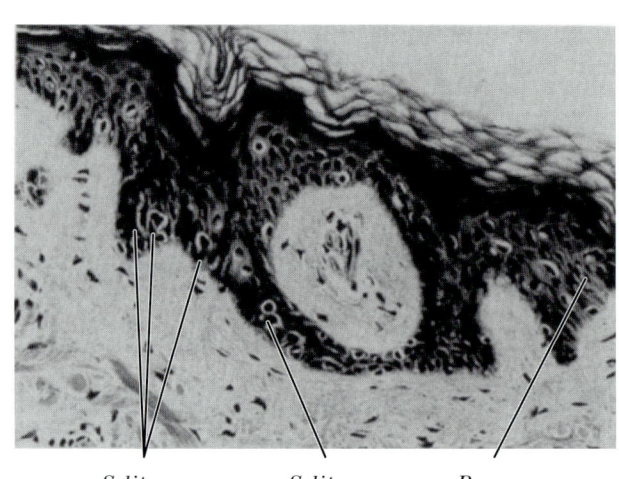

318   13 • Malignant melanoma in situ

Criteria for diagnosis of this melanoma in situ

This is a melanoma in situ because:

1. The lesion is asymmetric.
2. The proliferation of melanocytes is poorly circumscribed.
3. Nests of melanocytes within the epidermis and epithelial structures of adnexa are not equidistant from one another.
4. Nests of melanocytes vary in size and shape.
5. Some nests of melanocytes have peculiar shapes.
6. Some nests of melanocytes have become confluent.
7. Melanocytes disposed as solitary units predominate over nests in some foci.
8. Melanocytes arranged as solitary units and nests are dispersed diffusely throughout some rete ridges and some epithelial structures of adnexa.
9. Melanocytes arrayed as solitary units are present above the dermo-epidermal junction including the spinous, granular, and cornified layers.
10. Melanocytes, both those as solitary units and in nests, extend far down epithelial structures of adnexa.
11. Melanocytes in the form of solitary units are present above the basal layer of epithelial structures of adnexa.
12. Melanocytes disposed as solitary units are not set equidistant from one another.
13. Some melanocytes have atypical nuclei.

Pitfall in diagnosis

This melanoma in situ could be mistaken for a junctional "dysplastic" nevus because:

1. The lesion is small, i.e., less than 6.0 mm in greatest diameter.
2. Melanocytes arranged in nests predominate over melanocytes disposed as solitary units throughout most of the neoplasm.
3. Nests of melanocytes are situated mostly at the dermo-epidermal junction at bases of rete ridges.
4. In some foci, nests of melanocytes are relatively uniform in size and shape.
5. Elongated rete ridges resemble those of a "lentiginous" pattern.
6. Most of the melanocytes are relatively small and monomorphous.

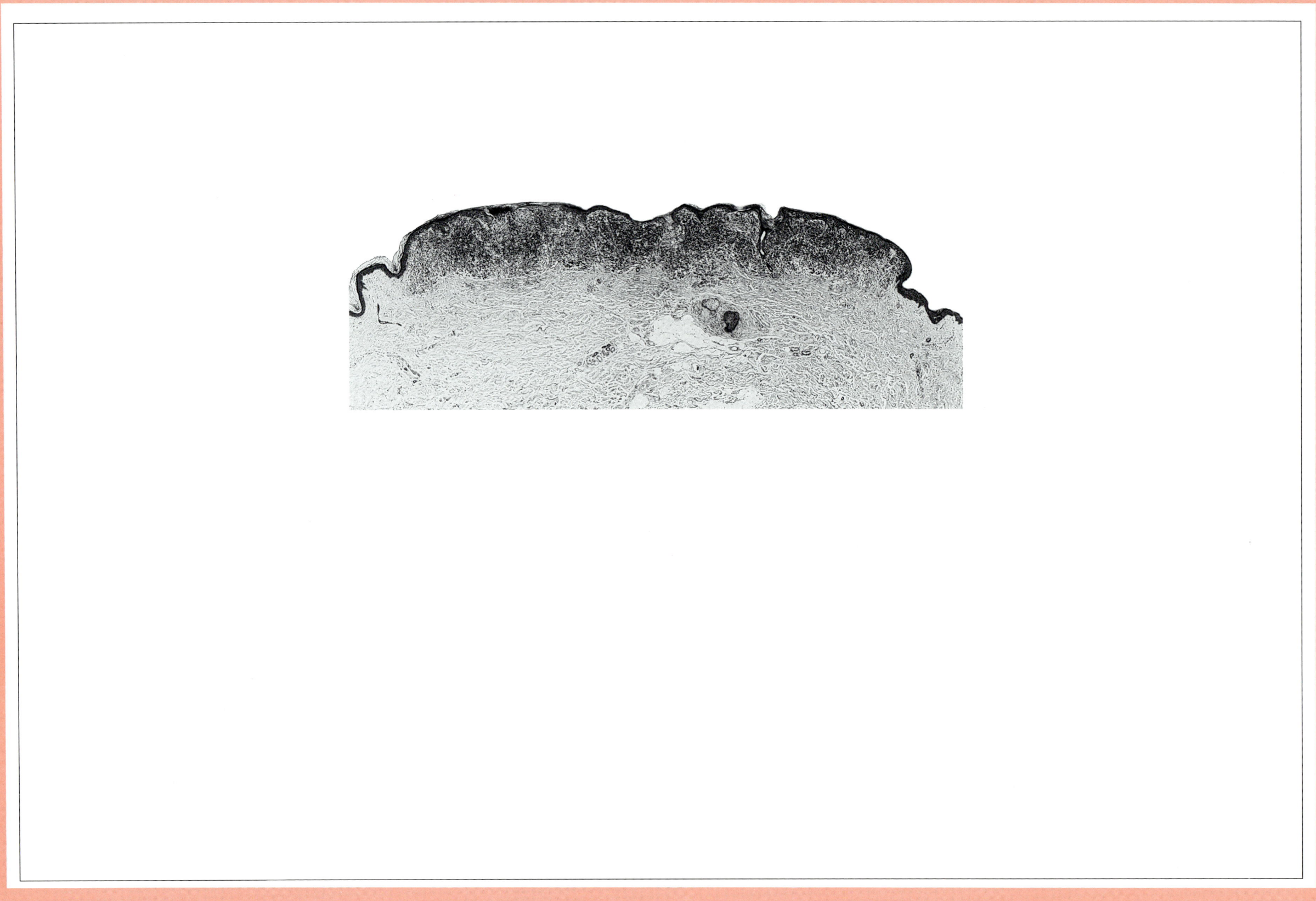

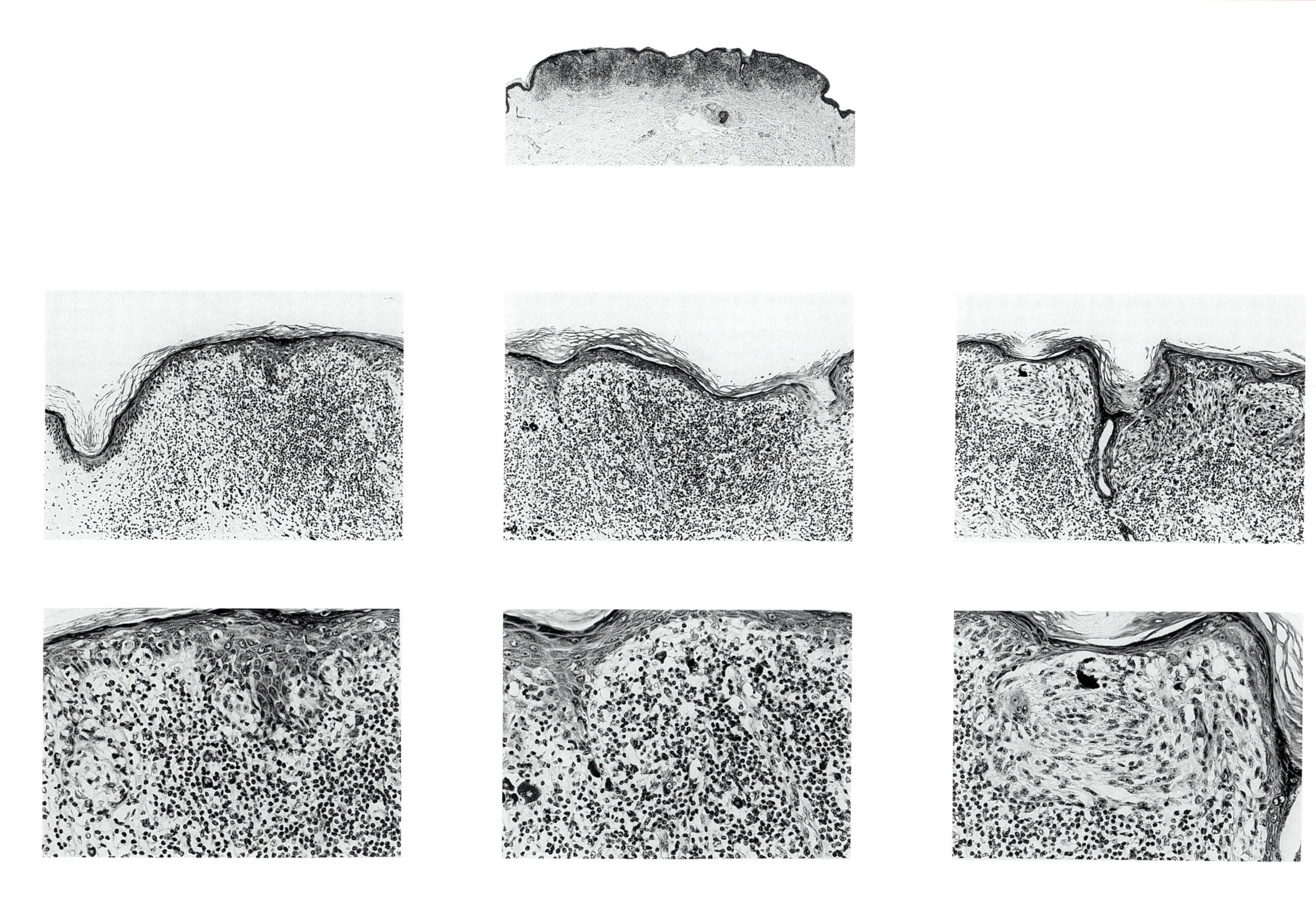

14. What is your diagnosis?

Irregularly shaped, slightly pigmented lesion on the right forearm of a 47-year-old woman that had changed during the previous year. Clinical diagnosis: melanoma. Patient was free of disease after 1 year.

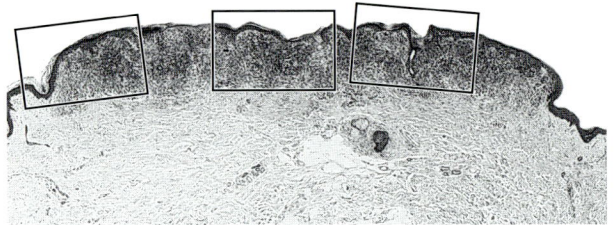

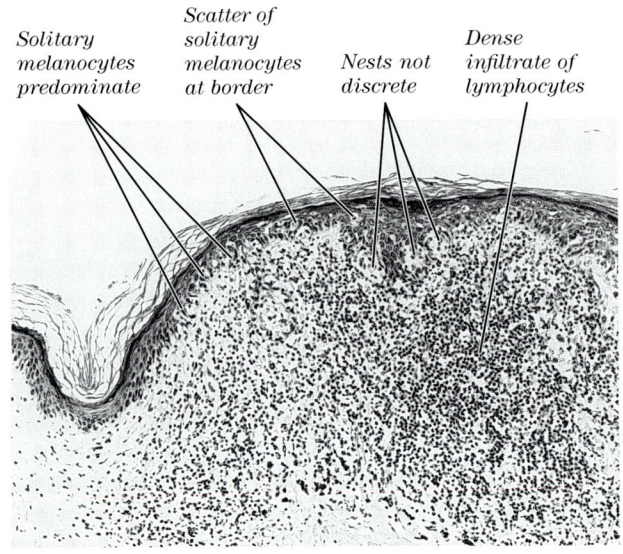
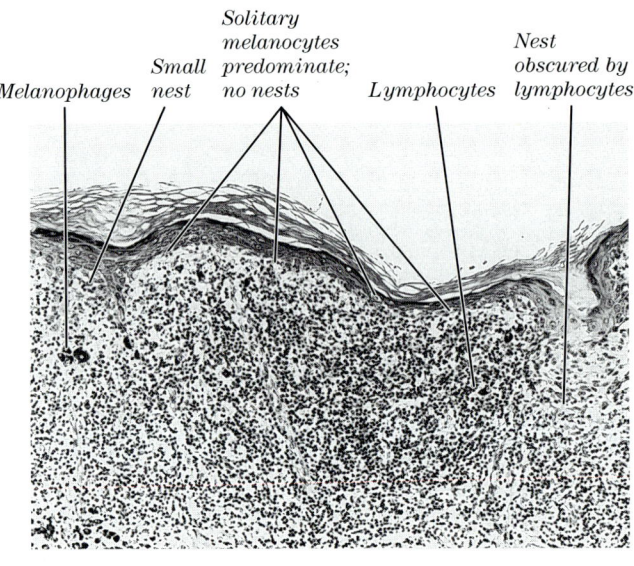
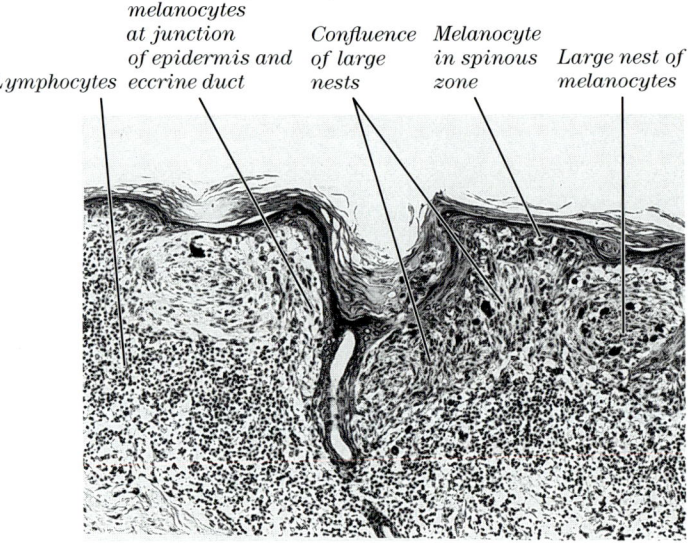

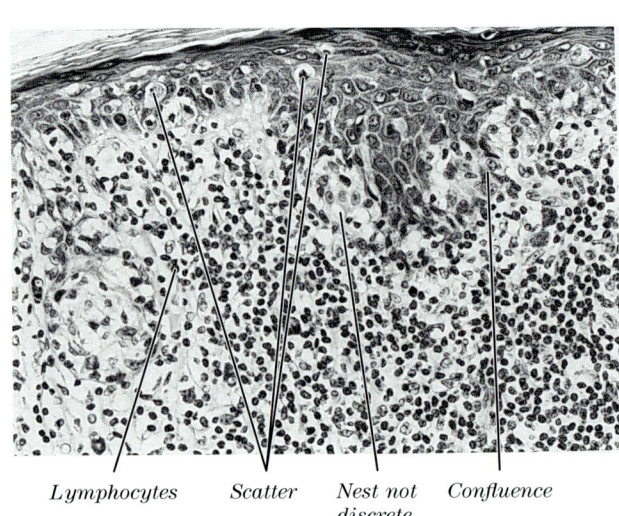
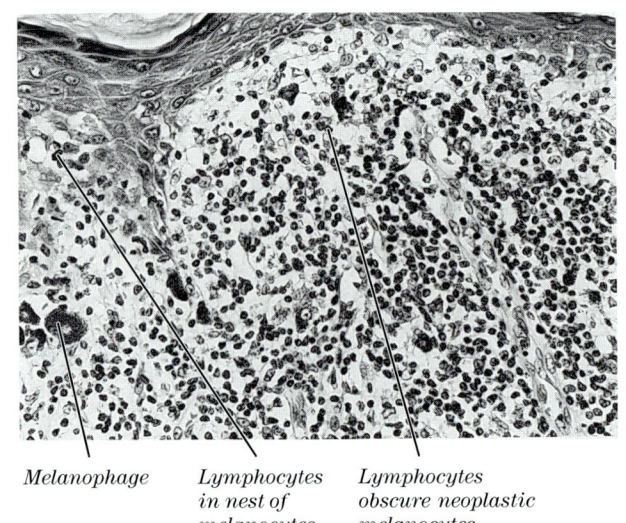
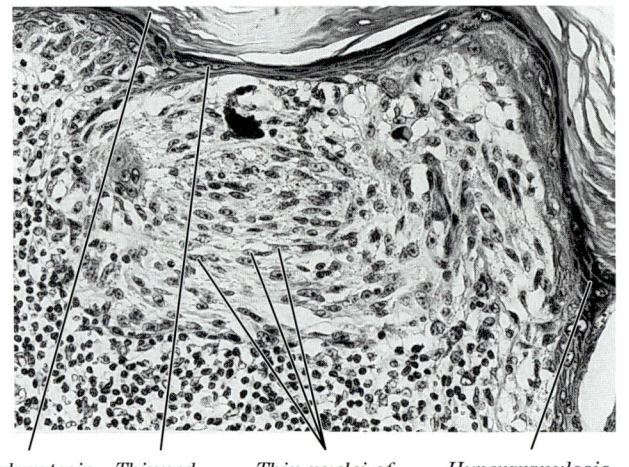

14 • Melanoma

Criteria for diagnosis of this melanoma

This is a melanoma because:

1. It is asymmetric, e.g., many more nests of melanocytes are present on the right side of the neoplasm than the left of it.

2. Nests of melanocytes within the epidermis are not equidistant from one another.

3. There is marked variation in size and shape of nests of melanocytes within the epidermis.

4. Melanocytes disposed as solitary units within the epidermis are more numerous than melanocytes in nests in some high-power fields.

5. Some melanocytes arranged as solitary units are situated far above the dermo-epidermal junction.

Pitfall in diagnosis

This melanoma could be misdiagnosed as a halo nevus because:

1. The process is confined to the epidermis and thickened papillary dermis.
2. It is slightly domed.
3. Circumscription is sharp.
4. Its bottom is relatively flat.
5. A dense infiltrate of lymphocytes is dispersed throughout much of the thickened papillary dermis.
6. Nests of melanocytes are seated only at the dermo-epidermal junction, not above it.
7. Nuclear atypia is hardly discernible.

At first glance at scanning magnification, this melanoma could be misconstrued as a halo nevus. As so often is the case, and in this case, judgment about symmetry and asymmetry is decisive. Note that there are many more large nests of melanocytes within the epidermis on the right side of the neoplasm than on the left side. Furthermore, the neoplasm is poorly circumscribed on the left, and melanocytes are scattered at all levels of the epidermis on the left. These findings of asymmetry indicate that the diagnosis is melanoma.

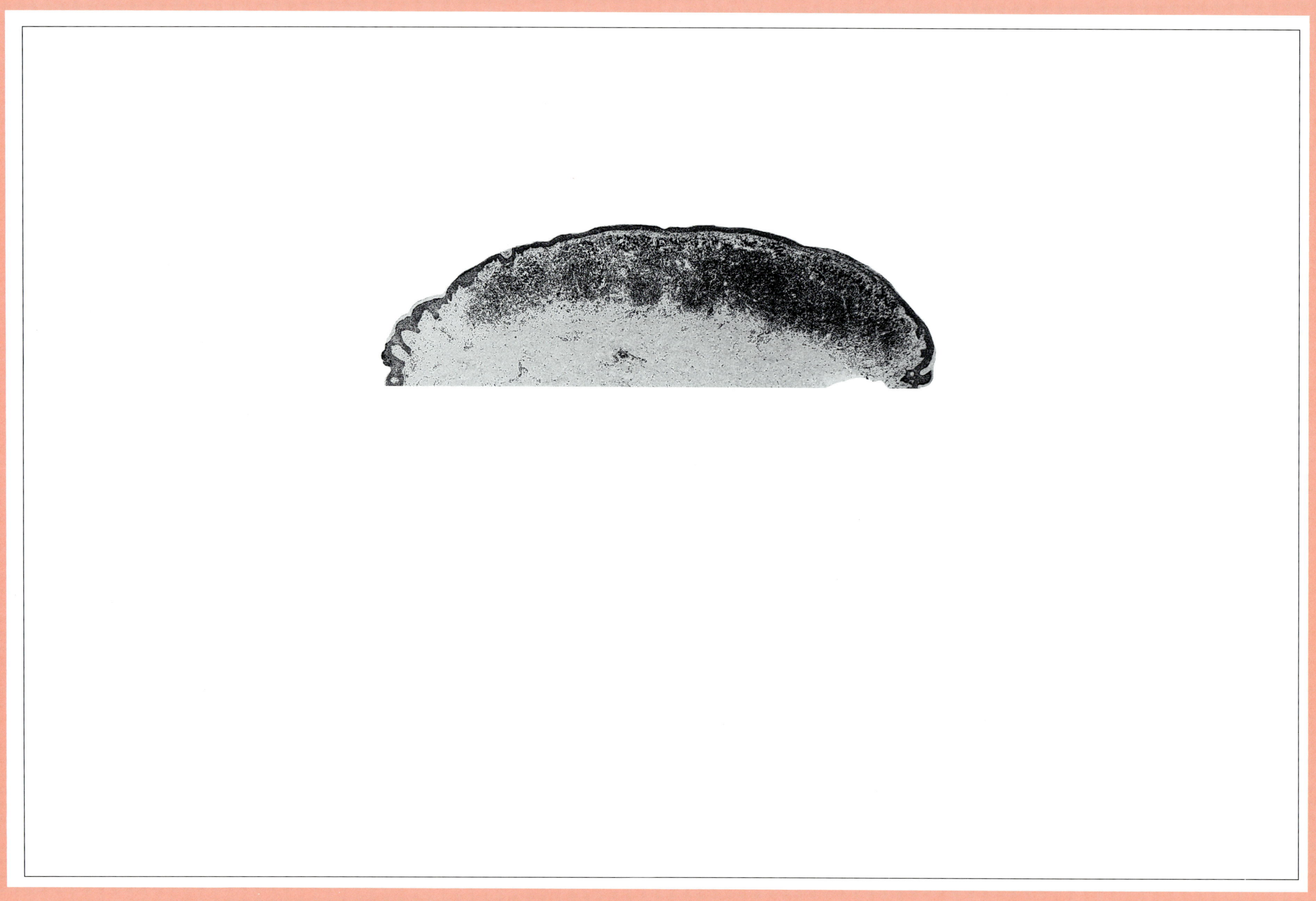

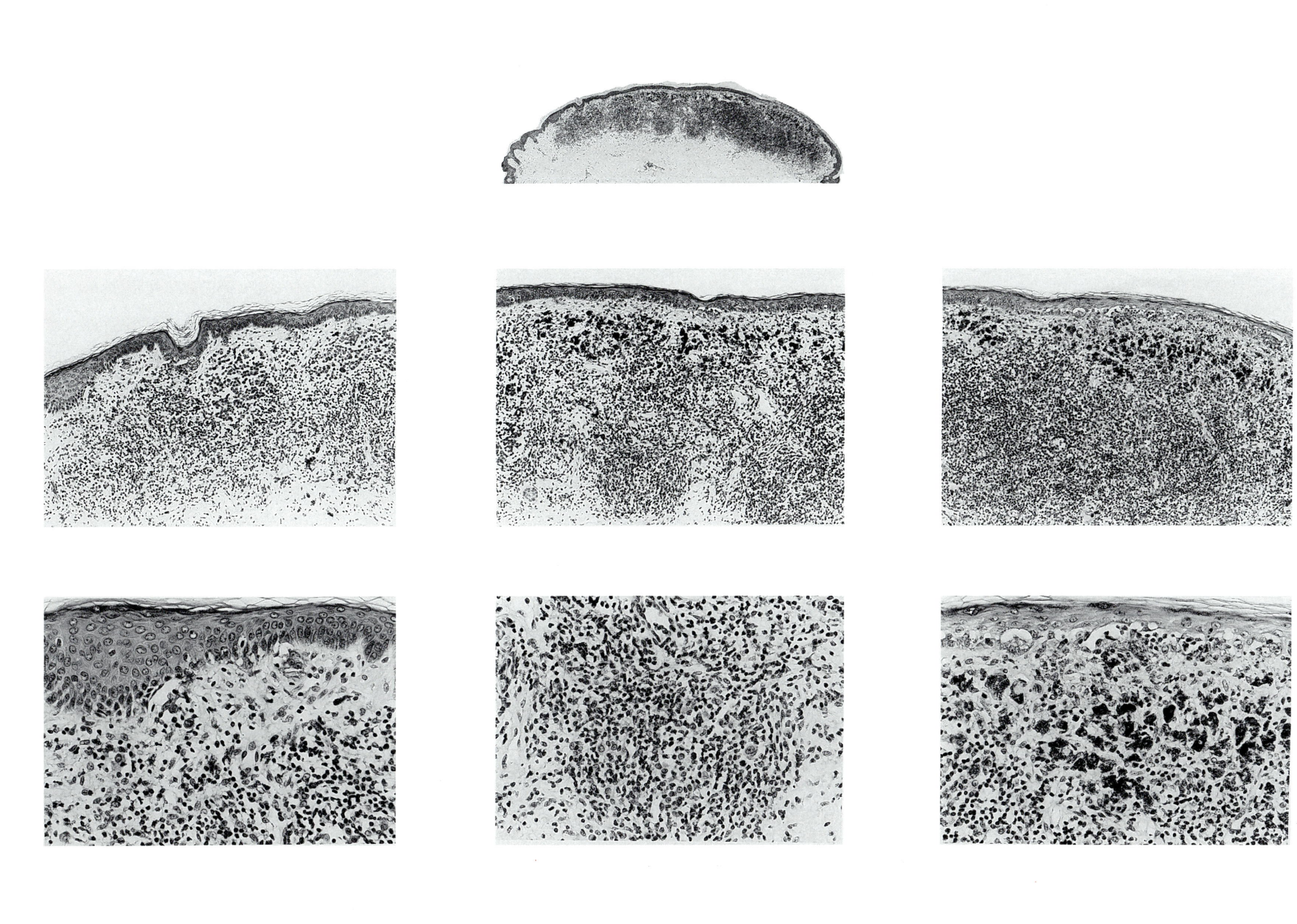

15. What is your diagnosis?

Unevenly pigmented and shaped macule on the right side of the chest of a 15-year-old man. Clinical diagnosis: dysplastic nevus, rule out melanoma. Patient had no evidence of disease after 7 years.

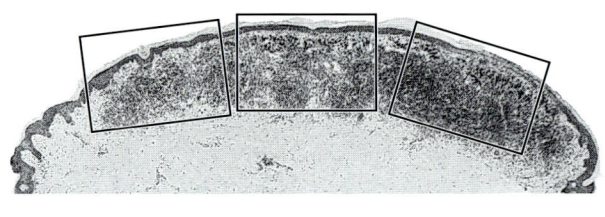

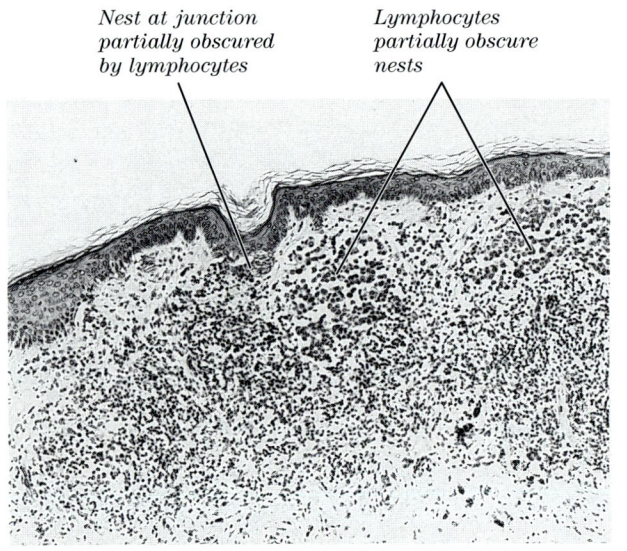

Nest at junction partially obscured by lymphocytes — *Lymphocytes partially obscure nests*

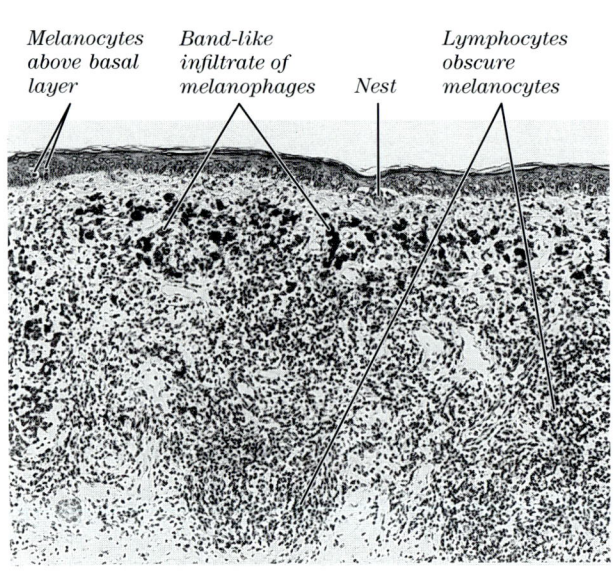

Melanocytes above basal layer — *Band-like infiltrate of melanophages* — *Nest* — *Lymphocytes obscure melanocytes*

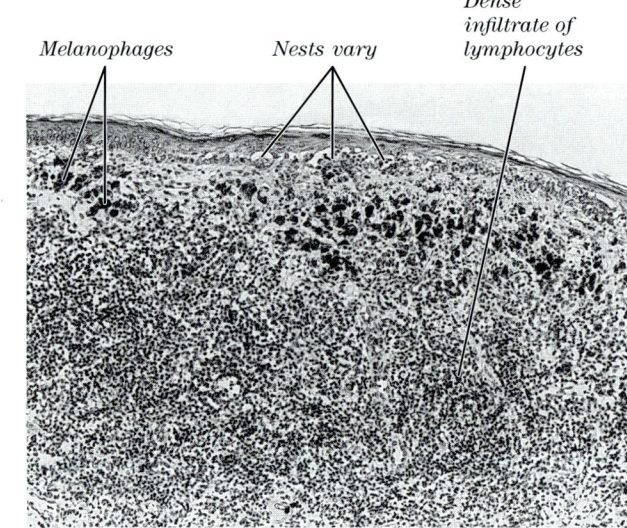

Melanophages — *Nests vary* — *Dense infiltrate of lymphocytes*

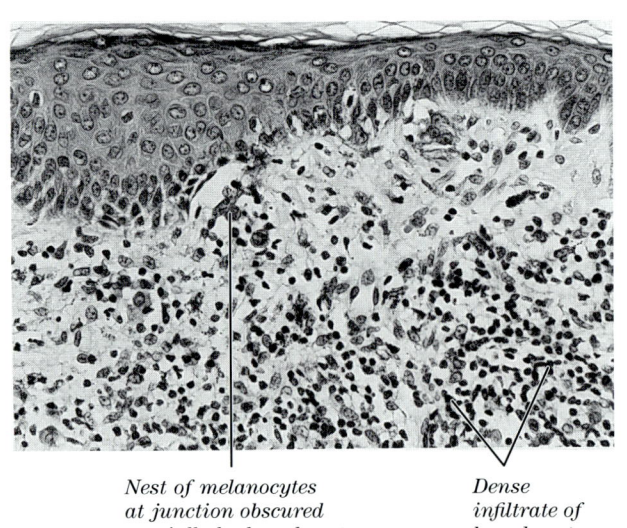

Nest of melanocytes at junction obscured partially by lymphocytes — *Dense infiltrate of lymphocytes*

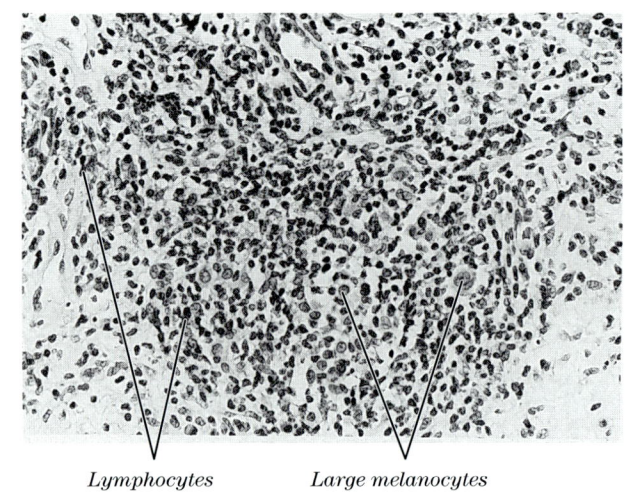

Lymphocytes — *Large melanocytes*

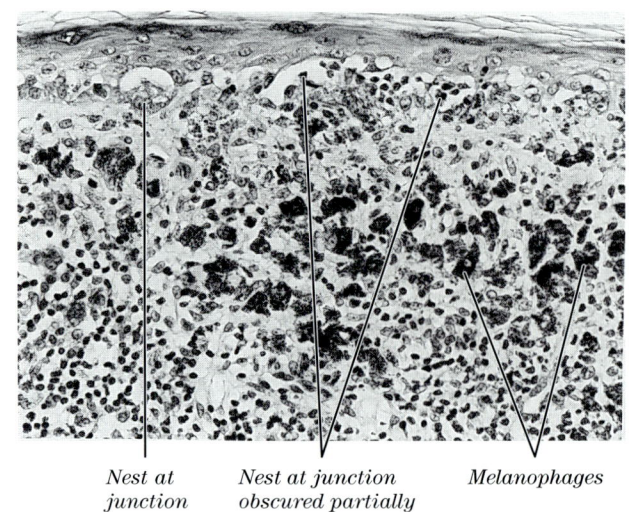

Nest at junction — *Nest at junction obscured partially by lymphocytes* — *Melanophages*

15 • Clark's Nevus *(halo type)*

Criteria for diagnosis of this Clark's nevus (halo type)

This is a nevus because:

1. The neoplasm is symmetric.
2. It is well-circumscribed.
3. Its base is relatively flat.
4. There is maturation of melanocytes.
5. Melanocytes within the epidermis, both those arranged as solitary units and those in nests, are situated at the dermo-epidermal junction, not above it.

This is a halo nevus because:

1. Melanocytes of a nevus, both within the epidermis and in the markedly thickened papillary dermis, are obscured by a dense infiltrate of lymphocytes.

Pitfall in diagnosis

This halo type of Clark's nevus could be misinterpreted as a melanoma because:

1. Nests of melanocytes within the epidermis are not equidistant from one another.
2. Nests of melanocytes at the dermo-epidermal junction vary in size and shape.
3. Some nests of melanocytes within the epidermis have become confluent.
4. Melanin is not distributed in uniform fashion throughout the neoplasm; more melanin is present on the right side of the neoplasm than on the left side of it.

This neoplasm is benign because of its architectural pattern and is a compound Clark's nevus because neoplastic melanocytes are confined to the dermo-epidermal junction and thickened papillary dermis of a gently domed lesion. The presence of a dense lymphocytic infiltrate throughout a Clark's nevus is consonant with a "halo" nevus, but such an infiltrate within a Clark's nevus is not associated consistently with a "halo" clinically. In short, a dense infiltrate of lymphocytes within a Clark's nevus does not necessarily signify a halo nevus. Nor does an infiltrate of lymphocytes, no matter how dense, necessarily indicate a melanoma. Lymphocytes are only important in the differentiation of nevus from melanoma when they are distributed asymmetrically. In that instance, they imply melanoma, but, as always, there is at least one exception—lymphocytes may be distributed asymmetrically when they are associated with one component of a combined nevus. In sum, density of lymphocytic infiltration is not an aid to distinguishing benign from malignant proliferations of melanocytes. In halo nevi, infiltrates of lymphocytes may be dense, and in many melanomas they may be sparse and even absent.

Parenthetically, although most halo nevi are Clark's nevi, not all are.

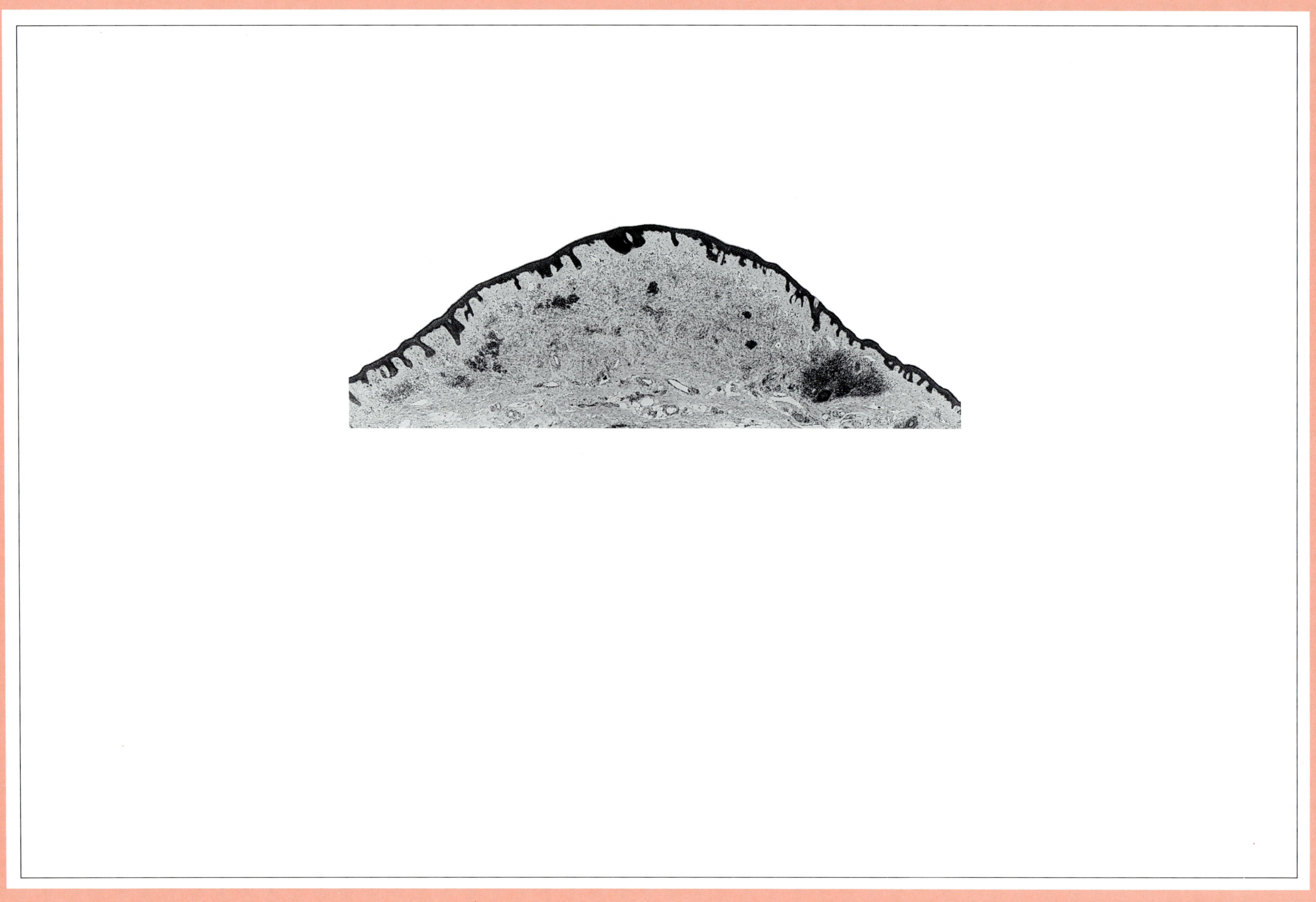

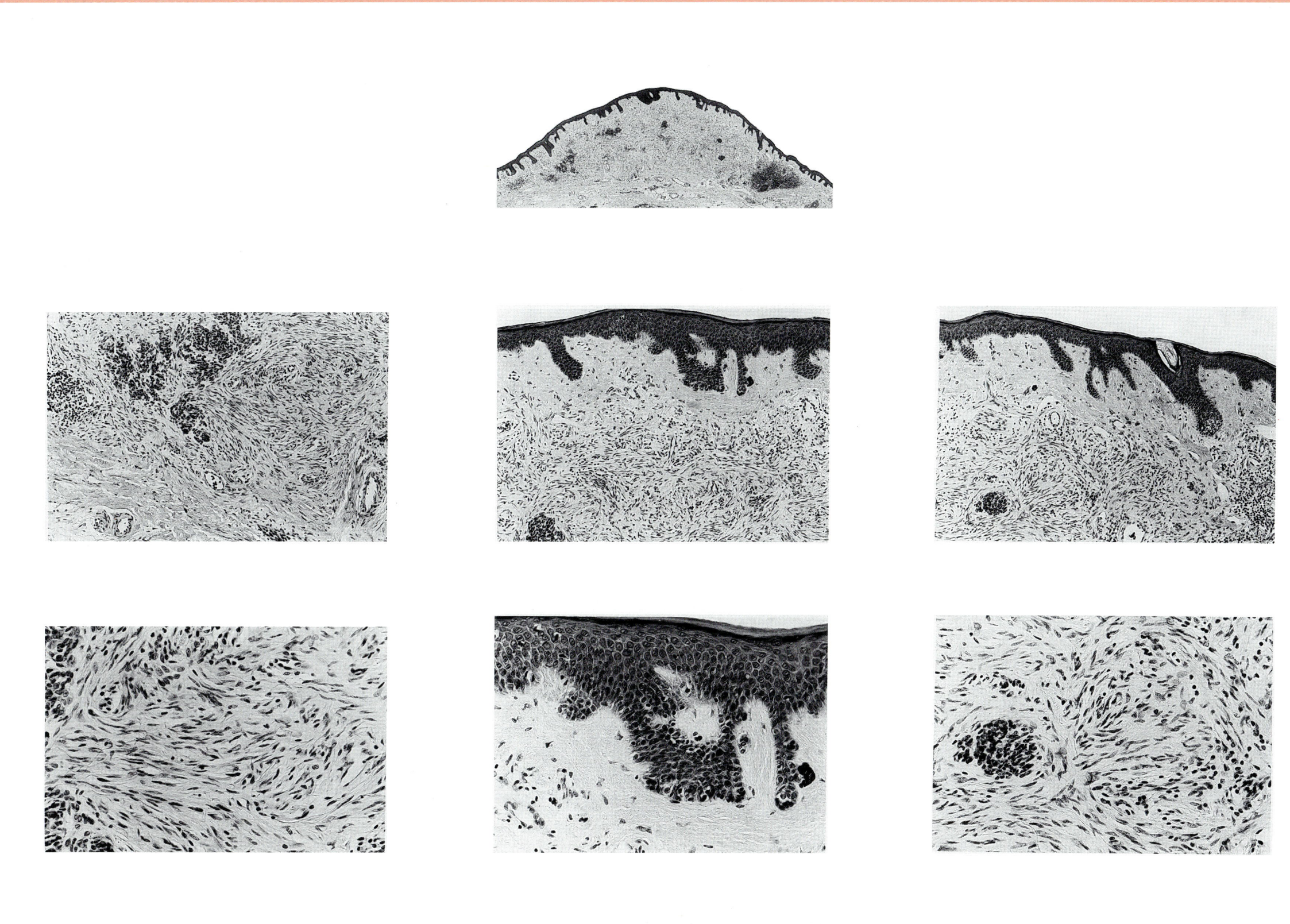

16. What is your diagnosis?

Skin-colored lesion on the left ear of a 63-year-old man. Clinical diagnosis: nevus. The site was excised completely. No follow-up data are available.

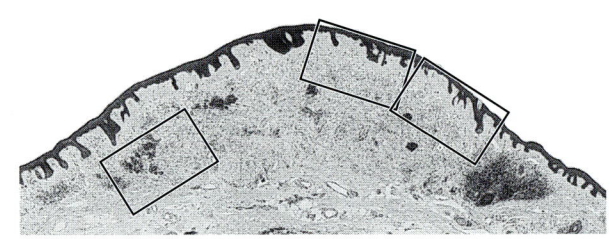

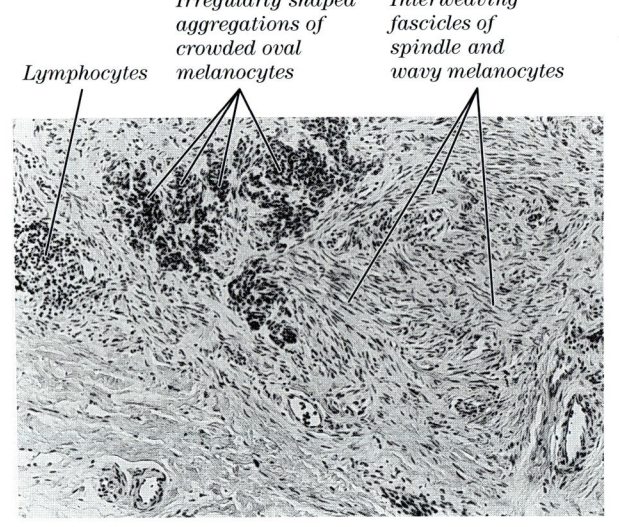

Lymphocytes — *Irregularly shaped aggregations of crowded oval melanocytes* — *Interweaving fascicles of spindle and wavy melanocytes*

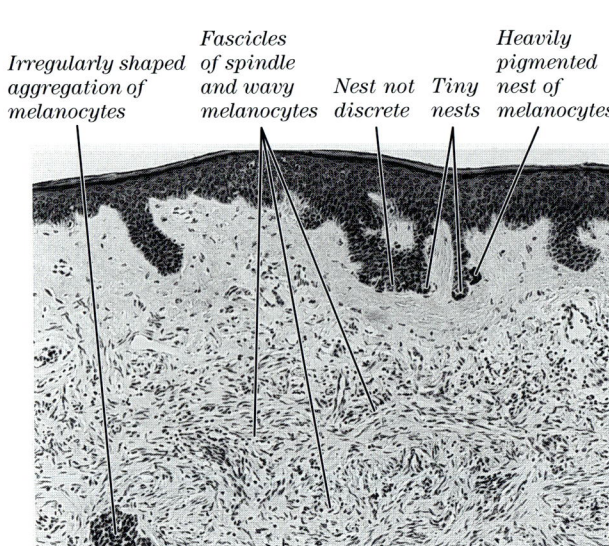

Irregularly shaped aggregation of melanocytes — *Fascicles of spindle and wavy melanocytes* — *Nest not discrete* — *Tiny nests* — *Heavily pigmented nest of melanocytes*

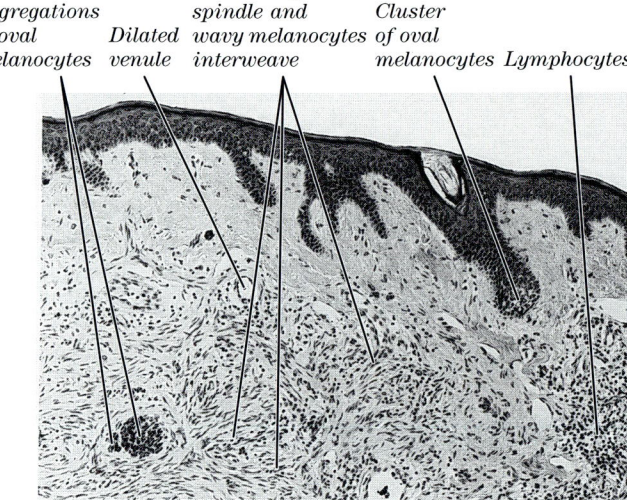

Aggregations of oval melanocytes — *Dilated venule* — *Fascicles of spindle and wavy melanocytes interweave* — *Cluster of oval melanocytes* — *Lymphocytes*

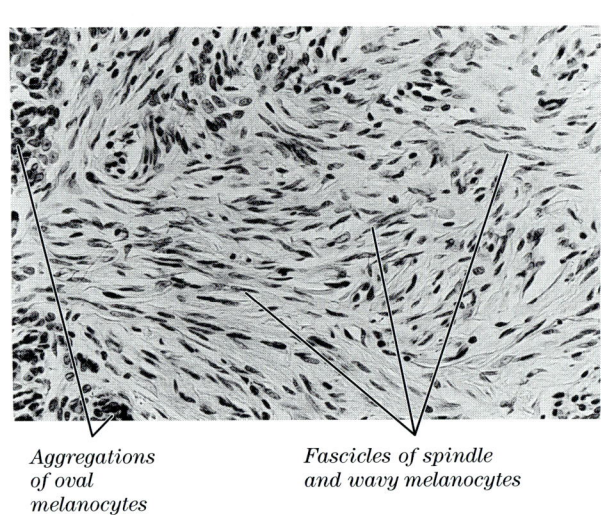

Aggregations of oval melanocytes — *Fascicles of spindle and wavy melanocytes*

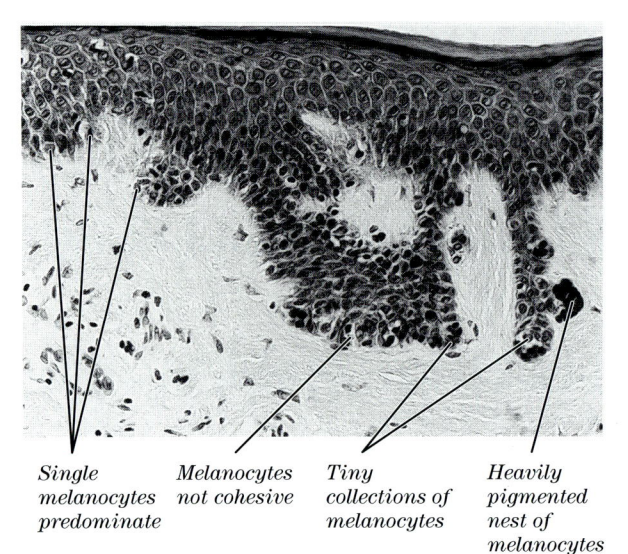

Single melanocytes predominate — *Melanocytes not cohesive* — *Tiny collections of melanocytes* — *Heavily pigmented nest of melanocytes*

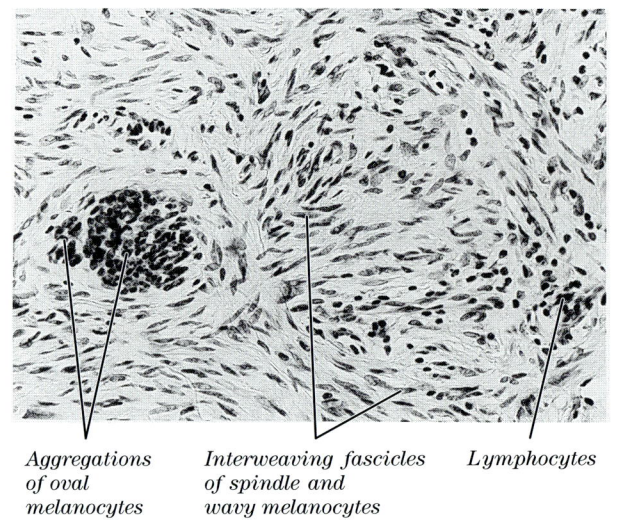

Aggregations of oval melanocytes — *Interweaving fascicles of spindle and wavy melanocytes* — *Lymphocytes*

16 • Melanoma *(with neural differentiation)*

Criteria for diagnosis of this melanoma (with neural differentiation)

This is a melanoma with neural differentiation because:

1. The neoplasm is asymmetric, e.g., large collections of dark-staining cells on the left are more numerous than those on the right, and the infiltrate of lymphocytes on the left is more dense than that on the right.

2. Subtle signs of melanoma in situ, namely, melanocytes disposed as solitary units, predominate overwhelmingly over melanocytes arranged in nests, many individual melanocytes are scattered far above the dermo-epidermal junction, nests of melanocytes are not equidistant from one another, and melanin is distributed in uneven fashion.

3. There are two populations of neoplastic cells, namely, those with large plump nuclei and those with elongated wavy nuclei, the latter, a sign of neural differentiation, are distributed randomly.

4. Fascicles of neoplastic cells with wavy nuclei are arranged in disorderly fashion.

Pitfall in diagnosis

This melanoma with neural differentiation could be misinterpreted as a neurofibroma beneath a junctional nevus because:

1. Nests of melanocytes are positioned at the dermo-epidermal junction.

2. There are fascicles of neoplastic cells.

3. Nuclei of neoplastic cells are relatively monomorphous.

4. Few mitotic figures are encountered.

An important clue to diagnosis of desmoplastic melanoma and melanoma with neural differentiation is the presence of dense infiltrates of lymphocytes around blood vessels throughout the neoplasm. In this instance, the infiltrate is asymmetric, being more dense on the right. Another evidence of asymmetry is the presence of irregularly shaped clusters of atypical melanocytes on the left, and not on the right. In the epidermis, there are subtle signs of melanoma in situ. The presence within a melanoma of wavy melanocytes, some of them organized in fascicles, is a sign of neural differentiation of that melanoma.

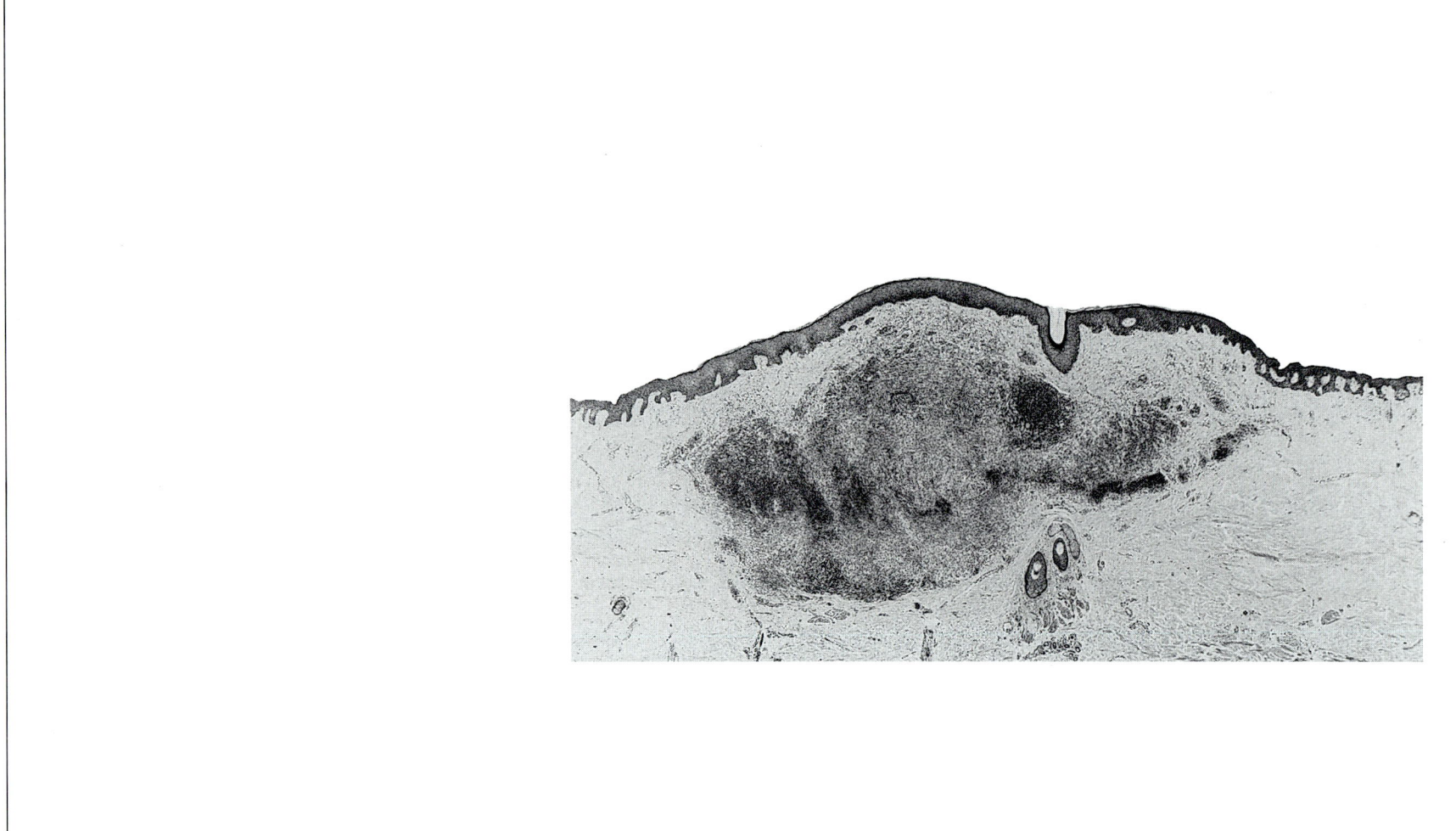

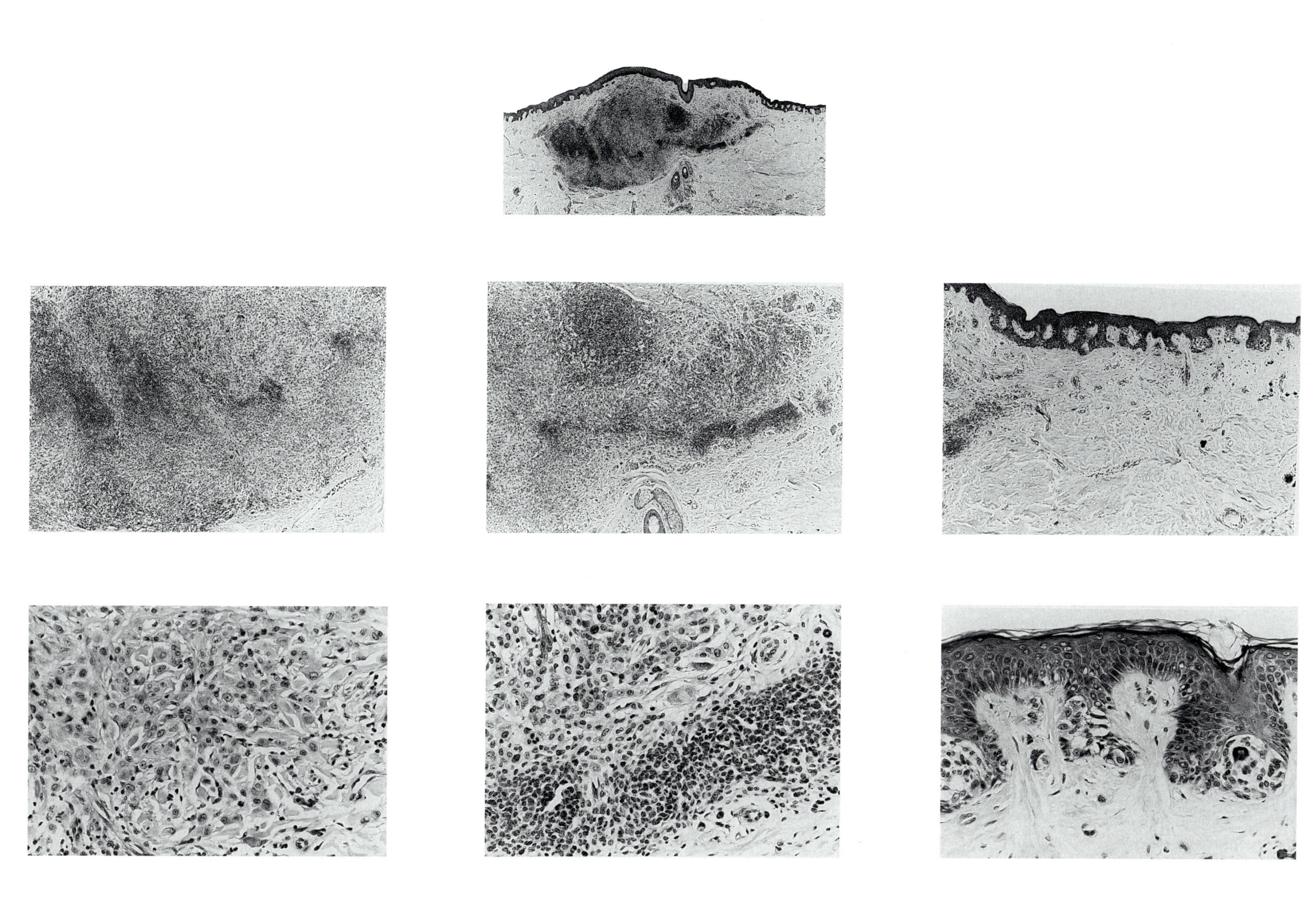

17. What is your diagnosis?

Pigmented lesion on the left side of the back of a 39-year-old man. Clinical diagnosis: combined Spitz's nevus. Simple excision of the site was performed. Patient was well after 2 years.

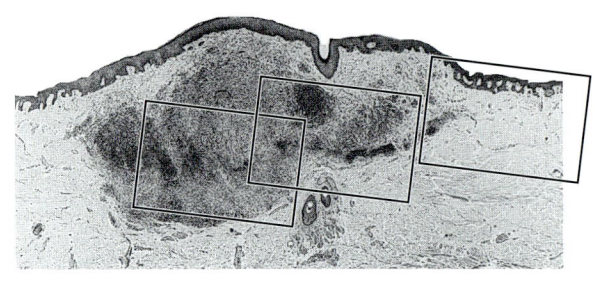

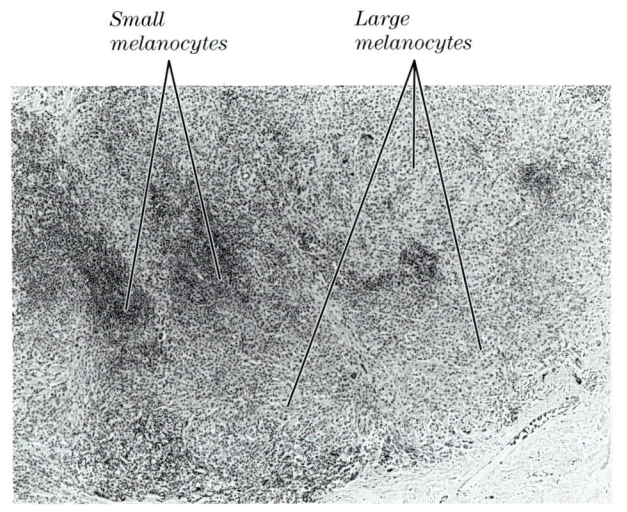

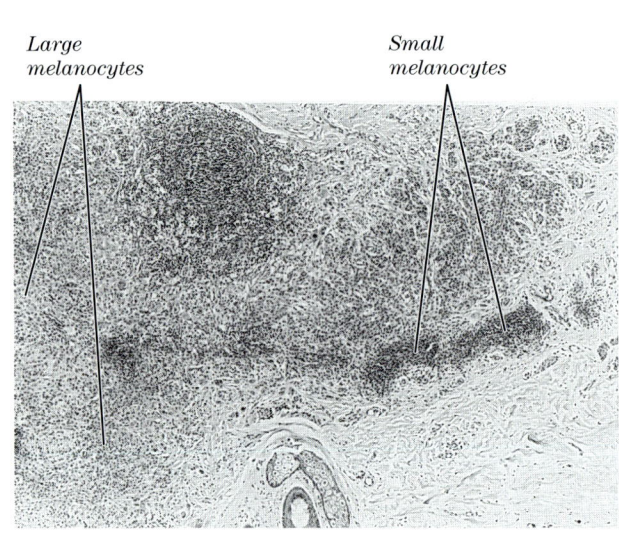

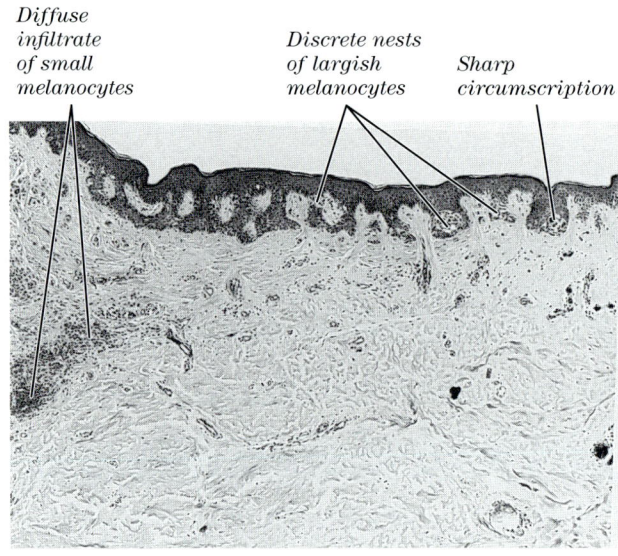

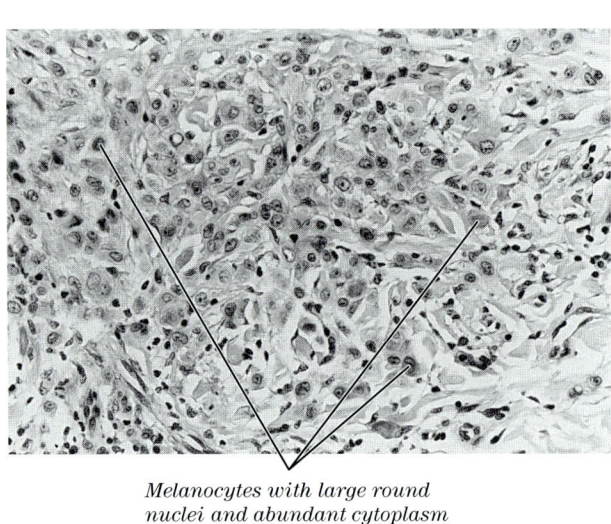

Melanocytes with large round nuclei and abundant cytoplasm

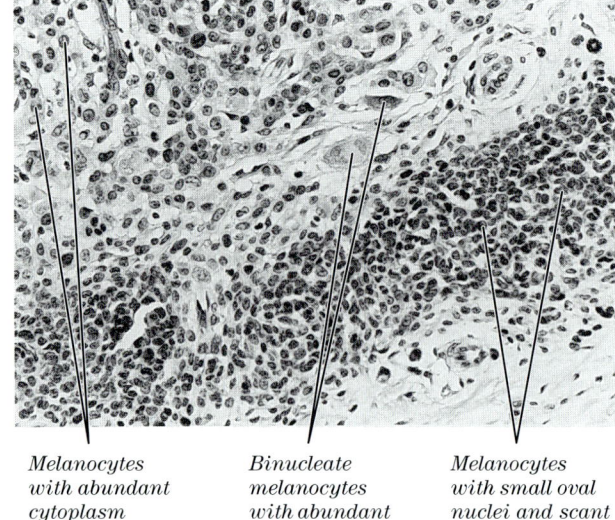

Melanocytes with abundant cytoplasm · Binucleate melanocytes with abundant cytoplasm · Melanocytes with small oval nuclei and scant cytoplasm

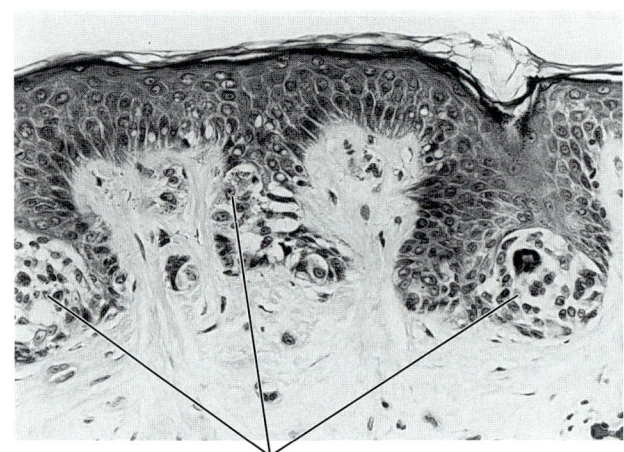

Discrete nests of plump oval melanocytes

334

17 • Combined Nevus *(Spitz's and Clark's)*

Criteria for diagnosis of this combined nevus (Spitz's and Clark's)

This is a combined nevus because:

1. There is no sign of melanoma in situ above the nodular infiltrate of melanocytes on the left.

2. Melanocytes show maturation with progressive descent into the dermis.

3. Neoplastic cells in the nodule possess rather monomorphous nuclei, i.e., large round ones, and abundant pale cytoplasm.

4. A patchy lymphocytic infiltrate is seen throughout the nodular (Spitz's) component.

5. The vertical component of the nodule is almost as great as the horizontal component.

Pitfall in diagnosis

This combined (Spitz's and Clark's) nevus could be misdiagnosed as a melanoma in a pre-existing Clark's nevus because:

1. The neoplasm is asymmetric.

2. The base of the neoplasm is irregular, being neither flat nor wedge-shaped.

3. More than two populations of melanocytes are present within the neoplasm.

4. There is a dense, patchy infiltrate of lymphocytes.

5. Many large melanocytes are found within the nodule.

6. A compound Clark's nevus is situated to the right of the nodule, as happens in about 20% of all melanomas in Caucasians.

In attempting to differentiate a combined nevus, such as this one, from a melanoma in association with a nevus, it is valuable to study each of the components separately and come to decisions about each of them. When that method is applied here, the lesion on the right can be determined to fulfill criteria for Clark's nevus, and the one on the left for Spitz's nevus. For obvious reasons, asymmetry is an expected finding in combined nevi.

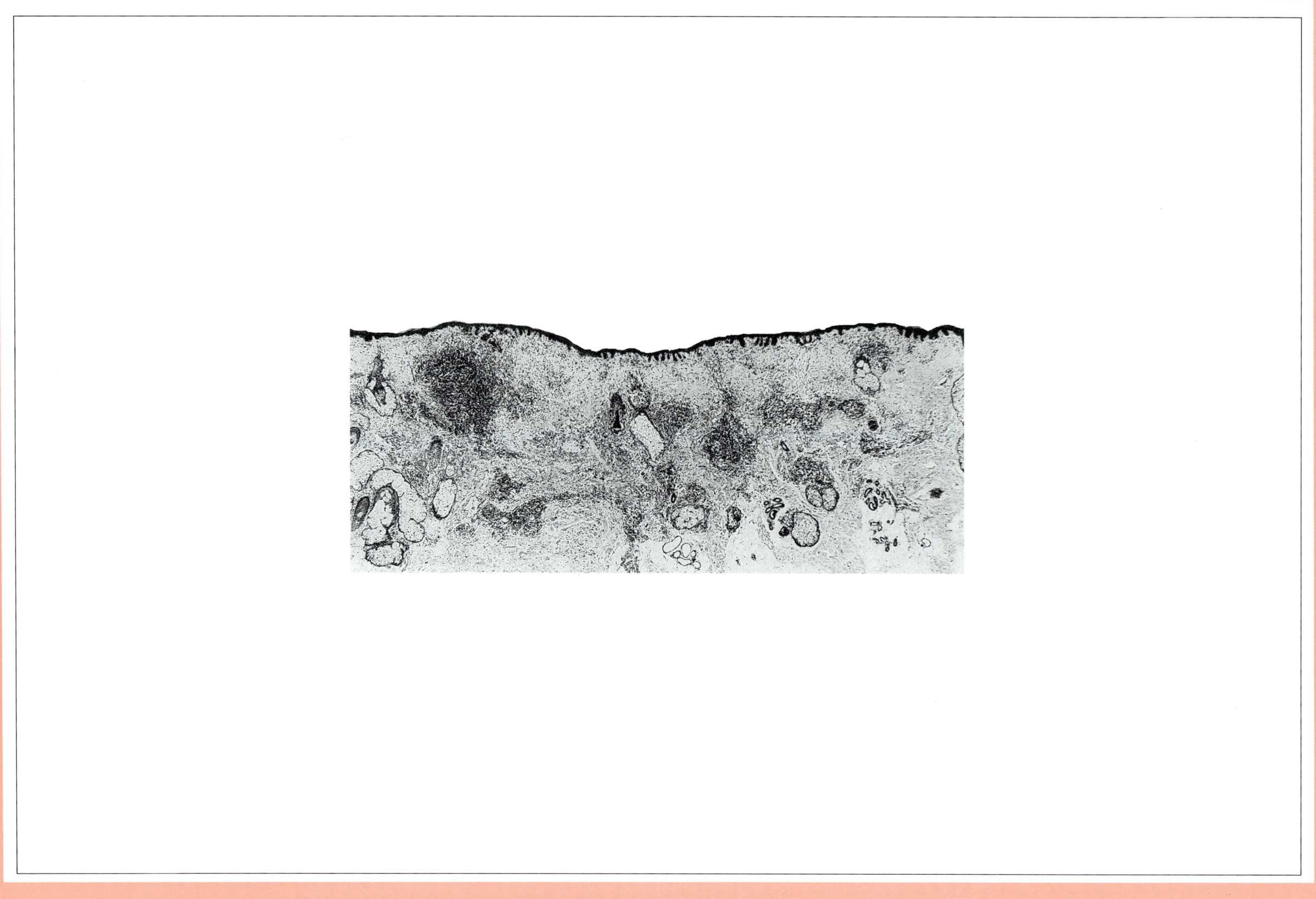

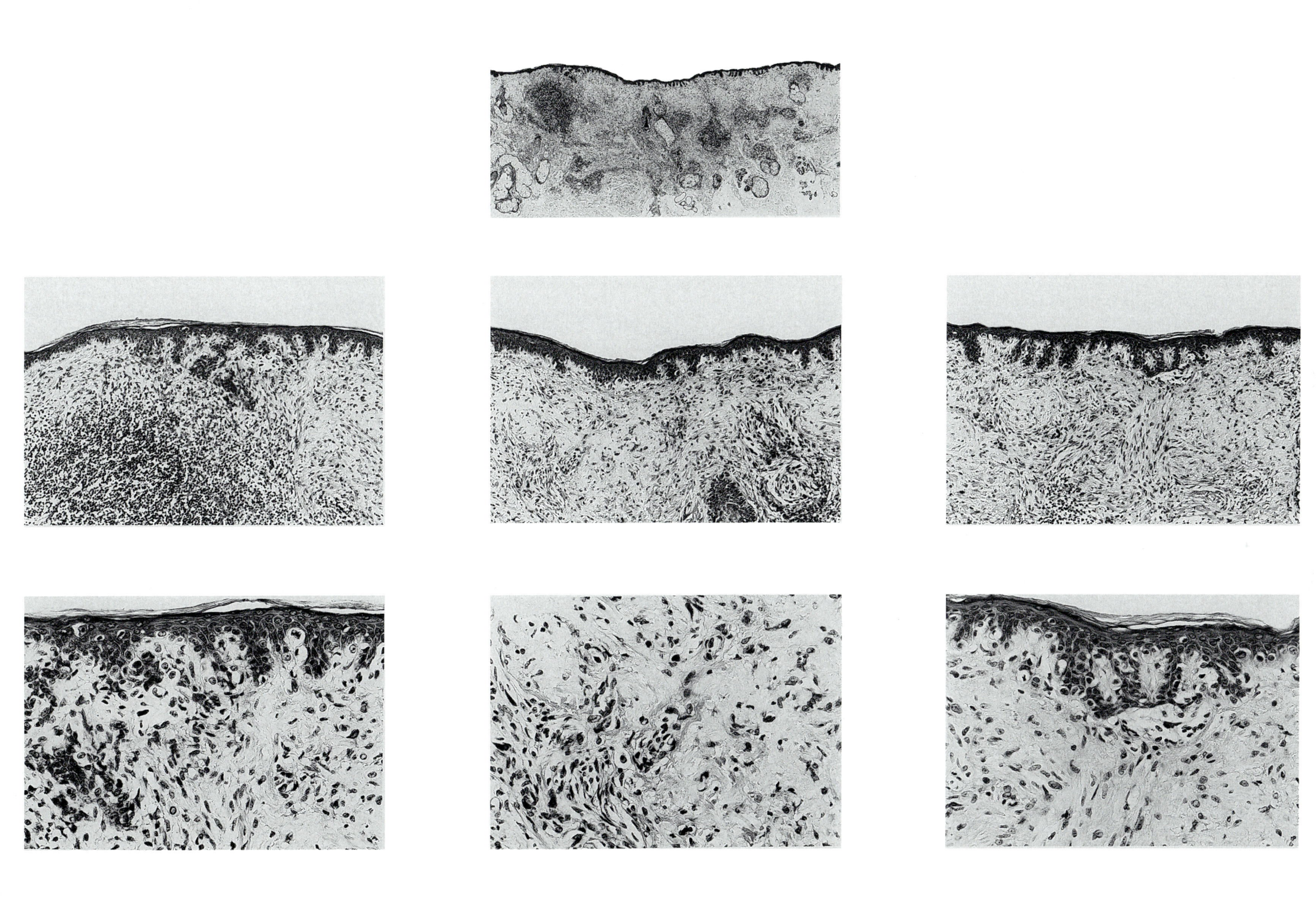

18. What is your diagnosis?

Pigmented lesion on the right cheek of a 54-year-old woman. Clinical diagnosis: basal-cell carcinoma. Wide excision of the site was performed. No follow-up data are available.

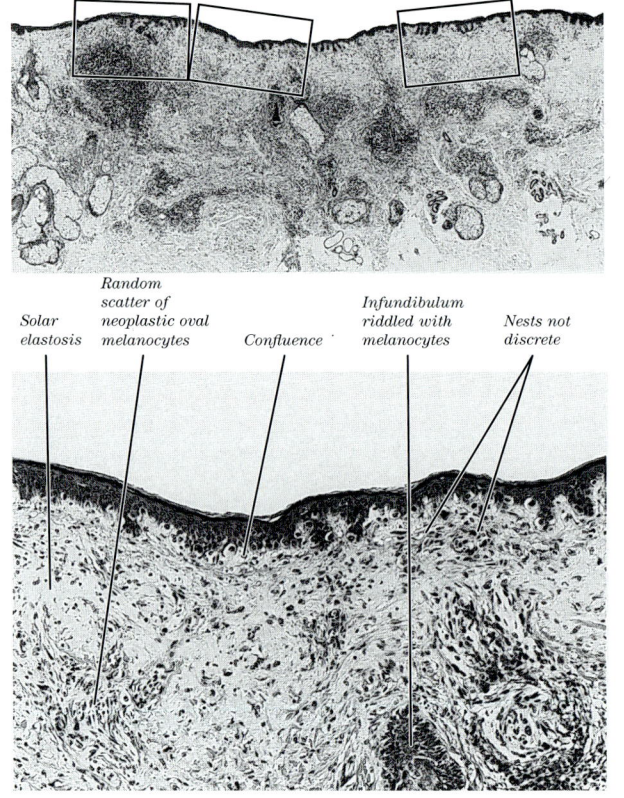

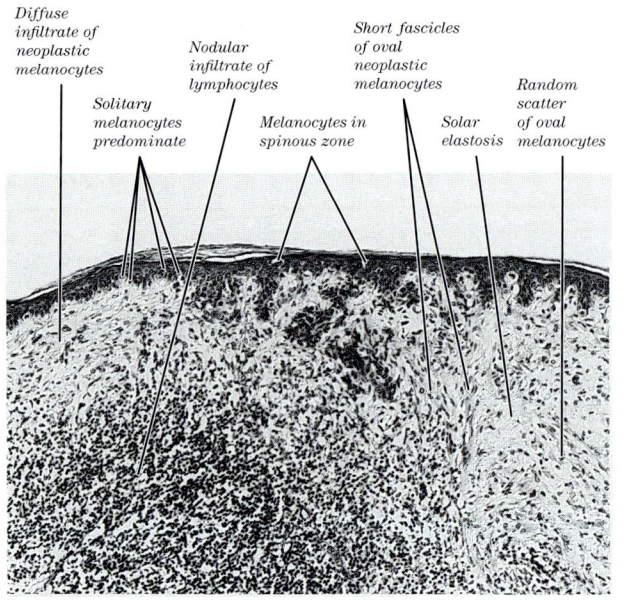

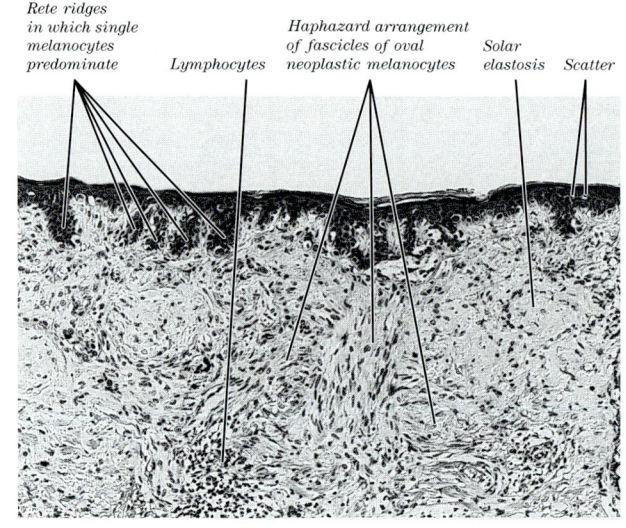

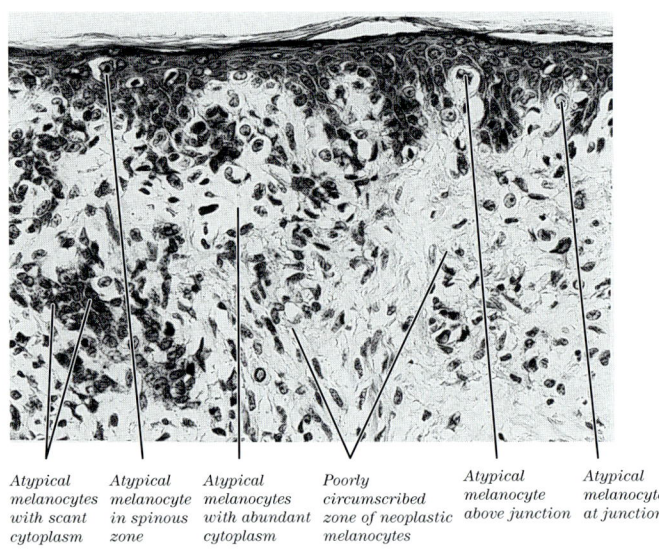

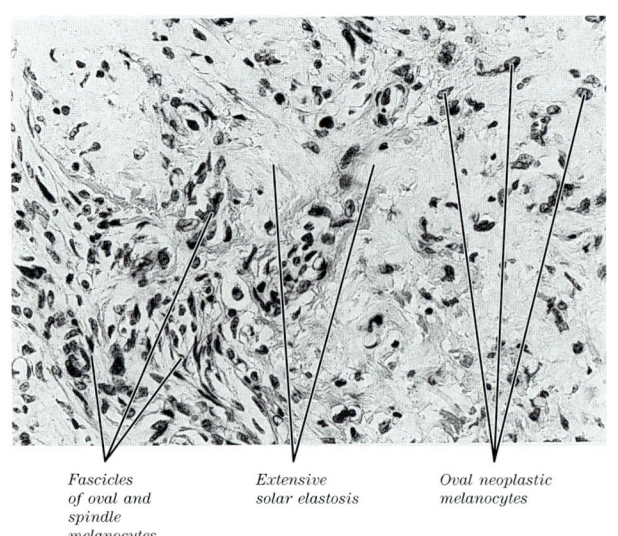

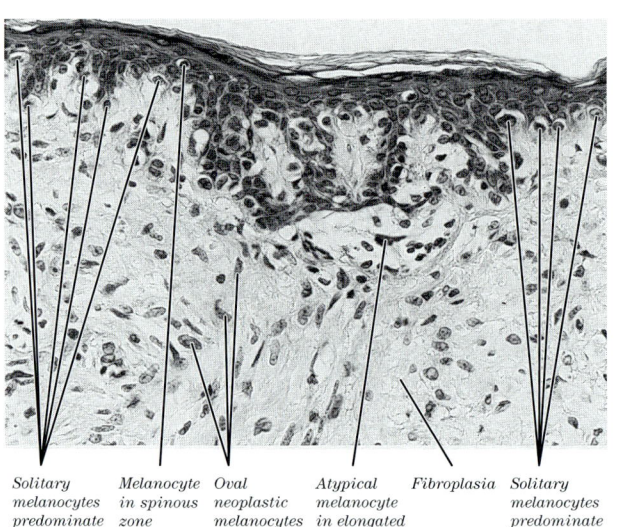

18 • Melanoma *(desmoplastic type)*

Criteria for diagnosis of this melanoma (desmoplastic type)

This is a desmoplastic melanoma because:

1. It is asymmetric.
2. Melanocytes within the epidermis are disposed mostly as solitary units.
3. Nests within the epidermis are not equidistant from one another.
4. No polygonal melanocytes are seen within nests.
5. Many neoplastic melanocytes have thin nuclei.

Pitfall in diagnosis

This desmoplastic melanoma could be misinterpreted as a desmoplastic Spitz's nevus because:

1. There are atypical melanocytes with oval, spindle, and round shapes.
2. Fibroplasia is prominent.
3. Patchy lymphocytic infiltrates are present throughout the entire neoplasm.
4. Melanocytes are arranged in fascicles, as well as in nests.
5. Most melanocytes are stationed at the dermo-epidermal junction and not above it.

That a lymphocytic infiltrate may be helpful to diagnosis of melanoma is illustrated well in this section. The dense nodule of lymphocytes in the upper part of the dermis on the left has no counterpart on the right, which indicates that the lesion is asymmetric. The lymphocytic infiltrate is deeper on the left than it is on the right, another aspect of asymmetry. A more important clue to recognition of this neoplasm as melanoma, rather than as Spitz's nevus, is the presence of extensive solar elastosis. For practical purposes, a compound Spitz's nevus, whether desmoplastic or not, will not be encountered on skin that has been damaged badly by sunlight.

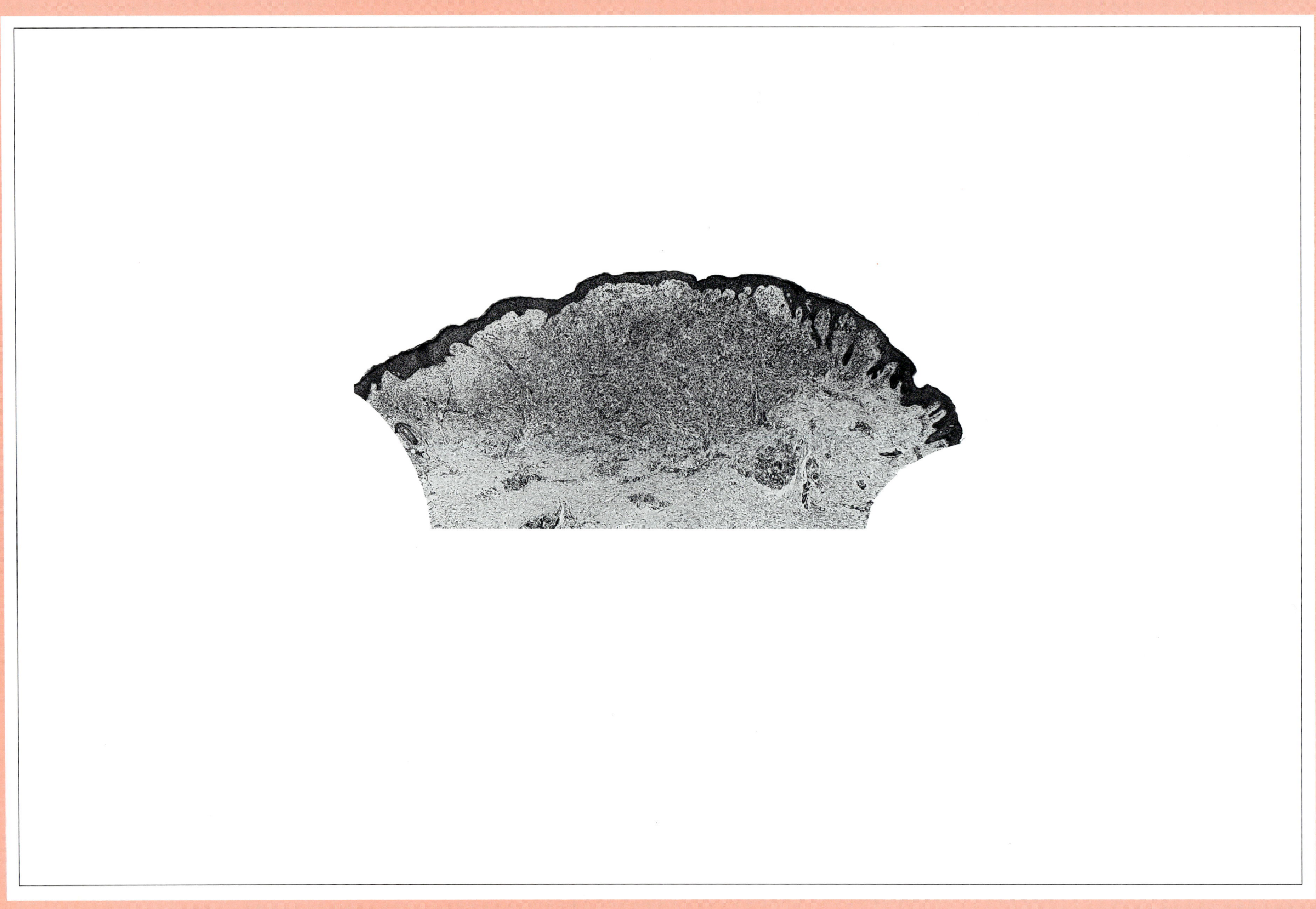

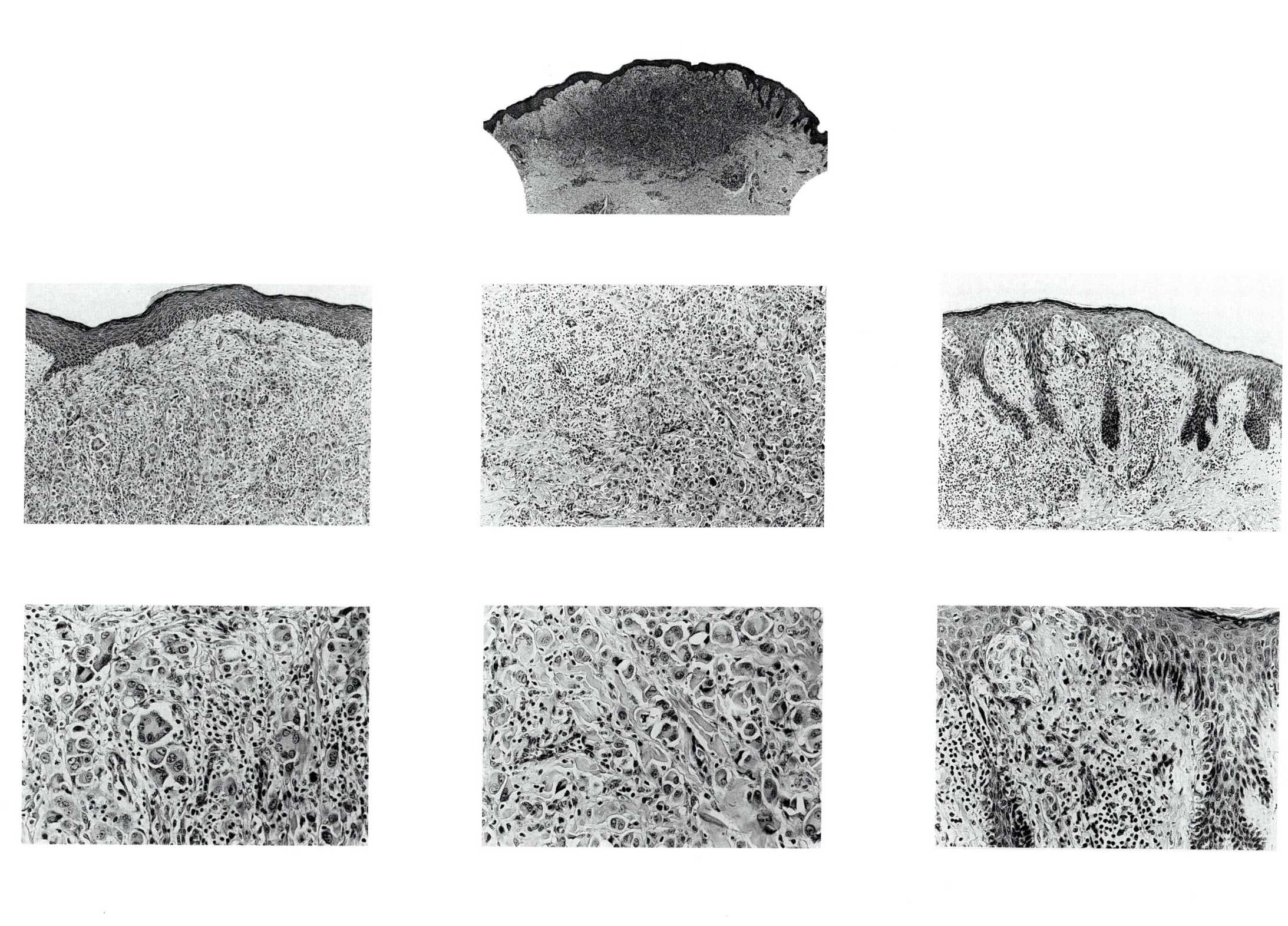

19. What is your diagnosis?

Round, red papule on the medial aspect of the right calf of a 5-year-old boy. Clinical diagnosis: Spitz's nevus. Patient had no persistence of the lesion after 3 years.

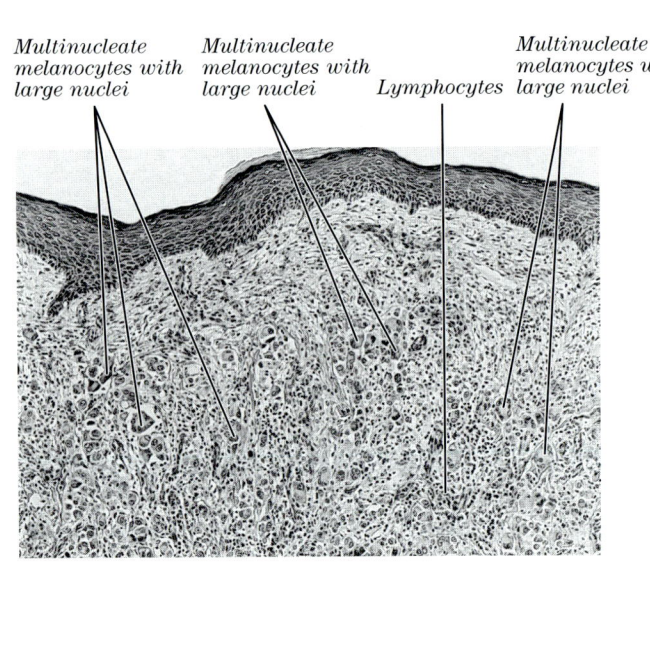

Multinucleate melanocytes with large nuclei   *Multinucleate melanocytes with large nuclei*   *Lymphocytes*   *Multinucleate melanocytes with large nuclei*

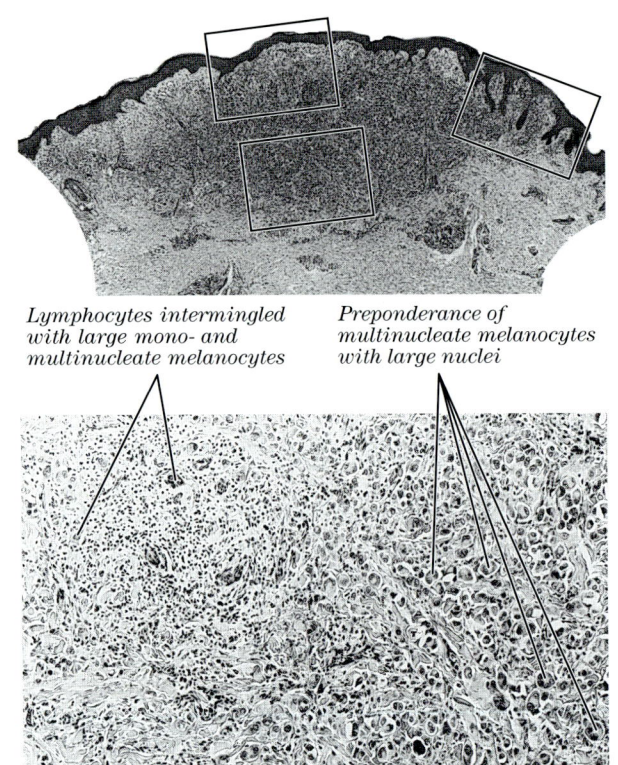

Lymphocytes intermingled with large mono- and multinucleate melanocytes   *Preponderance of multinucleate melanocytes with large nuclei*

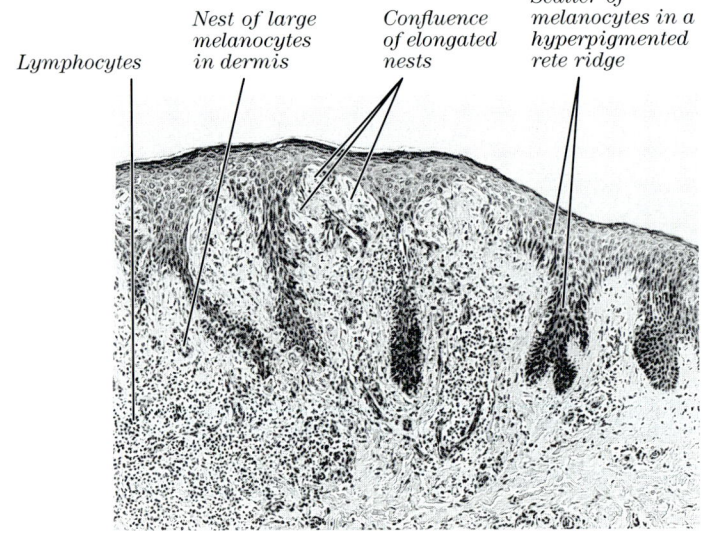

Lymphocytes   *Nest of large melanocytes in dermis*   *Confluence of elongated nests*   *Scatter of melanocytes in a hyperpigmented rete ridge*

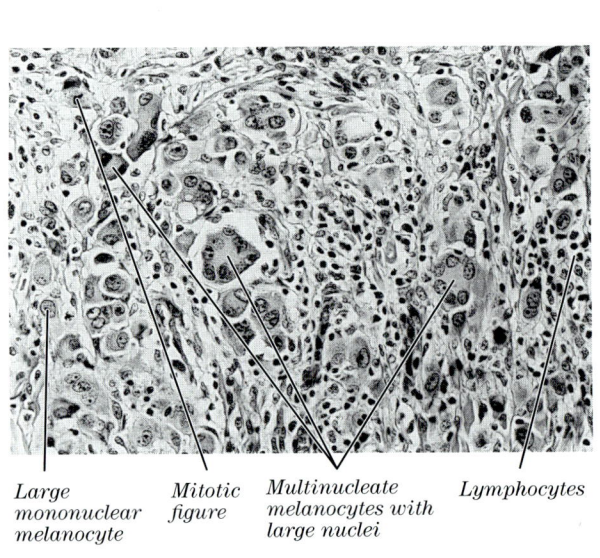

Large mononuclear melanocyte   *Mitotic figure*   *Multinucleate melanocytes with large nuclei*   *Lymphocytes*

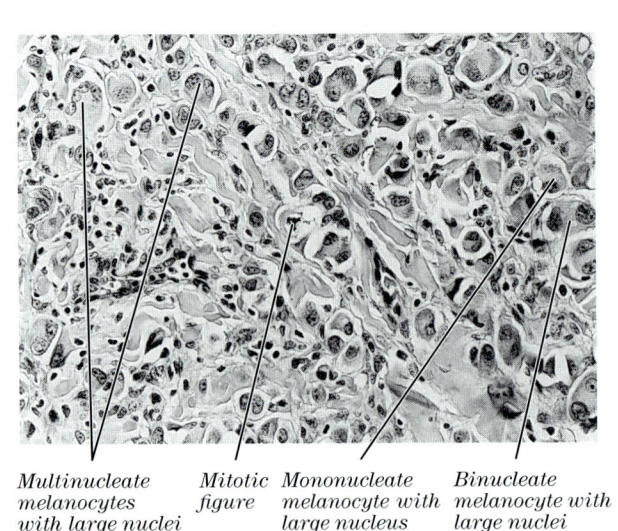

Multinucleate melanocytes with large nuclei   *Mitotic figure*   *Mononucleate melanocyte with large nucleus*   *Binucleate melanocyte with large nuclei*

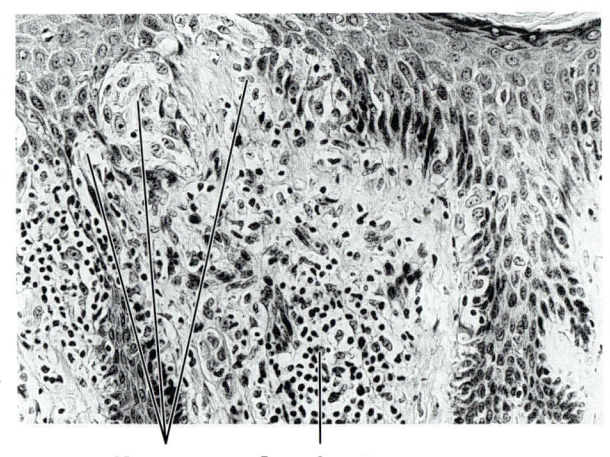

Nests vary   *Lymphocytes*

19 • Spitz's Nevus

Criteria for diagnosis of this Spitz's nevus

This neoplasm is benign because:

1. It is somewhat wedge-shaped.
2. Binucleate and multinucleate melanocytes predominate throughout most of the neoplasm.
3. Melanocytes within the epidermis, both those arranged as solitary units and those in nests, are seated mostly at the dermo-epidermal junction, not above it.

This is a Spitz's nevus because:

1. Most melanocytes have large nuclei, abundant cytoplasm, and round, oval, and polygonal shapes.
2. Most melanocytes are binucleate and multinucleate.
3. Some melanocytes are in mitosis.
4. A patchy, perivascular lymphocytic infiltrate is present throughout the entire neoplasm.

Pitfall in diagnosis

This Spitz's nevus could be misinterpreted as a melanoma because:

1. The neoplasm is slightly asymmetric.
2. Circumscription of the neoplasm is not sharp.
3. There is no unequivocal maturation of melanocytes.
4. Some melanocytes have atypical nuclei.
5. Some melanocytes are in mitosis.

This neoplasm illustrates that asymmetry may be induced artifactually. This somewhat wedge-shaped Spitz's nevus was symmetric before a superficial biopsy specimen was taken from it. That surgical procedure left as residuum fibrosis in the upper part of the dermis, and that zone to the left of center causes the lesion to appear asymmetric when it was not originally. Another pitfall revealed by this neoplasm is an aberrant mitotic figure in an atypical melanocyte. That finding, in itself, is not synonymous with melanoma. It may be seen, on occasion, in a Spitz's nevus like this one. Last, when multinucleate melanocytes with atypical nuclei predominate throughout a neoplasm, Spitz's nevus is the likely diagnosis.

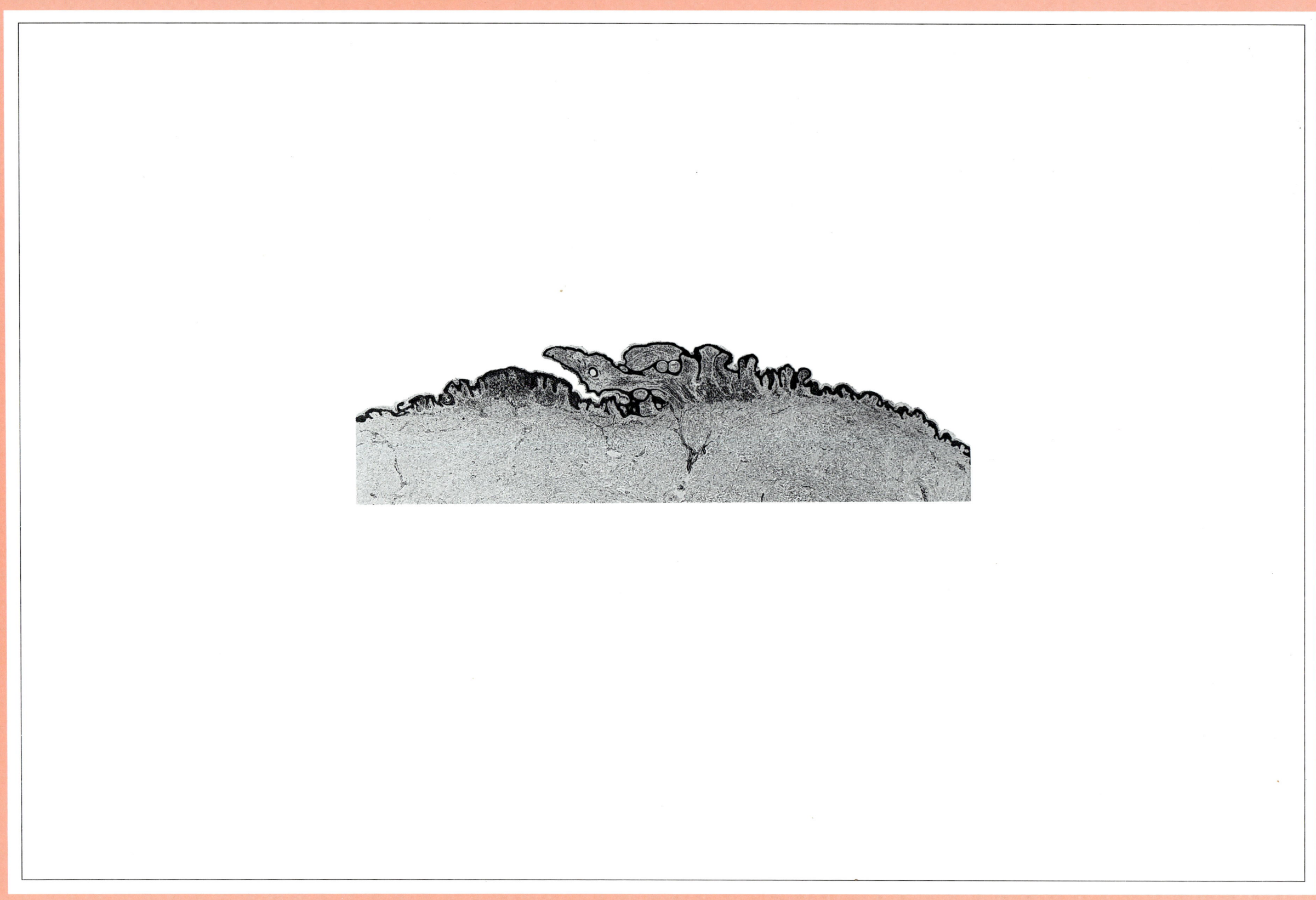

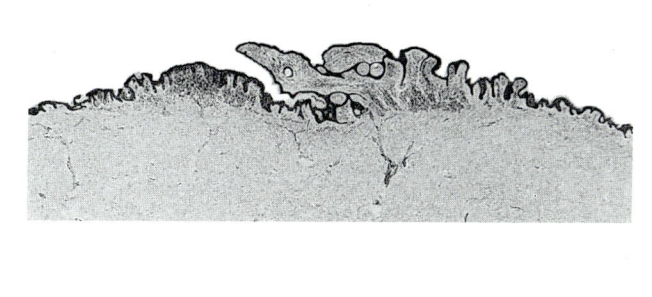

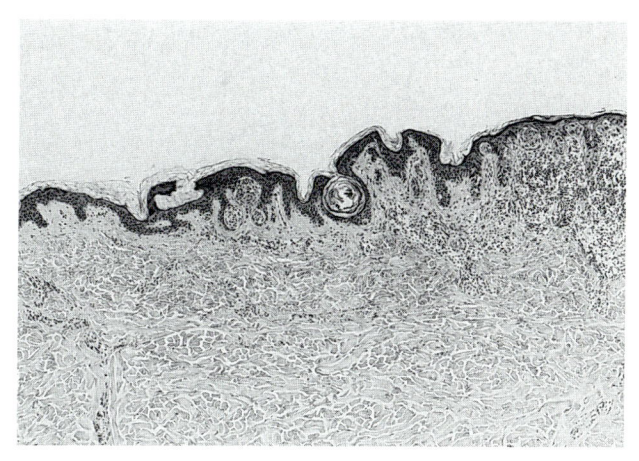
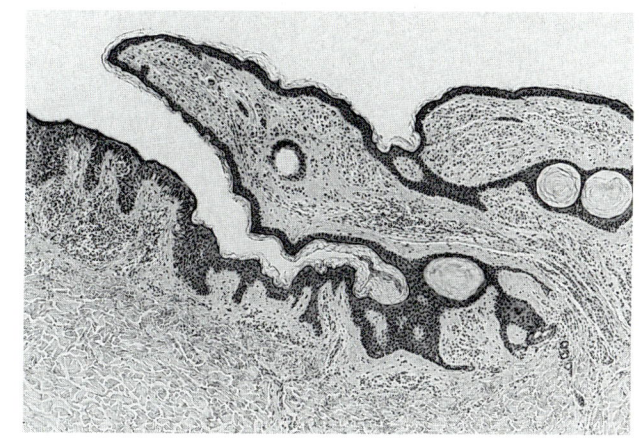
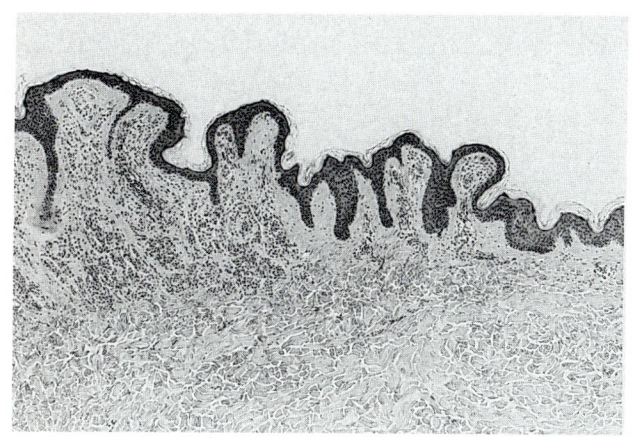

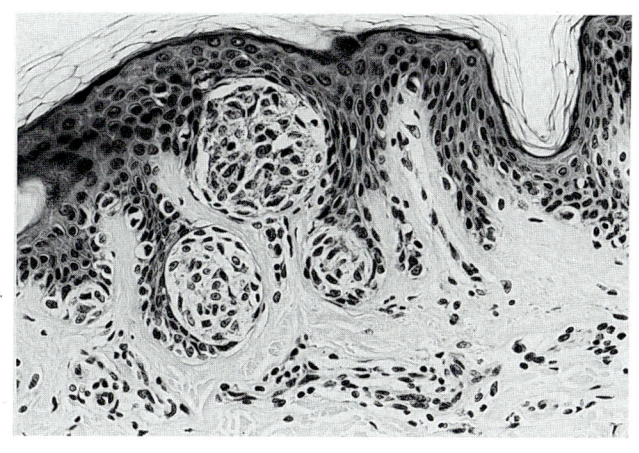
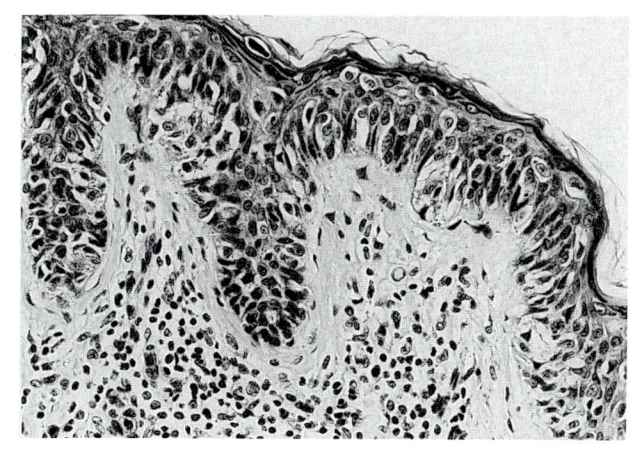
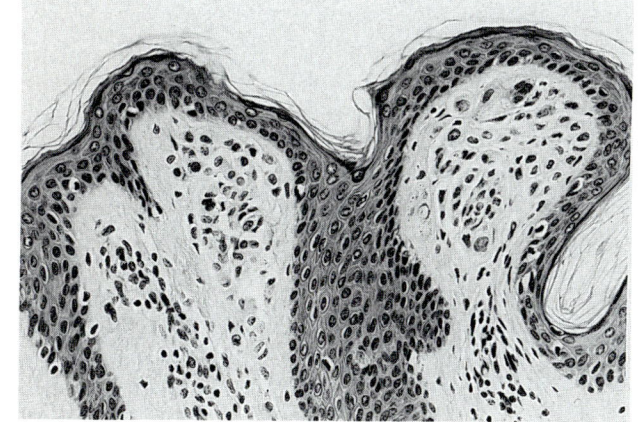

20. What is your diagnosis?

Pigmented lesion that housed a darker spot on the back of a 39-year-old woman. Clinical diagnosis: melanoma. Wide excision was performed. There was no evidence of disease after 2 years.

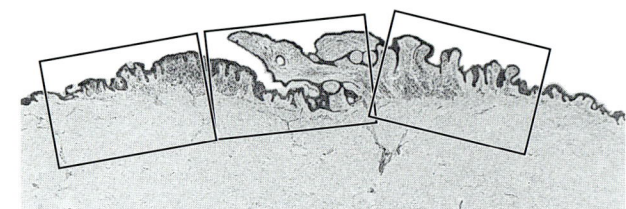

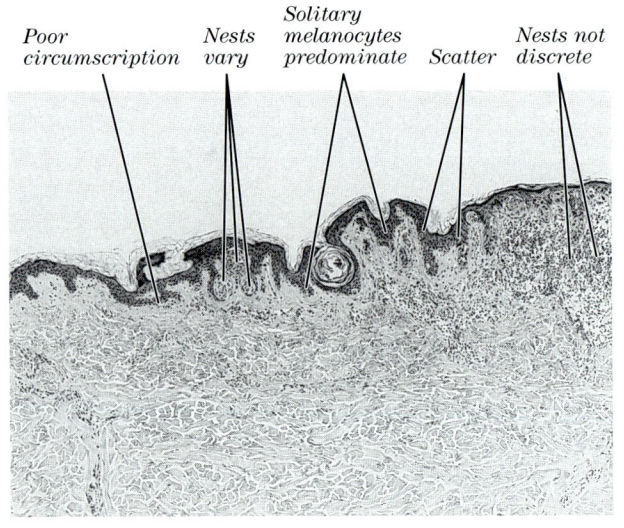

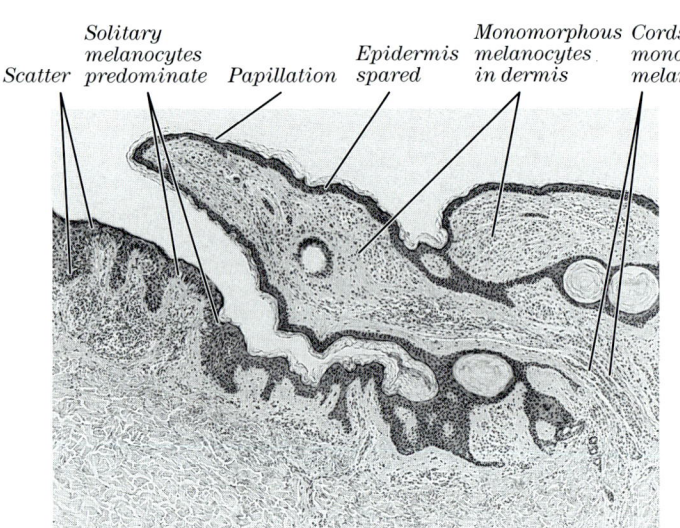

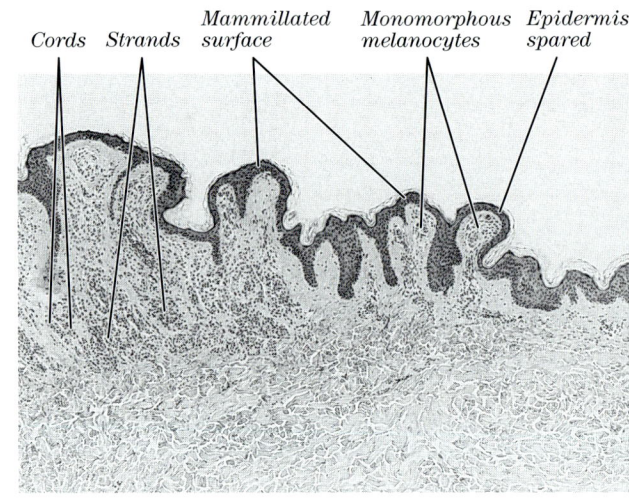

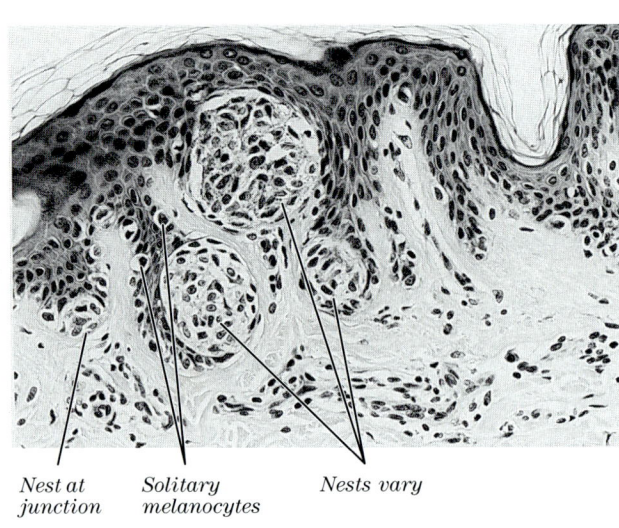

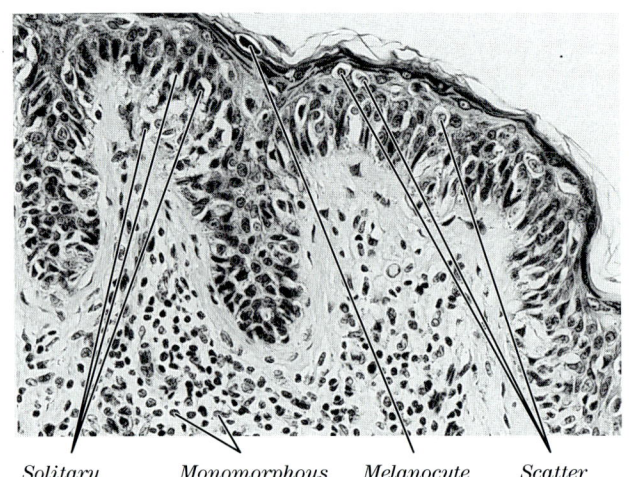

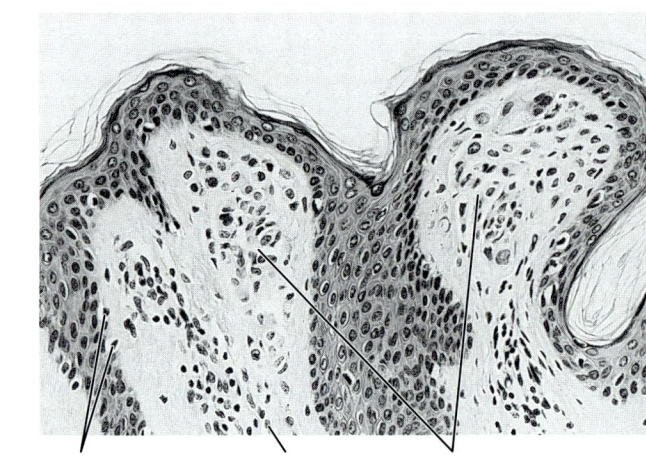

20 • Melanoma in situ and Combined Nevus (Clark's and Unna's)

Criteria for diagnosis of this melanoma in situ in association with a combined (Clark's and Unna's) nevus

The polypoid lesion in the center and the right is Unna's nevus because:

1. It is prominently exophytic.
2. It is constituted of orderly nests, cords, and strands of uniform melanocytes within a markedly thickened papillary dermis.

The lesion on the extreme left is a Clark's nevus because:

1. The lesion is slightly elevated and gently mammillated.
2. Melanocytes arranged as solitary units and in discrete nests are situated at the dermo-epidermal junction, not above it.
3. The melanocytes have round and ovoid, somewhat monomorphous, nuclei and abundant pale cytoplasm.

The changes within the epidermis to the left of Unna's nevus are those of melanoma in situ because:

1. Melanocytes arranged as solitary units are scattered at all levels of the epidermis, including the granular zone and cornified layer.
2. Melanocytes disposed as solitary units predominate over nests.
3. Nests of melanocytes are not discrete.
4. Some nests of melanocytes have become confluent.

Pitfall in diagnosis

This melanoma in situ in association with a combined nevus could be misread as "severe dysplasia" within a pre-existing nevus because:

1. The proliferation of atypical melanocytes is confined to the epidermis.
2. The proliferation of atypical melanocytes is sandwiched between components of a nevus.
3. The nuclei of melanocytes, although atypical, are not strikingly abnormal.
4. An indubitable melanocytic nevus is present on either side of the proliferation.

Two entirely different patterns are apparent in the neoplasm: one of a nevus and the other of a melanoma in situ. The nevus can be diagnosed accurately because it fulfills accepted criteria. The same should be true also of the melanoma in situ, and it is. That proliferation of melanocytes fulfills all criteria for melanoma confined to the epidermis. The diagnosis of this latter proliferation, therefore, should be melanoma in situ, rather than any variation on the theme of "dysplasia," pagetoid intra-epidermal proliferation, or atypical melanocytic hyperplasia. These three are not diagnoses conveyed in the language of clinical dermatology; they are severely flawed histopathologic descriptions.

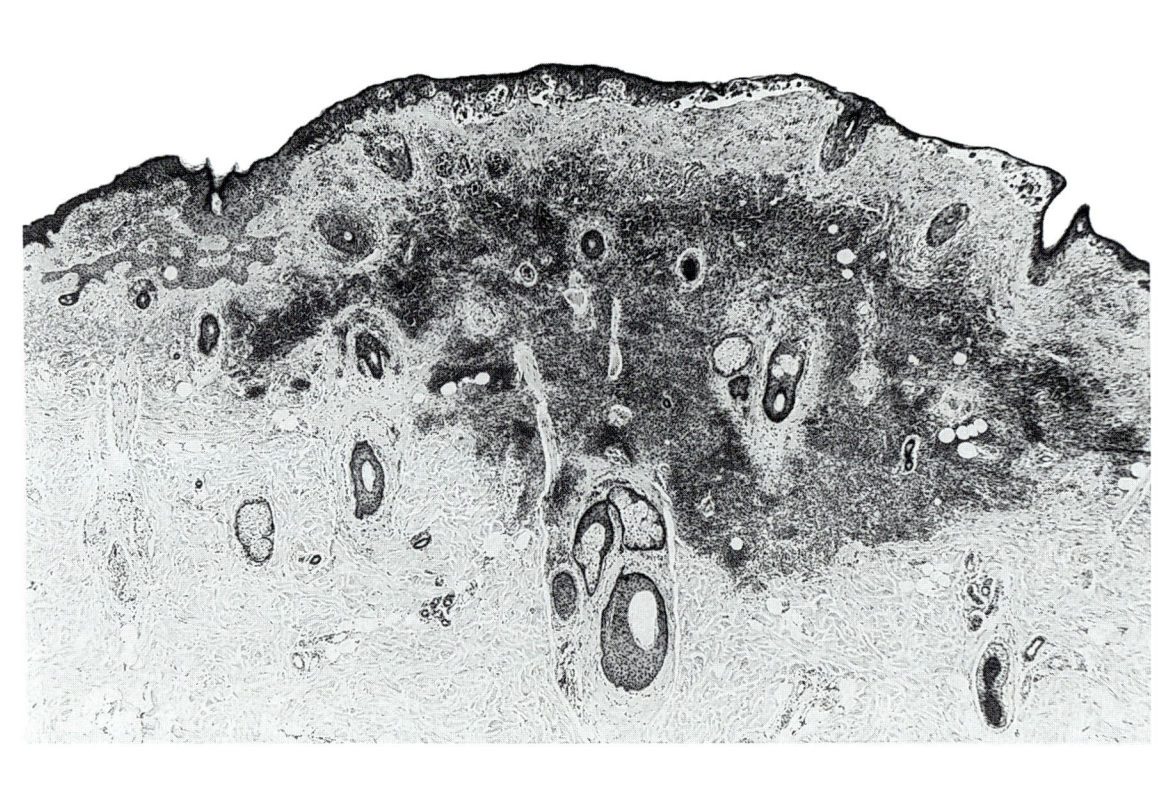

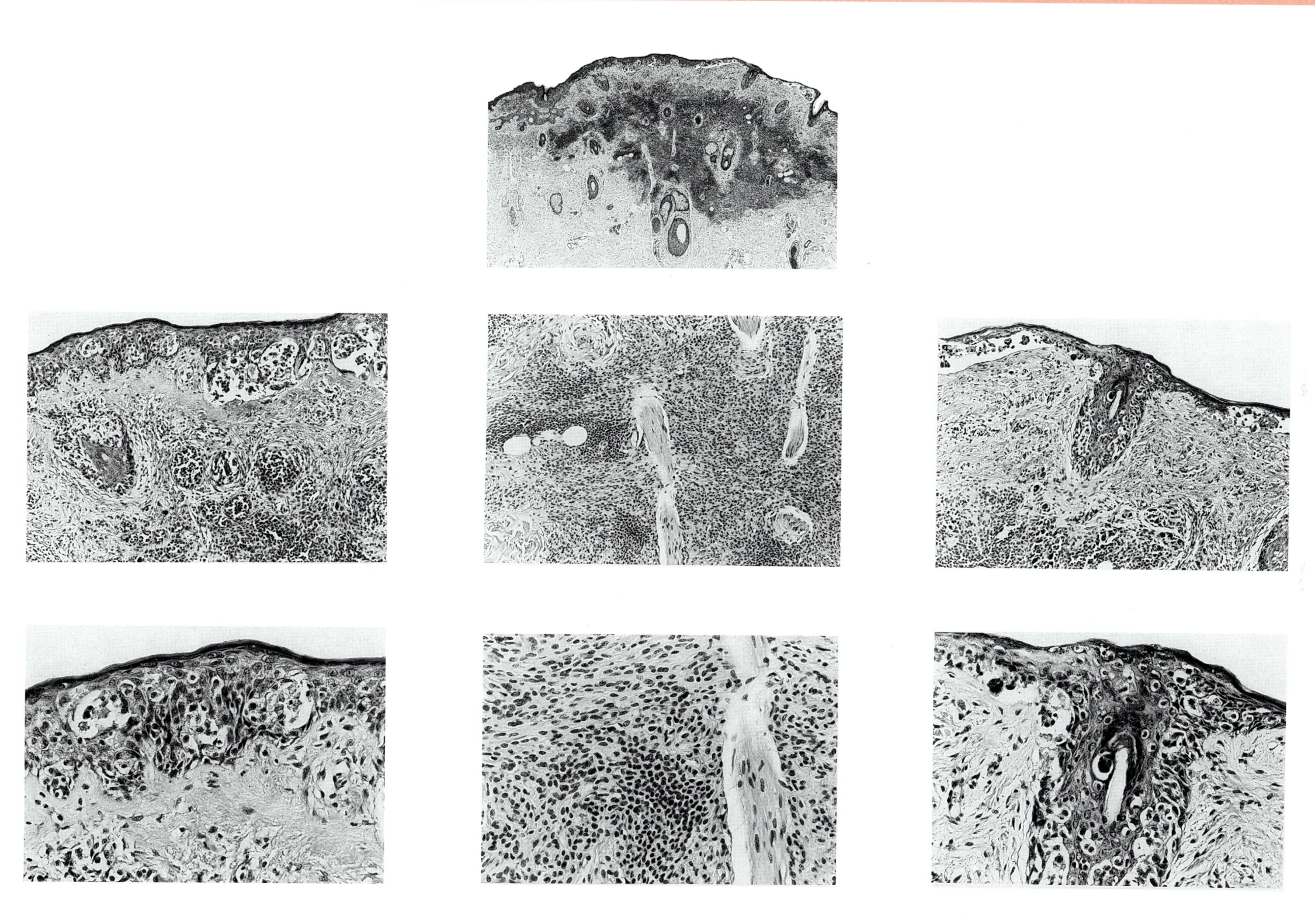

21. What is your diagnosis?

Pigmented lesion in a neonate. Clinical diagnosis: congenital nevus. No follow-up data available.

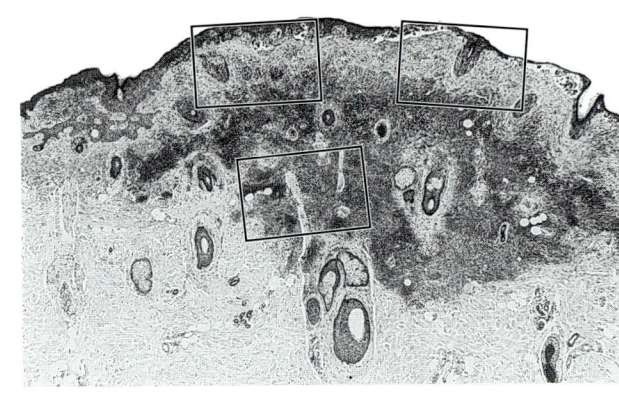

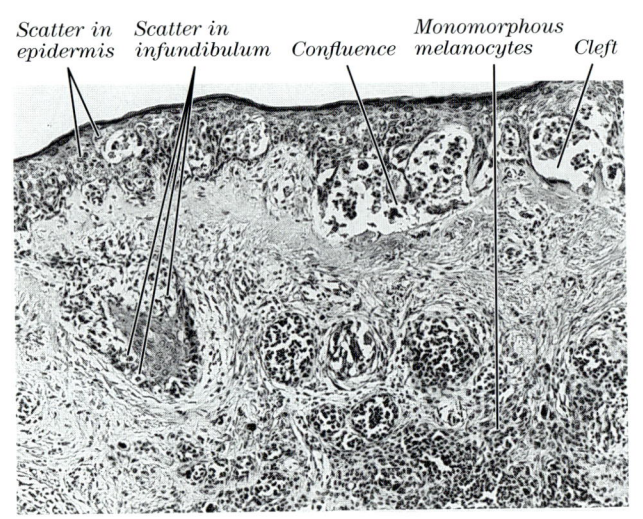
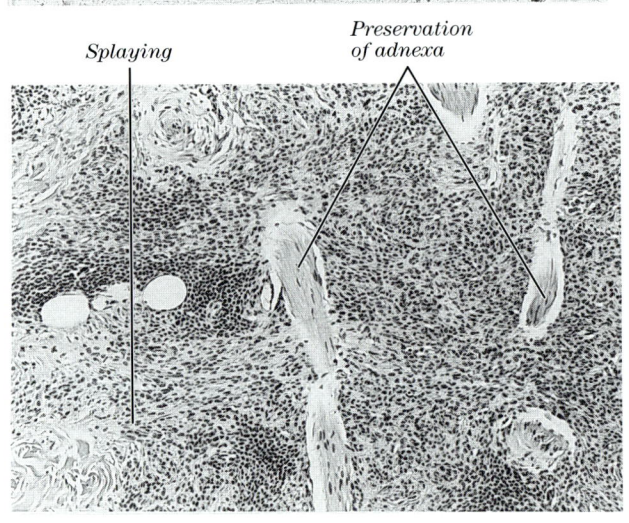
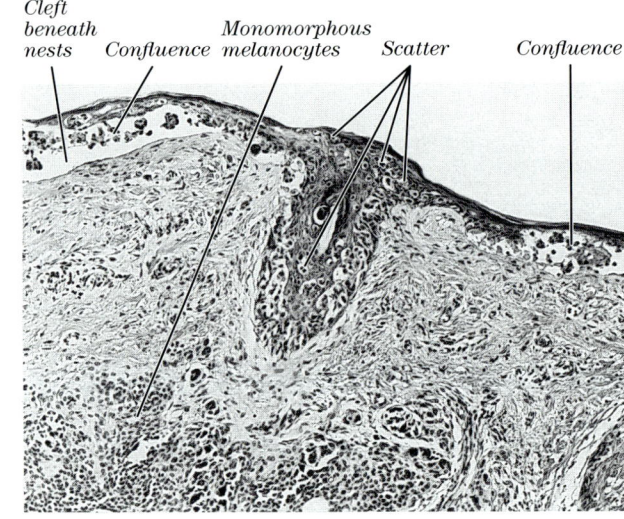

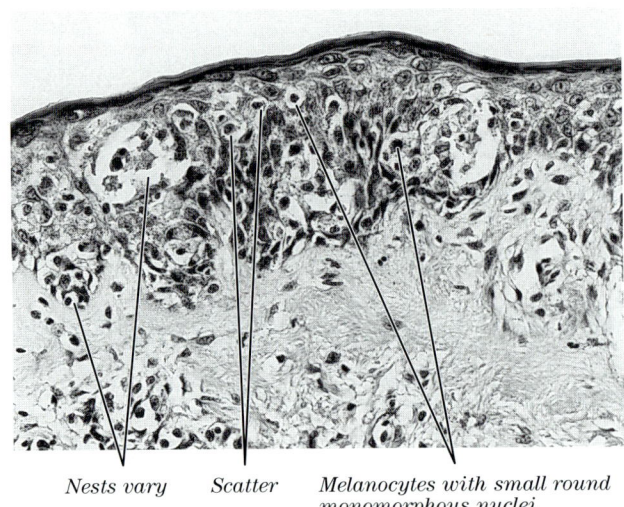
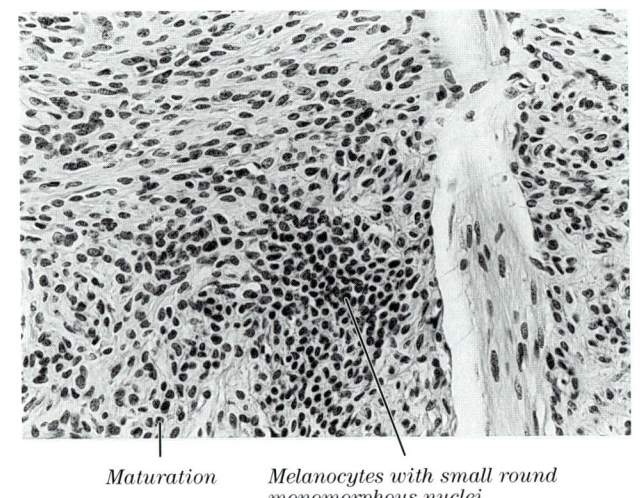
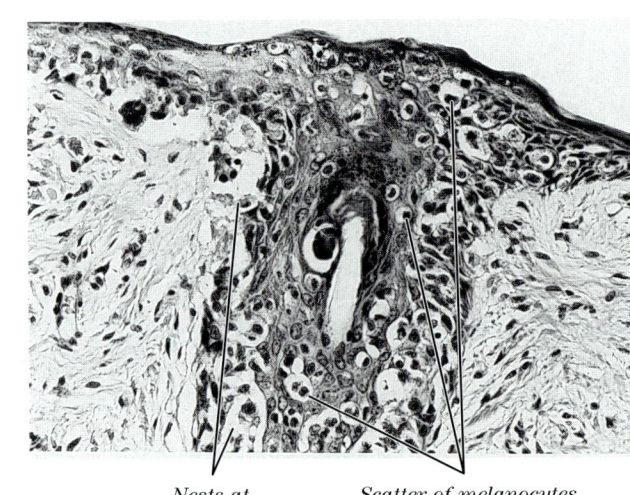

21 • Congenital Nevus *(superficial type)* Biopsied Shortly After Birth

Criteria for diagnosis of this congenital nevus (superficial type) biopsied shortly after birth

This is a nevus because:

1. The proliferation of melanocytes within the epidermis does not extend beyond the intradermal portion of the lesion.

2. The intra-epidermal portion of the neoplasm is relatively symmetric.

3. Nests of melanocytes within the epidermis predominate over melanocytes arranged as solitary units there.

4. The nuclei of melanocytes within the epidermis are mostly small, oval, and monomorphous.

This is a superficial congenital nevus because:

1. Melanocytes in the upper two thirds of the reticular dermis are arranged in angiocentric and adnexocentric fashion.

2. Melanocytes are splayed between collagen bundles in foci.

Pitfall in diagnosis

This superficial congenital nevus biopsied shortly after birth could be misinterpreted as a melanoma in situ above a superficial congenital nevus because:

1. Nests of melanocytes within the epidermis are not equidistant from one another.

2. Nests of melanocytes vary in size and shape.

3. Some nests of melanocytes have become confluent.

4. Clefts have formed beneath some aggregations of melanocytes that have become confluent within the epidermis.

5. Melanocytes arrayed as solitary units and in nests are present at all levels of the epidermis.

6. Changes such as those within the epidermis are present far down epithelial structures of adnexa.

The changes within the reticular dermis are typical of a superficial congenital nevus: a melanocytic nevus confined to the upper two thirds of that part of the dermis and associated with angiocentricity, adnexocentricity, and splaying of melanocytes between collagen bundles. It must be acknowledged that without a typical superficial congenital nevus within the dermis, it would be virtually impossible to differentiate the changes pictured here within the epidermis and epithelial structures of adnexa from melanoma in situ. Were the age of the patient not known, it must also be admitted that the changes within the epidermis and epithelial structures of adnexa easily could be misread as melanoma in situ.

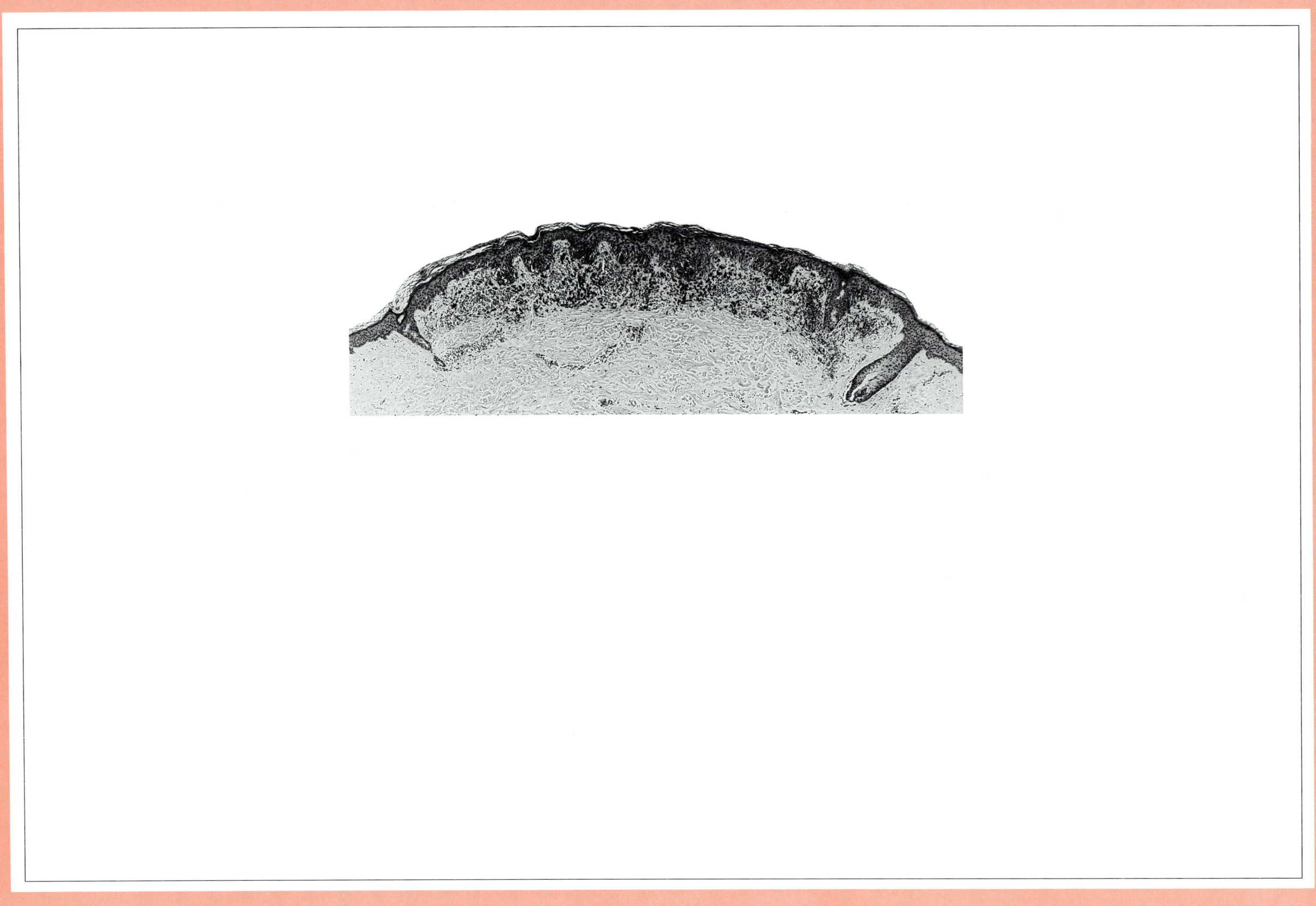

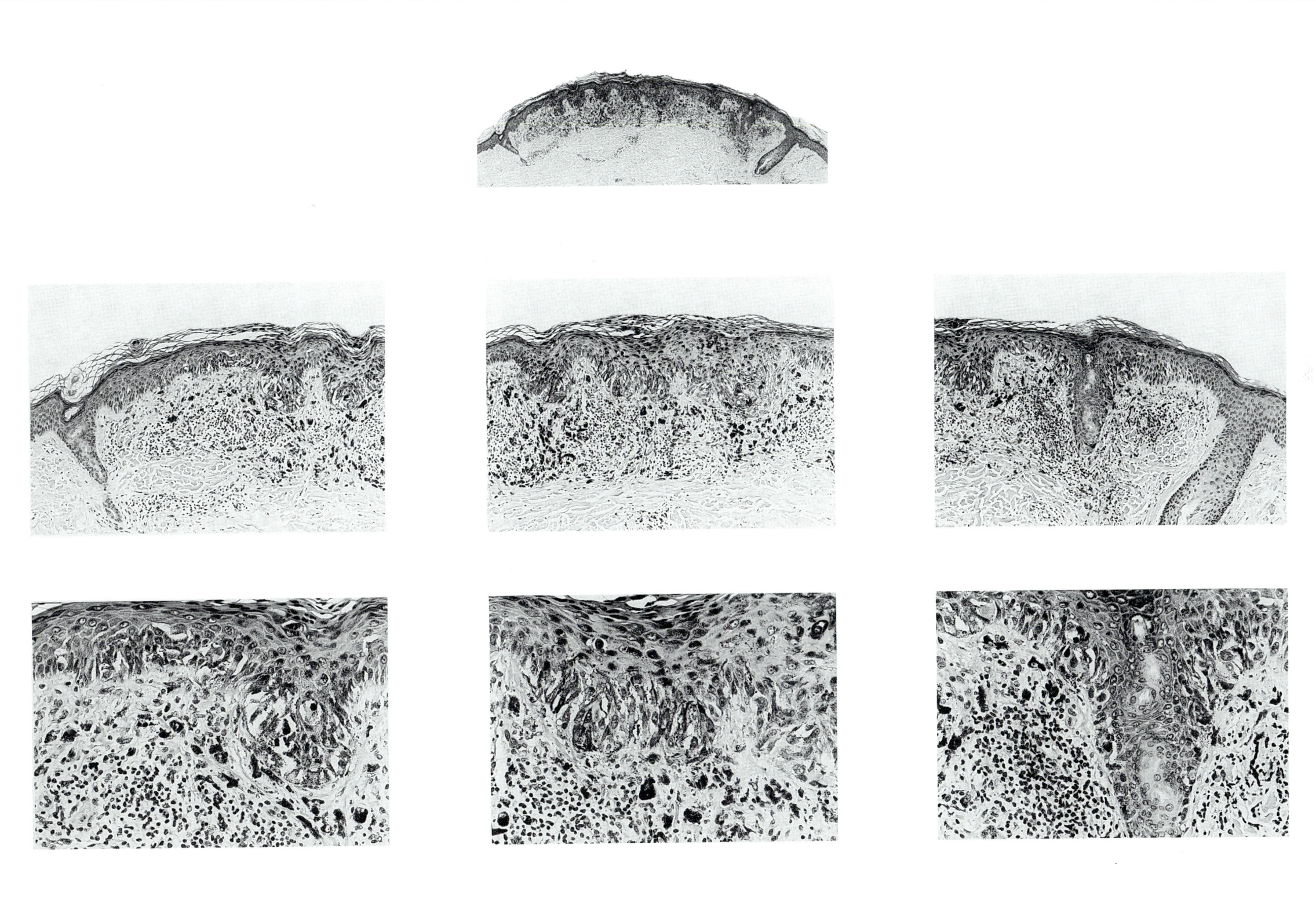

22. What is your diagnosis?

Dark brown, poorly circumscribed nodule on the posterior aspect of the left leg of a 40-year-old woman. Clinical diagnosis: dysplastic nevus vs. melanoma. Patient underwent a wide local excision, and no residual neoplasm was present in the specimen.

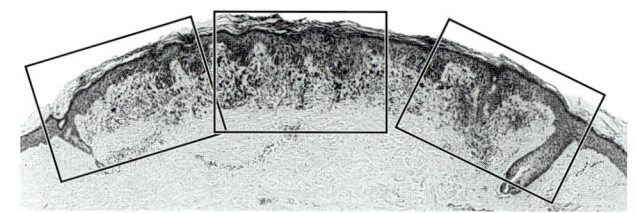

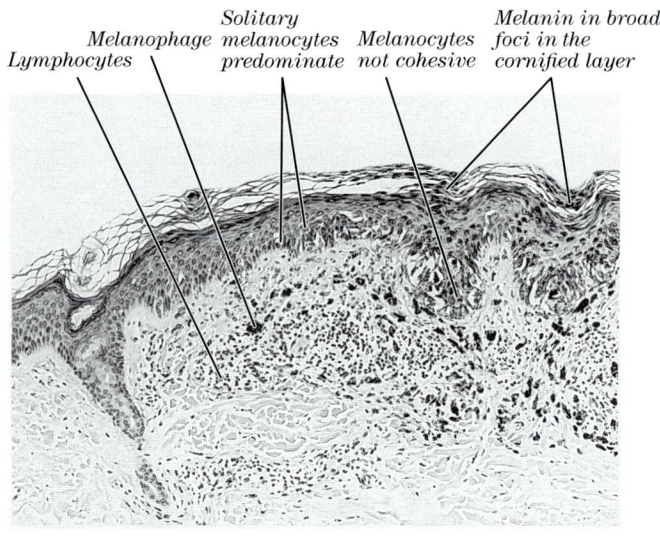

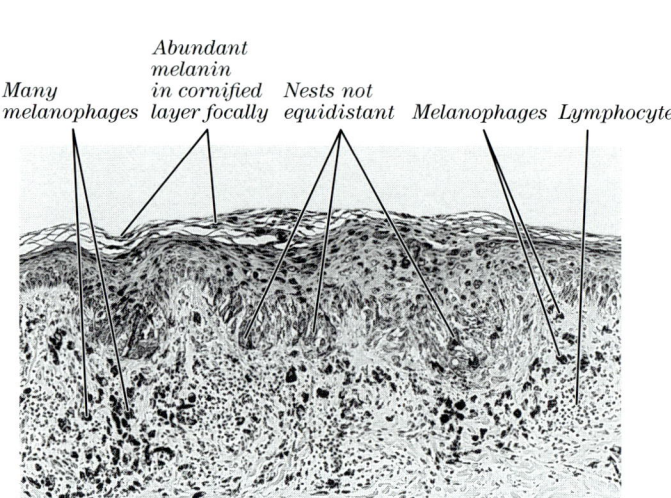

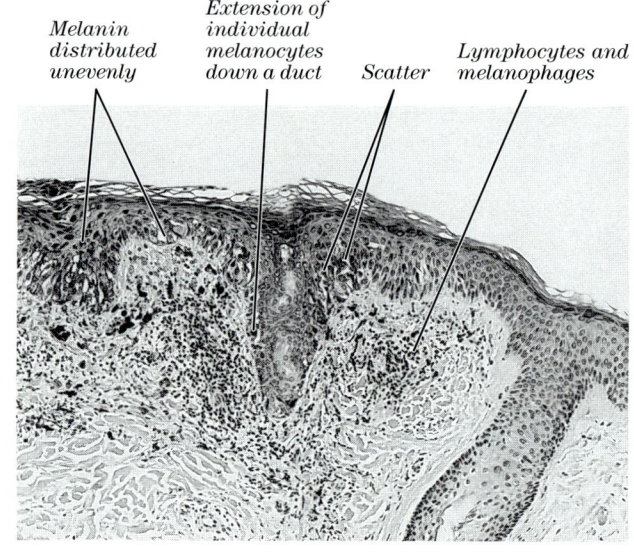

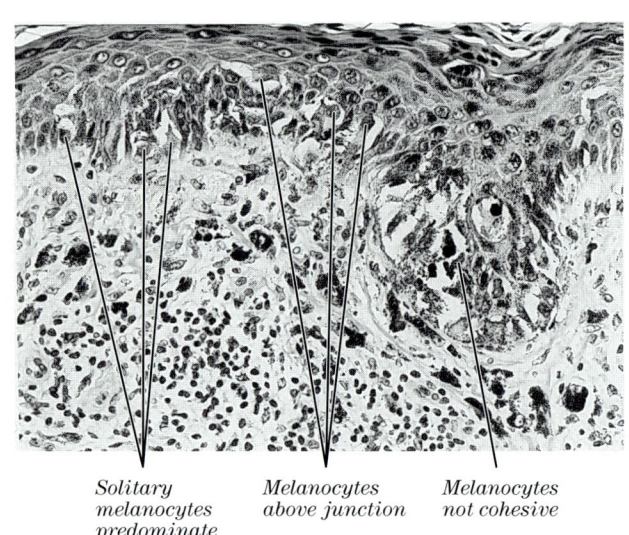

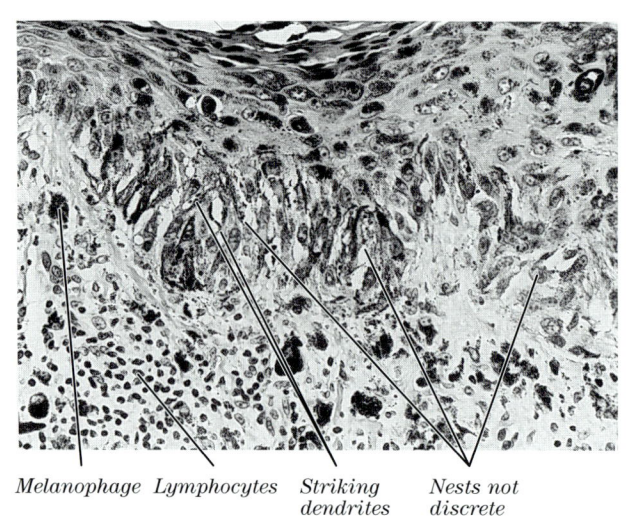

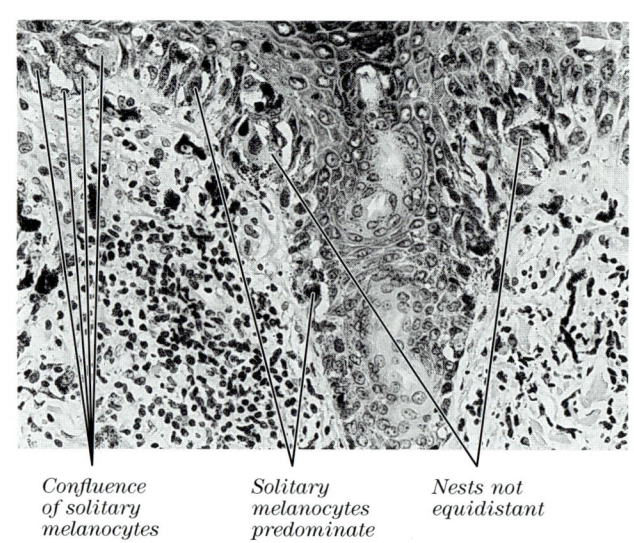

22 • Melanoma in situ

Criteria for diagnosis of this melanoma in situ

This is a melanoma in situ because:

1. The lesion is poorly circumscribed.
2. Atypical melanocytes disposed as solitary units within the epidermis predominate over nests of them in several high-power fields.
3. Melanocytes arranged as solitary units extend far down epithelial structures of adnexa.
4. Nests of melanocytes are not equidistant from one another.
5. Neoplastic melanocytes arrayed as solitary units within the epidermis are not equidistant from one another.
6. Melanocytes arranged as solitary units are scattered far above the dermo-epidermal junction.
7. Some melanocytes have pagetoid attributes.
8. Melanocytes in some "nests" are not cohesive.

Pitfall in diagnosis

This melanoma in situ could be misinterpreted as a pigmented spindle-cell variant of Spitz's nevus because:

1. The neoplasm is small.
2. The neoplasm seems to be symmetric.
3. Nests of melanocytes within the epidermis are seated at the dermo-epidermal junction and not above it.
4. Melanin is distributed in relatively uniform fashion throughout the neoplasm.

It is difficult to diagnose this melanoma in situ at scanning magnification. At higher magnification, however, melanocytes disposed as solitary units are seen to predominate over nests of melanocytes in some high-power fields, melanocytes as solitary units are scattered above the dermo-epidermal junction, and melanocytes arranged as solitary units extend far down epithelial structures of adnexa. These findings, each of which pertains to melanocytes arranged as solitary units, are definitive signs of melanoma in situ. The numerous dendritic melanocytes within the epidermis are not, in themselves, indicative of melanoma. They also may be seen in Spitz's nevi, especially in Asians.

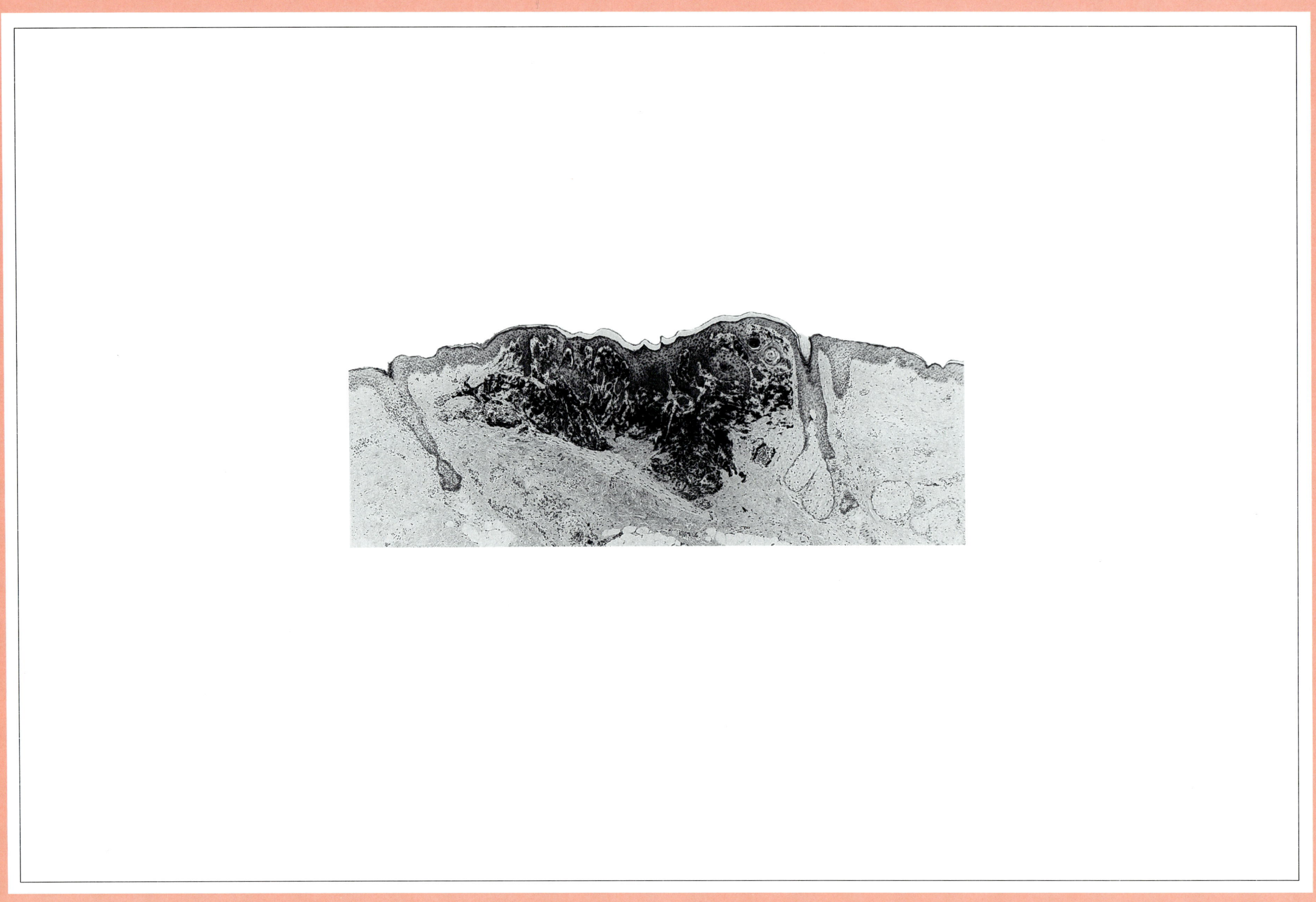

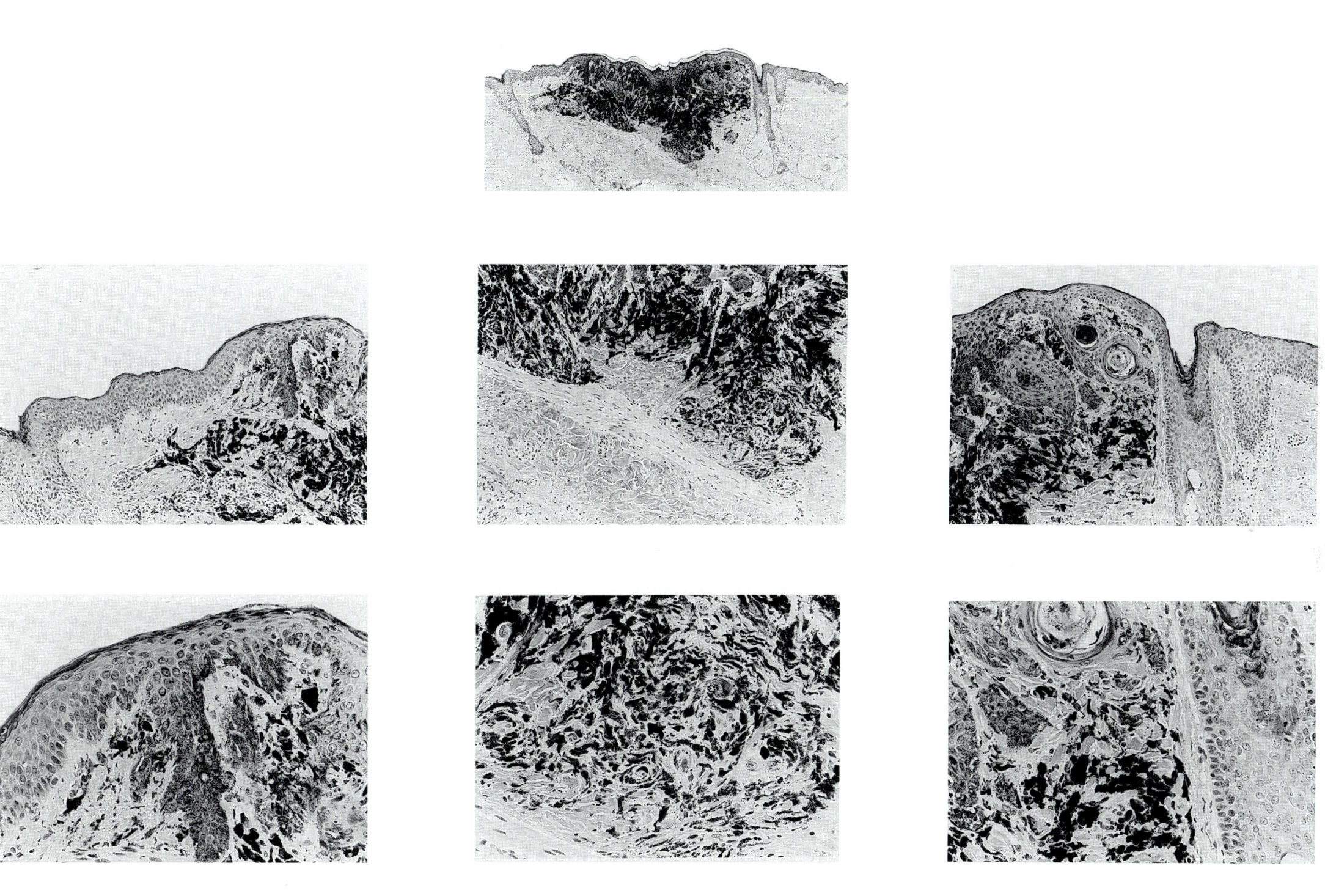

23. What is your diagnosis?

Pigmented lesion in the right supraorbital region of a 15-year-old girl. Clinical diagnosis: combined nevus. The patient was free of disease after 1 year.

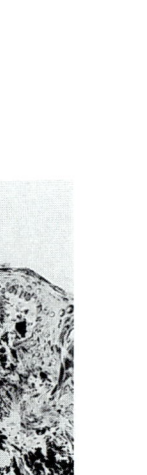

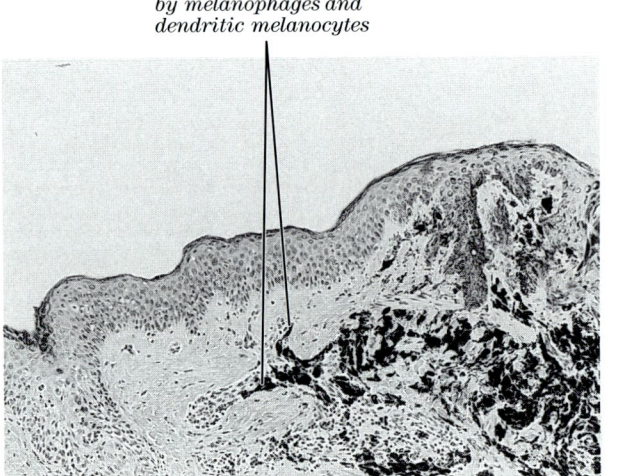

Jagged outline formed by melanophages and dendritic melanocytes

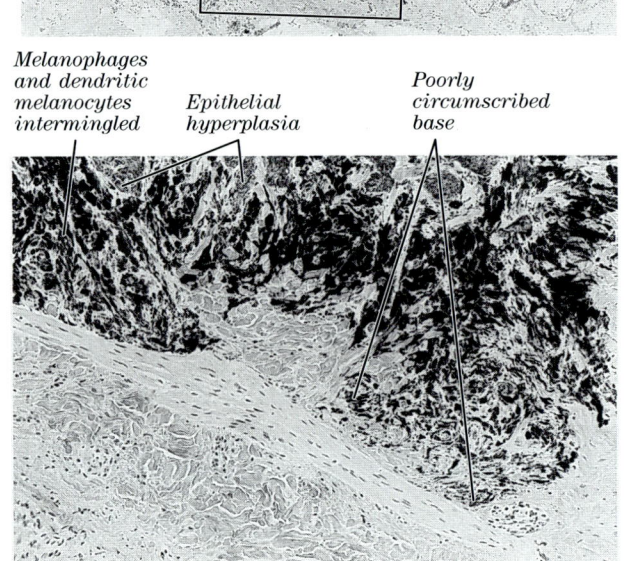

Melanophages and dendritic melanocytes intermingled / Epithelial hyperplasia / Poorly circumscribed base

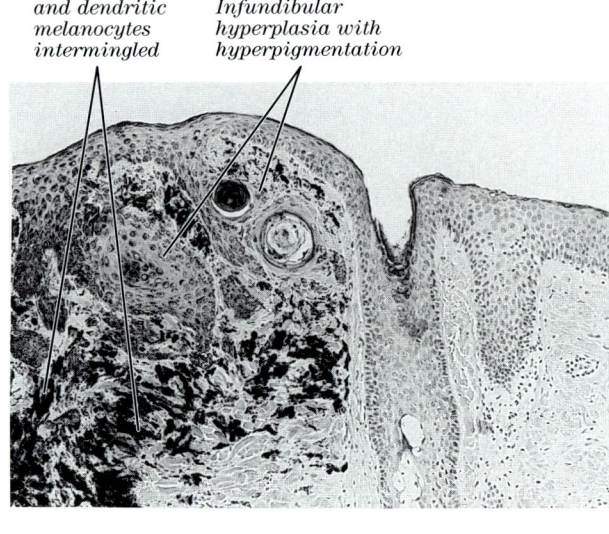

Melanophages and dendritic melanocytes intermingled / Infundibular hyperplasia with hyperpigmentation

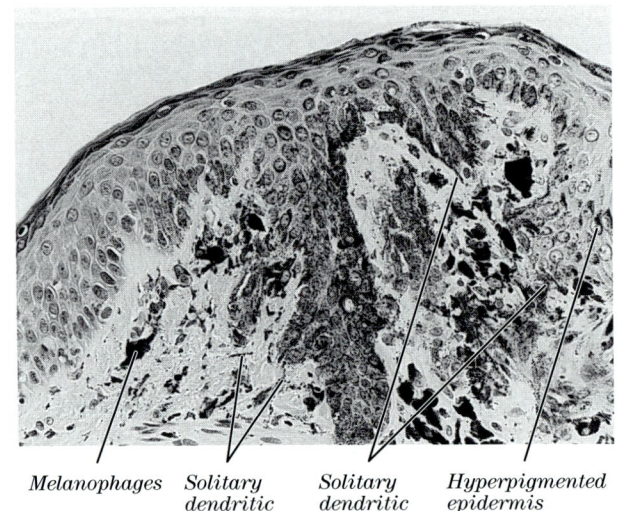

Melanophages / Solitary dendritic melanocyte in dermis / Solitary dendritic melanocytes in epidermis / Hyperpigmented epidermis

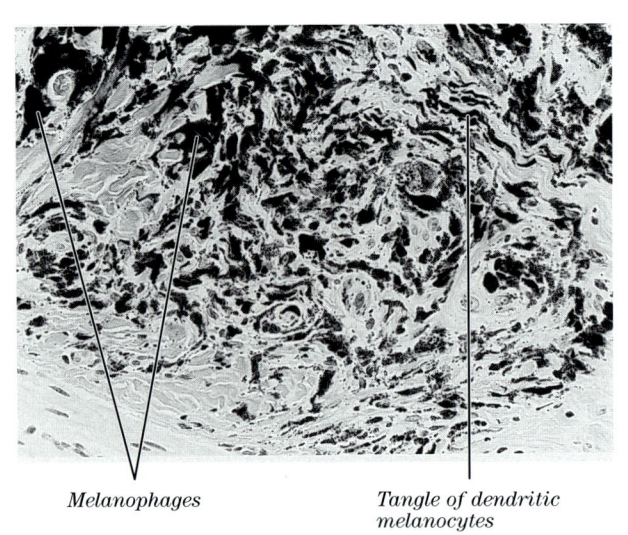

Melanophages / Tangle of dendritic melanocytes

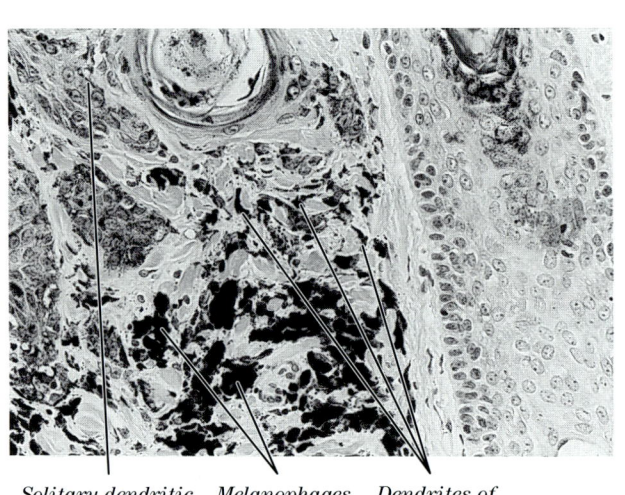

Solitary dendritic melanocyte within epithelium / Melanophages / Dendrites of melanocytes

23 • Blue Nevus *(superficial dendritic type)*

Criteria for diagnosis of this blue nevus (superficial dendritic type)

This is a superficial dendritic blue nevus because:

1. The neoplasm has a wedge shape.
2. The lesion is well-circumscribed.
3. All of the melanocytes within the epidermis are arranged as solitary units; none are in nests.
4. At the base of the neoplasm there are dendritic melanocytes and melanophages.
5. Melanin is distributed in uniform fashion throughout the neoplasm.

Pitfall in diagnosis

This blue nevus could be misinterpreted as a primary melanoma because:

1. The neoplasm appears to be asymmetric.
2. The melanocytes are strikingly dendritic, markedly pigmented, and disposed as solitary units within the epidermis.
3. The epidermis and the dermis are pigmented extensively by melanocytes.

This blue nevus is a variant in which numerous, dramatically dendritic, markedly pigmented melanocytes are disposed as solitary units within the epidermis. The situation is analogous to that in some examples of intradermal Miescher's nevi in which large oval and round melanocytes arranged as solitary units equidistant from one another are positioned at the dermo-epidermal junction. This nevus cannot be considered to be compound because none of the melanocytes within the epidermis are organized into nests.

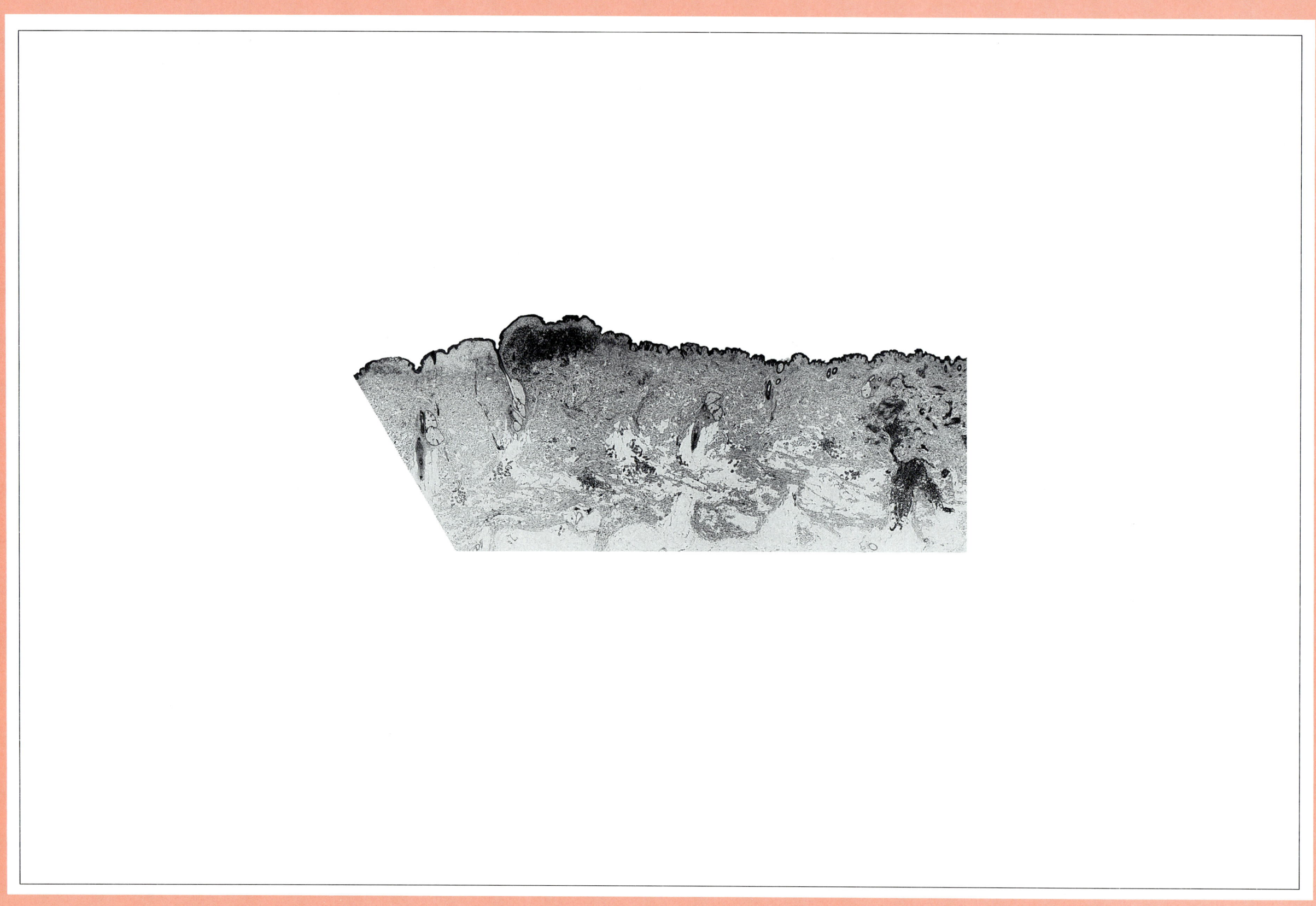

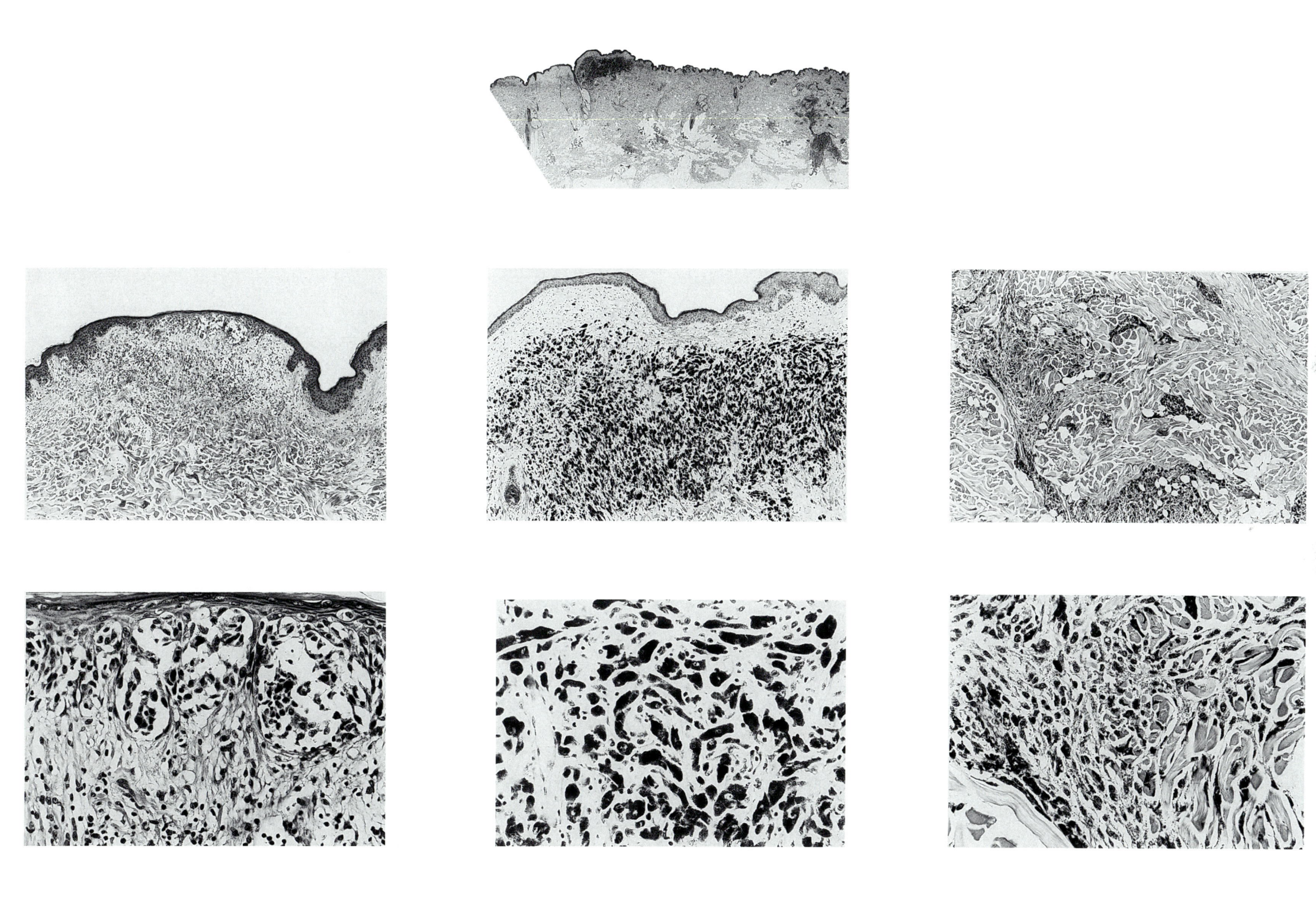

24. What is your diagnosis?

Pigmented lesion on the trunk of a 37-year-old man. Clinical diagnosis: Melanoma. Patient died within months of metastatic melanoma.

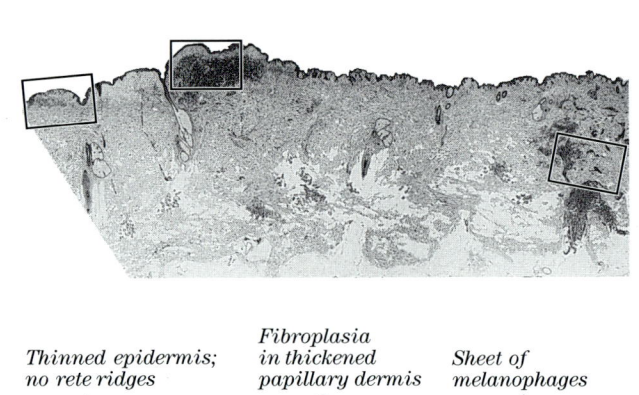

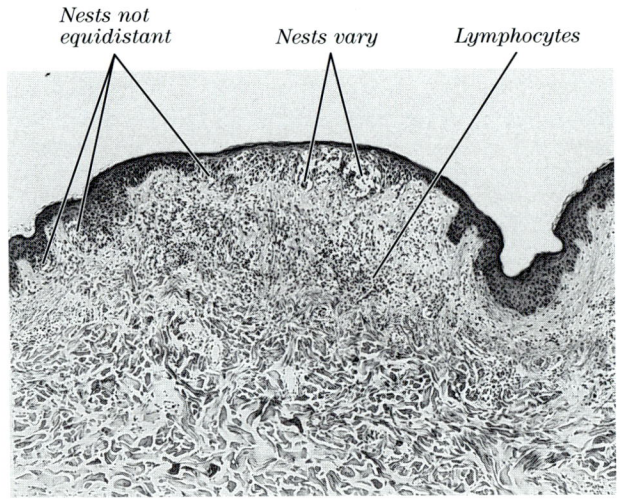

Nests not equidistant — Nests vary — Lymphocytes

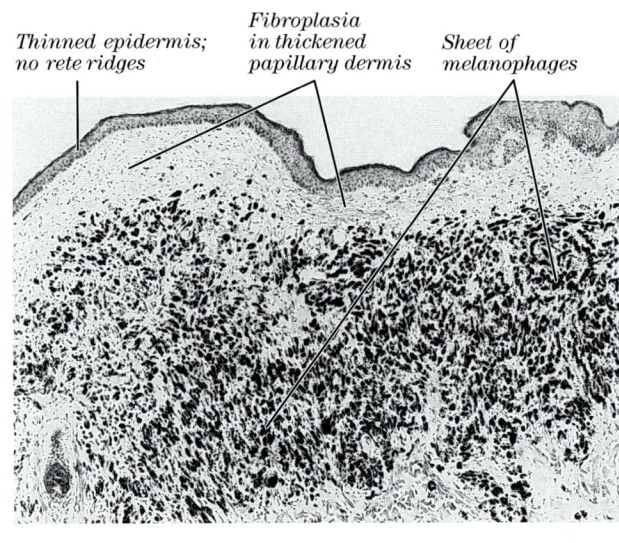

Thinned epidermis; no rete ridges — Fibroplasia in thickened papillary dermis — Sheet of melanophages

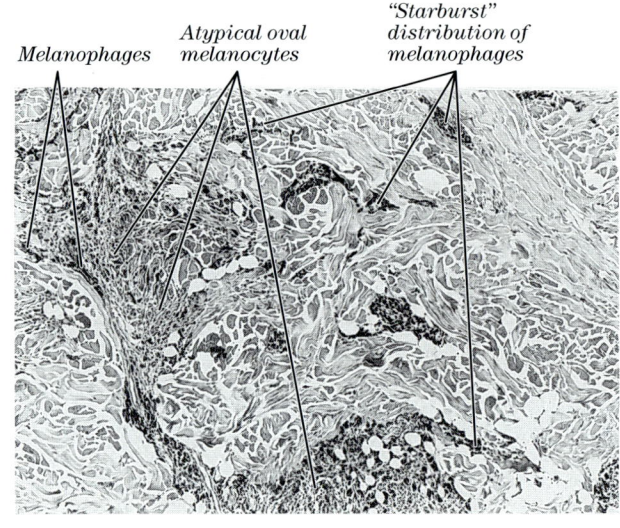

Melanophages — Atypical oval melanocytes — "Starburst" distribution of melanophages

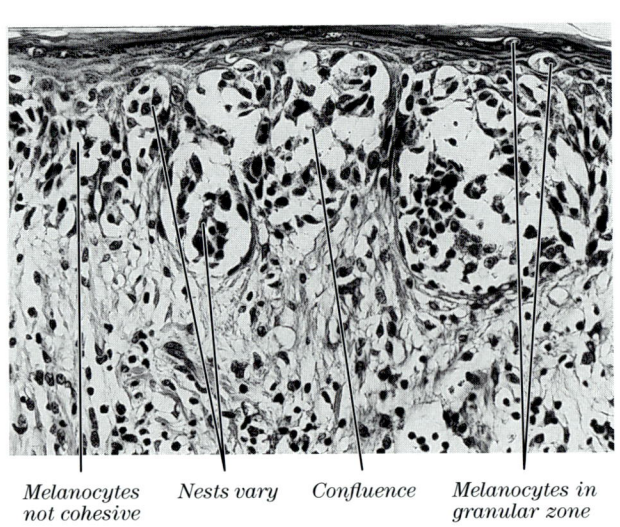

Melanocytes not cohesive — Nests vary — Confluence — Melanocytes in granular zone

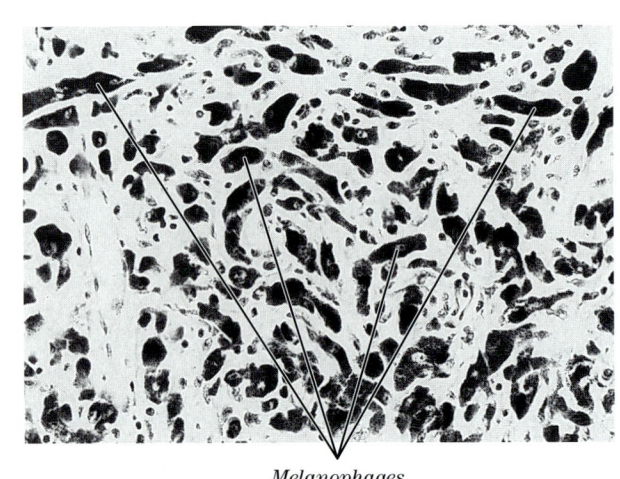

Melanophages

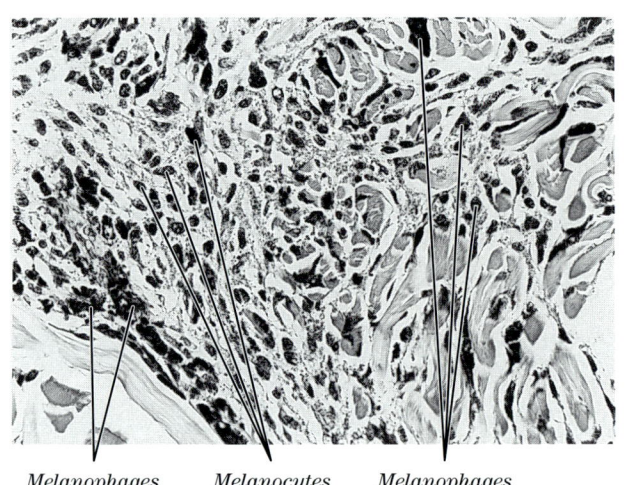

Melanophages — Melanocytes — Melanophages

24 • Primary Melanoma *(with regression)* and Satellite Metastasis *(with regression)*

Criteria for diagnosis of this primary melanoma (with focal regression) and satellite metastases (with complete regression)

This is a primary melanoma because:

In a focus on the extreme left are seen indubitable signs of melanoma in situ: atypical melanocytes are arranged as solitary units and nests, and nests are not equidistant from one another, vary in size and shape, have been confluent in foci, and are situated at all levels of the epidermis.

A prominent zone of regression of primary melanoma is evidenced by:

A broad, band-like zone of melanophages is present in a markedly thickened papillary dermis (melanosis) in the center of the lesion.

Complete regression of satellite metastases of melanoma is apparent because:

On the right side of the photomicrograph taken at scanning magnification, irregularly shaped aggregations of melanophages are positioned in the dermis and subcutaneous fat.

Pitfall in diagnosis

Complete regression of this satellite metastasis could be misinterpreted as a blue nevus to the side of a melanoma because:

1. Innumerable melanophages are present in patchy distribution in the reticular dermis and in the upper part of the subcutaneous fat.

2. The zone of pigmentation is oriented vertically.

3. There is no nuclear atypia.

4. There are no mitotic figures.

This lesion illustrates the importance of studying an entire section. On the far left is a melanoma in situ, to the left of center is a zone of melanosis (a sign of focal regression of primary melanoma), and on the far right are irregularly shaped deposits of melanophages that represent complete regression of a metastasis of melanoma. In essence, all of the melanophages in zones of regression, both those of the focally regressed primary melanoma and those of the totally regressed satellite metastasis, represent postinflammatory changes. Neoplastic melanocytes were destroyed by the effects on them of inflammatory cells, to wit, lymphocytes.

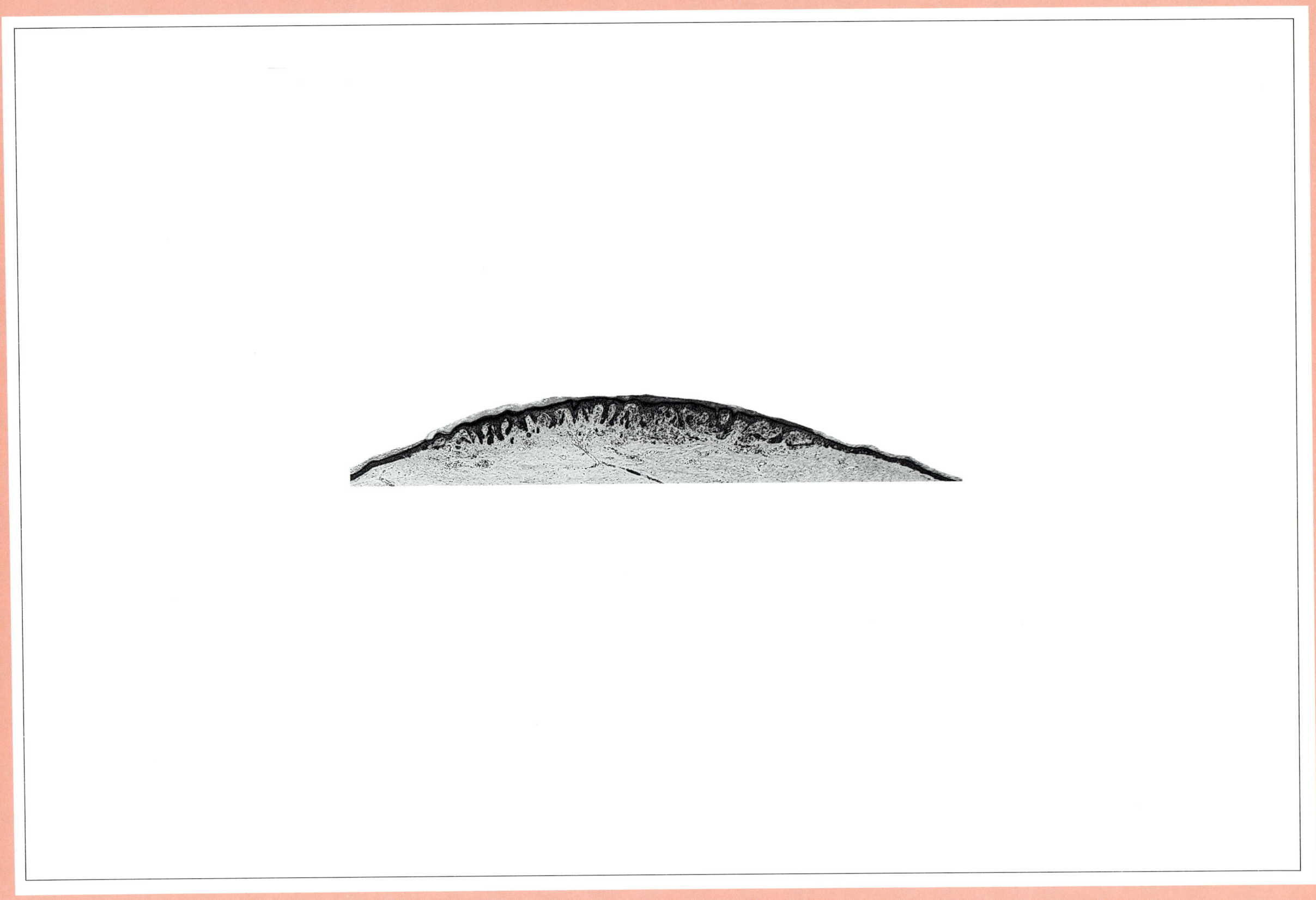

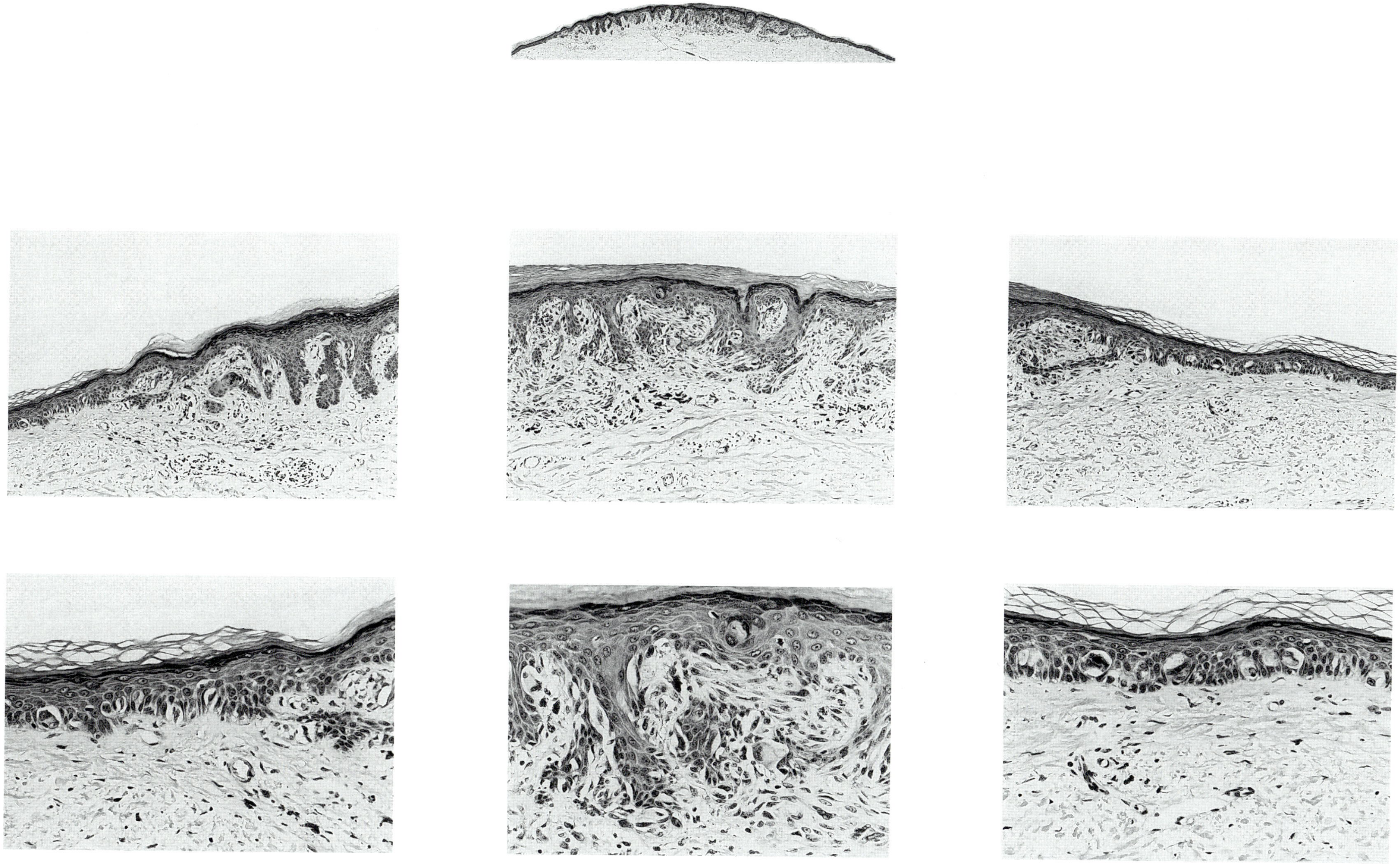

25. What is your diagnosis?

Black, slightly raised, angulated, asymptomatic papule of 2 months duration on the left leg of a 72-year-old woman. Clinical diagnosis: nevus vs. seborrheic keratosis. Wide and deep excision eventually was performed. No residual neoplasm was found in the specimen and no evidence of disease after 1 year.

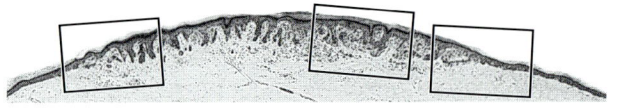

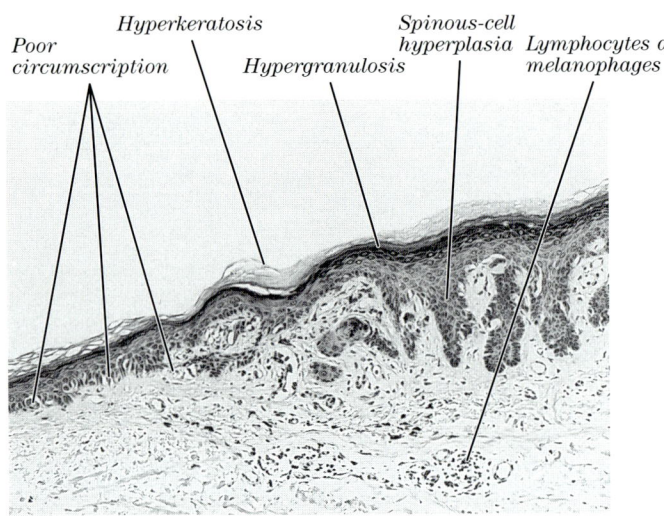

Poor circumscription — *Hyperkeratosis* — *Spinous-cell hyperplasia* — *Lymphocytes and melanophages* — *Hypergranulosis*

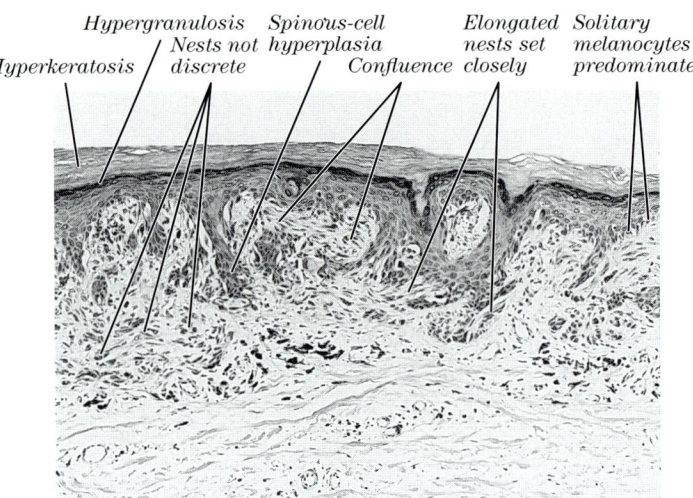

Hyperkeratosis — *Hypergranulosis* — *Nests not discrete* — *Spinous-cell hyperplasia* — *Confluence* — *Elongated nests set closely* — *Solitary melanocytes predominate*

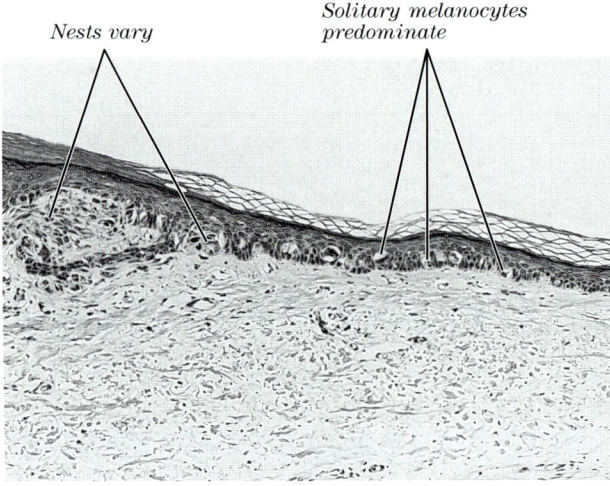

Nests vary — *Solitary melanocytes predominate*

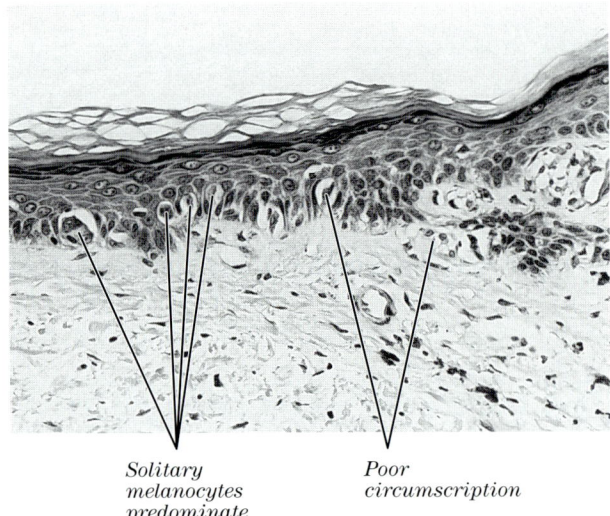

Solitary melanocytes predominate — *Poor circumscription*

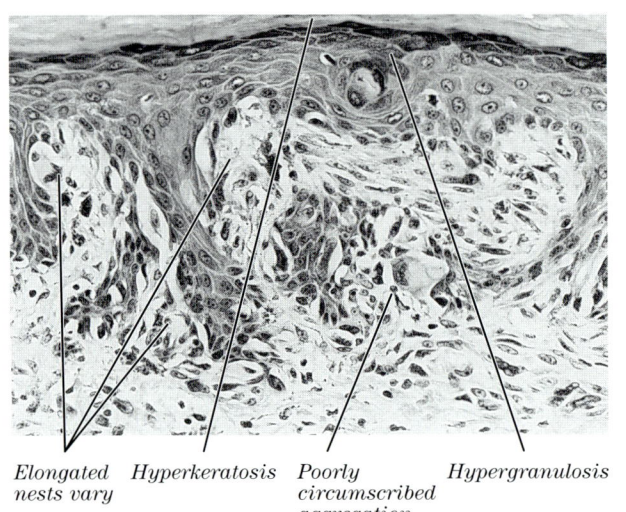

Elongated nests vary — *Hyperkeratosis* — *Poorly circumscribed aggregation* — *Hypergranulosis*

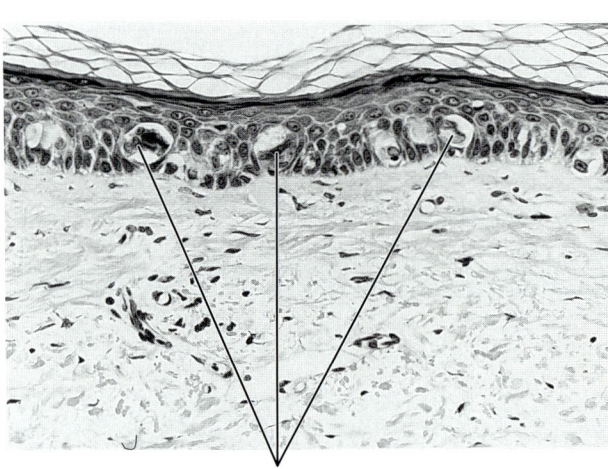

Atypical melanocytes above junction

25 • Melanoma

Criteria for diagnosis of this melanoma

This is a melanoma because:

1. The neoplasm is asymmetric, e.g., melanocytes in the "shoulder" on the right extend for a far greater distance beyond the intradermal component than in the "shoulder" on the left.

2. Melanocytes disposed as solitary units are more numerous than nests in many high-power fields within the epidermis.

3. Nests of melanocytes within the epidermis are not equidistant from one another.

4. There is variation in size and shape of nests of melanocytes within the epidermis.

5. Some nests of melanocytes within the epidermis have become confluent.

Pitfall in diagnosis

This melanoma could be misread as a compound Spitz's nevus because:

1. There are hyperkeratosis, hypergranulosis, and irregular spinous-cell hyperplasia.

2. Atypical nuclei are found in many melanocytes.

3. Melanocytes are oval, spindle, and polygonal.

4. Many melanocytes are binucleate and multinucleate.

5. Some nests of melanocytes are elongated.

6. Some elongated nests of melanocytes are oriented perpendicularly to the skin surface.

7. The neoplasm is gently domed.

The changes in the center of this neoplasm could be misconstrued as those of Spitz's nevus. However, characteristic findings of melanoma in situ are present at the "shoulders" of the neoplasm. At the "shoulders," the neoplasm may be seen to be poorly circumscribed, atypical melanocytes arranged as solitary units may be observed to predominate overwhelmingly over nests of melanocytes, and some melanocytes may be noted well above the dermo-epidermal junction.

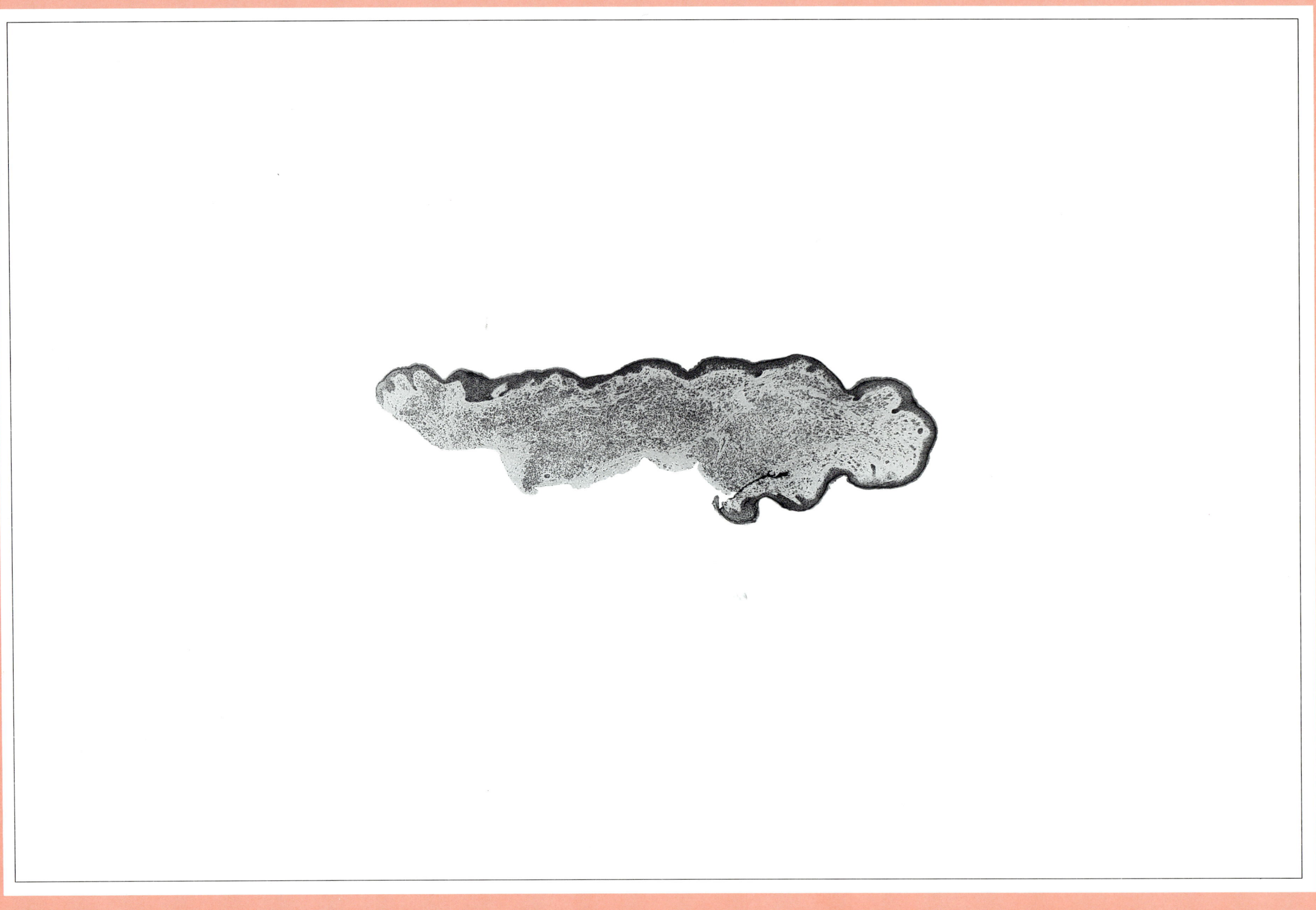

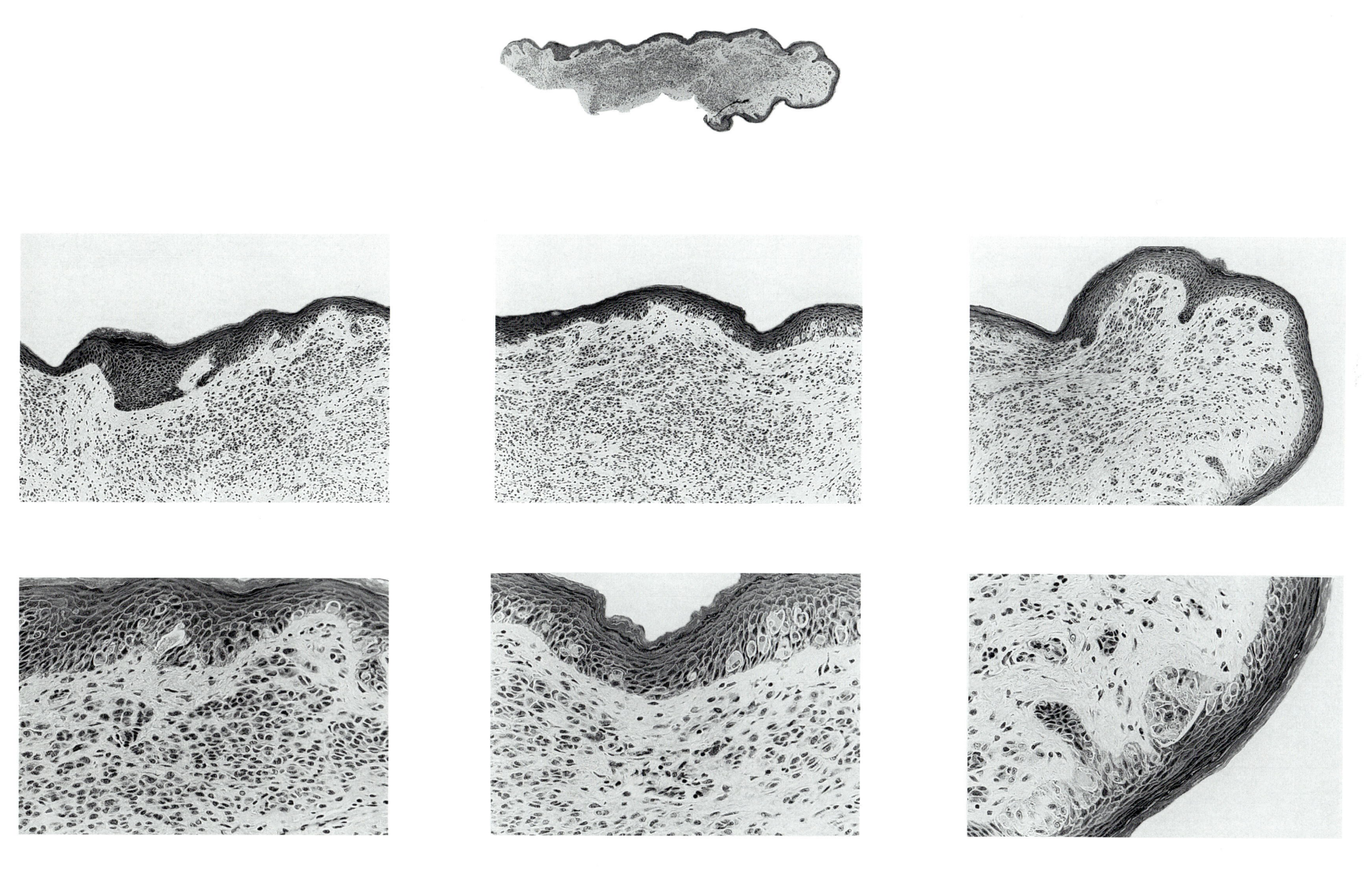

26. What is your diagnosis?

Pigmented lesion on the vulva of a 21-year-old removed incidentally following parturition. Clinical diagnosis: Mole. Patient is well five years later.

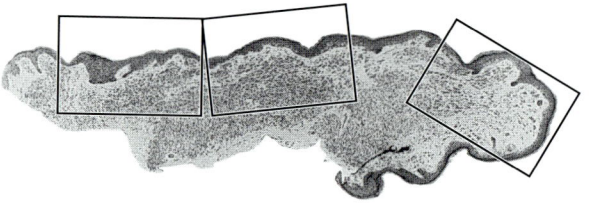

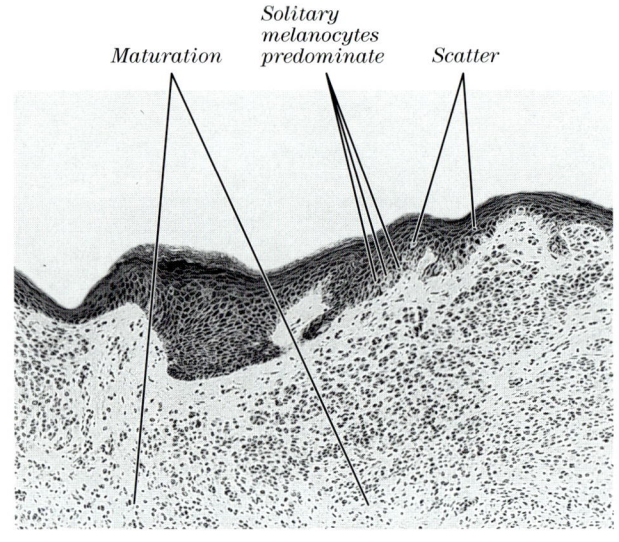
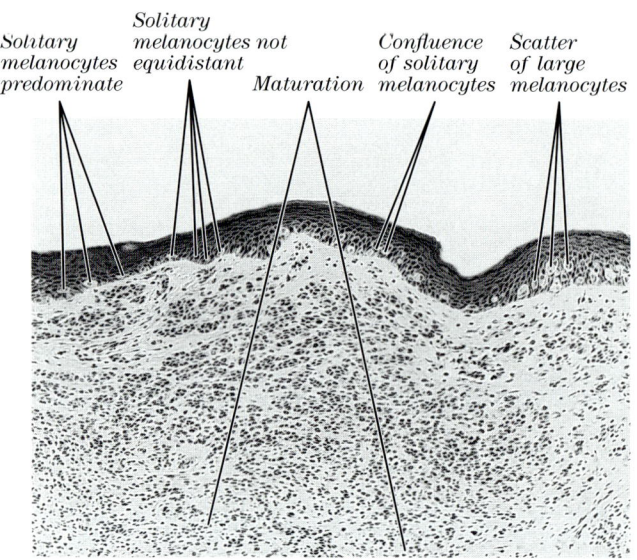
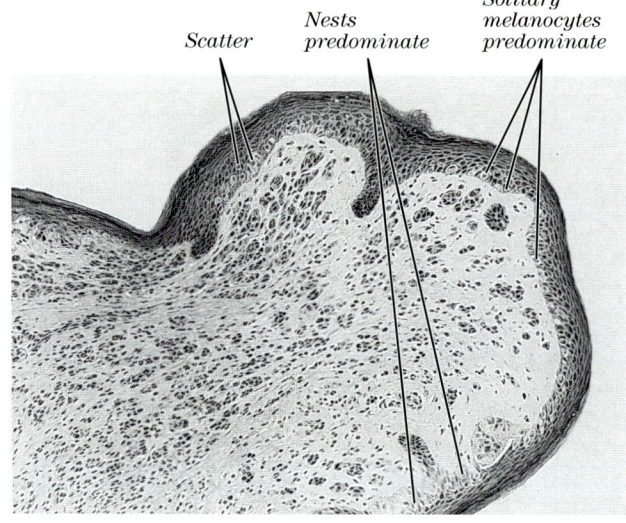

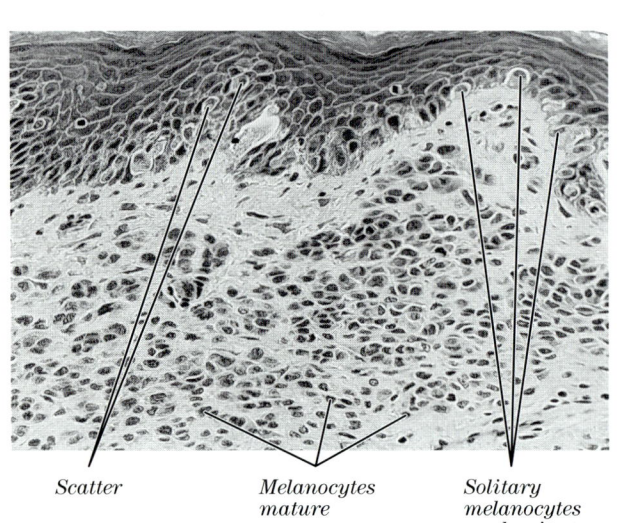
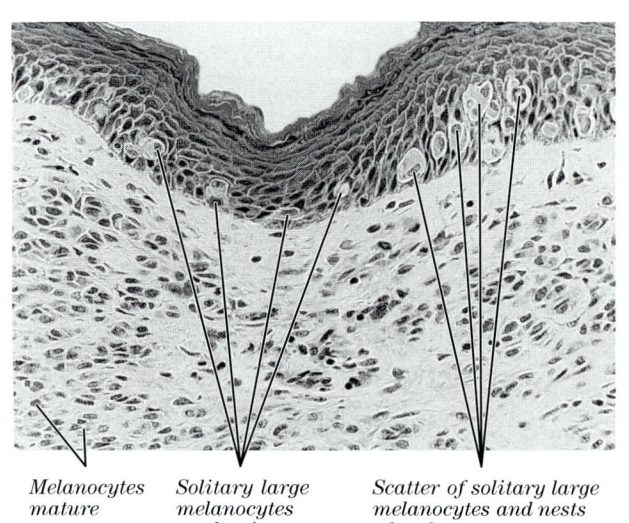
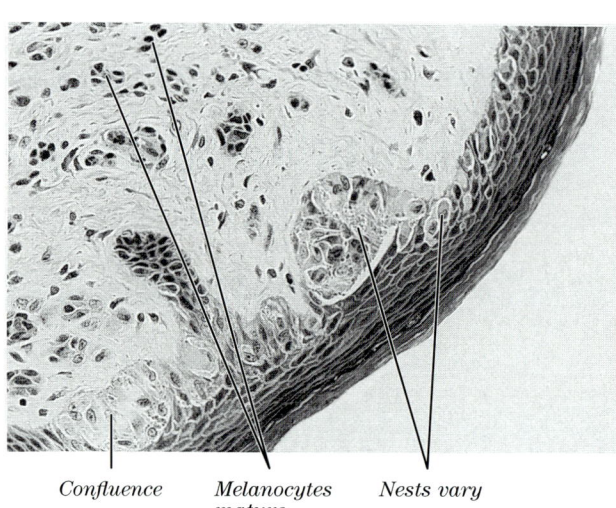

26 • Clark's Nevus on Genital Skin

Criteria for diagnosis of this Clark's nevus on genital skin

The neoplasm is benign because:

1. Maturation of melanocytes is striking.
2. Orderly nests, cords, and strands of melanocytes are found within the dermis.
3. Nuclei of melanocytes within the epidermis and the dermis are typical.

This is a compound nevus because:

Nests of melanocytes are present in both the epidermis and the dermis.

This is a Clark's nevus because:

Nests of melanocytes are confined to the epidermis and the equivalent of a markedly thickened papillary dermis.

Pitfall in diagnosis

This compound nevus from a vulva could be misdiagnosed as melanoma in situ in association with a pre-existing intradermal nevus because:

1. Nests of melanocytes are not equidistant from one another.
2. Melanocytes arranged as solitary units predominate over nests in many high-power fields.
3. Melanocytes disposed both as solitary units and small nests are scattered above the dermo-epidermal junction.
4. Nests of melanocytes vary in size and shape.
5. Melanocytes within the epidermis are much larger than those within the dermis.

Just as is the case in certain persistent (recurrent) nevi where changes in the epidermis resemble closely those of melanoma in situ, the same is true often for melanocytic nevi on the genitalia, such as this one. Although the findings in the epidermis are nearly indistinguishable from those of melanoma in situ, the presence of an obvious nevus within the dermis is a clue to the fact that this lesion is benign, just as the situation is in some recurrent nevi. In brief, there tends to be a major disparity between the expected epidermal and dermal patterns of melanocytes in a Clark's nevus and the histopathologic appearance of that nevus on genital skin. In addition, the dermal component of a Clark's nevus usually is confined to the papillary dermis, which may be thickened enormously by it. On genital skin, there is no sharp demarcation between papillary and reticular dermis, so that a compound type of Clark's nevus at that site, although superficial, does not have a well-defined inferior boundary.

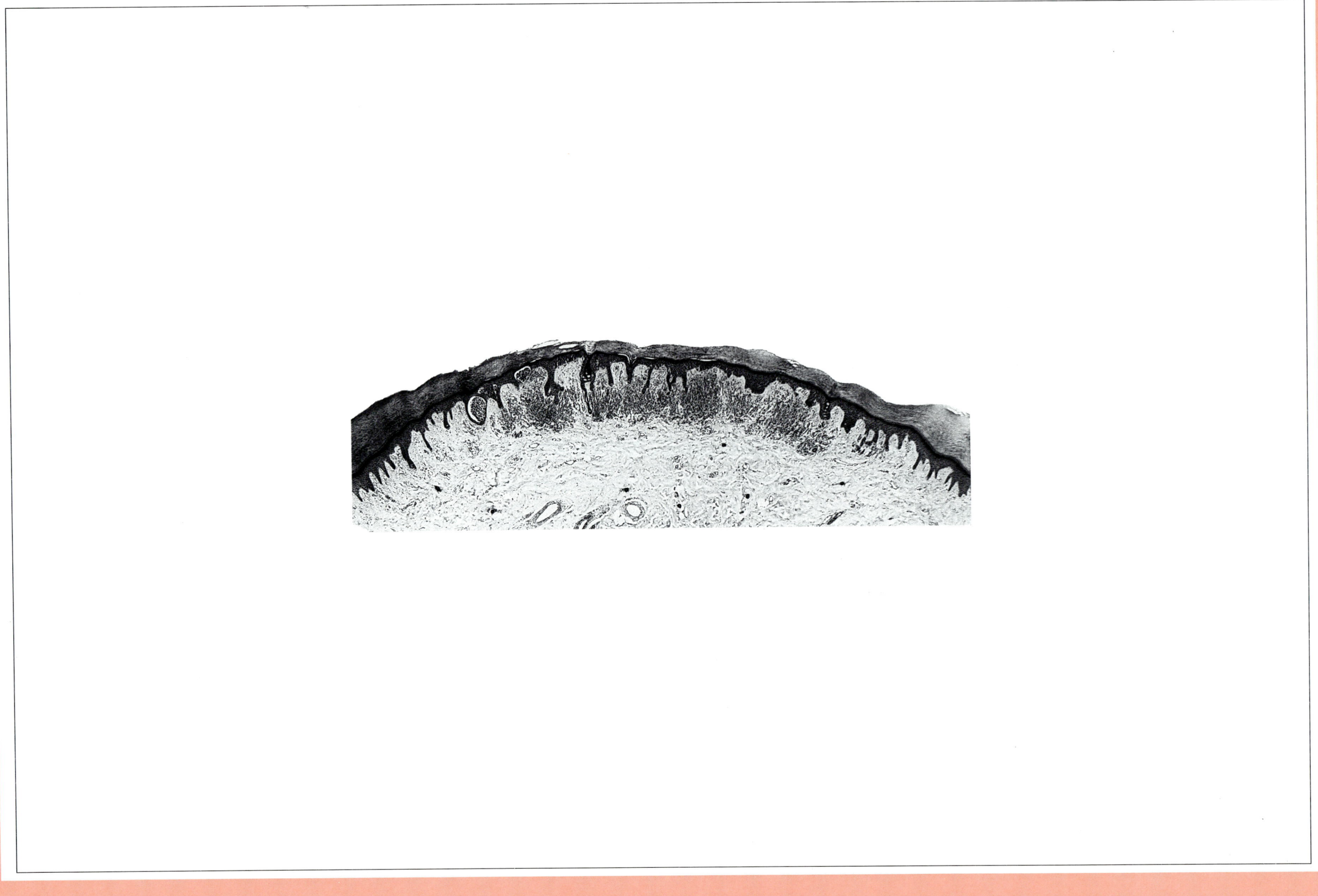

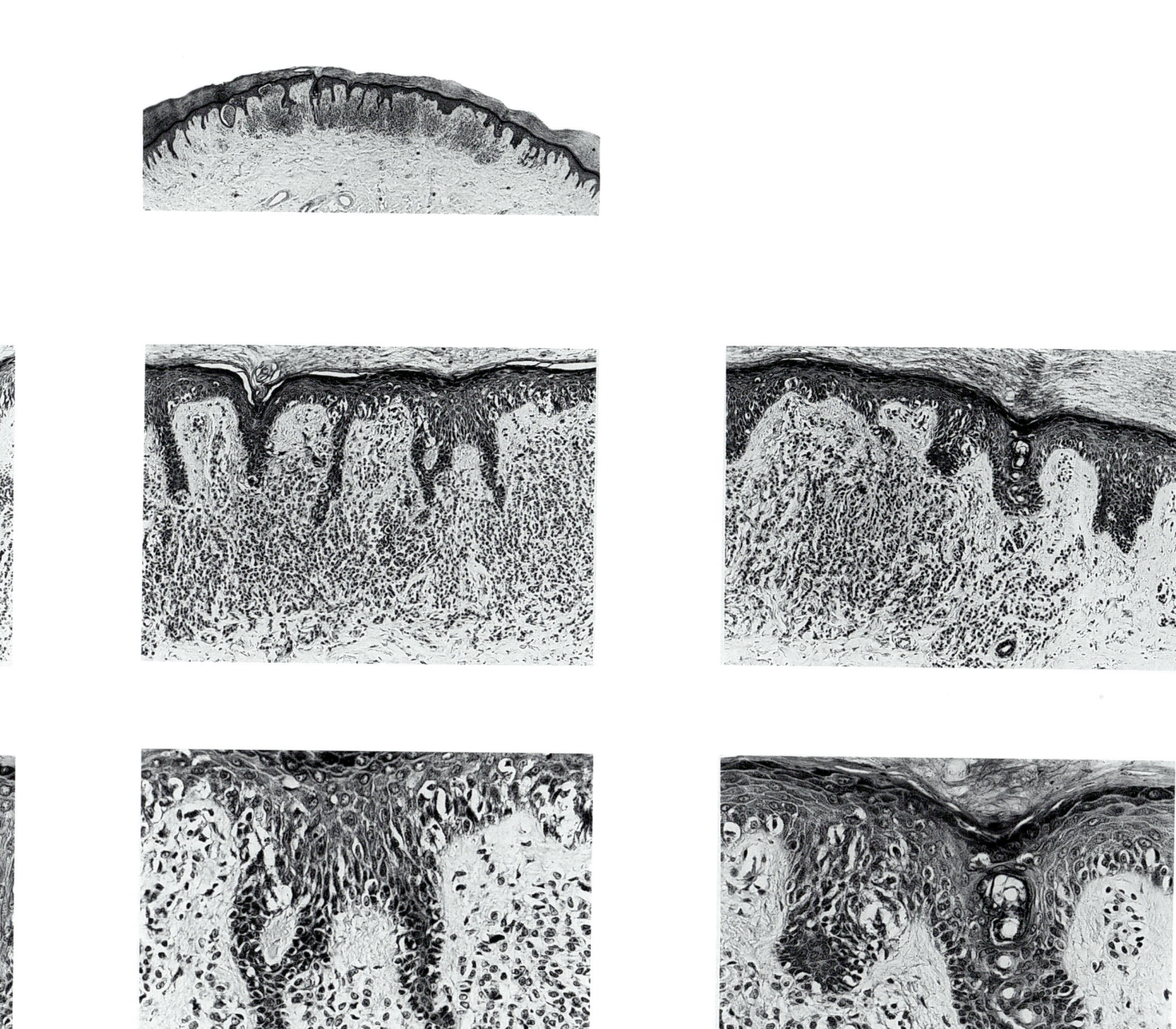

27. What is your diagnosis?

Pigmented lesion of 20 years duration from the lateral aspect of the right foot of a 46-year-old woman. Clinical diagnosis: nevus. No follow-up information is available.

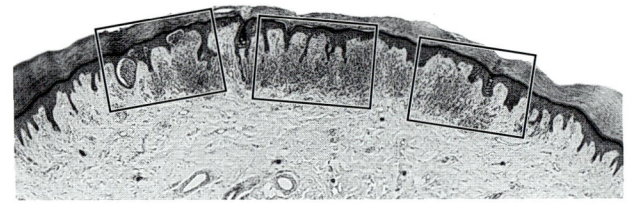

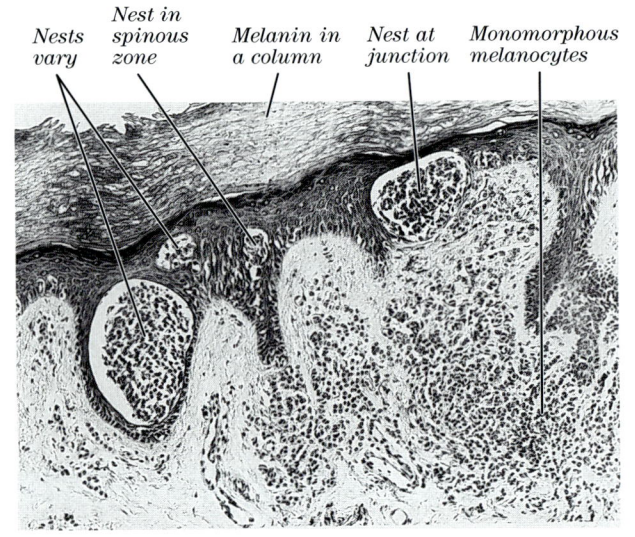

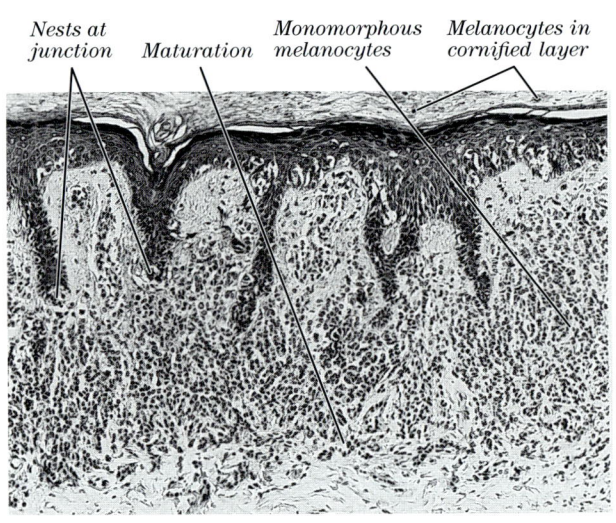

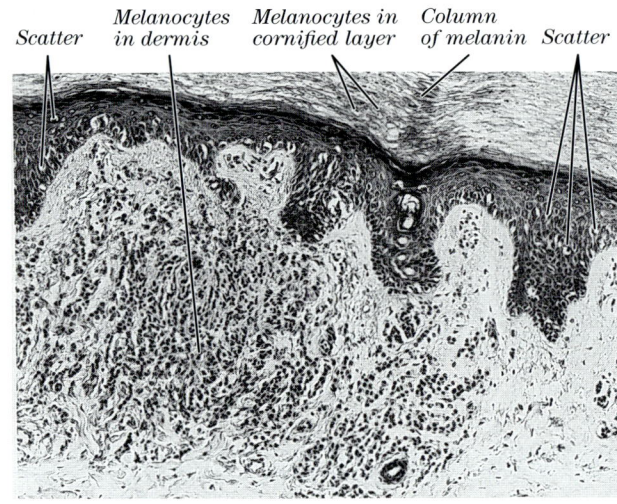

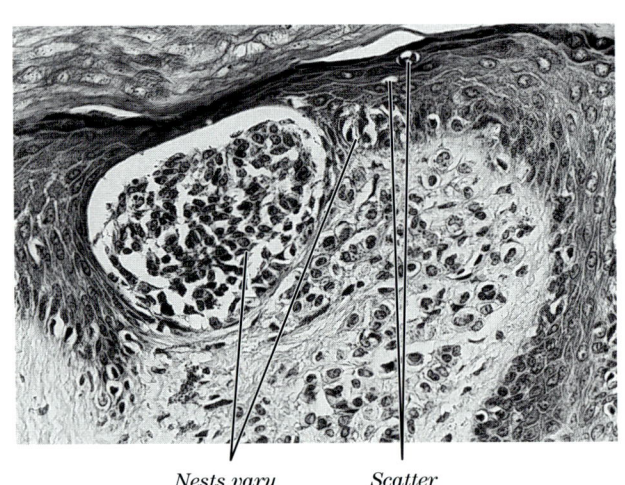

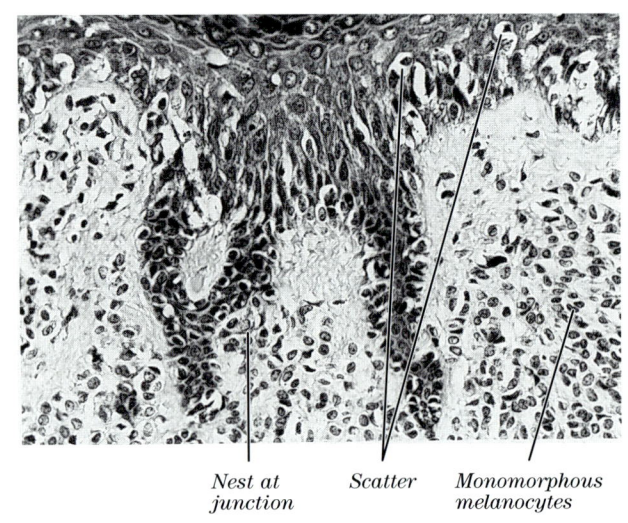

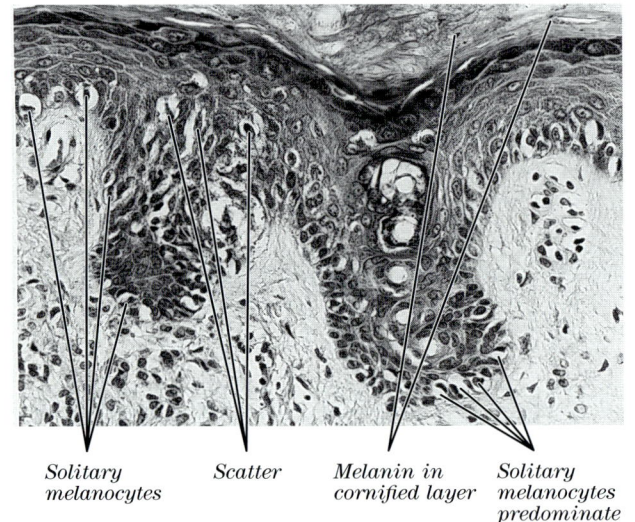

27 • Clark's Nevus

Criteria for diagnosis of this Clark's nevus (compound type) on volar skin

This is a nevus because:

1. It is well-circumscribed.
2. Melanocytes mature.
3. Most of the nests of melanocytes within the epidermis are situated at the dermo-epidermal junction, not above it.
4. The melanocytes themselves are small, oval, and monomorphous.

This is a Clark's nevus because:

1. The slightly domed lesion is confined mostly to the dermo-epidermal junction and thickened papillary dermis.

Pitfall in diagnosis

This compound Clark's nevus on volar skin could be misinterpreted as a melanoma in situ in association with an intradermal nevus because:

1. Melanocytes, especially those disposed as solitary units but also those arranged in nests, are present not only at the dermo-epidermal junction but considerably above it.
2. The neoplasm is asymmetric, e.g., many more nests of melanocytes are seen within the epidermis on the left side than on the right.
3. Melanocytes arranged as solitary units extend far down eccrine ducts.
4. Nests of melanocytes are not equidistant from one another.
5. Melanocytes arranged as solitary units predominate over nests in many high-power fields.

A remarkable pitfall in diagnosis of melanocytic nevi on volar skin is the strong tendency to scatter of melanocytes, both as solitary units and in nests, above the dermo-epidermal junction, sometimes in the upper reaches of the epidermis. If a melanocytic neoplasm, such as this one, fulfills all architectural criteria for a nevus, then presence of melanocytes above the dermo-epidermal junction should be interpreted as an expected finding in junctional and compound nevi on volar skin.

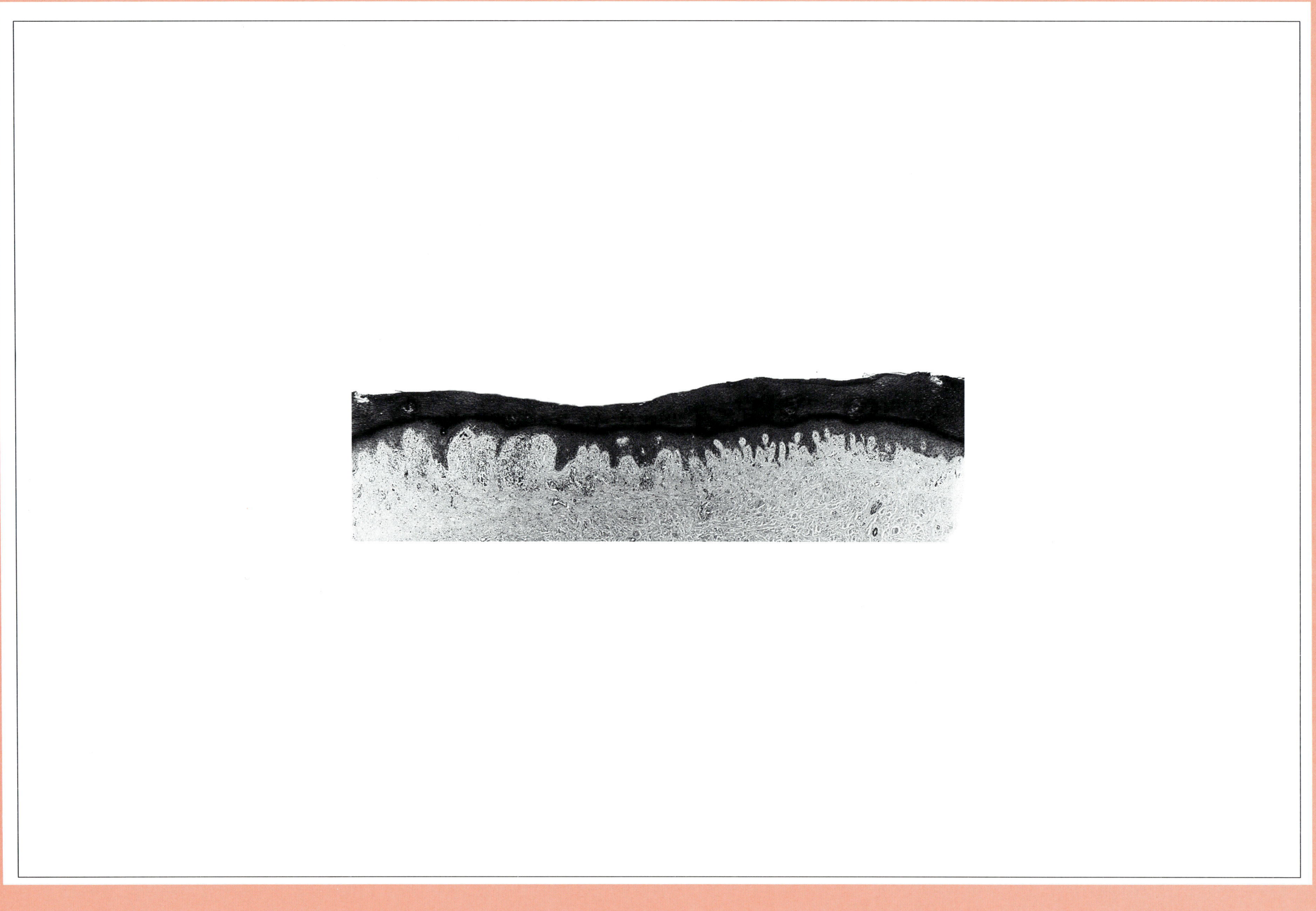

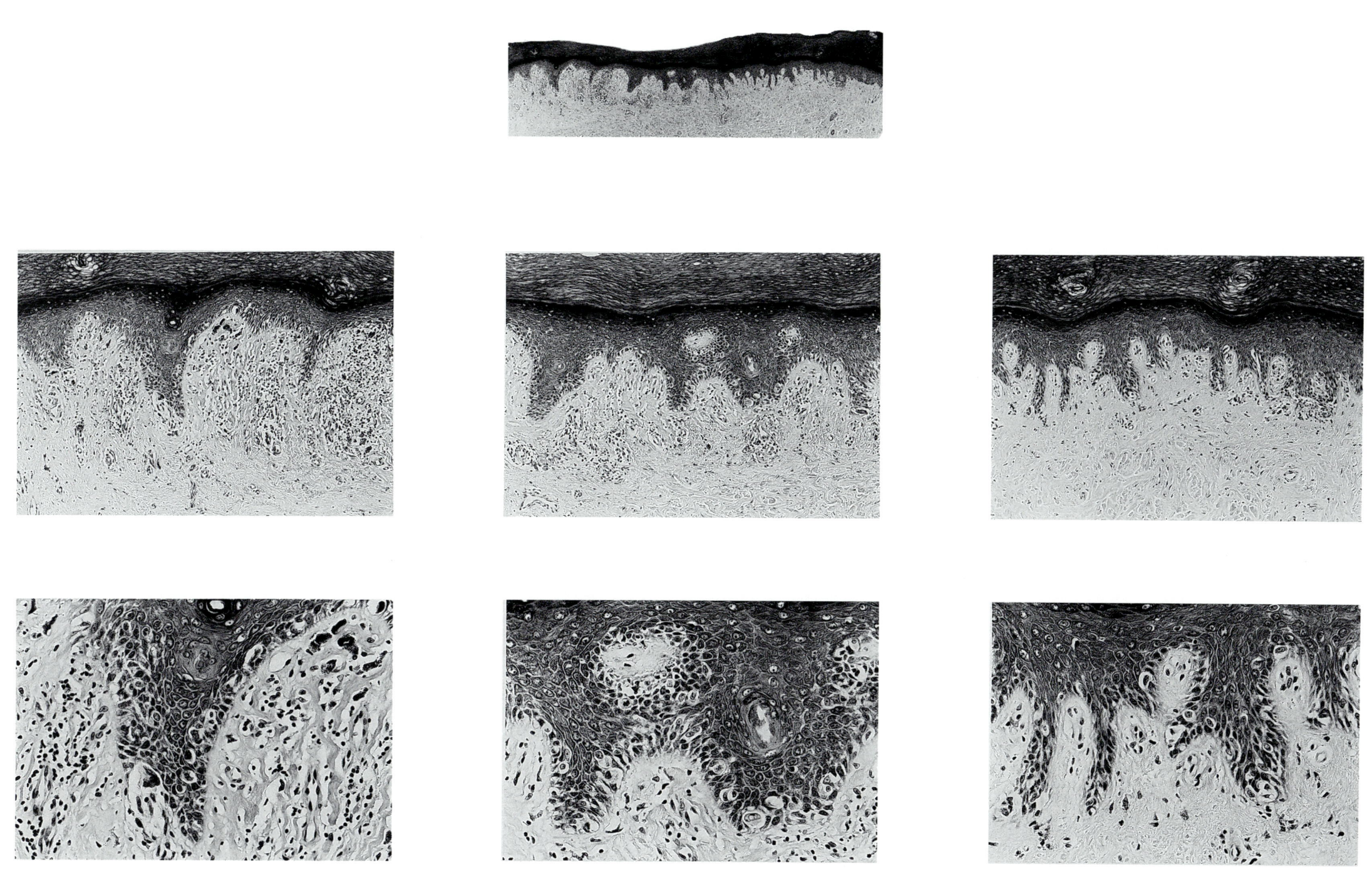

28. What is your diagnosis?

Pigmented lesion on the plantar surface of a 68-year-old woman. The lesion was removed by excision and covered by a graft. The patient was free of disease after 9 years.

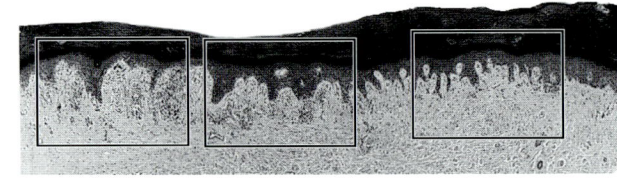

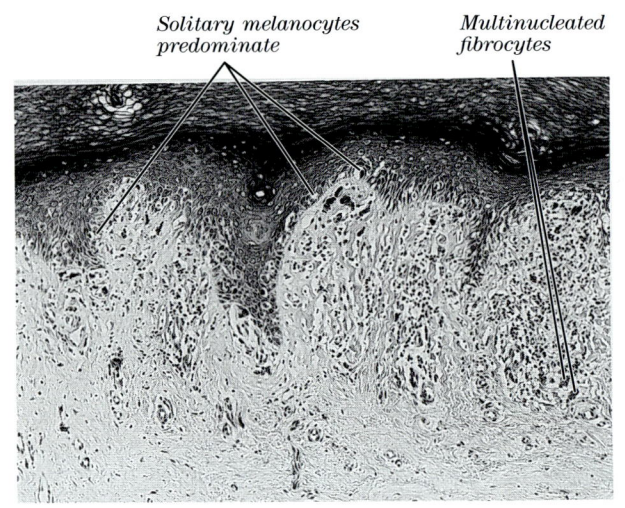

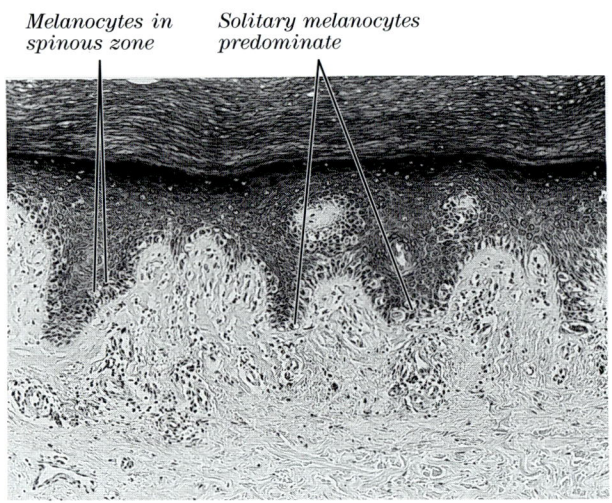

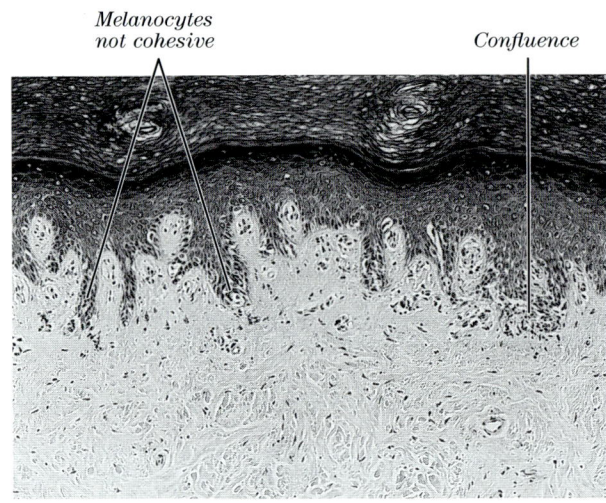

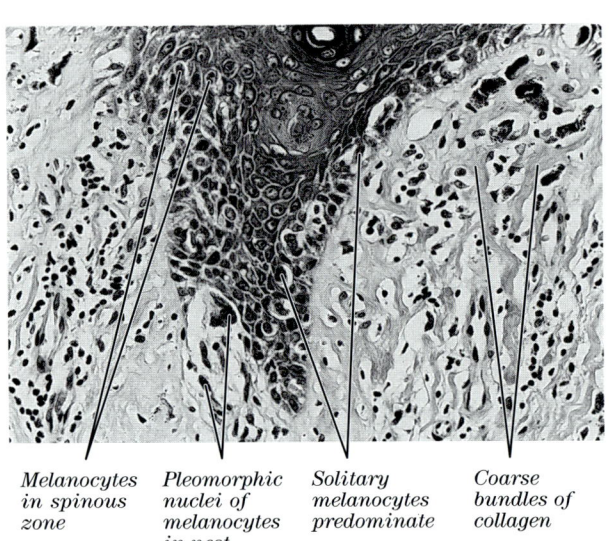

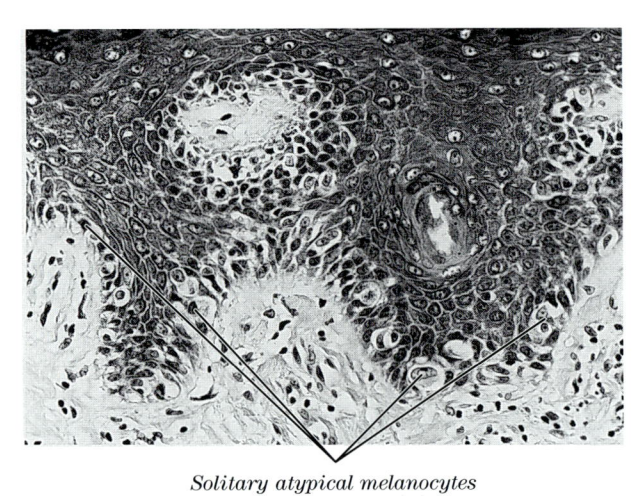

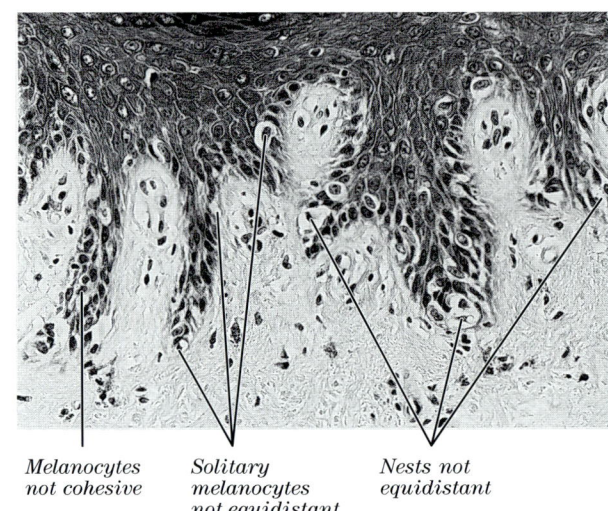

28 • Melanoma

Criteria for diagnosis of this melanoma

This is a melanoma because:

1. The neoplasm is broad (more than 1.5 cm in greatest diameter).

2. Melanocytes disposed as solitary units are more numerous within the epidermis than as nests there.

3. Nests of melanocytes within the epidermis are not equidistant from one another.

4. Melanocytes arrayed as solitary units are situated well above the dermo-epidermal junction.

5. Nuclei of many neoplastic melanocytes are atypical.

6. Changes like those in the epidermis also are present far down eccrine ducts.

Pitfall in diagnosis

This melanoma in situ on volar skin could be misinterpreted as "severe dysplasia," but it should not be read as anything other than melanoma in situ because the findings are stereotypical of that stage in the evolution of melanoma.

Differential diagnosis is a valuable exercise when lesions look so much alike that they resemble identical twins. That circumstance is as uncommon in dermatopathology as monozygotic twins are in the general population of human beings. In short, there is no authentic differential diagnosis for most melanocytic neoplasms, and this melanoma in situ is an example of that proposition. In any event, it is far preferable to acknowledge that one does not know a diagnosis than to pretend that one does with meaningless evasions like "severe dysplasia." Clinicians and patients are served well by the diagnosis "melanoma in situ."

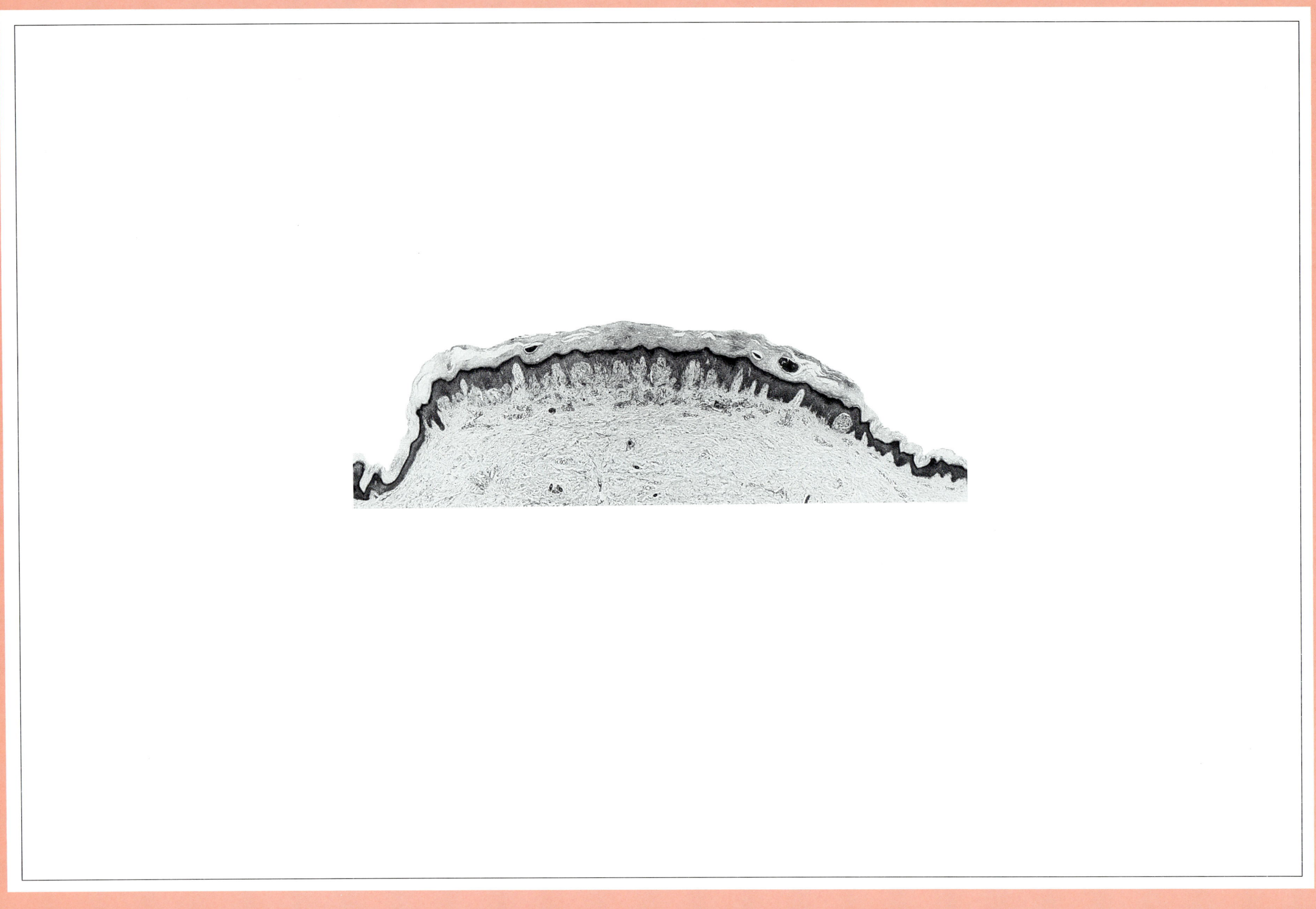

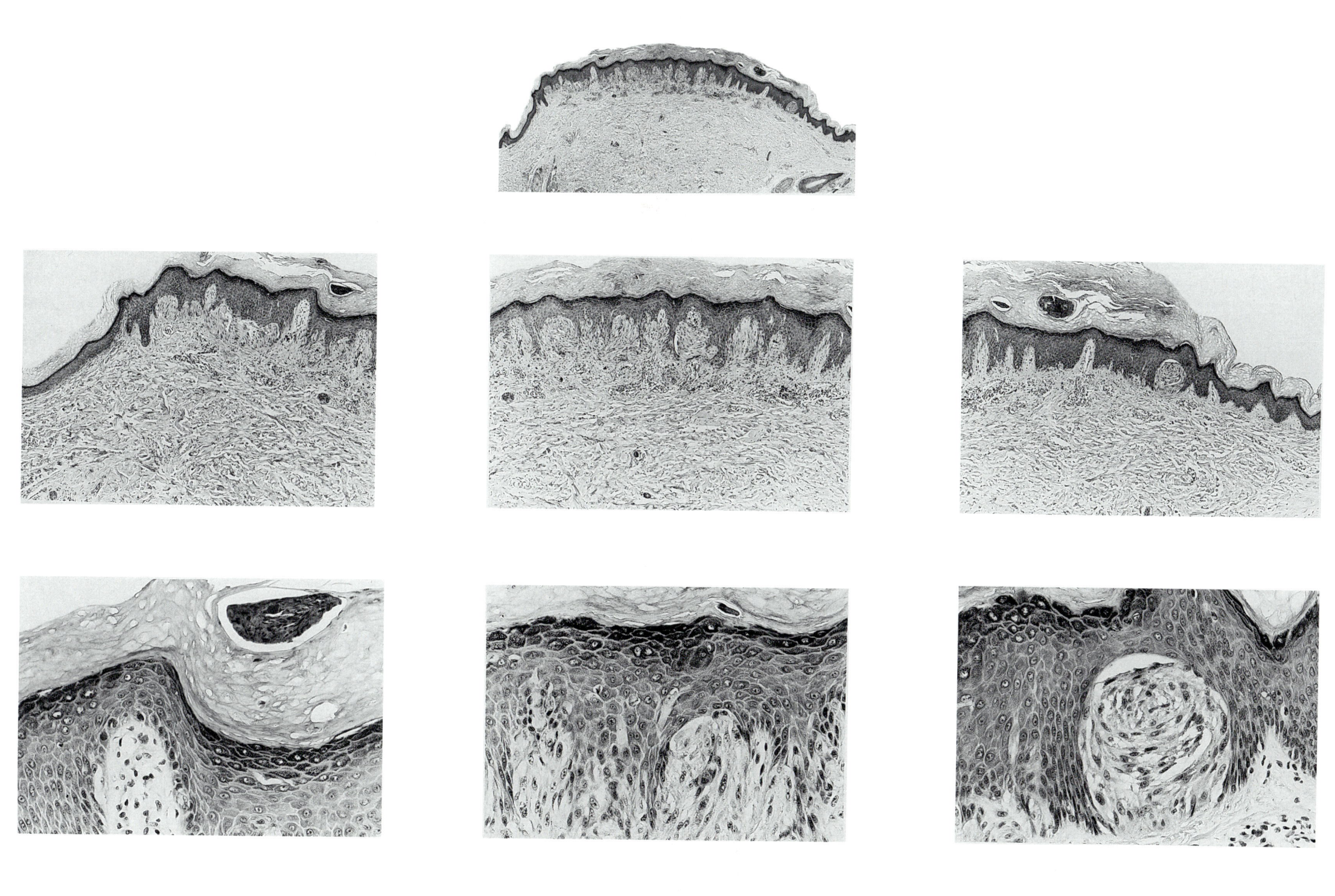

29. What is your diagnosis?

Pigmented lesion on the thigh of a 19-year-old woman. Clinical diagnosis: nevus. Patient well a decade after the procedure.

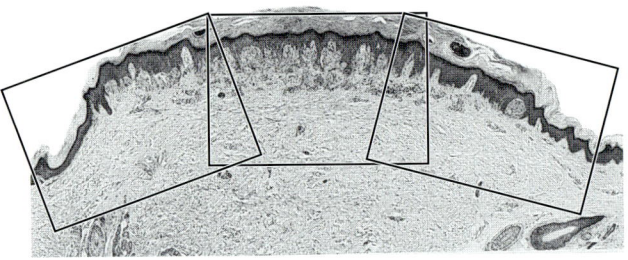

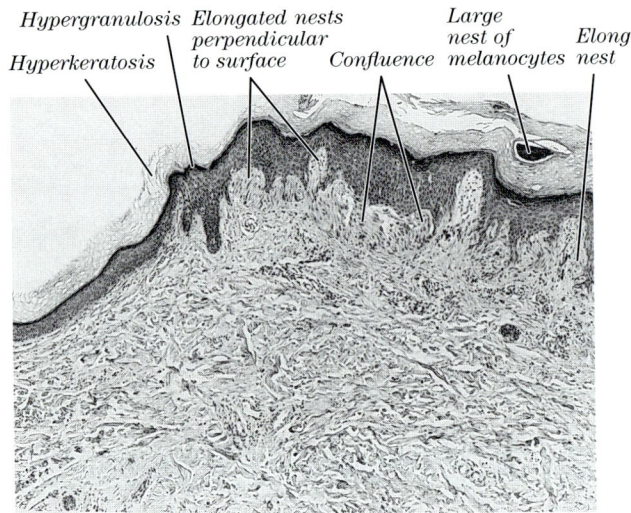

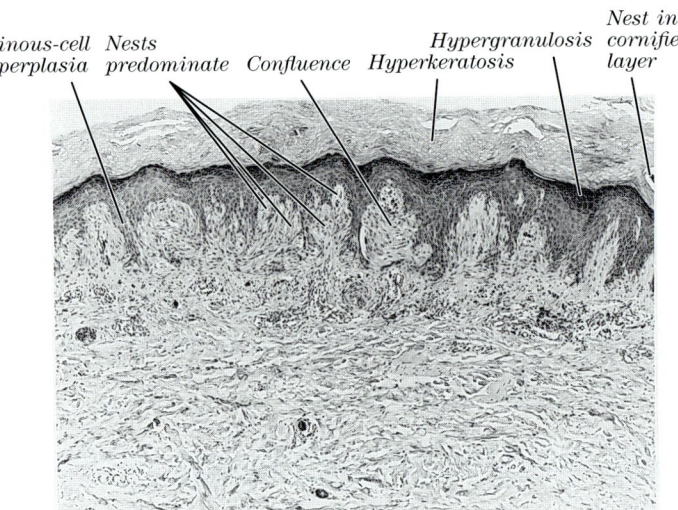

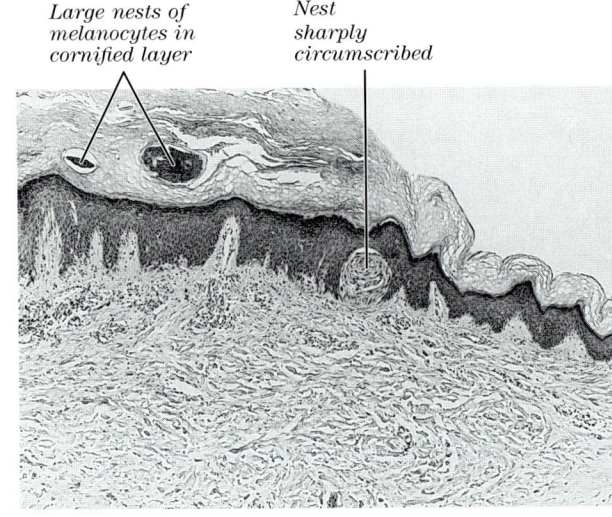

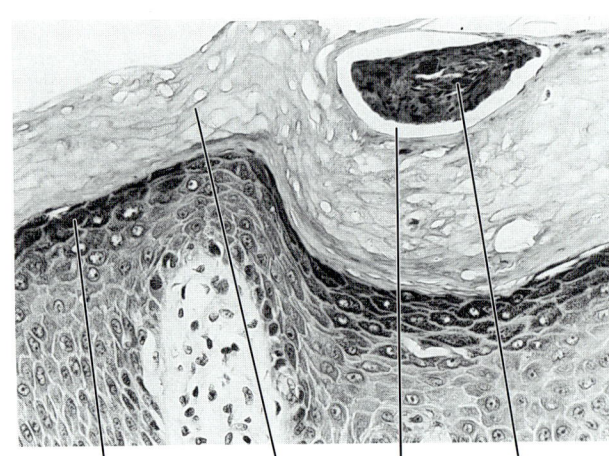

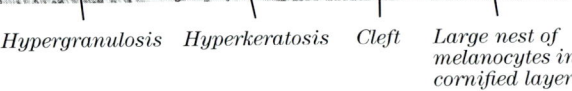

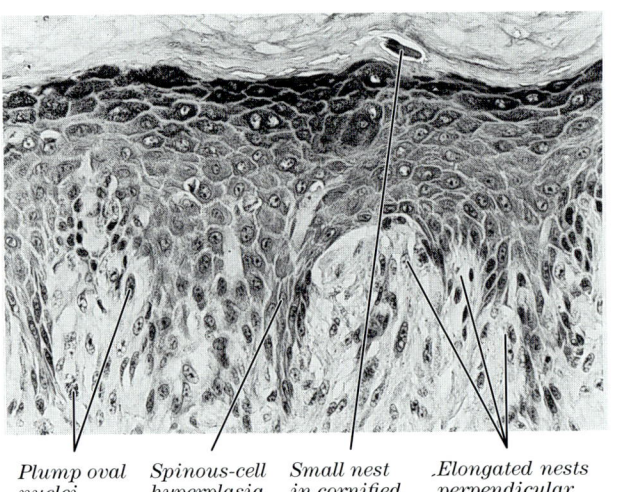

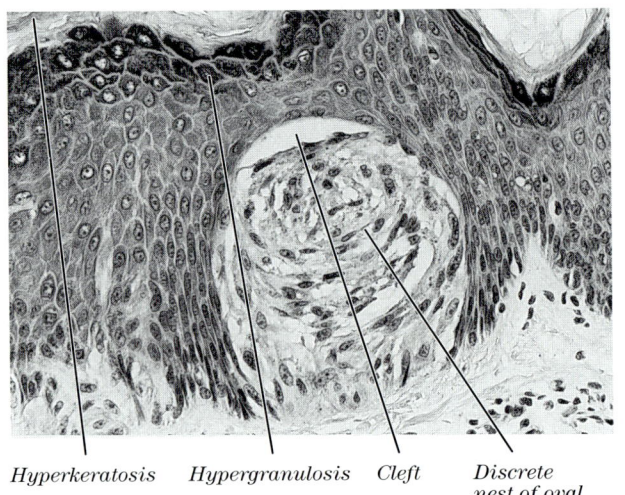

29 • Spitz's Nevus

Criteria for diagnosis of this Spitz's nevus

This is a nevus because:

1. The neoplasm is symmetric.
2. It is well-circumscribed.
3. It consists of melanocytes arranged mostly in nests, rather than as solitary units.
4. Nests of melanocytes are situated mostly at the dermo-epidermal junction, rather than above it.
5. Nuclei of melanocytes are relatively monomorphous.

This is a Spitz's nevus because:

1. Some of the melanocytes have largish nuclei, abundant cytoplasm, and oval shape.
2. There are marked hyperkeratosis, hypergranulosis, and hyperplasia of spinous cells.
3. Clefts separate some nests of melanocytes from adjacent keratinocytes.
4. Some nests of melanocytes are oriented perpendicularly to the skin surface.
5. Melanocytes disposed both as solitary units and in nests are present throughout the entire thickness of the epidermis, including the cornified layer.

Pitfall in diagnosis

This Spitz's nevus could be misconstrued as a melanoma because:

1. Nests of melanocytes, both small and large ones, are scattered throughout the cornified layer.
2. Some nests of melanocytes within the epidermis have become confluent.

Perhaps the greatest pitfall in overdiagnosis of melanoma is misinterpretation of scatter of melanocytes in the upper reaches of the epidermis, especially in the cornified layer, as synonymous with melanoma. In short, the two are not synonymous. Nests of melanocytes throughout the entire thickness of the epidermis are seen commonly in junctional and compound Spitz's nevi, as pictured, in nevi situated on palms and soles, and in congenital nevi biopsied shortly after birth, to mention but a few examples. In sum, a diagnosis of Spitz's nevus is made best at scanning magnification on the basis of criteria predicated upon silhouette. The presence of nests of melanocytes within the cornified layer is an expected finding in Spitz's nevi. That diagnosis should never be changed to melanoma because of the presence of nests of melanocytes within the cornified layer alone, no matter how many or how large the nests, or because of the age of a patient alone.

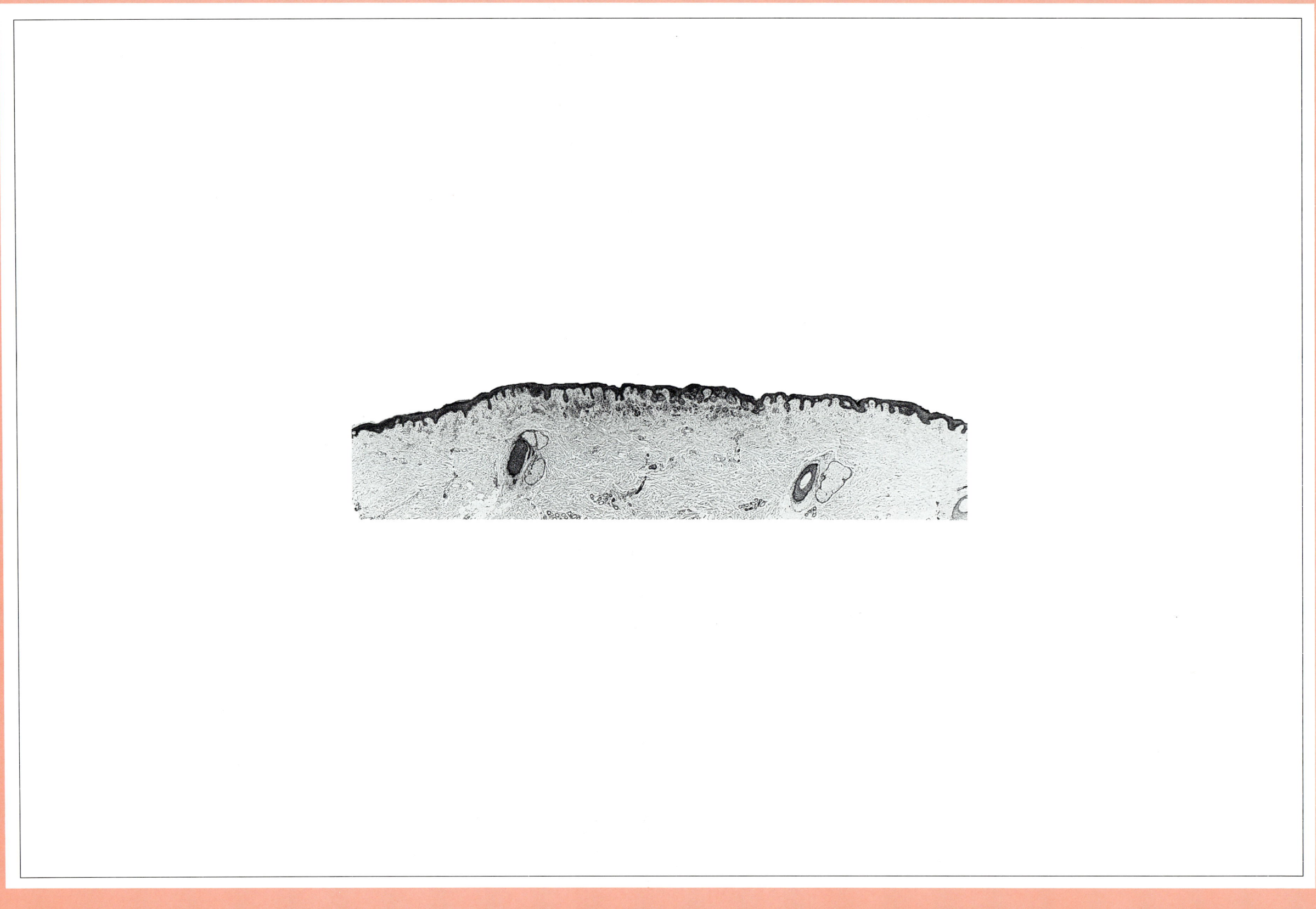

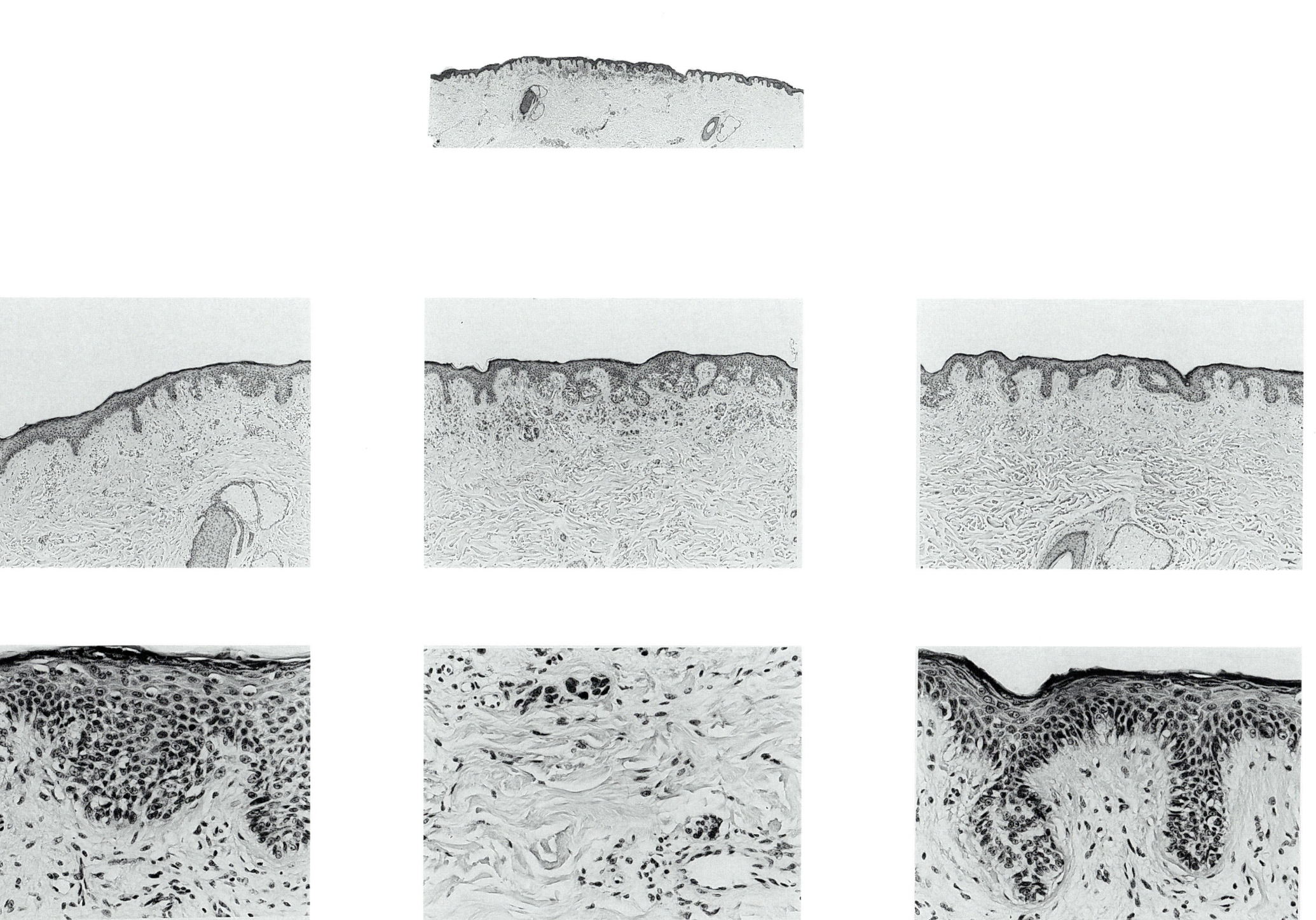

30. What is your diagnosis?

Pigmented lesion on the left forearm of 35-year-old man. Clinical diagnosis: regressed melanoma. One year after surgical excision, the patient was well.

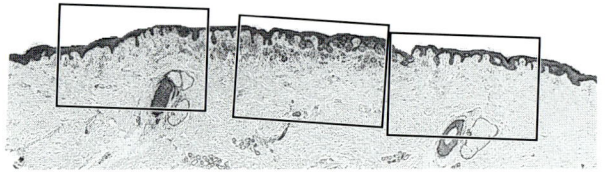

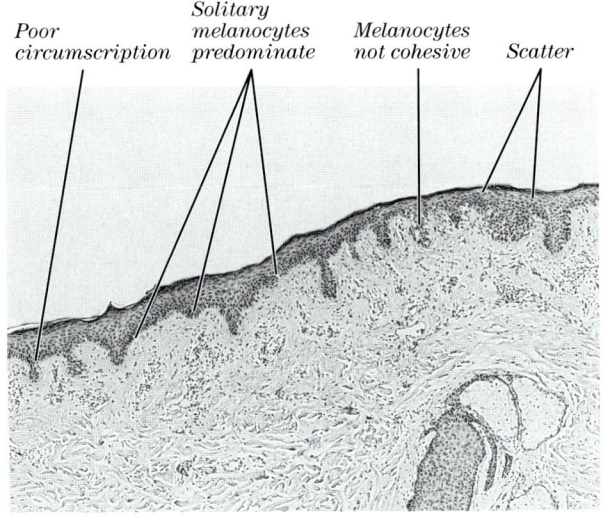

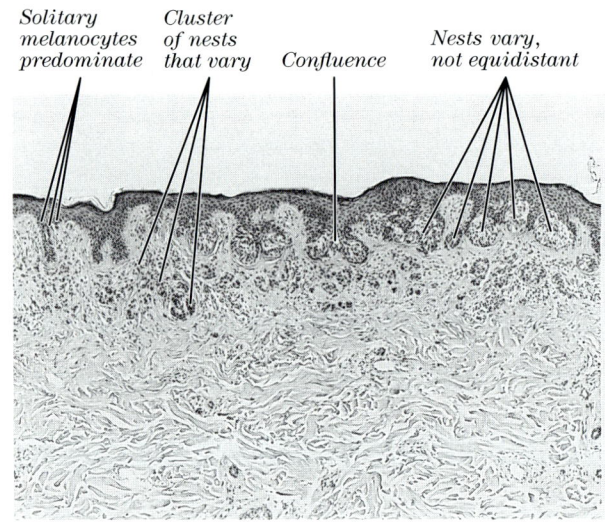

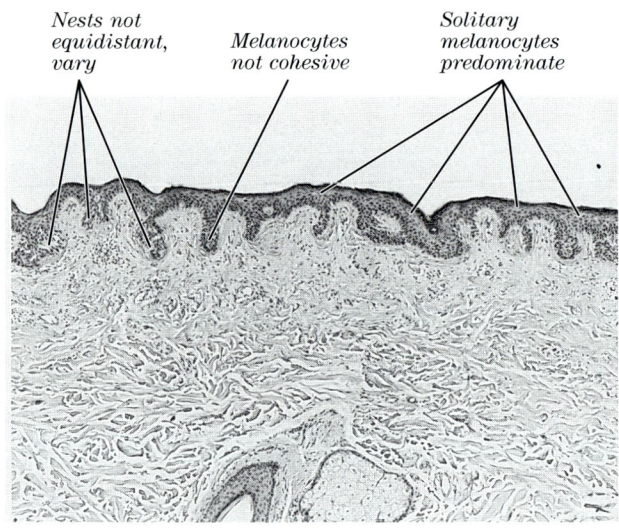

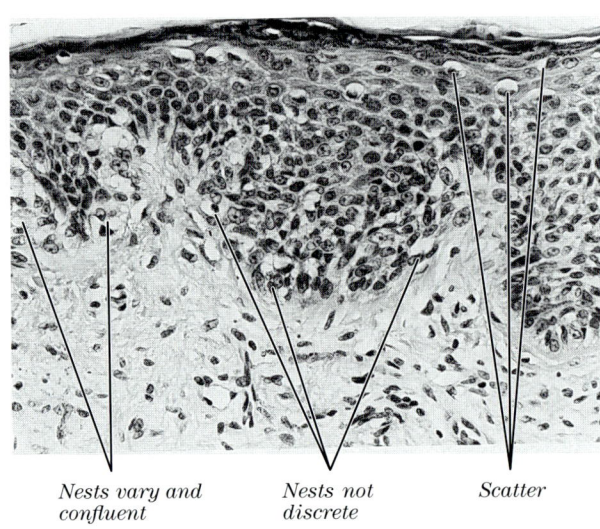

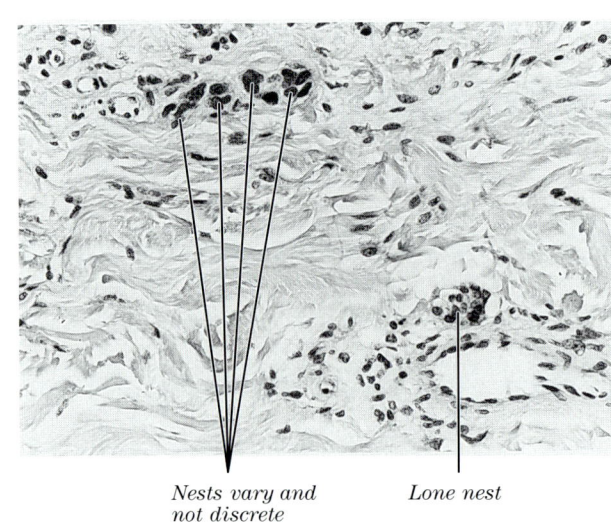

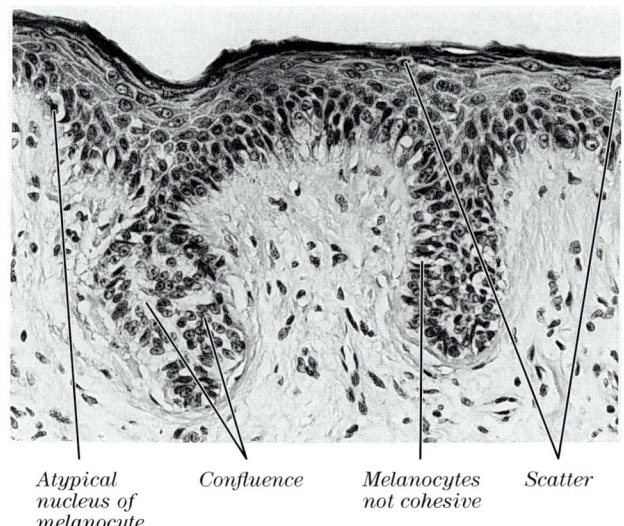

30 • Melanoma

Criteria for diagnosis of this melanoma

This is a melanoma because:

1. The neoplasm is poorly circumscribed.
2. Melanocytes disposed as solitary units, especially at the periphery, predominate over melanocytes arranged in nests.
3. Melanocytes are scattered at all levels of the epidermis, including the granular and cornified layers.
4. Nests of melanocytes, especially at the periphery, are not equidistant from one another.
5. Some nests of melanocytes have become confluent.
6. Melanocytes in some "nests" are not cohesive.
7. Melanin, especially within melanocytes in nests within the dermis, is not distributed in uniform fashion.

Pitfall in diagnosis

This melanoma could be misinterpreted as a compound type of Clark's nevus because:

1. The neoplasm is relatively symmetric.
2. Nests of melanocytes within the epidermis, especially in the center of the lesion, predominate over melanocytes arranged as solitary units.
3. Nests of melanocytes are situated mostly at the dermo-epidermal junction.
4. The neoplasm is slightly elevated in its center.
5. Nests of melanocytes are confined to the epidermis and thickened papillary dermis.

Although this neoplasm could be misinterpreted at scanning magnification as a compound Clark's nevus, scrutiny at higher magnifications reveals that it is not that nevus because, among other findings, melanocytes disposed as solitary units are scattered throughout the entire thickness of the epidermis. As a rule, melanocytes arranged both as solitary units and in nests within the epidermis of Clark's nevi are seated at the dermo-epidermal junction and not above it. If any melanocytes in that nevus are present above the junction, they are found only in the lower part of the spinous zone. When melanocytes are scattered in the upper reaches of the epidermis, as shown here, the lesion must be melanoma, at least in part, e.g., a melanoma in situ in association with a Clark's nevus. In this instance, however, the entire neoplasm is a melanoma.

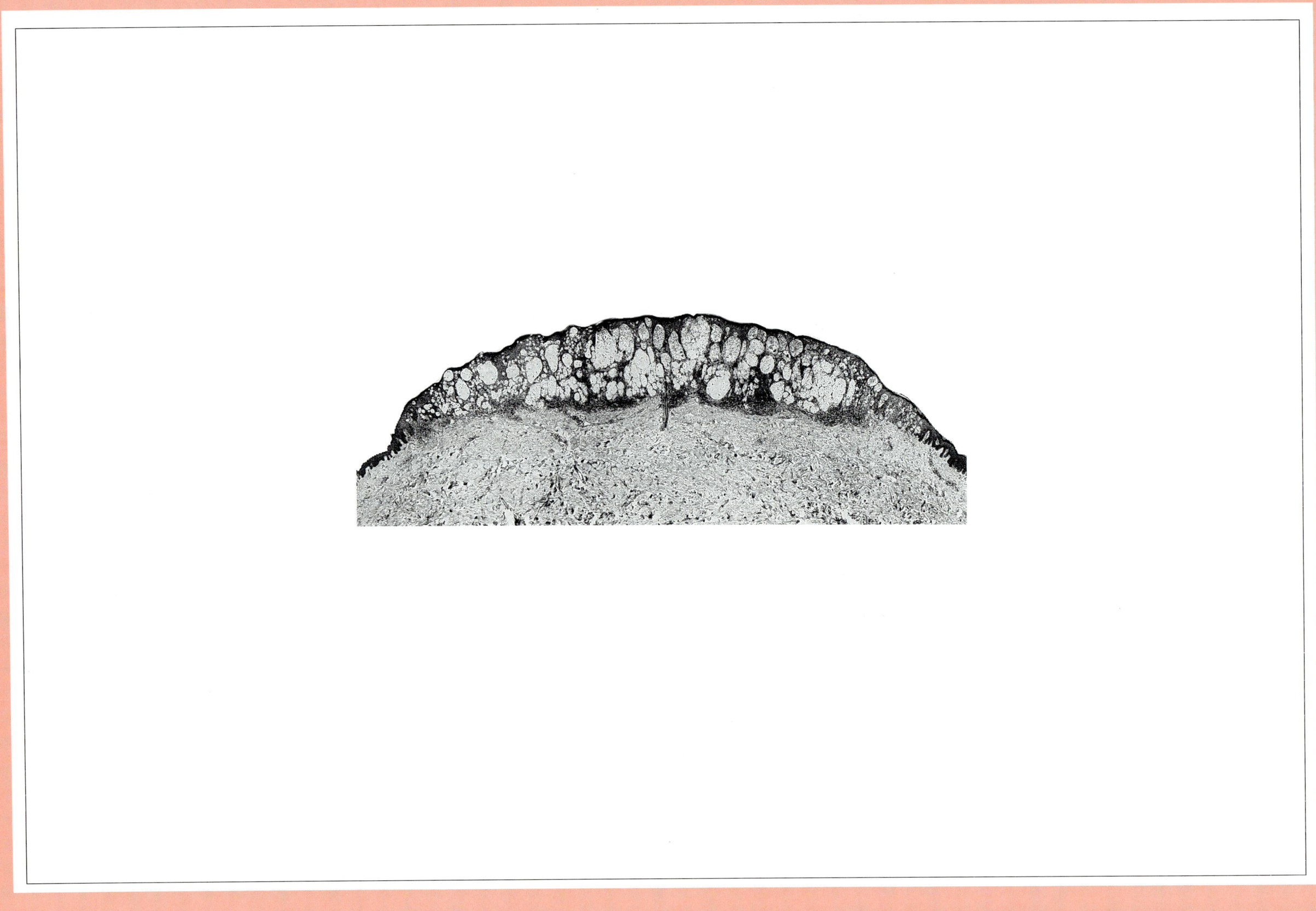

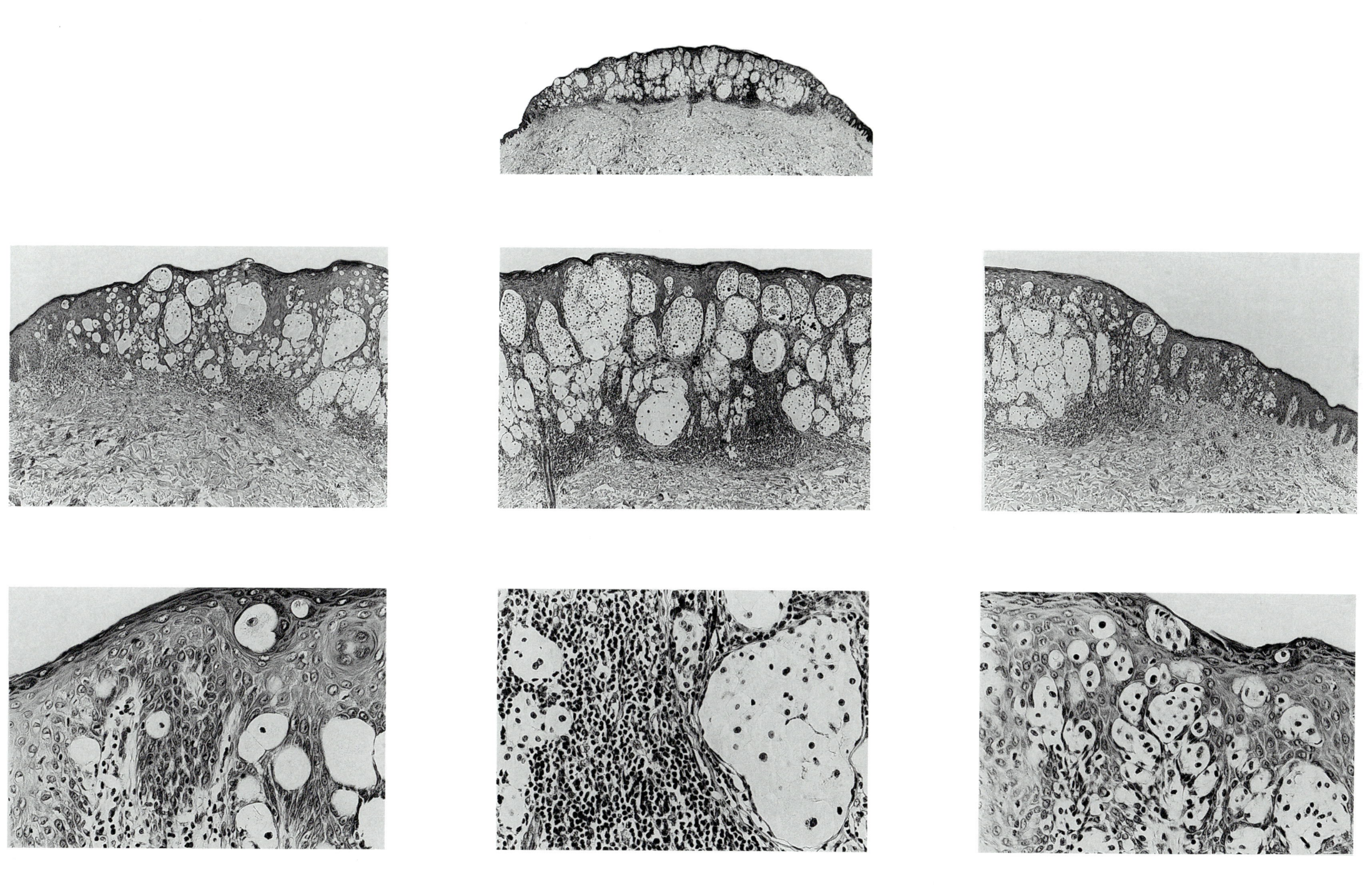

31. What is your diagnosis?

Lesion on the left thigh of a 43-year-old man present for years without any change. Clinical diagnosis: melanoma. Patient had no evidence of disease after 8 years.

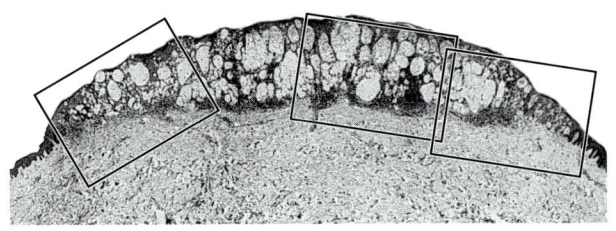

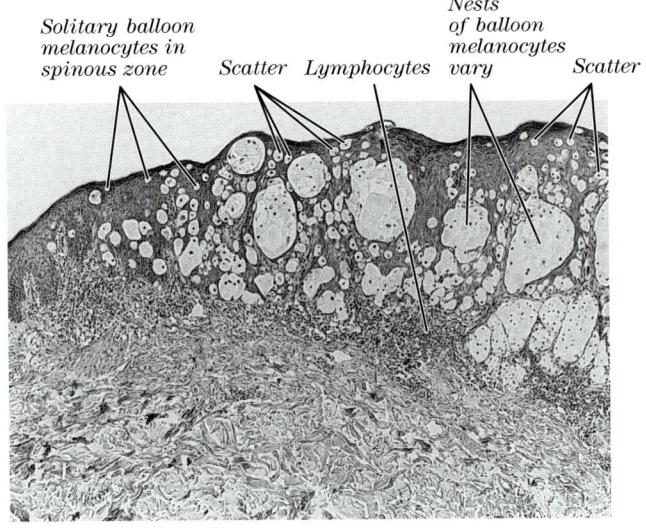

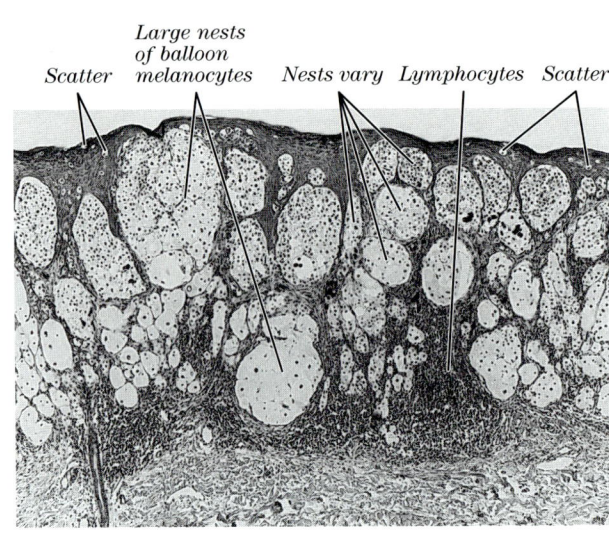

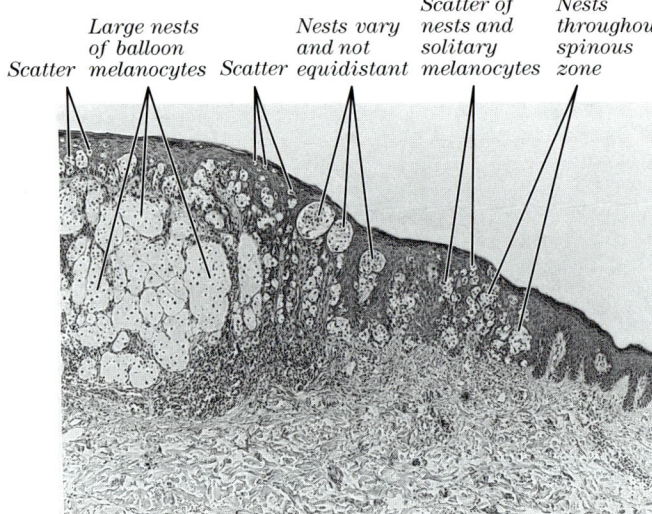

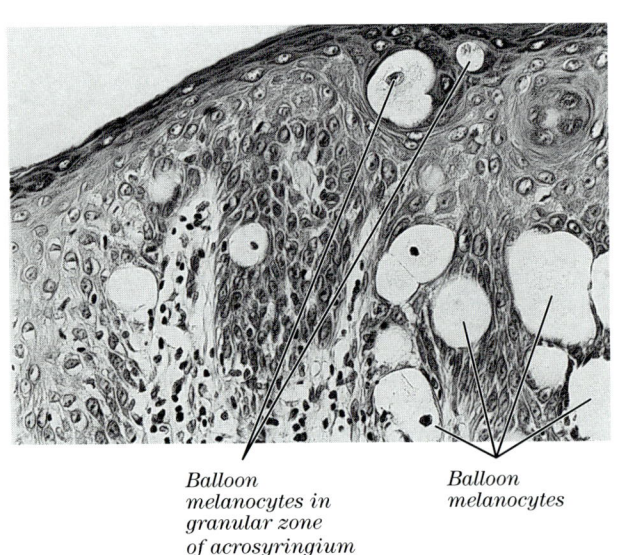

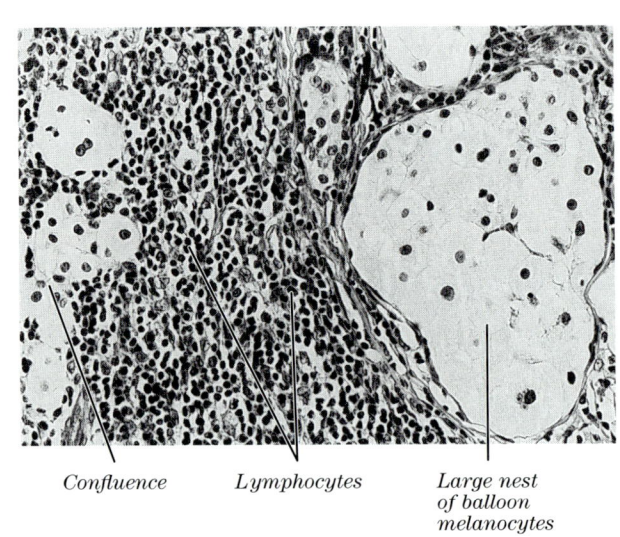

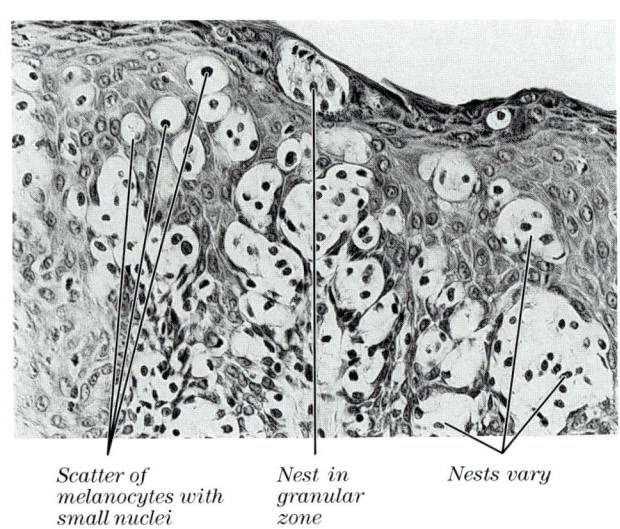

31 • Melanoma *(balloon-cell type)*

Criteria for diagnosis of this melanoma (balloon-cell type)

This is a melanoma because:

1. The lesion is asymmetric.
2. Circumscription is not sharp.
3. Variation in size and shape of nests of melanocytes is striking.
4. Some nests of melanocytes have become confluent.
5. Some nests of melanocytes have bizarre shapes.
6. Melanocytes are scattered at all levels of the epidermis.
7. Nests of melanocytes are not equidistant from one another.

Pitfall in diagnosis

This balloon-cell melanoma could be misinterpreted as a balloon-cell nevus because:

1. The lesion is confined to the epidermis and papillary dermis, as in a Clark's nevus.
2. Individual balloon cells are indistinguishable cytologically from those in a balloon-cell nevus, i.e., the nuclei are small and round, and the cytoplasm is strikingly abundant and pale or clear.
3. The base of the neoplasm is relatively flat.
4. There are hints of maturation.

This balloon-cell melanoma could be misinterpreted as a balloon-cell nevus because both are constituted, at least in part, of balloon melanocytes whose nuclei are not atypical, and both are domed and confined to the dermo-epidermal junction and thickened papillary dermis. The two neoplasms, however, are diametric in terms of architectural pattern. The nevus has the silhouette of a benign neoplasm, whereas the melanoma has that of a malignant one. The two should not be confused if heed is paid to those architectural features.

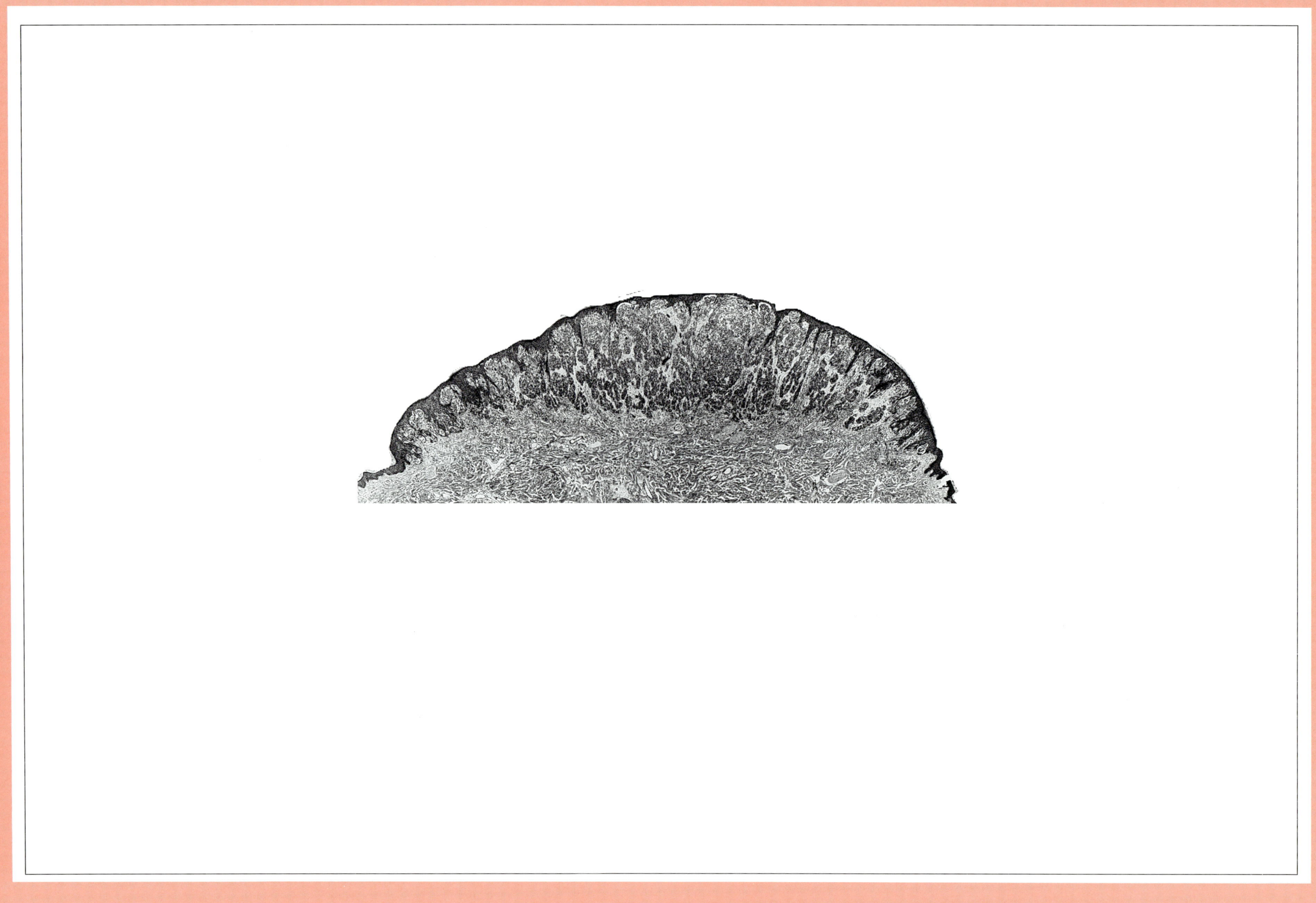

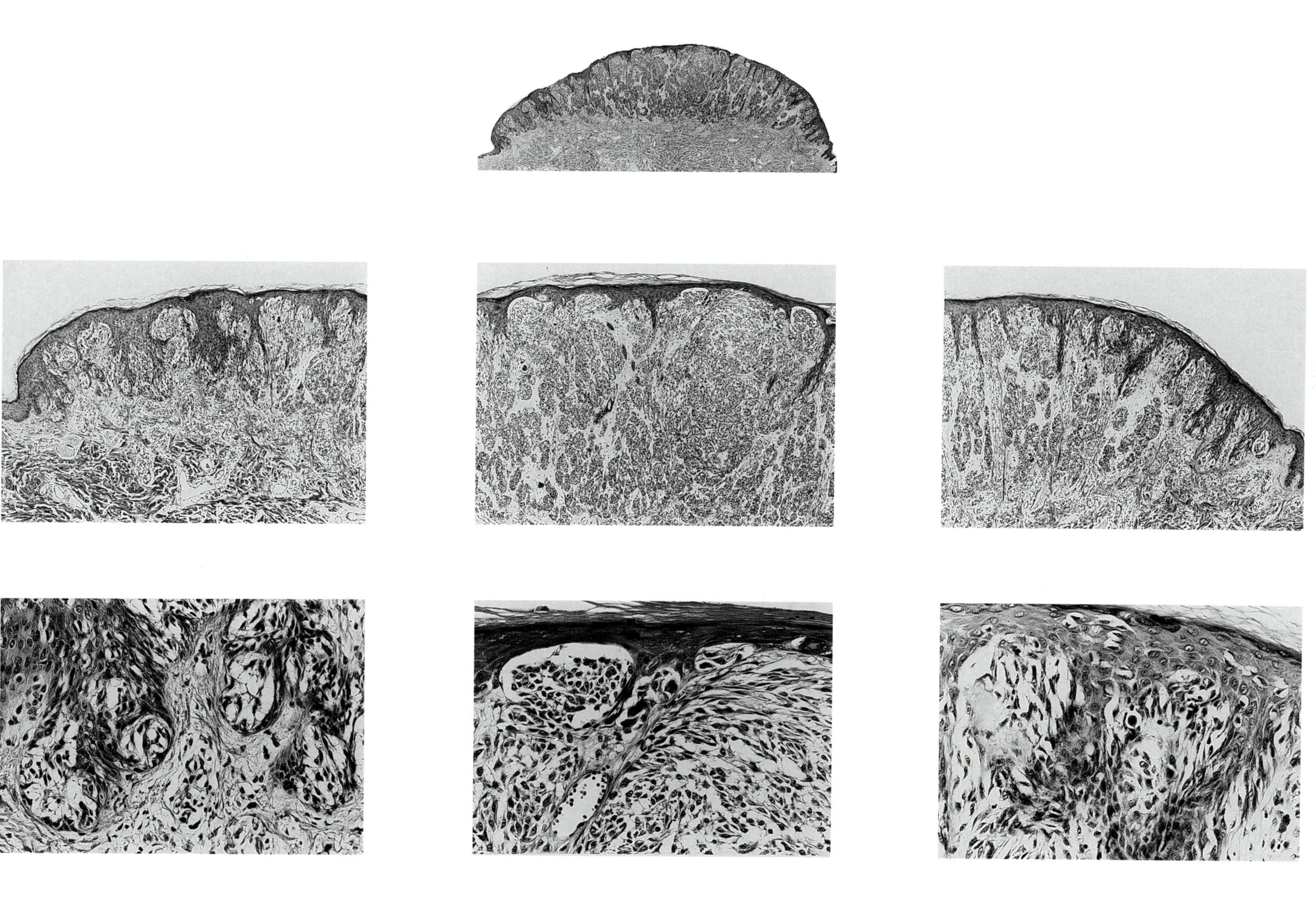

32. What is your diagnosis?

Dome-shaped red-brown lesion on the right buttock of a 20-year-old woman. Clinical diagnosis: nevus. The site was excised completely and the patient was free of disease after 4 years.

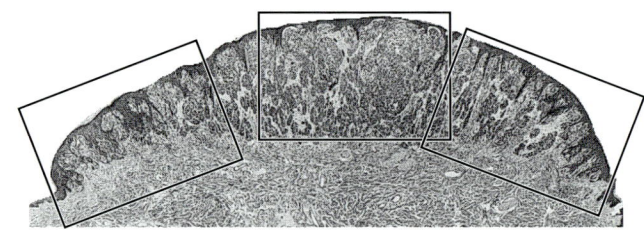

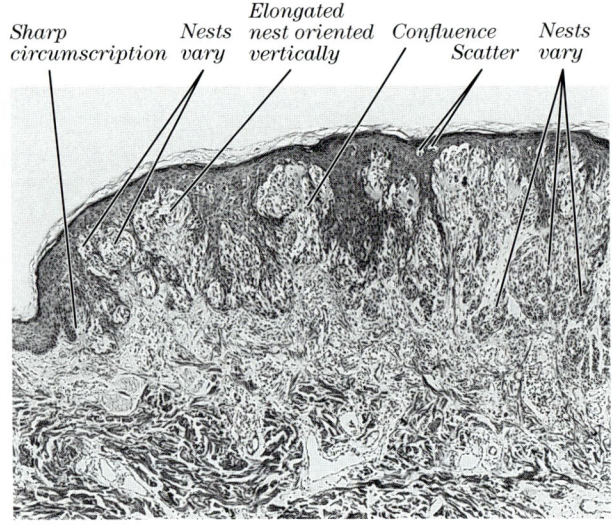

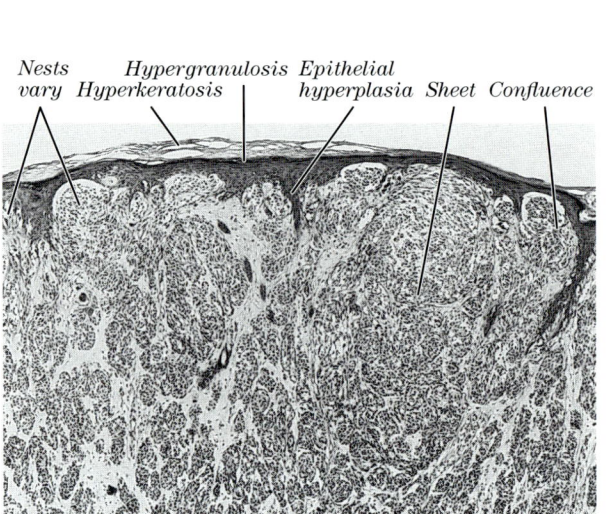

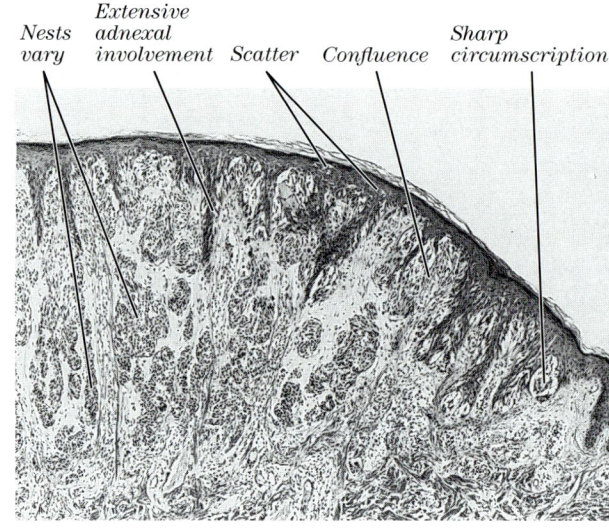

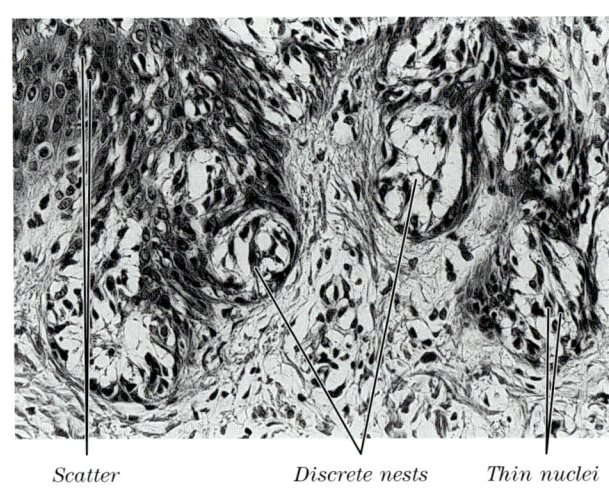

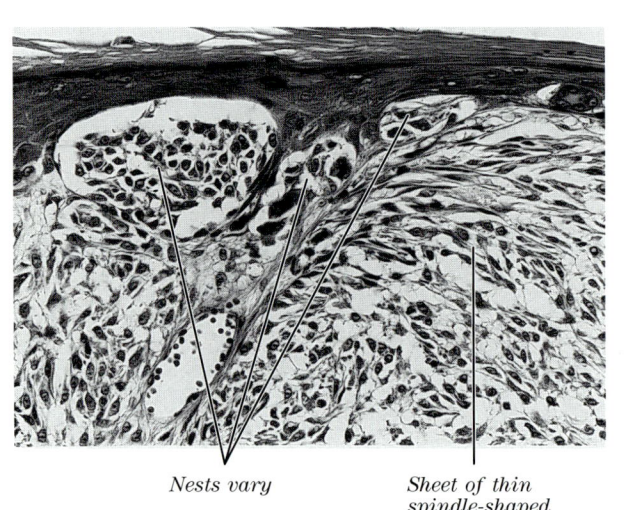

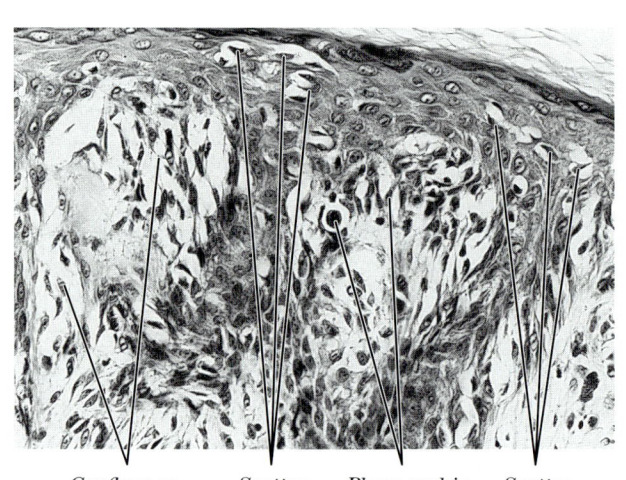

32 • Melanoma

Criteria for diagnosis of this melanoma

This is a melanoma because:

1. There is asymmetry.
2. Nests of melanocytes within the epidermis are not equidistant from one another.
3. Nests of melanocytes within the epidermis differ in size and shape.
4. Melanocytes in the upper reaches of the epidermis are disposed mostly as solitary units.
5. Nests of melanocytes within the dermis vary in size and shape.
6. Many nests of melanocytes within the dermis have become confluent to form sheets.
7. There is no distinct maturation of melanocytes.

Pitfall in diagnosis

This melanoma could be misconstrued as a compound Spitz's nevus because:

1. It is dome-shaped.
2. Its circumscription is sharp.
3. The base of the neoplasm is relatively flat.
4. Melanocytes within the epidermis are arranged mostly in nests.
5. The epidermis is irregularly hyperplastic.
6. Clefts have formed between some nests of melanocytes and adjacent keratinocytes.
7. Some elongated nests of melanocytes are perpendicular to the skin surface.

At scanning magnification, it is apparent that the differential diagnosis is between Spitz's nevus and melanoma. It also is obvious that the neoplasm is asymmetric, many more neoplastic melanocytes being present on the right side than on the left side. Also at scanning magnification, it can be appreciated that nests of melanocytes within the dermis have become confluent to form sheets. These two findings, noticeable at scanning magnification, are indispensable for differentiation of this melanoma from a Spitz's nevus. In some high-power fields, especially in the upper part of the dermis at the periphery of the lesion, differentiation between the two neoplasms is nearly impossible.

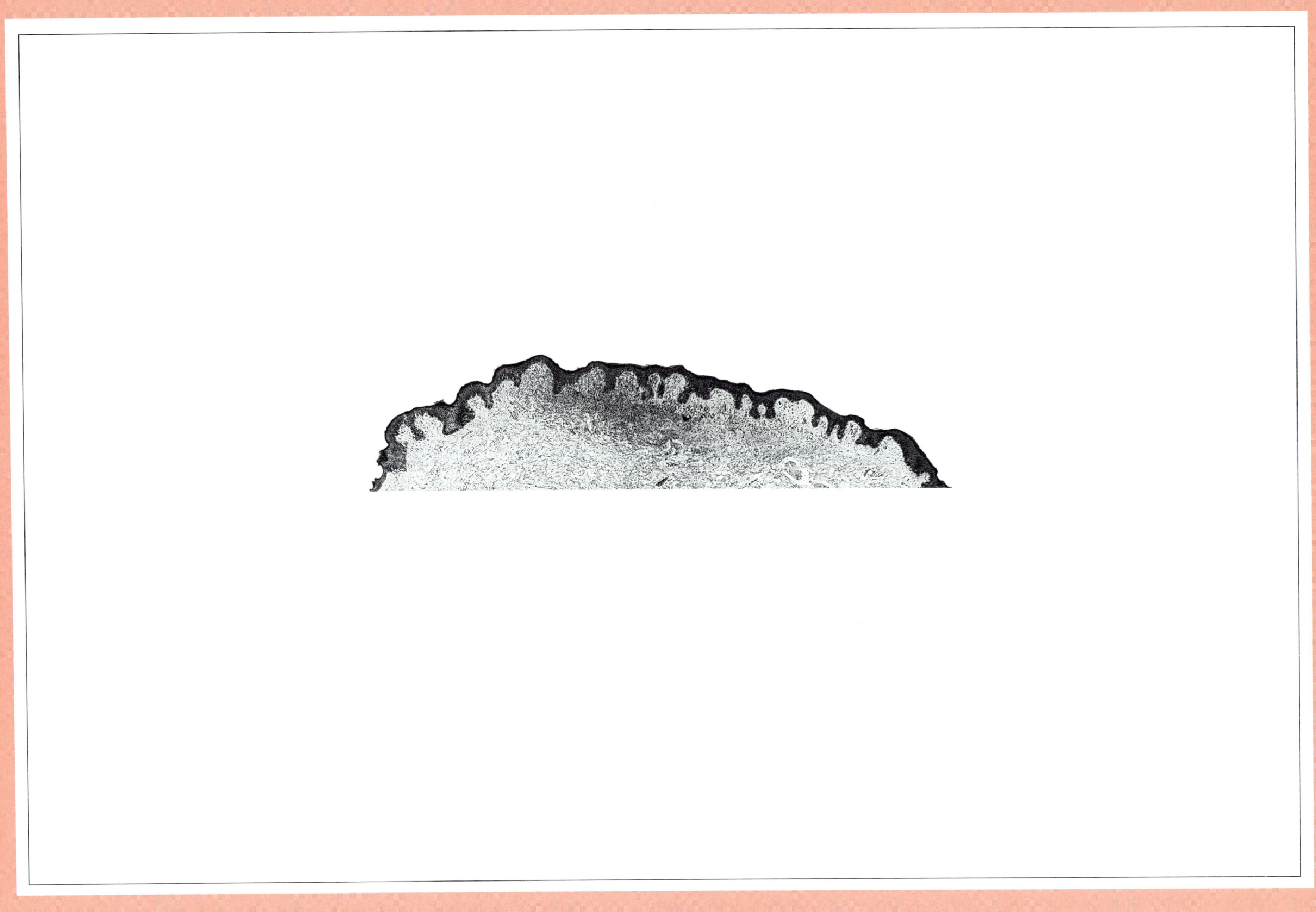

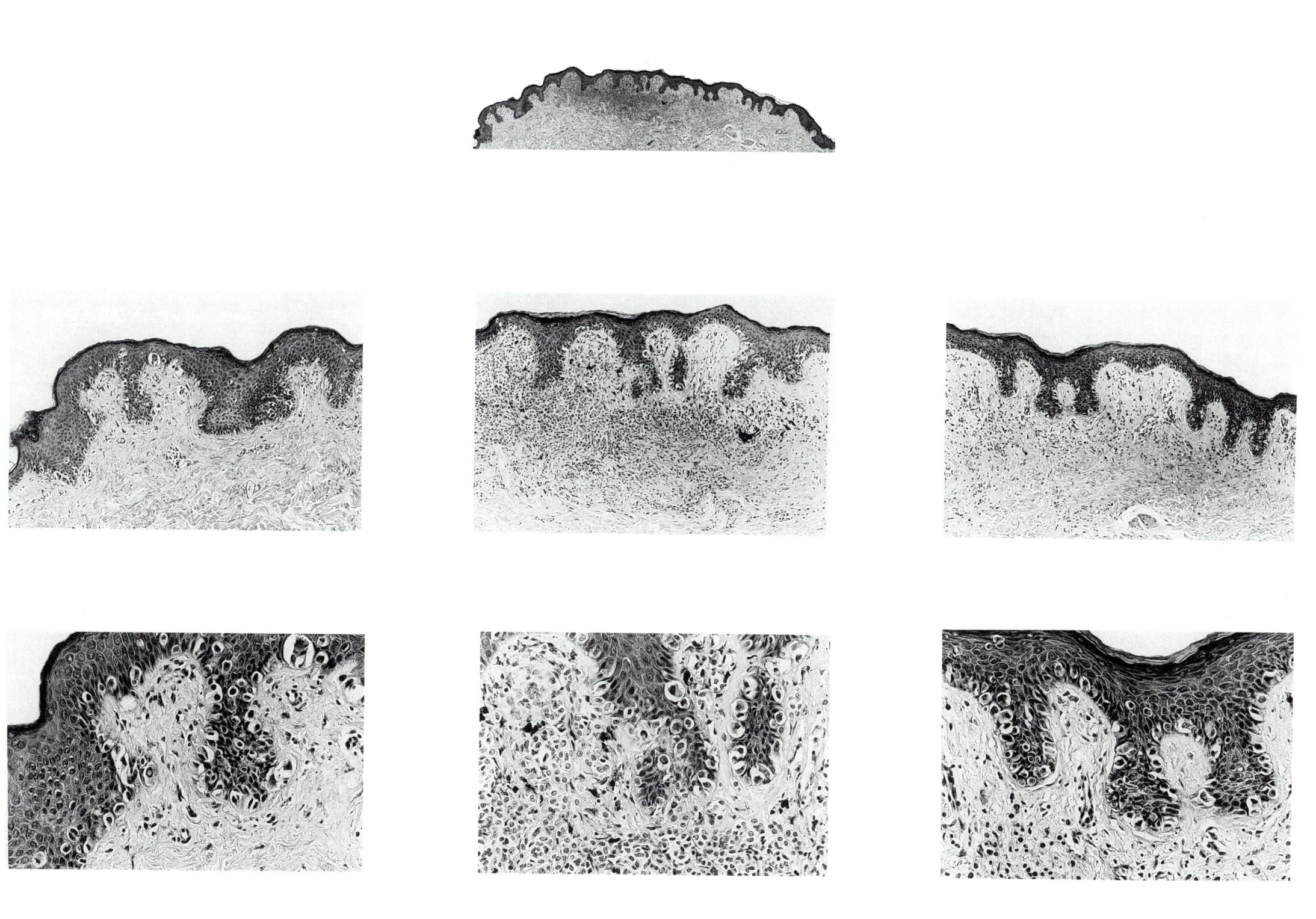

33. What is your diagnosis?

Lesion on the left arm of a 42-year-old woman. The lesion was excised completely. Patient had no evidence of disease after 1 year.

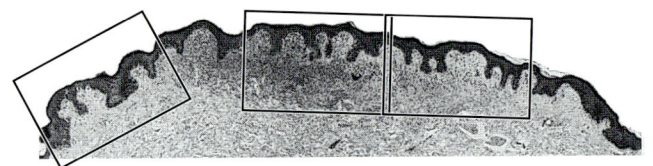

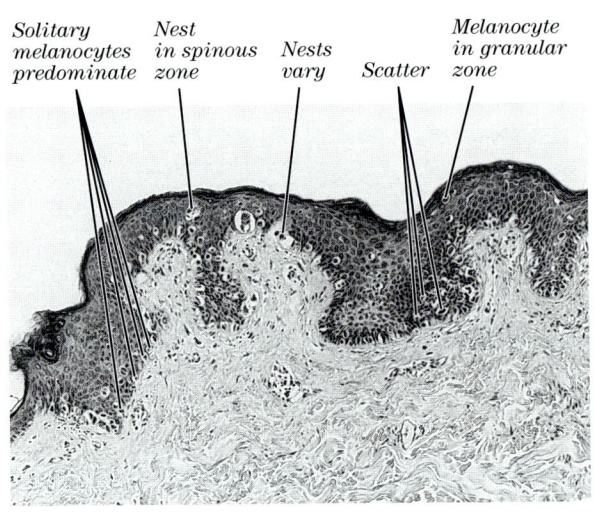
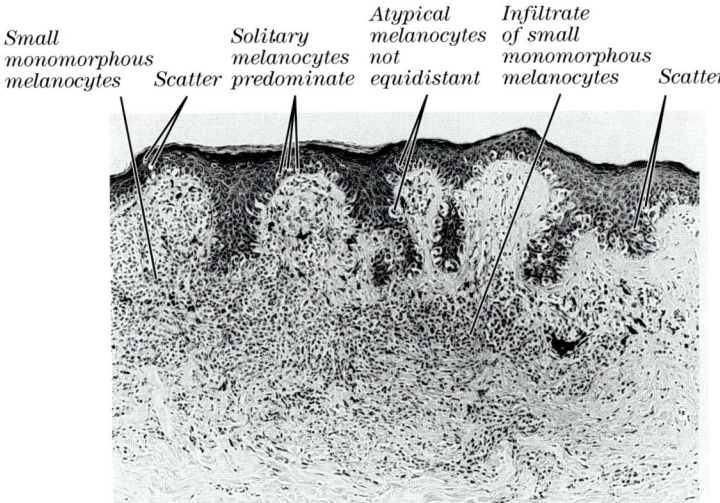
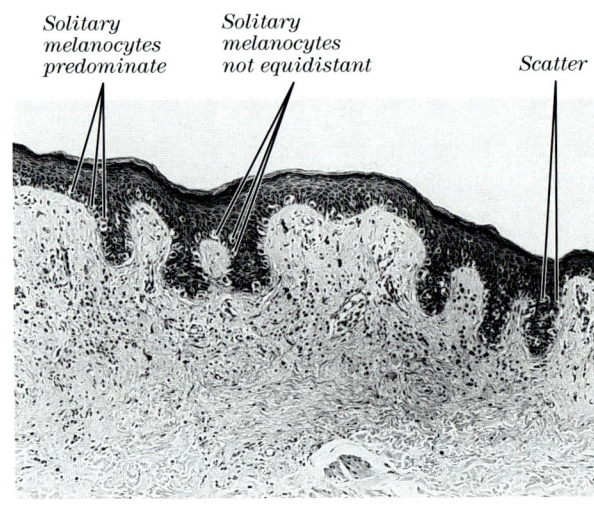
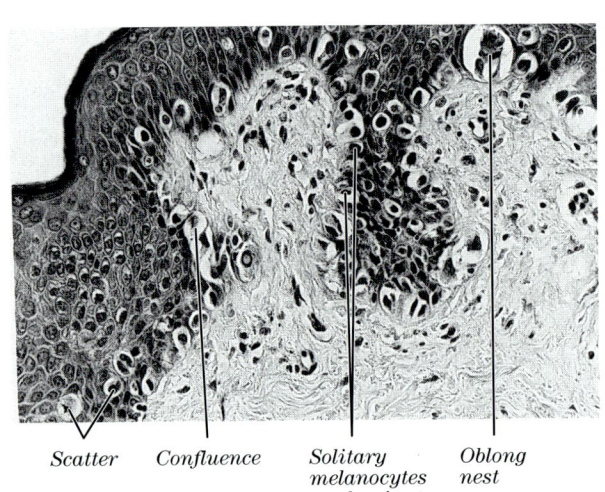
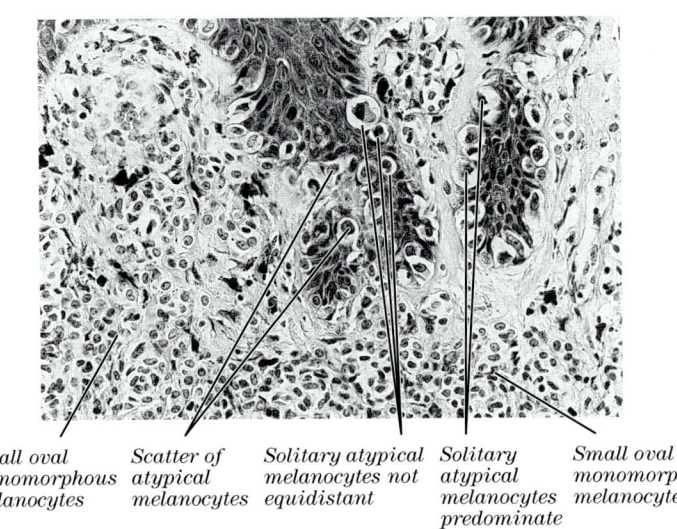
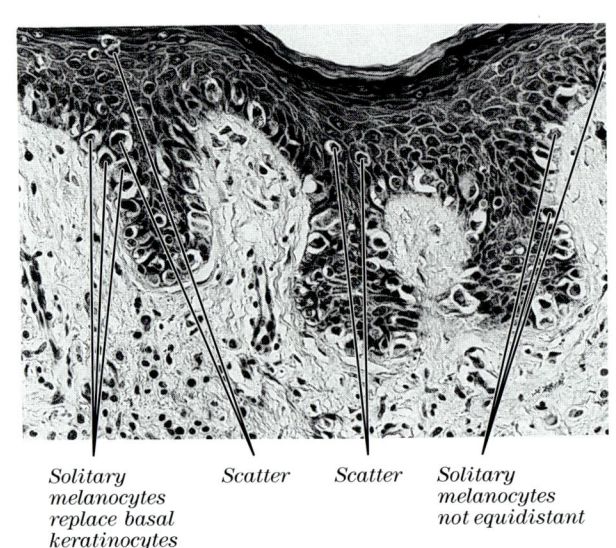

398   33 • Melanoma in situ and Clark's Nevus

Criteria for diagnosis of this melanoma in situ above a Clark's nevus (intradermal type)

This is a melanoma because:

1. Melanocytes within the epidermis are not positioned entirely at the dermo-epidermal junction, but far above it in the spinous and granular zones.//
2. Melanocytes disposed as solitary units within the epidermis are not equidistant from one another.
3. Small nests of melanocytes within the epidermis are not equidistant from one another.
4. Nuclear atypia of melanocytes within the epidermis is striking.
5. Many pagetoid melanocytes are seen within the epidermis.
6. Some solitary melanocytes within the epidermis have become confluent.
7. Cytologic aspects of intra-epidermal melanocytes differ from those in the dermis, to wit, atypical in the epidermis, but not in the dermis.

Pitfall in diagnosis

This melanoma in situ in association with an intradermal Clark's nevus could be misinterpreted as a compound Clark's nevus because:

1. It is small (less than 4.0 mm in greatest diameter).
2. It is symmetric.
3. An intradermal nevus is present in the center of the lesion.
4. The junctional component of the neoplasm extends beyond the intradermal component of the neoplasm.
5. Most melanocytes in the "shoulder" are situated at the dermo-epidermal junction.
6. An increased number of melanocytes arranged as solitary units are present mostly within elongated, hyperpigmented rete ridges in the "shoulder."
7. Nests of melanocytes are connected at the bases of some rete ridges.
8. Hints of both "concentric" and "lamellar" fibroplasia can be noted in the papillary dermis.
9. Telangiectases, scattered lymphocytes, and melanophages are housed in the papillary dermis.

When a melanoma in situ occurs above an intradermal nevus, as above the Clark's nevus pictured, the entire lesion could be misconstrued as either a melanoma or a nevus. When the changes in the epidermis are assessed alone, such as in this example, they are seen to fulfill criteria for melanoma in situ. When the findings in the thickened papillary dermis are scrutinized alone, they can be seen to fulfill criteria for an intradermal nevus. The conclusion, therefore, is that in this section, a melanoma in situ is present in association with an intradermal Clark's nevus.

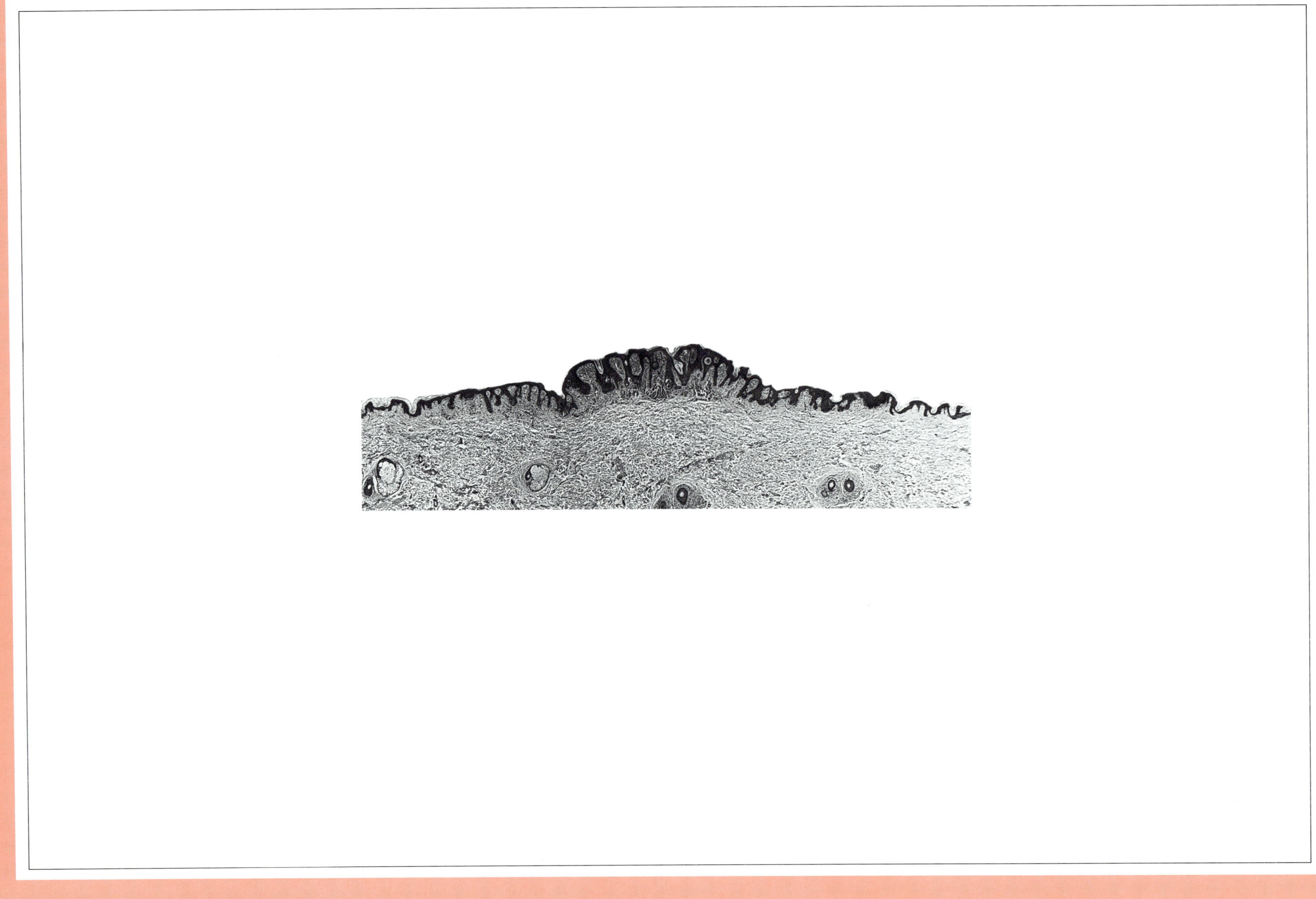

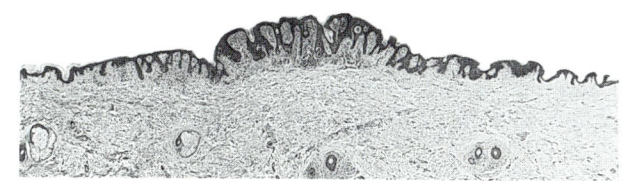
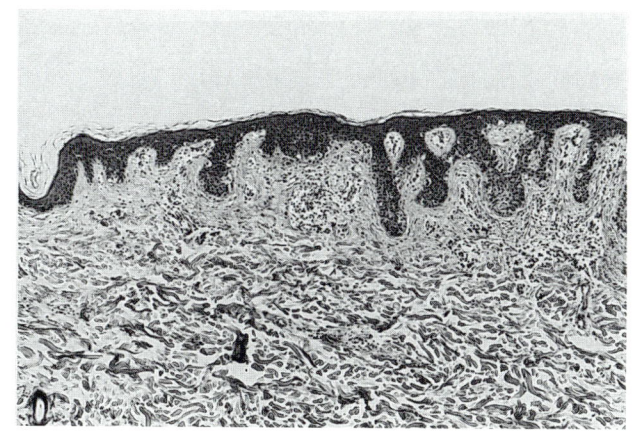
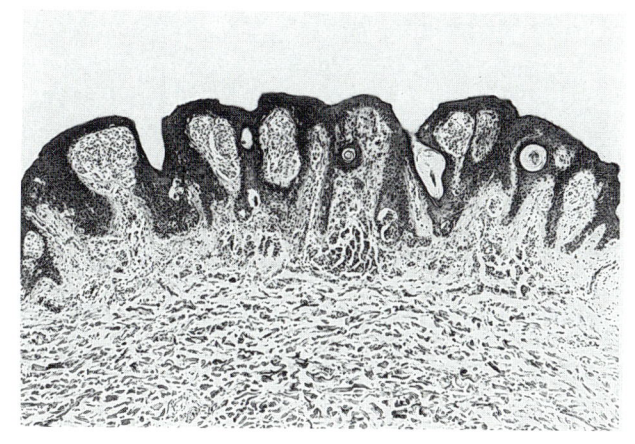
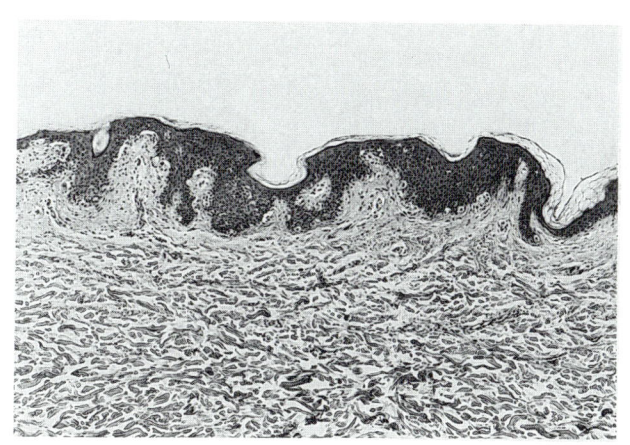
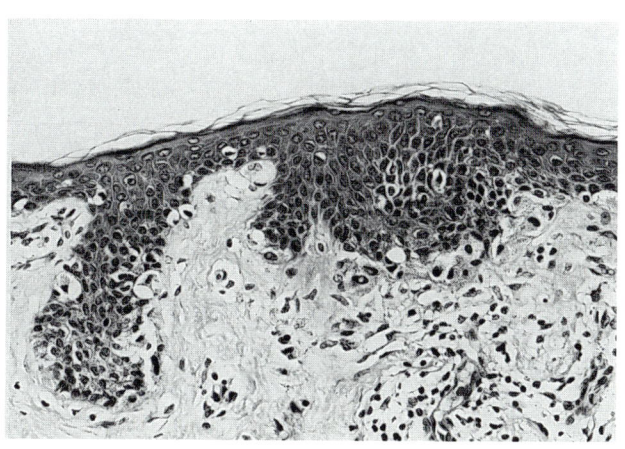
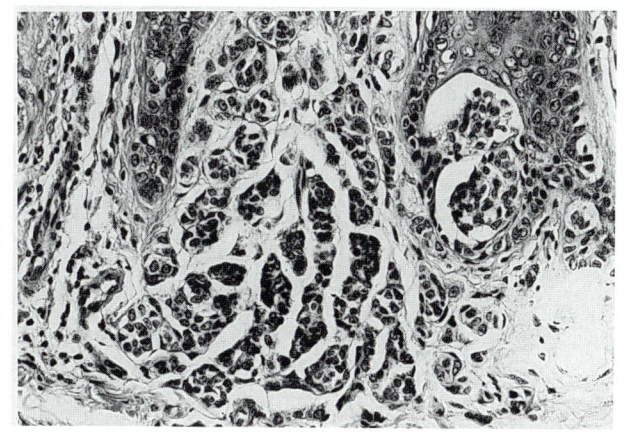
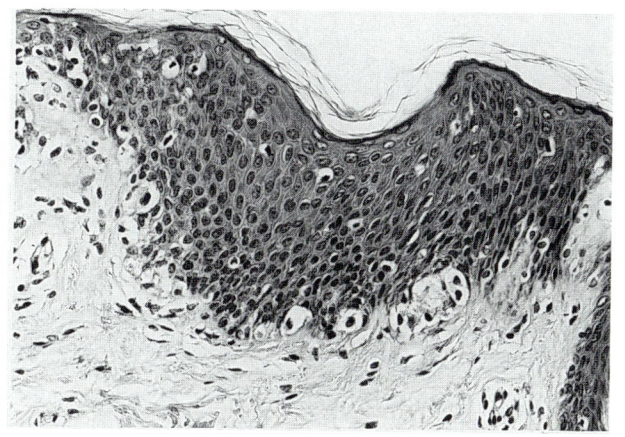

34. What is your diagnosis?

Lesion on the midchest of a 31-year-old woman. Clinical diagnosis: B-K mole. The site was excised completely. The patient was lost to follow-up after 1 year.

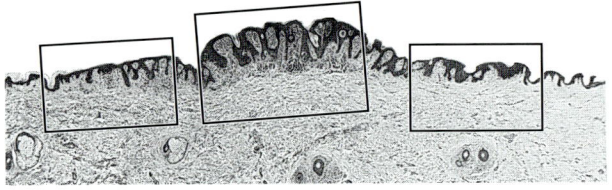

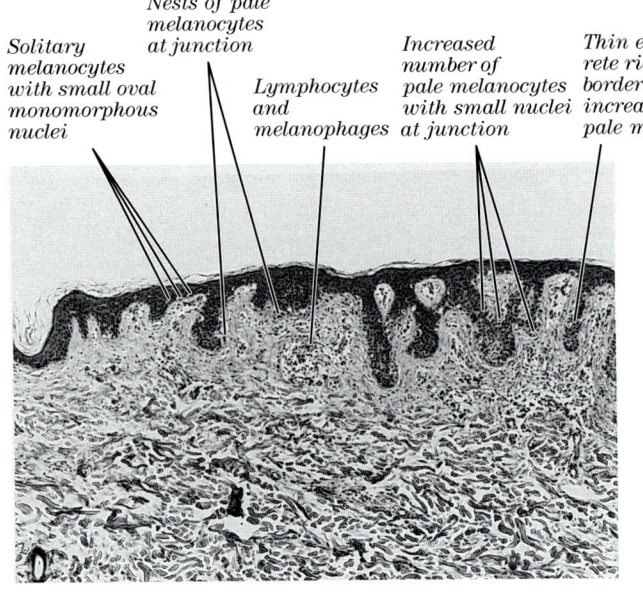

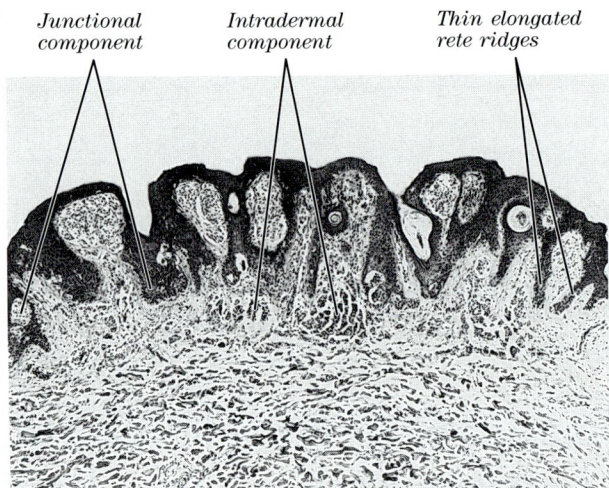

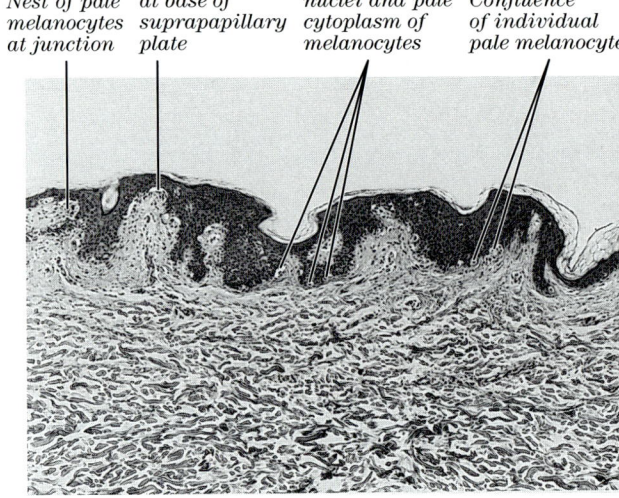

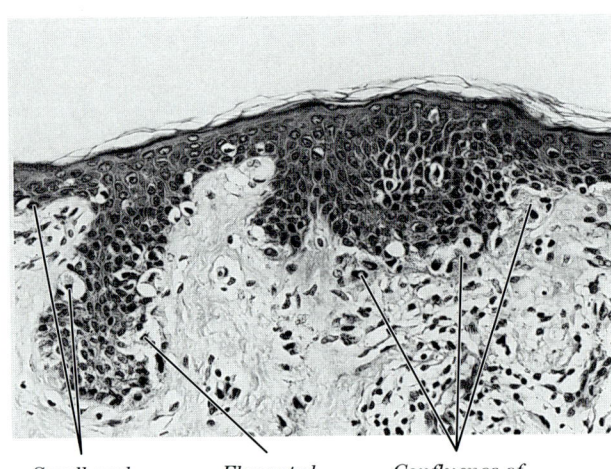

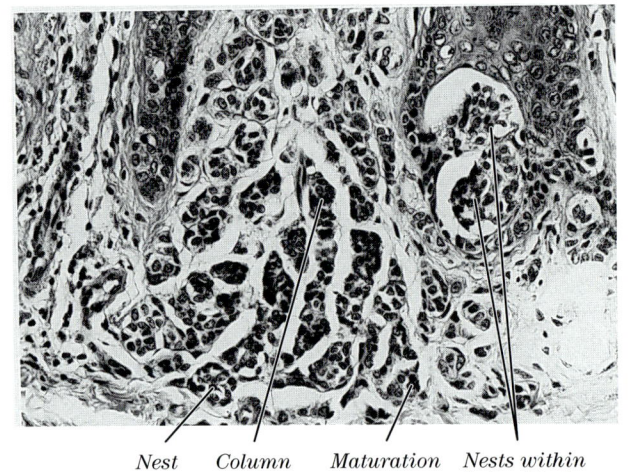

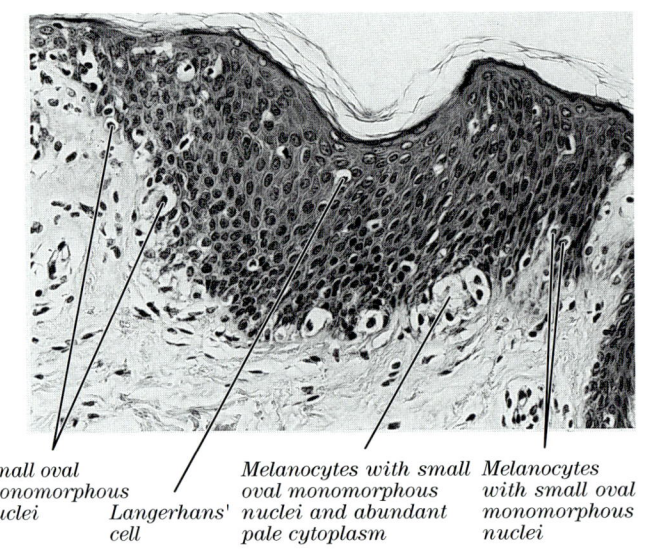

34 • Clark's Nevus

Criteria for diagnosis of this Clark's nevus (compound type)

This is a nevus because:

1. The neoplasm is symmetric.
2. It is rather well-circumscribed.
3. Melanocytes mature slightly.
4. Virtually all of the melanocytes, both those disposed as solitary units and those in nests, are situated at the dermo-epidermal junction, not above it.
5. Nuclei of melanocytes are relatively monomorphous.

This is a Clark's nevus because:

1. The lesion is slightly elevated and mammillated in its center.
2. Melanocytes arranged as solitary units and in nests are confined almost entirely to the dermo-epidermal junction and thickened papillary dermis.
3. The junctional component of the nevus extends beyond the intradermal component, i.e., there are "shoulders."
4. Melanocytes at the "shoulders" have small, oval, monomorphous nuclei and abundant pale cytoplasm.

Pitfall in diagnosis

This compound Clark's nevus could be misinterpreted as melanoma in situ (or some variation on the theme of "dysplasia") in association with a nevus because:

1. Pagetoid melanocytes are present at the "shoulders" of the lesion.
2. Pagetoid melanocytes are not equidistant from one another, and some have become confluent, thereby forming elongated nests.
3. Langerhans' cells, present as solitary units in the upper part of the spinous zone, may be interpreted incorrectly as "high level melanocytes."

The changes in the "shoulders" of this compound Clark's nevus are expected findings in that nevus. This interpretation results from equating pagetoid melanocytes with pagetoid melanoma (they are unrelated), from assuming that extension of the junctional component of the nevus beyond the intradermal component of it implies transformation into melanoma (it does not), and from designating as "dysplastic" changes that do not conform to conventional notions of a nevus (the concept of dysplasia has no place in diagnostic dermatopathology). Other faulty concepts that could lead to misdiagnosis of this nevus as a melanoma are "architectural atypia" and "cytoplasmic atypia." There is only one atypia in classic histopathology and that is nuclear atypia, of which there is none in this or hardly any other Clark's nevus. In conclusion, the entire neoplasm shown here is a stereotypical Clark's nevus.

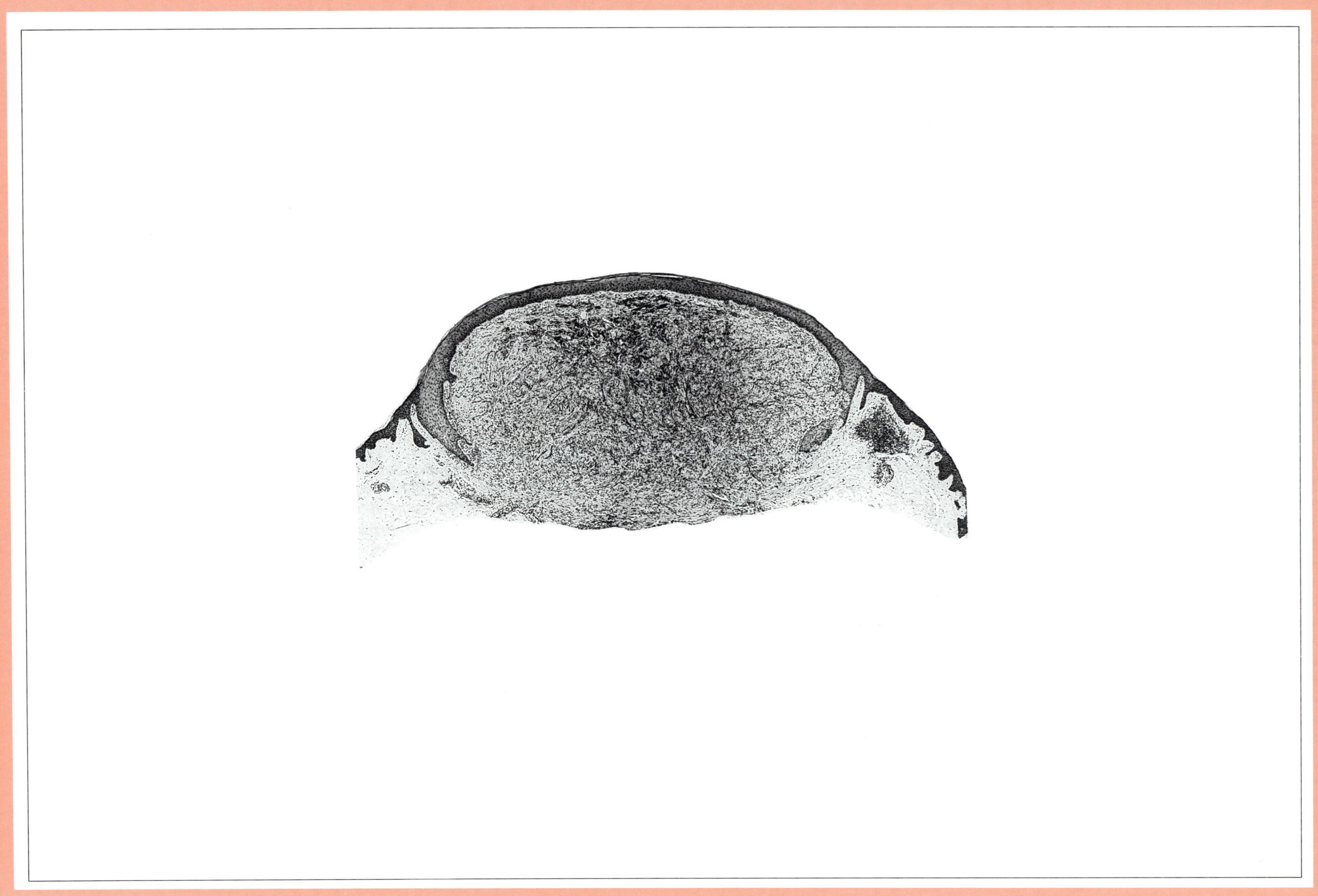

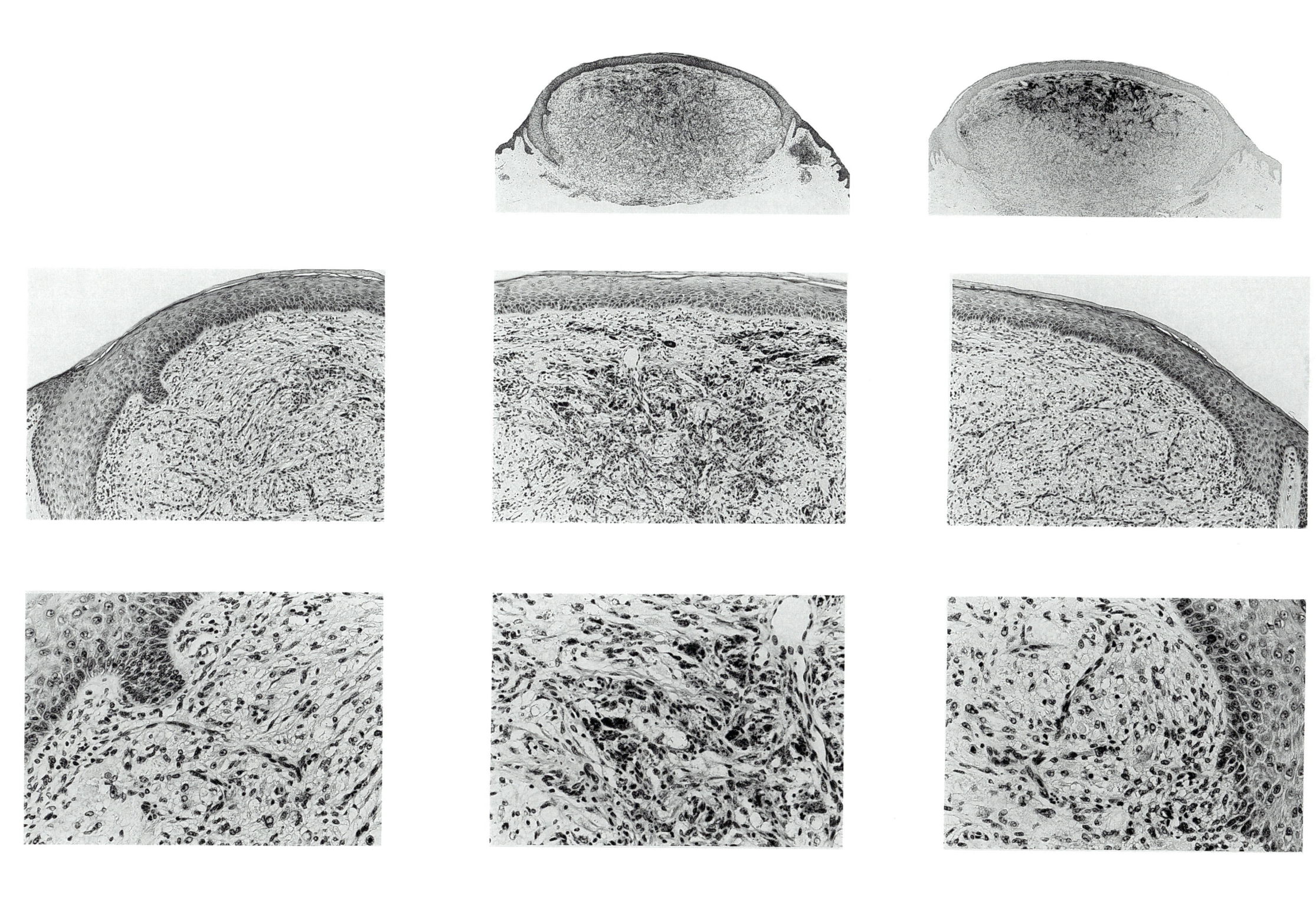

35. What is your diagnosis?

Pigmented lesion on the right shoulder of a 31-year-old man. Clinical diagnosis: angioma vs. atypical nevus. Patient had no evidence of disease after more than 1 year.

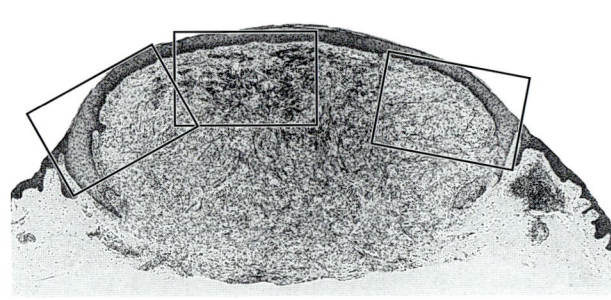

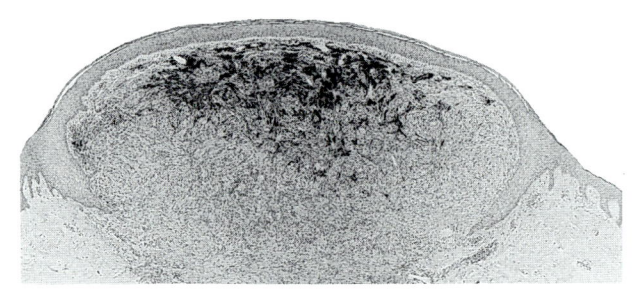
Perls' stain

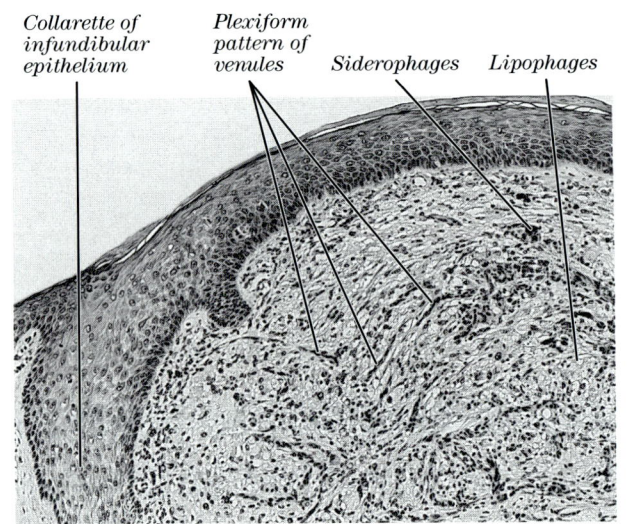
Collarette of infundibular epithelium — *Plexiform pattern of venules* — *Siderophages* — *Lipophages*

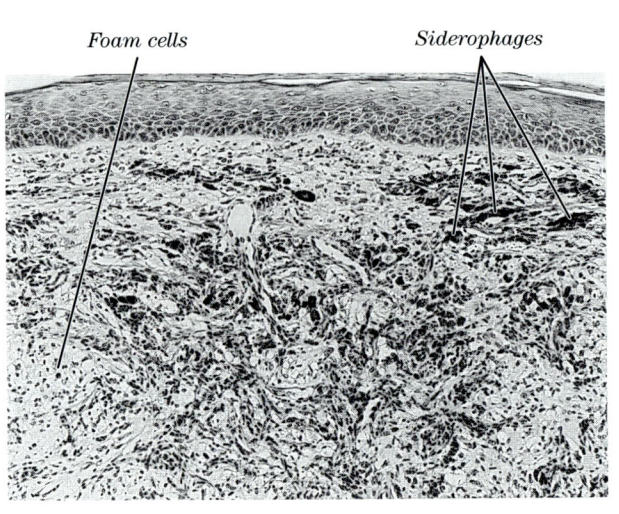
Foam cells — *Siderophages*

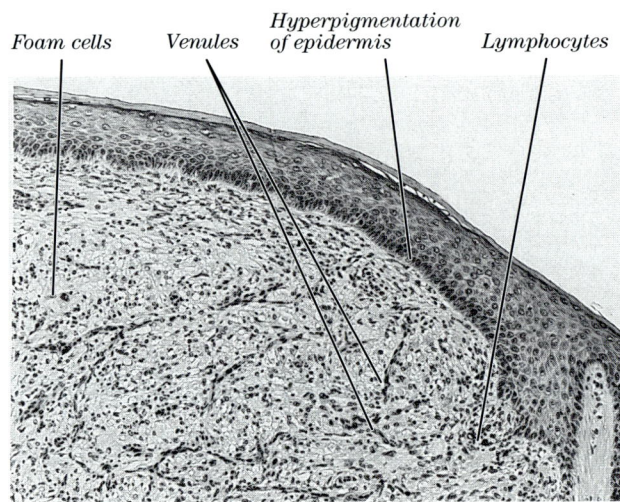
Foam cells — *Venules* — *Hyperpigmentation of epidermis* — *Lymphocytes*

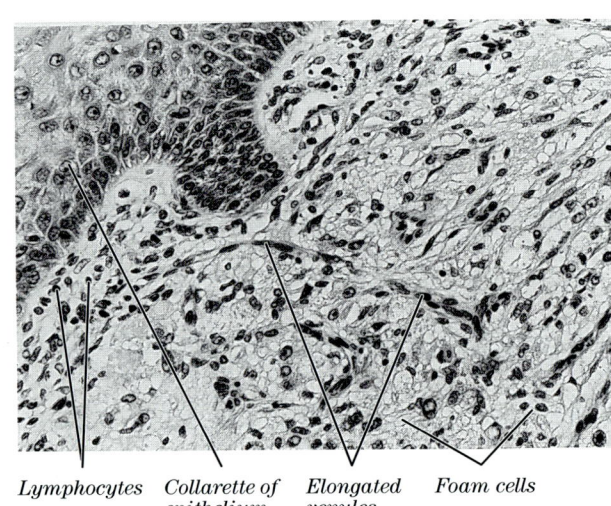
Lymphocytes — *Collarette of epithelium* — *Elongated venules* — *Foam cells*

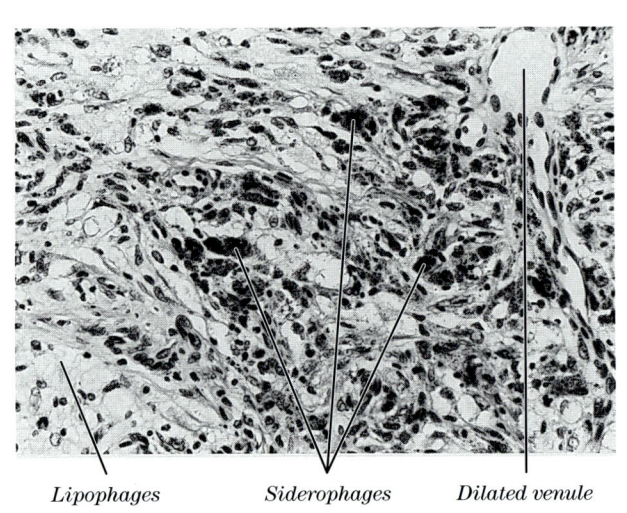
Lipophages — *Siderophages* — *Dilated venule*

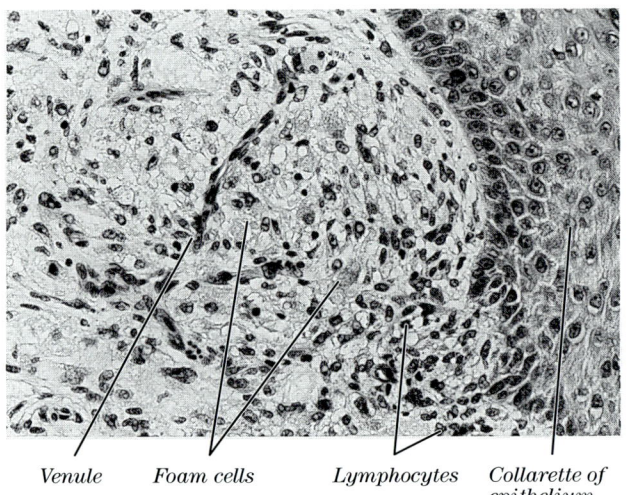
Venule — *Foam cells* — *Lymphocytes* — *Collarette of epithelium*

35 • Dermatofibroma

Criteria for diagnosis of this dermatofibroma

This is a dermatofibroma because:

1. The infiltrate consists mostly of foam cells.

2. The vasculature is striking with numerous venules lined by plump endothelial cells arranged in linear fashion.

Pitfall in diagnosis

This dermatofibroma could be misinterpreted as a metastasis of melanoma because:

1. Abundant, brown, granular pigment is present throughout the lesion (but in sections stained by hematoxylin and eosin, that pigment has a refractile quality and is golden brown).

2. Collarettes of adnexal epithelium embrace the infiltrate partially.

3. The lesion is slightly asymmetric, being associated with a nodular infiltrate of lymphocytes on the right, but not on the left.

Note the scanning photomicrograph on upper right. It is a Perls' stain that reveals abundant hemosiderin.

This lesion demonstrates how cytologic features can confound a histopathologist. The architectural pattern is of a benign condition (it even is an inflammatory, rather than a neoplastic process), but the abundant brown granular pigment scattered randomly within it could be misperceived as melanin and the lesion misinterpreted as a metastasis of melanoma. Abundant brown granular pigment in the skin is not always melanin!

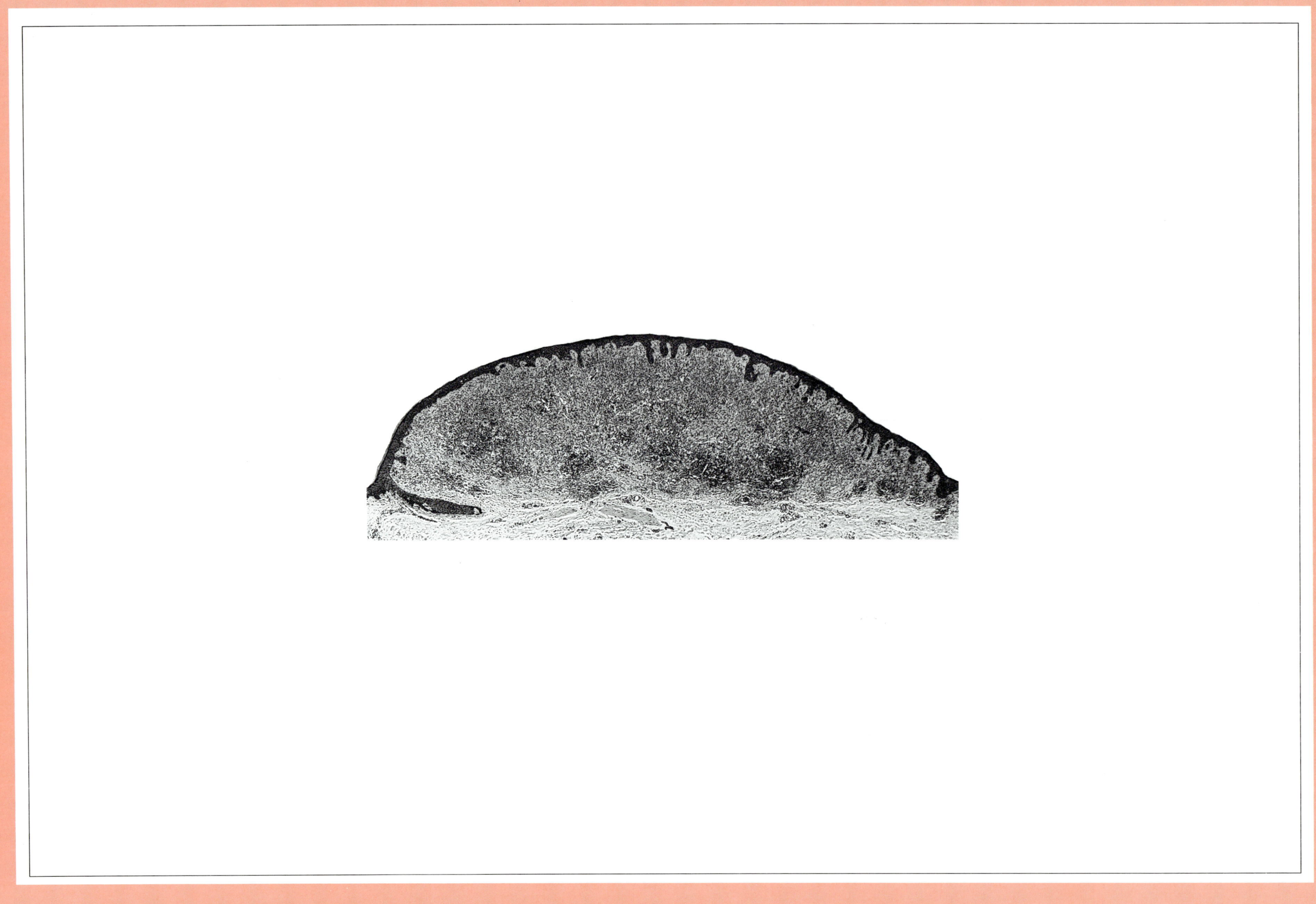

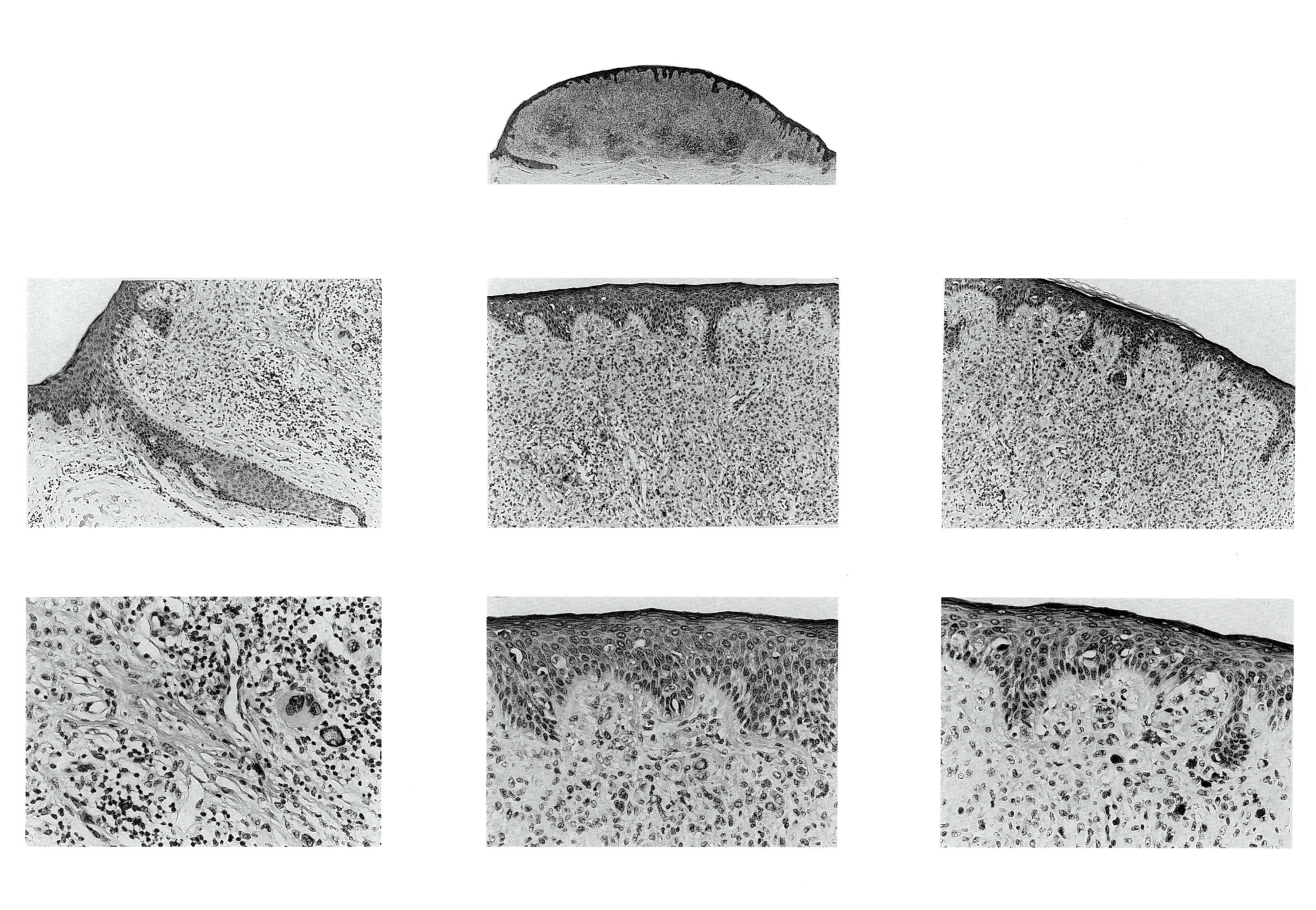

36. What is your diagnosis?

Blue-brown smooth-surfaced lesion from the right anterior thigh of a 47-year-old woman became elevated. Clinical diagnosis: nevus. Histopathologic examination of a wide excision of the site revealed a scar only. Patient was in good health 6 years later.

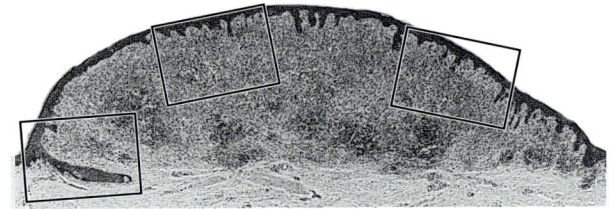

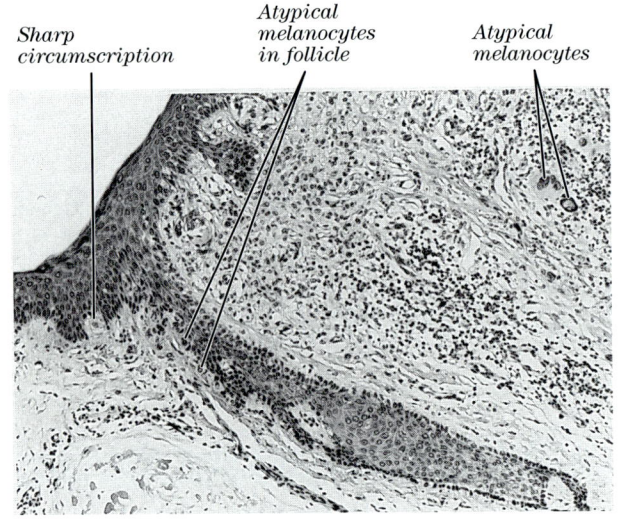

Sharp circumscription — Atypical melanocytes in follicle — Atypical melanocytes

Lymphocytes — Multinucleate atypical melanocyte — Atypical melanocytes

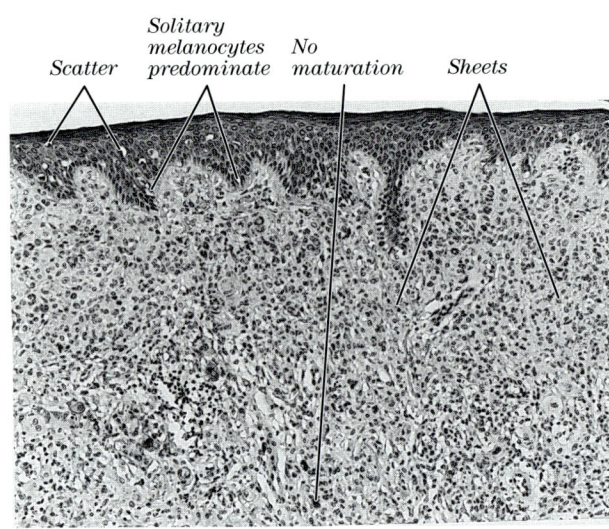

Scatter — Solitary melanocytes predominate — No maturation — Sheets

Scatter — Sheet — Atypical melanocytes

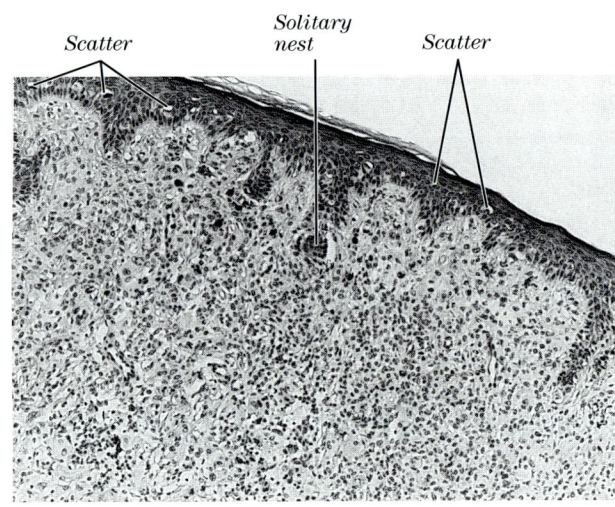

Scatter — Solitary nest — Scatter

Scatter — Sheet — Atypical melanocytes in nest — Melanophages

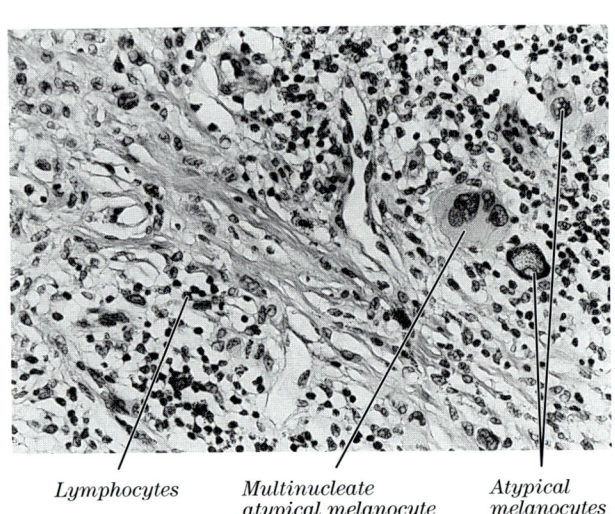

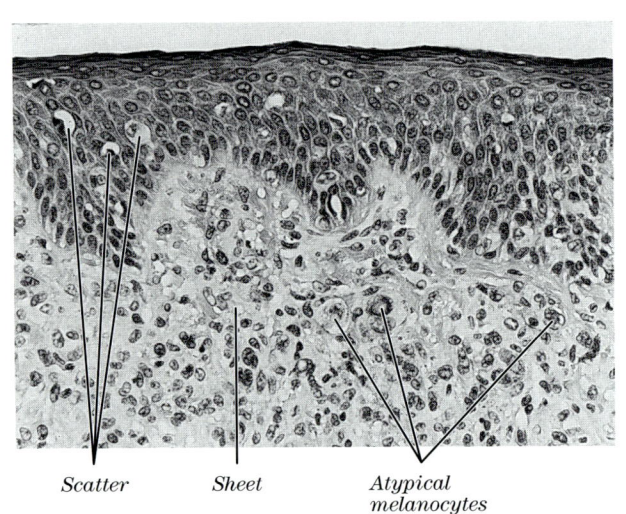

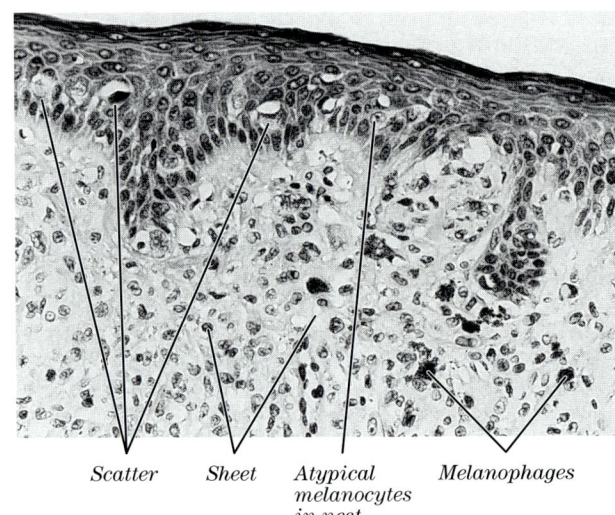

36 • Melanoma

Criteria for diagnosis of this melanoma

This is a melanoma because:

1. It is asymmetric.

2. Melanocytes are scattered across the epidermis and far down epithelial structures of adnexa.

3. There is no maturation of melanocytes.

4. Nuclei of many melanocytes are strikingly atypical.

Pitfall in diagnosis

This melanoma could be misinterpreted as a halo type of Clark's nevus because:

1. It is dome-shaped.

2. Its circumscription is sharp.

3. Neoplastic cells are present both within the epidermis and the upper part of the dermis.

4. Some neoplastic melanocytes have large nuclei.

5. Dense, patchy infiltrates of lymphocytes are found throughout the neoplasm.

As is often the case, the clue to diagnosis of this melanoma is its asymmetry as seen at scanning magnification. Note the collarette of adnexal epithelium on the left, but not on the right, the snub-nosed appearance of the neoplasm on the left, but not on the right, and the denser infiltrate of lymphocytes on the right than on the left. Cytologic features noted at higher magnification confirm the diagnosis of melanoma.

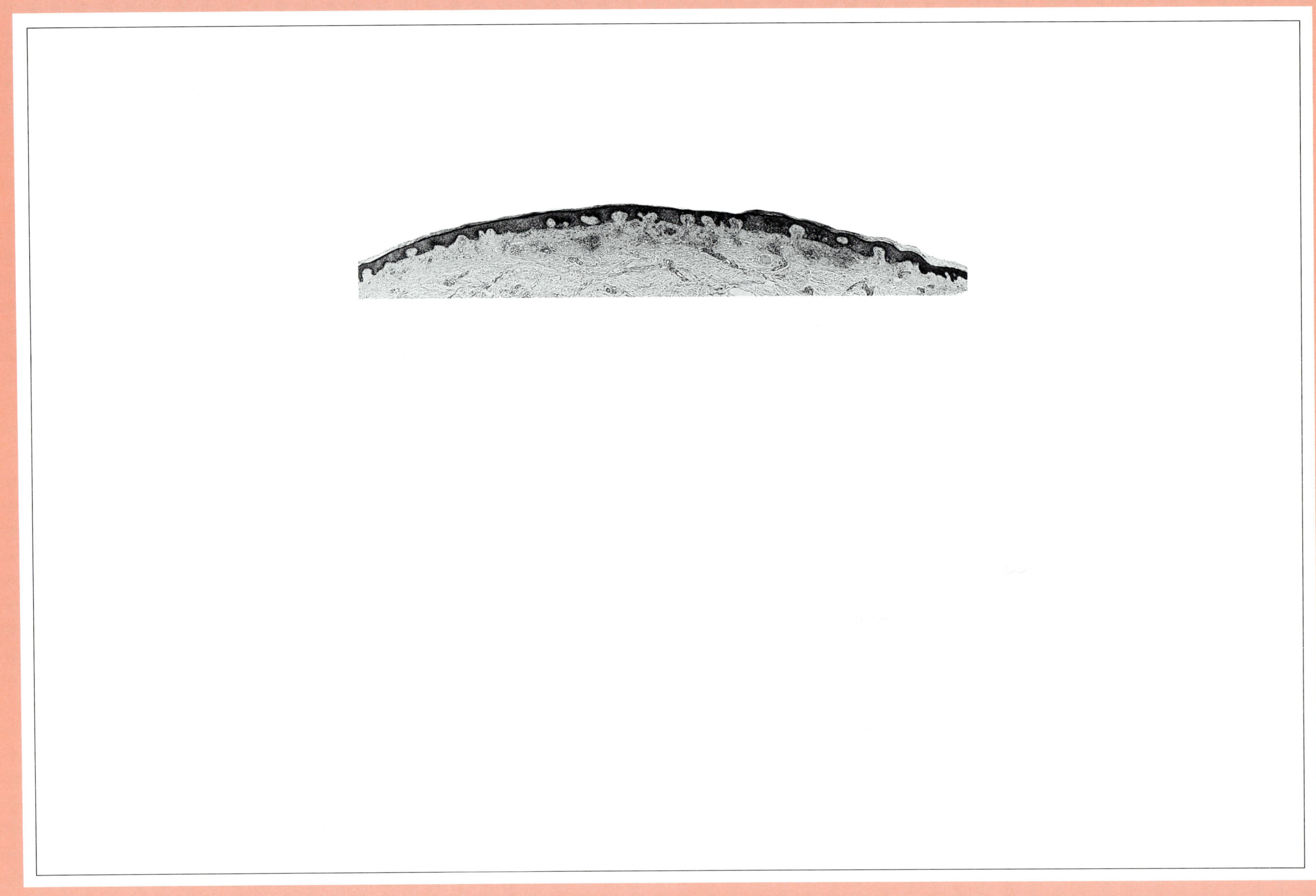

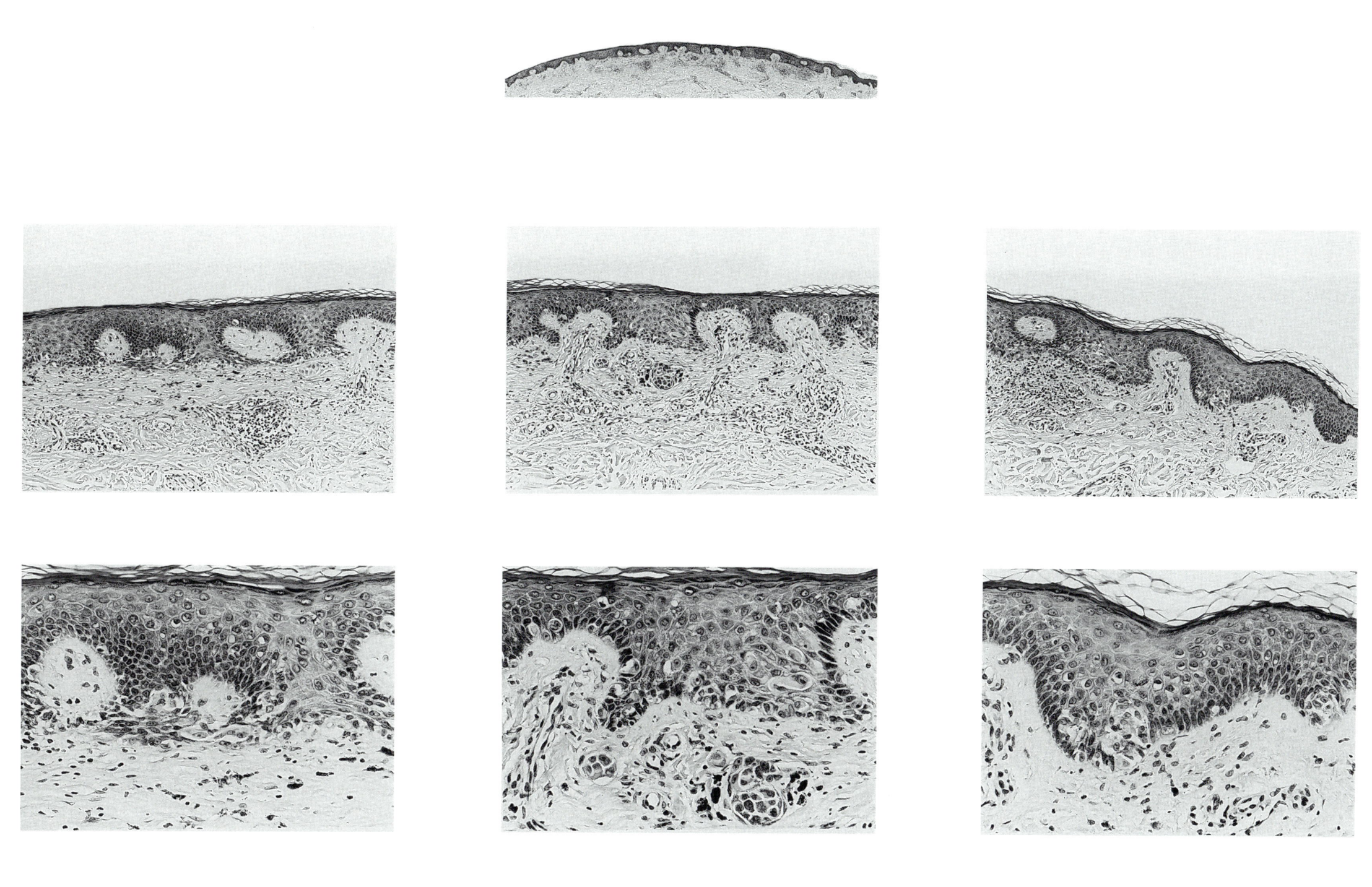

37. What is your diagnosis?

Brown plaque with a black center on the leg of a 34-year-old woman increased in size recently. Clinical diagnosis: dysplastic nevus vs. melanoma. No follow-up data were available.

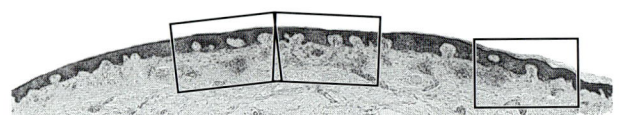

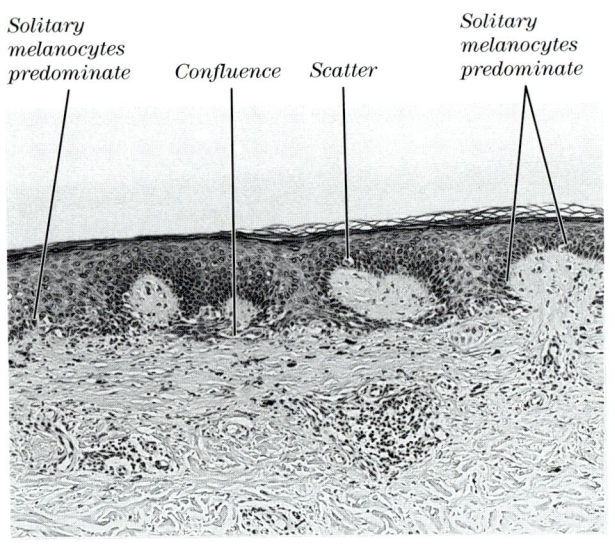

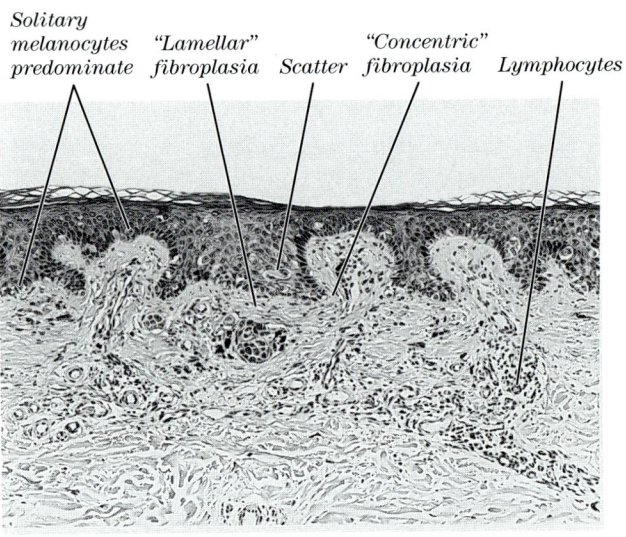

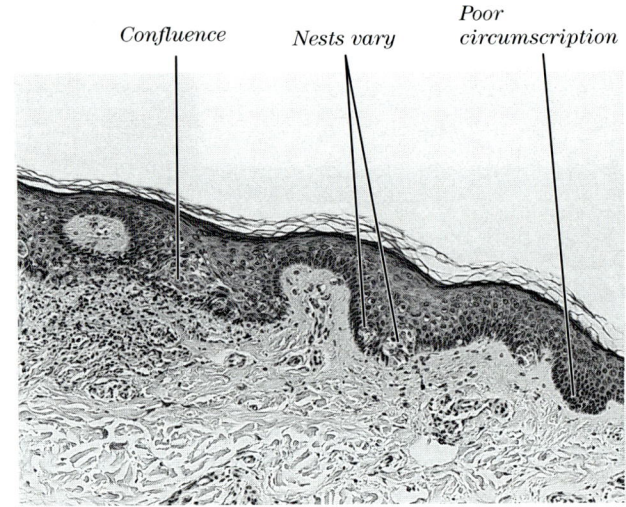

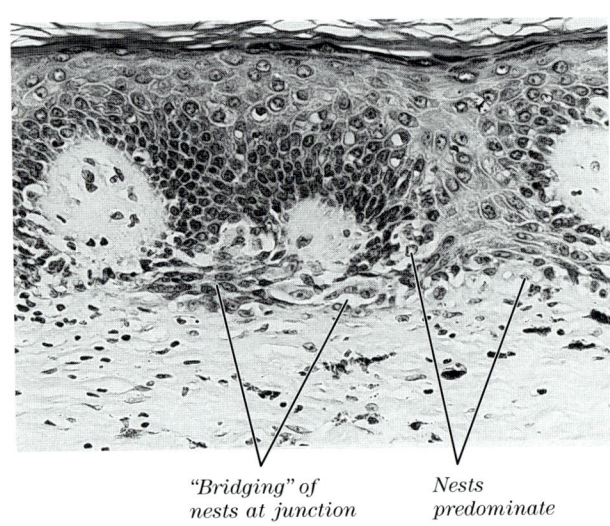

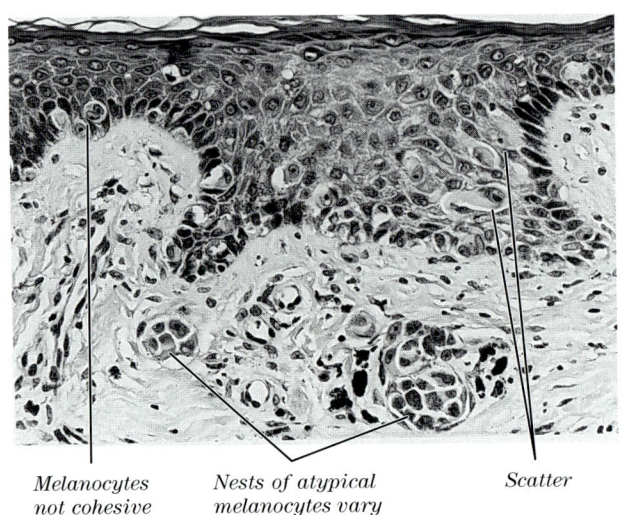

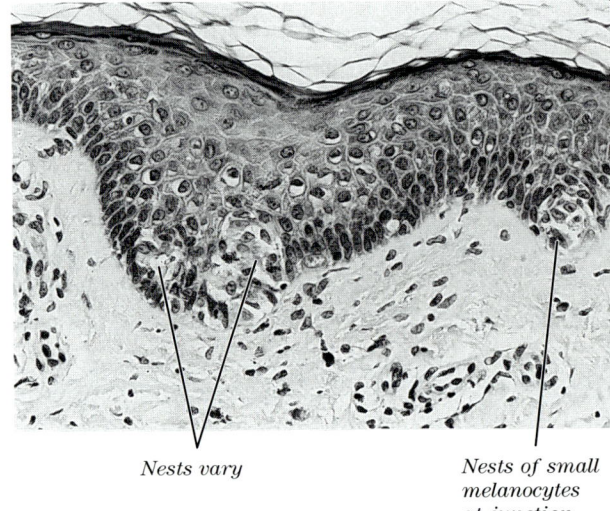

37 • Melanoma

Criteria for diagnosis of this melanoma

This is a melanoma because:

1. The neoplasm is poorly circumscribed.
2. Nests of melanocytes within the epidermis are not equidistant from one another.
3. Nests of melanocytes within the epidermis vary in size and shape.
4. Some nests of melanocytes within the epidermis have become confluent.
5. Melanocytes within the epidermis disposed as solitary units predominate over nests in some high-power fields.
6. Melanocytes within the epidermis, especially those arrayed as solitary units, are scattered throughout the entire thickness of the epidermis.
7. Nests of melanocytes within the dermis vary in size and shape.
8. Some nests of melanocytes at the base of the thickened papillary dermis are larger than nests above them.
9. Nuclei of melanocytes are atypical.
10. Melanin is not distributed in uniform fashion within the intradermal portion of the neoplasm.

Pitfall in diagnosis

This melanoma could be misinterpreted as a compound Clark's nevus because:

1. The neoplasm is relatively symmetric.
2. There is "bridging" of nests of melanocytes at the base of the epidermis.
3. The lesion is slightly elevated in its center.
4. Melanocytes are confined to the epidermis and thickened papillary dermis.
5. There are both "lamellar" and "concentric" fibroplasia.
6. Perivascular lymphocytic infiltrates are apparent.
7. Telangiectases are present.

This neoplasm is a melanoma for the reasons given. Despite the fact that it shares some features with a Clark's nevus, nothing about it is "dysplastic"; everything about it is melanoma.

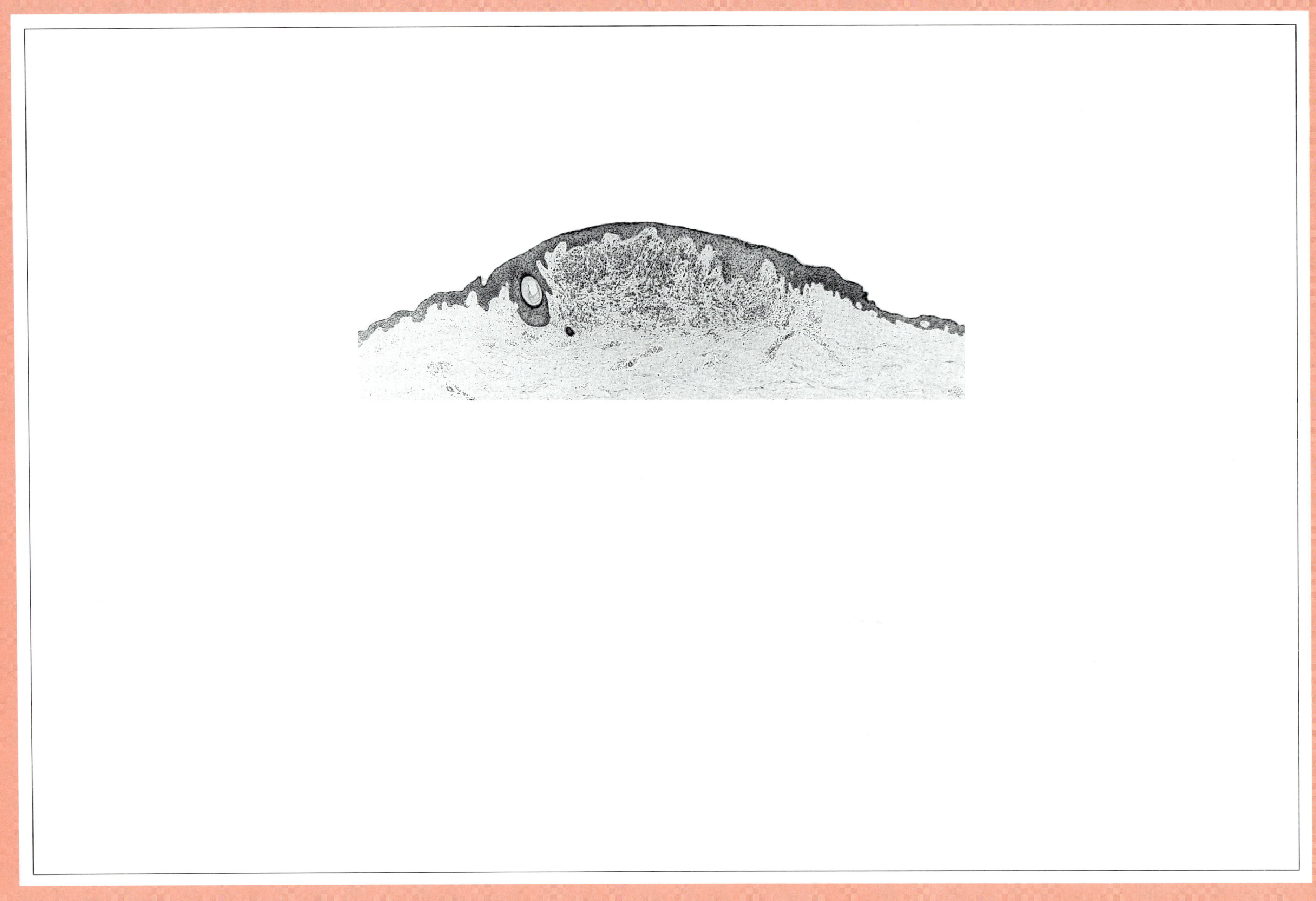

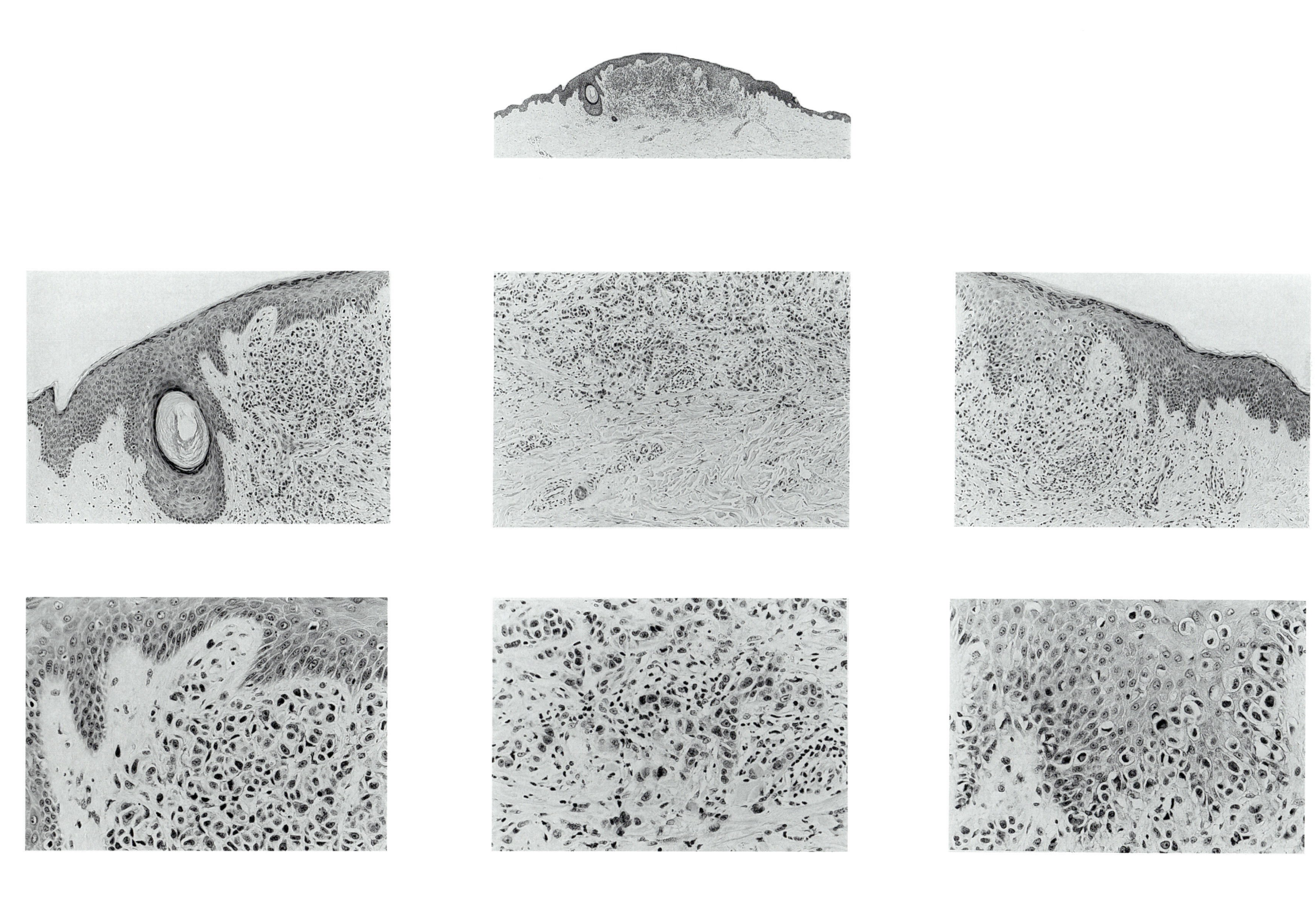

38. What is your diagnosis?

Pigmented lesion of 2 months duration was removed from the left medial thigh of a 52-year-old man with a history of melanoma. Clinical diagnosis: metastatic melanoma. Patient subsequently developed numerous metastases.

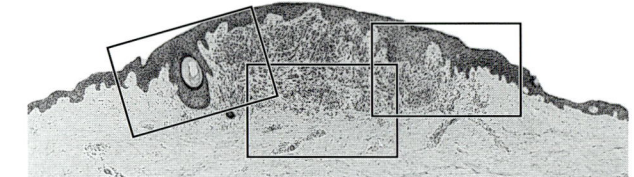

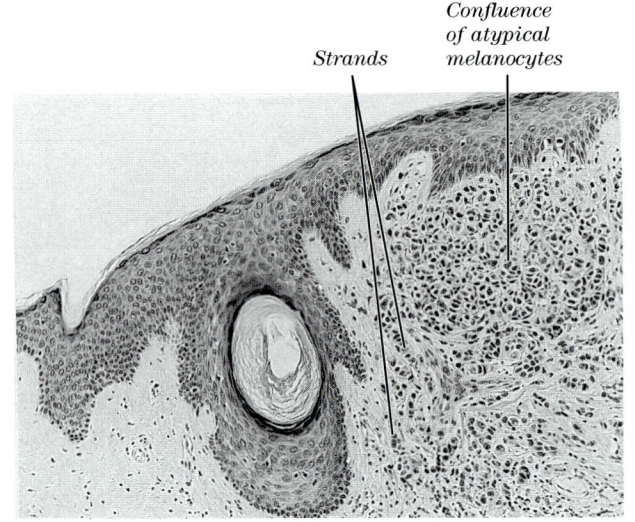

Strands — *Confluence of atypical melanocytes*

Confluence

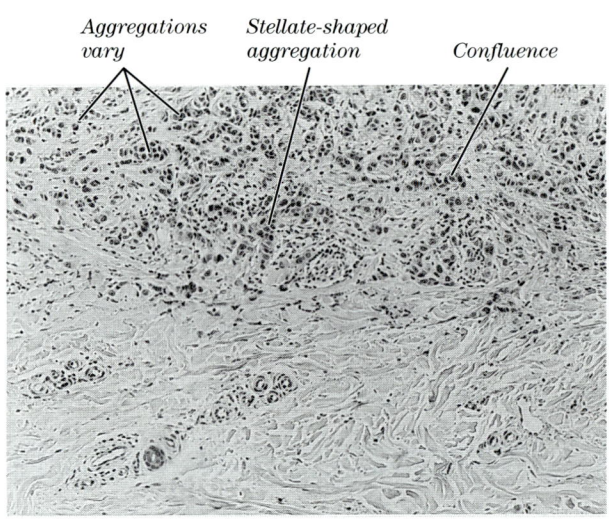

Aggregations vary — *Stellate-shaped aggregation* — *Confluence*

Peculiar shapes of aggregations — *Stellate-shaped aggregation* — *Few lymphocytes*

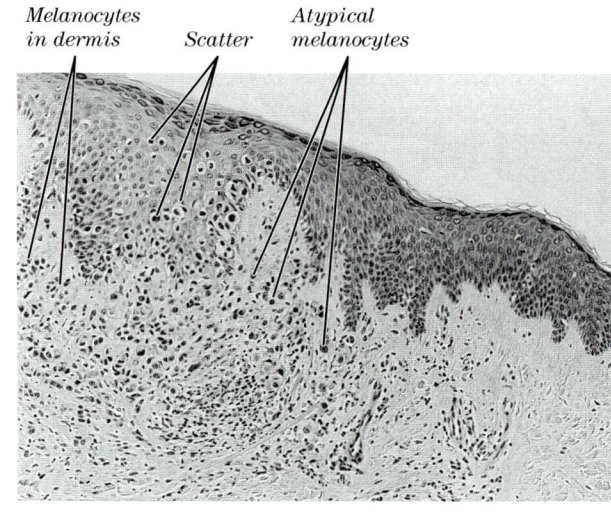

Melanocytes in dermis — *Scatter* — *Atypical melanocytes*

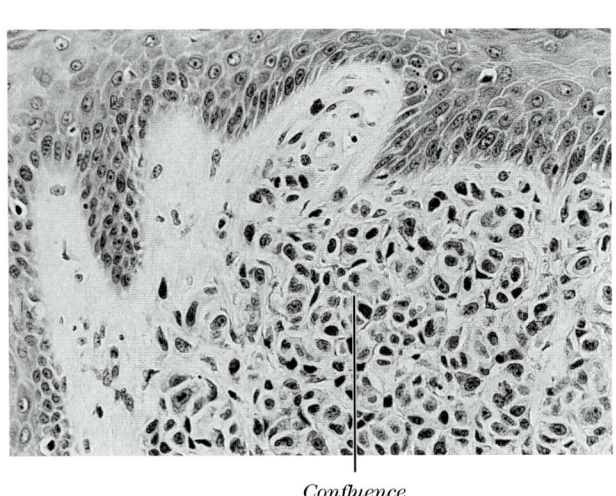

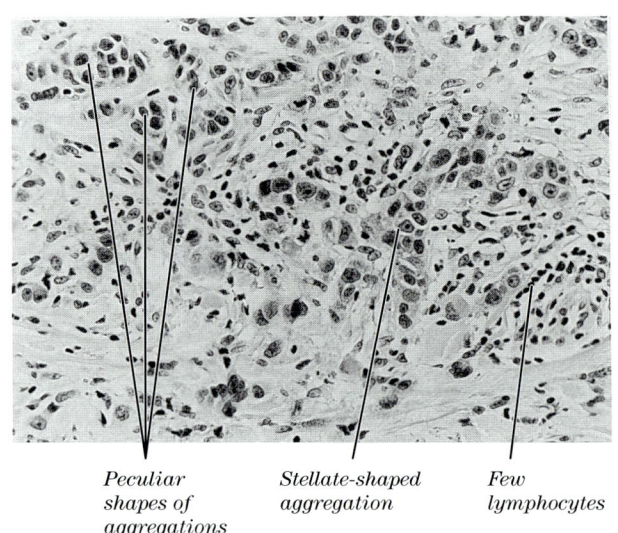

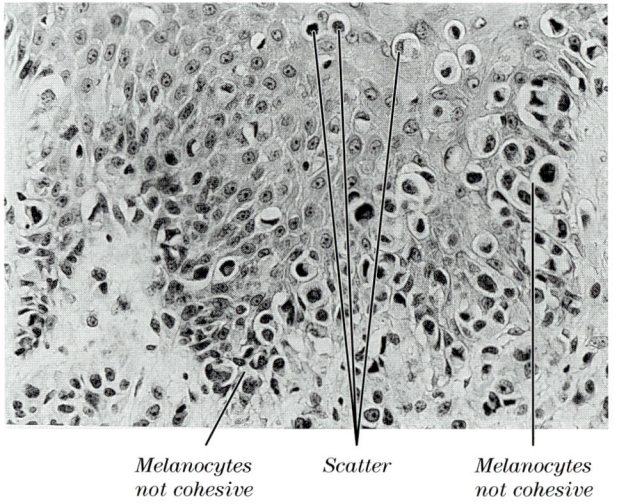

Melanocytes not cohesive — *Scatter* — *Melanocytes not cohesive*

38 • Metastasis of Melanoma *(epidermotropic)*

Criteria for diagnosis of this metastatic melanoma (epidermotropic)

This neoplasm is a melanoma because:

1. It is asymmetric.
2. Atypical melanocytes are present within the epidermis and the dermis.
3. Sheets of neoplastic melanocytes are situated in the upper part of the dermis.
4. There is scatter of atypical melanocytes throughout the epidermis on one side of the neoplasm.
5. Melanocytes do not mature.

This is an epidermotropically metastatic melanoma because:

1. Although the neoplasm is tiny, neoplastic melanocytes are present well within the upper part of the reticular dermis.
2. The intradermal component of the neoplasm extends beyond the intra-epidermal component.
3. No atypical melanocytes are arranged either as solitary units or in nests at the dermo-epidermal junction across most of this neoplasm.

Pitfall in diagnosis

This metastasis of melanoma could be misconstrued as a primary melanoma because:

1. The neoplasm is asymmetric, poorly circumscribed, and constituted of atypical melanocytes.
2. The neoplasm consists of atypical melanocytes within the epidermis and the dermis.

This epidermotropic metastasis of melanoma can be differentiated from primary melanoma because it is so small (only about 2.0 mm in greatest diameter), yet neoplastic cells are present not only in the papillary dermis but also in the reticular dermis. It is virtually impossible biologically for a primary melanoma to be so small and to reach into the reticular dermis. Although epidermotropically metastatic melanomas may simulate primary melanomas closely, the two types of melanoma usually can be differentiated if the criteria listed are applied scrupulously.

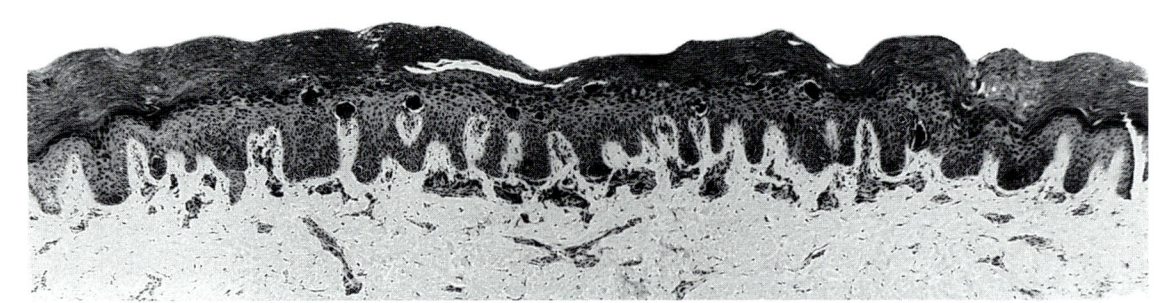

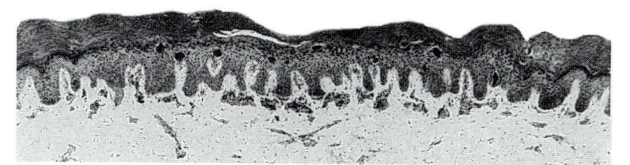
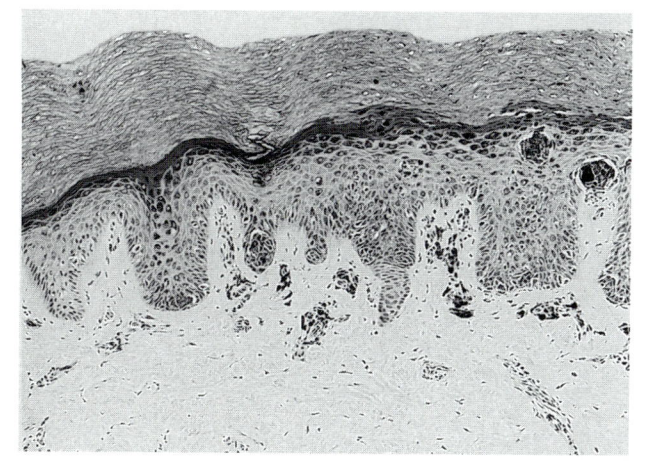
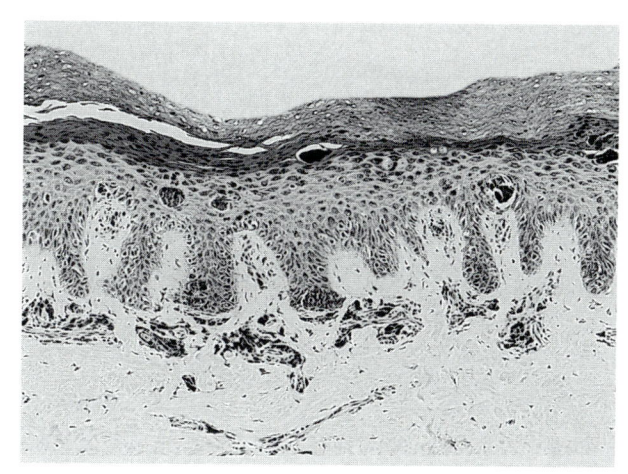
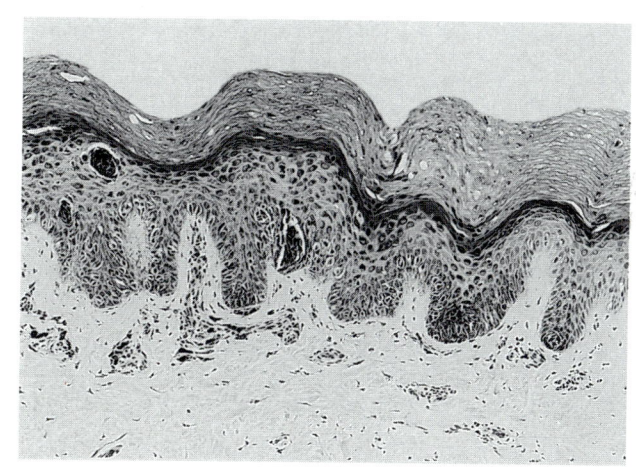
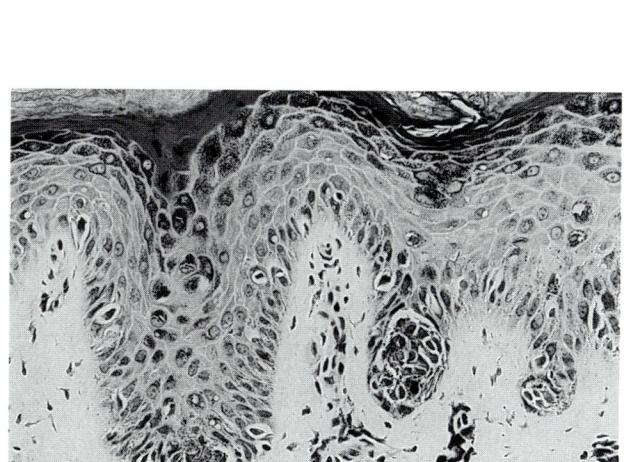
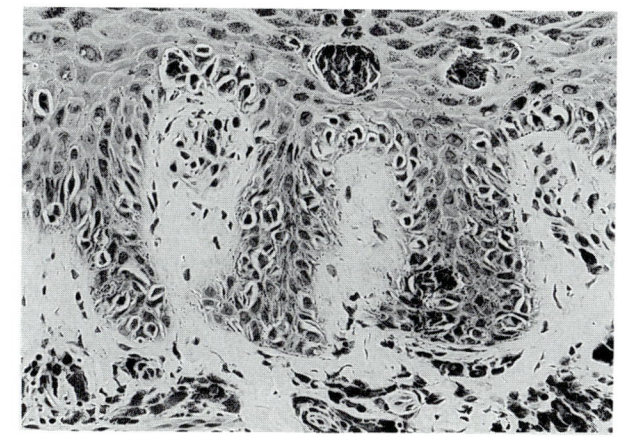
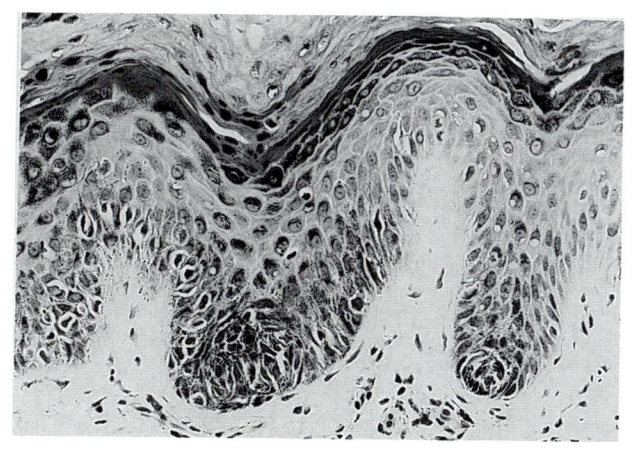

39. What is your diagnosis?

Lesion on the right fifth toe of a 2-year-old boy. Clinical diagnosis: junctional nevus.

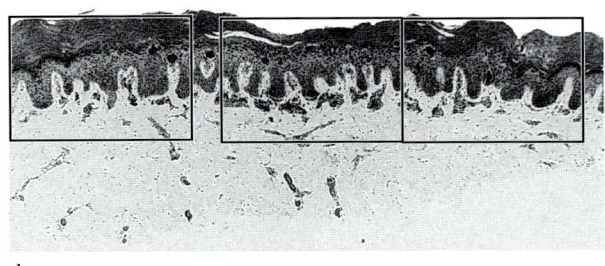

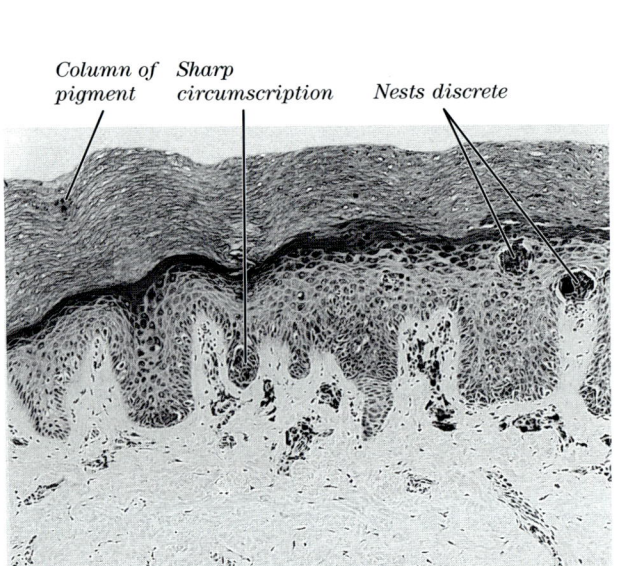

Column of pigment — *Sharp circumscription* — *Nests discrete*

Individual melanocytes predominate — *Nests in spinous zone* — *Nest in cornified layer* — *Nest in spinous zone* — *Nest in granular zone*

Scatter of nests — *Scatter of solitary cells* — *Nests vary* — *Melanin distributed differently in contiguous rete ridges* — *Column of pigment*

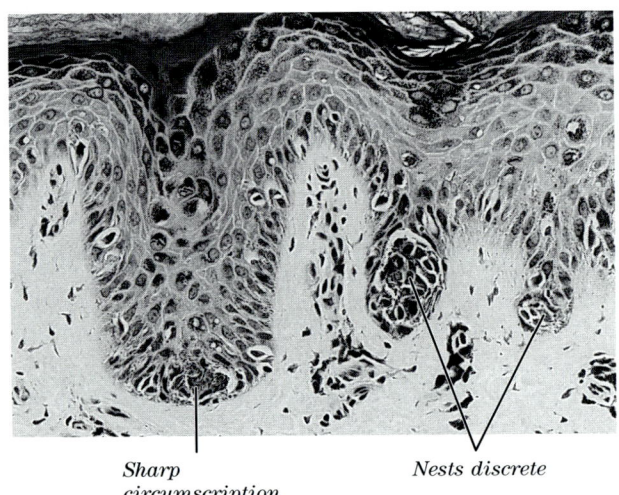

Sharp circumscription — *Nests discrete*

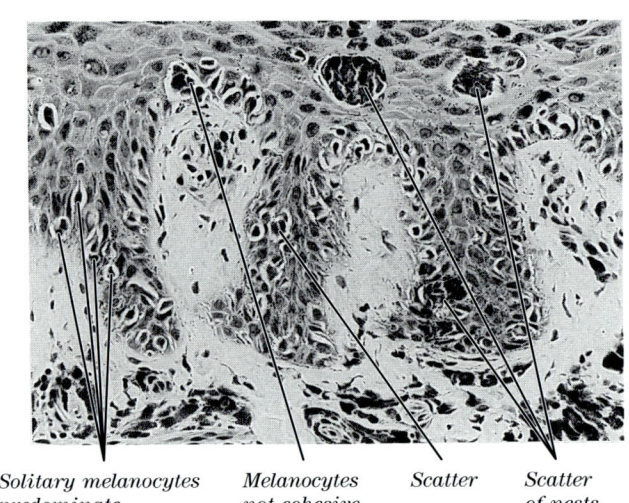

Solitary melanocytes predominate — *Melanocytes not cohesive* — *Scatter* — *Scatter of nests*

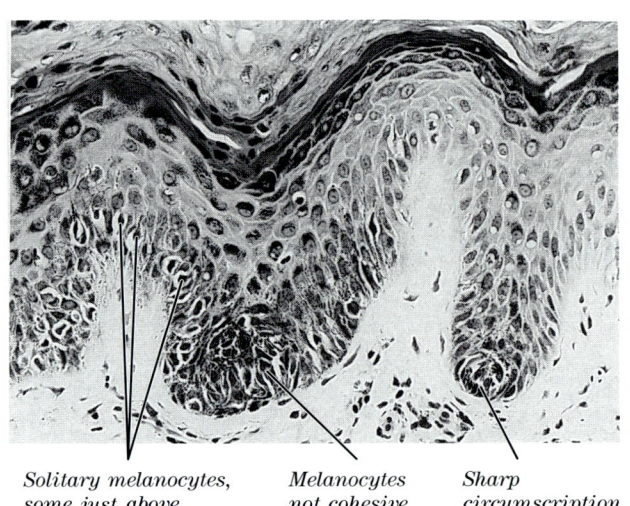

Solitary melanocytes, some just above junction, predominate — *Melanocytes not cohesive* — *Sharp circumscription by a discrete nest*

39 • Congenital nevus *(junctional type)* in a youngster

Criteria for diagnosis of this junctional congenital nevus

This is a junctional nevus because:

1. The neoplasm is sharply circumscribed.
2. Columns of pigment are present in the cornified layer.
3. Nests of melanocytes are discrete.
4. Nuclei of melanocytes are monomorphous.
5. Melanin is distributed in relatively uniform fashion throughout the lesion.

Pitfall in diagnosis

This junctional congenital nevus in a youngster could be misinterpreted as melanoma in situ because:

1. Nests of melanocytes are not equidistant from one another.
2. Melanocytes disposed as solitary units are more numerous than nests of melanocytes in many high-power fields.
3. Melanocytes, both those arrayed as solitary units and those in nests, are scattered above the dermo-epidermal junction, including the granular zone and cornified layer.
4. Melanocytes arranged as solitary units are not equidistant from one another.
5. Some dendrites of melanocytes are elongated and some of them extend to about the mid-spinous zone.

At times a junctional congenital nevus on volar skin may be difficult to distinguish from a melanoma in situ at that site. If reliable criteria for differentiating nevi from melanoma are employed, however, the neoplasm pictured here can be identified as a junctional nevus. Pitfalls in diagnosis of nevi and melanoma, in general, result when particular lesions, such as those on volar skin, have features of both neoplasms in common, as is the case here. Despite that coincidence, a particular neoplasm can be diagnosed as a nevus, a melanoma, or a melanoma in association with a nevus if the criteria set forth in this text are applied scrupulously and rigorously. It is inevitable, however, that as occasional melanocytic neoplasm may be disguised so effectively that it eludes Sherlockian application of criteria, and mistakes in diagnosis will then occur.

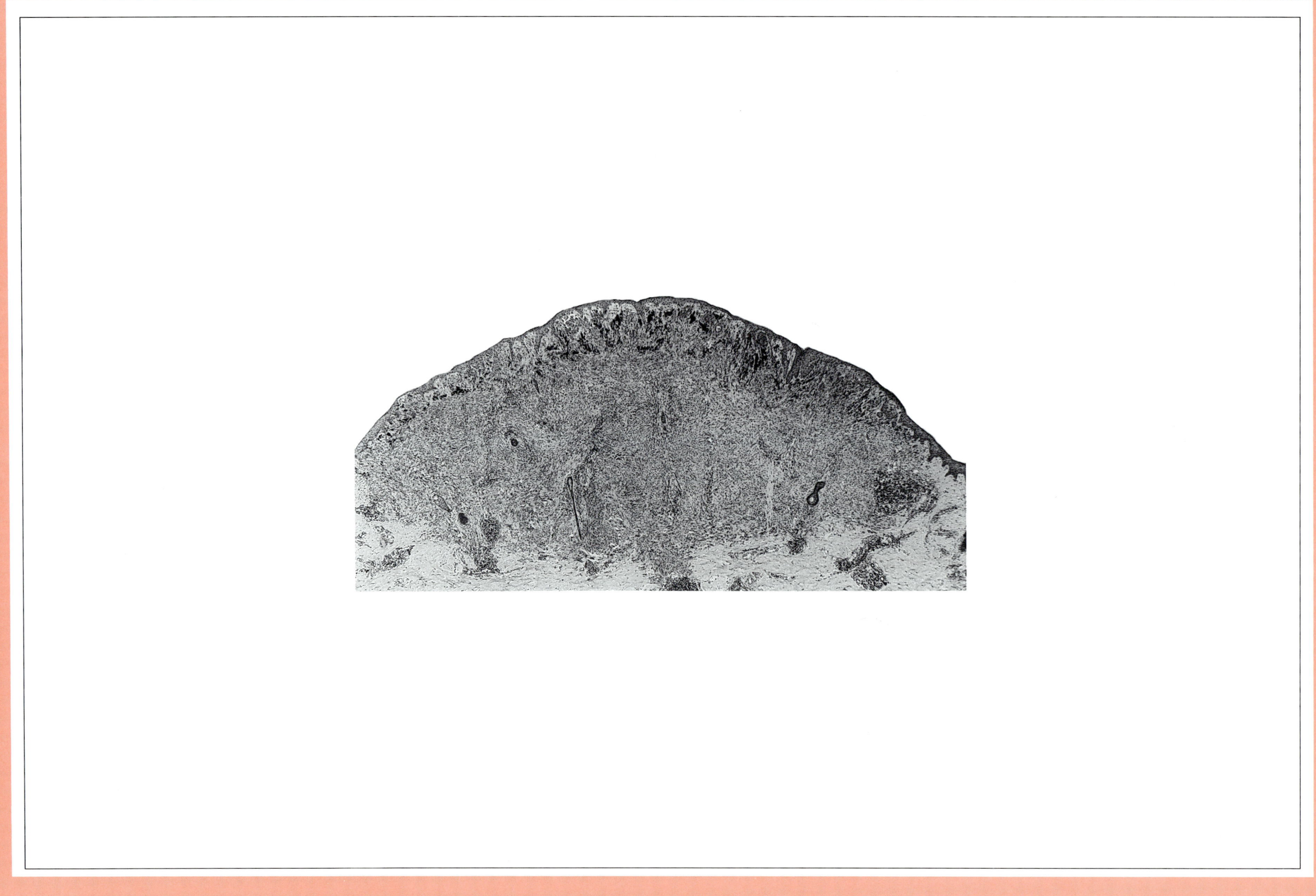

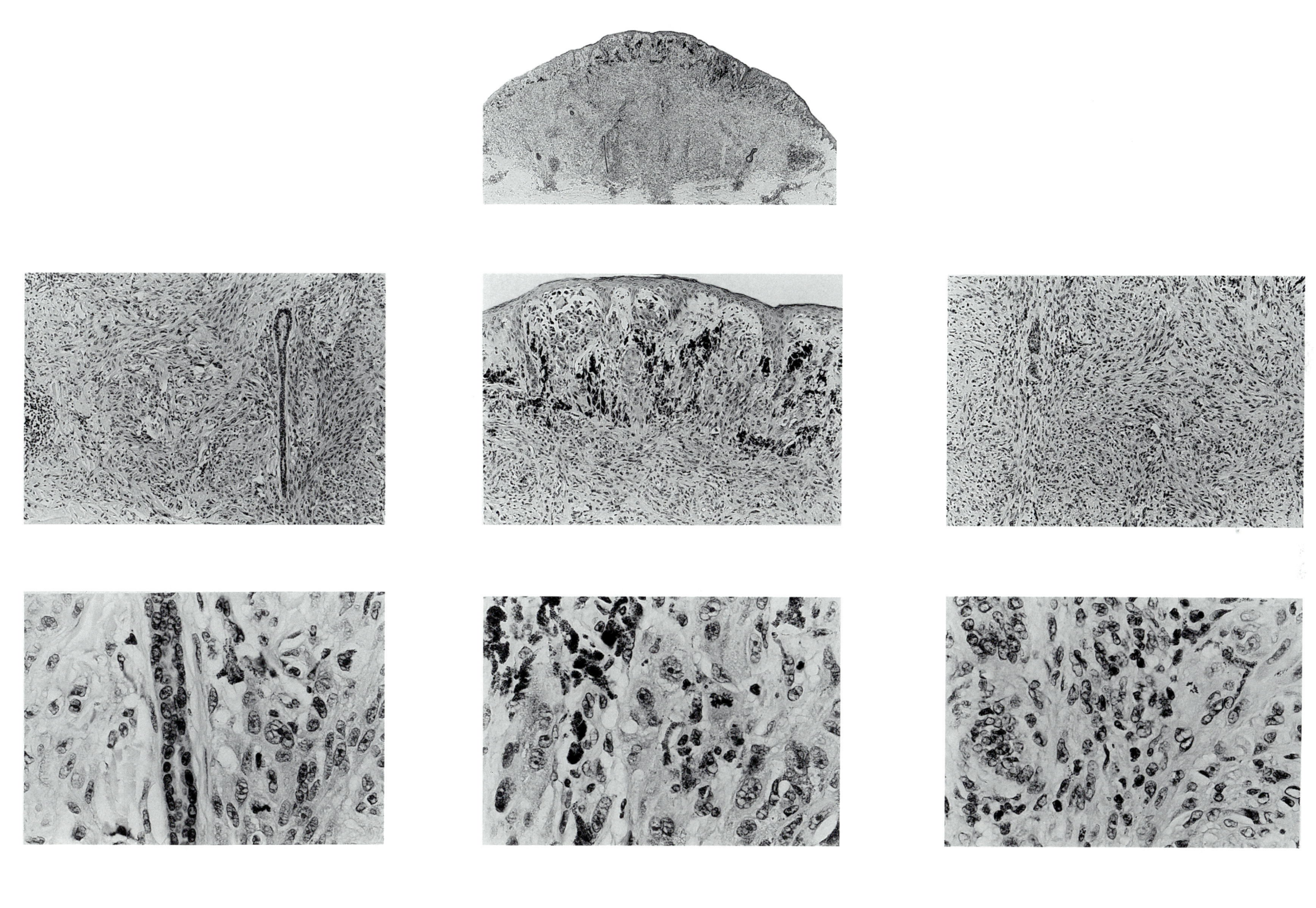

40. What is your diagnosis?

Raised pigmented lesion on the left cheek of a 25-year-old woman had increased in size and become darker over the previous several months. Clinical diagnosis: Spitz's nevus. Patient was in good health after 3 years.

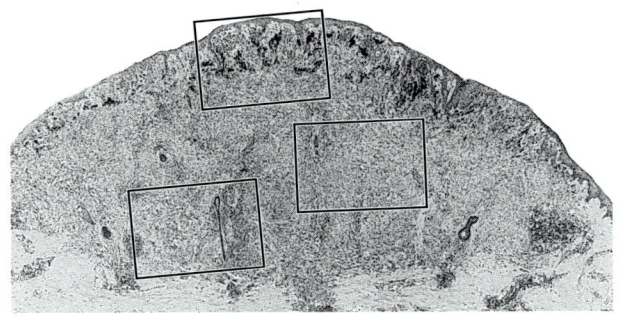

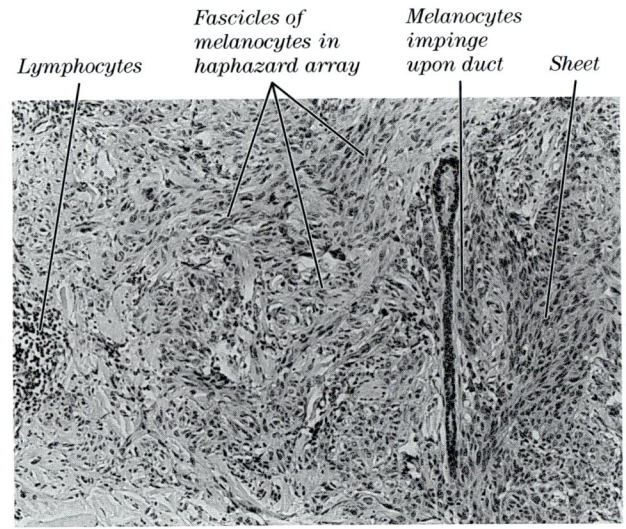
Lymphocytes / Fascicles of melanocytes in haphazard array / Melanocytes impinge upon duct / Sheet

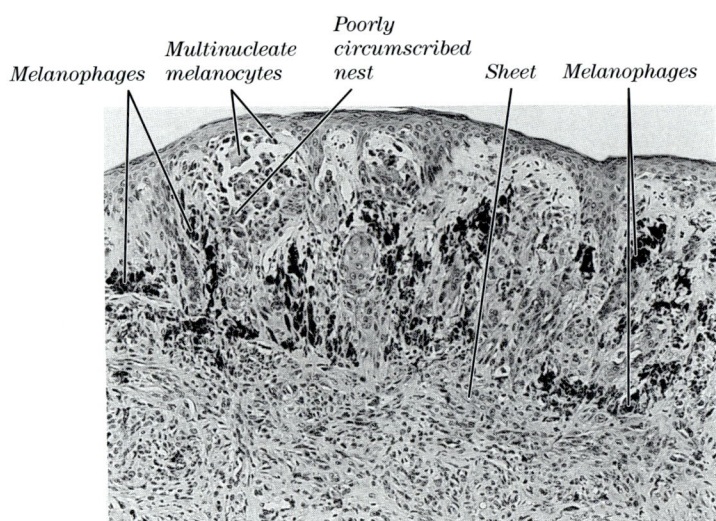
Melanophages / Multinucleate melanocytes / Poorly circumscribed nest / Sheet / Melanophages

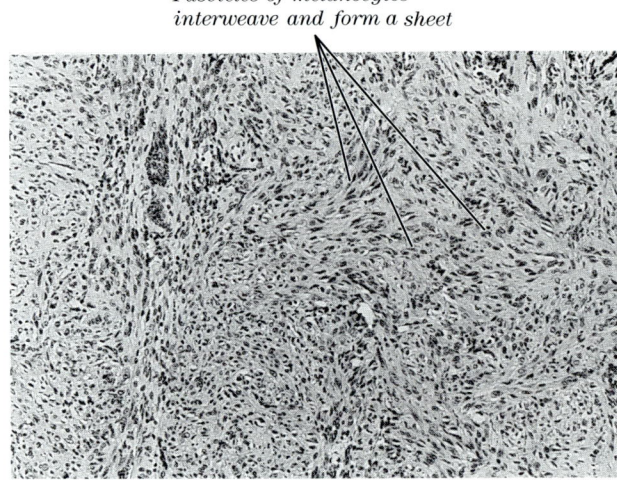
Fascicles of melanocytes interweave and form a sheet

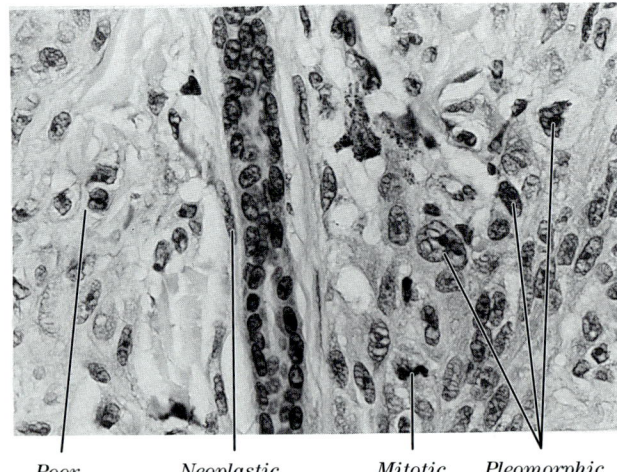
Poor cohesion / Neoplastic melanocyte contiguous to eccrine duct / Mitotic figure / Pleomorphic nuclei

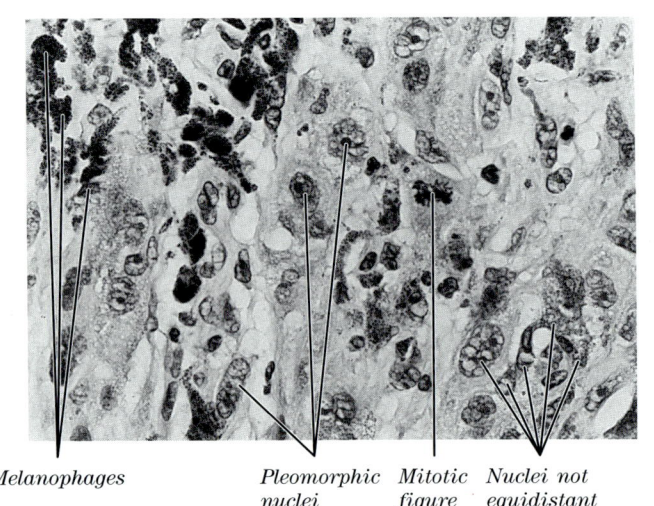
Melanophages / Pleomorphic nuclei / Mitotic figure / Nuclei not equidistant

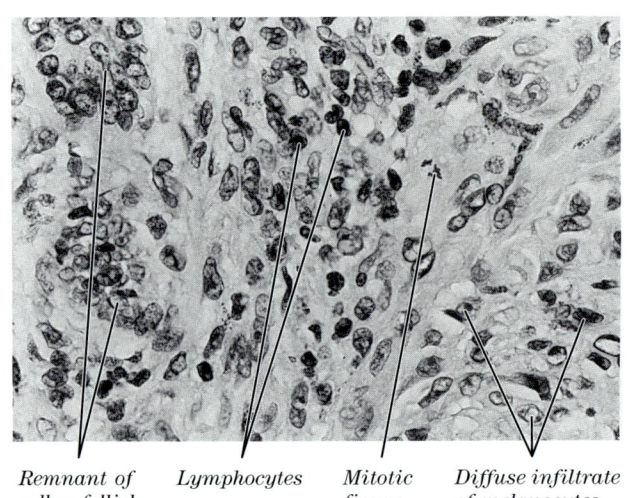
Remnant of vellus follicle / Lymphocytes / Mitotic figure / Diffuse infiltrate of melanocytes

40 • Melanoma

Criteria for diagnosis of this melanoma

This is a melanoma because:

1. It is asymmetric; melanophages are preponderant on one side of it.
2. Sheets of neoplastic melanocytes are present in the reticular dermis.
3. Nuclei of melanocytes are strikingly pleomorphic.
4. Mitotic figures, many of them in the lower half of the neoplasm, are numerous.
5. Some mitotic figures are abnormal.
6. Many nuclei of melanocytes are thin.
7. Some neoplastic melanocytes are pagetoid.

Pitfall in diagnosis

This melanoma could be misjudged as a Spitz's nevus because:

1. It has a dome shape.
2. Melanocytes mature.
3. Many melanocytes have large nuclei and abundant cytoplasm.
4. The neoplasm, at first glance at scanning magnification, seems to be symmetric.
5. Numerous melanocytes are multinucleate.
6. Some epithelial structures of adnexa are preserved.
7. A perivascular infiltrate of lymphocytes is disposed within the substance of the neoplasm.

Of all the cytopathologic features important for differentiation of Spitz's nevus from melanoma, the single most compelling is the presence of numerous mitotic figures near the base of a neoplasm. This neoplasm shows those findings and, therefore, is a melanoma. Episodically, a "thick" Spitz's nevus may be associated with an occasional mitotic figure near its base, but practically never are many of them detected there, unlike the situation in this melanoma.

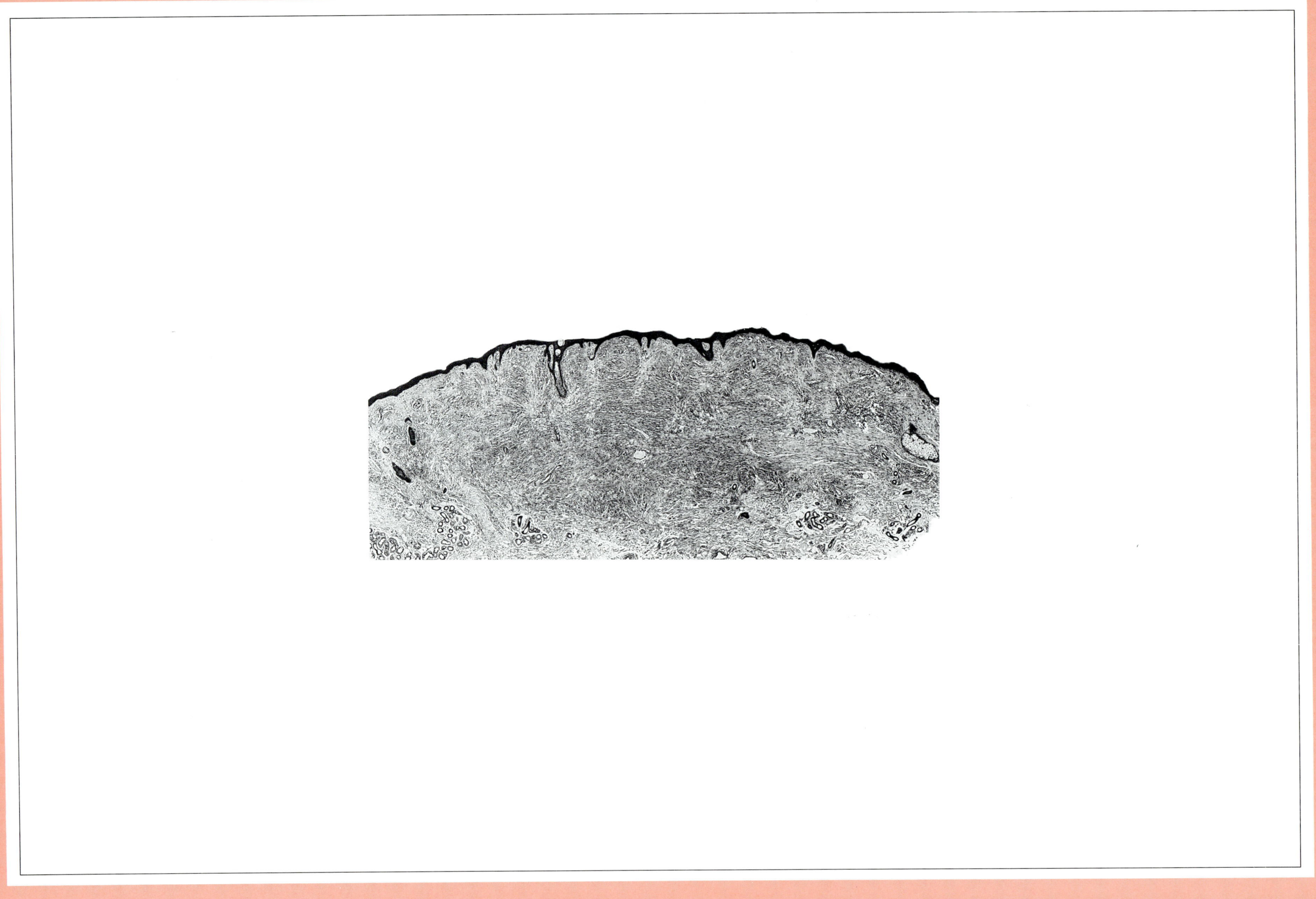

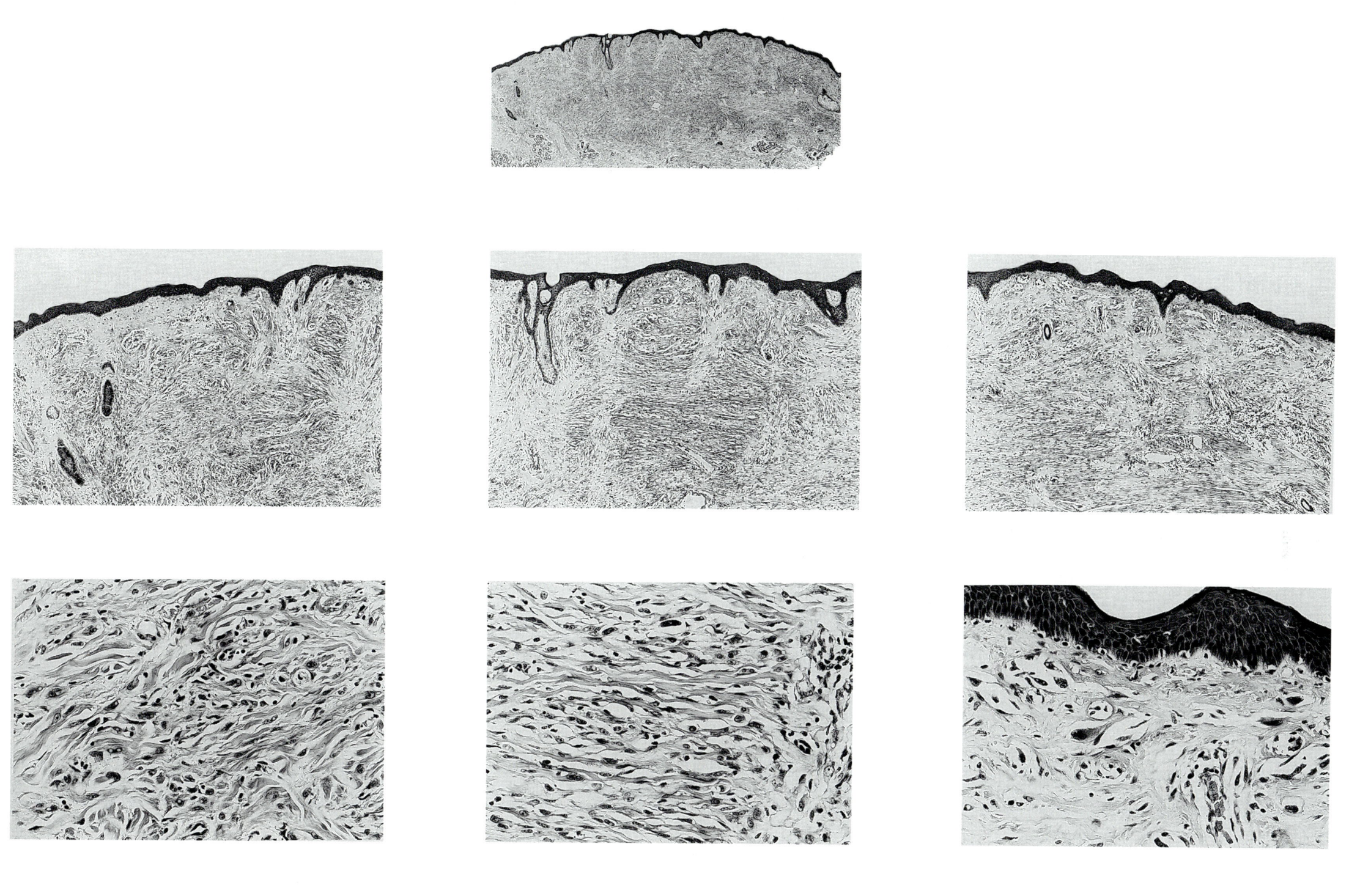

41. What is your diagnosis?

Lesion in a 27-year-old man, site unknown. No follow-up data available.

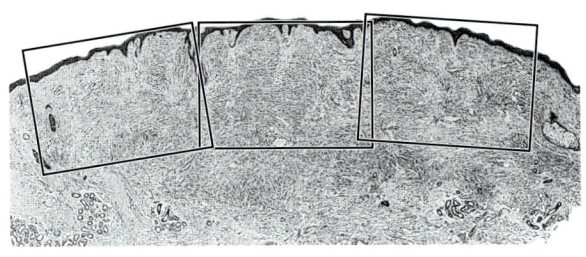

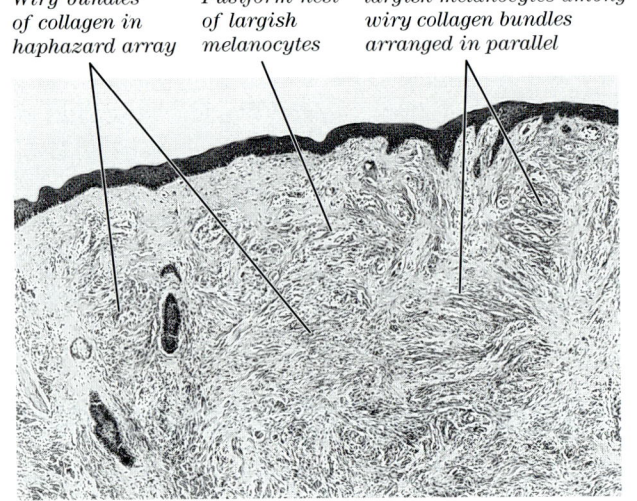
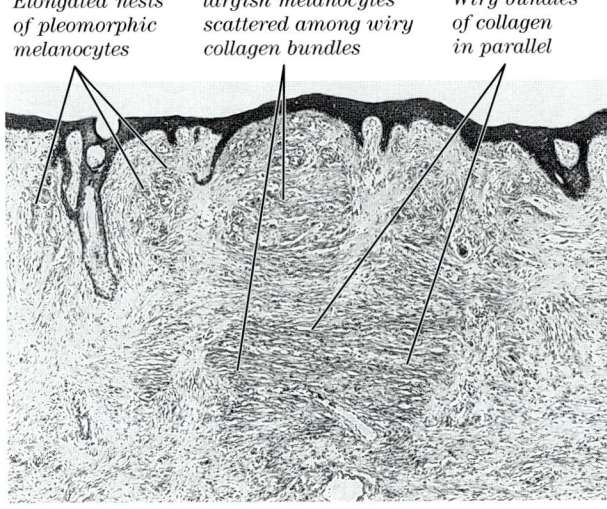
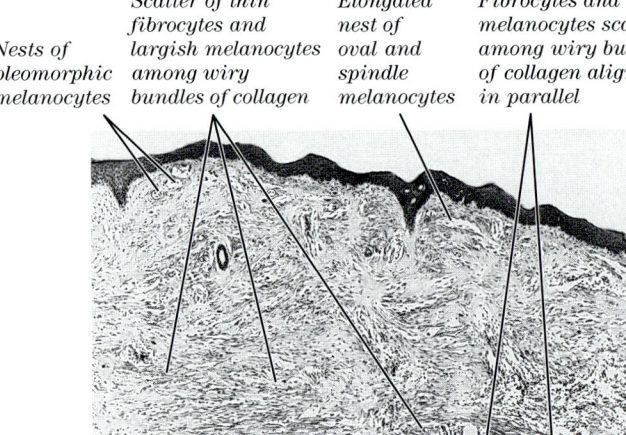

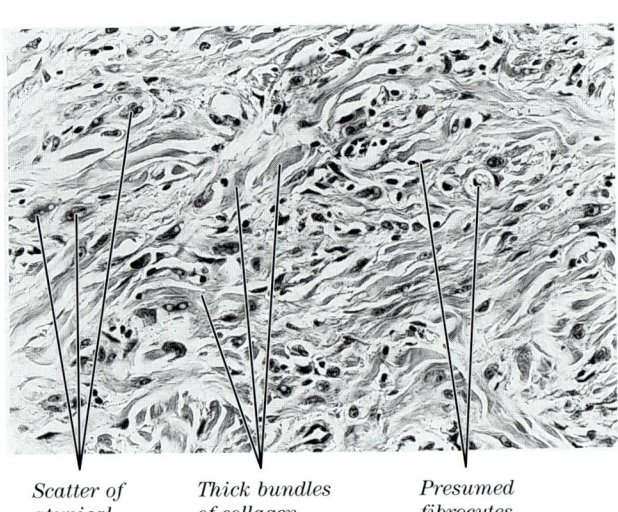
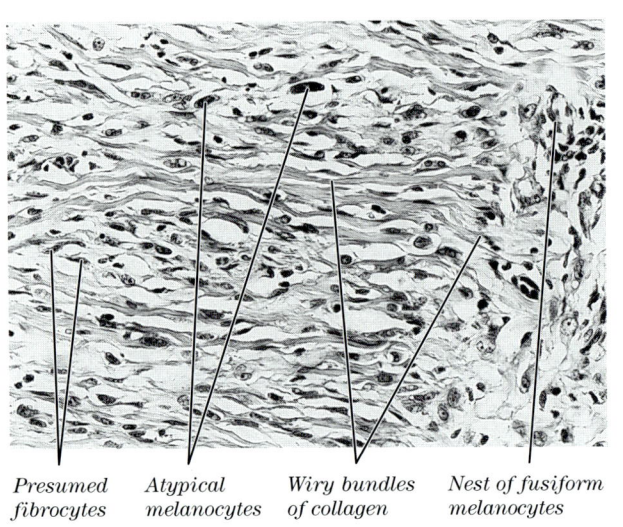
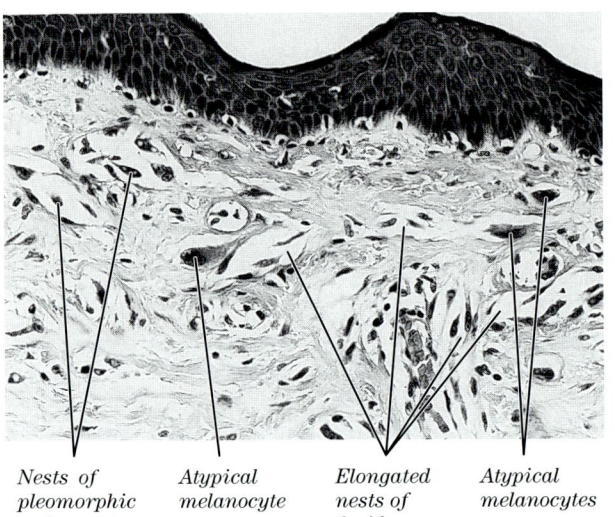

41 • Spitz's Nevus *(desmoplastic type)*

Criteria for diagnosis of this Spitz's nevus (desmoplastic type)

This is a nevus because:

1. The neoplasm is symmetric.
2. Melanocytes mature.
3. Neoplastic melanocytes are confined wholly to the dermis; none are present within the epidermis, i.e., there are no signs of melanoma in situ.
4. Epithelial structures of adnexa are spared.

This is a desmoplastic Spitz's nevus because:

1. Numerous melanocytes have large nuclei, abundant cytoplasm, and plump oval, polygonal, and round shapes.
2. Many nests in the upper part of the lesion consist of polygonal melanocytes that are not cohesive.
3. Desmoplasia is extensive.
4. A patchy, perivascular infiltrate of lymphocytes is present throughout the neoplasm.
5. Bundles of collagen are wiry and arranged parallel to one another and to the skin surface.

Pitfall in diagnosis

This desmoplastic Spitz's nevus could be misinterpreted as desmoplastic melanoma because:

1. Some nuclei of melanocytes are atypical.
2. Desmoplasia is striking.

Desmoplastic Spitz's nevus and desmoplastic melanoma have little in common except for proliferation of melanocytes and for desmoplasia. That is exemplified well in this lesion. This desmoplastic Spitz's nevus has the silhouette of a benign neoplasm, it is wholly intradermal, and many of its melanocytes have large nuclei. In contrast, desmoplastic melanoma has the silhouette of a malignant neoplasm, shows signs of melanoma in situ, if only subtle ones, and is constituted of melanocytes with small oval and thin wavy nuclei. Neurotropism is practically never observed in desmoplastic Spitz's nevus, whereas it is exceedingly common in desmoplastic melanoma.

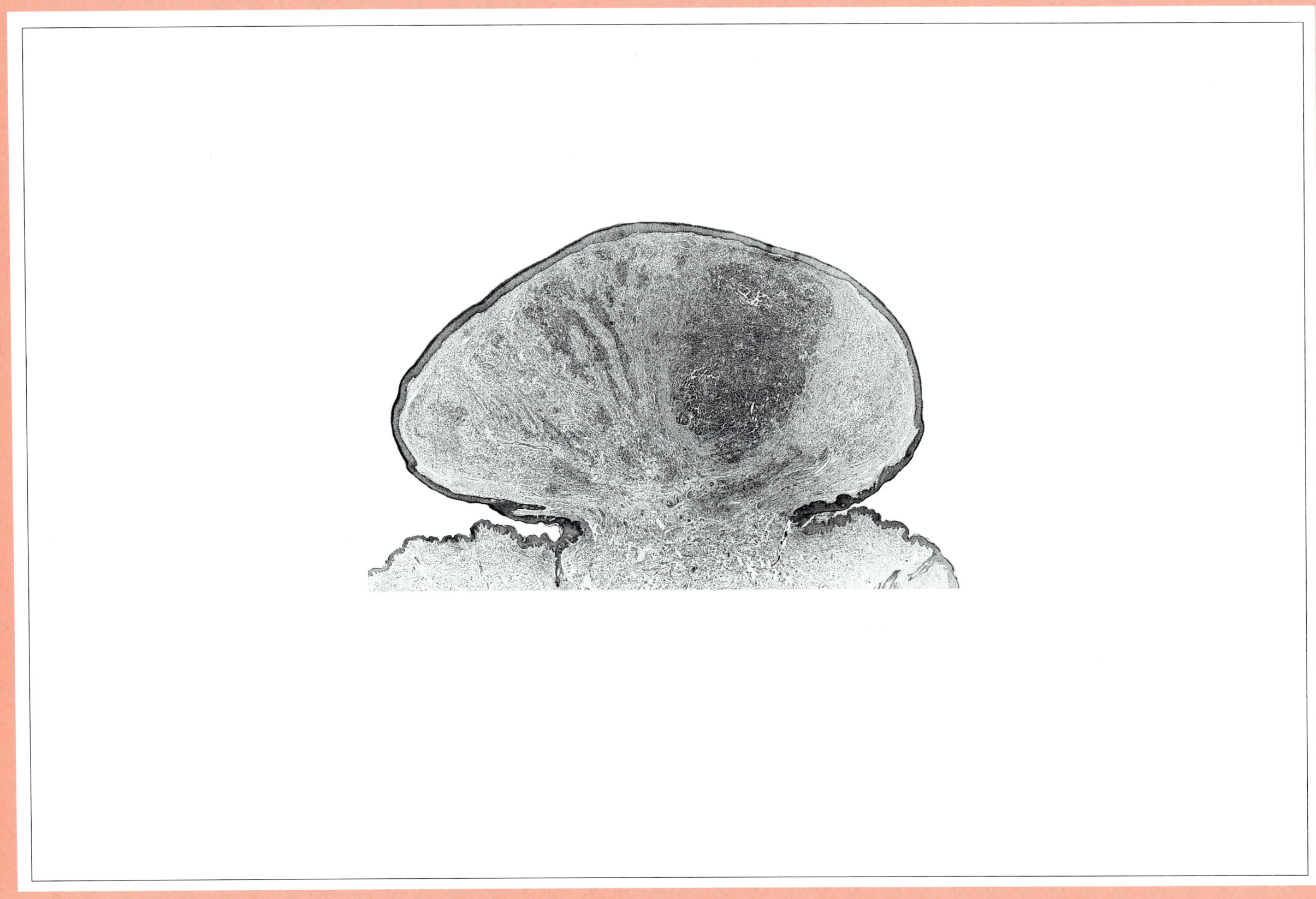

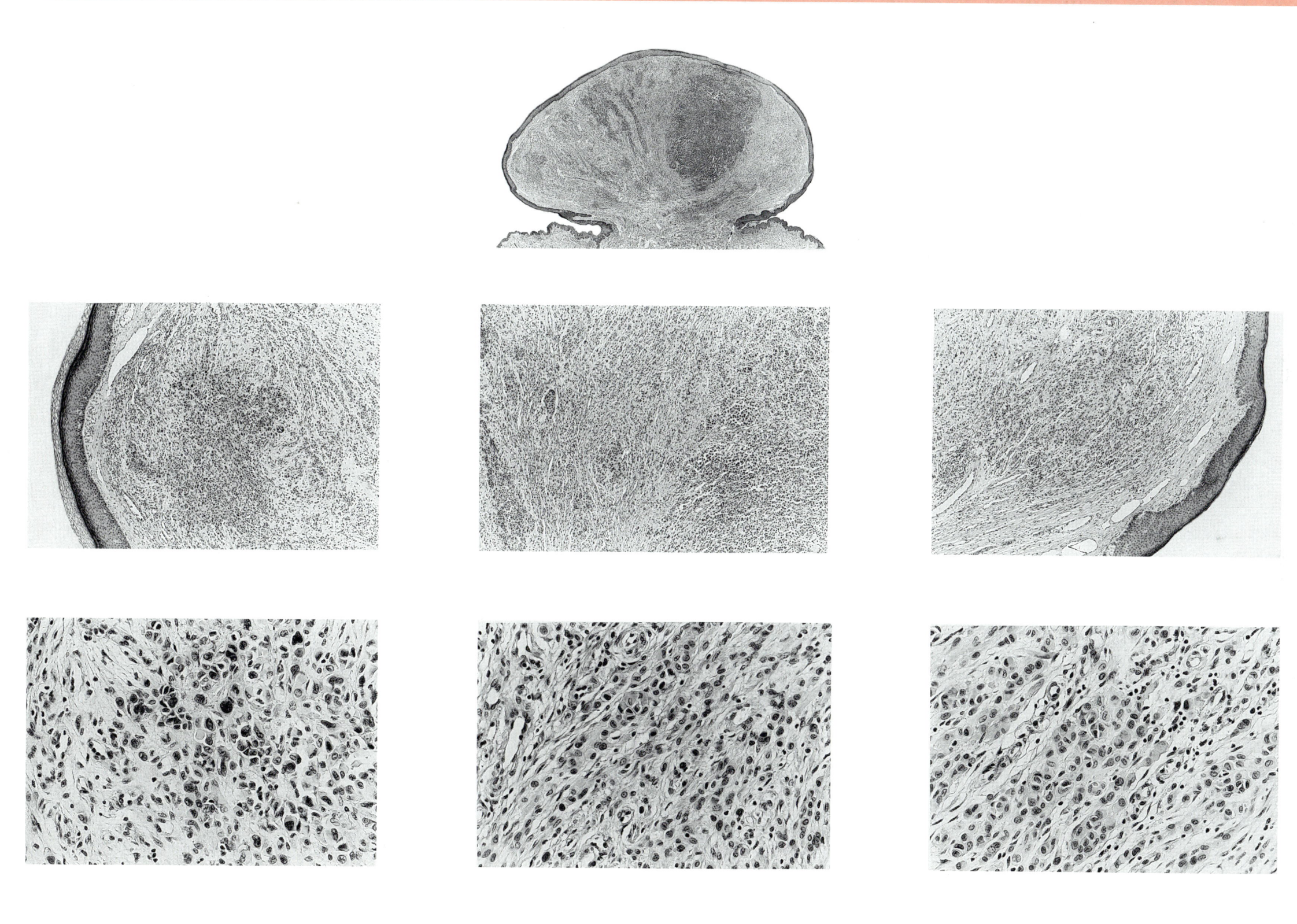

42. What is your diagnosis?

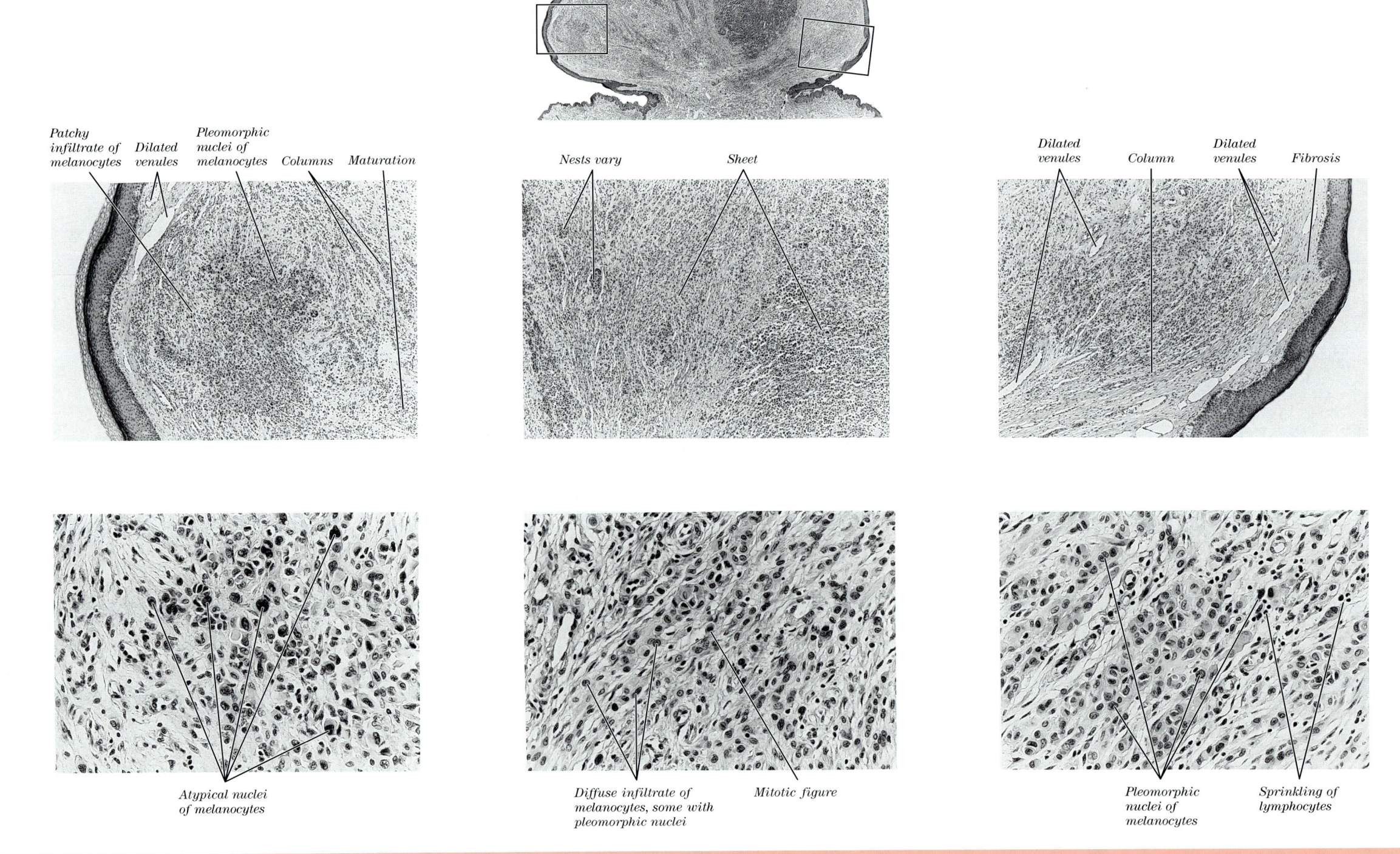

42 • Unna's Nevus (ancient)

Criteria for diagnosis of this Unna's nevus (ancient)

This is an ancient Unna's nevus because:

1. Topographically, the neoplasm is relatively symmetric.
2. The neoplasm is well-circumscribed.
3. Melanocytes mature.
4. Beneath the epidermis, in addition to telangiectases, there is fibroplasia, a sign of chronicity.
5. Mitotic figures are rare.

Pitfall in diagnosis

This ancient Unna's nevus could be misinterpreted as a metastasis of melanoma because:

1. The silhouette of the intradermal components is asymmetric.
2. Many neoplastic melanocytes have atypical nuclei.
3. There is more than one cytologic population of melanocytes, and those populations are intermingled.
4. Nests of melanocytes vary in size and shape.
5. Many nests of melanocytes have become confluent to form sheets.
6. An occasional melanocyte is in mitosis.

Topographically, this polypoid lesion is symmetric, but the distribution of melanocytes within it is not. That finding is characteristic of ancient nevi of both Unna's and Miescher's types. The maturation of melanocytes with progressive descent into the dermis in the absence of signs of melanoma in situ make this lesion a nevus.

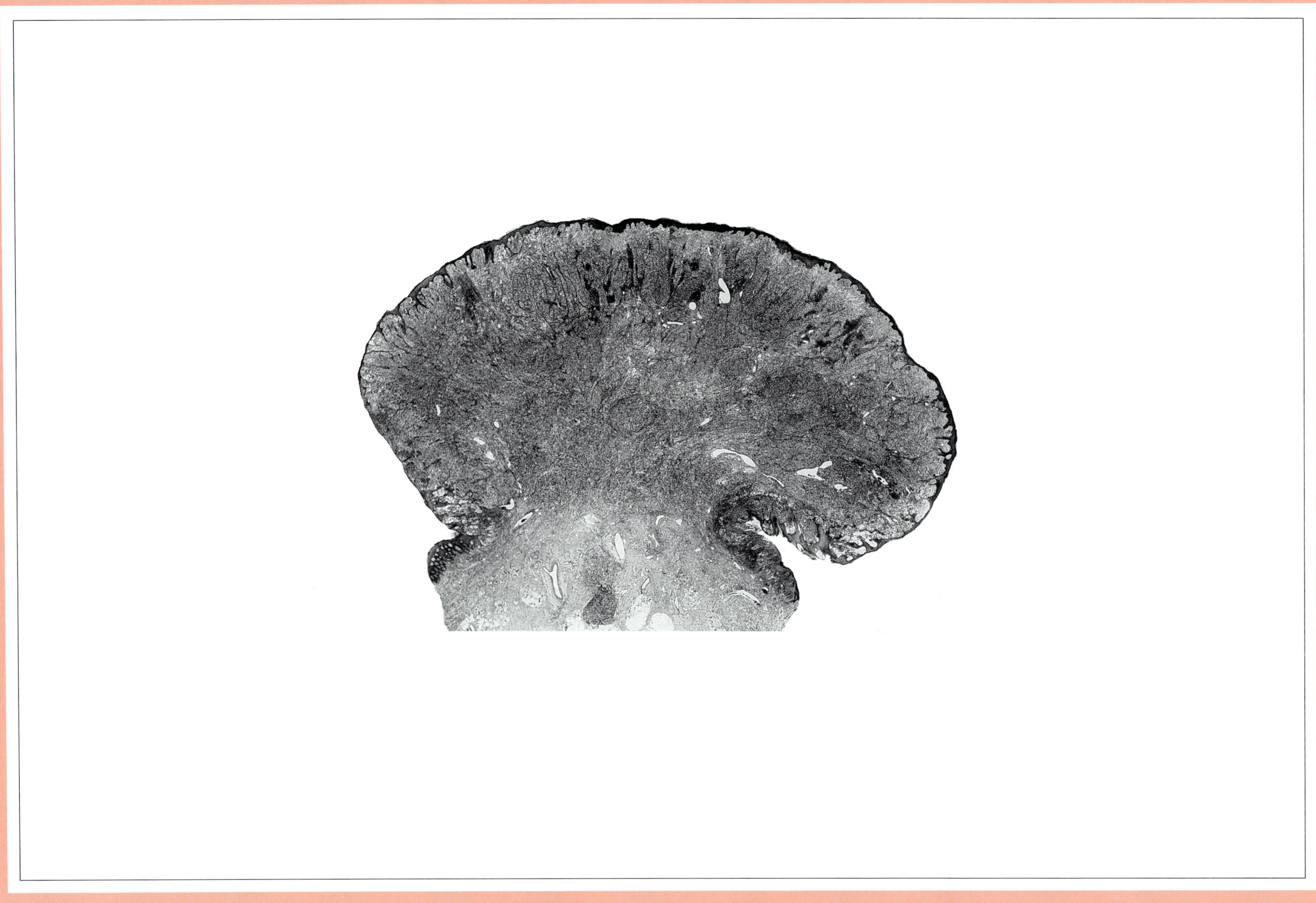

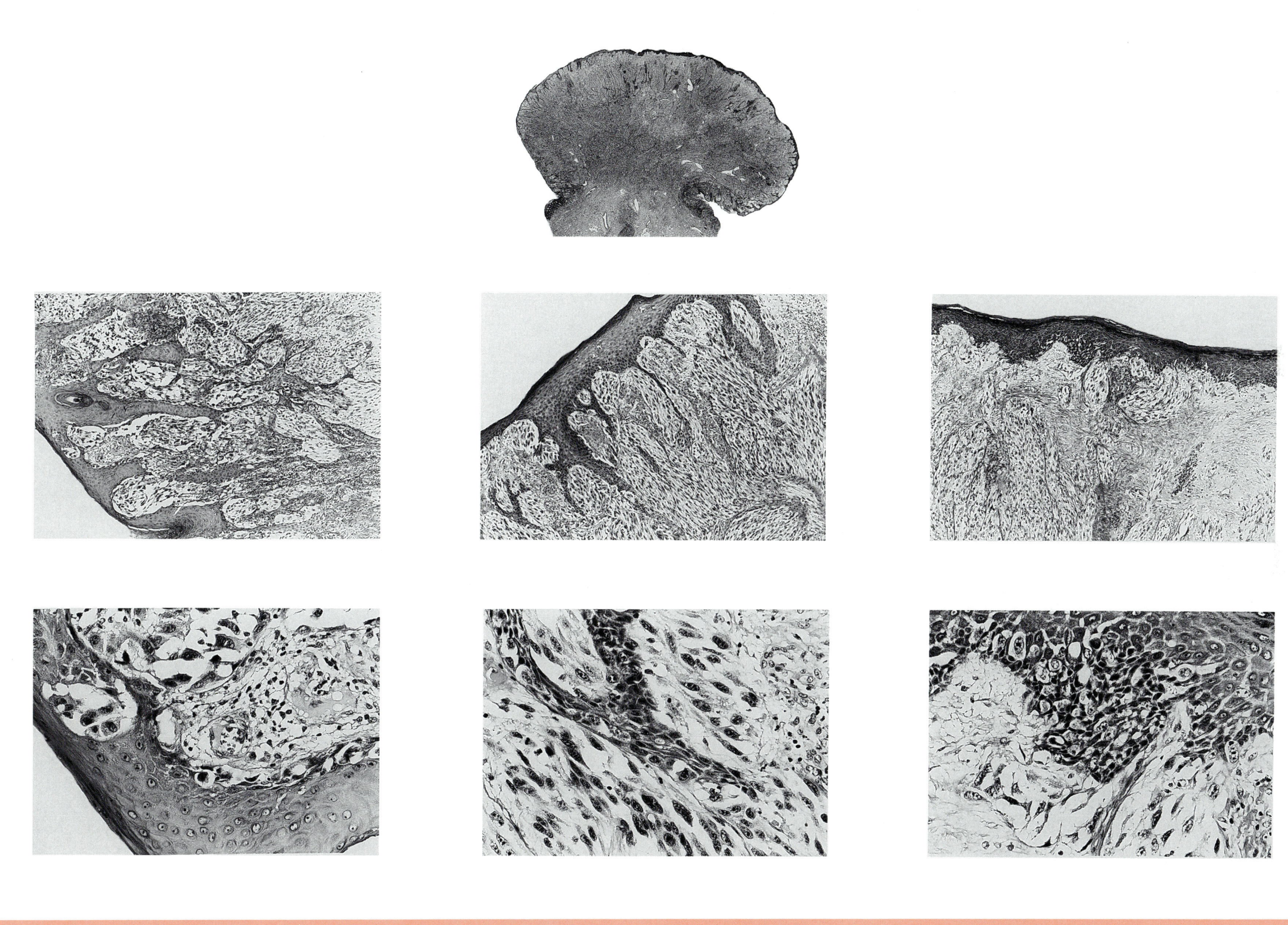

43. What is your diagnosis?

Pigmented lesion on the left elbow of a 61-year-old man. Clinical diagnosis: nodular melanoma. The lesion was excised completely and axillary lymph nodes were dissected. Patient developed a metastasis in 1 year.

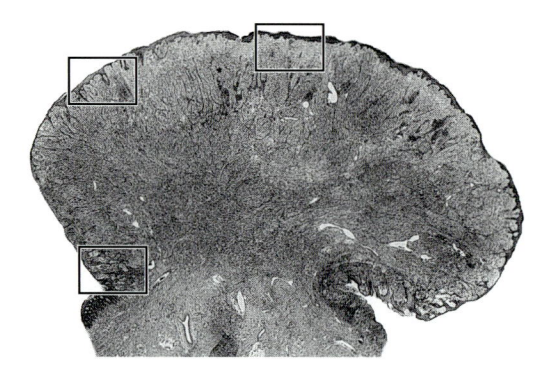

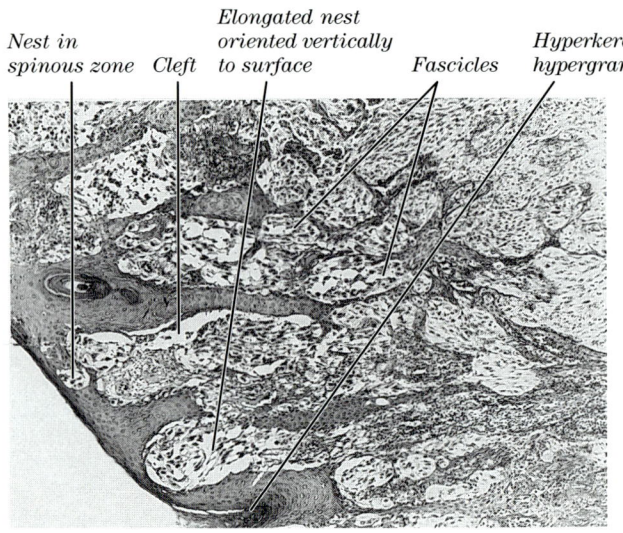

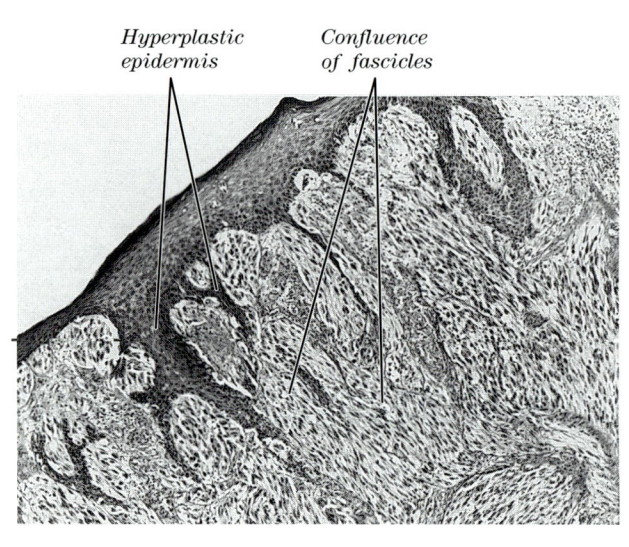

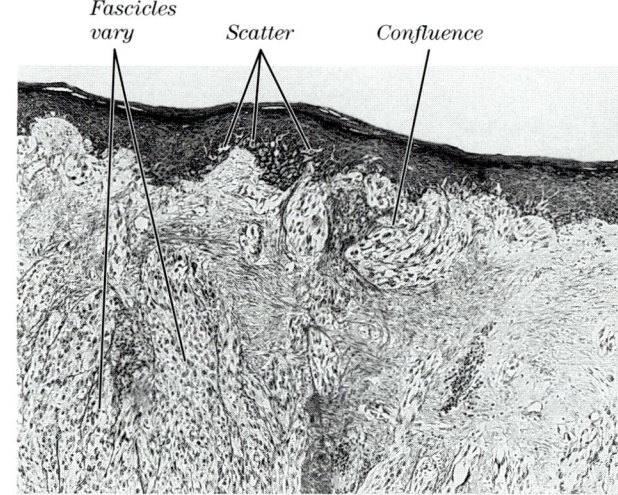

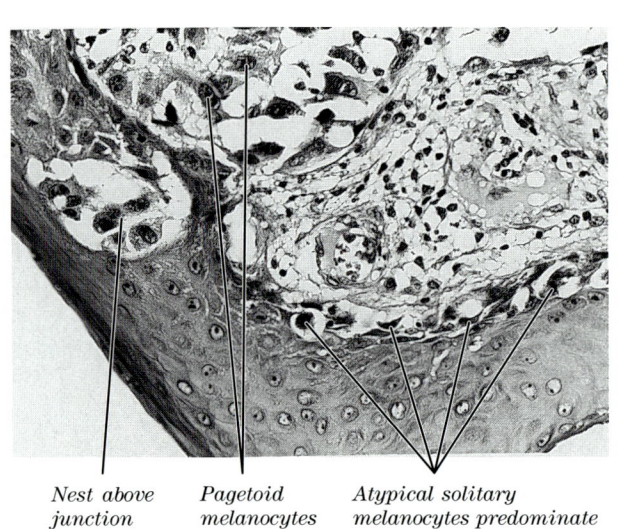

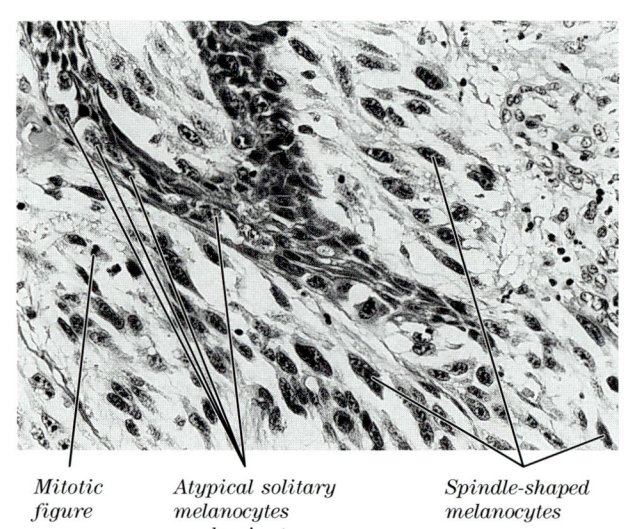

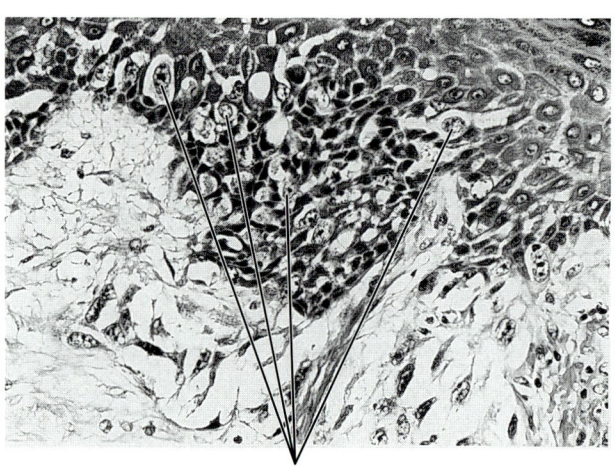

43 • Melanoma

Criteria for diagnosis of this melanoma

This is a melanoma because:

1. The neoplasm is asymmetric.
2. Melanocytes disposed as solitary units predominate over nests of melanocytes in some high-power fields.
3. Melanocytes arranged as solitary units are scattered at all levels of the epidermis in some foci.
4. Nests of melanocytes within the epidermis are not equidistant from one another.
5. Nests of melanocytes within the epidermis vary in size and shape.
6. Some nests of melanocytes within the epidermis have jagged outlines.
7. Fascicles of spindle-shaped melanocytes within the dermis have become confluent and formed sheets.

Pitfall in diagnosis

This melanoma could be misinterpreted as a Spitz's nevus because:

1. The neoplasm is exo-endophytic.
2. It is well-circumscribed.
3. There are hyperkeratosis, hypergranulosis, and irregular spinous-cell hyperplasia.
4. Clefts separate elongated nests of melanocytes within the epidermis from adjacent keratinocytes.
5. The nuclei of neoplastic melanocytes are large and mostly oval or spindle.
6. The cytoplasm of melanocytes is abundant.
7. Melanin is not distributed in uniform fashion within the dermis, as can be seen at scanning magnification.

That this neoplasm is malignant can be determined at scanning magnification because of asymmetry and sheets of neoplastic cells. At higher magnification, features like those of Spitz's nevi can be recognized at the dermo-epidermal junction in many high-power fields. The changes are not those of Spitz's nevus, however, for reasons apparent at scanning magnification; they are those of spitzoid melanoma.

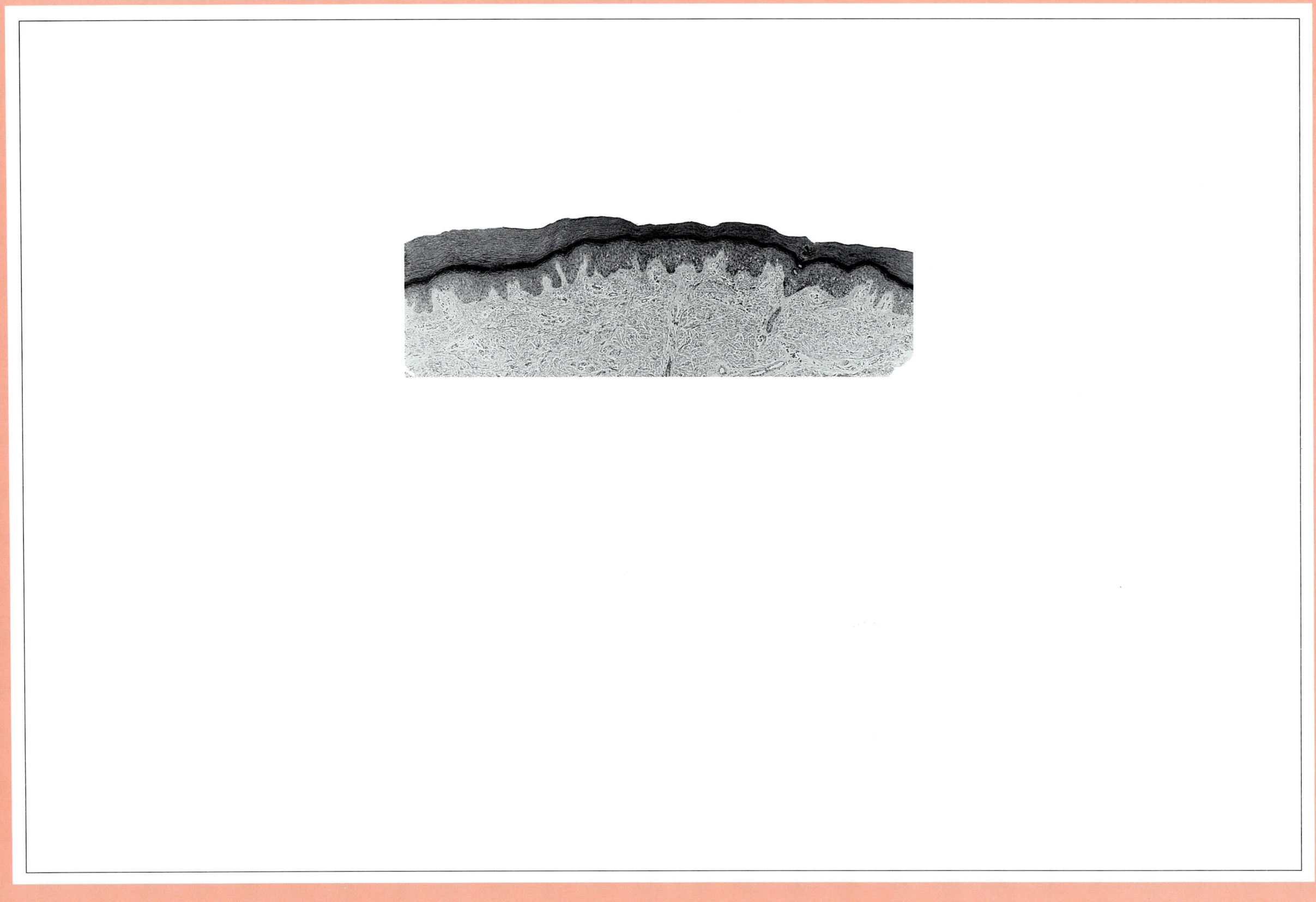

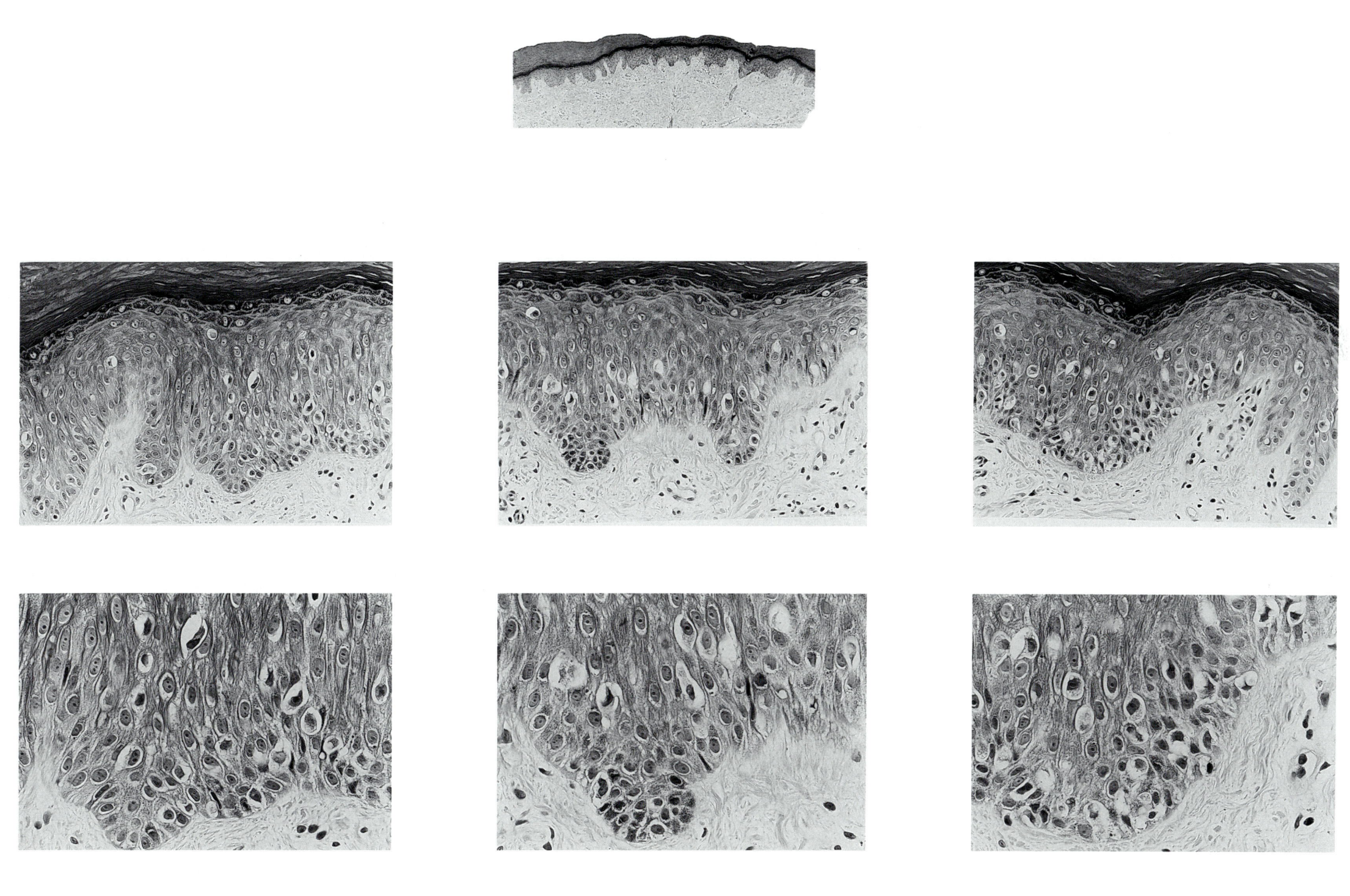

44. What is your diagnosis?

Small pigmented lesion on the medial aspect of the left foot of a 47-year-old woman that had increased in size over a 3-month period. Clinical diagnosis: junctional nevus vs. melanoma in situ. Wide local resection was performed. Patient was free of disease after 1 year.

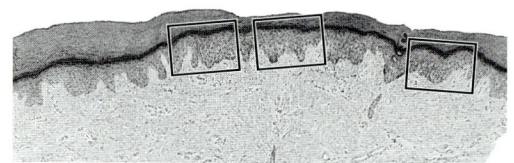

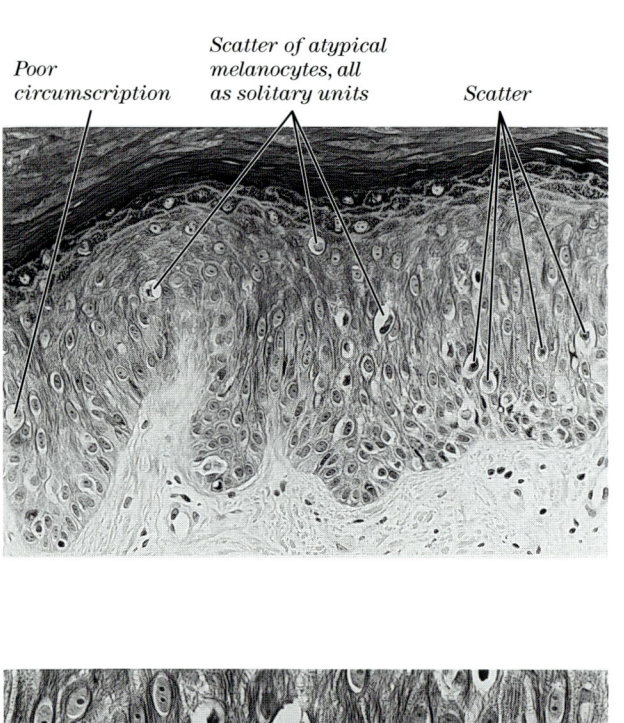

Poor circumscription — *Scatter of atypical melanocytes, all as solitary units* — *Scatter*

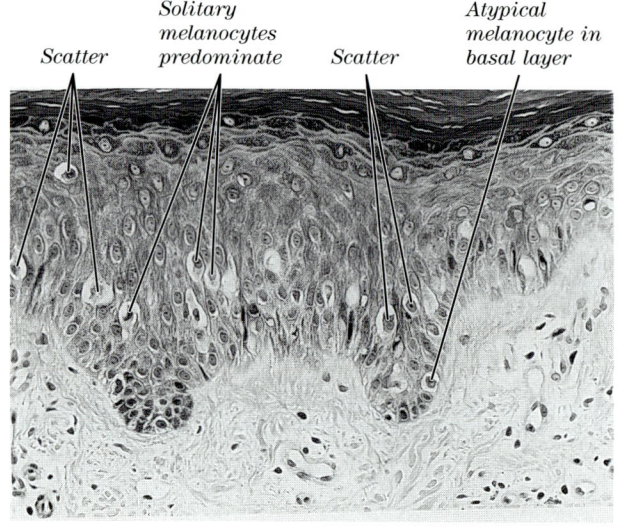

Scatter — *Solitary melanocytes predominate* — *Scatter* — *Atypical melanocyte in basal layer*

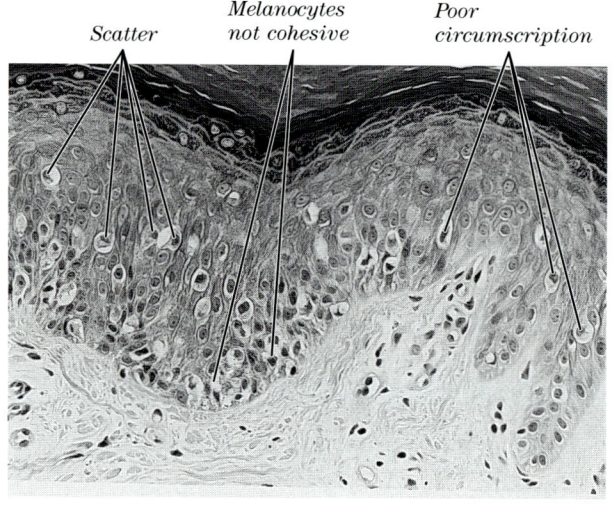

Scatter — *Melanocytes not cohesive* — *Poor circumscription*

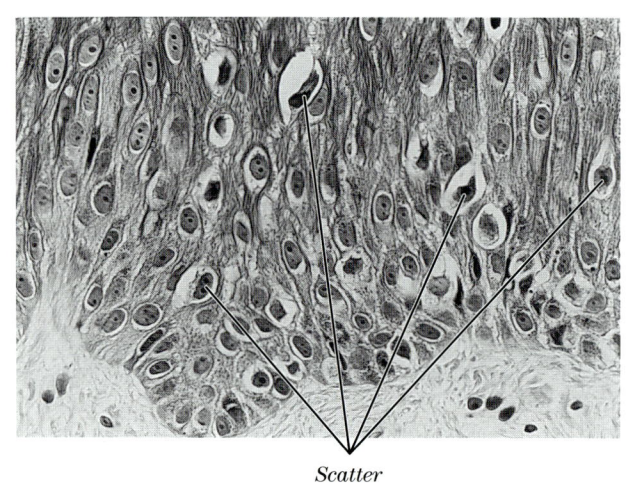

Scatter

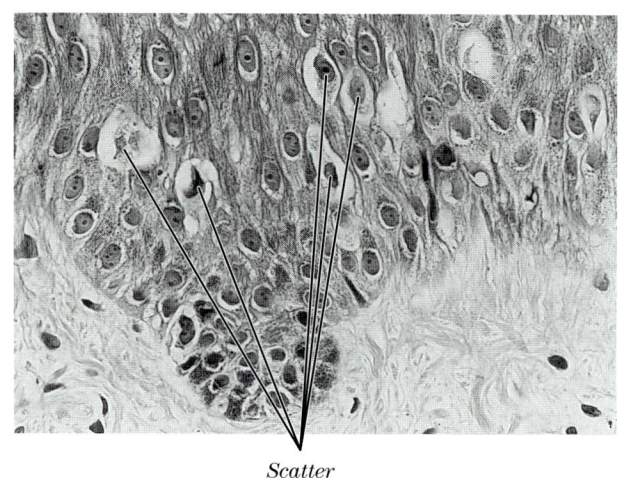

Scatter

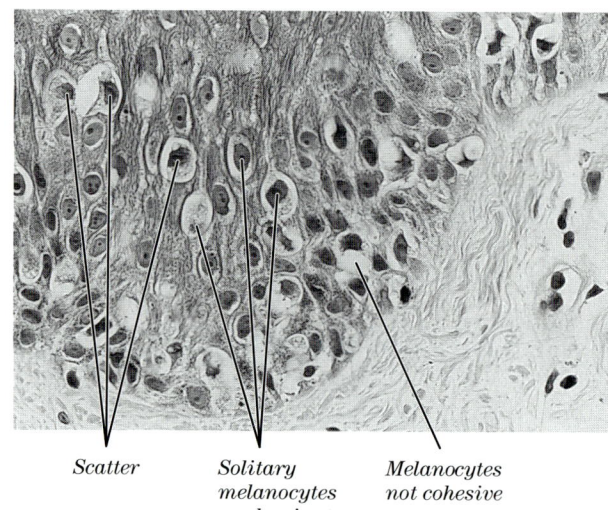

Scatter — *Solitary melanocytes predominate* — *Melanocytes not cohesive*

44 • Melanoma in situ

Criteria for diagnosis of this melanoma in situ

This is a melanoma in situ because:

1. Many melanocytes arranged as solitary units are scattered far above the dermo-epidermal junction.
2. Melanocytes arrayed as solitary units are not equidistant from one another.
3. Nuclei of melanocytes are atypical, i.e., they are pleomorphic and are stained differently from one another.
4. The number of melanocytes in the epidermis differs markedly from high-power field to high-power field.

Pitfall in diagnosis

This melanoma in situ could be misread as an early stage in the evolution of a Spitz's nevus because:

1. All the neoplastic melanocytes within the epidermis are arranged as solitary units.
2. Solitary melanocytes are present not only at the dermo-epidermal junction, but far above it.
3. Nuclei of melanocytes are large.
4. Some melanocytes have abundant pale cytoplasm.

A vexing problem in differential diagnosis of melanocytic neoplasms is the early intra-epidermal stage of Spitz's nevus versus the early intra-epidermal stage of melanoma. In both neoplasms, melanocytes arranged as solitary units predominate overwhelmingly. The crucial differentiating feature is the monomorphous appearance of the melanocytes in Spitz's nevus in contrast to the pleomorphic guise of melanocytes in melanoma in situ. Apart from that distinction, it may be nearly impossible at times to distinguish the benign from the malignant neoplasm. Criteria such as symmetry, circumscription, and maturation usually are not applicable in evolving proliferations of melanocytes confined to the epidermis across a front of but 2.0 or 3.0 mm.

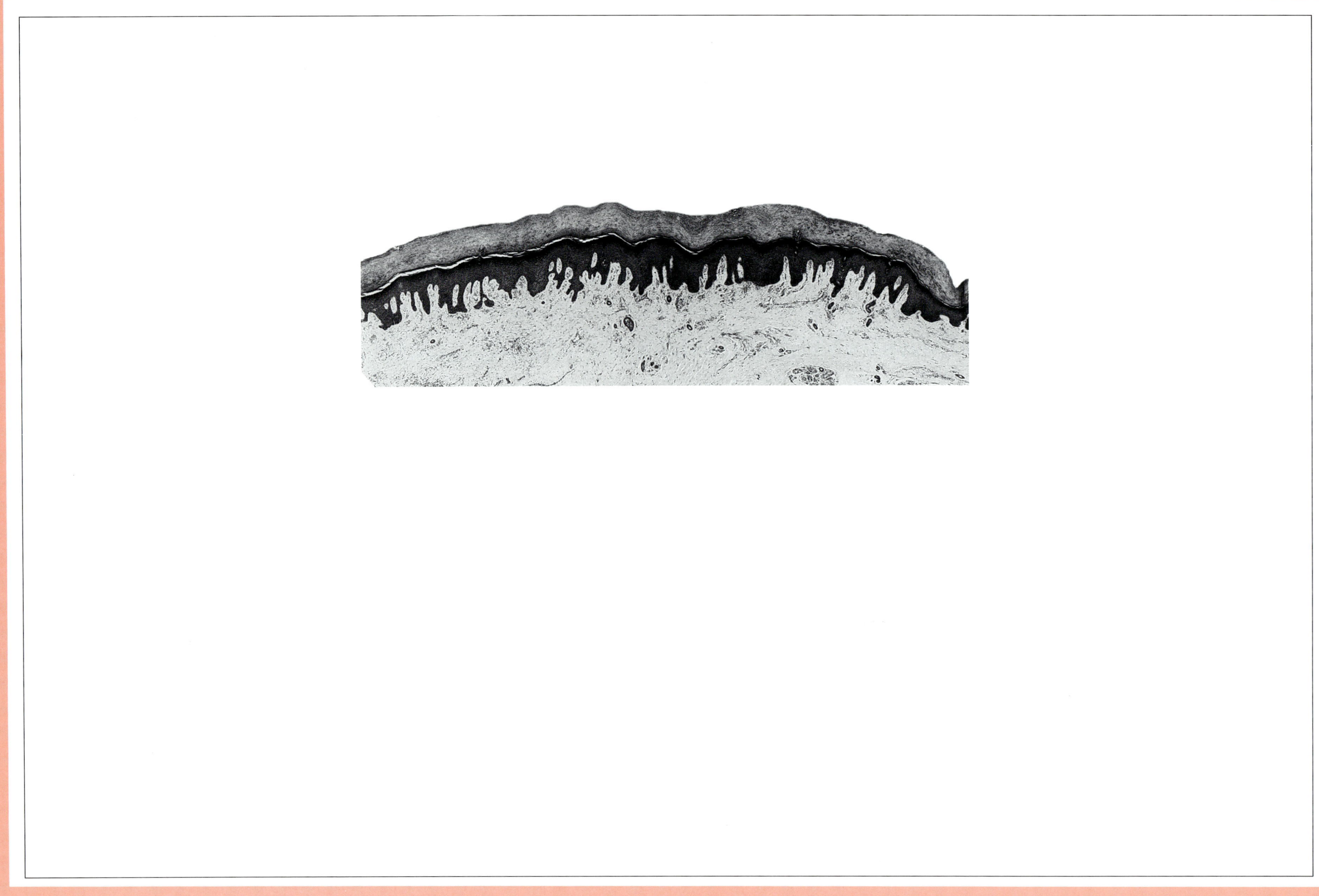

45. What is your diagnosis?

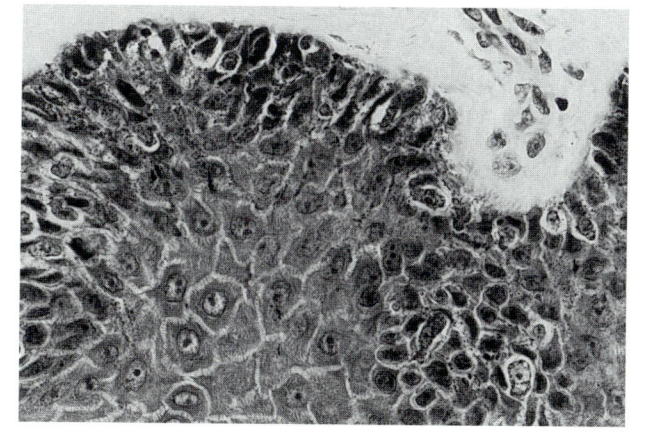
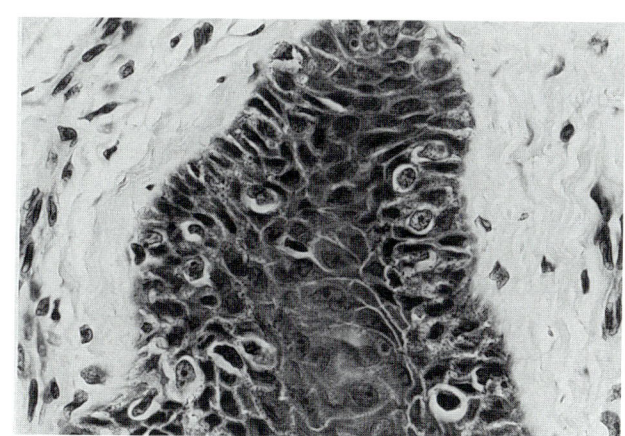
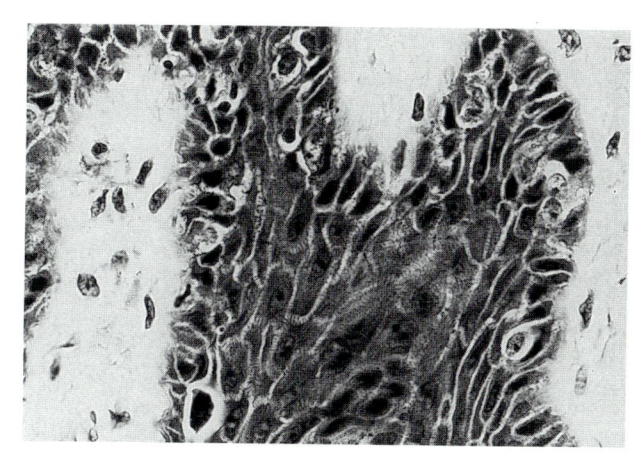
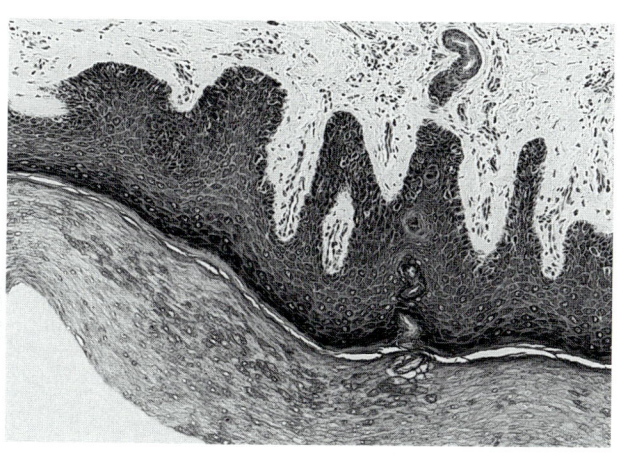
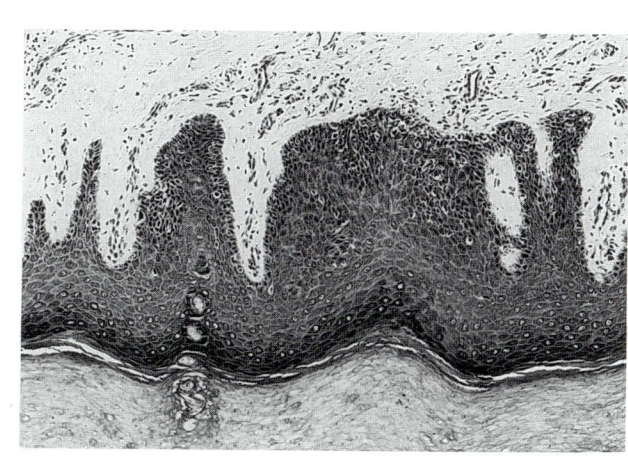
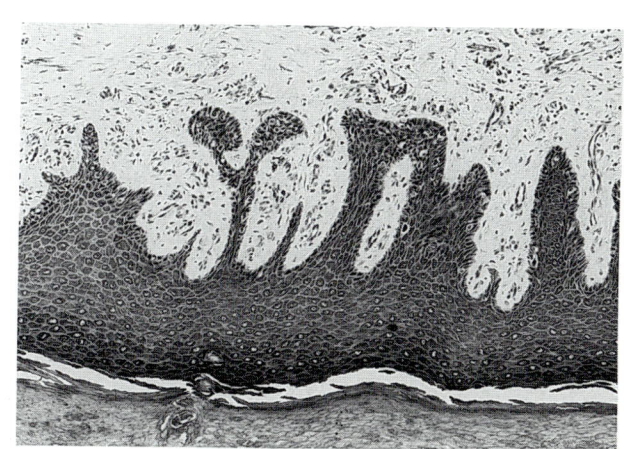
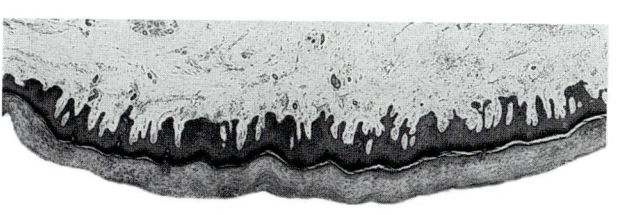

45 • Melanoma in situ

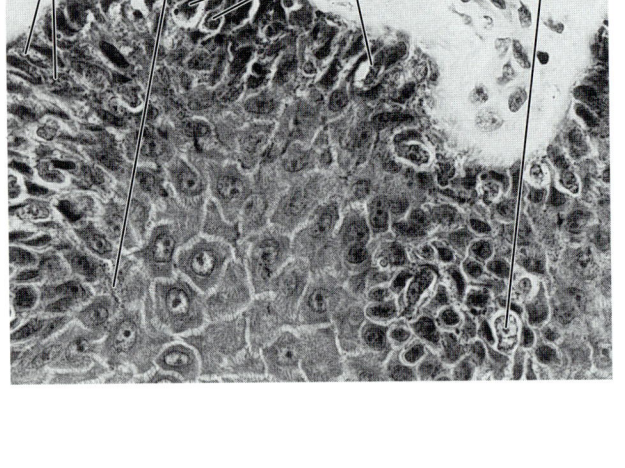

- Tangle of dendrites
- Strikingly elongated dendrite
- Increased number of melanocytes, some above junction
- Atypical melanocyte in spinous zone

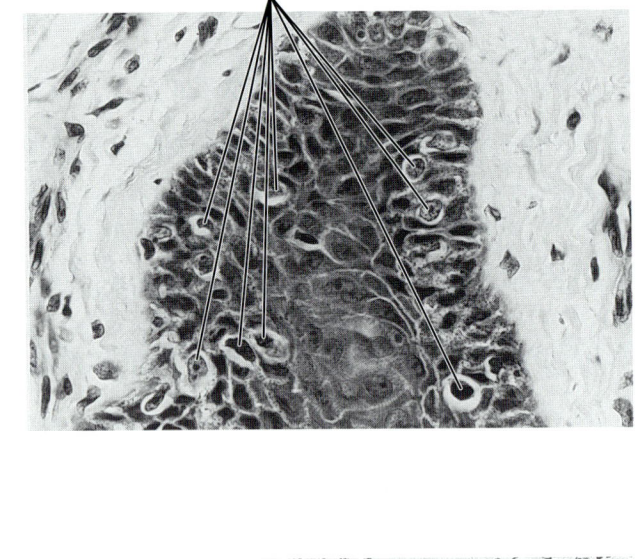

Scatter

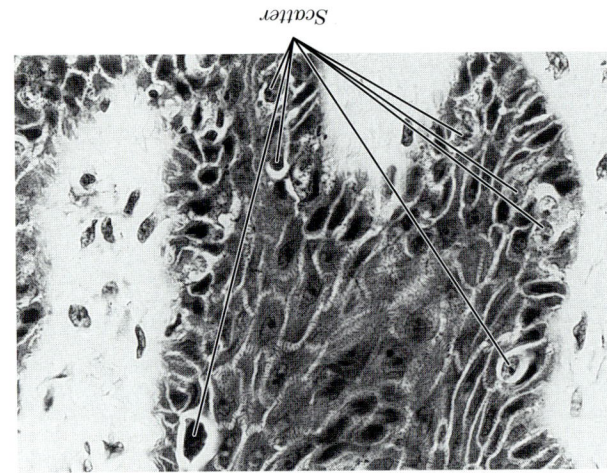

Scatter

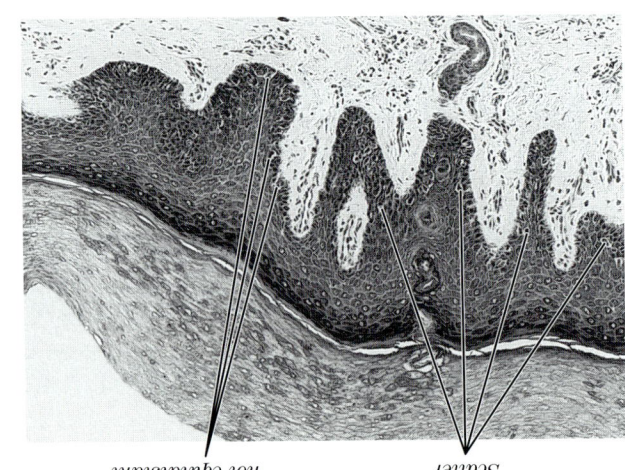

- Solitary melanocytes not equidistant
- Scatter

Scatter

- Solitary melanocytes not equidistant

- Atypical melanocytes not equidistant
- Scatter
- Scatter

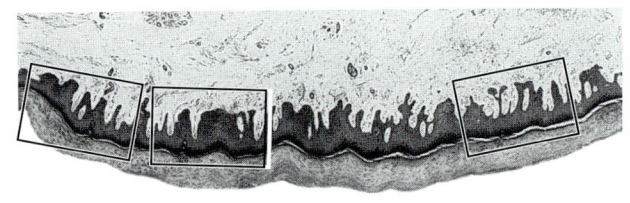

Well-circumscribed, uniformly pigmented lesion on the plantar surface of the right fifth toe of an 81-year-old man. Clinical diagnosis: simple lentigo. No persistence of this lesion was observed after 2 years.

Criteria for diagnosis of this melanoma in situ

This is a melanoma in situ because:

1. The neoplasm is more than 1.5 cm in diameter.
2. Many melanocytes are disposed as solitary units far above the dermo-epidermal junction.
3. Neoplastic melanocytes arranged as solitary units are not equidistant from one another.
4. Some neoplastic melanocytes exhibit strikingly elongated dendrites that extend to at least the mid-spinous zone.
5. Nuclei of melanocytes are pleomorphic; some nucleoli are prominent.

Pitfall in diagnosis

This melanoma in situ could be misconstrued as a simple lentigo because:

1. Melanocytes often are present above the dermo-epidermal junction of benign proliferations on volar skin.
2. Melanocytes are disposed entirely as solitary units.
3. Some dendrites of melanocytes are apparent.
4. Upper segments of some eccrine ducts are involved.

A challenging problem in differential diagnosis is posed by the distinction between junctional nevi, including the stage of simple lentigines, on volar skin from melanomas in situ there. In both neoplasms, there may be scatter of melanocytes arrayed as solitary units and in nests within the epidermis. In melanoma in situ, in contrast to junctional nevi, melanocytes arranged as solitary units tend to predominate over nests in some high-power fields, melanocytes arranged as solitary units are not equidistant from one another, and nuclei of melanocytes are atypical. Another helpful sign for identification of melanoma in situ is solitary melanocytes with exceptionally long dendrites that extend far into the spinous zone and sometimes even into the granular zone. Such dramatic dendrites are not encountered in simple lentigines and fully formed junctional nevi as a rule.

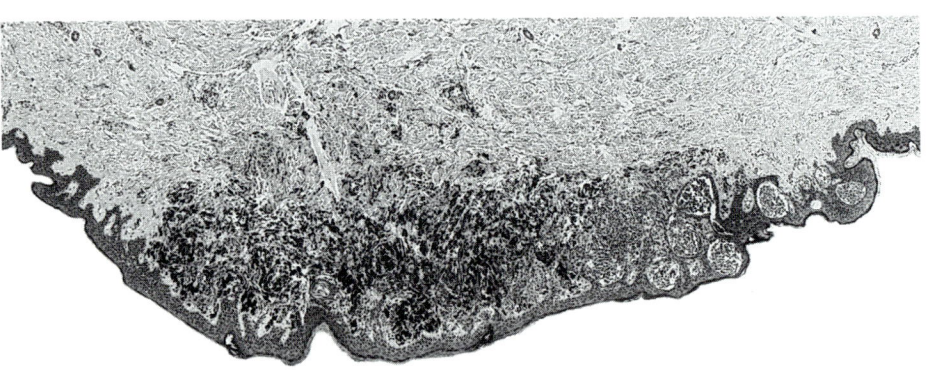

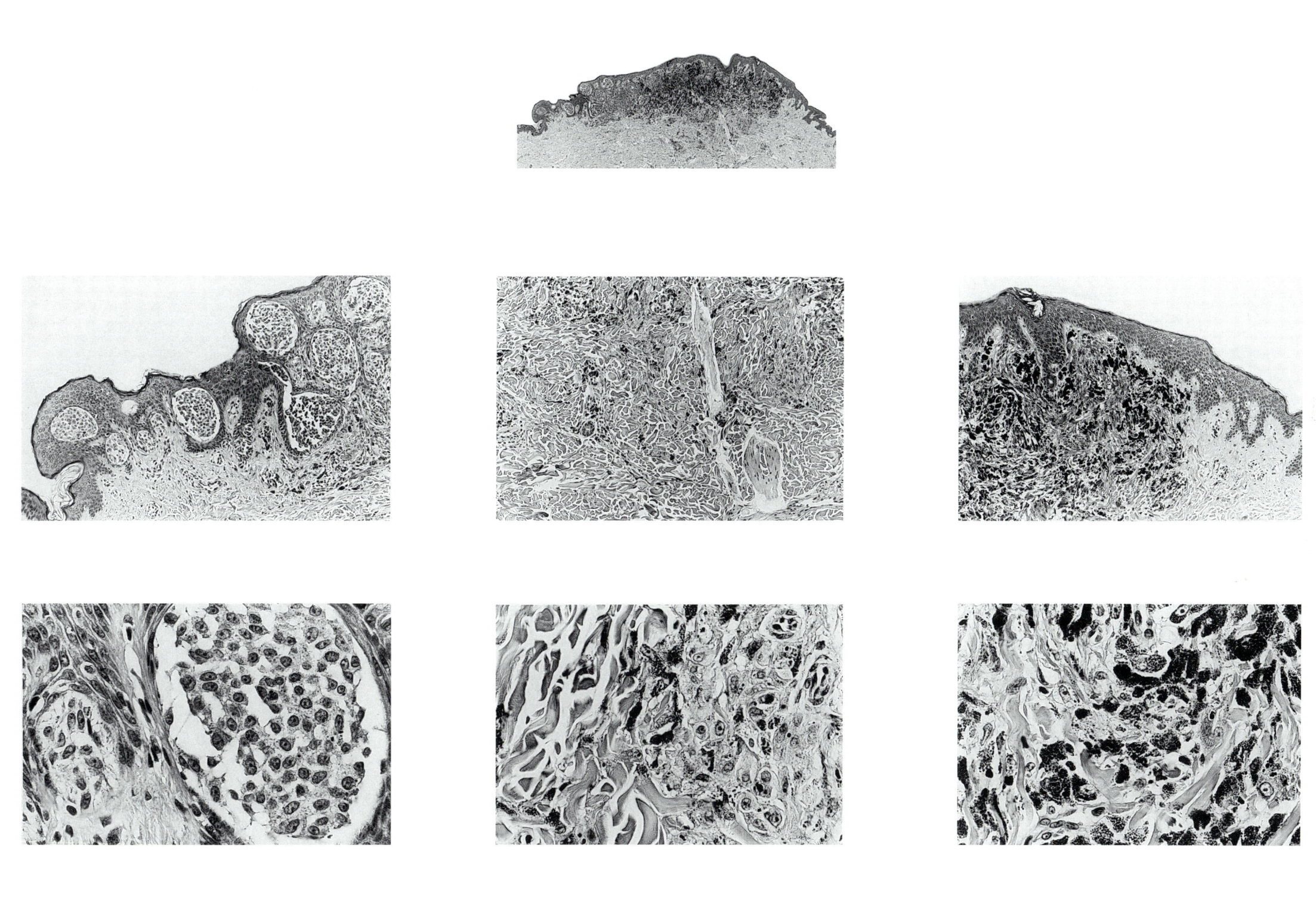

46. What is your diagnosis?

Black papule surrounded by a brown macular rim on the back of an 8-year-old boy had increased in size recently. Clinical diagnosis: melanoma or Spitz's nevus. No follow-up data were available.

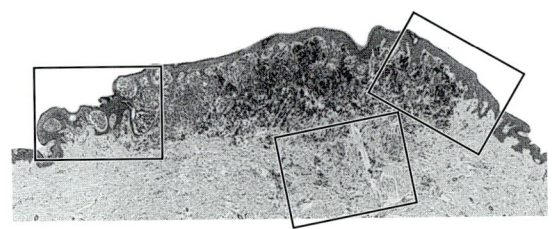

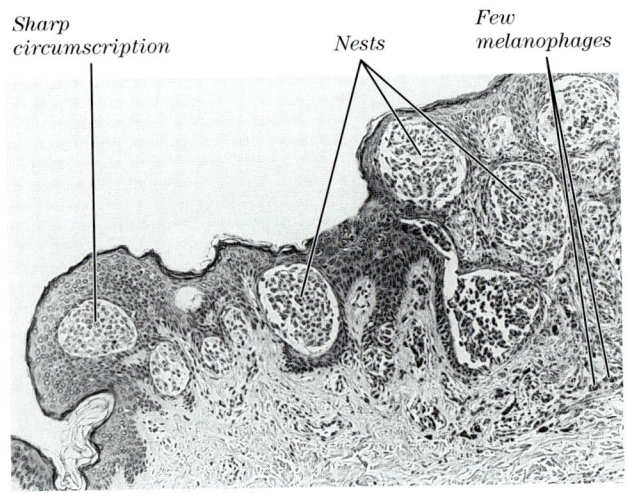

Sharp circumscription — *Nests* — *Few melanophages*

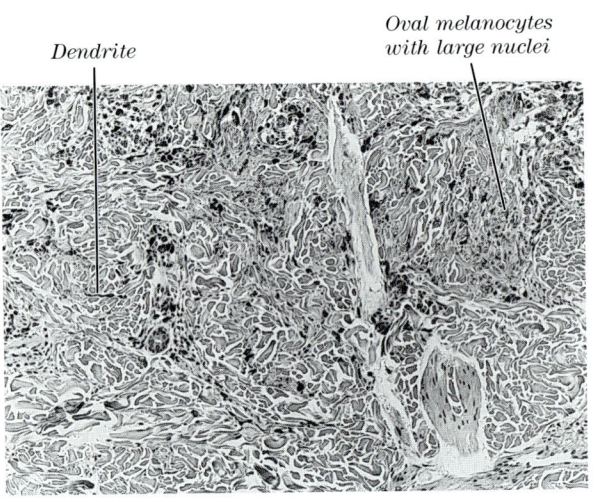

Dendrite — *Oval melanocytes with large nuclei*

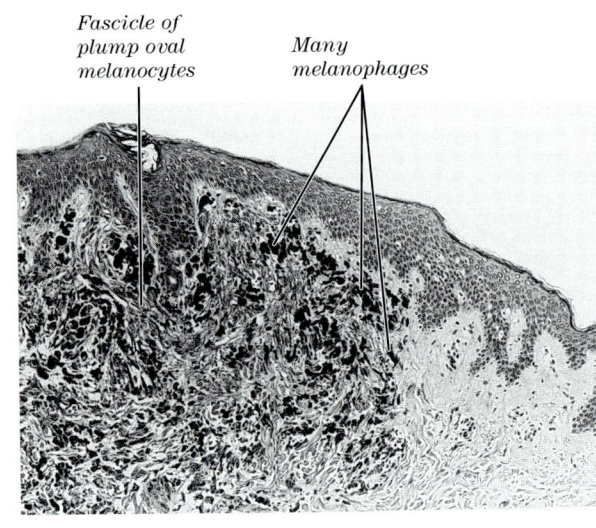

Fascicle of plump oval melanocytes — *Many melanophages*

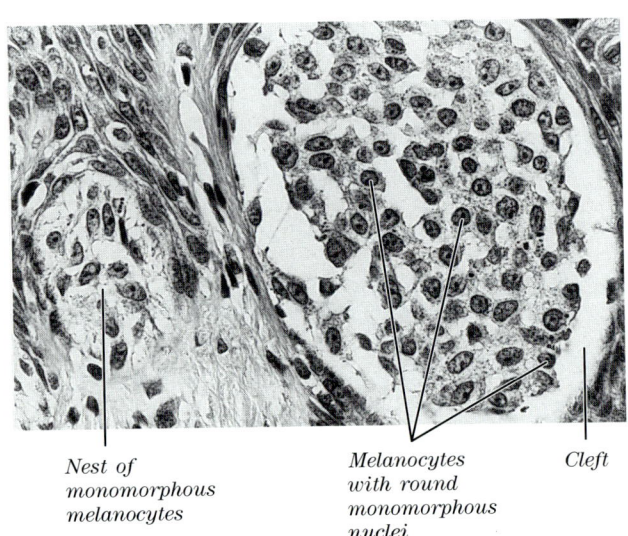

Nest of monomorphous melanocytes — *Melanocytes with round monomorphous nuclei* — *Cleft*

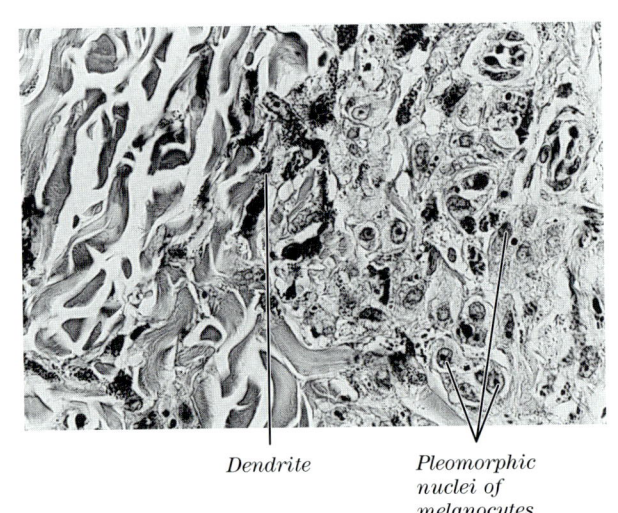

Dendrite — *Pleomorphic nuclei of melanocytes*

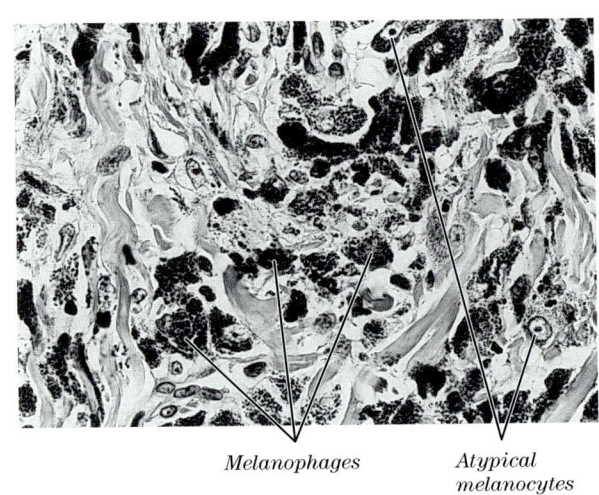

Melanophages — *Atypical melanocytes*

46 • Combined Nevus *(Clark's and Spitz's)*

Criteria for diagnosis of this combined nevus (Clark's and Spitz's)

This neoplasm is benign because:

1. It is well-circumscribed.

2. The component of the lesion on the left has a relatively flat bottom, whereas that on the right is wedge-shaped.

3. All of the melanocytes within the epidermis, both those disposed as solitary units and those in nests, are situated at the dermo-epidermal junction, not above it.

4. The pigmented lesion on the right is but little more than 2.0 mm in greatest diameter and extends far into the reticular dermis.

The neoplasm on the left is a Clark's nevus because:

1. The lesion is but slightly elevated and gently mammillated.

2. Nests of melanocytes within the epidermis and the dermis are confined to the dermo-epidermal junction and thickened papillary dermis.

3. Nuclei of melanocytes are small, oval, and monomorphous.

The pigmented lesion on the right is a Spitz's nevus because:

1. Many of the melanocytes within the dermis have large nuclei, abundant cytoplasm, and round and oval shapes.

Pitfall in diagnosis

This combined (Clark's and Spitz's) nevus could be misinterpreted as a melanoma in association with a Clark's nevus because:

1. The neoplasm is asymmetric.

2. Melanin is not distributed in uniform fashion.

3. Many of the nuclei on the right side of the neoplasm are atypical.

4. An indubitable Clark's nevus is positioned on the left side.

A major exception to the precept that asymmetry is the cardinal feature for distinguishing melanomas from nevi is found in combined nevi such as this one. It is inevitable that combinations of types of nevi, such as Clark's nevus and Spitz's nevus in this instance, produce a silhouette that is asymmetric. When other features of architectural pattern, such as circumscription and maturation, are taken into account, however, a correct diagnosis can be reached.

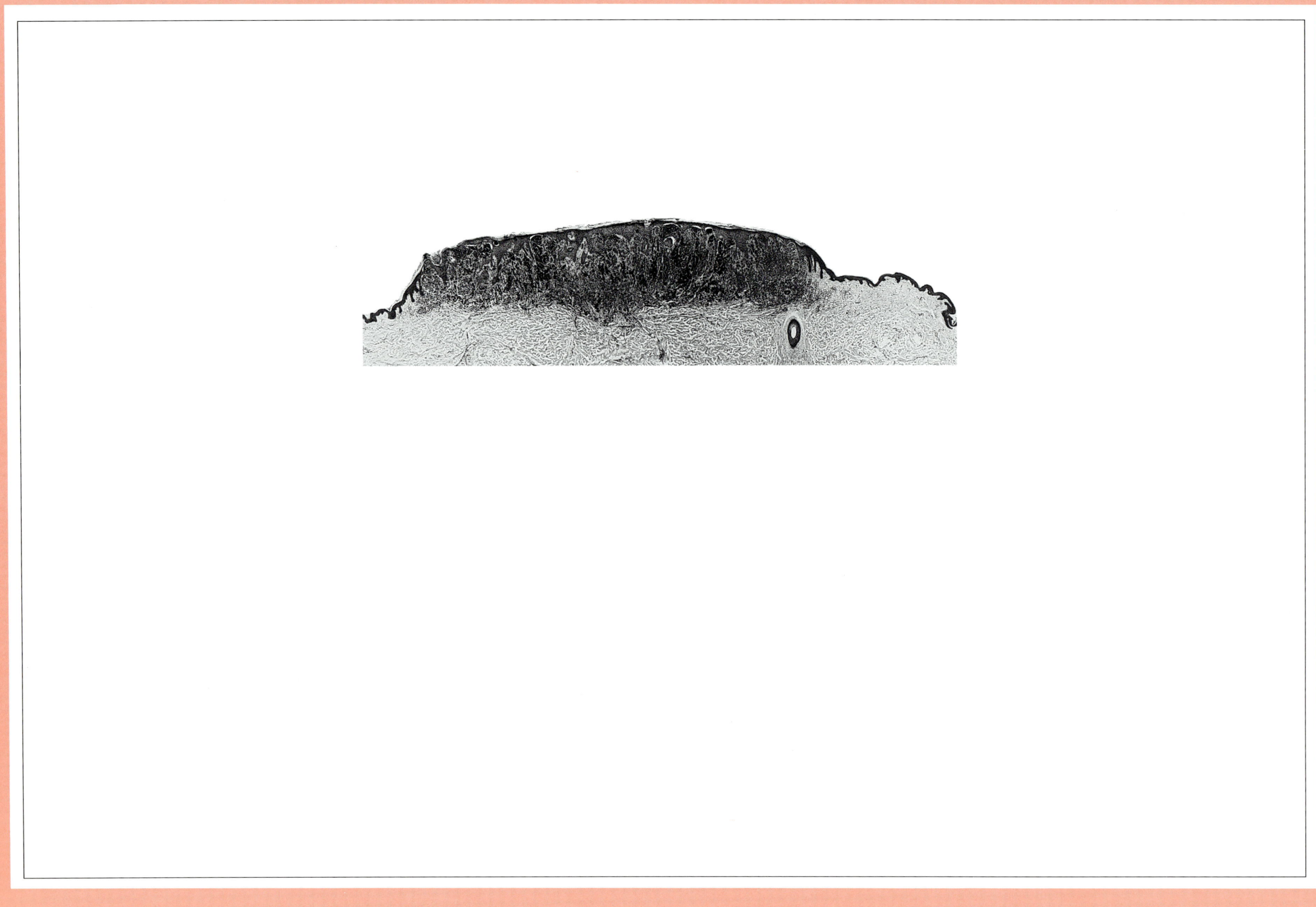

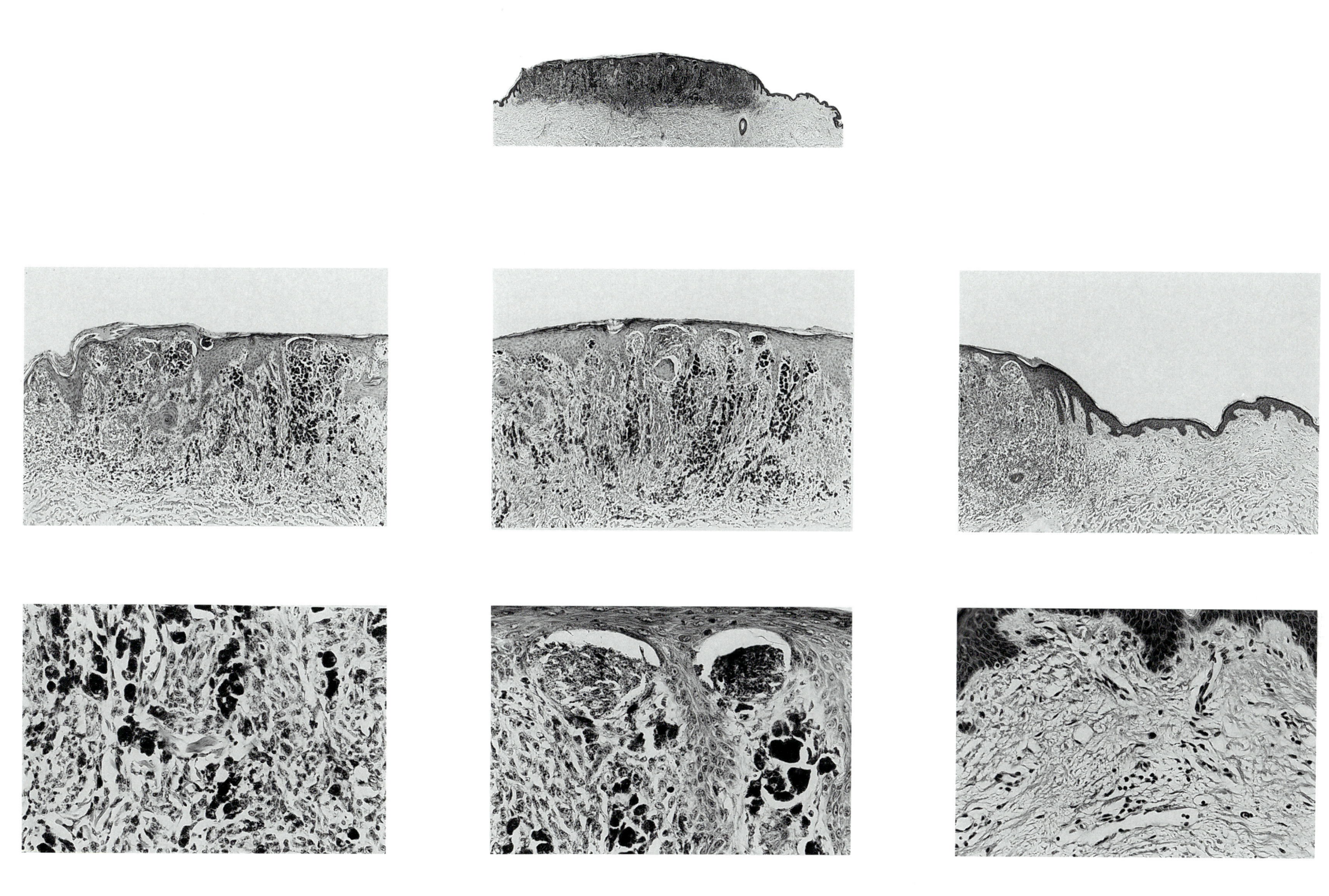

47. What is your diagnosis?

Blue-black lesion on the left side of the back of a 33-year-old man. Clinical diagnosis: melanoma. A wide excision revealed no residual neoplasm. Left axillary dissection produced 23 lymph nodes that were free of metastases. Patient was well after 3 years.

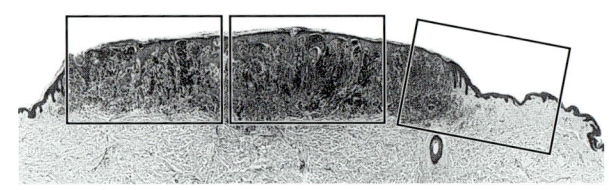

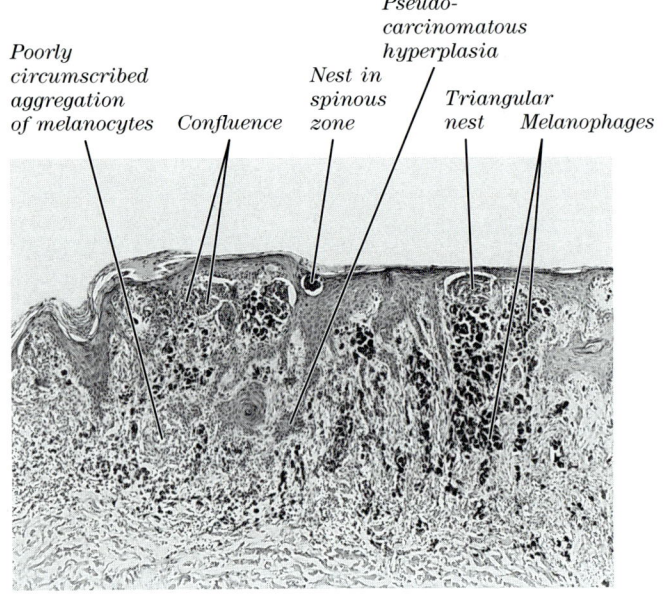

Poorly circumscribed aggregation of melanocytes — Confluence — Nest in spinous zone — Pseudo-carcinomatous hyperplasia — Triangular nest — Melanophages

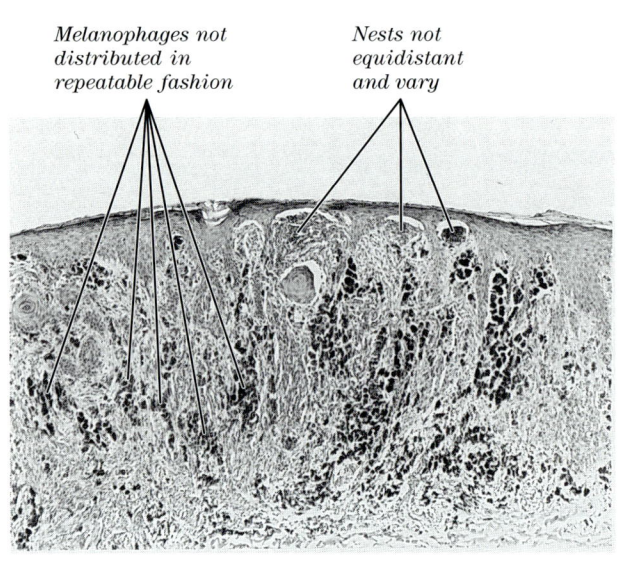

Melanophages not distributed in repeatable fashion — Nests not equidistant and vary

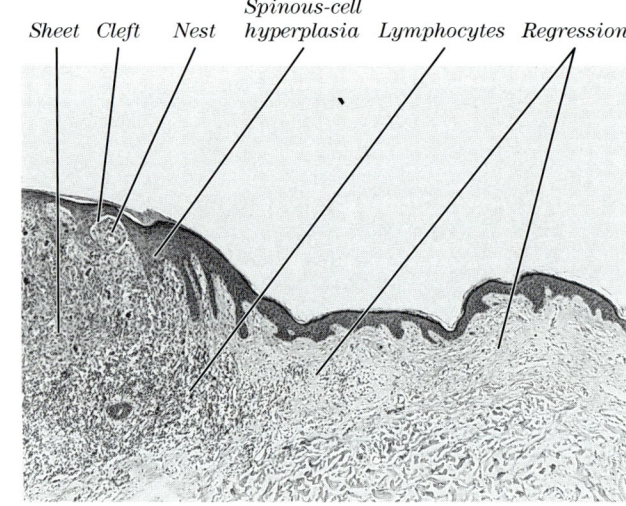

Sheet — Cleft — Nest — Spinous-cell hyperplasia — Lymphocytes — Regression

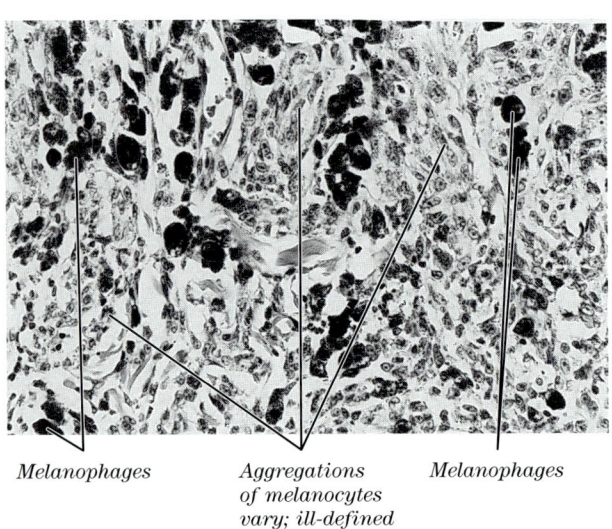

Melanophages — Aggregations of melanocytes vary; ill-defined — Melanophages

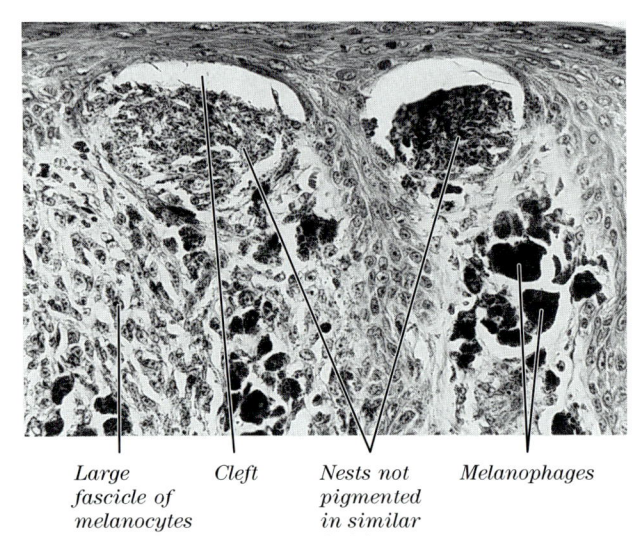

Large fascicle of melanocytes — Cleft — Nests not pigmented in similar fashion — Melanophages

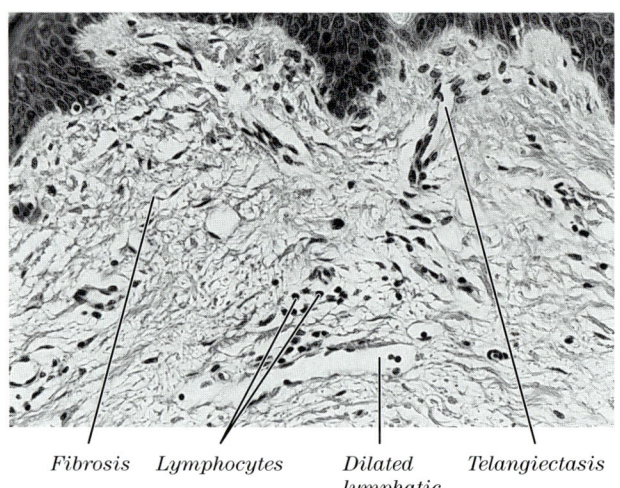

Fibrosis — Lymphocytes — Dilated lymphatic — Telangiectasis

47 • Melanoma

Criteria for diagnosis of this melanoma

This is a melanoma because:

1. The neoplasm is asymmetric.

2. A zone of regression on the right of the neoplasm is characterized by a papillary dermis thickened by fibroplasia, a sparse lymphocytic infiltrate, and telangiectases.

3. Melanin is not distributed in uniform fashion throughout the neoplasm.

4. Nests of melanocytes within the epidermis and the dermis vary in size and shape.

5. Many nests of melanocytes within the epidermis and the dermis have become confluent.

6. The base of the neoplasm is neither flat nor wedge-shaped.

Pitfall in diagnosis

This melanoma could be misinterpreted as a compound pigmented spindle-cell variant of Spitz's nevus because:

1. It is a richly pigmented neoplasm confined to the epidermis and upper part of the dermis.

2. The neoplasm is rather well-circumscribed.

3. There are hyperkeratosis, hypergranulosis, and irregular epidermal hyperplasia.

4. Clefts are present between nests of melanocytes seated at the dermoepidermal junction and adjacent keratinocytes.

5. Some nests of melanocytes are elongated and oriented vertically to the skin surface.

6. Nuclei of melanocytes are oval and monomorphous.

At scanning magnification, this neoplasm could be considered to be symmetric, but, in actuality, it is not. Note that, on the left, nests of melanocytes are discernible at scanning magnification, whereas hardly any nests can be appreciated on the right. Note also that melanin is much less on the left than it is on the right. Last, the infiltrate of lymphocytes does not obscure the left side of the neoplasm to the same extent that it does the right side. This constellation of findings stamps the neoplasm as melanoma.

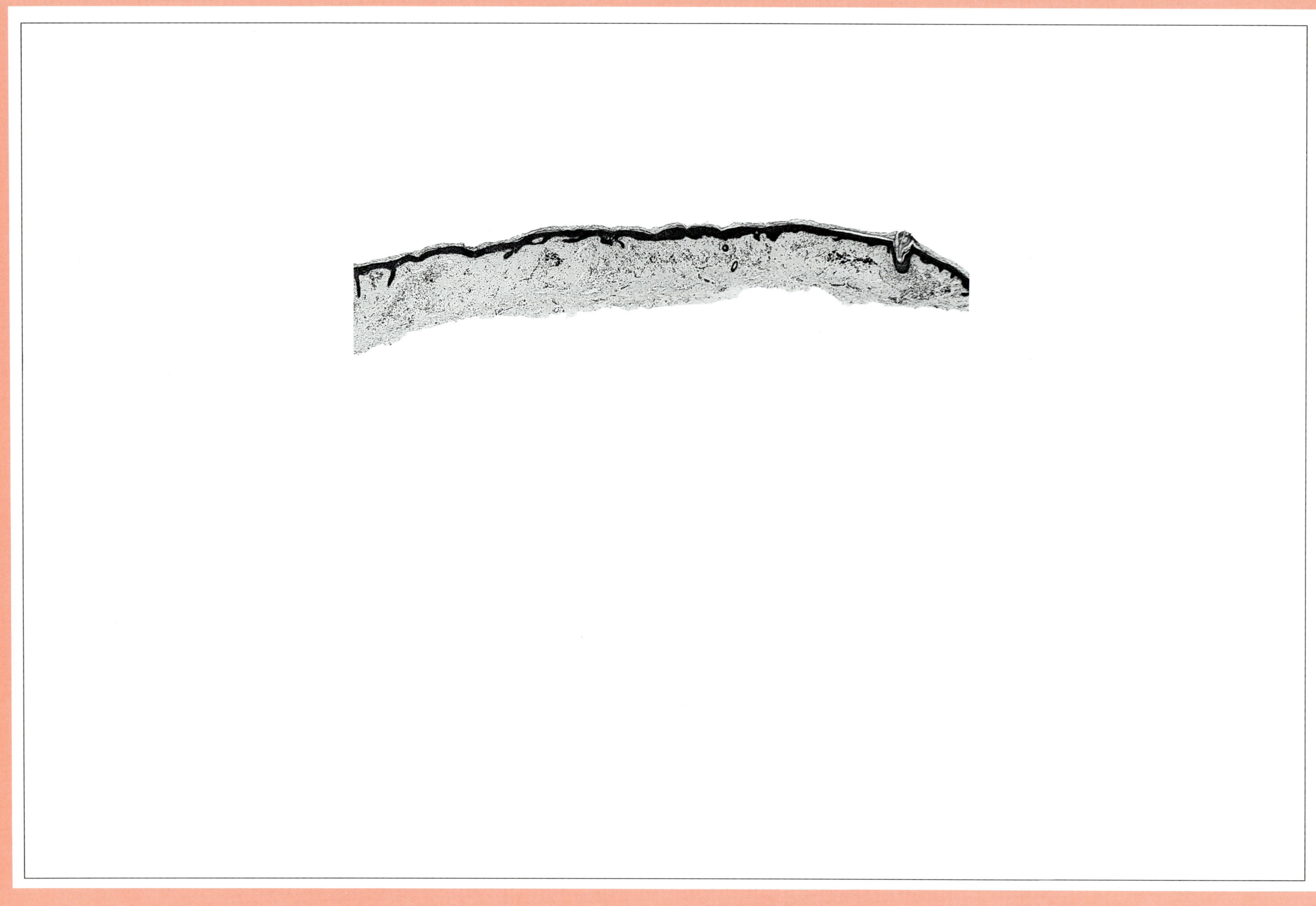

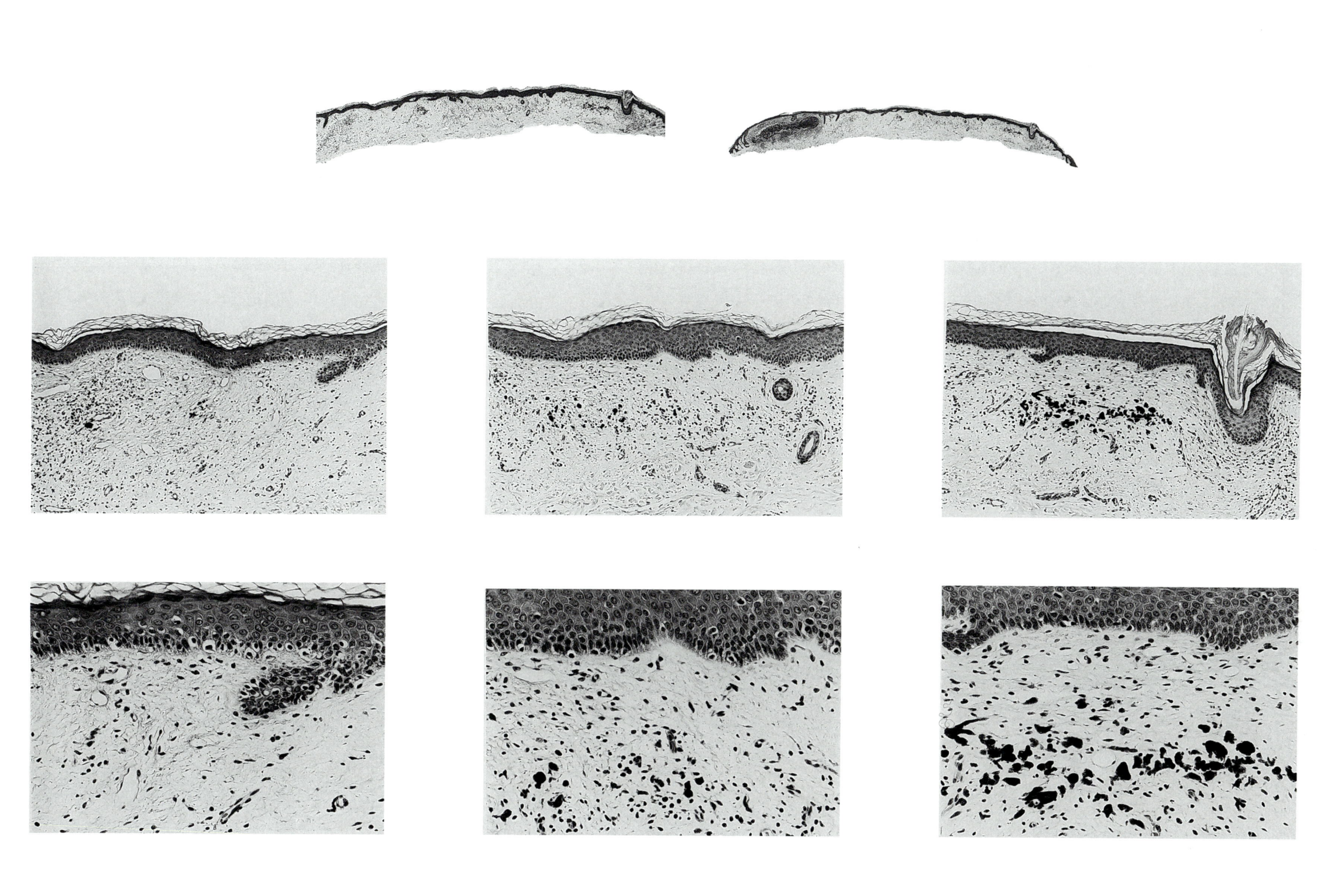

48. What is your diagnosis?

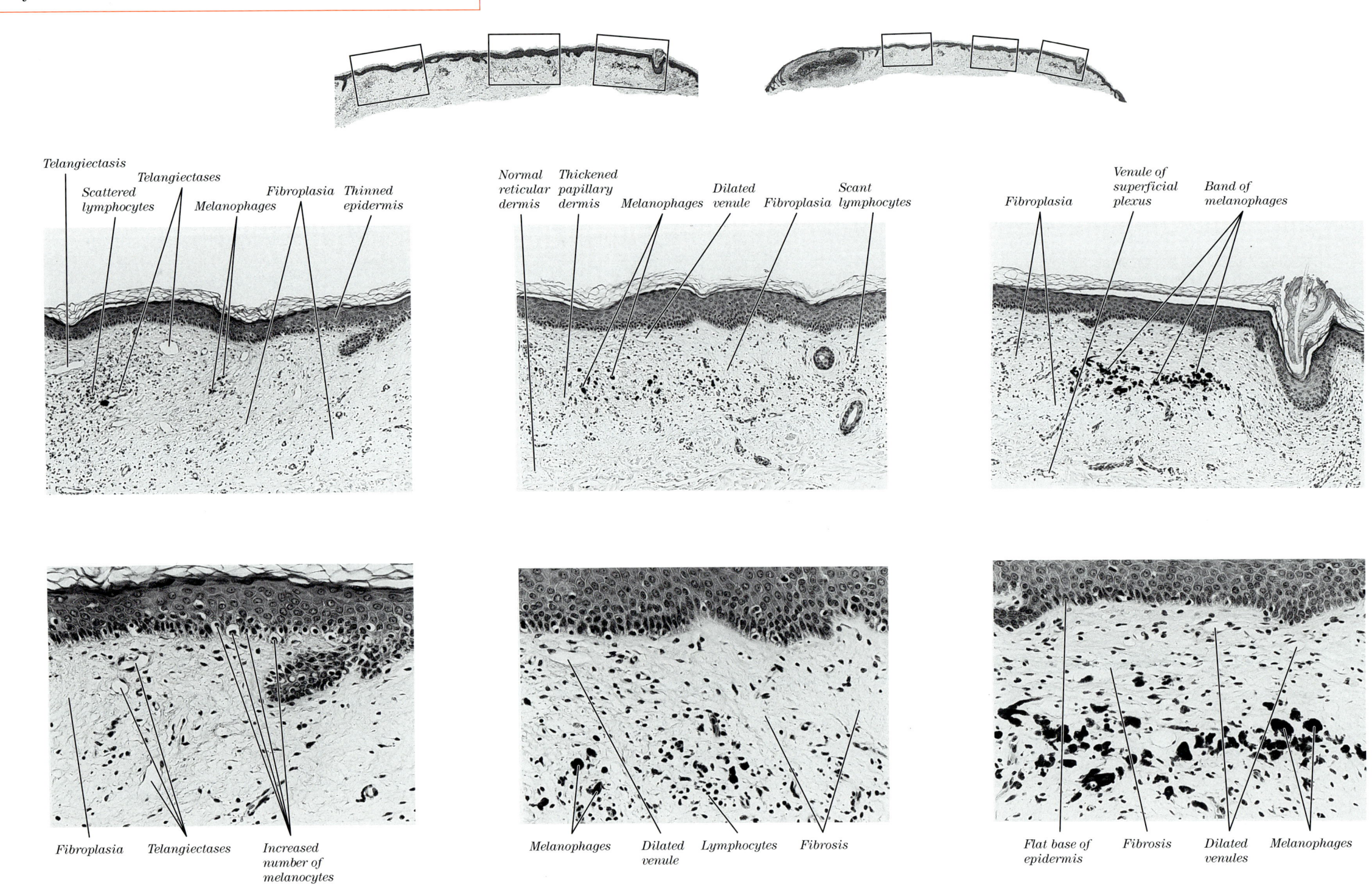

48 • Basal-Cell Carcinoma (with partial regression)

Criteria for diagnosis of this basal-cell carcinoma (with partial regression)

This is a basal-cell carcinoma because:

A basal-cell carcinoma is detected.

Apart from the finding of a basal-cell carcinoma, the changes pictured in a thickened papillary dermis beneath an epidermis largely devoid of rete ridges are indistinguishable from those of regression of primary melanoma. Those findings of regression are a papillary dermis thickened markedly by fibroplasia, melanophages, a patchy lymphocytic infiltrate, and telangiectases. As a rule, epidermal rete ridges are muted or flattened.

Pitfall in diagnosis

The extensive regression in association with this superficial basal-cell carcinoma could be misinterpreted as regression of melanoma because:

The thickened papillary dermis is marked by fibroplasia, telangiectases, and a sprinkling of lymphocytes.

From features of regression alone characterized mostly by fibroplasia, a histopathologist cannot determine what kind of neoplasm has undergone regression. Only if residual changes of melanoma, superficial basal-cell carcinoma, or lichen planus-like keratosis are detected can a specific diagnosis be rendered. In the case of this lesion, step sections uncovered a basal-cell carcinoma. If no residual findings of the primary neoplasm are detected, the histopathologic diagnosis can be only "regression of a primary neoplasm," and the differential diagnosis appended in a note.

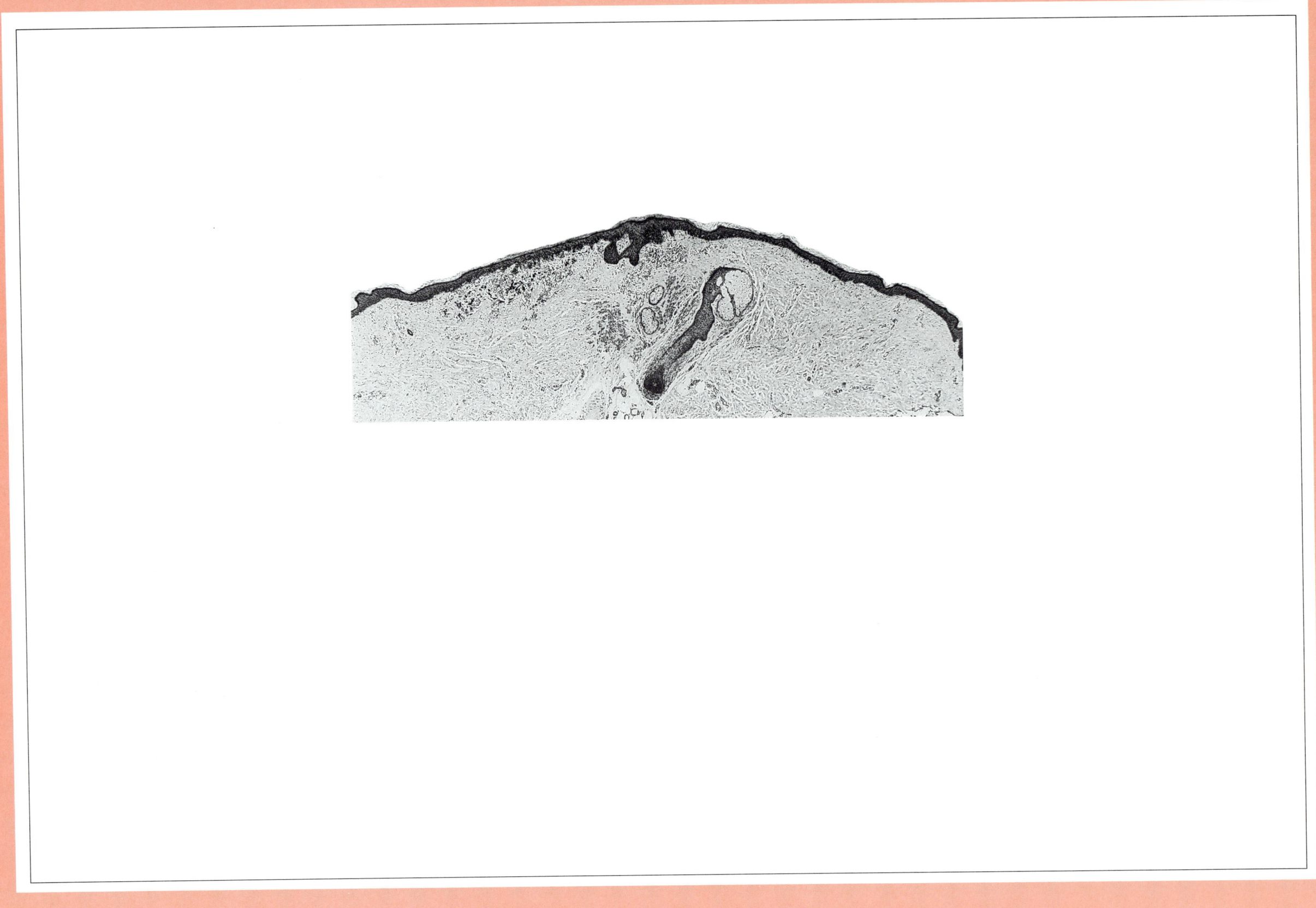

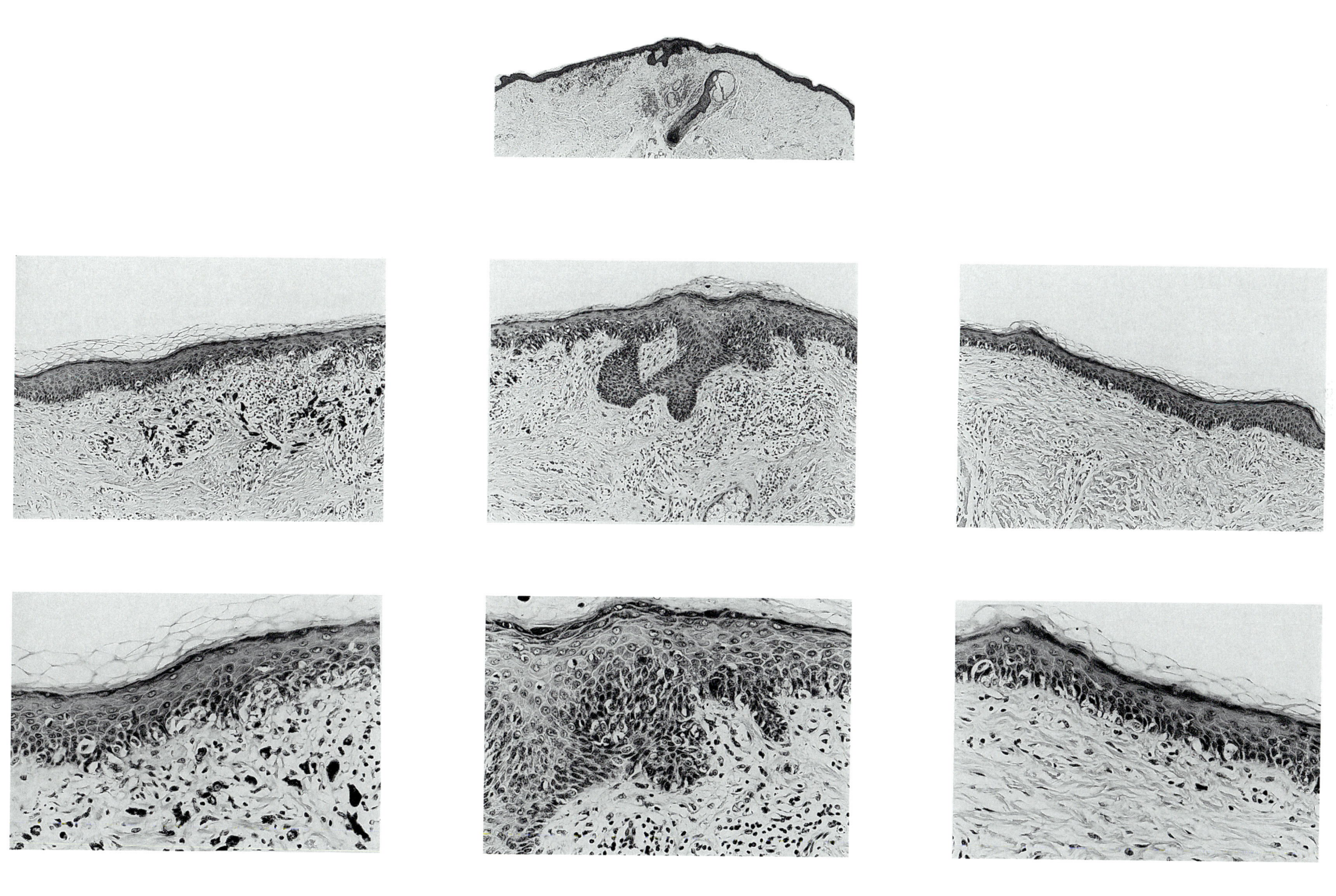

49. What is your diagnosis?

Pigmented lesion on the posterior calf of a 28-year-old woman. Clinical diagnosis: nevus. No follow-up data were available.

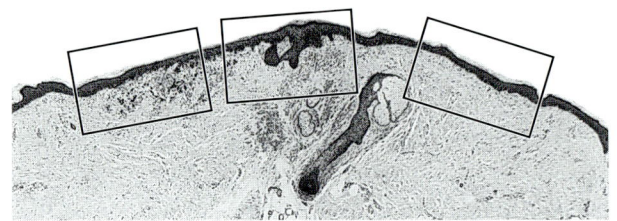

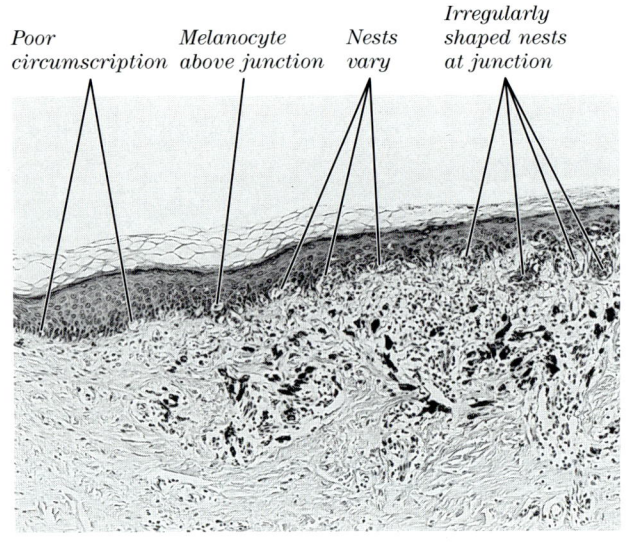

Poor circumscription — Melanocyte above junction — Nests vary — Irregularly shaped nests at junction

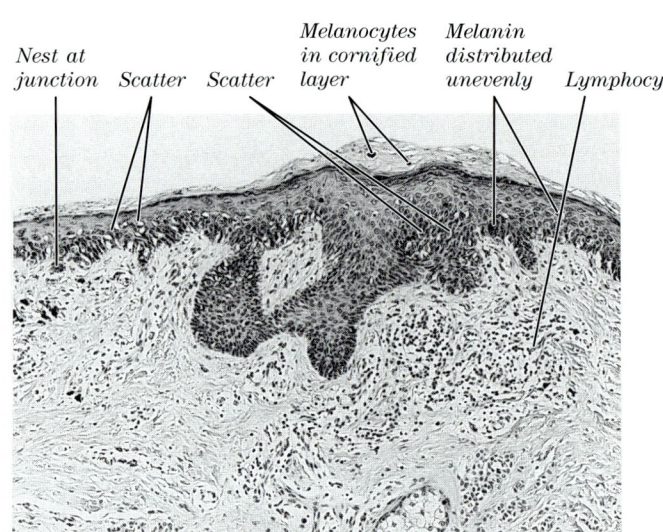

Nest at junction — Scatter — Scatter — Melanocytes in cornified layer — Melanin distributed unevenly — Lymphocytes

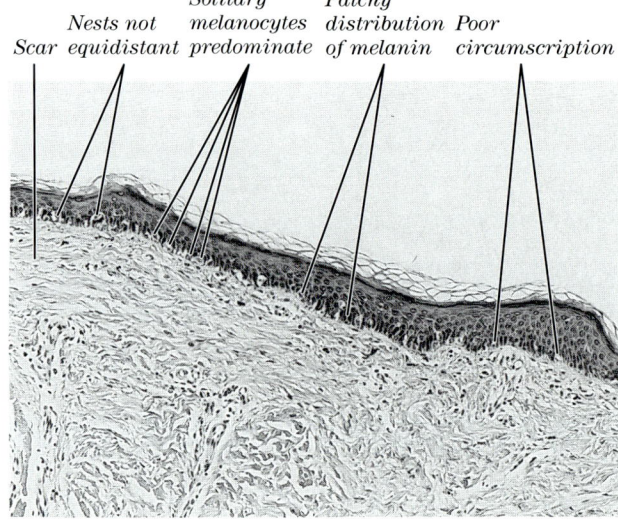

Scar — Nests not equidistant — Solitary melanocytes predominate — Patchy distribution of melanin — Poor circumscription

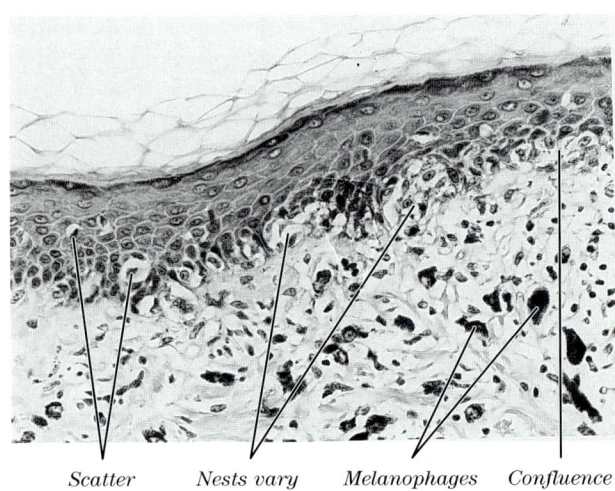

Scatter — Nests vary — Melanophages — Confluence

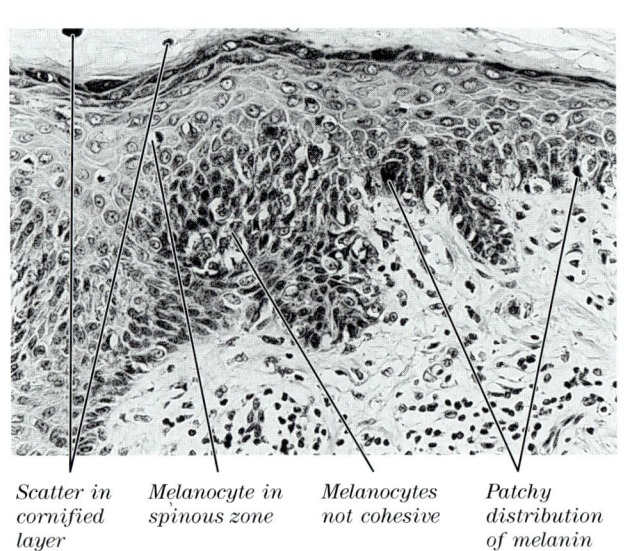

Scatter in cornified layer — Melanocyte in spinous zone — Melanocytes not cohesive — Patchy distribution of melanin

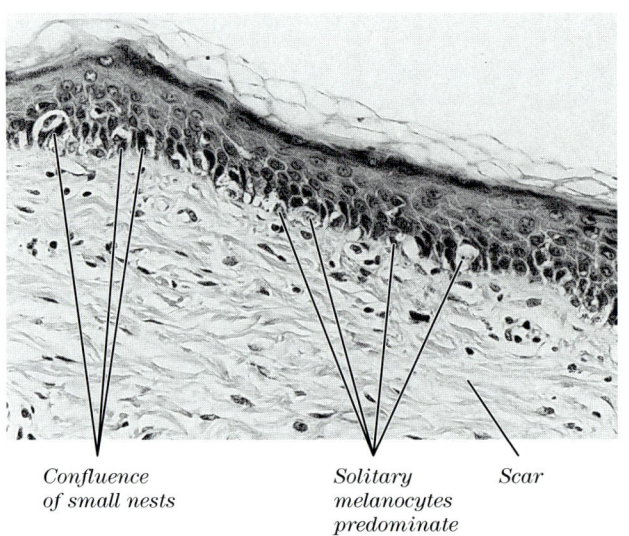

Confluence of small nests — Solitary melanocytes predominate — Scar

49 • Congenital Nevus (*superficial, persistent*)

Criteria for diagnosis of this persistent (recurrent) congenital nevus (superficial type)

This is a nevus because:

1. At scanning magnification, there are small monomorphous melanocytes arranged in nests, cords, and strands in the upper part of the reticular dermis.
2. Virtually all the nests of melanocytes within the epidermis are seated at the dermo-epidermal junction, not above it.
3. The melanocytes, both those disposed as solitary units and those in nests within the epidermis, have small, oval, monomorphous nuclei.
4. The proliferation of melanocytes within the epidermis does not extend beyond the scar in the upper part of the dermis.

This is a superficial congenital nevus because:

1. Melanocytes in the upper part of the reticular dermis are present around adnexal structures, especially sebaceous units, and also are splayed between collagen bundles.

This is a compound nevus because:

1. Nests of melanocytes are present within the epidermis and the dermis.

This is a recurrent nevus because:

1. There is a scar in the upper part of the dermis, an indication of a previous surgical procedure at this site.
2. Above the scar, melanocytes are arrayed as solitary units, not only at the dermo-epidermal junction, but far above it, including the granular zone and cornified layer.
3. Beneath the scar in the upper part of the dermis, in a focus, are melanocytes of a congenital nevus.

Pitfall in diagnosis

This recurrent congenital nevus could be misinterpreted as a melanoma in situ in association with a congenital nevus because:

1. The lesion is asymmetric with both melanocytes and melanophages being more numerous on the left side of it than on the right.
2. Melanocytes disposed as solitary units predominate over nests of melanocytes in many high-power fields.
3. Melanocytes arranged as solitary units are scattered far above the dermo-epidermal junction.
4. Nests of melanocytes within the epidermis are not equidistant from one another.
5. Nests of melanocytes within the epidermis vary in size and shape.
6. Some nests of melanocytes within the epidermis have become confluent.
7. Melanocytes in some foci within the epidermis are clustered, but are not cohesive.

This persistent nevus could be misconstrued as a melanoma in situ. In fact, it has more features in common with melanoma in situ than it displays differences from it. Not always is it possible to distinguish on histopathologic grounds alone a melanoma in situ from a persistent nevus. For that reason, review of sections from the original biopsy specimen is mandatory. Almost always that exercise enables resolution of the quandary.

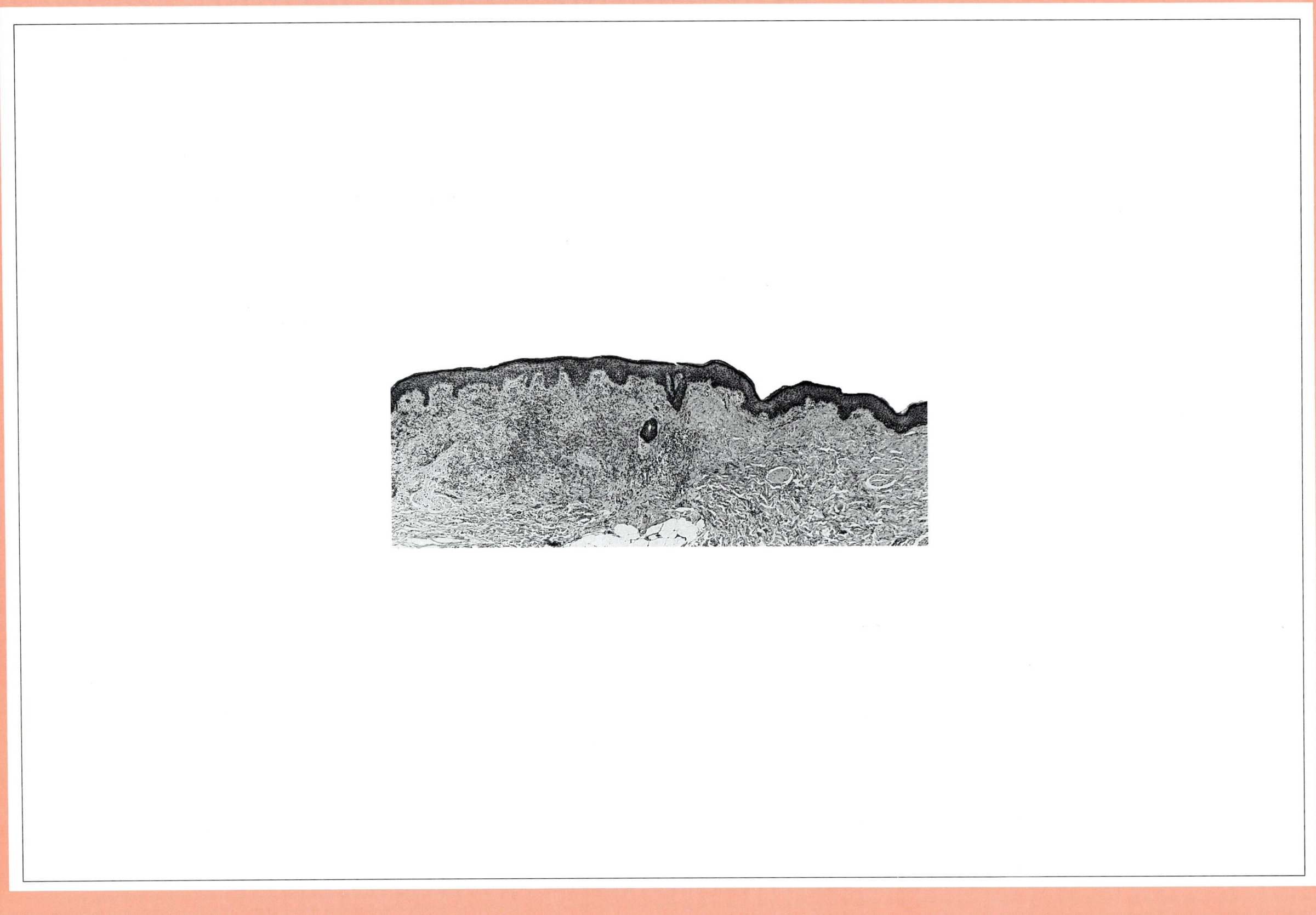

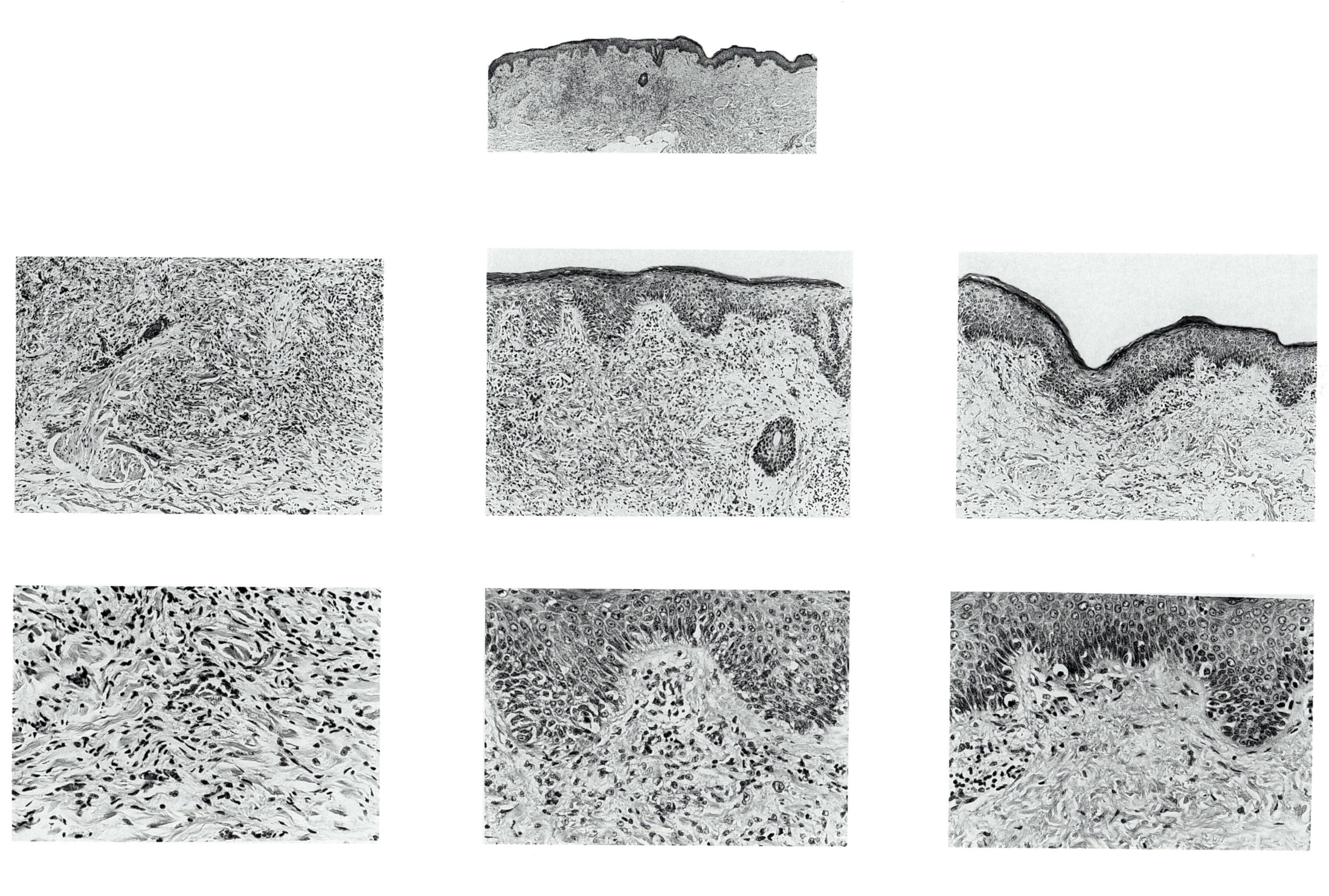

50. What is your diagnosis?

Lesion on the left arm of a 67-year-old woman. Clinical diagnosis: pigmented basal-cell carcinoma. Patient was free of disease after 3 years.

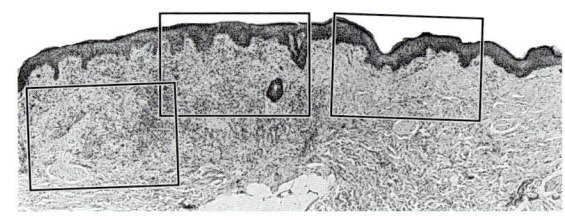

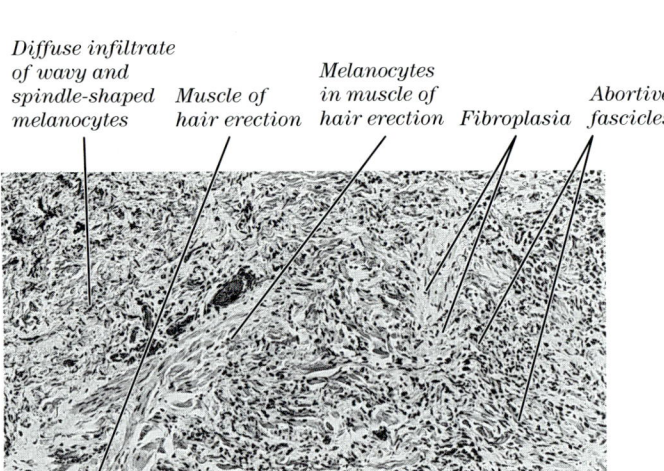

Diffuse infiltrate of wavy and spindle-shaped melanocytes — *Muscle of hair erection* — *Melanocytes in muscle of hair erection* — *Fibroplasia* — *Abortive fascicles*

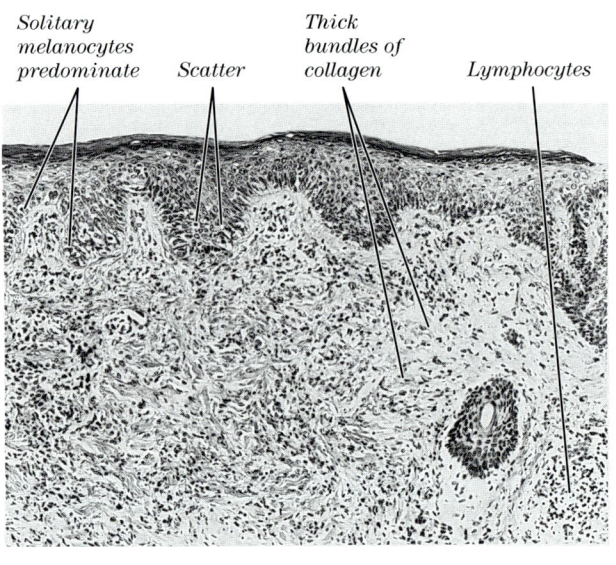

Solitary melanocytes predominate — *Scatter* — *Thick bundles of collagen* — *Lymphocytes*

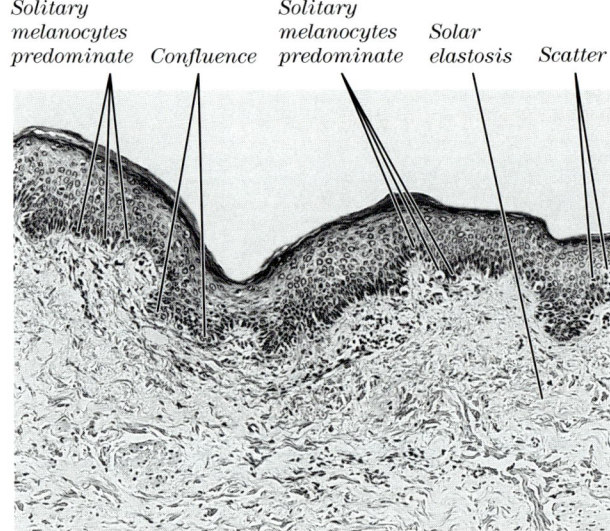

Solitary melanocytes predominate — *Confluence* — *Solitary melanocytes predominate* — *Solar elastosis* — *Scatter*

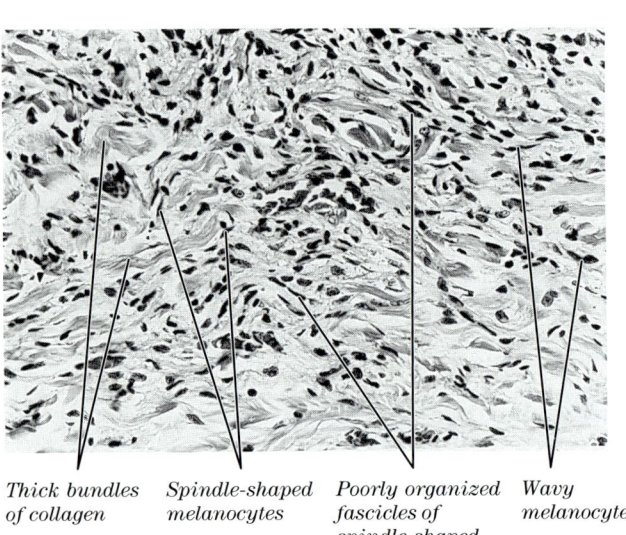

Thick bundles of collagen — *Spindle-shaped melanocytes* — *Poorly organized fascicles of spindle-shaped melanocytes* — *Wavy melanocytes*

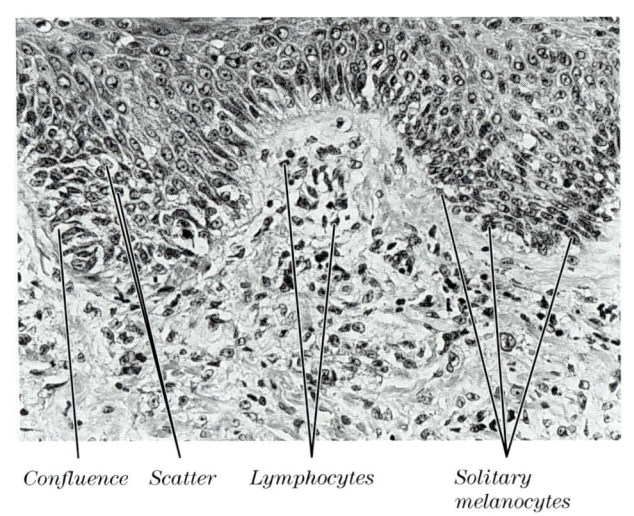

Confluence — *Scatter* — *Lymphocytes* — *Solitary melanocytes predominate*

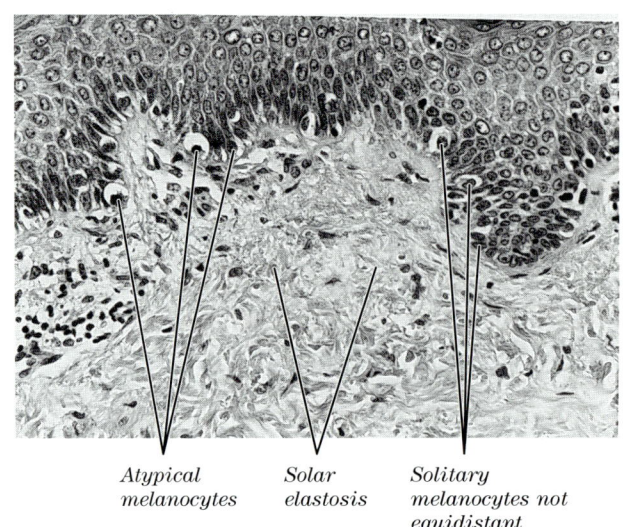

Atypical melanocytes — *Solar elastosis* — *Solitary melanocytes not equidistant*

50 • Melanoma *(desmoplastic type)*

Criteria for diagnosis of this melanoma (desmoplastic type)

This is a melanoma because:

1. It is asymmetric.
2. It is poorly circumscribed.
3. Melanocytes disposed as solitary units within the epidermis are much more numerous than melanocytes in nests there.
4. Melanocytes are distributed diffusely within the dermis; no discrete nests are present there.
5. Neoplastic melanocytes are found within smooth muscles of hair erection.
6. No polygonal melanocytes are detected within the dermis.

Pitfall in diagnosis

This desmoplastic melanoma could be misdiagnosed as a desmoplastic Spitz's nevus because:

1. The predominant findings are within the dermis, rather than the epidermis.
2. Some melanocytes have large nuclei.
3. Fibroplasia is prominent.
4. A patchy, perivascular, lymphocytic infiltrate is present throughout the neoplasm.

Desmoplastic Spitz's nevi may be wholly intradermal, unlike desmoplastic melanoma that invariably involves the epidermis and the dermis. Furthermore, characteristic polygonal cells nearly always are present in at least the upper part of the dermis in a desmoplastic Spitz's nevus, in contrast to desmoplastic melanoma in which nuclei tend to be thin and often wavy, as they are in this neoplasm. Most important in the differentiation, a Spitz's nevus, whether desmoplastic or not, has the silhouette of a benign neoplasm, whereas a melanoma, whether desmoplastic or not, has the silhouette of a malignant neoplasm.

Another pitfall in diagnosis of desmoplastic melanoma is misconstruction of wavy melanocytes of a melanoma as those of a benign neoplasm with neural differentiation. That inclination can be rectified by attention to the epidermis for signs of melanoma in situ, as are shown here, and to the reticular dermis for evidences of neurotropism.

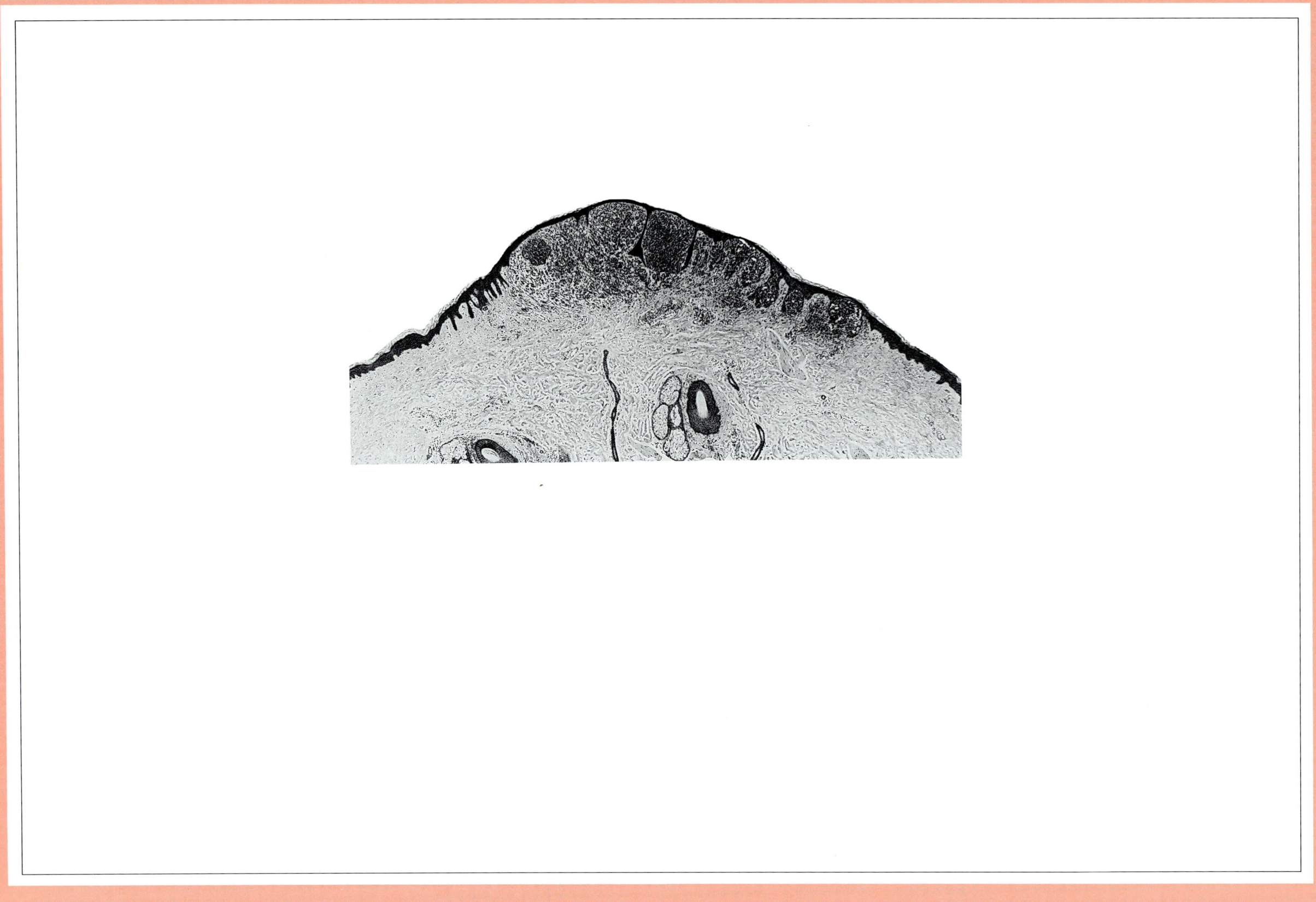

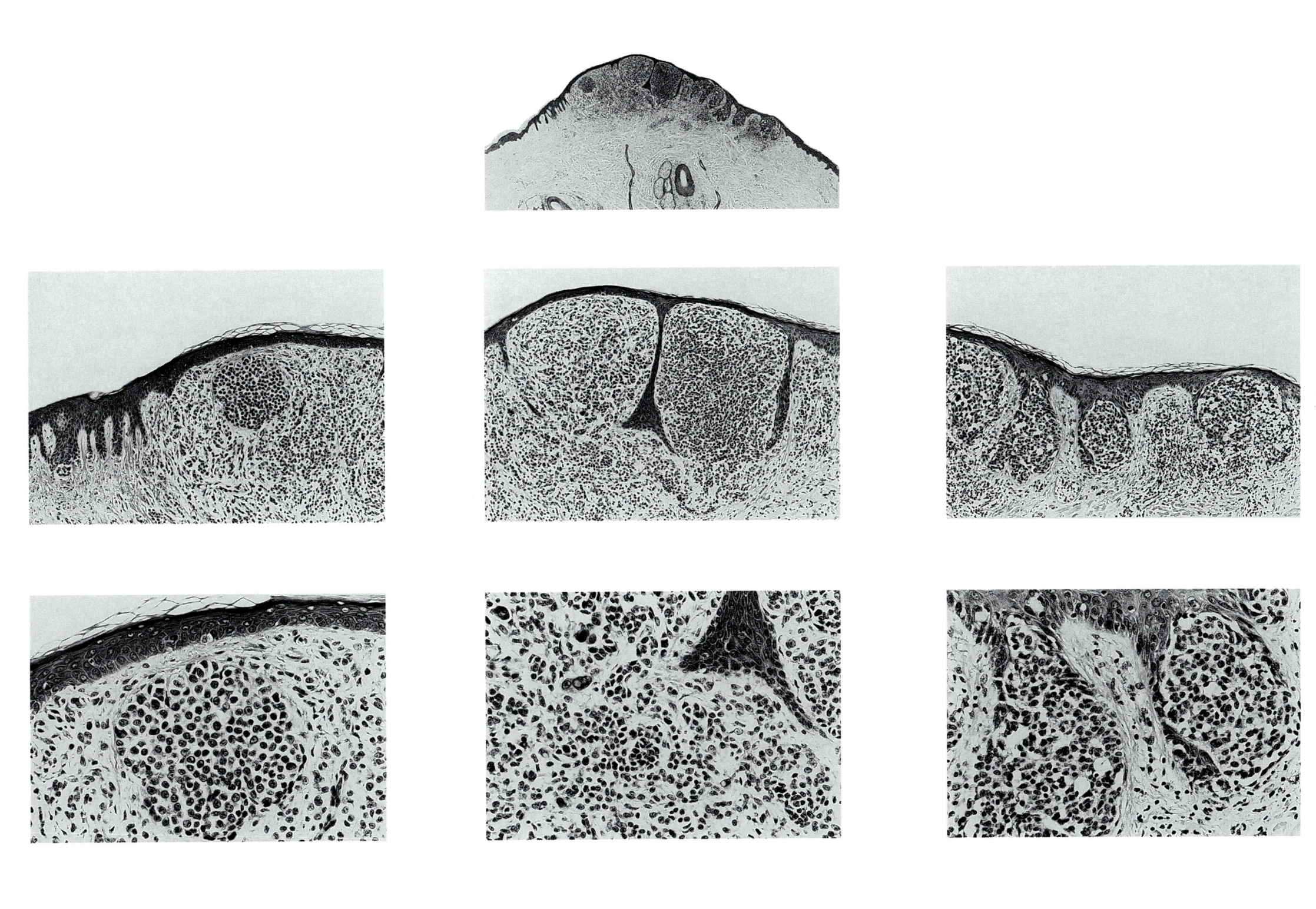

51. What is your diagnosis?

Raised, tan-brown, circular papule on the left forearm of a 37-year-old man was present for many years, but became slightly more elevated 1 month prior to biopsy. Clinical diagnosis: nevus. Wide and deep excision was performed. Patient was free of disease 7 years later.

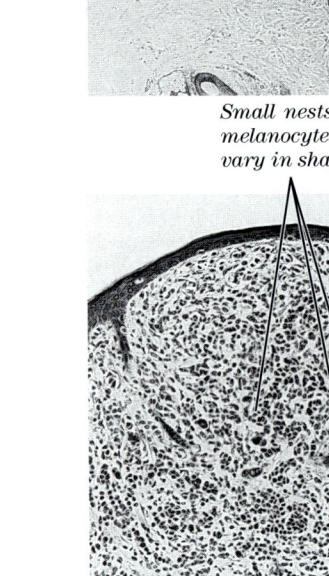

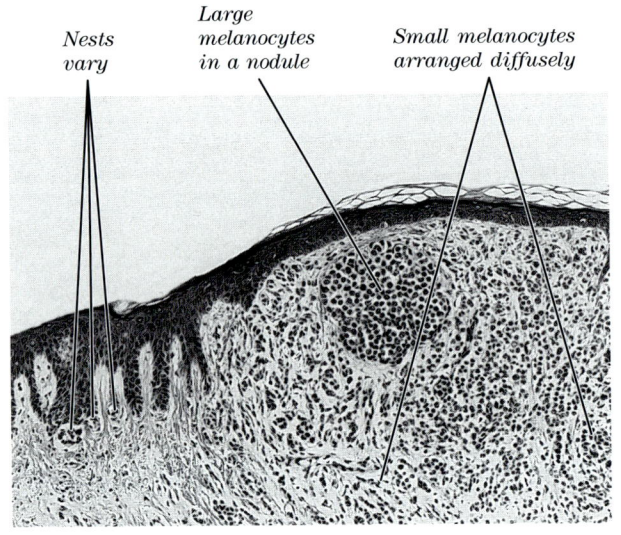

Nests vary · Large melanocytes in a nodule · Small melanocytes arranged diffusely

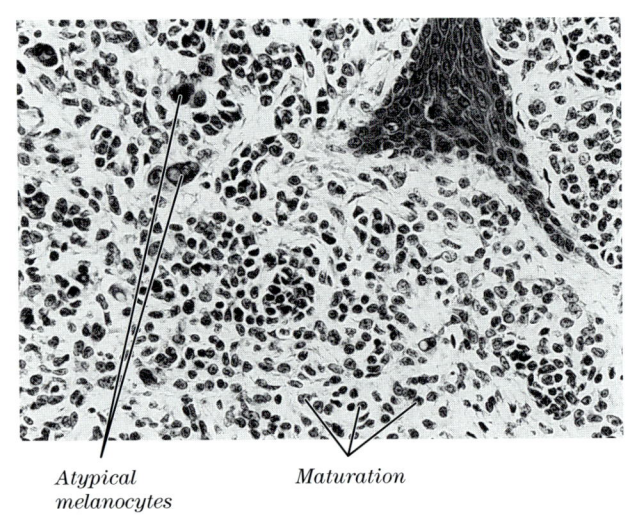

Small nests of melanocytes vary in shape · Sheet

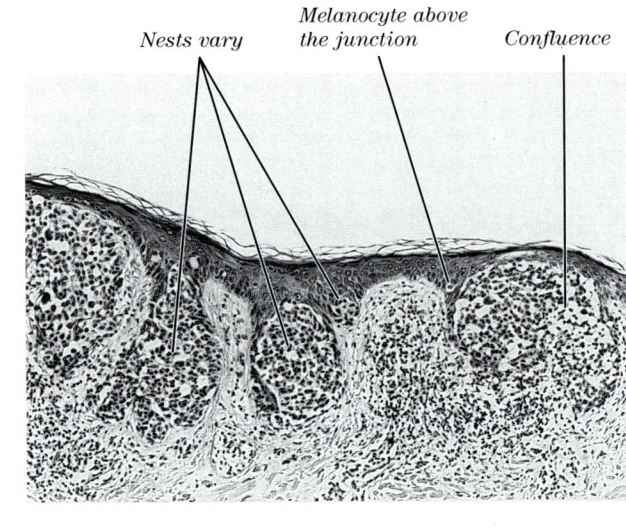

Nests vary · Melanocyte above the junction · Confluence

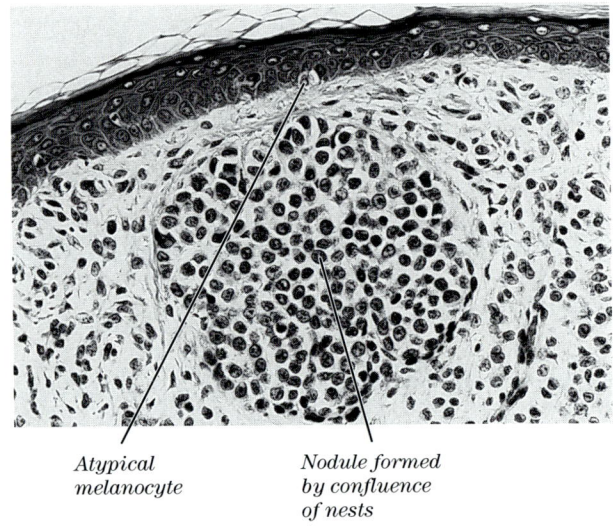

Atypical melanocyte · Nodule formed by confluence of nests

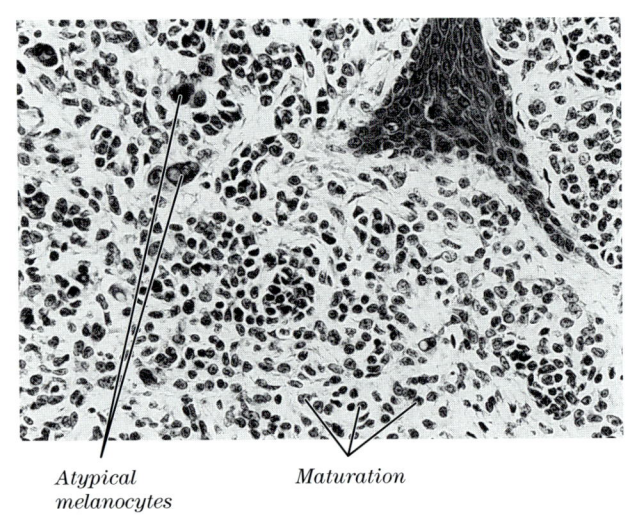

Atypical melanocytes · Maturation

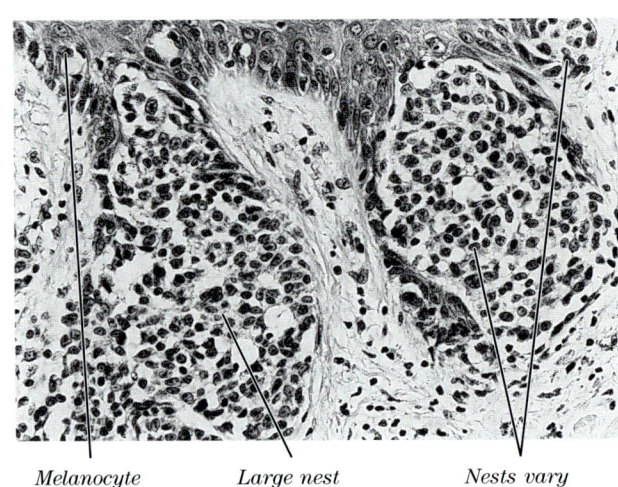

Melanocyte above junction · Large nest · Nests vary

51 • Melanoma

Criteria for diagnosis of this melanoma

This is a melanoma because:

1. The neoplasm is asymmetric.
2. Nests of melanocytes within the epidermis and the dermis vary in size and shape.
3. Neoplastic melanocytes in the dermis have become confluent with formation of sheets.
4. Nests of melanocytes within the epidermis are not equidistant from one another.
5. Some melanocytes are scattered above the dermo-epidermal junction.
6. Nuclei of most melanocytes are notably atypical.

Pitfall in diagnosis

This melanoma could be misinterpreted as a compound Miescher's nevus because:

1. The neoplasm has a dome shape.
2. The neoplasm is exo-endophytic with extension of melanocytes into the reticular dermis in somewhat wedge-shaped fashion.
3. Melanocytes mature with progressive descent into the dermis.
4. Most neoplastic melanocytes within the epidermis are situated at the dermo-epidermal junction.

This neoplasm could be confused with a compound Miescher's nevus because it is domed, exo-endophytic, and vaguely wedge-shaped. Observations made at scanning magnification, however, dispel the possibility of a nevus of any kind. The lesion is asymmetric and poorly circumscribed, nests of melanocytes within it are not equidistant from one another, nests vary markedly in size and shape, and some nests have become confluent and formed sheets of melanocytes within the dermis. In short, this is a melanoma.

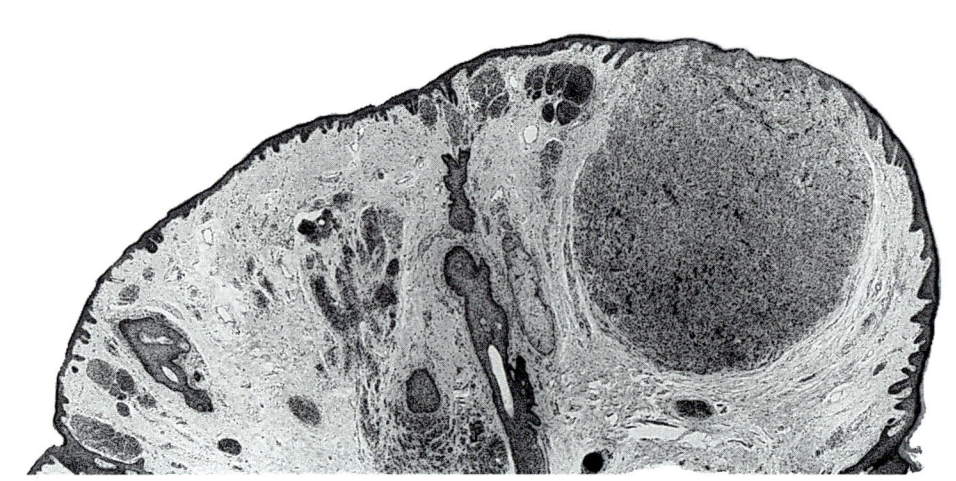

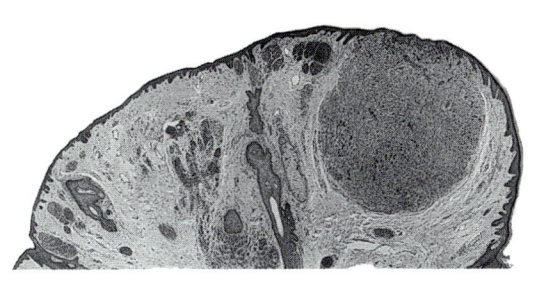
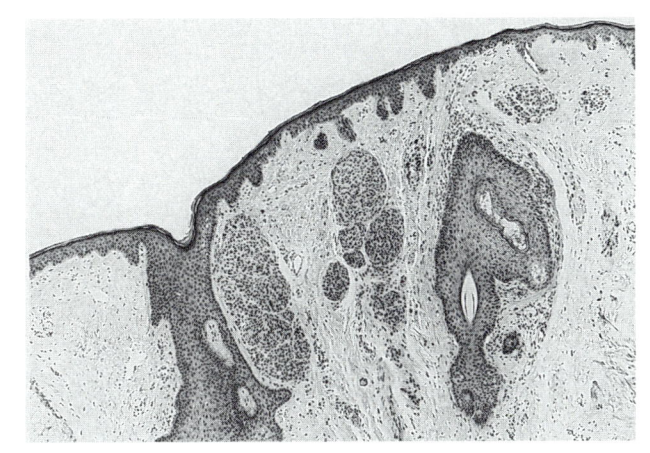
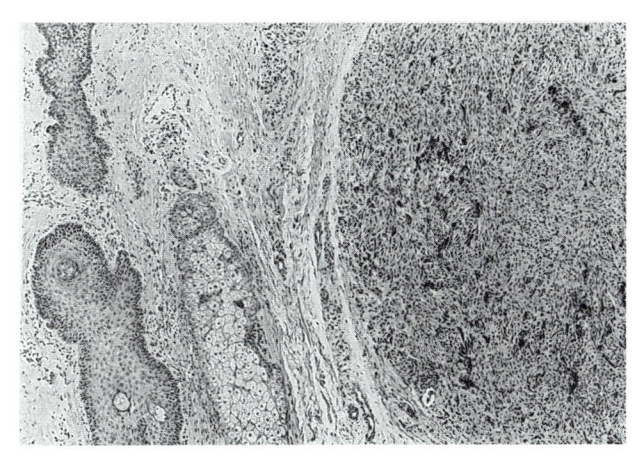
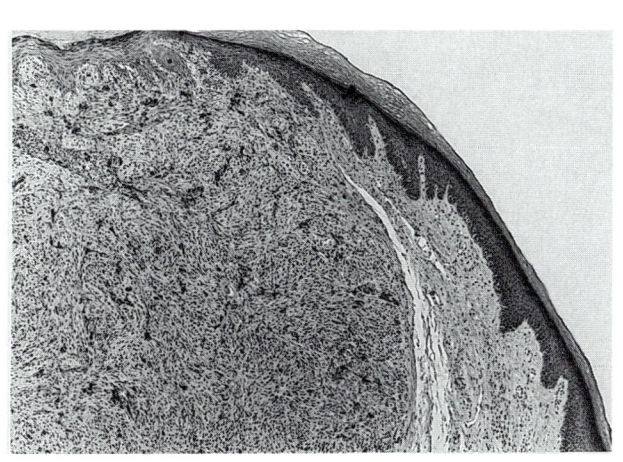
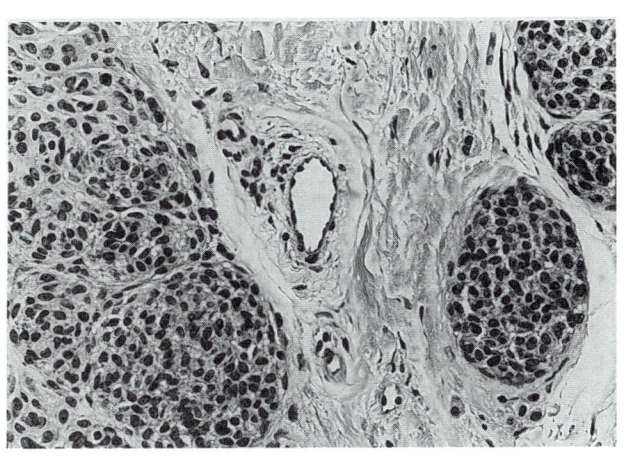
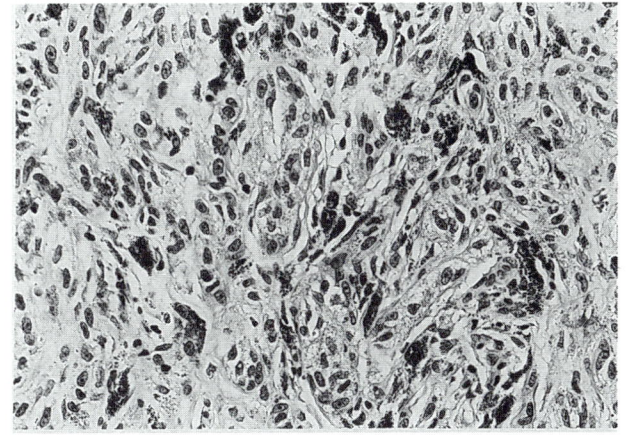
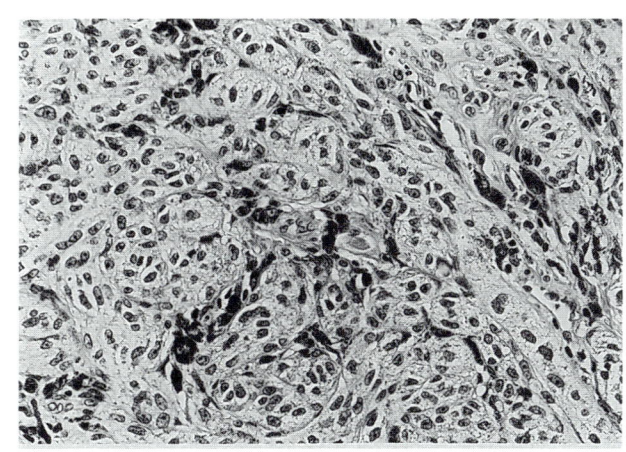

52. What is your diagnosis?

Mole on the nose of a 67-year-old man that had enlarged recently and bled. Clinical diagnosis: Spitz's nevus. Site was re-excised. Patient had no evidence of recurrence of this lesion or of any other skin cancers after 6 years.

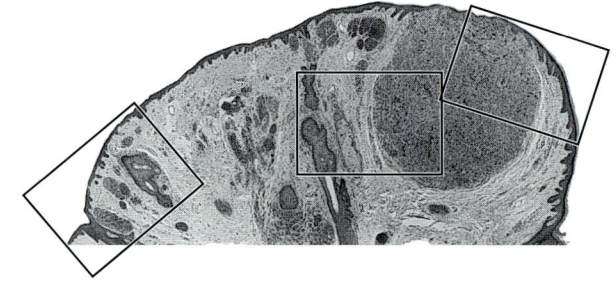

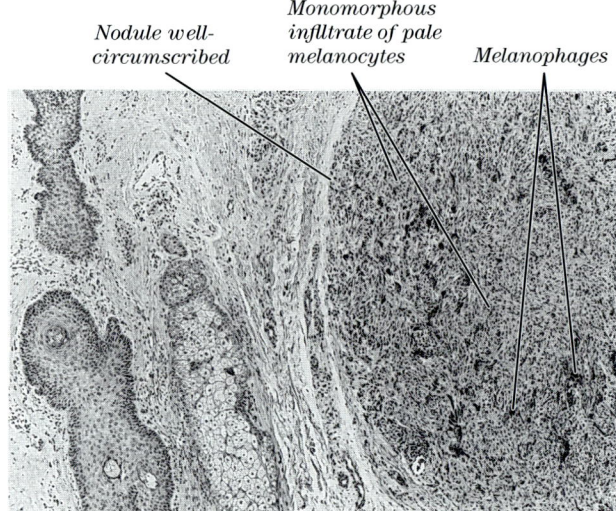

Nests of melanocytes with monomorphous nuclei and scant cytoplasm

Nodule well-circumscribed

Monomorphous infiltrate of pale melanocytes

Melanophages

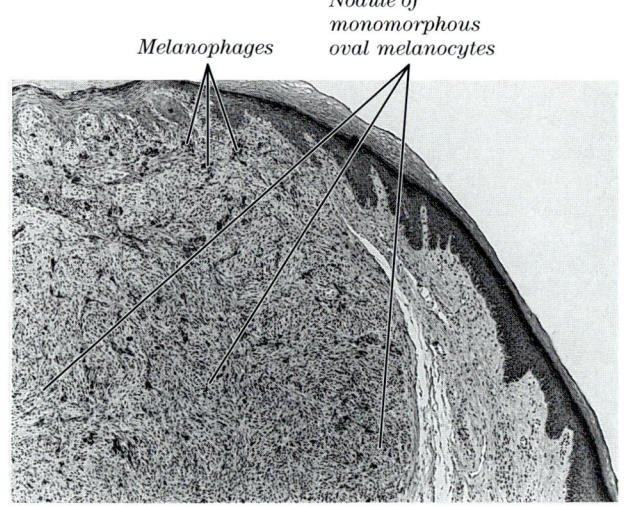

Melanophages

Nodule of monomorphous oval melanocytes

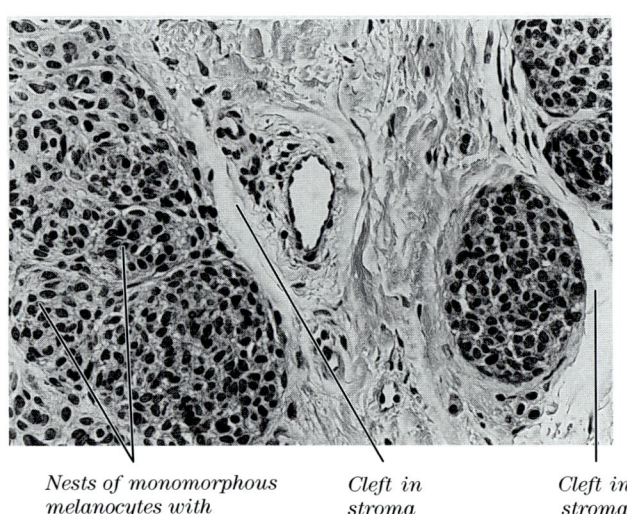

Nests of monomorphous melanocytes with oval nuclei and scant cytoplasm

Cleft in stroma

Cleft in stroma

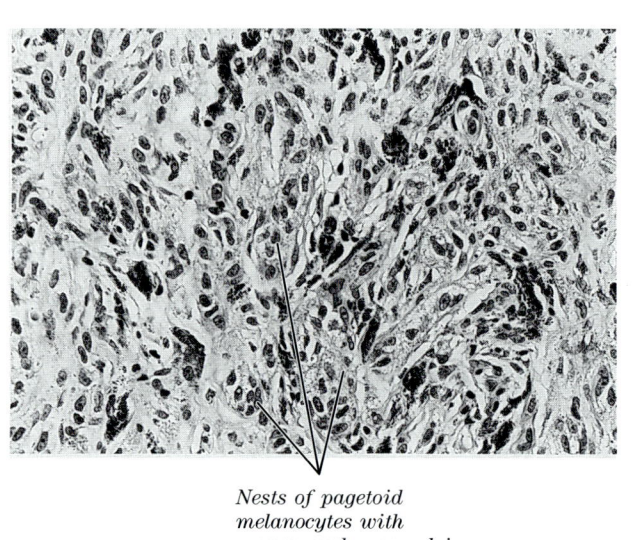

Nests of pagetoid melanocytes with monomorphous nuclei

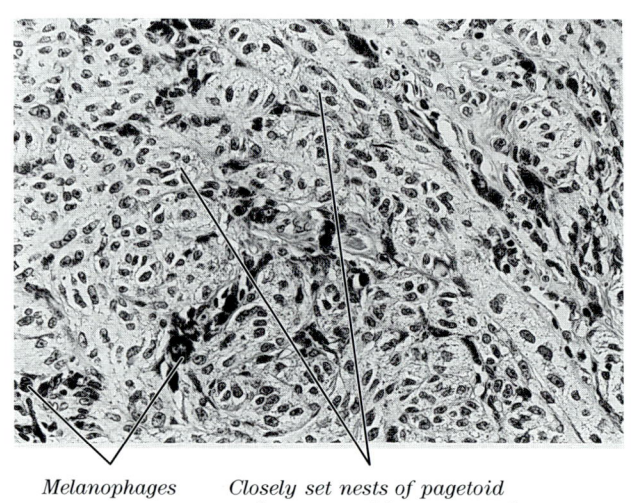

Melanophages

Closely set nests of pagetoid melanocytes with monomorphous oval nuclei

52 • Combined Nevus (*Miescher's and blue*)

Criteria for diagnosis of this combined nevus (Miescher's and blue)

This is a nevus because:

1. The neoplasm is well-circumscribed.
2. Melanocytes mature.
3. Melanocytes have monomorphous oval nuclei.
4. There are no mitotic figures.

This is a combined nevus because:

Features of a Miescher's nevus are seen on the left and of a blue nevus on the right.

Pitfall in diagnosis

This combined nevus could be misinterpreted as a nodule of melanoma that arose in association with a pre-existing nevus because:

1. The neoplasm is asymmetric.
2. The nodule of blue nevus is large.
3. Several types of cells constitute the nodule of blue nevus: dendritic, pagetoid, and oval.

Striking asymmetry of a neoplasm, such as this one, does not exclude the possibility of its being a nevus. Combined nevi (whether of types of nevi or types of melanocytes), like melanomas, are asymmetric. The large nodule can be diagnosed as benign because it is symmetric, well-circumscribed by smooth borders, and associated with clefts in the stroma that surrounds it. In short, if each of the components of a combined nevus is assessed separately, a correct conclusion about its benign nature can be reached. Combined nevi of the type illustrated here tend to be congenital.

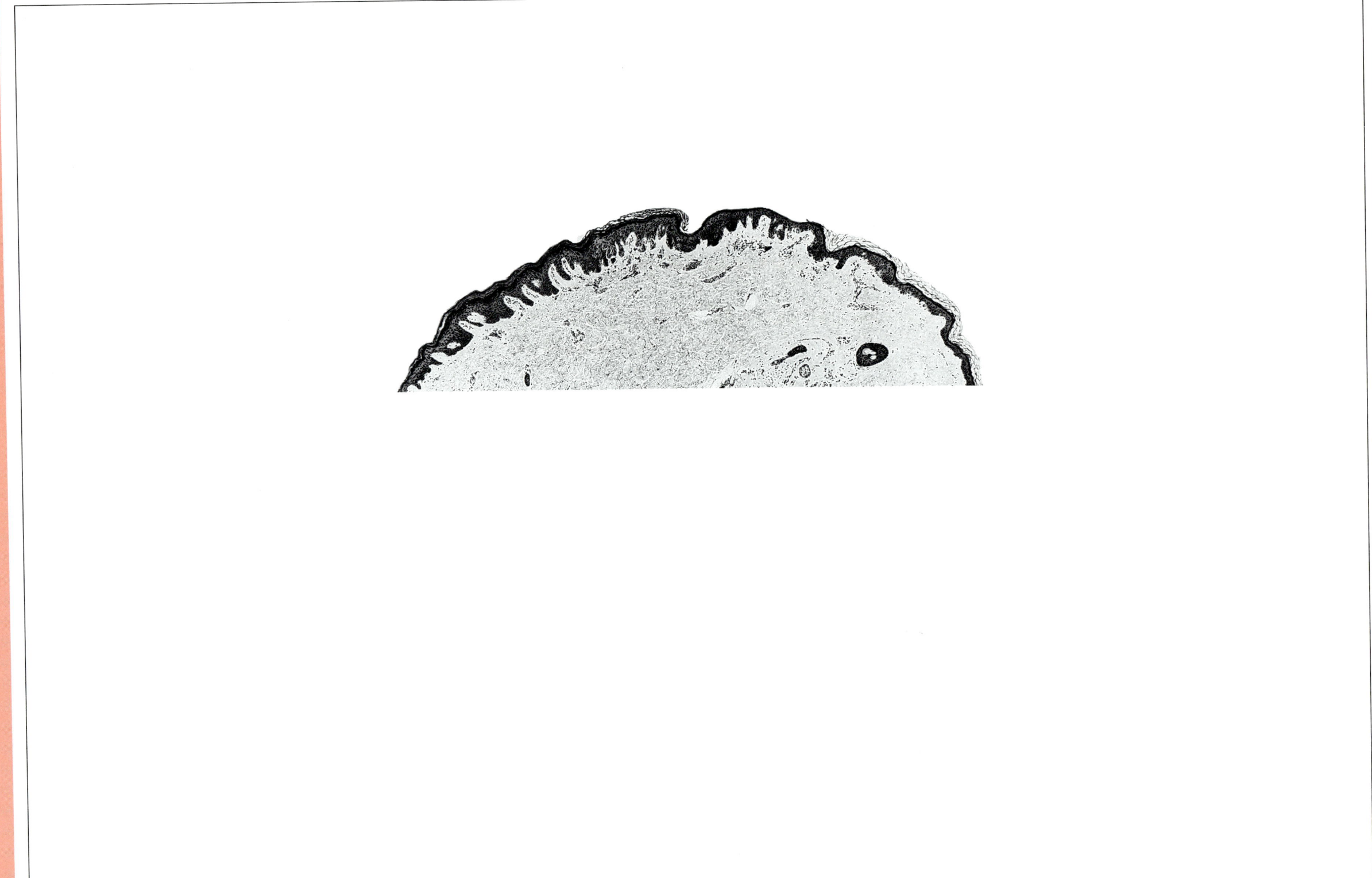

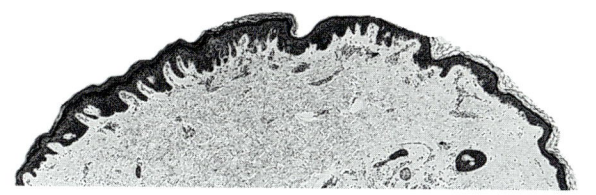
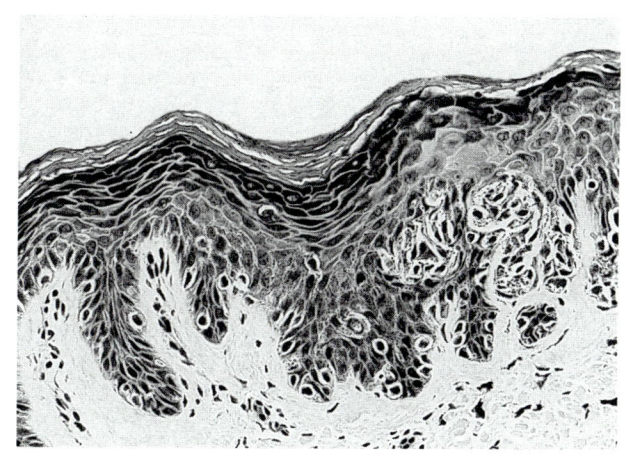
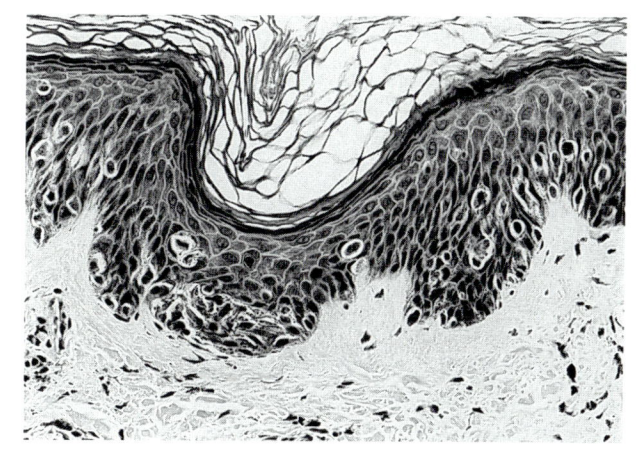
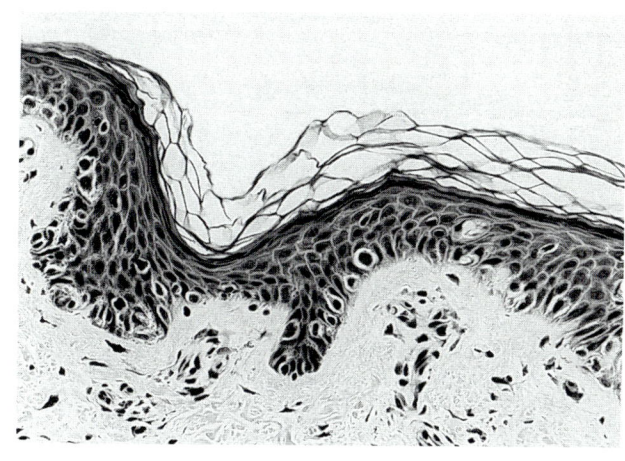
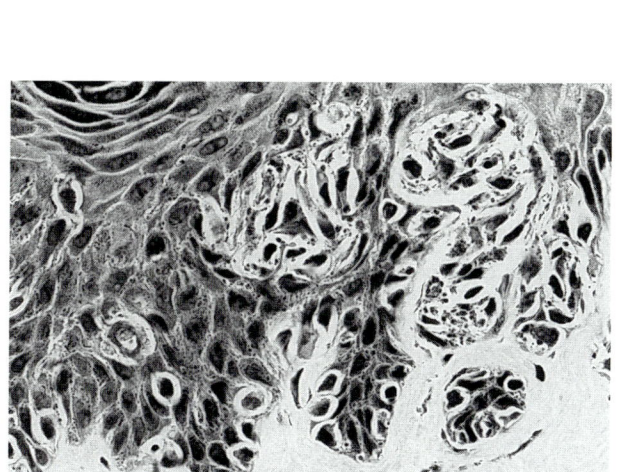
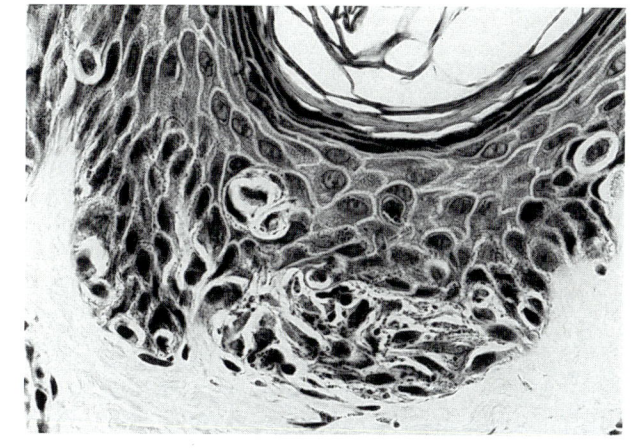
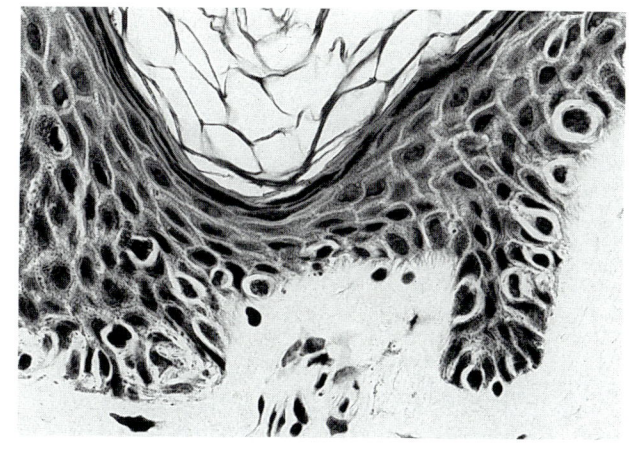

53. What is your diagnosis?

Pigmented lesion on the left leg of a 68-year-old woman. Clinical diagnosis: nevus. No follow-up information was available.

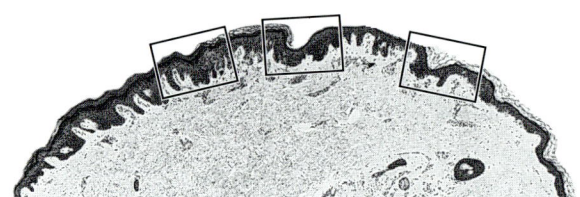

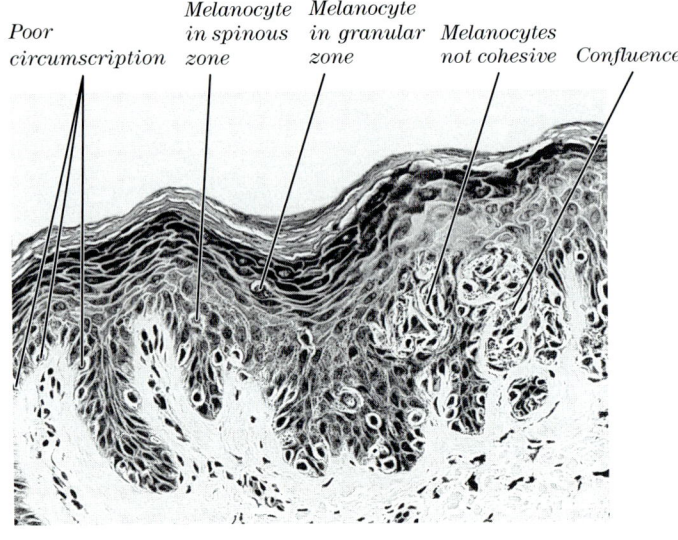

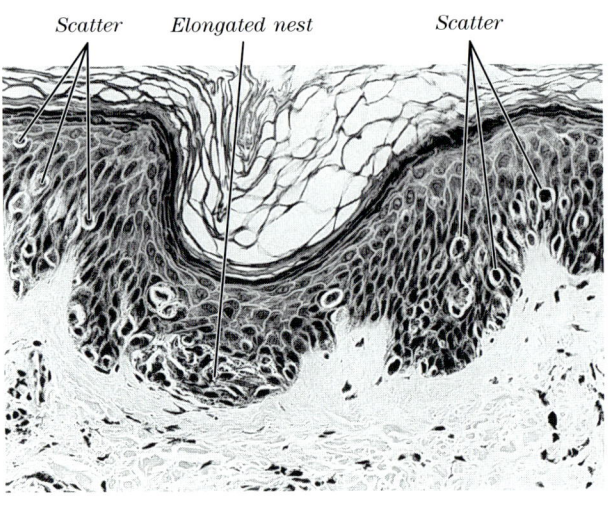

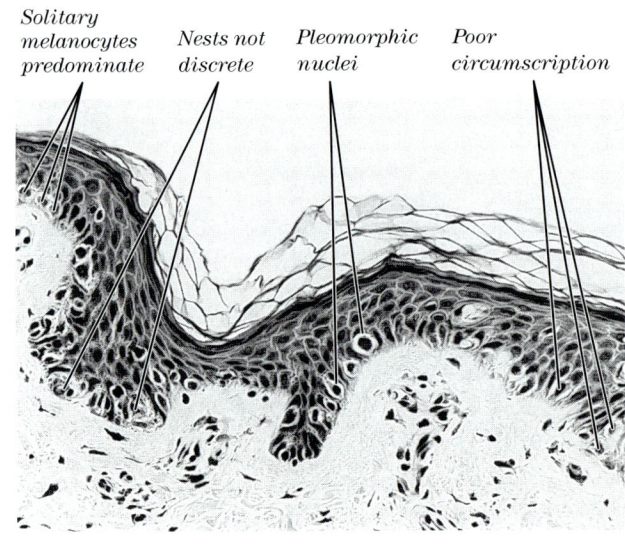

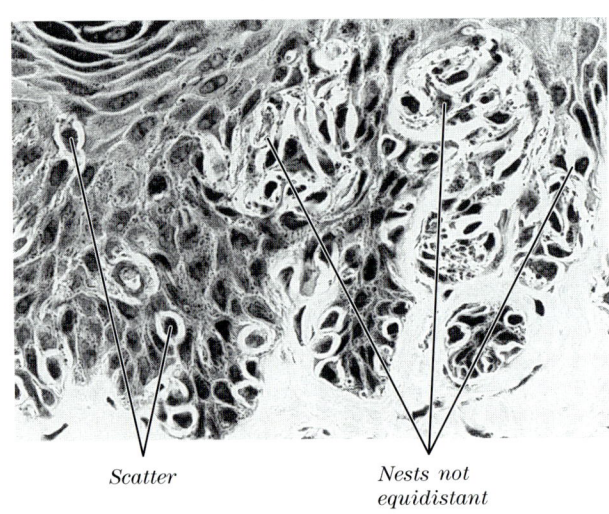

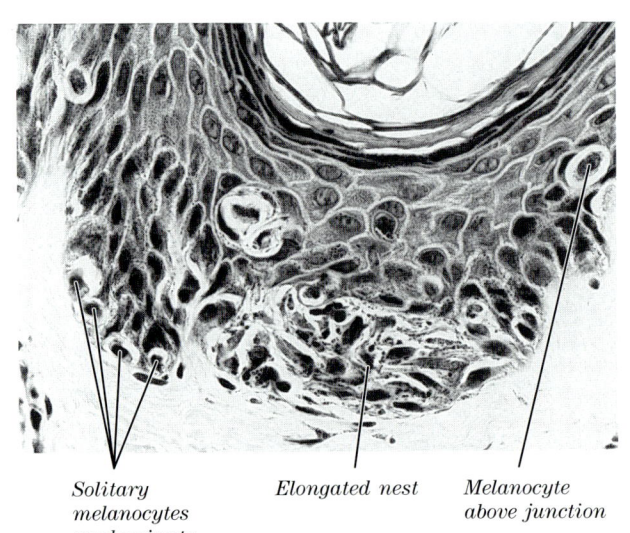

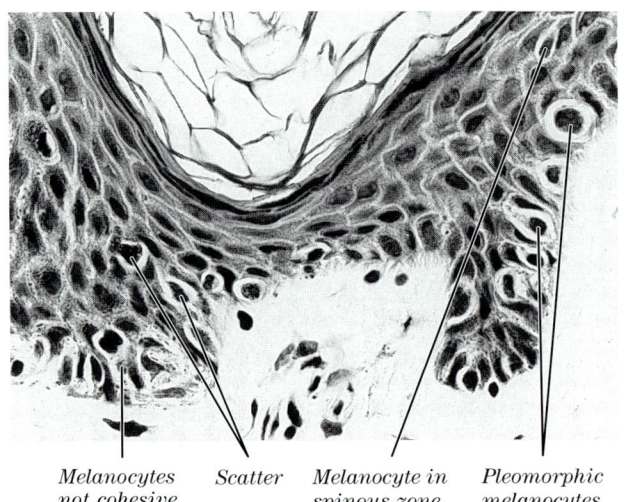

53 • Melanoma in situ

Criteria for diagnosis of this melanoma in situ

This is a melanoma in situ because:

1. The neoplasm is asymmetric, e.g., there are many more melanocytes on the left side of it than on the right side.
2. Nests of melanocytes are not equidistant from one another.
3. Nests of melanocytes vary in size and shape.
4. Some nests of melanocytes have become confluent.
5. Some nests of melanocytes have jagged outlines.
6. Melanocytes arranged as solitary units predominate over nests of melanocytes in many high-power fields.
7. Melanocytes arrayed both as solitary units and in nests are present far above the dermo-epidermal junction.
8. Melanocytes disposed as solitary units are not equidistant from one another.
9. Some melanocytes have atypical nuclei.

Pitfall in diagnosis

This small melanoma in situ could be misjudged as a junctional Spitz's nevus because:

1. The melanocytes have largish nuclei, abundant cytoplasm, and oval, spindle, polygonal, and dendritic shapes.
2. Melanocytes arranged as solitary units and in nests are present not only at the dermo-epidermal junction, but far above it.
3. There are hyperkeratosis, hypergranulosis, and spinous-cell hyperplasia.

A melanoma in situ, such as this one, can be distinguished from a junctional Spitz's nevus if attention is paid to lack of symmetry, poor circumscription, predominance of melanocytes arranged as solitary units over those arranged in nests in some high-power fields, and nests of melanocytes that are not equidistant from one another, vary in size and shape, and, in some instances, have jagged outlines. For the aforementioned criteria to be decisive, they must be applied rigorously and, preferably, in nearly the same sequence every time.

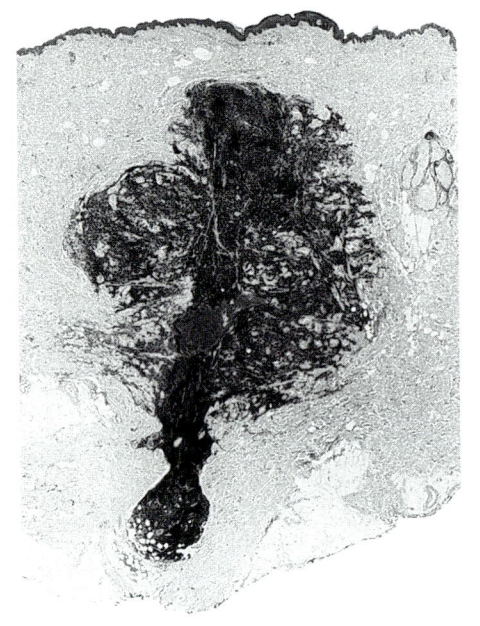

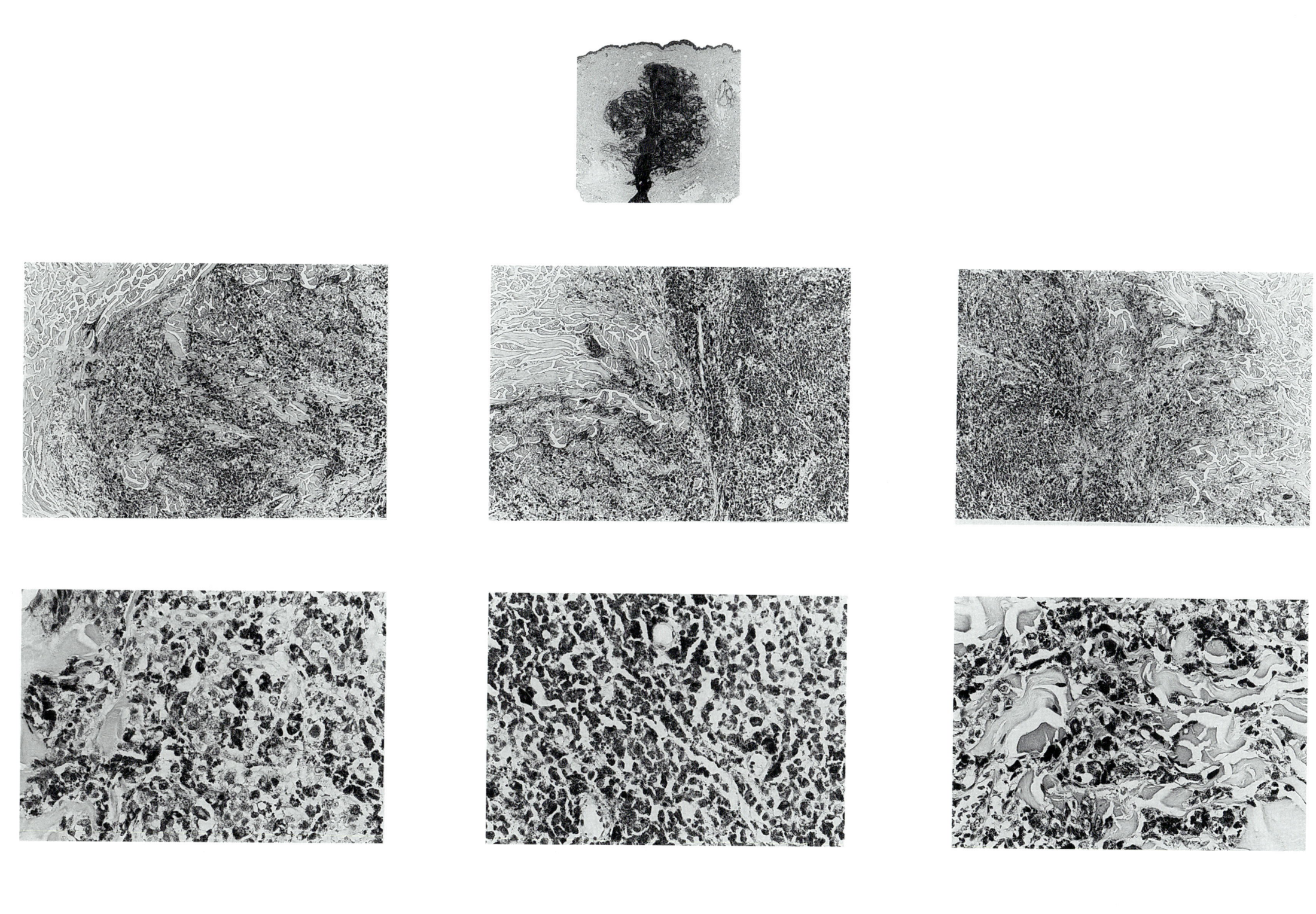

54. What is your diagnosis?

Lesion on the back of a 29-year-old man who had a history of melanoma. Clinical diagnosis: metastatic melanoma. Evidence of metastases of melanoma developed subsequently, and the patient became disabled by metastases to the central nervous system. He died 6 months after the histopathologic diagnosis had been made.

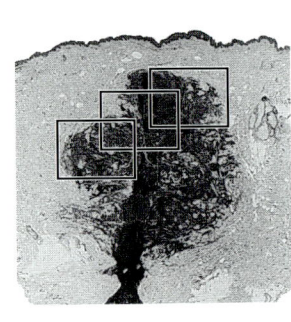

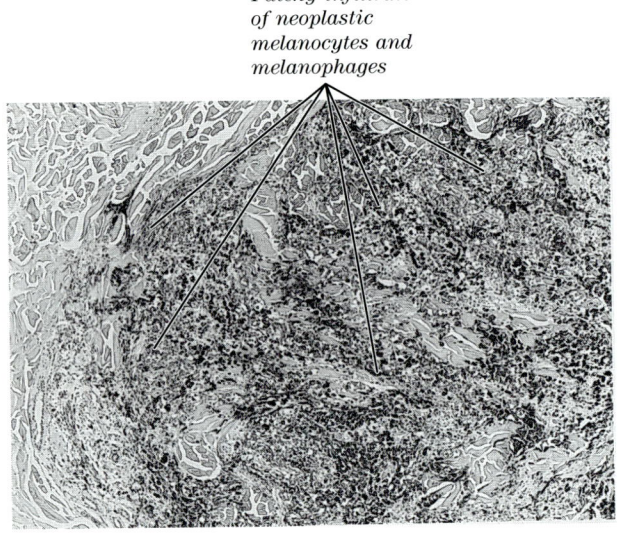

Patchy infiltrate of neoplastic melanocytes and melanophages

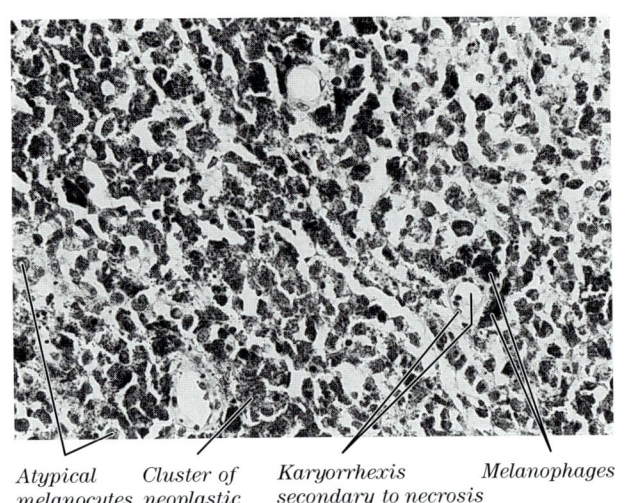

Melanophages and melanocytes — *Collagen bundles thickened* — *Sheets of neoplastic melanocytes*

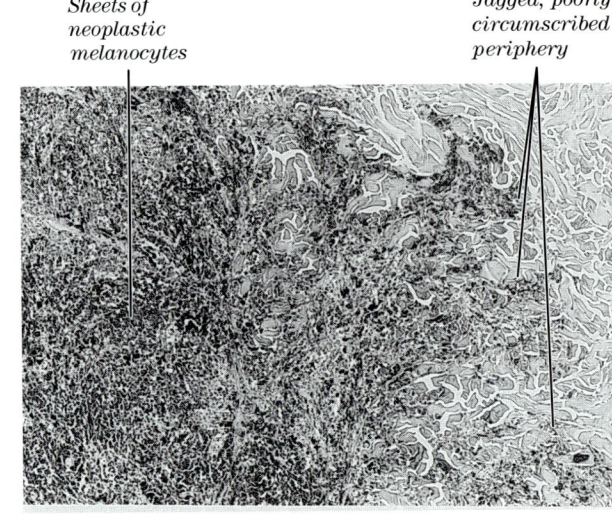

Sheets of neoplastic melanocytes — *Jagged, poorly circumscribed periphery*

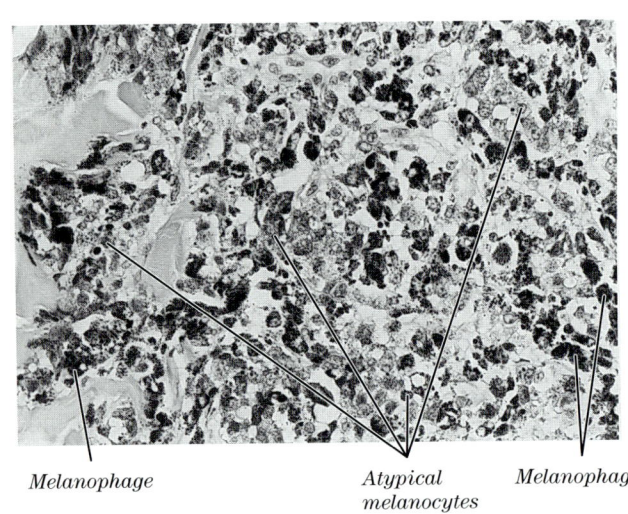

Melanophage — *Atypical melanocytes* — *Melanophages*

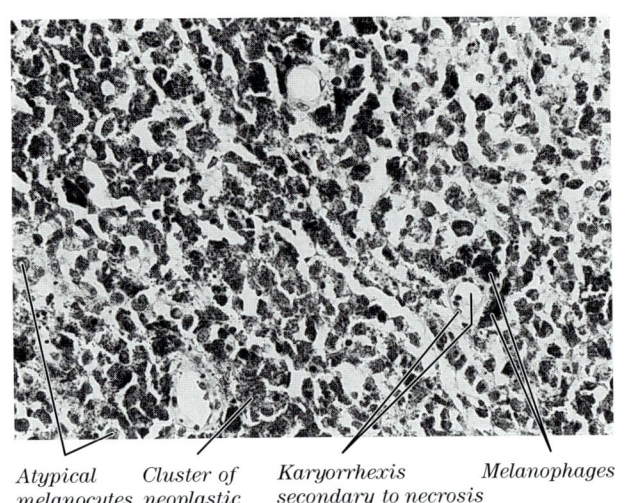

Atypical melanocytes — *Cluster of neoplastic melanocytes* — *Karyorrhexis secondary to necrosis of melanocytes* — *Melanophages*

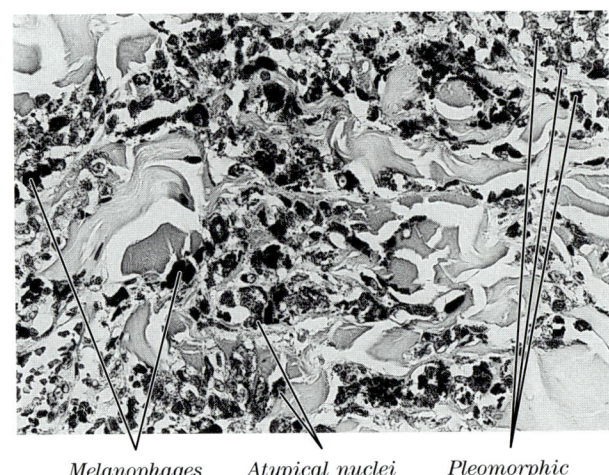

Melanophages — *Atypical nuclei of melanocytes* — *Pleomorphic nuclei of melanocytes*

54 • Metastasis of Melanoma

Criteria for diagnosis of this metastasis of melanoma

This is a metastasis of melanoma because:

1. The neoplasm is asymmetric.
2. Numerous neoplastic cells are necrotic, as evidenced by karyorrhexis.
3. The nuclei of many viable melanocytes are atypical and contain prominent nucleoli.
4. Melanophages predominate overwhelmingly over viable melanocytes.

Pitfall in diagnosis

This metastasis of melanoma could be misinterpreted as a blue nevus because:

1. The neoplasm is oriented vertically.
2. The neoplastic cells and melanophages are interspersed between collagen bundles at the periphery.
3. Both neoplastic melanocytes and melanophages are present.
4. The neoplasm is pigmented by melanin.
5. Collagen bundles at the periphery of the neoplasm are thickened.

It is easy for a microscopist to misinterpret this metastasis of melanoma as a blue nevus. Vertical orientation is to no avail in the attempt to resolve the diagnostic dilemma because metastases of melanoma, unlike primary melanomas, may be oriented vertically. In a circumstance such as this one, these cytopathologic features are important: atypia of melanocytes, mitotic figures in melanocytes, and necrosis of melanocytes. As a rule, those three findings are not seen in blue nevi of any kind.

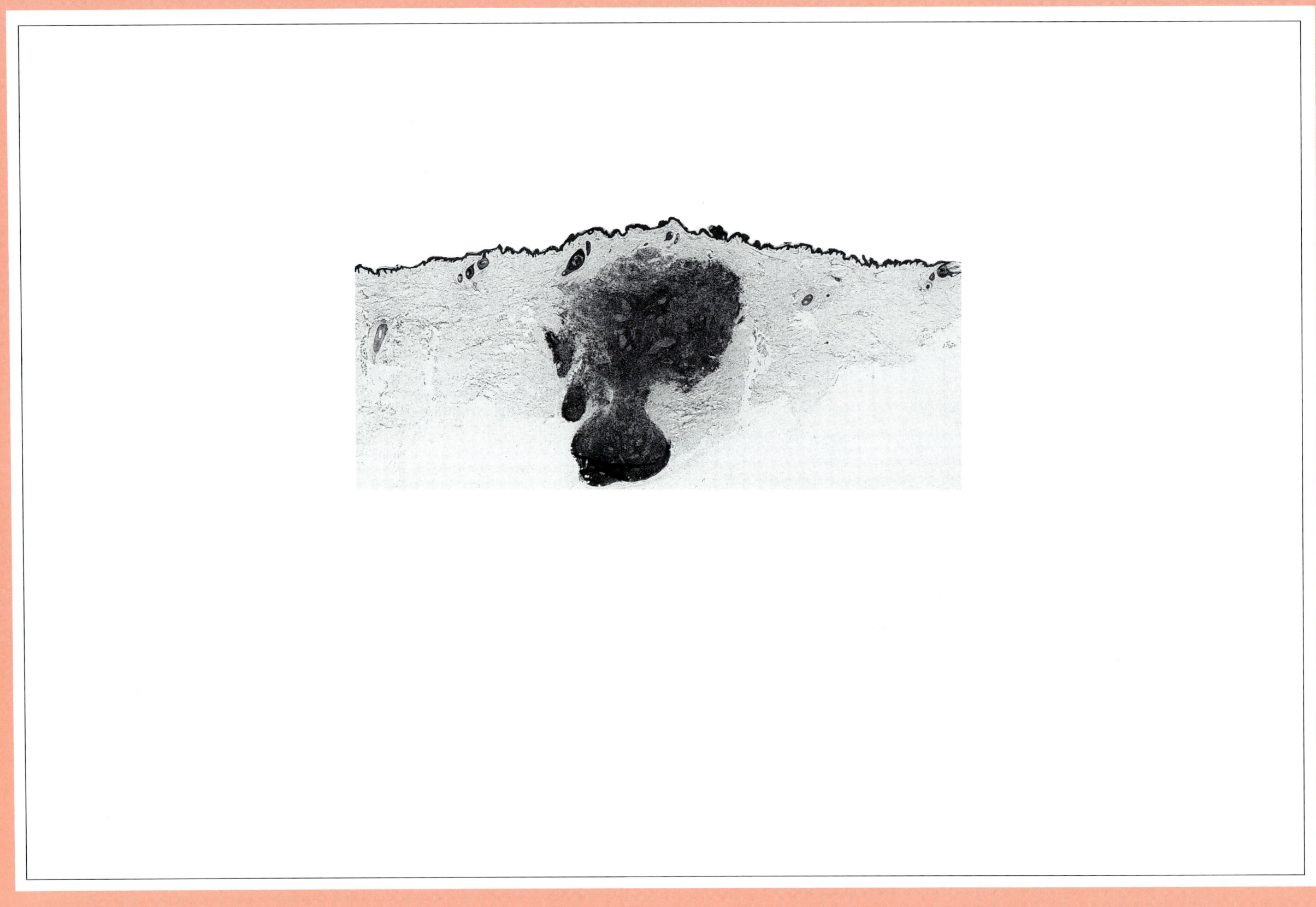

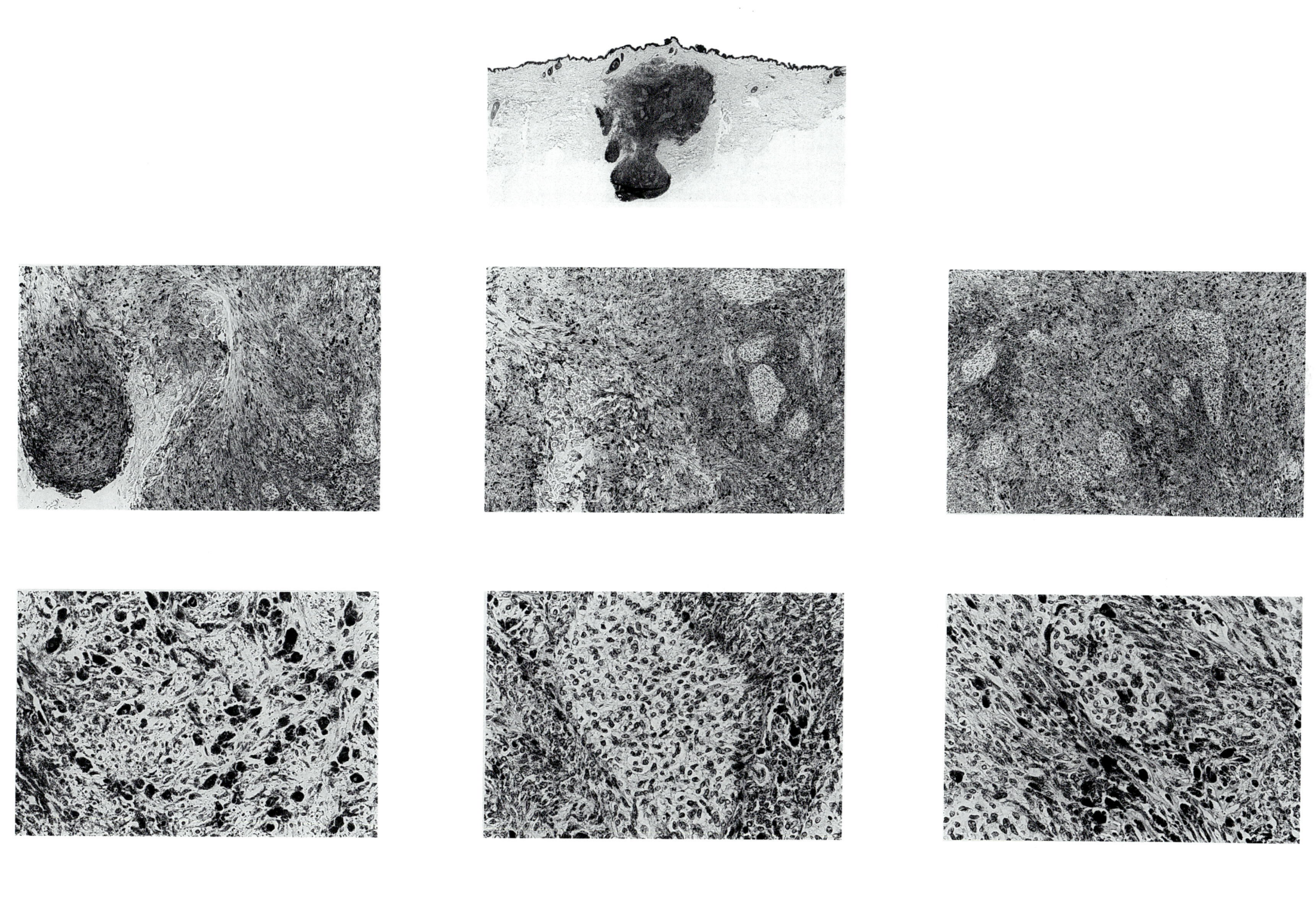

55. What is your diagnosis?

No clinical information was available.

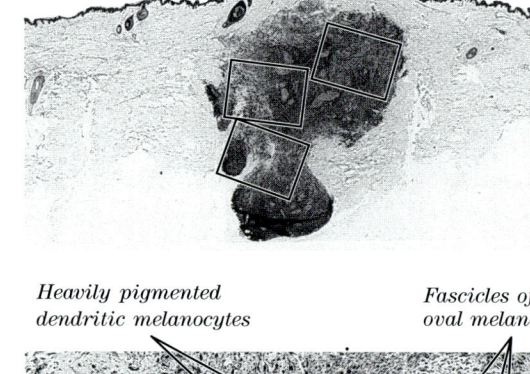

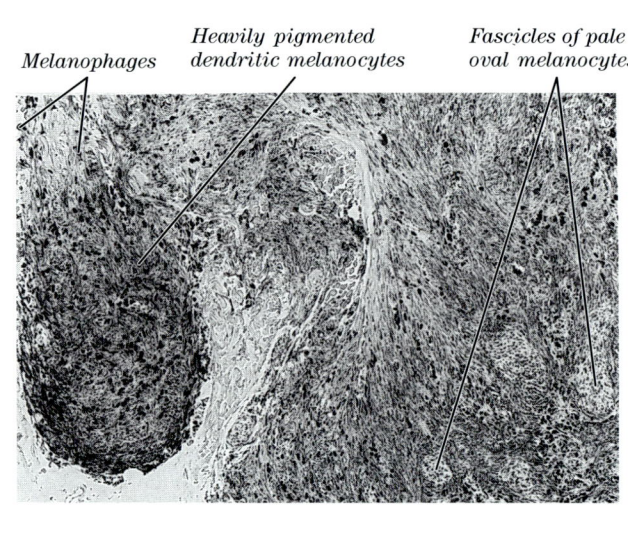

Melanophages — Heavily pigmented dendritic melanocytes — Fascicles of pale oval melanocytes

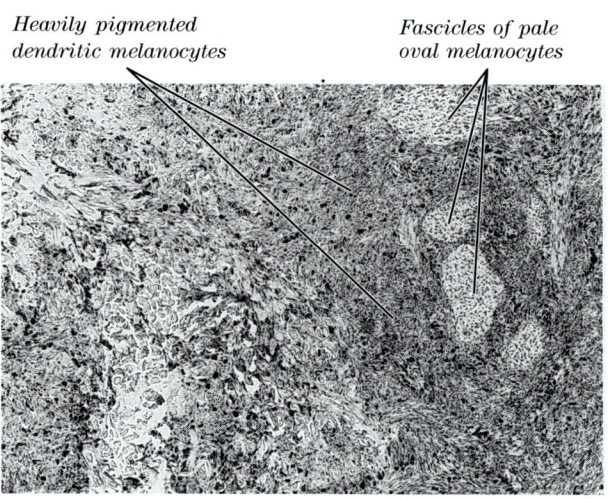

Heavily pigmented dendritic melanocytes — Fascicles of pale oval melanocytes

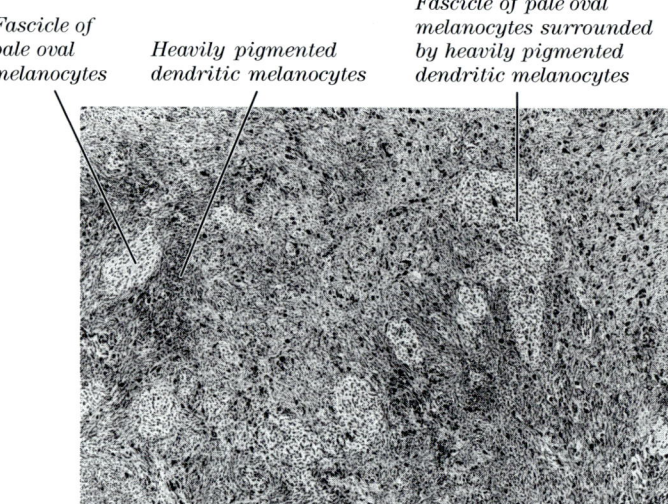

Fascicle of pale oval melanocytes — Heavily pigmented dendritic melanocytes — Fascicle of pale oval melanocytes surrounded by heavily pigmented dendritic melanocytes

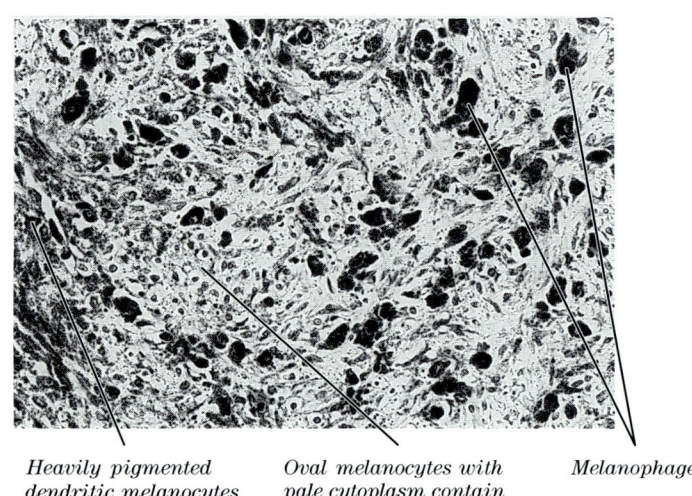

Heavily pigmented dendritic melanocytes — Oval melanocytes with pale cytoplasm contain "dusty" melanin — Melanophages

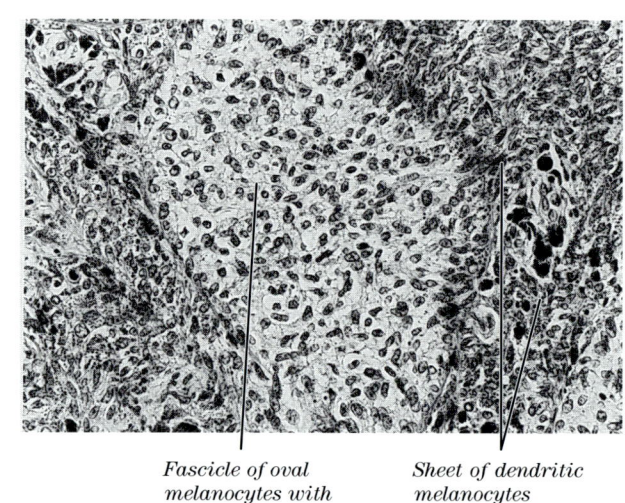

Fascicle of oval melanocytes with pale cytoplasm — Sheet of dendritic melanocytes

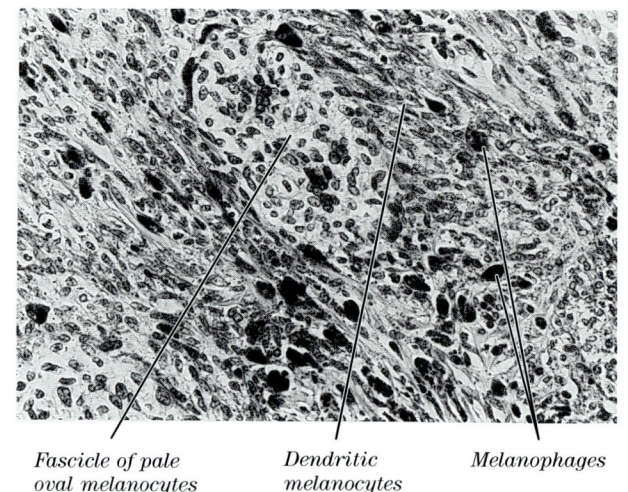

Fascicle of pale oval melanocytes — Dendritic melanocytes — Melanophages

55 • Blue Nevus (*deep, dendritic type*)

Criteria for diagnosis of this blue nevus (deep, mostly dendritic type)

This is a blue nevus because:

1. The neoplasm is oriented vertically.
2. The lower half of the neoplasm is well-circumscribed by smooth borders.
3. Two populations of melanocytes are seen throughout the neoplasm: heavily pigmented mostly dendritic melanocytes in sheets, and lightly pigmented non-dendritic melanocytes in nests and fascicles.
4. Nuclei of melanocytes, irrespective of cytologic type, are small, oval, and monomorphous.
5. Within nests themselves, fascicles themselves, and sheets of melanocytes, melanin is distributed relatively evenly.
6. There are no mitotic figures.
7. There are no necrotic cells.

Pitfall in diagnosis

This blue nevus could be misinterpreted as a metastasis of melanoma because:

1. Both may be oriented vertically.
2. The epidermis and upper part of the dermis are not involved.
3. Neoplastic cells extend into the subcutaneous fat.
4. The neoplasm is asymmetric.
5. The neoplasm is pigmented extensively by melanin.
6. Distribution of melanin is patchy.
7. Melanophages are numerous.

At scanning magnification, this neoplasm resembles closely the metastasis of melanoma in Figure 54. It differs, however, by smooth margins of its bulbous base, signs of benignancy. At higher magnification, the two patterns formed by the two cytologic types of melanocytes are apparent and they mark this lesion as a blue nevus of Masson's type.

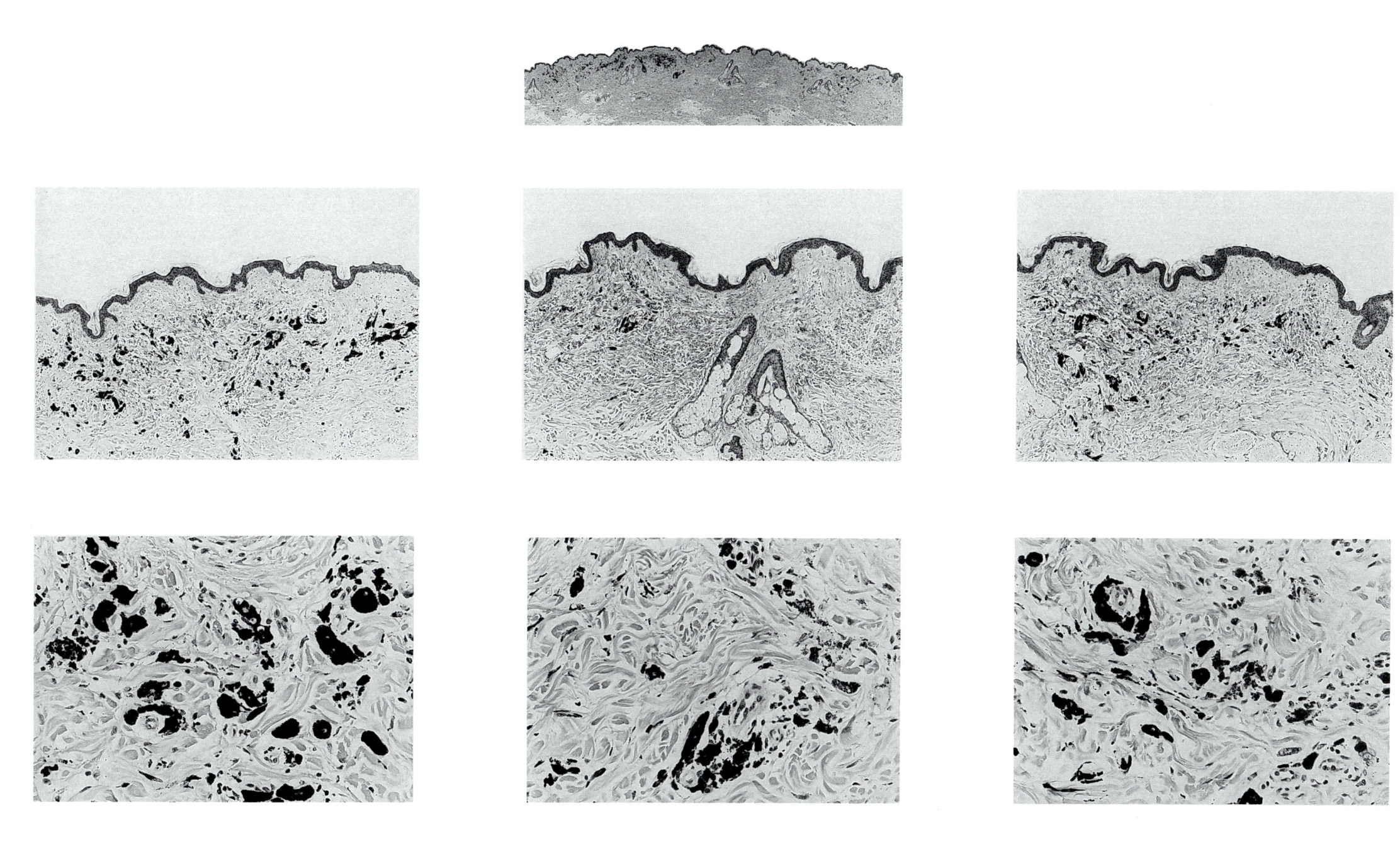

56. What is your diagnosis?

Lesion on the left arm of a 35-year-old woman. Clinical description: "large tattoo."

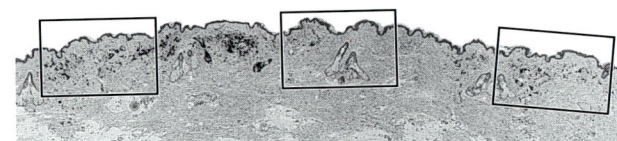

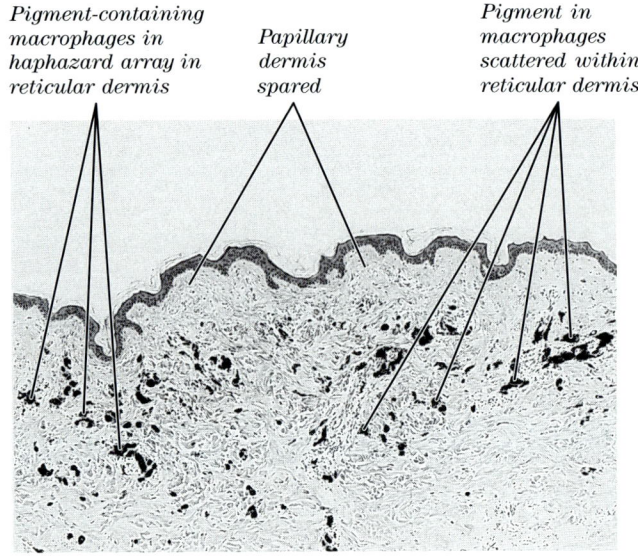

Pigment-containing macrophages in haphazard array in reticular dermis — *Papillary dermis spared* — *Pigment in macrophages scattered within reticular dermis*

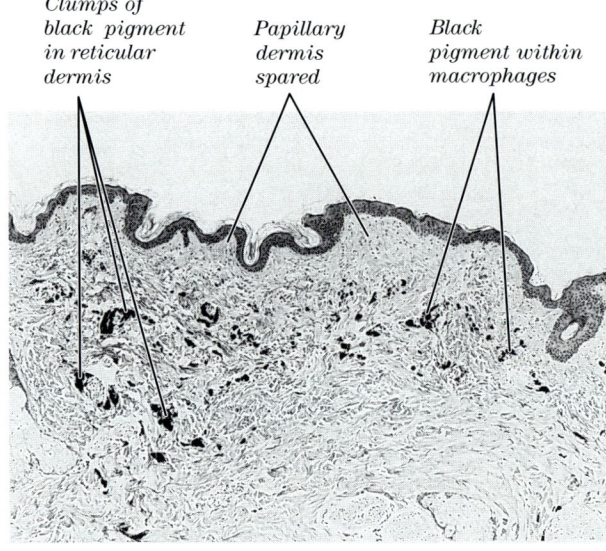

Clumps of black pigment within macrophages — *Papillary dermis spared*

Clumps of black pigment in reticular dermis — *Papillary dermis spared* — *Black pigment within macrophages*

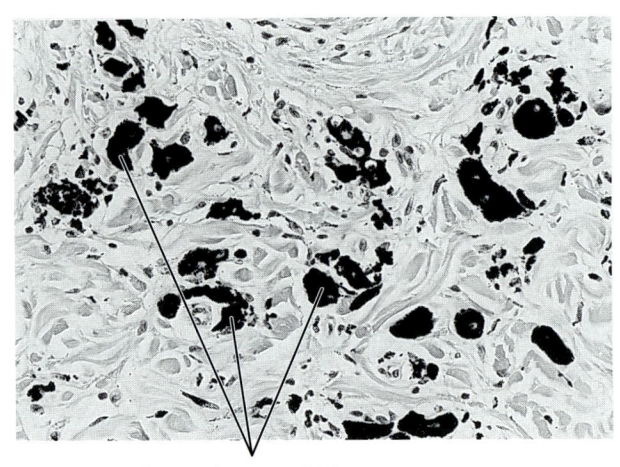

Black pigment within macrophages in reticular dermis; no melanocytes

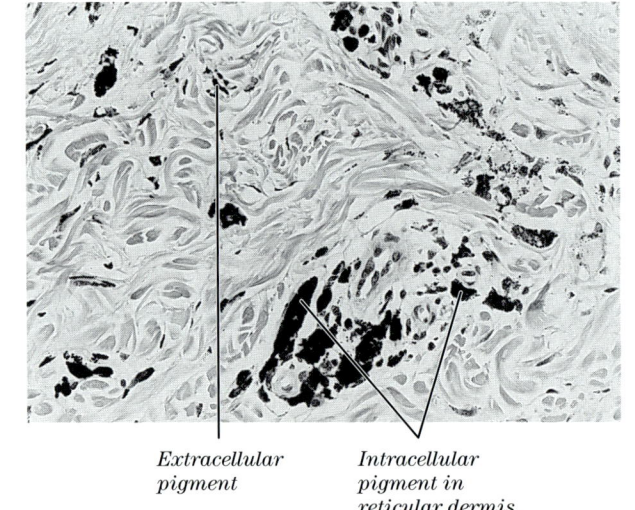

Extracellular pigment — *Intracellular pigment in reticular dermis*

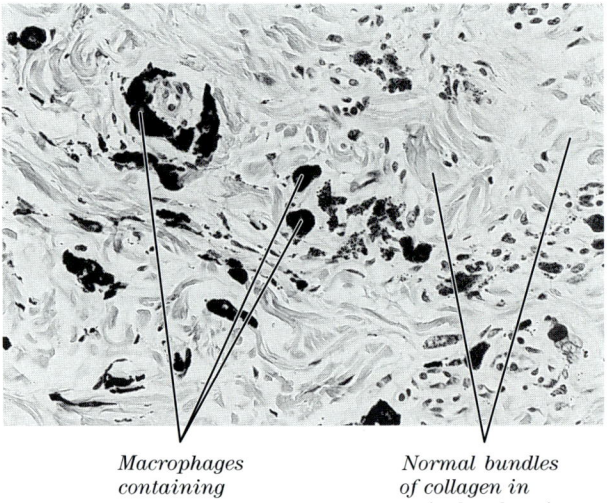

Macrophages containing black pigment — *Normal bundles of collagen in reticular dermis*

56 • Tattoo by Carbon

Criteria for diagnosis of this tattoo by carbon

This is a tattoo because:

1. Pigment in clumps is distributed throughout the upper part of the dermis.
2. The pigment is black.
3. There is no infiltrate of lymphocytes in association with the pigment.
4. The epidermis is normal.

Pitfall in diagnosis

This tattoo by carbon could be misdiagnosed as melanosis, i.e., complete regression of a primary melanoma, because:

1. Abundant dark pigment resides in the upper part of the dermis.
2. Clumps of carbon resemble melanophages.

Even in black and white photomicrography, this lesion can be diagnosed as a tattoo and not a blue nevus because melanin in blue nevi is housed within dendritic melanocytes and macrophages, There are no dendritic cells in tattoos. In sections stained by hematoxylin and eosin and visualized in color, carbon in a tattoo appears black, whereas melanin in blue nevi is brown.

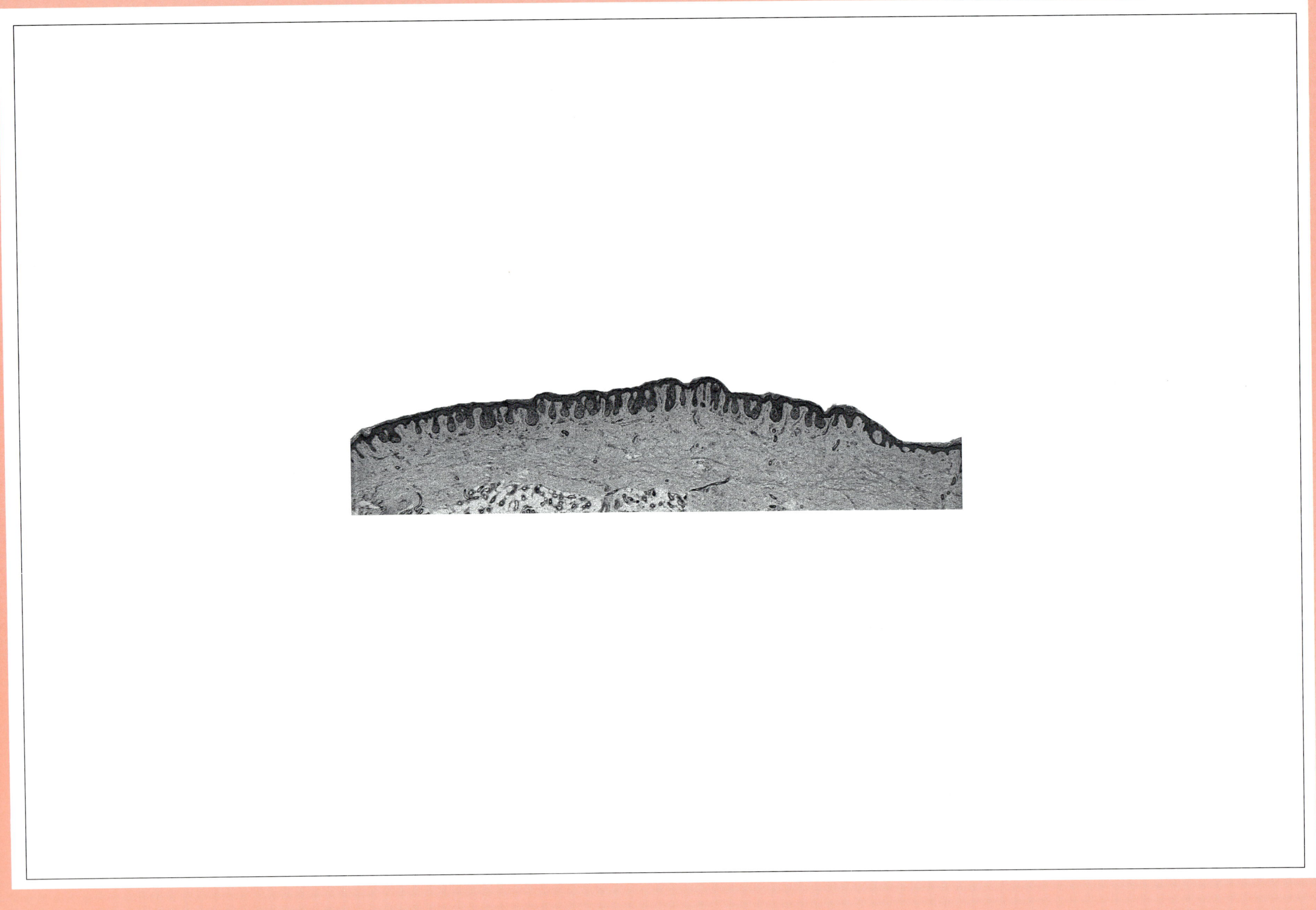

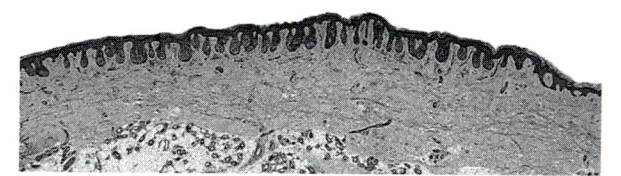
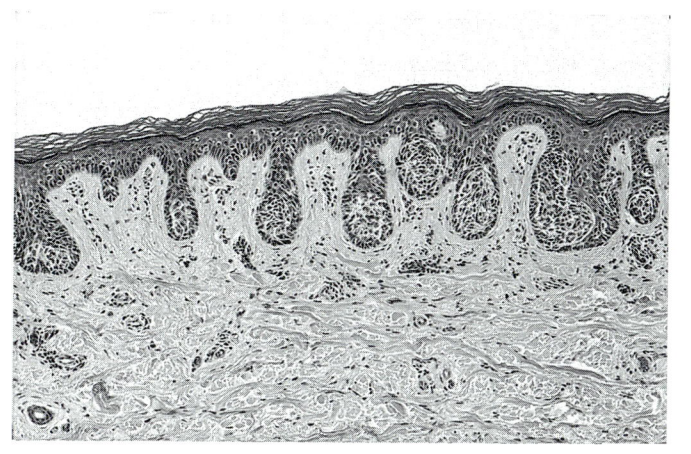
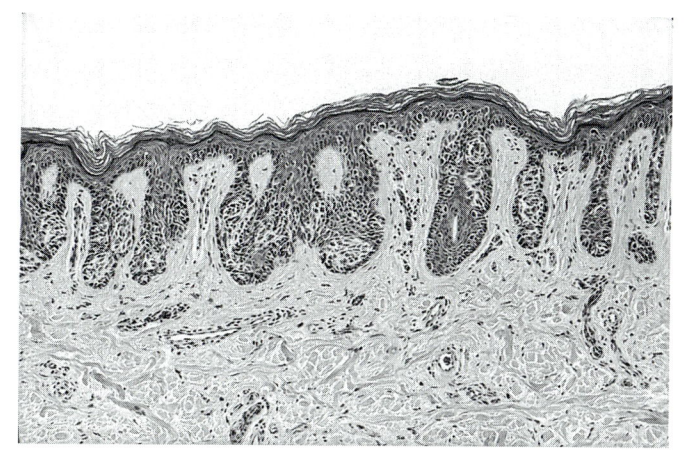
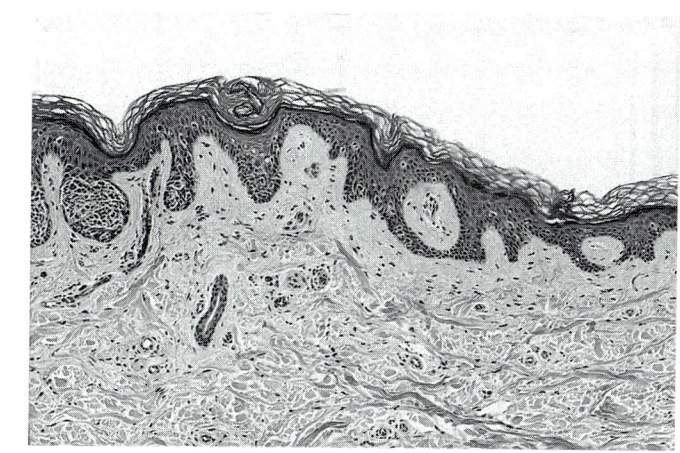
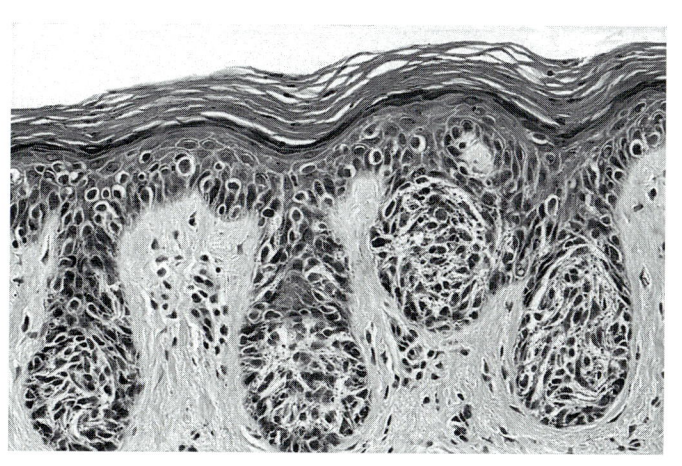
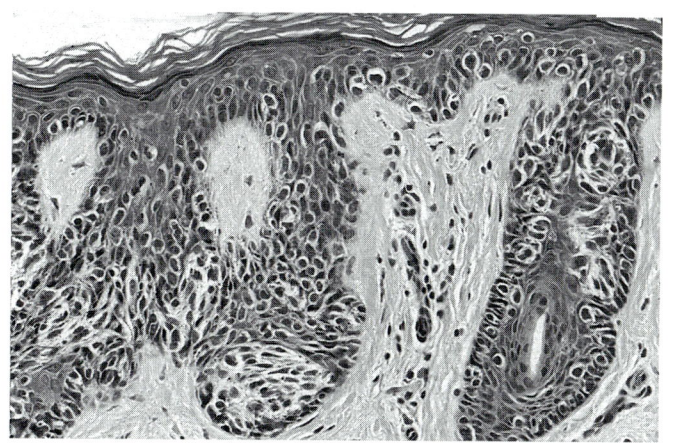
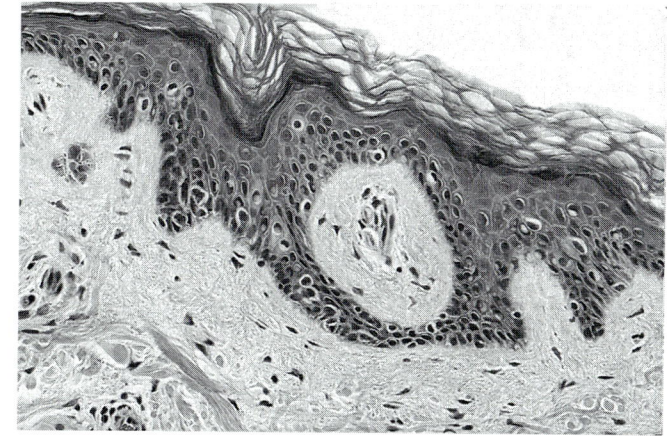

57. What is your diagnosis?

Pigmented lesion on the third toe of the left foot of a 72-year-old man. No clinical diagnosis or follow-up was available.

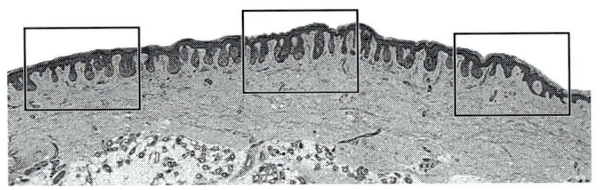

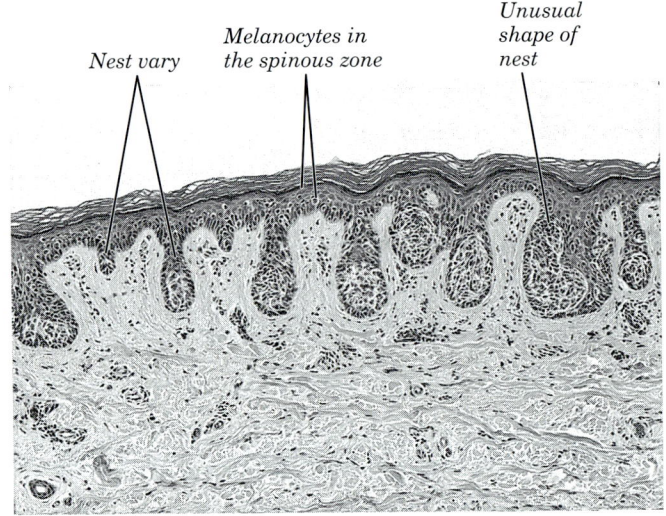

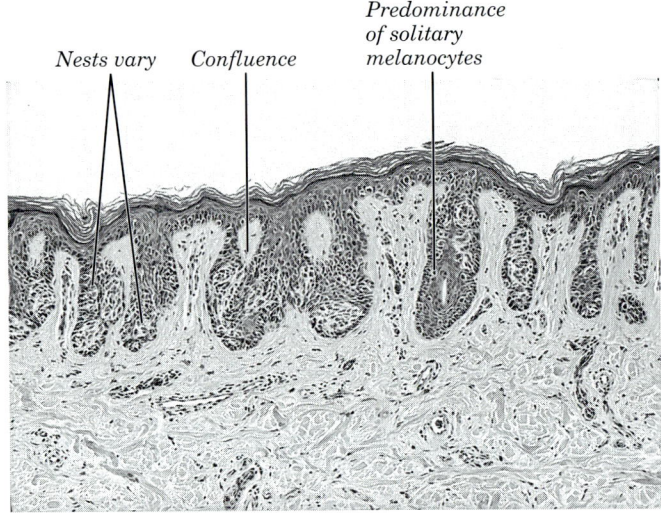

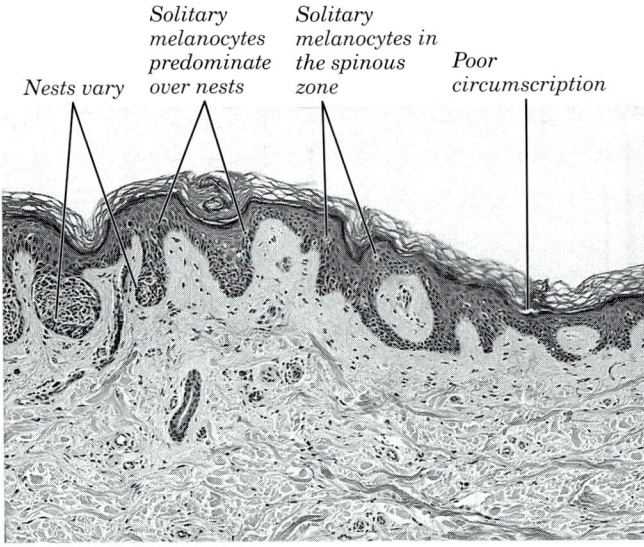

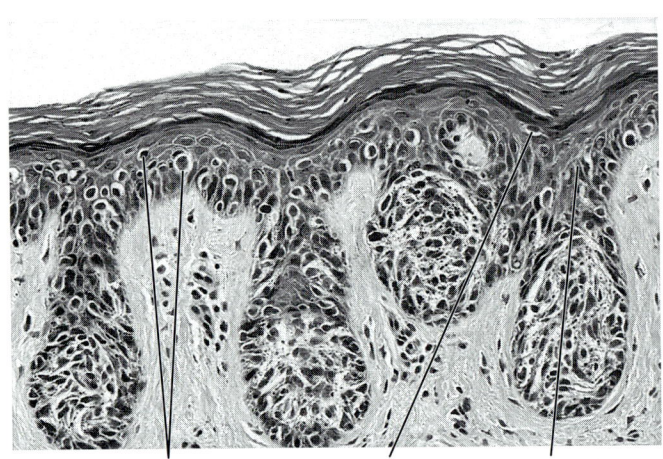

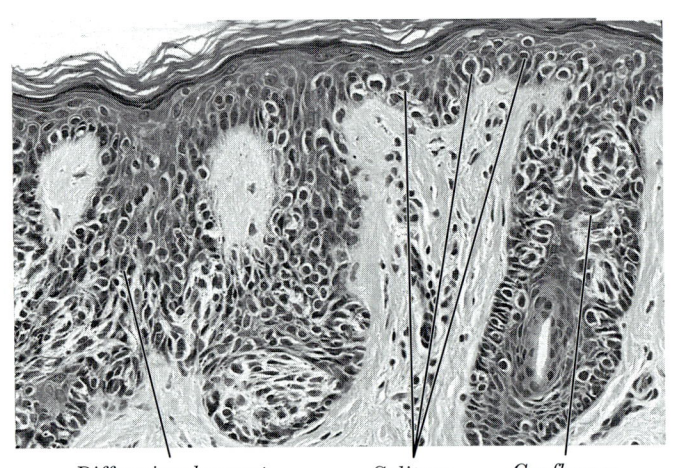

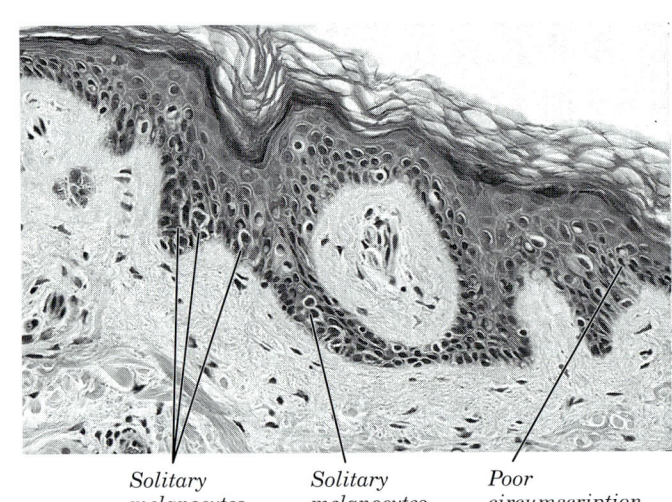

57 • Melanoma in situ

Criteria for diagnosis of this melanoma in situ

This is a melanoma in situ because:

1. The lesion is asymmetric.
2. The proliferation of melanocytes is poorly circumscribed.
3. Nests of melanocytes within the epidermis and epithelial structures of adnexa are not equidistant from one another.
4. Nests of melanocytes vary in size and shape.
5. Some nests of melanocytes have peculiar shapes.
6. Some nests of melanocytes have become confluent.
7. Melanocytes disposed as solitary units predominate over nests in some foci.
8. Melanocytes arranged as solitary units and nests are dispersed diffusely throughout some rete ridges and some epithelial structures of adnexa.
9. Melanocytes arrayed as solitary units are present above the dermo-epidermal junction including the spinous, granular, and cornified layers.
10. Melanocytes, both those as solitary units and in nests, extend far down epithelial structures of adnexa.
11. Melanocytes in the form of solitary units are present above the basal layer of epithelial structures of adnexa.
12. Melanocytes disposed as solitary units are not set equidistant from one another.
13. Some melanocytes have atypical nuclei.

Pitfall in diagnosis

This melanoma in situ could be mistaken for a junctional "dysplastic" nevus because:

1. The lesion is small, i.e., less than 6.0 mm in greatest diameter.
2. Melanocytes arranged in nests predominate over melanocytes disposed as solitary units throughout most of the neoplasm.
3. Nests of melanocytes are situated mostly at the dermo-epidermal junction at bases of rete ridges.
4. In some foci, nests of melanocytes are relatively uniform in size and shape.
5. Elongated rete ridges resemble those of a "lentiginous" pattern.
6. Most of the melanocytes are relatively small and monomorphous.

The differential diagnosis of this neoplasm is a junctional Clark's nevus versus a melanoma in situ. It is a melanoma in situ for the reasons stated here. A histopathologic diagnosis of "dysplastic nevus" not only is an evasion, but also it is wrong.

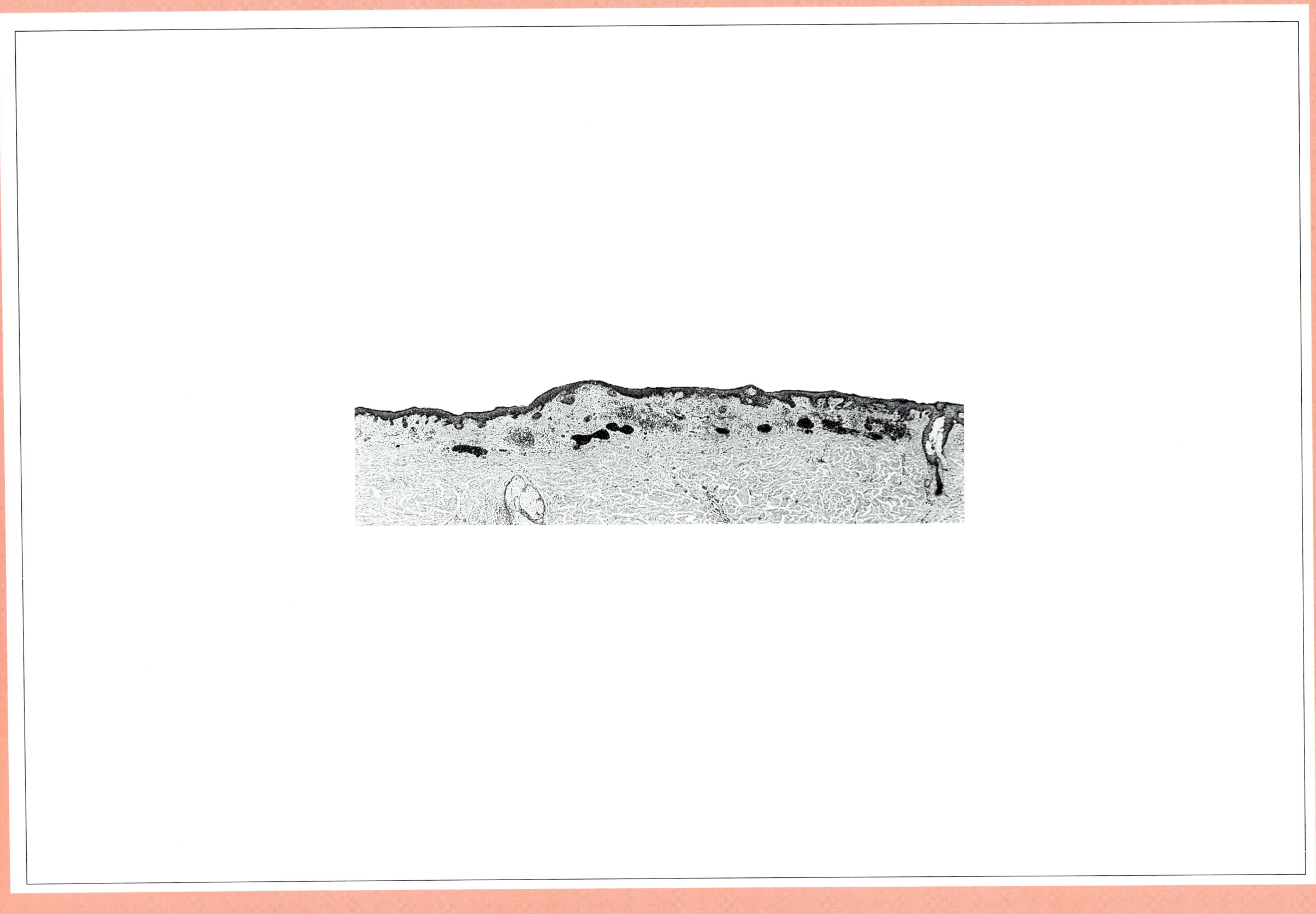

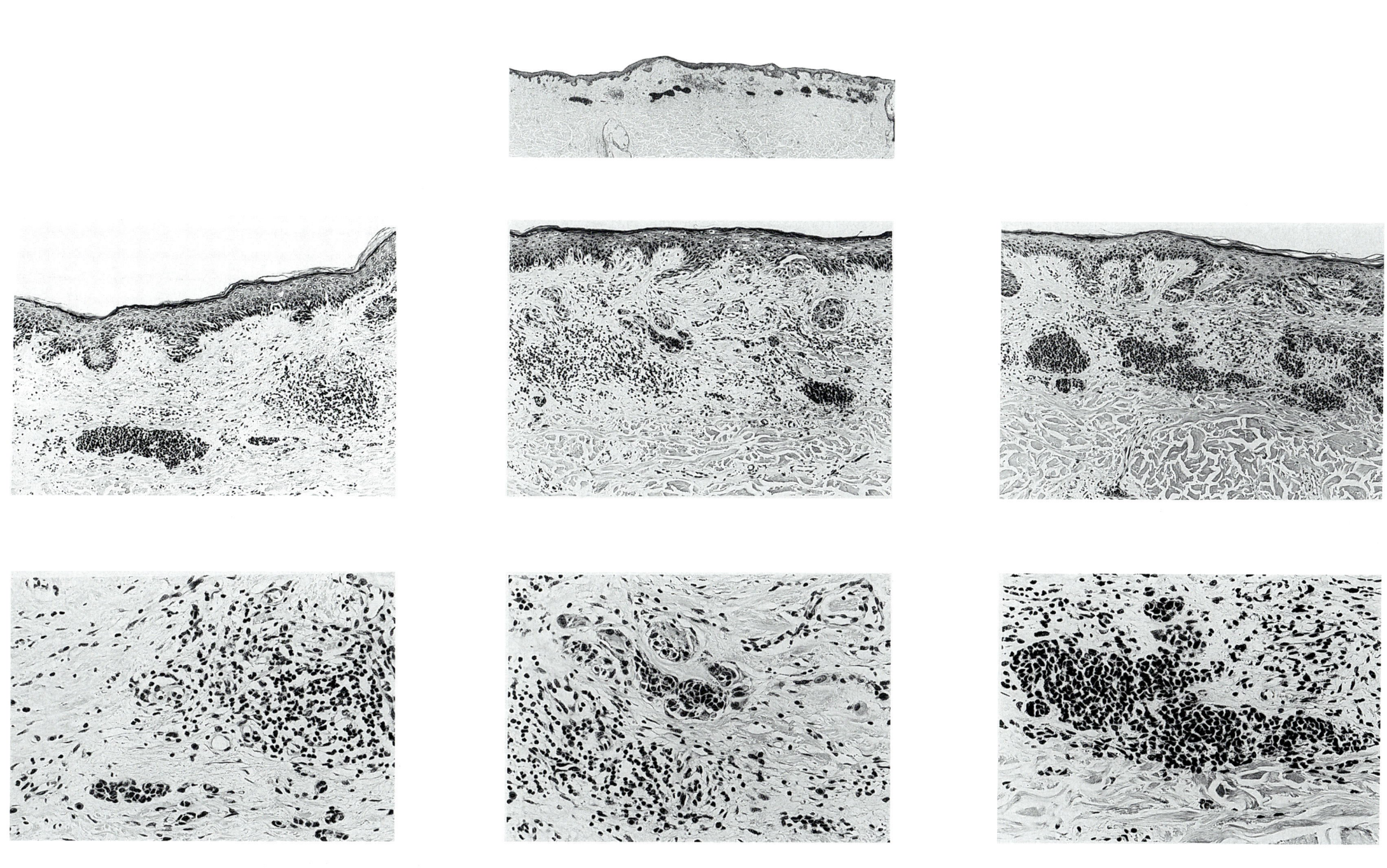

58. What is your diagnosis?

Lesion on the back of a 61-year-old man. Clinical diagnosis: dysplastic nevus. Wide and deep excision eventually was performed. Patient exhibited no evidence of disease after 2 years.

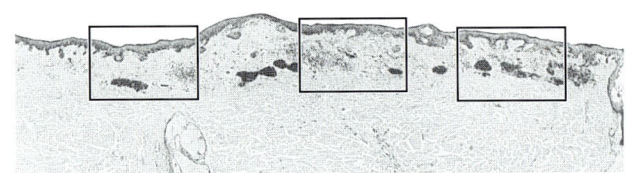

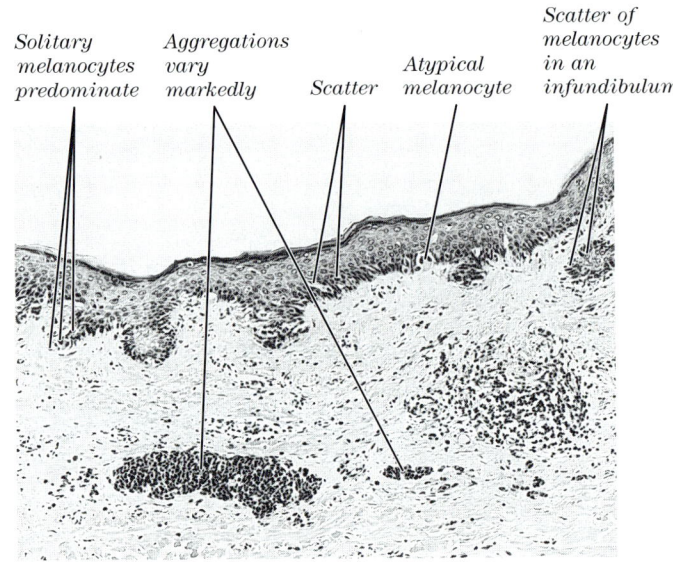

Solitary melanocytes predominate — *Aggregations vary markedly* — *Scatter* — *Atypical melanocyte* — *Scatter of melanocytes in an infundibulum*

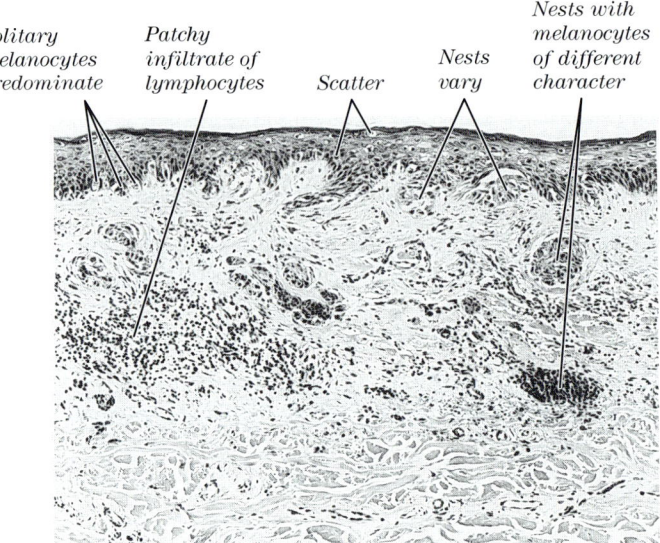

Solitary melanocytes predominate — *Patchy infiltrate of lymphocytes* — *Scatter* — *Nests vary* — *Nests with melanocytes of different character*

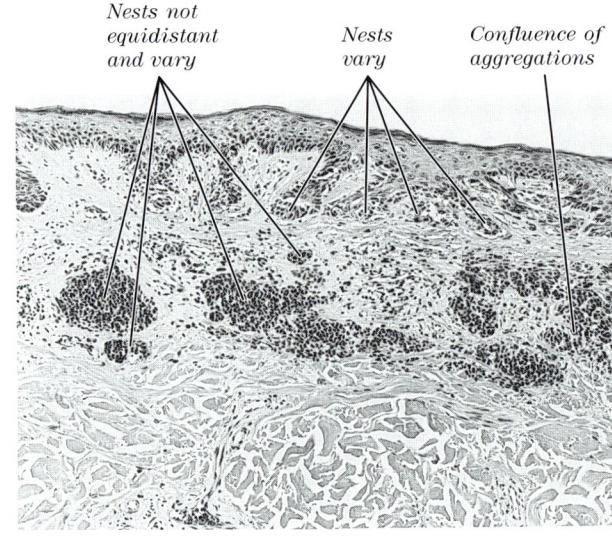

Nests not equidistant and vary — *Nests vary* — *Confluence of aggregations*

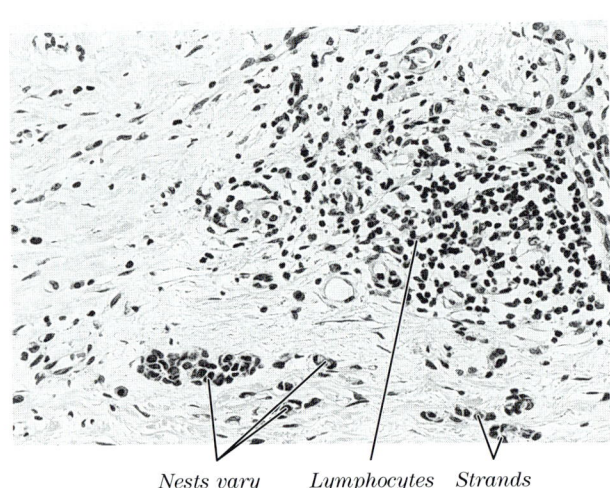

Nests vary — *Lymphocytes* — *Strands*

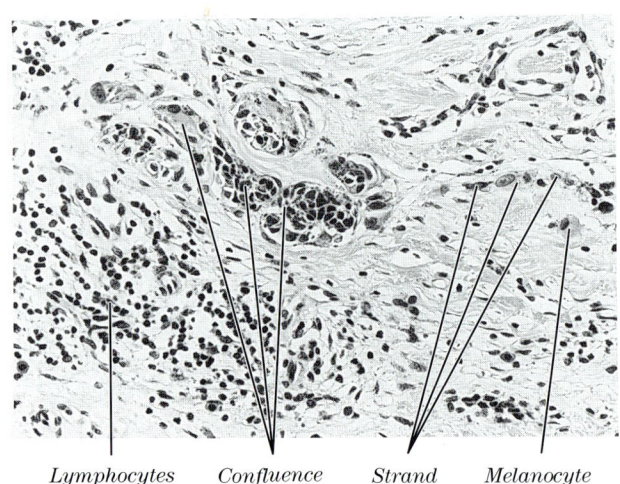

Lymphocytes — *Confluence* — *Strand* — *Melanocyte*

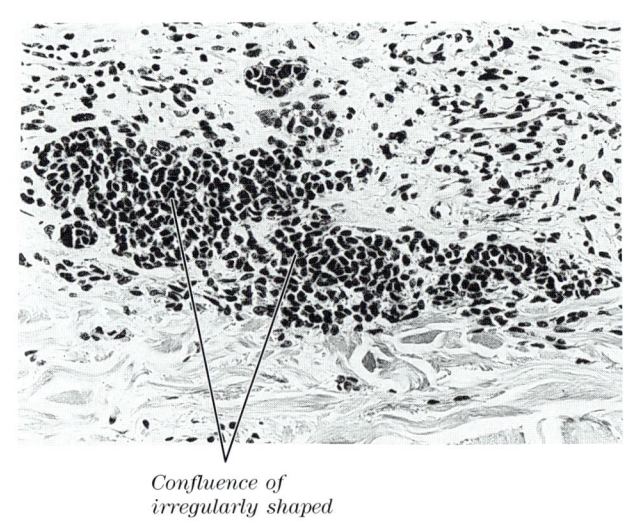

Confluence of irregularly shaped aggregations

58 • Melanoma

Criteria for diagnosis of this melanoma

This is a melanoma because:

1. The neoplasm is asymmetric.
2. Nests of melanocytes within the epidermis and the dermis are not equidistant from one another.
3. Melanocytes are scattered far above the dermo-epidermal junction, including the granular zone and cornified layer.
4. Nests of melanocytes vary in size and shape.
5. Melanocytes disposed as solitary units within the epidermis predominate over those in nests in some high-power fields.
6. Nuclei of many melanocytes are atypical.

Pitfall in diagnosis

This melanoma could be misdiagnosed as a compound Clark's nevus because:

1. Melanocytes with small dark nuclei are set in discrete nests at the base of the reticular dermis.
2. Melanocytes mature with progressive descent into the thickened papillary dermis.
3. Nests of melanocytes within the epidermis are situated mostly at the dermo-epidermal junction.
4. The base of the neoplasm is flat.

The problem posed by this melanocytic neoplasm is vexing. Is the neoplasm melanoma in situ in association with an intradermal Clark's nevus or is the entire neoplasm a melanoma? The latter diagnosis is correct because, as can be seen at scanning magnification, nests of melanocytes in the lower portion of the thickened papillary dermis are not equidistant from one another, they vary in size and shape, some have peculiar shapes, and several have become confluent. Therefore, despite the maturation of melanocytes with progressive descent into a thickened papillary dermis, the entire neoplasm is a melanoma.

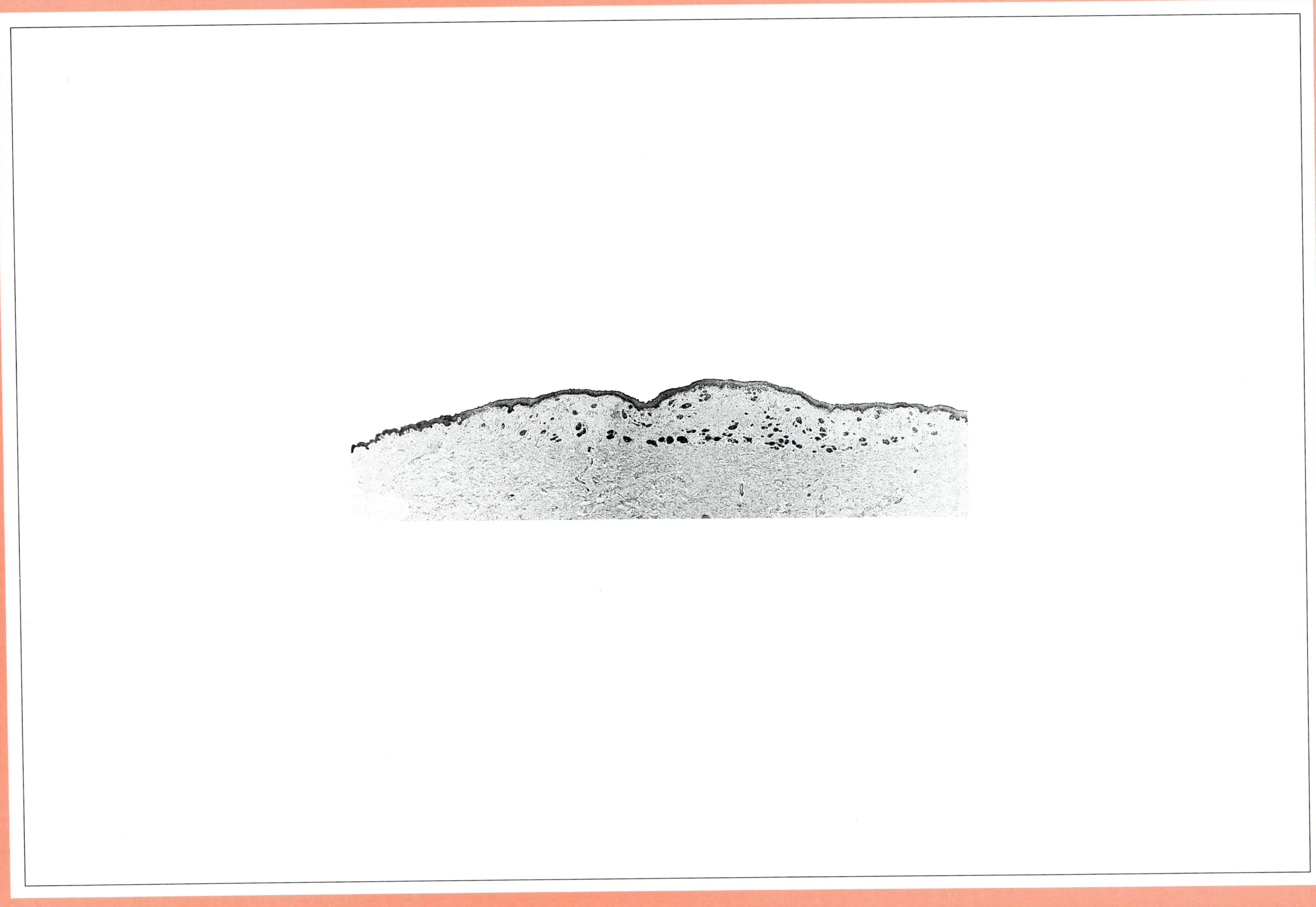

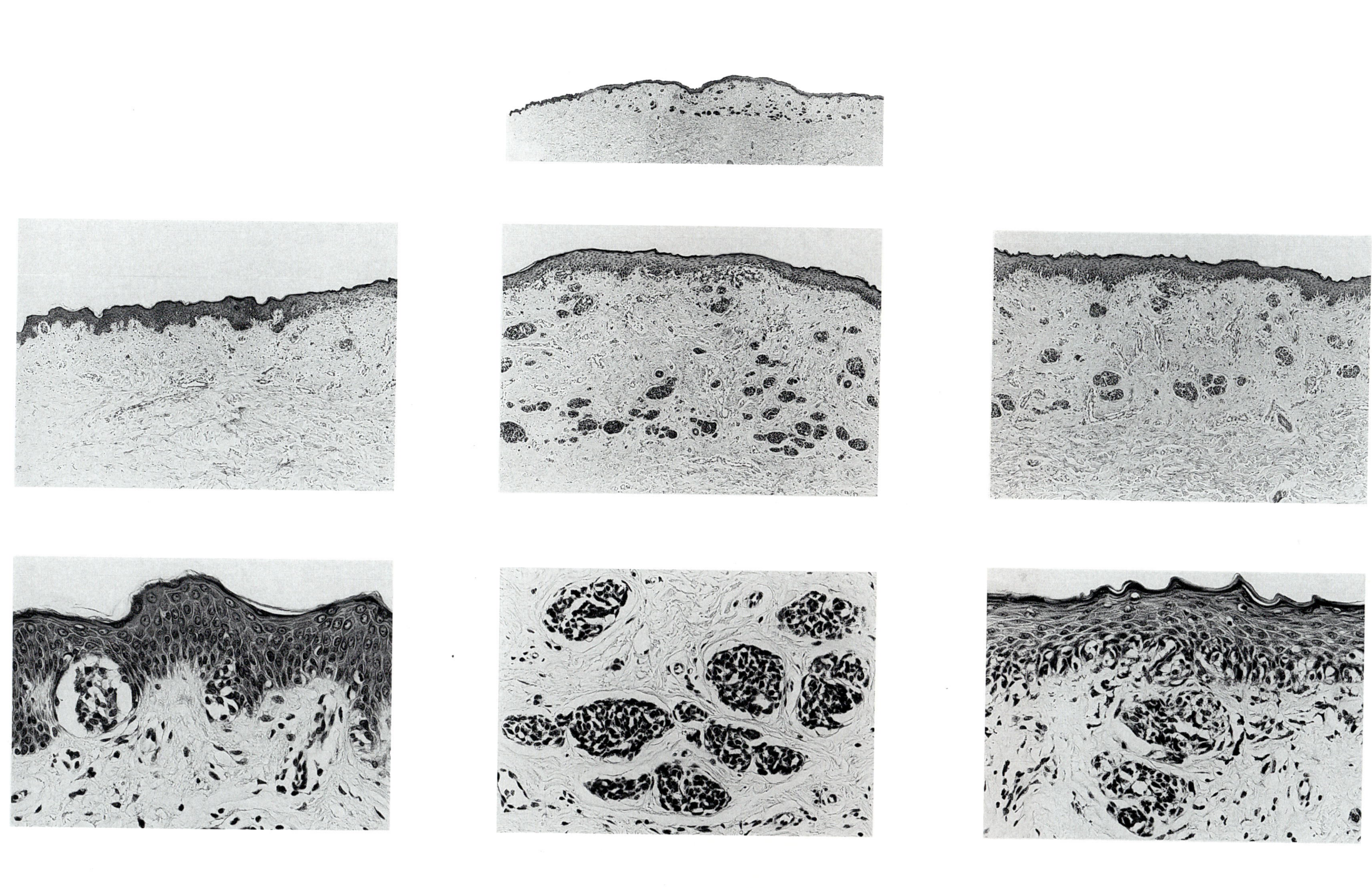

59. What is your diagnosis?

No clinical information was available.

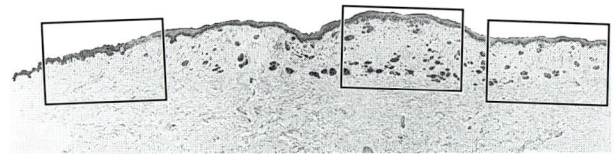

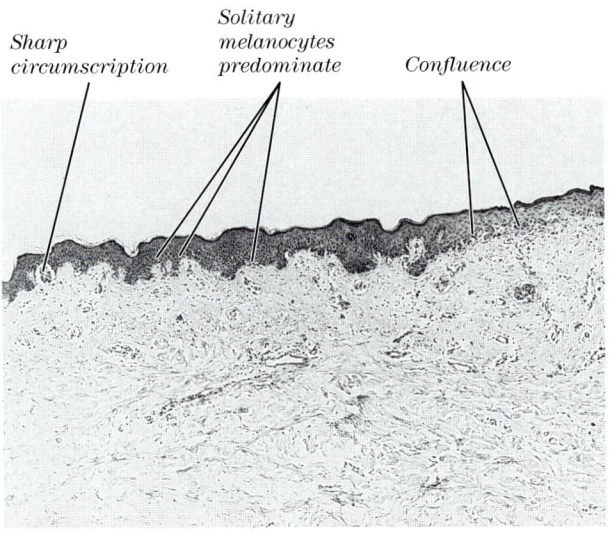

Sharp circumscription   *Solitary melanocytes predominate*   *Confluence*

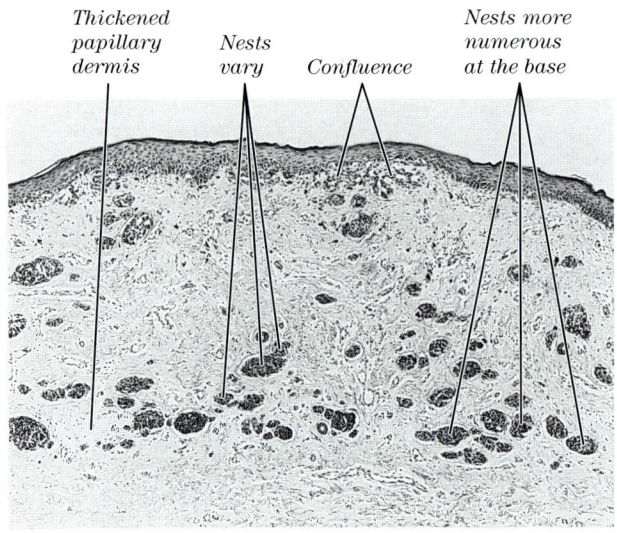

Thickened papillary dermis   *Nests vary*   *Confluence*   *Nests more numerous at the base*

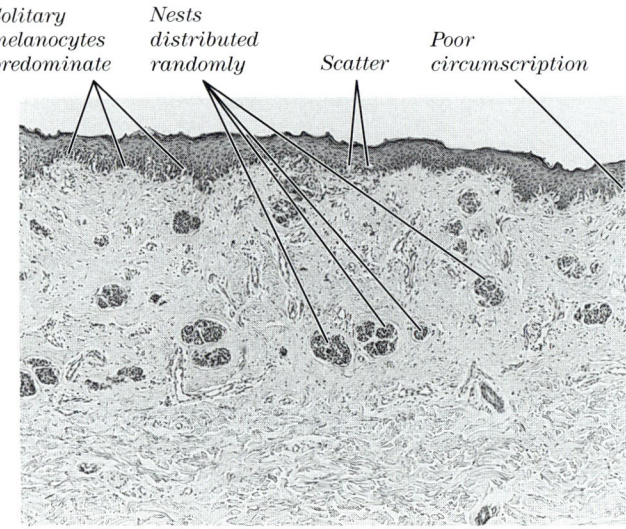

Solitary melanocytes predominate   *Nests distributed randomly*   *Scatter*   *Poor circumscription*

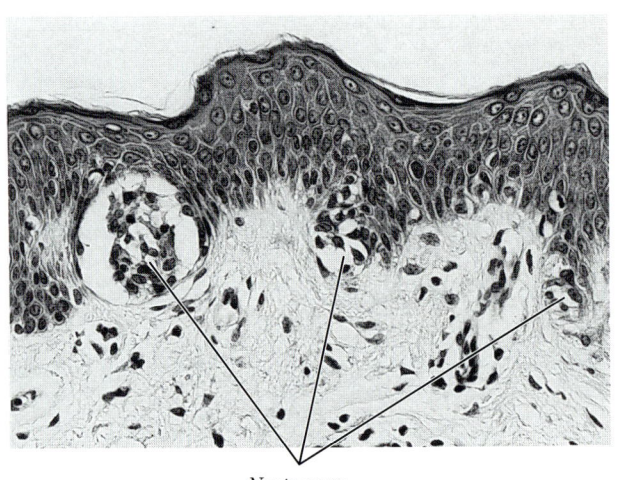

Nests vary

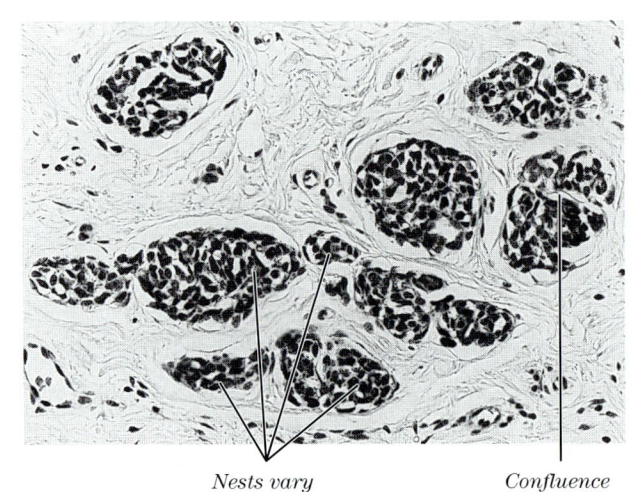

Nests vary   *Confluence*

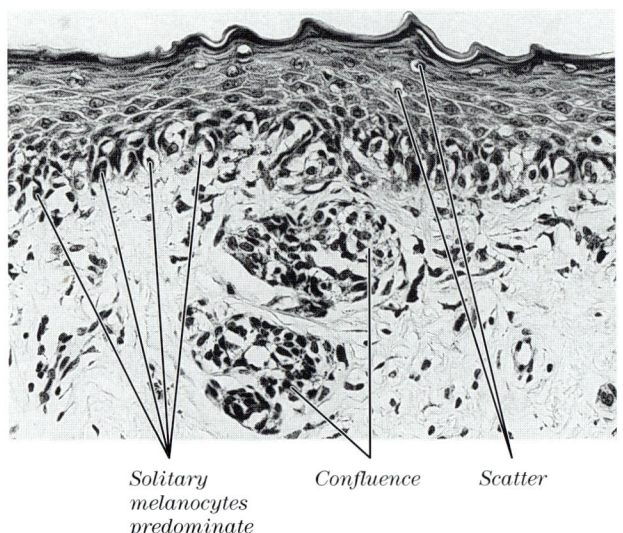

Solitary melanocytes predominate   *Confluence*   *Scatter*

59 • Melanoma

Criteria for diagnosis of this melanoma

This is a melanoma because:

1. Melanocytes within the epidermis disposed as solitary units predominate over nests in many high-power fields.

2. Nests of melanocytes within the epidermis are not equidistant from one another.

3. Some nests of melanocytes within the epidermis have irregular jagged shapes.

4. Some nests of melanocytes within the epidermis have become confluent.

5. Melanocytes within the epidermis, especially those arranged as solitary units, are scattered above the dermo-epidermal junction, some in the upper reaches of the epidermis.

6. Nests of melanocytes within the dermis vary markedly in size and shape.

7. Nests of melanocytes within the dermis are not equidistant from one another.

Pitfall in diagnosis

This melanoma could be misinterpreted as a compound Clark's nevus because:

1. The neoplasm is relatively symmetric.

2. It is relatively well-circumscribed.

3. There is some maturation of melanocytes with progressive descent into the dermis.

4. Some nests of melanocytes within the epidermis are discrete.

5. The neoplasm is confined to the epidermis and markedly thickened papillary dermis.

6. The central portion of the neoplasm is slightly domed.

7. There is little nuclear atypia, most of the nuclei being small and oval.

The thorny problem in differential diagnosis posed by a neoplasm such as this one is "compound Clark's nevus, melanoma in situ in association with a nevus, or melanoma"? The scatter of melanocytes within the epidermis militates against Clark's nevus. The asymmetric distribution of nests and the marked variation in size and shape of nests within the thickened papillary dermis argue against a Clark's nevus. In sum and for these reasons, this entire neoplasm is a melanoma.

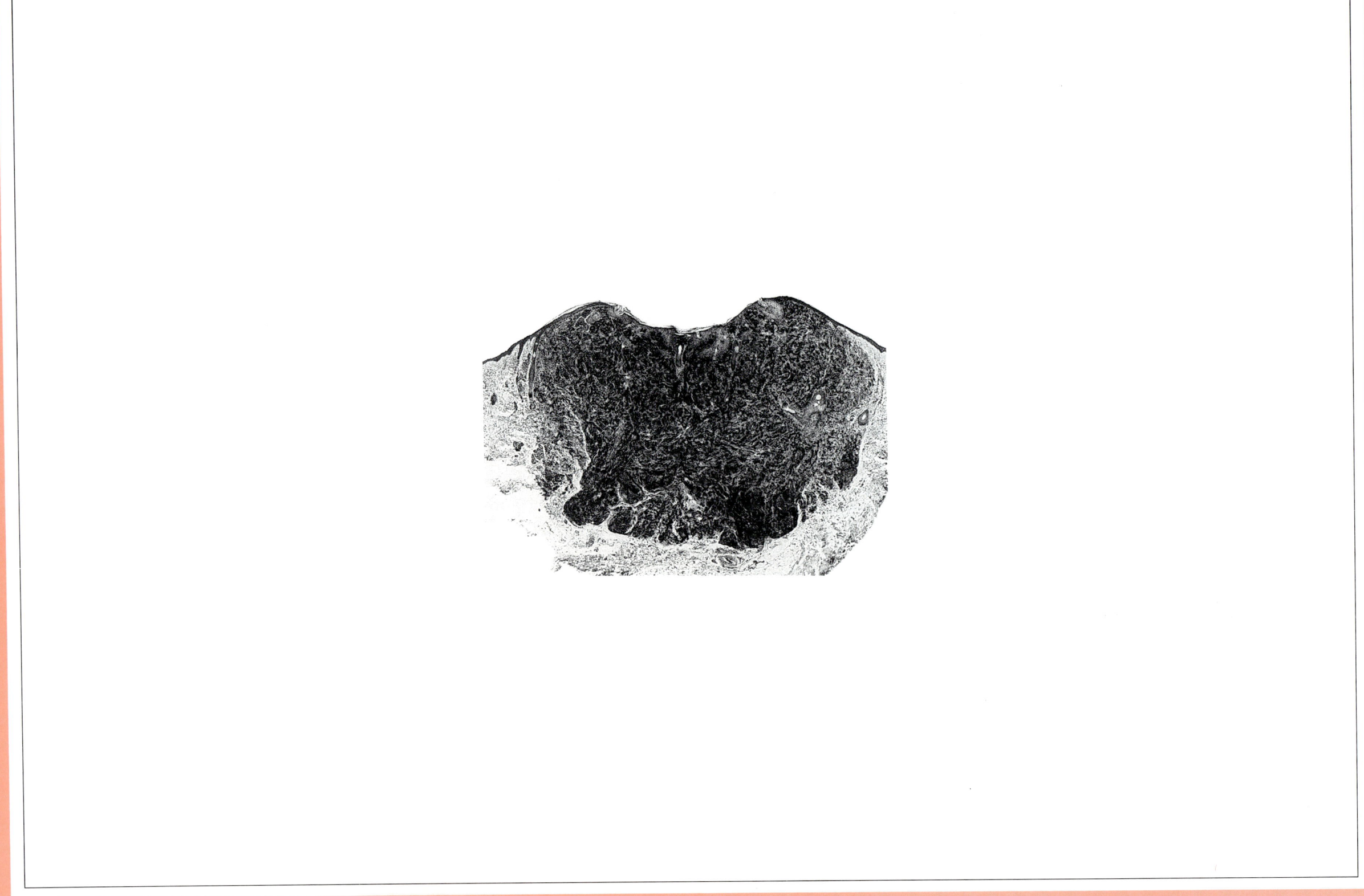

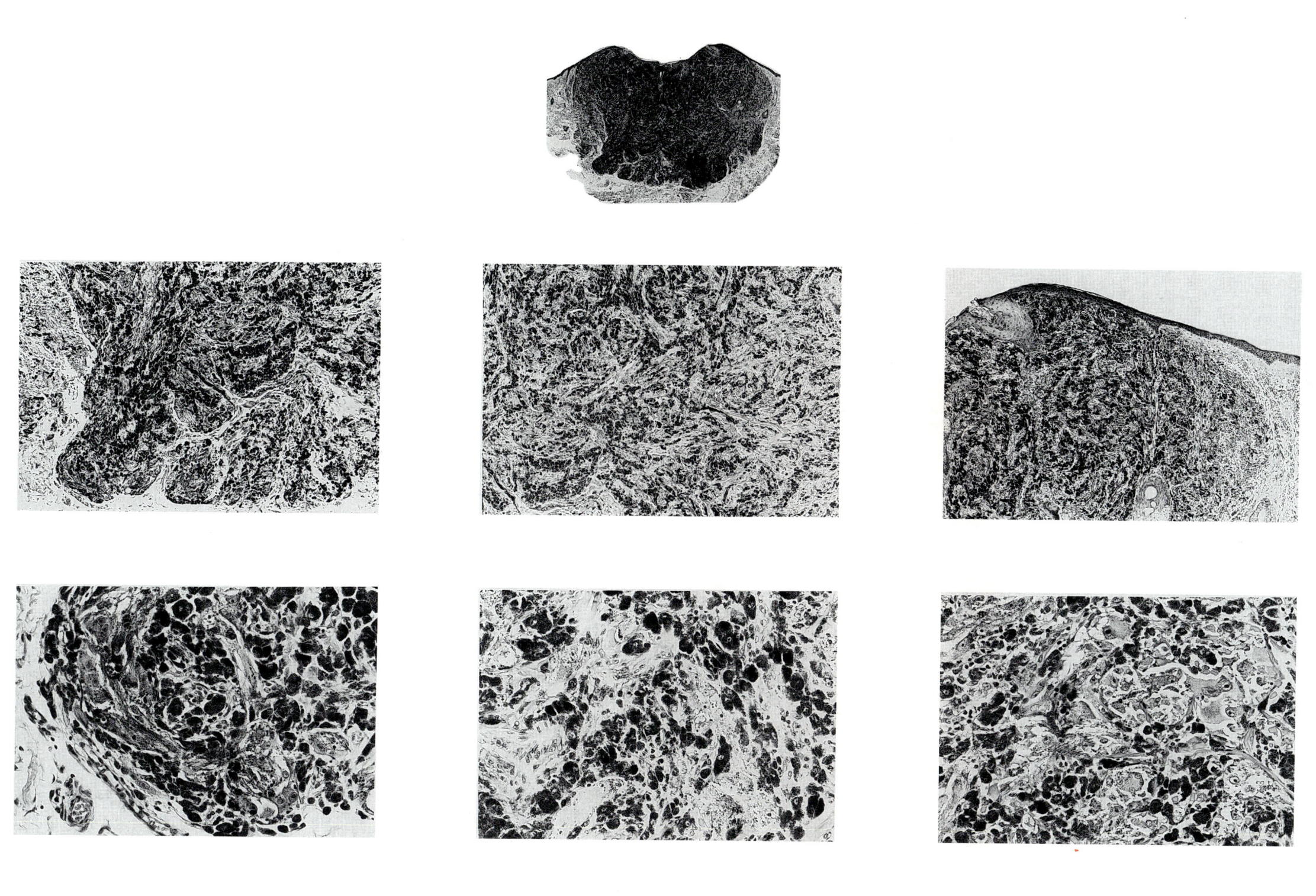

60. What is your diagnosis?

No clinical information was available.

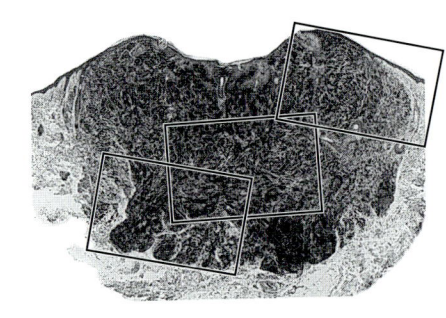

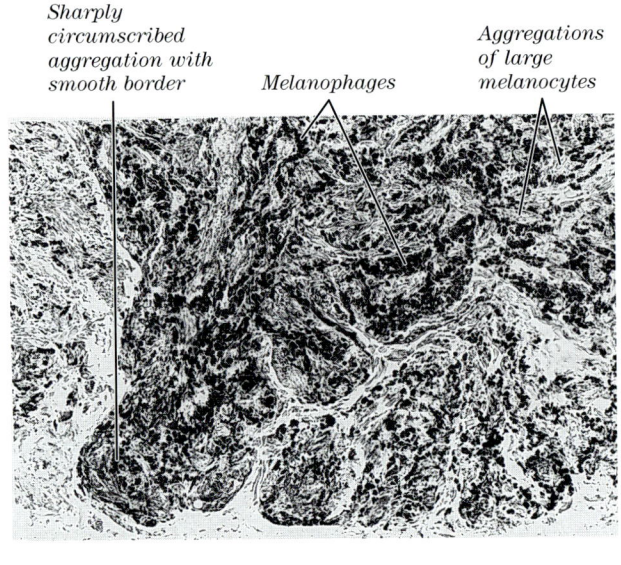

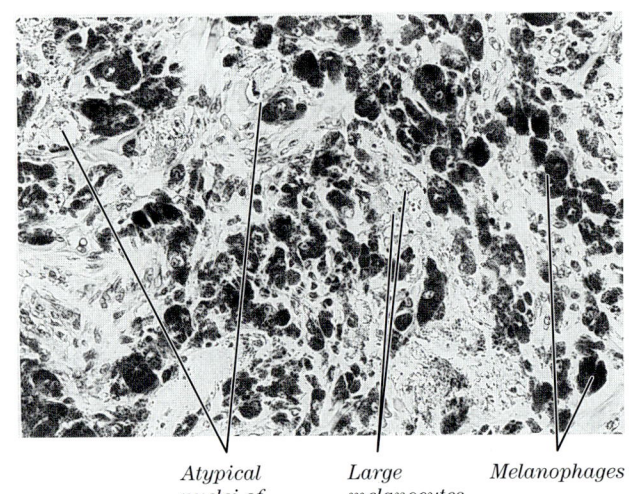

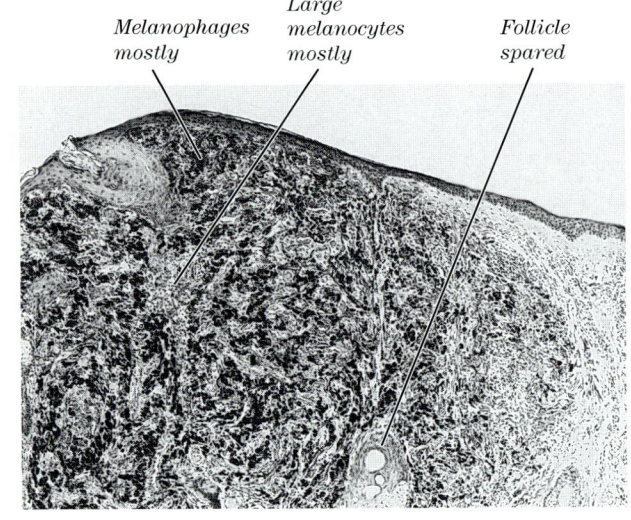

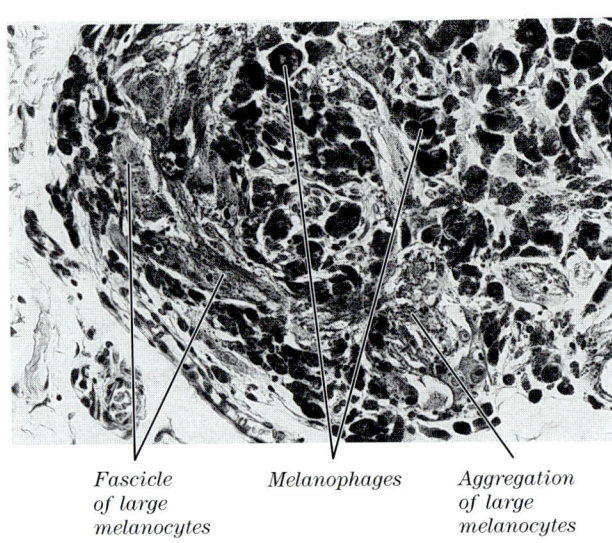

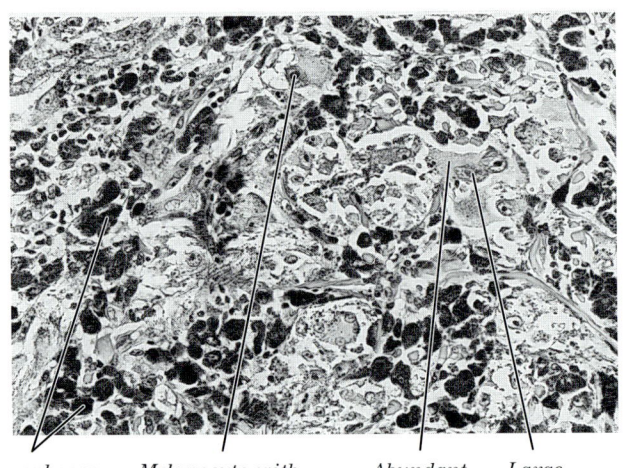

60 • Spitz's Nevus

Criteria for diagnosis of this Spitz's nevus

This neoplasm is benign because:

1. It is sharply circumscribed.
2. It is almost as deep as it is broad.
3. Melanin is distributed uniformly throughout it.

This is a Spitz's nevus because:

Nuclei of melanocytes are large, cytoplasm of melanocytes is abundant, and shapes of melanocytes are oval and round.

Pitfall in diagnosis

This Spitz's nevus could be misinterpreted as a melanoma because:

1. The neoplasm is slightly asymmetric.
2. Melanocytes with atypical nuclei are present in the dermis.
3. Abundant pigment in melanocytes and macrophages is distributed throughout the entire extent of neoplasm, even at the base of it.

The benign nature of this neoplasm is apparent at scanning magnification: it is symmetric and well-circumscribed, and it has smooth borders. The presence of atypical melanocytes within a Spitz's nevi is expected. Note that melanin, especially within macrophages, is distributed in relatively uniform fashion throughout the neoplasm, another sign of benignancy.

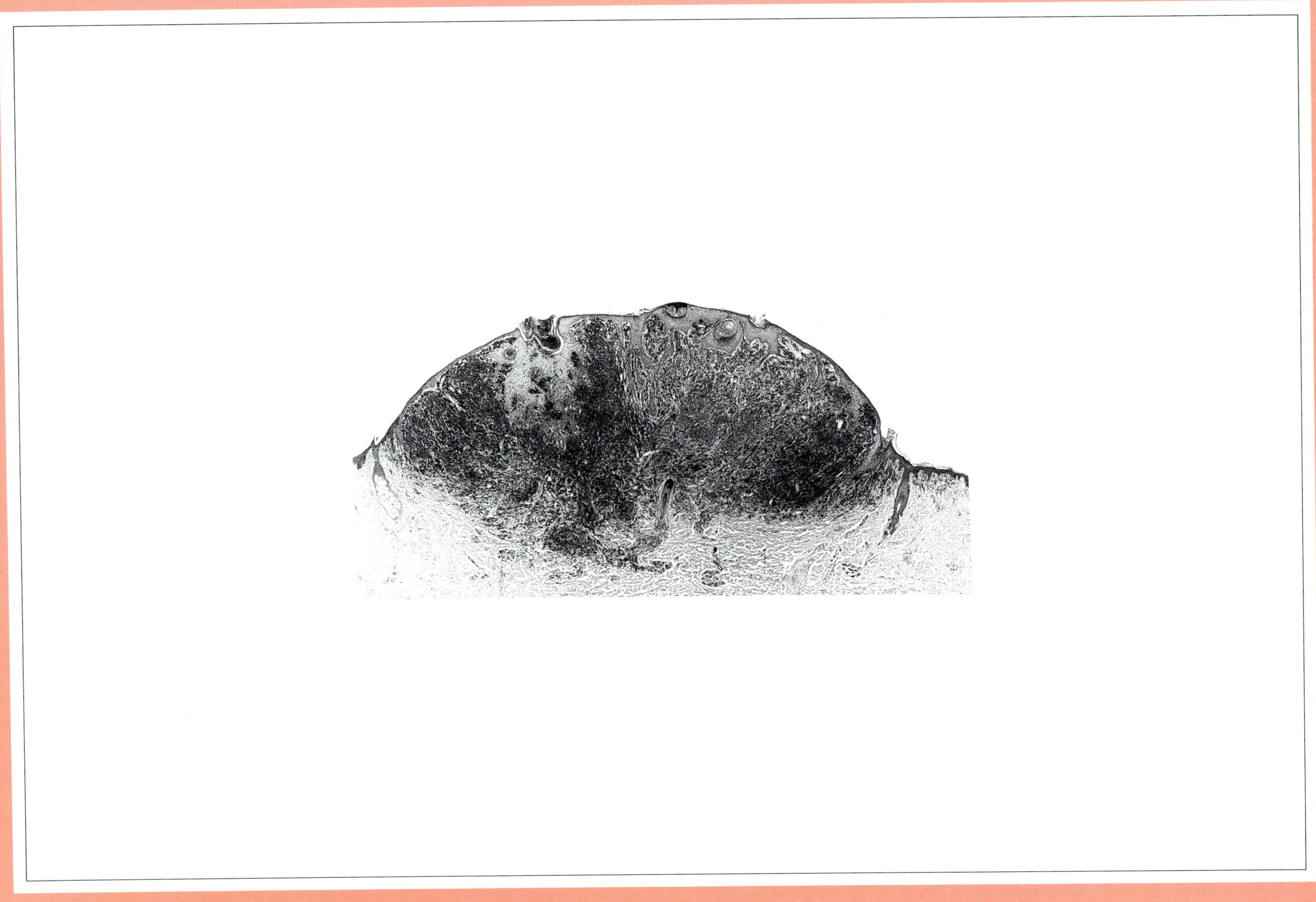

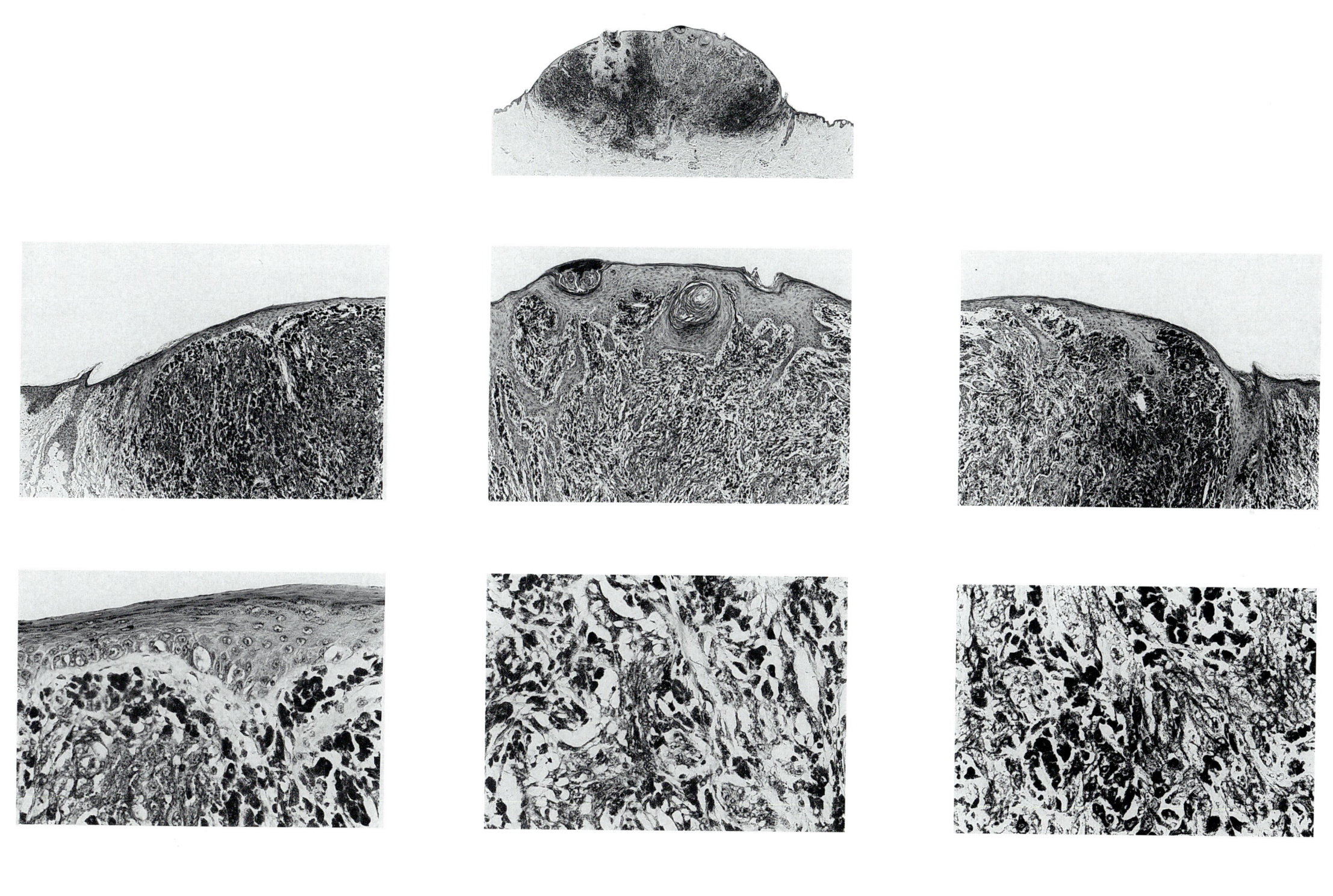

61. What is your diagnosis?

Lesion on the left cheek of a 31-year-old woman. Clinical diagnosis: melanoma. No follow-up information was available.

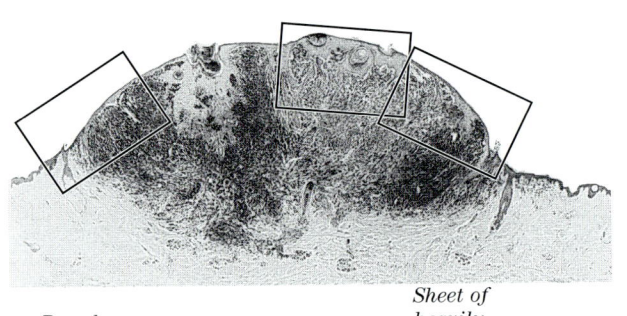

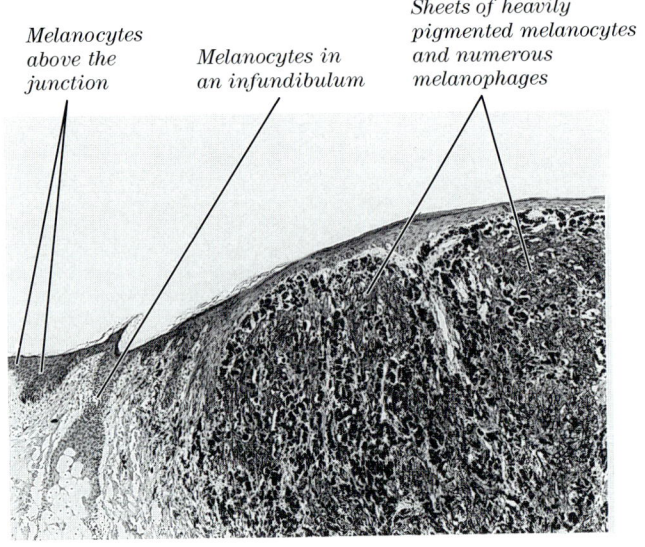

Melanocytes above the junction — *Melanocytes in an infundibulum* — *Sheets of heavily pigmented melanocytes and numerous melanophages*

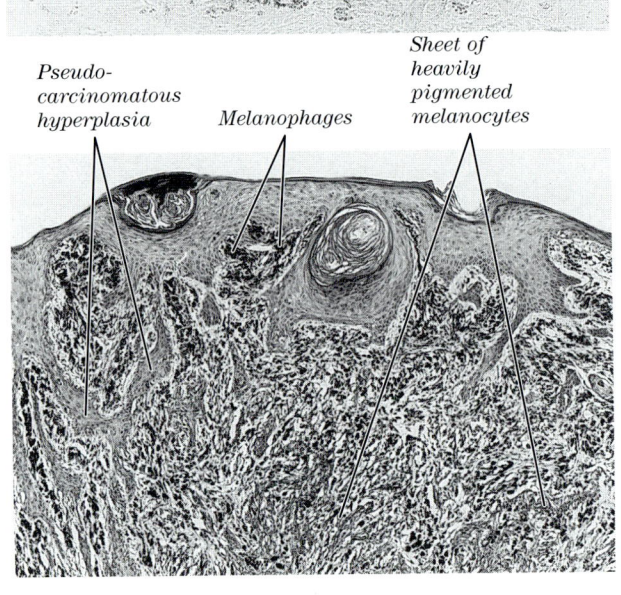

Pseudo-carcinomatous hyperplasia — *Melanophages* — *Sheet of heavily pigmented melanocytes*

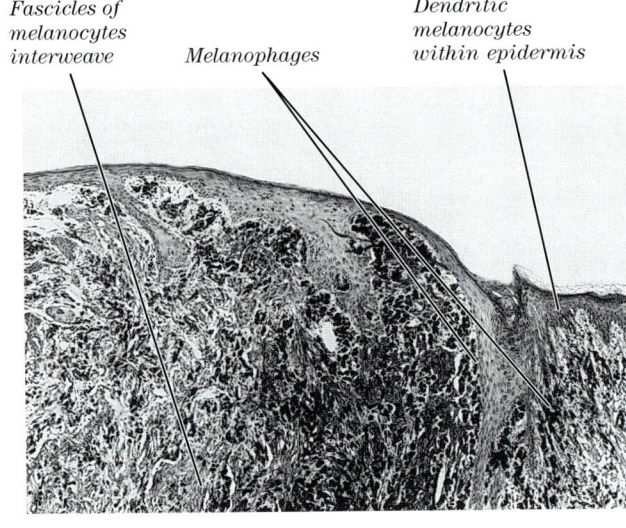

Fascicles of melanocytes interweave — *Melanophages* — *Dendritic melanocytes within epidermis*

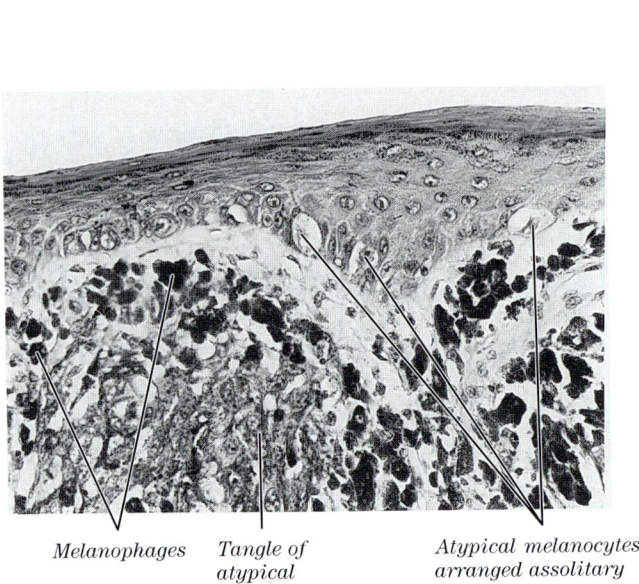

Melanophages — *Tangle of atypical melanocytes* — *Atypical melanocytes arranged as solitary units*

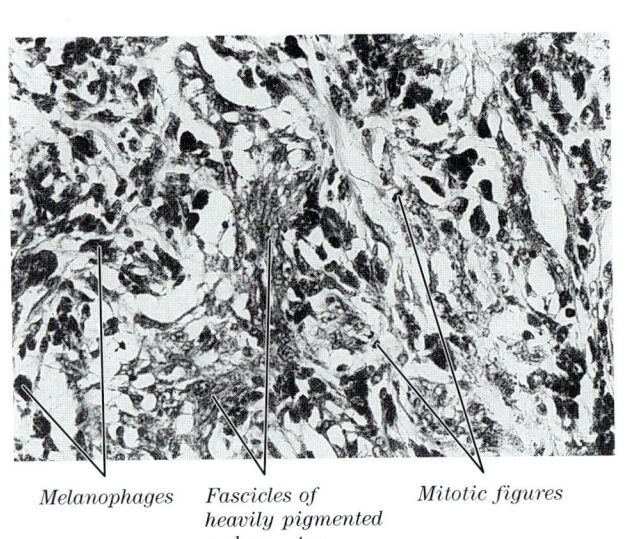

Melanophages — *Fascicles of heavily pigmented melanocytes* — *Mitotic figures*

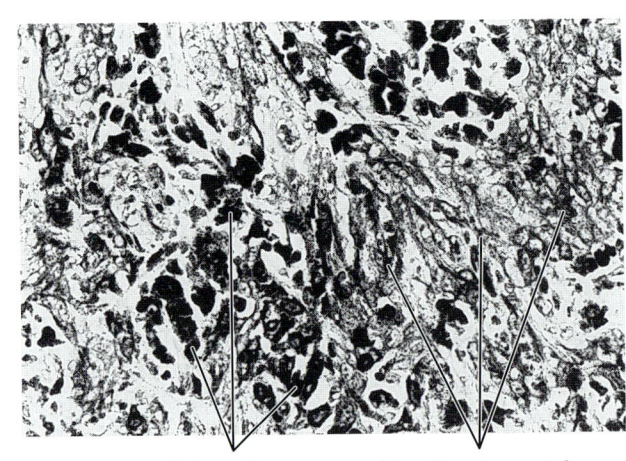

Melanophages — *Heavily pigmented dendritic melanocytes*

61 • Melanoma

Criteria for diagnosis of this melanoma

This is a melanoma because:

1. The neoplasm is asymmetric, e.g., it is mostly dark on the left and mostly pale on the right.
2. It is poorly circumscribed.
3. Melanocytes disposed as solitary units within the epidermis predominate over nests in many high-power fields.
4. Sheets of neoplastic melanocytes are present throughout the dermis.
5. Melanin is not distributed in uniform fashion throughout the neoplasm.
6. Nuclei of neoplastic cells are atypical.
7. Many neoplastic cells are in mitosis.

Pitfall in diagnosis

This melanoma could be misread as a "compound" blue nevus because:

1. Topographically, the dome-shaped lesion is symmetric (although in distribution of melanin, it is strikingly asymmetric).
2. The vast majority of melanocytes within the dermis are markedly pigmented and dendritic.
3. Some dendritic melanocytes are present as solitary units within the epidermis.
4. There are numerous melanophages.

This neoplasm illustrates the importance of factors other than topography in assessing the issue of symmetry versus asymmetry. Topographically, this neoplasm is symmetric, but the distribution of melanin within it is strikingly asymmetric. For that reason, even at scanning magnification, it can be diagnosed as a melanoma and not a blue nevus. An exception to this "rule" is combined nevi, especially that kind in which "pagetoid" melanocytes within the dermis are surrounded by clusters of melanophages. Parenthetically, so-called compound blue nevus is truly an intradermal blue nevus because markedly pigmented dendritic melanocytes are present as solitary units only, not nests, within the epidermis.

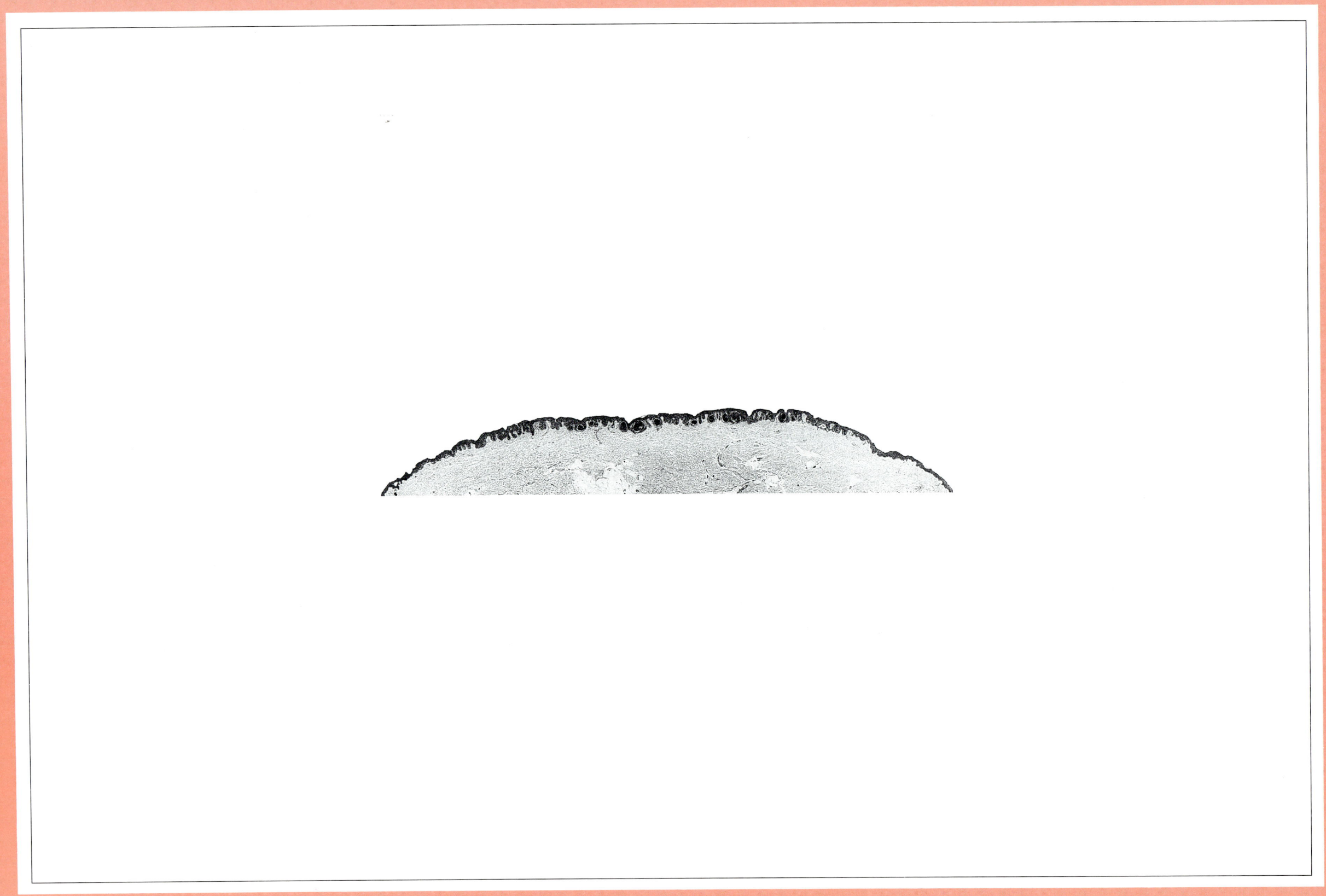

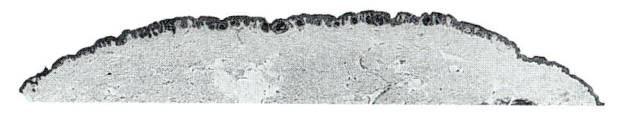
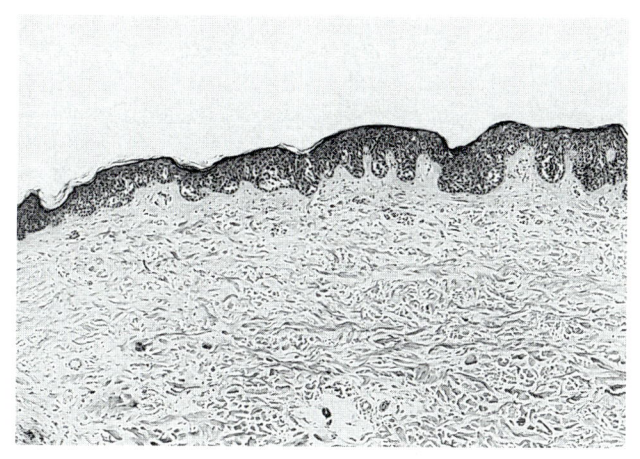
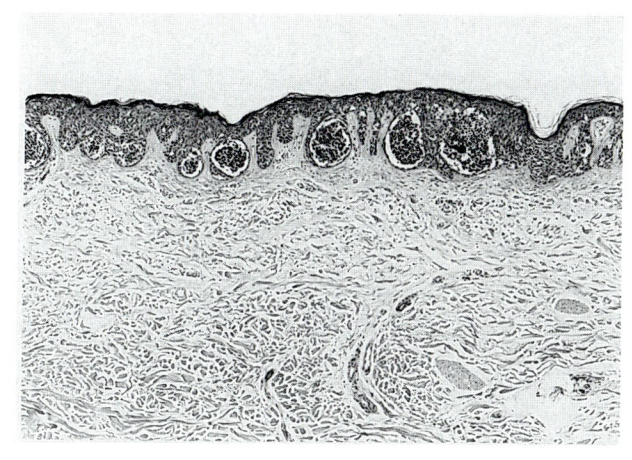
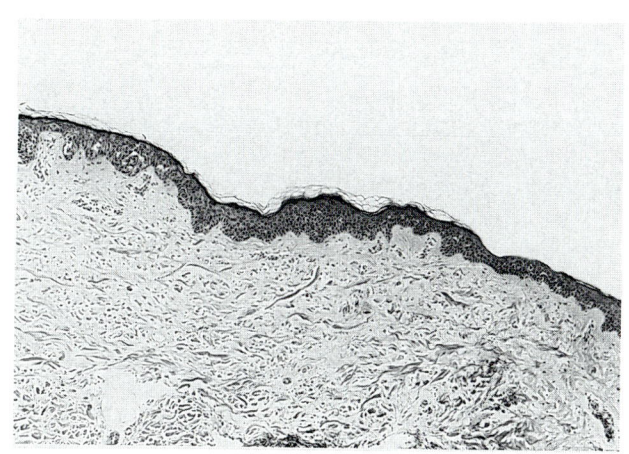
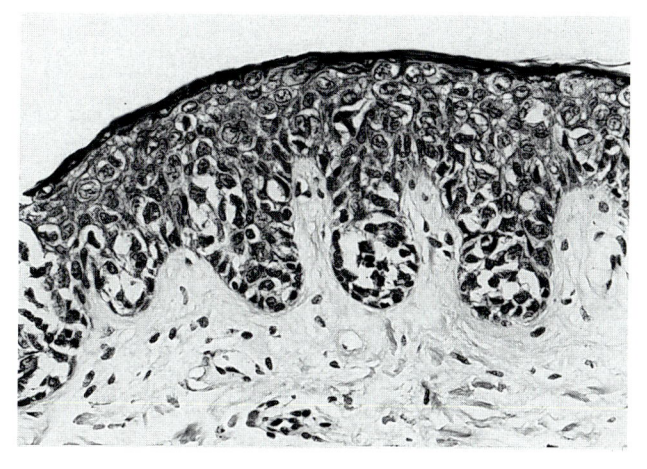
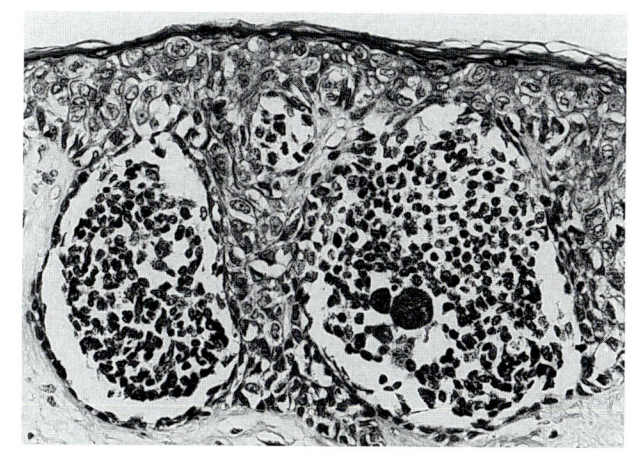
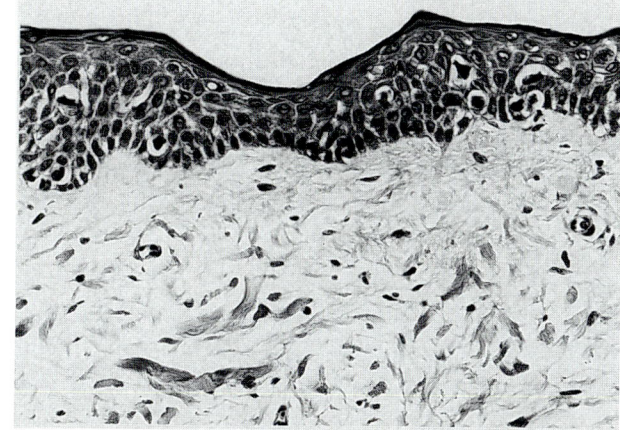

62. What is your diagnosis?

Irregularly pigmented papule on the left calf of a 65-year-old woman that had increased in size recently. There was a family history of melanoma. Clinical diagnosis: melanoma. Patient had no evidence of persistence of the neoplasm after 7 years.

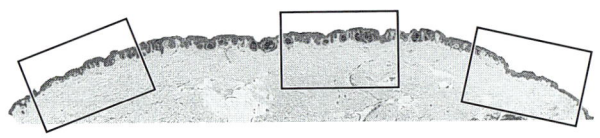

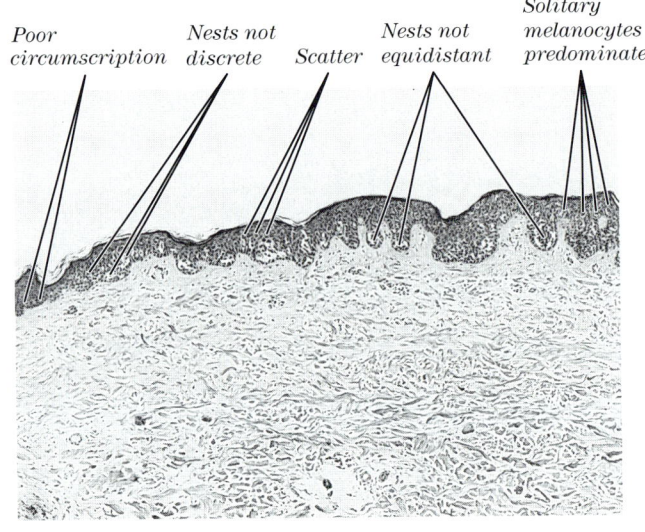
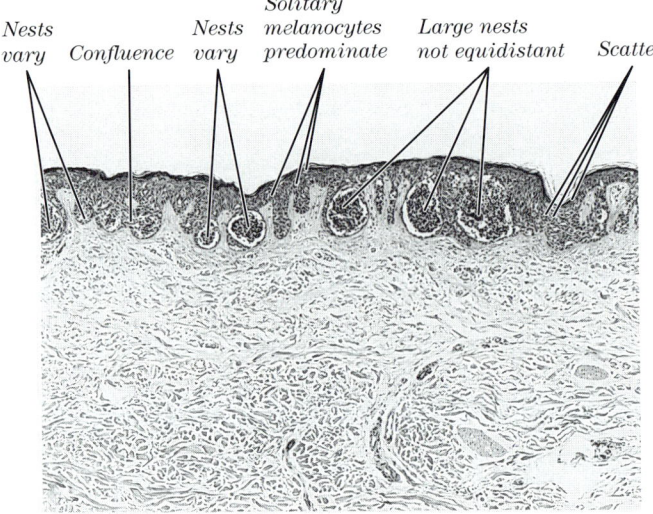
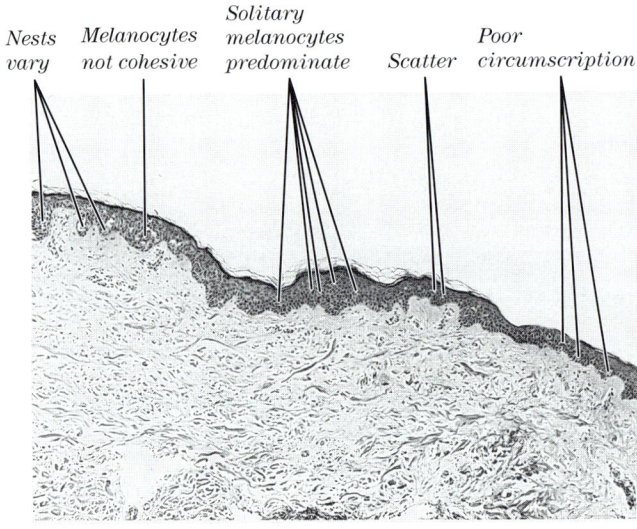

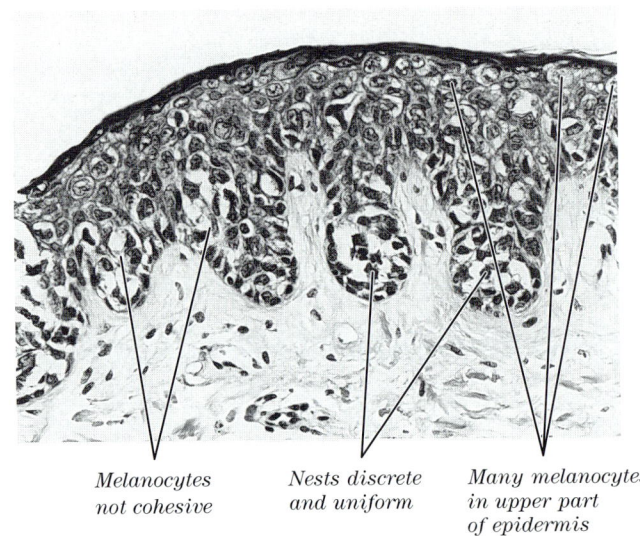
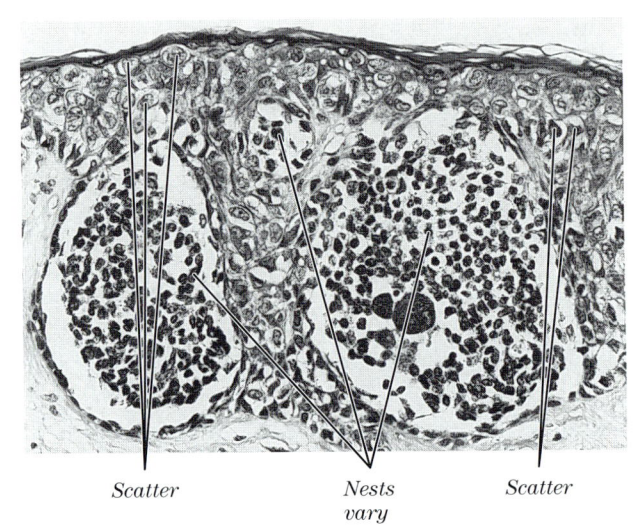
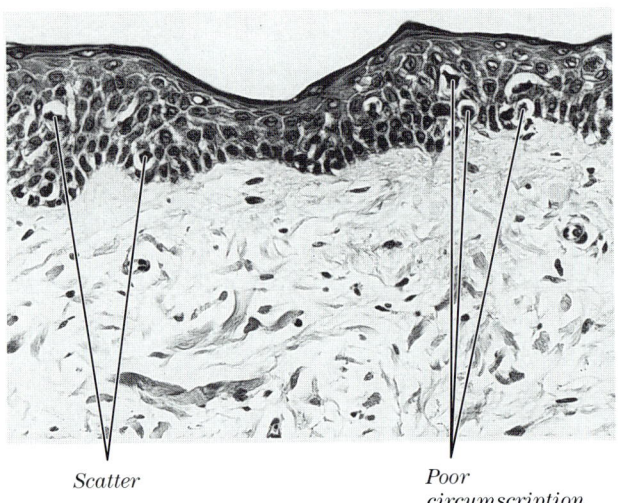

62 • Melanoma in situ

Criteria for diagnosis of this melanoma in situ

This is a melanoma in situ because:

1. The neoplasm is broad, i.e., more than 1.5 cm in diameter.
2. Nests of melanocytes within the epidermis are not equidistant from one another.
3. Nests of melanocytes within the epidermis differ markedly in size and shape.
4. Some nests of melanocytes within the epidermis have become confluent.
5. Neoplastic melanocytes are not cohesive in some "nests."
6. Melanocytes disposed as solitary units within the epidermis predominate over nests of melanocytes in some high-power fields.
7. Melanocytes arranged as solitary units, and to a lesser extent in nests, are scattered throughout the entire thickness of the epidermis.
8. The neoplasm is poorly circumscribed.

Pitfall in diagnosis

This melanoma in situ could be misdiagnosed as a junctional Clark's nevus because:

1. Melanocytes in nests are more numerous than melanocytes disposed as solitary units throughout much of the neoplasm.
2. Most nests of melanocytes are discrete.
3. Nuclei of melanocytes in nests are small, roundish, and monomorphous.
4. Most nests of melanocytes are situated either at the dermo-epidermal junction or just above it.

At scanning magnification, this neoplasm could easily be misread as a junctional nevus, characterized as it is by numerous discrete nests of melanocytes within the epidermis. Those nests, however, are not equidistant from one another, they vary in size and shape, and some have become confluent. At higher magnification, indubitable signs of melanoma in situ become apparent: melanocytes dispersed as solitary units throughout the entire thickness of the epidermis across the entire front of the epidermis.

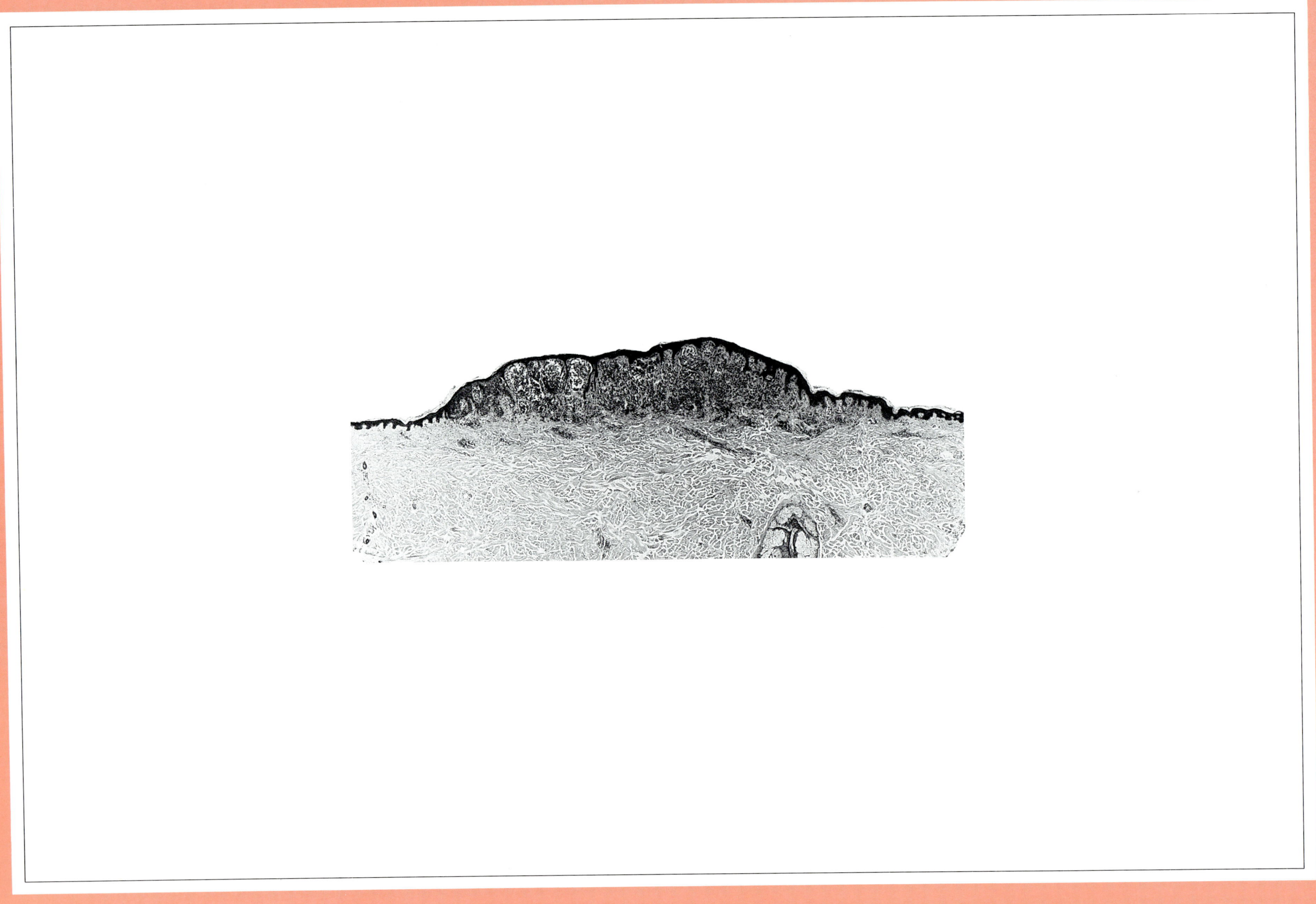

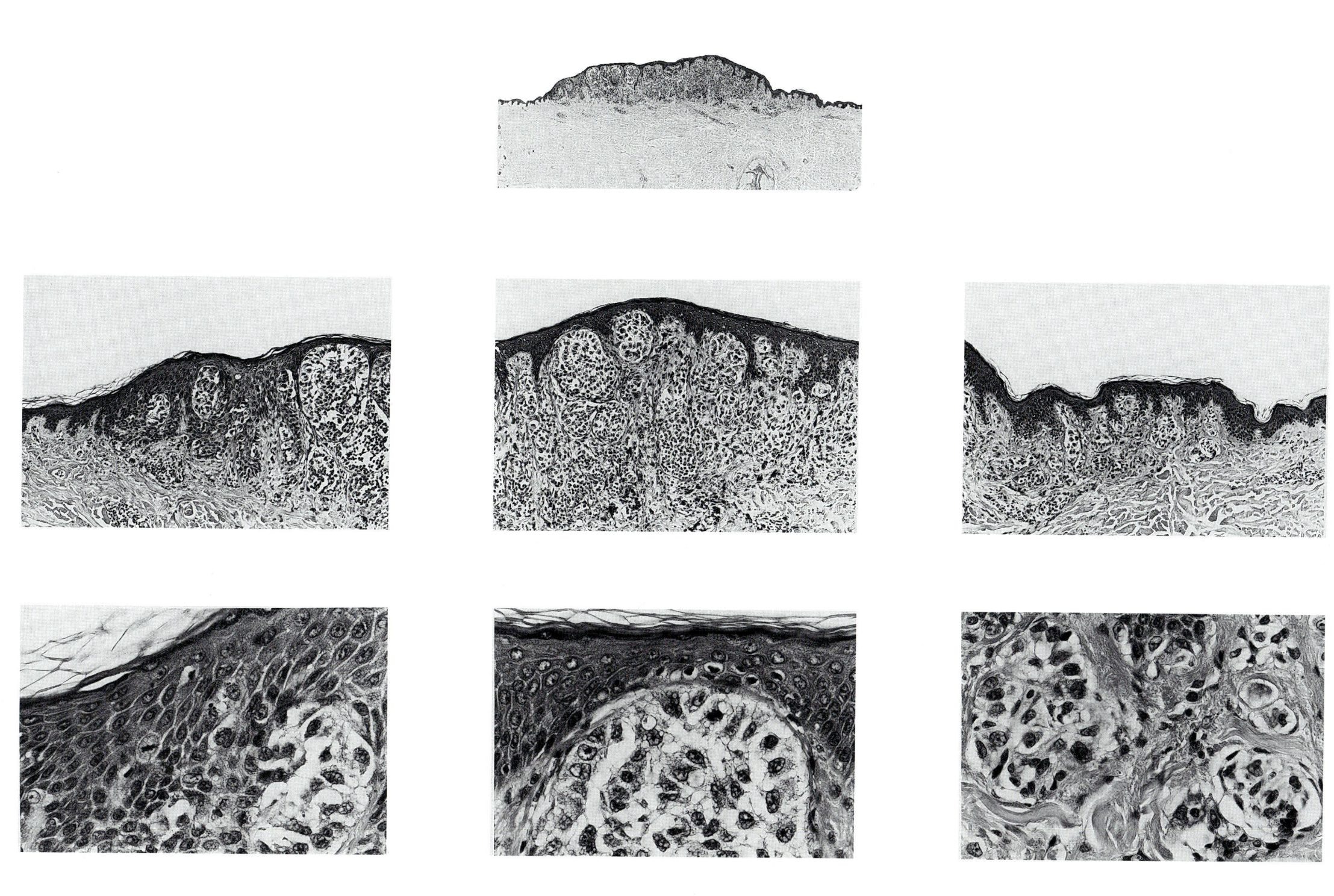

63. What is your diagnosis?

Lesion on the midback of a 61-year-old man. Clinical diagnosis: atypical nevus vs. melanoma. The site was re-excised with borders of 1 cm. Only foreign body reaction and scar were seen in sections from the re-excised specimen. Patient was well after 3 years.

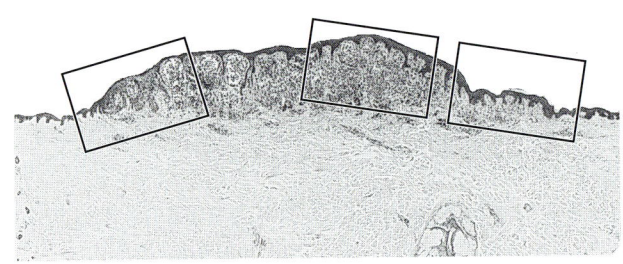

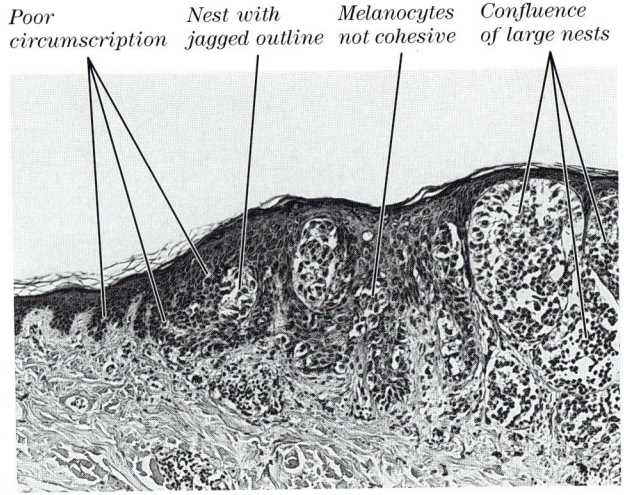

Poor circumscription — *Nest with jagged outline* — *Melanocytes not cohesive* — *Confluence of large nests*

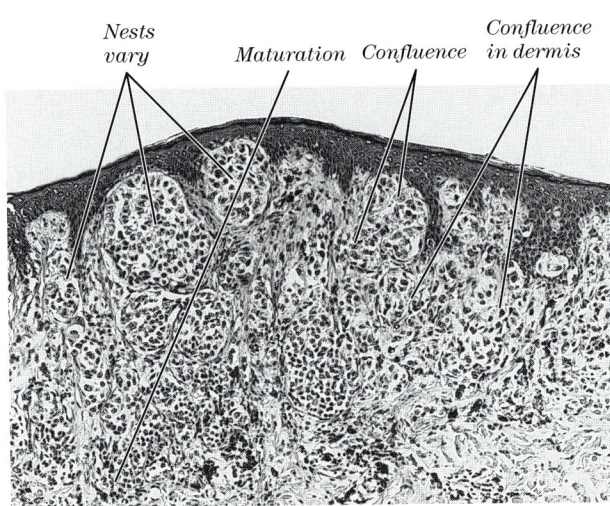

Nests vary — *Maturation* — *Confluence* — *Confluence in dermis*

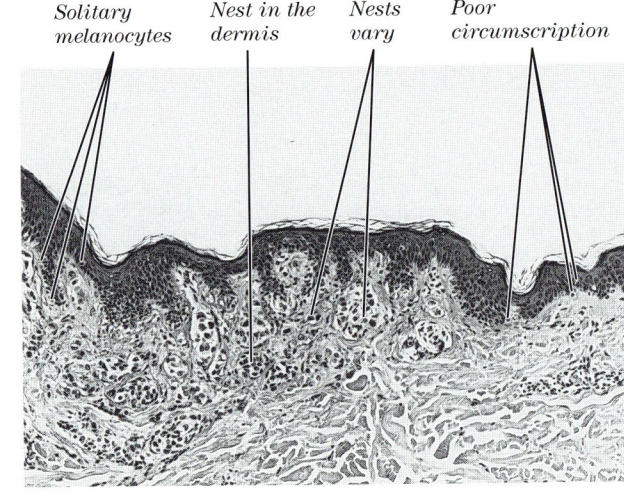

Solitary melanocytes — *Nest in the dermis* — *Nests vary* — *Poor circumscription*

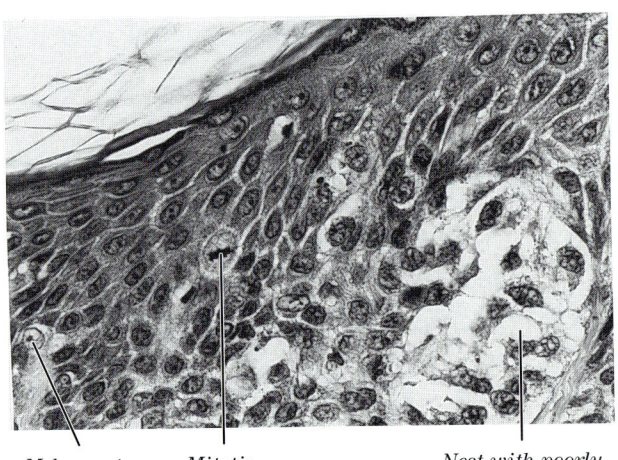

Melanocyte in spinous zone — *Mitotic figure in keratinocyte* — *Nest with poorly circumscribed borders*

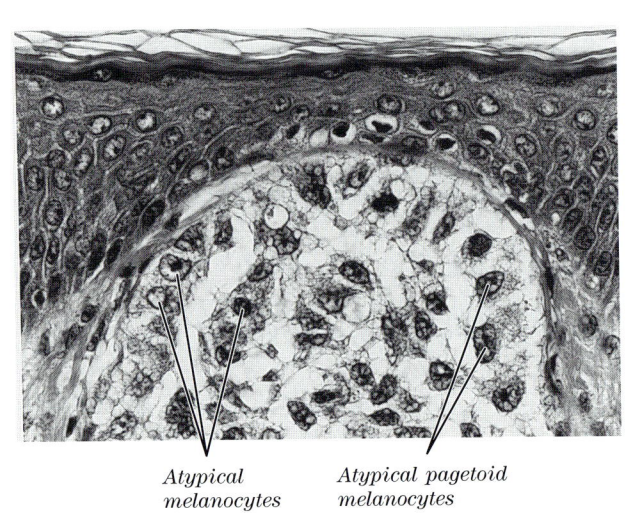

Atypical melanocytes — *Atypical pagetoid melanocytes*

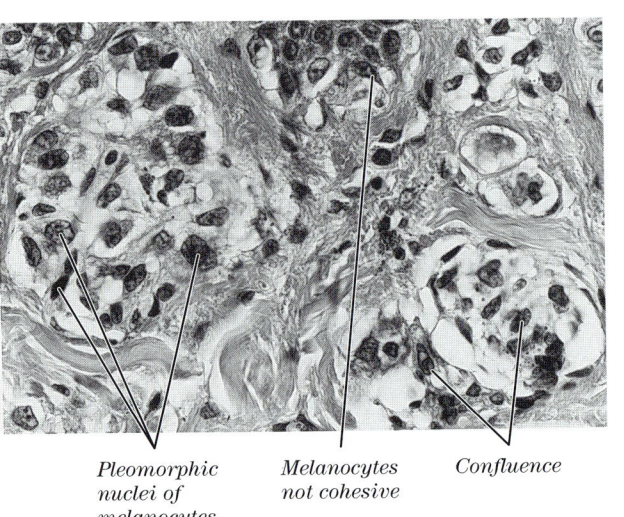

Pleomorphic nuclei of melanocytes — *Melanocytes not cohesive* — *Confluence*

63 • Melanoma

Criteria for diagnosis of this melanoma

This is a melanoma because:

1. The neoplasm is asymmetric.
2. It is poorly circumscribed on one side.
3. Nests of melanocytes within the epidermis and the dermis vary in size and shape.
4. Nests of melanocytes within the epidermis are not equidistant from one another.
5. Many nests of melanocytes within the epidermis and the dermis have become confluent.
6. Some melanocytes disposed as solitary units and others in nests are scattered far above the dermo-epidermal junction in some foci.
7. Pagetoid melanocytes in pagetoid pattern are present in some high-power fields.
8. Nuclei of melanocytes are atypical.

Pitfall in diagnosis

This small melanoma could be mistaken for a Spitz's nevus because:

1. The neoplasm is small.
2. It is well-circumscribed on one side.
3. Melanocytes within the epidermis are arranged mostly in nests rather than as solitary units.
4. Most of the nests of melanocytes are situated at the dermo-epidermal junction, not above it.
5. Melanocytes mature with progressive descent into the dermis.

Despite several features in common, this neoplasm is a melanoma and not a Spitz's nevus because it is poorly circumscribed on one side, nests of melanocytes within the epidermis vary in size and shape, nests have become confluent, nests are not equidistant from one another, and many of the melanocytes, if not most of them, are pagetoid, that is, they have large roundish nuclei and abundant pale cytoplasm. Pagetoid melanocytes are seen commonly in melanomas but hardly ever in Spitz's nevi.

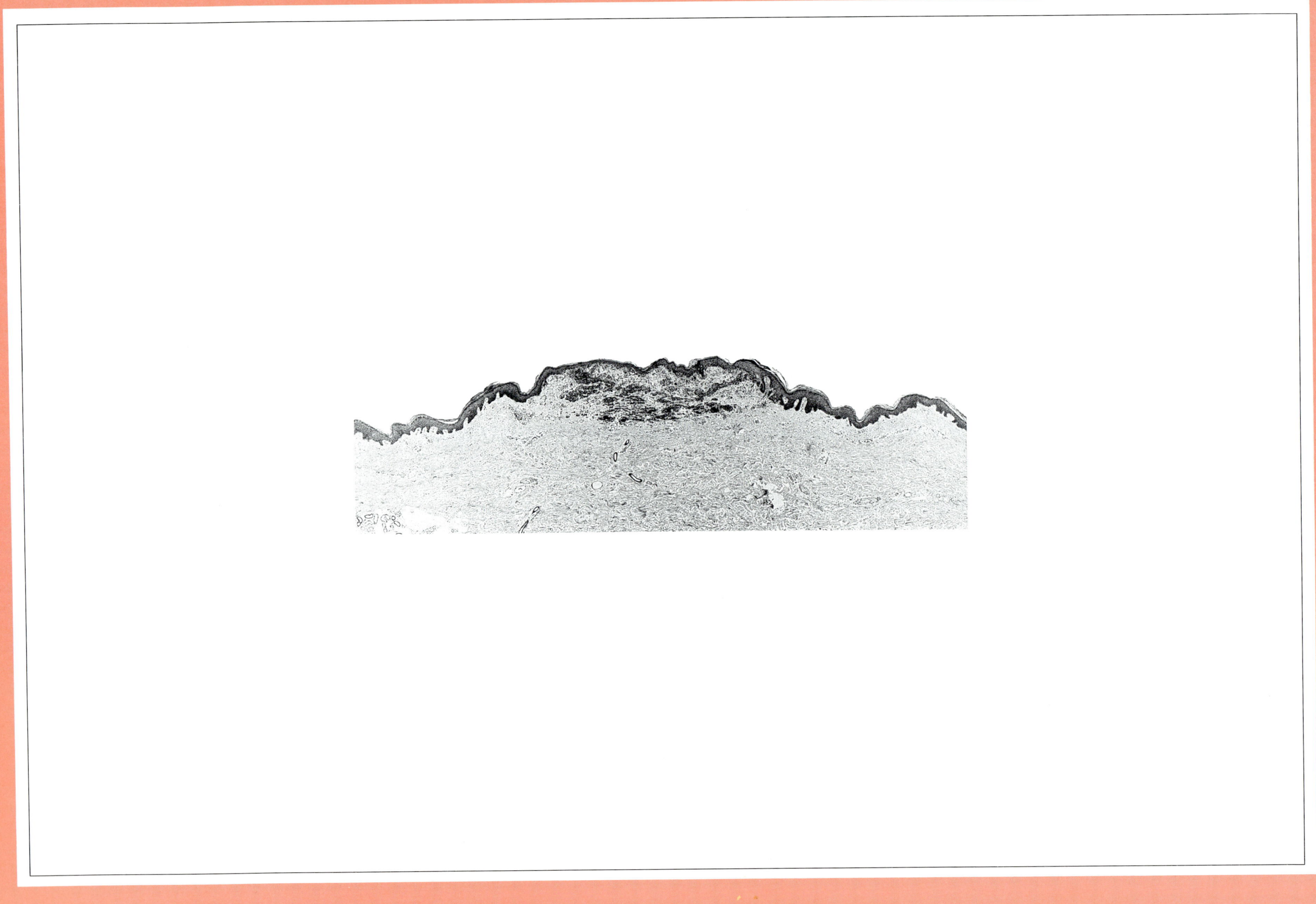

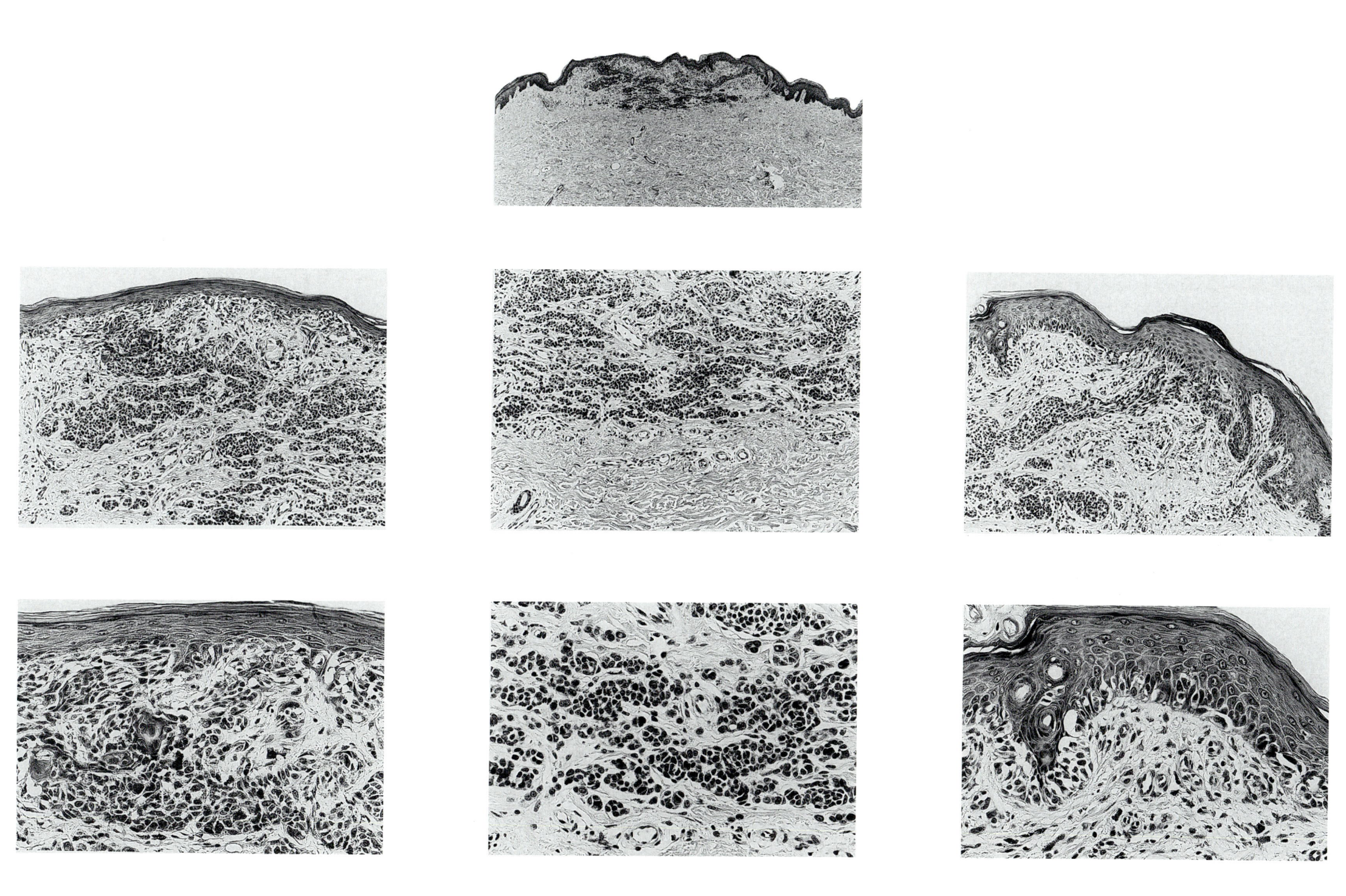

64. What is your diagnosis?

Pigmented lesion on the lower part of the left leg of a 46-year-old man. Clinical diagnosis: nevus. The site was excised completely and the patient was free of disease after 4 years.

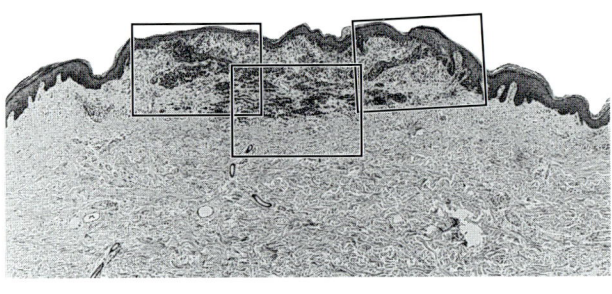

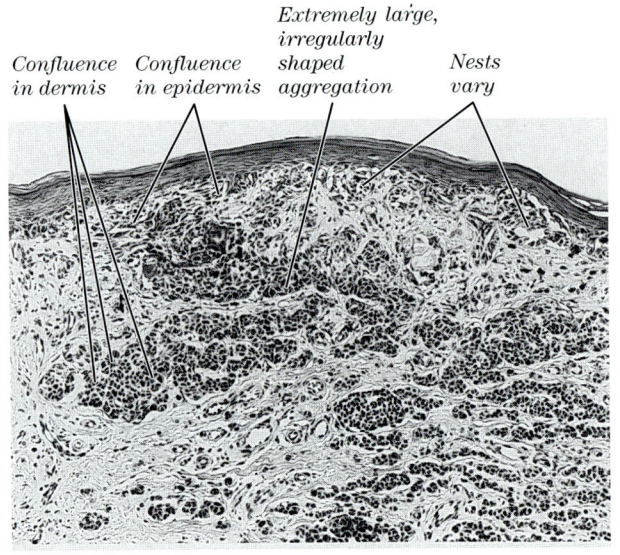

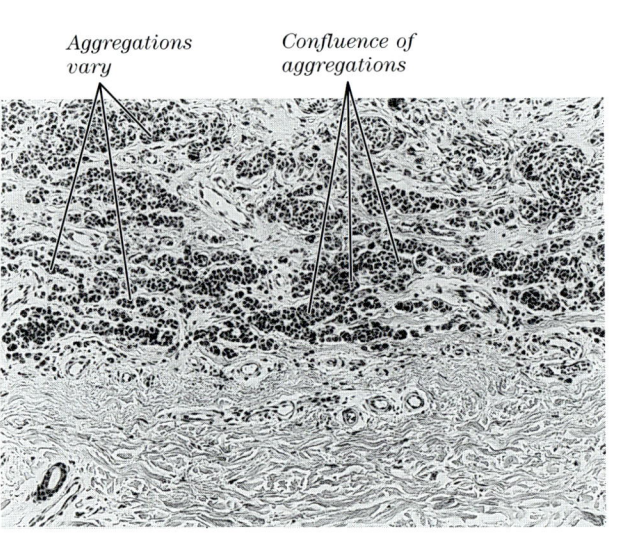

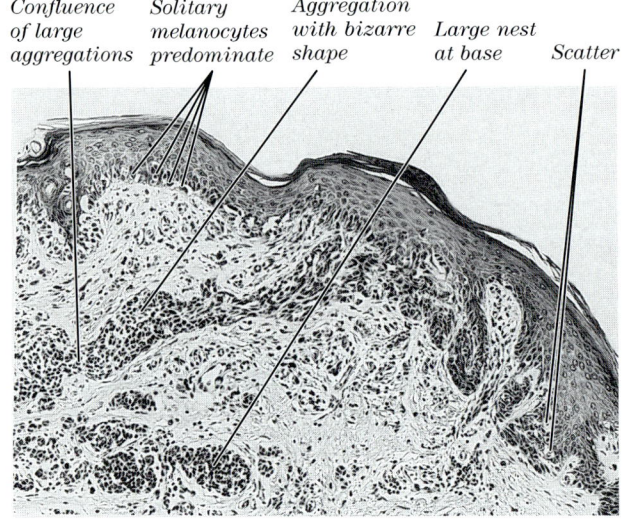

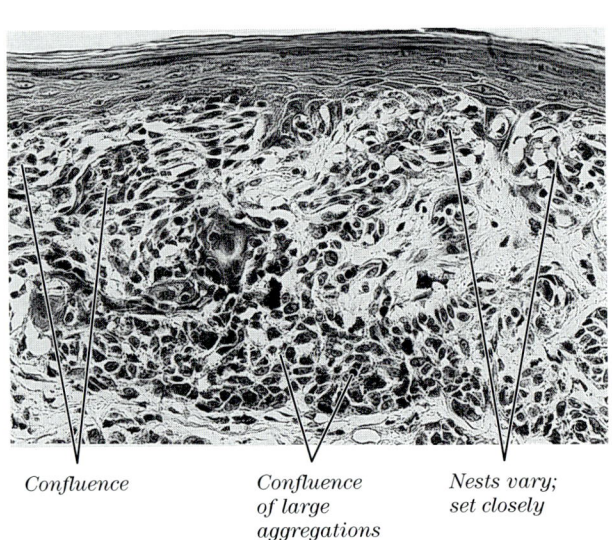

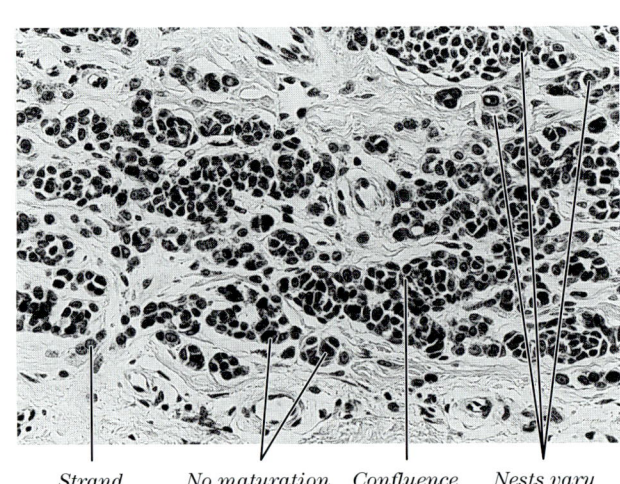

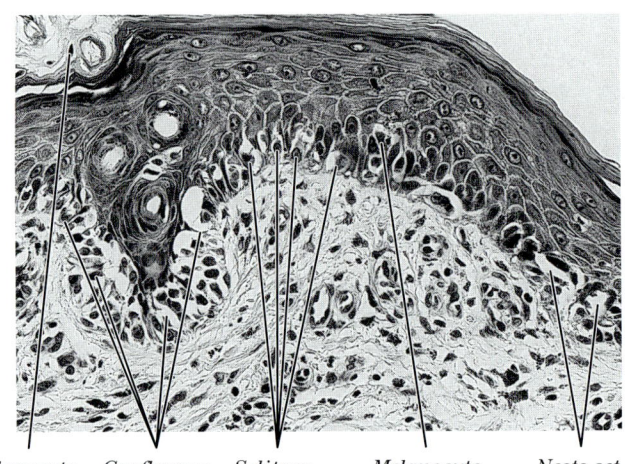

64 • Melanoma

Criteria for diagnosis of this melanoma

This is a melanoma because:

1. Some neoplastic melanocytes are positioned for above the dermo-epidermal junction, including within the cornified layer.

2. Melanocytes disposed as solitary units are more numerous than nests of them within the epidermis in some high-power fields.

3. Nests of melanocytes within the epidermis are not equidistant from one another.

4. Neoplastic melanocytes are present not only in a thickened papillary dermis, but well within the reticular dermis.

5. Some extremely elongated fascicles of melanocytes are situated within the dermis.

6. There is marked variation in size and shape of aggregations of melanocytes within the dermis.

7. Some aggregations of melanocytes within the dermis have bizarre shapes, i.e., jagged outlines.

Pitfall in diagnosis

This melanoma could be misconstrued as a compound Clark's nevus because:

1. It is relatively symmetric.

2. It is rather sharply circumscribed.

3. Melanocytes mature slightly.

4. Most melanocytes within the epidermis are organized into nests that are seated mostly at the dermo-epidermal junction.

5. Very few mitotic figures can be detected.

At scanning magnification, this neoplasm could be misjudged a superficial congenital nevus. It is not a superficial congenital nevus because of the absence of splaying of melanocytes, angiocentricity of melanocytes, and adnexocentricity of melanocytes in the reticular dermis. Of the many features that permit differentiation of melanoma from Clark's nevus, none is more important than scatter of melanocytes in the upper reaches of the epidermis as is witnessed so often in melanoma. That finding marks this neoplasm as a melanoma and not a Clark's nevus in which melanocytes are practically never spotted in the upper part of the epidermis.

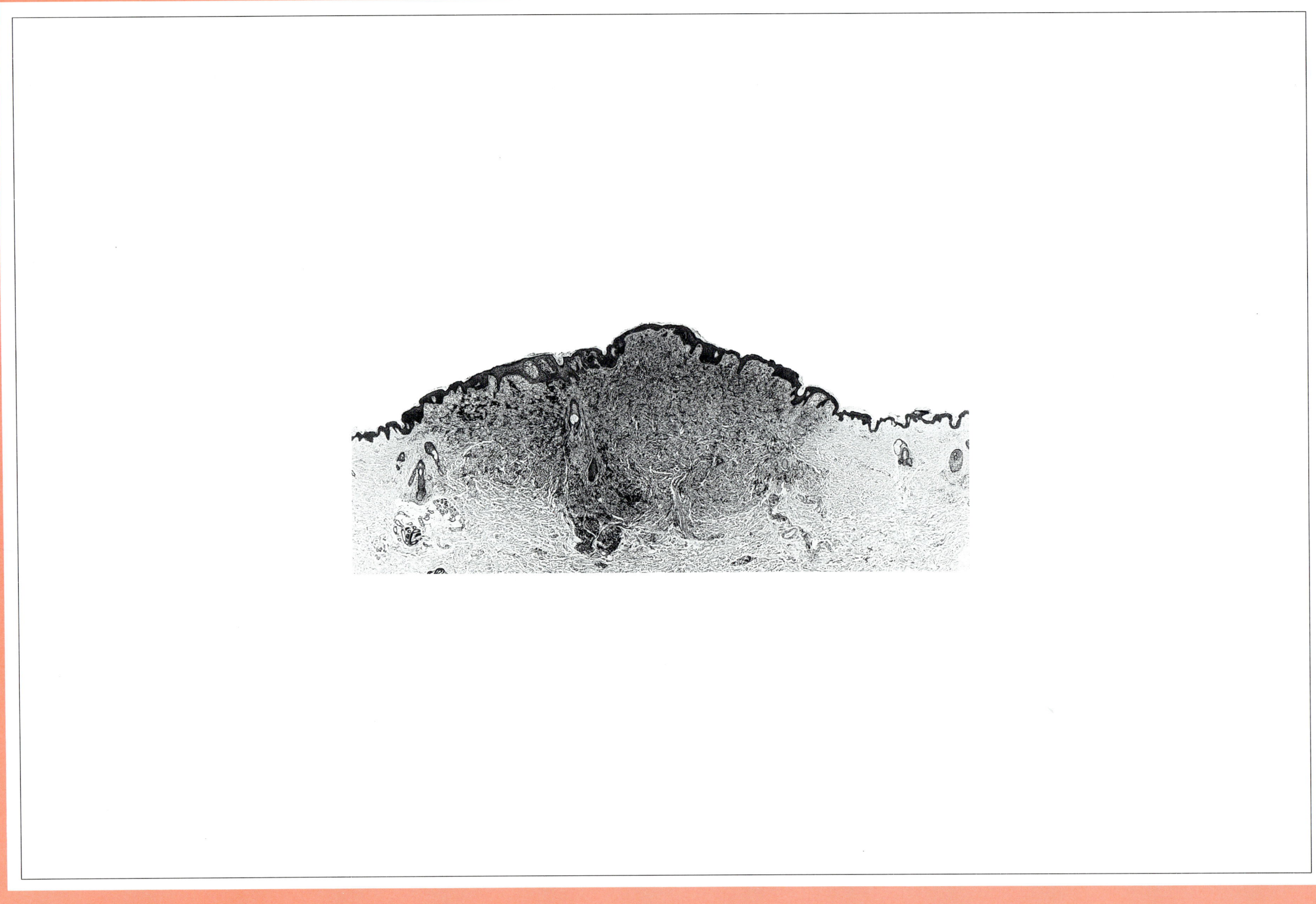

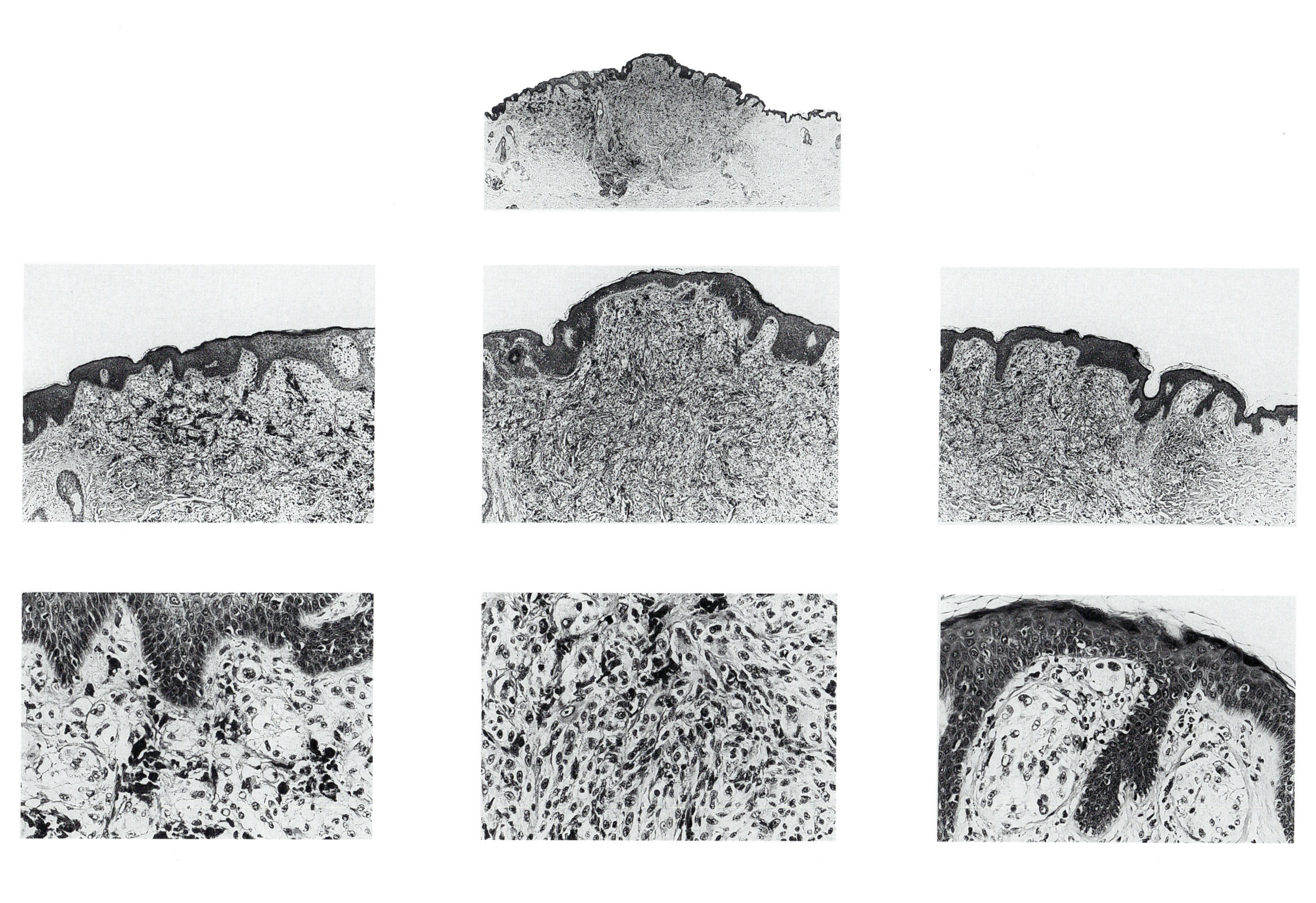

65. What is your diagnosis?

Black papule, 8 to 10 mm in diameter, on the left breast of a 35-year-old woman that in the previous months had changed from a brown macule. Clinical diagnosis: melanoma. A wide and deep excision was performed. No residual melanocytic neoplasm was detected in the re-excised specimen. No additional follow-up was available.

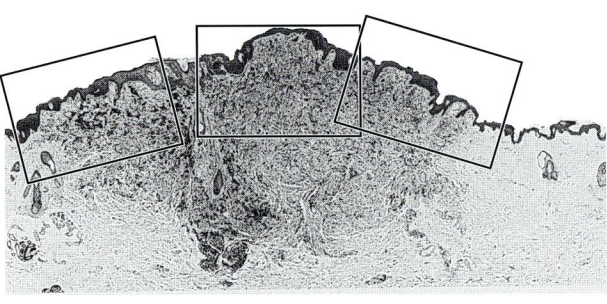

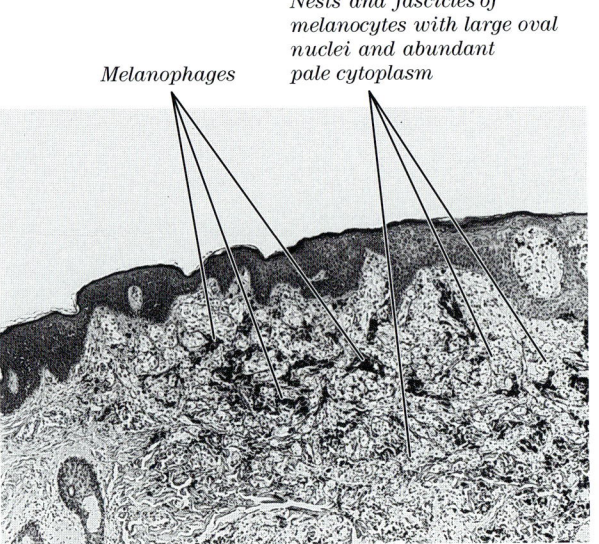

Melanophages

Nests and fascicles of melanocytes with large oval nuclei and abundant pale cytoplasm

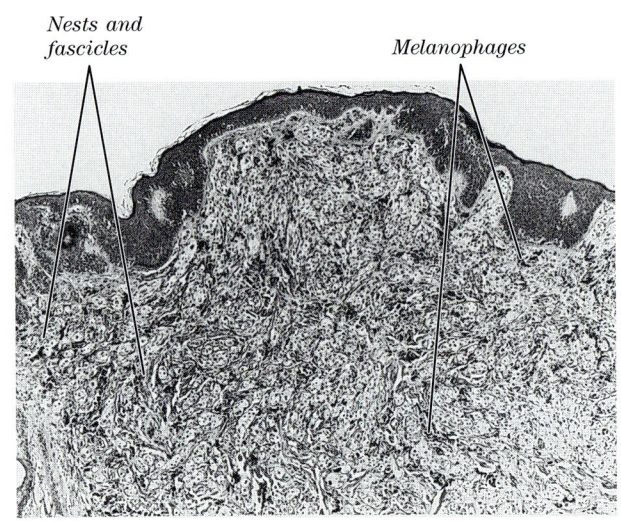

Nests and fascicles   *Melanophages*

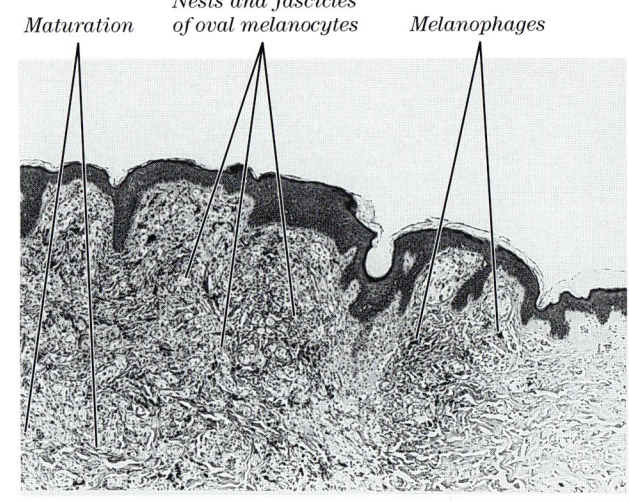

Maturation   *Nests and fascicles of oval melanocytes*   *Melanophages*

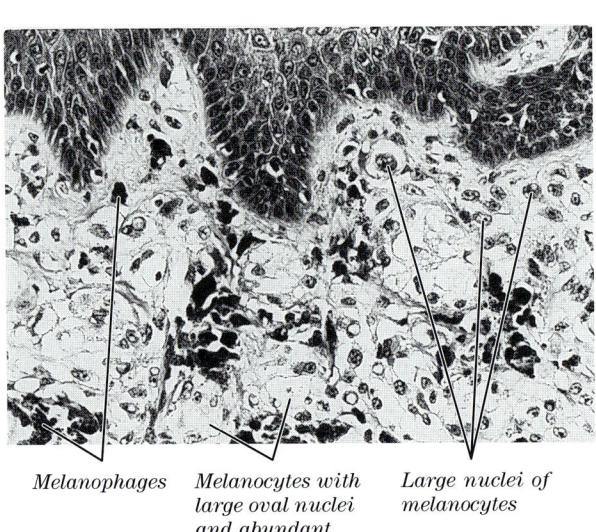

Melanophages   *Melanocytes with large oval nuclei and abundant pale cytoplasm*   *Large nuclei of melanocytes*

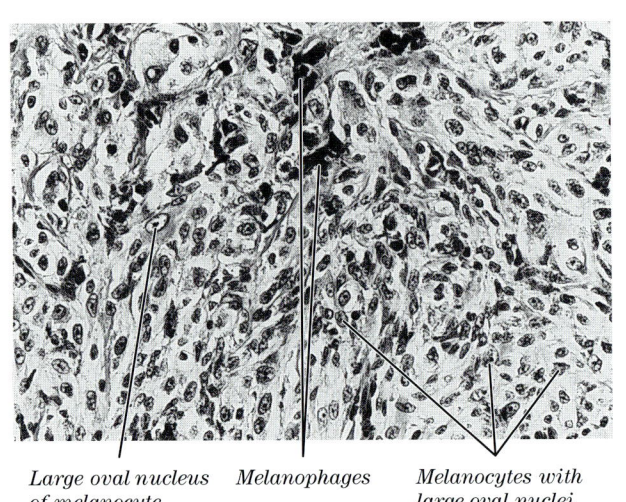

Large oval nucleus of melanocyte   *Melanophages*   *Melanocytes with large oval nuclei in fascicles that interweave*

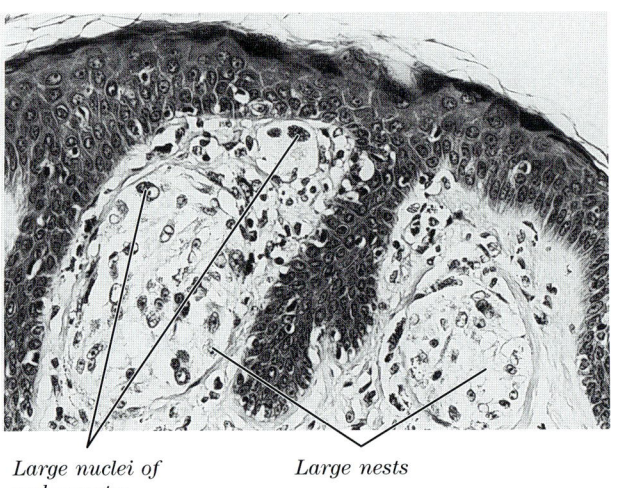

Large nuclei of melanocytes   *Large nests*

65 • "Deep Penetrating" Nevus

Criteria for diagnosis of this "deep penetrating" nevus

This neoplasm is benign because:

1. It has a rather wedge shape.

2. Melanocytes mature.

3. No mitotic figures are detected.

This is a "deep penetrating" nevus because:

1. The neoplasm is somewhat wedge-shaped.

2. Most of the melanocytes that constitute it have either large oval nuclei and abundant cytoplasm that houses "dusty" melanin, or large round nuclei and scant cytoplasm.

3. Many nuclei are pleomorphic.

Pitfall in diagnosis

This "deep penetrating" nevus could be misinterpreted as a primary cutaneous melanoma because:

1. The neoplasm is asymmetric.

2. Melanin is not distributed in uniform fashion, being much more prominent on the left side than on the right side of it.

3. Some neoplastic cells have atypical nuclei, i.e., they are large and pleomorphic with prominent nucleoli.

4. Some of the melanocytes disposed as solitary units within the epidermis are present above the dermo-epidermal junction.

This benign neoplasm fulfills criteria for "deep penetrating" nevus. The majority of the melanocytes have oval nuclei and abundant pale cytoplasm that contains dust-like particles of melanin. Some have distinct, markedly pigmented dendrites. Many have large pleomorphic nuclei. There is no sign of melanoma in situ. In short, this is a nevus and not a melanoma. Parenthetically, as can be intuited, not all "deep penetrating" nevi are deep. Most of them, however, have architectural features of a blue nevus (wedge-shaped, bulbous bases, periadnexal distribution), nuclear ones of a Spitz's nevus (pleomorphism), and cytoplasmic ones of a blue nevus (subtle but heavily pigmented, bipolar, dendritic melanocytes).

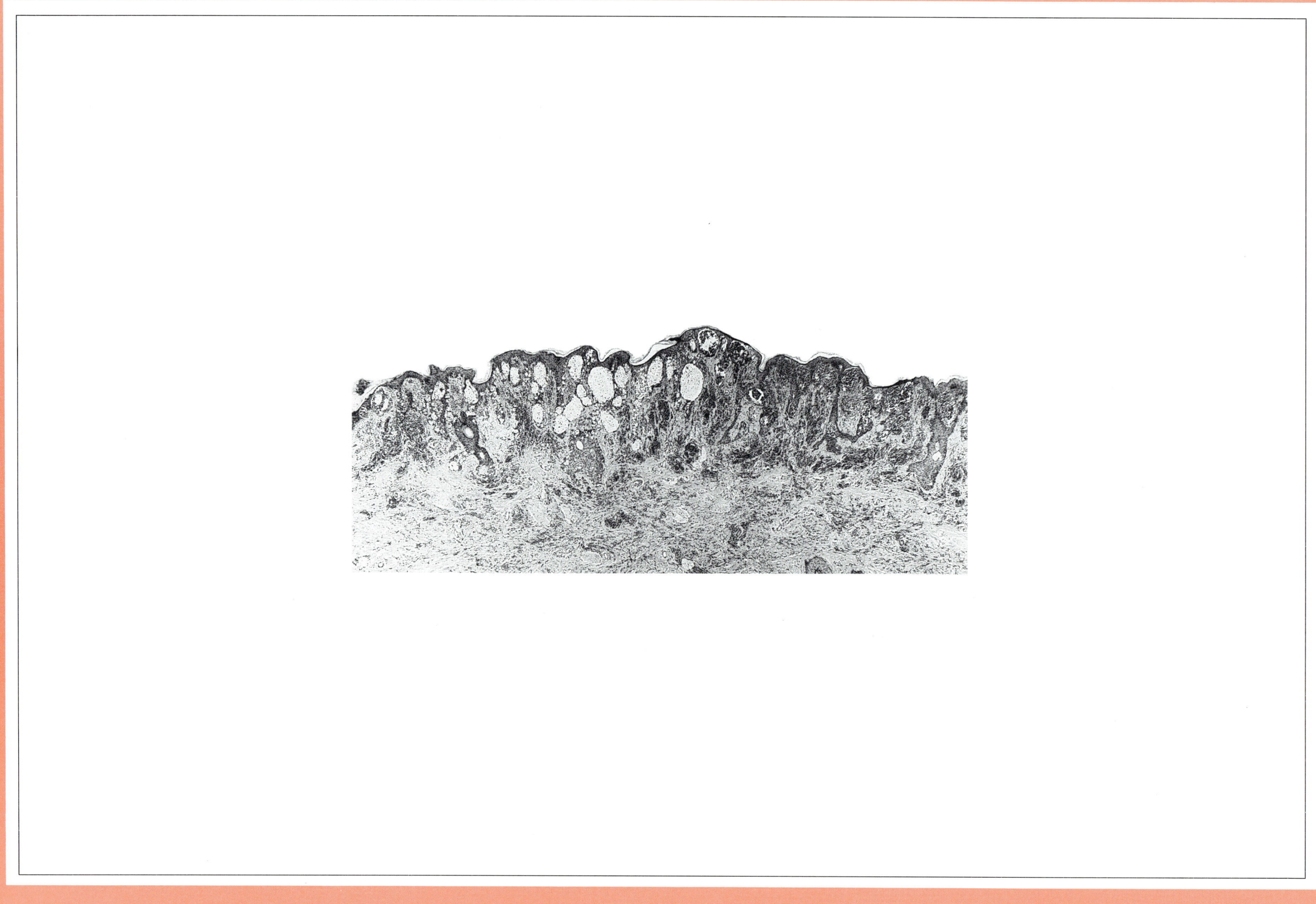

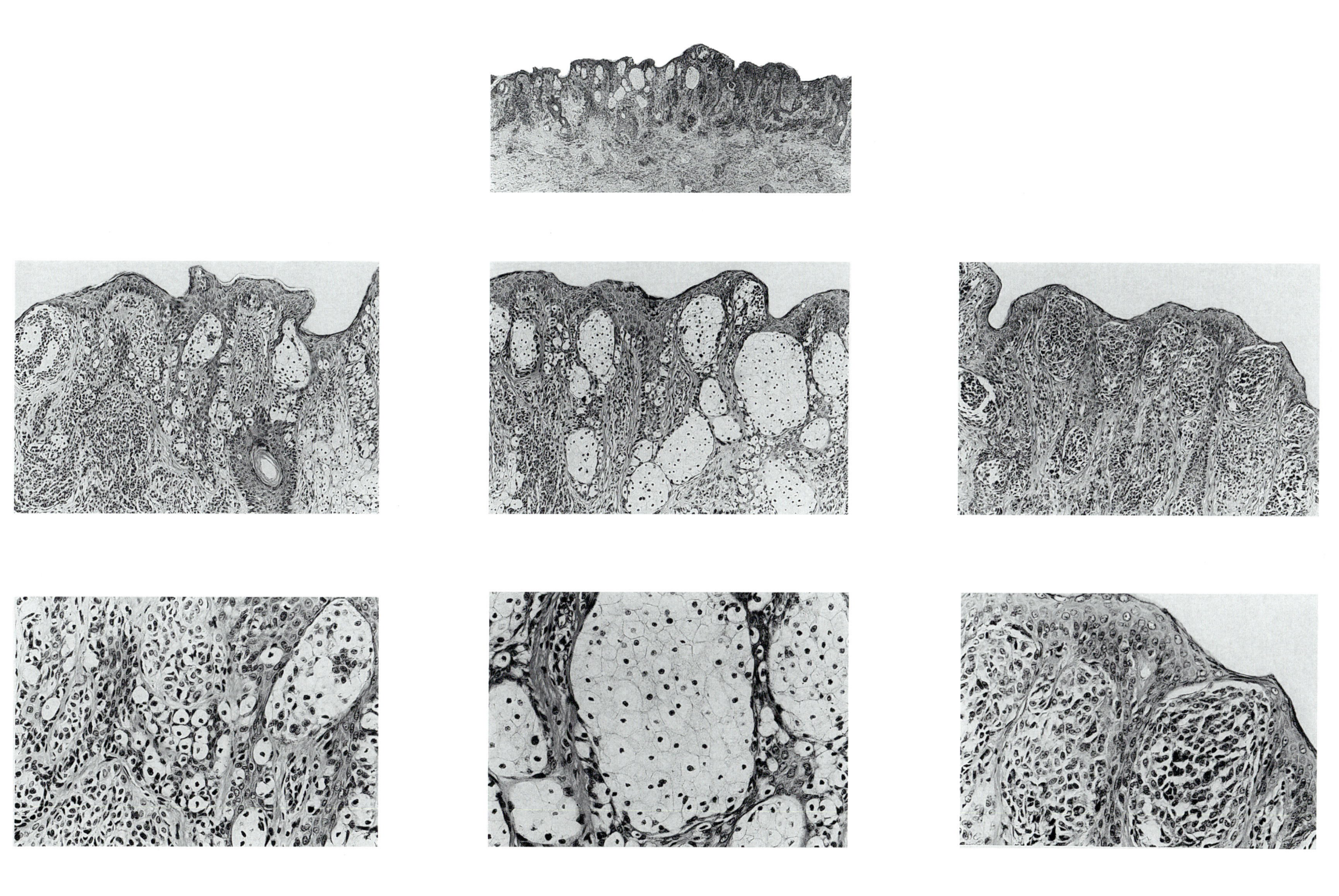

66. What is your diagnosis?

Lesion that recently changed color on the thigh of a 5-year-old boy. Clinical diagnosis: congenital nevus. No follow-up data were available.

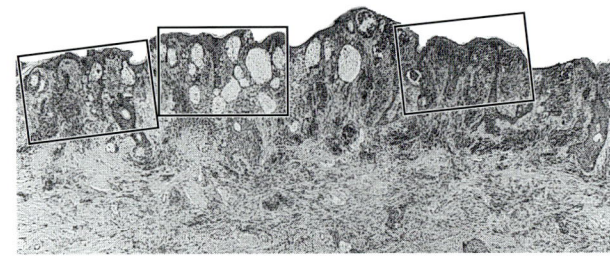

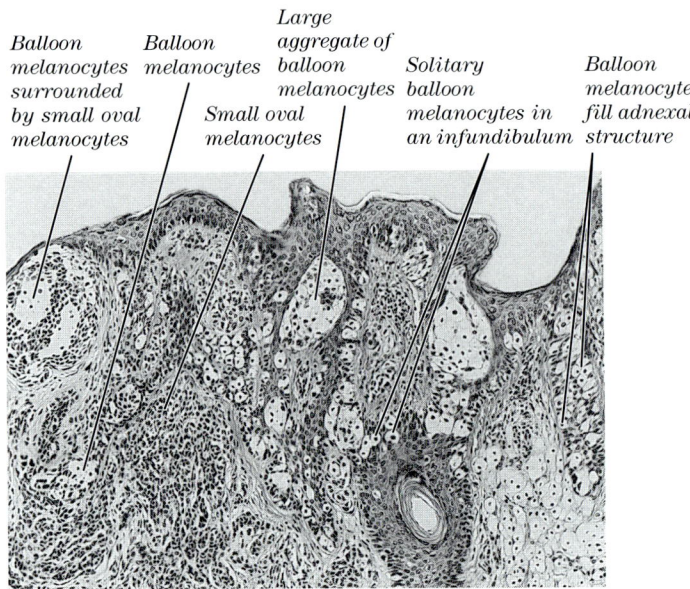

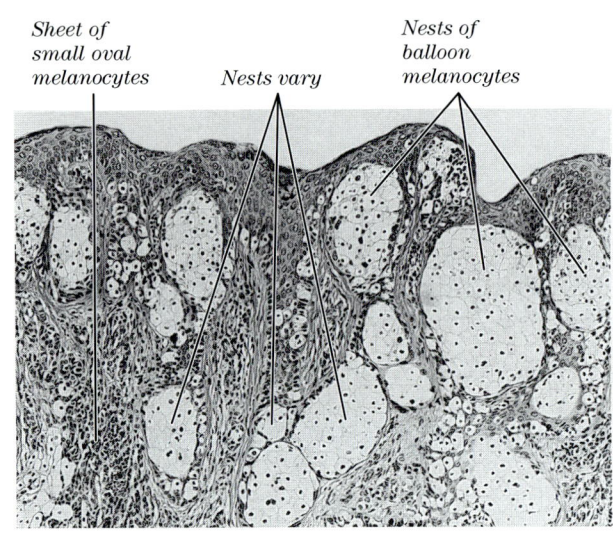

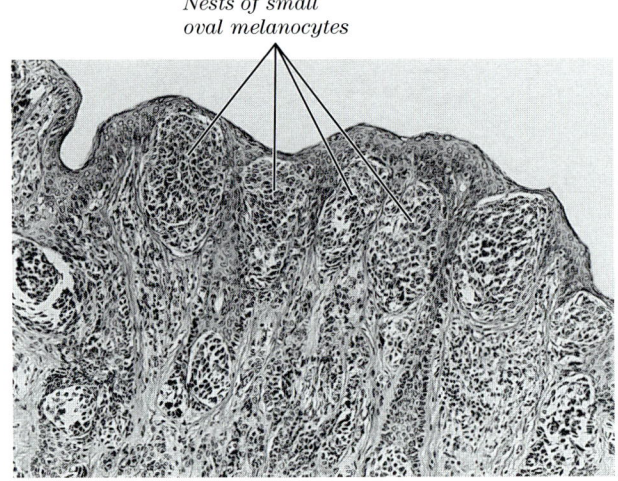

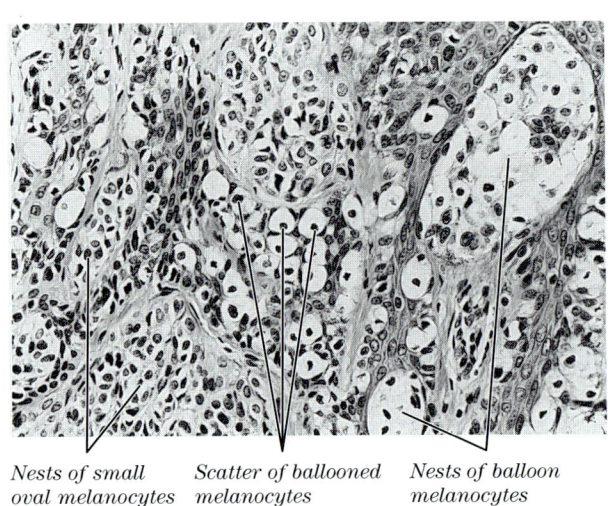

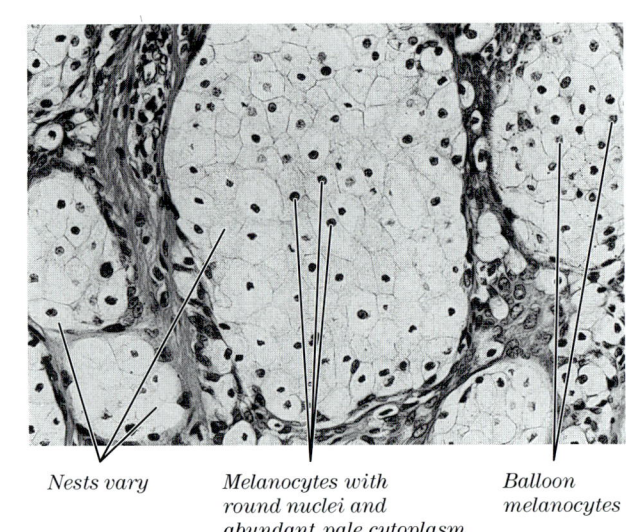

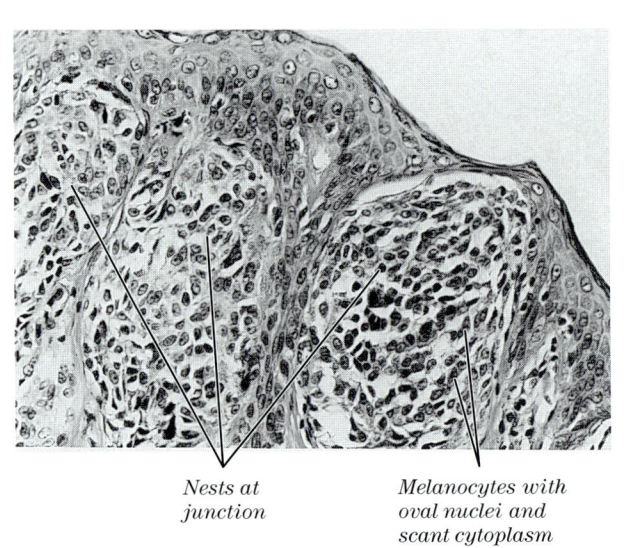

66 • Congenital Nevus *(superficial type with balloon cells)*

Criteria for diagnosis of this congenital nevus (superficial type with many balloon cells)

This is a nevus because:

1. Melanocytes within the epidermis, disposed both as solitary units and in nests, are situated mostly at the dermo-epidermal junction.
2. Melanocytes mature.
3. Nests of melanocytes within the epidermis predominate over melanocytes arranged as solitary units there.
4. Nuclei of melanocytes are small, round, and monomorphous.

This is a congenital nevus because:

1. Melanocytes are splayed in foci between collagen bundles in the reticular dermis.
2. Some melanocytes in the reticular dermis are arrayed in angiocentric and adnexocentric fashion.

Pitfall in diagnosis

This congenital nevus with numerous balloon cells could be misinterpreted as a melanoma with balloon cells because:

1. The neoplasm is asymmetric.
2. Nests of balloon melanocytes are distributed in uneven fashion throughout the neoplasm.
3. Nests of balloon melanocytes are not equidistant from one another.
4. Nests of balloon melanocytes vary in size and shape.
5. Some nests of balloon melanocytes have become confluent.
6. Balloon melanocytes disposed as solitary units predominate over nests of balloon cells within the epidermis and epithelial structures of adnexa.
7. A few balloon melanocytes are present above the dermo-epidermal junction, some of them in the spinous and granular zones.

Balloon-cell nevus always is a "combined" nevus, i.e., a combination of balloon melanocytes and at least one other cytologic type of melanocyte, e.g., small round or oval with scant cytoplasm. For that reason, it is nearly inevitable that the neoplasm will be asymmetric. Differentiation of balloon-cell nevus from balloon-cell melanoma is accomplished by application of the usual criteria for distinguishing a benign from a malignant neoplasm of melanocytes. This neoplasm fulfills all the criteria for a combined nevus, including asymmetry. Asymmetry in this setting is the "exception that proves the rule."

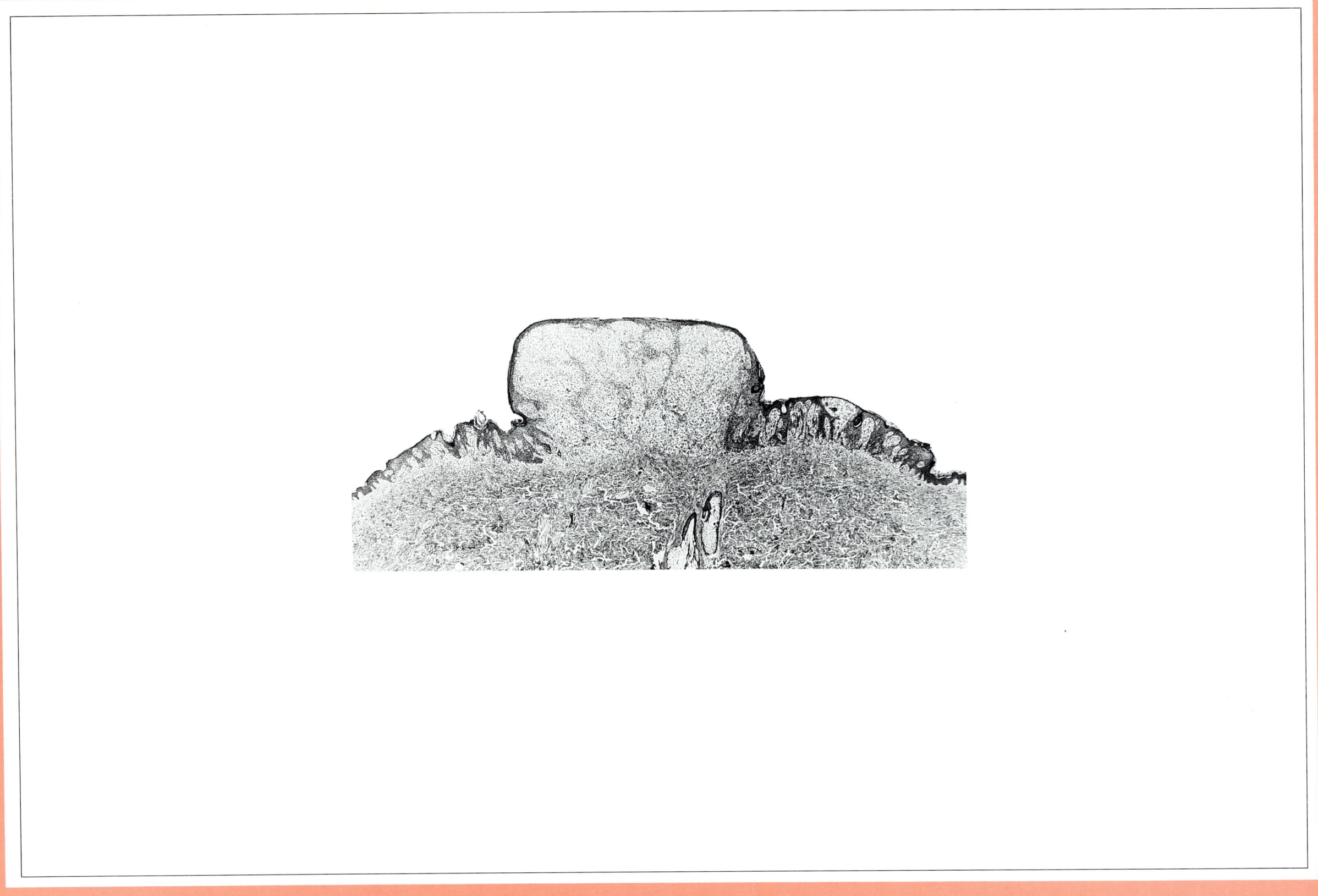

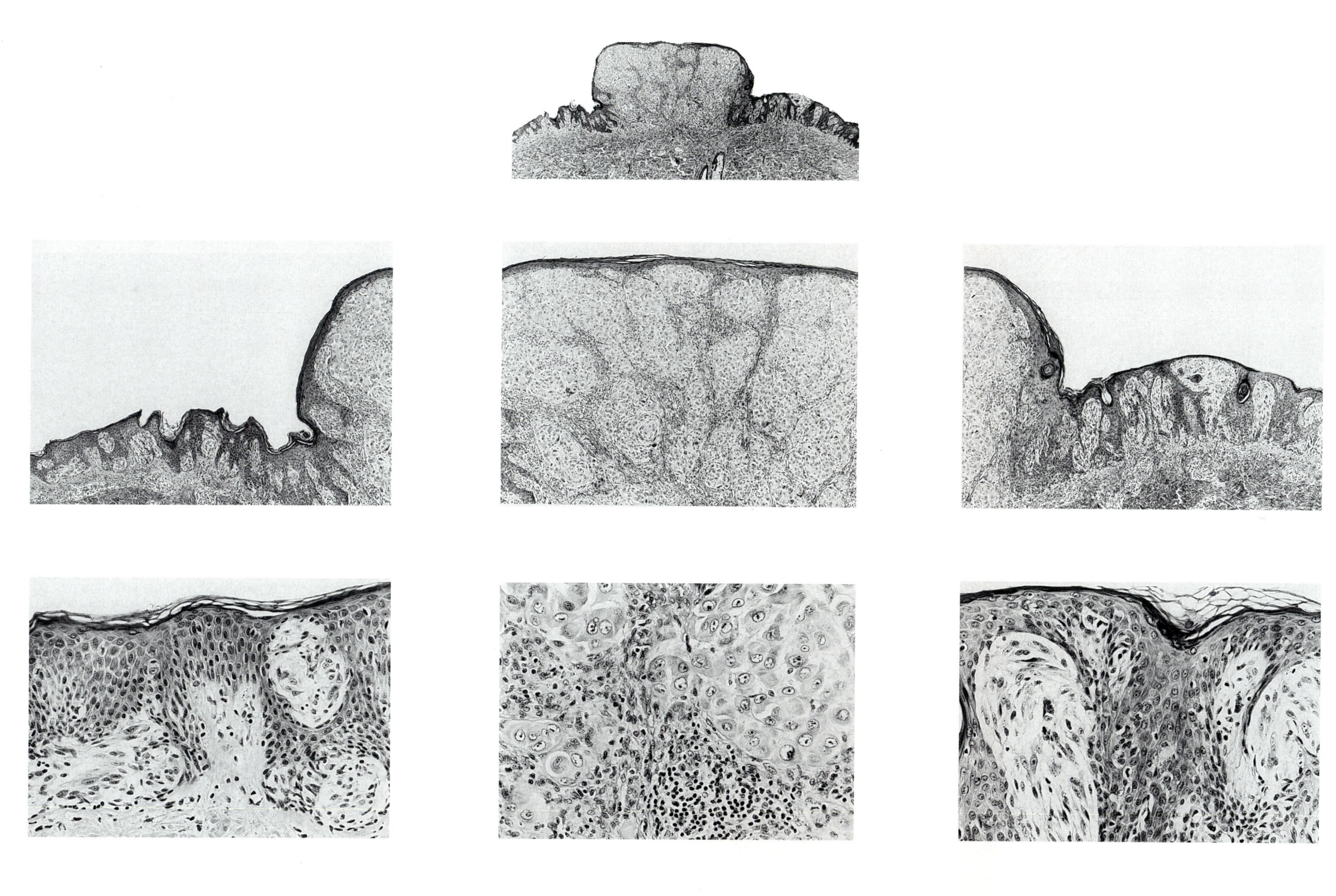

67. What is your diagnosis?

Pigmented lesion on the back of a 22-year-old woman. There were signs of inflammation. Clinical diagnosis: nevus. Patient was free of disease after 2 years.

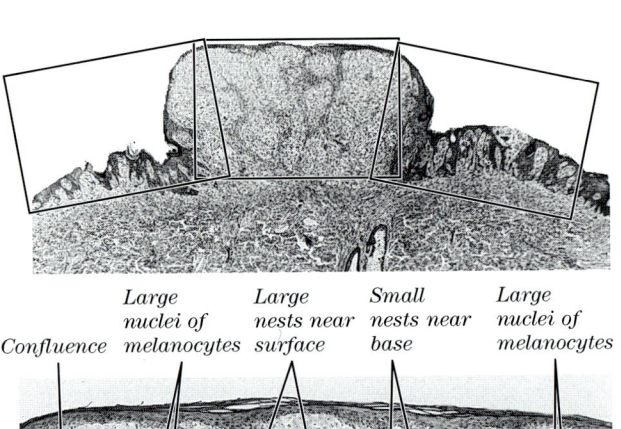
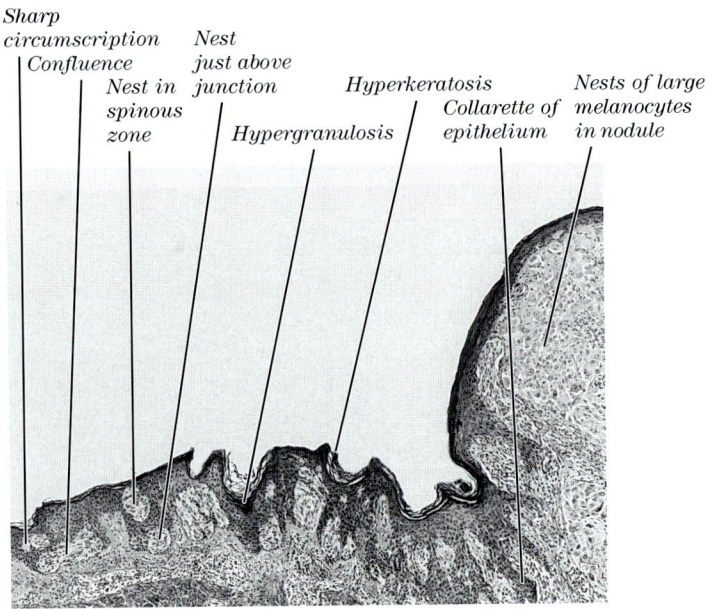
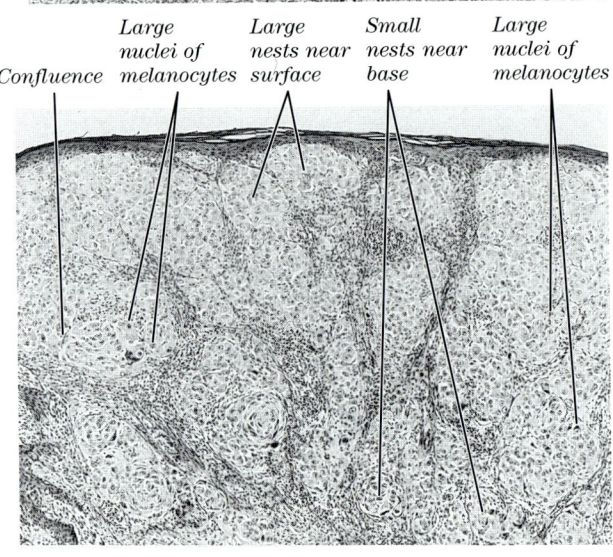
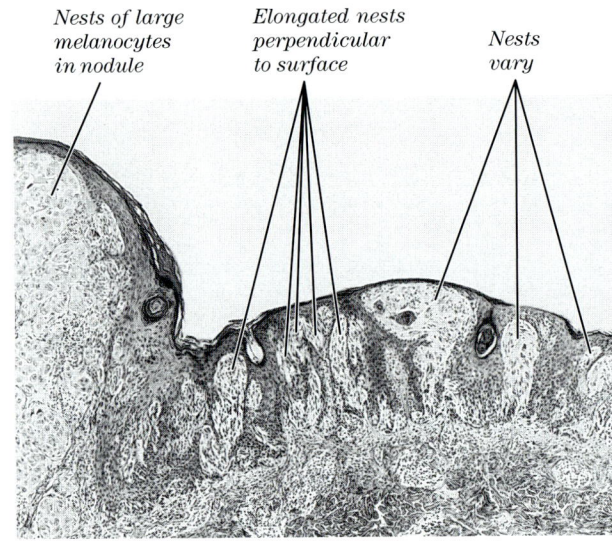
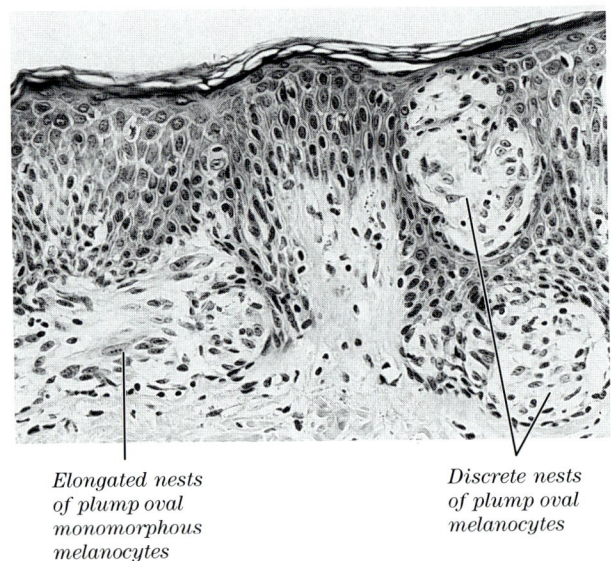
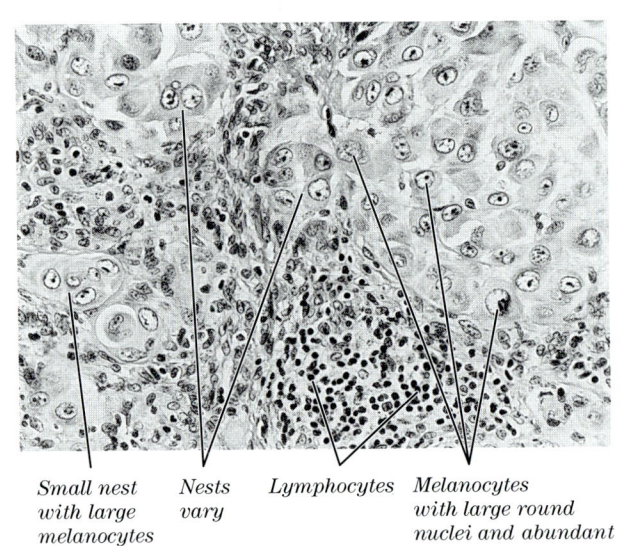
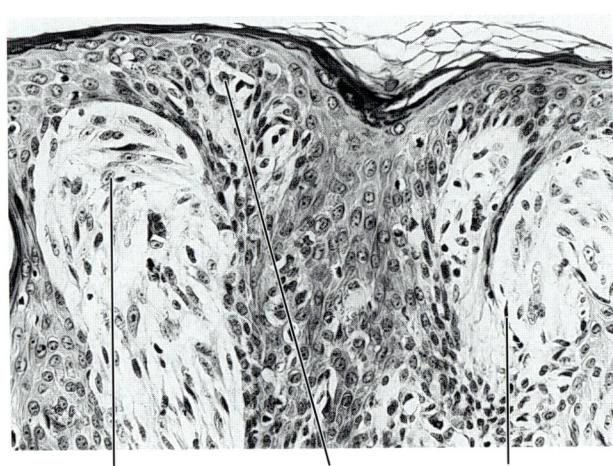

67 • Spitz's Nevus *(combined type)*

Criteria for diagnosis of this Spitz's nevus (combined type)

The neoplasm is benign because:

1. It is relatively symmetric.
2. It is well circumscribed.
3. Melanocytes within the epidermis and the dermis are arranged mostly in nests, rather than as solitary units.
4. Nuclei of melanocytes in particular high-power fields are relatively monomorphous.

This is a Spitz's nevus because:

1. The neoplastic melanocytes have large nuclei, abundant cytoplasm, and mostly round-polygonal and oval-spindle shapes.
2. There are hyperkeratosis, hypergranulosis, and epidermal hyperplasia in some foci.
3. Many nests of melanocytes within the epidermis are elongated.
4. Many nests of melanocytes within the epidermis are perpendicular to the skin surface.
5. A perivascular lymphocytic infiltrate is present throughout the neoplasm.

This is a combined Spitz's nevus because:

There are two different populations of melanocytes: round-polygonal in the dome-shaped center of the neoplasm and oval-spindle at the "shoulders" of it. The former have abundant cytoplasm, the latter much less.

Pitfall in diagnosis

This compound combined Spitz's nevus could be misread as a melanoma in association with a pre-existing nevus because:

1. Melanocytes within the papule have a round-polygonal shape, whereas melanocytes at the "shoulders" have an oval-spindle shape.
2. There is little, if any, maturation of melanocytes with progressive descent into the dermis.
3. It is slightly asymmetric because the "shoulder" on the right is broader than that on the left.

This neoplasm is a Spitz's nevus that exhibits different topographic and cytologic features. The central dome-shaped papule consists of large round-polygonal melanocytes, whereas the slightly elevated "shoulders" consist of oval-spindle melanocytes with much less cytoplasm. These attributes of the cellular components were responsible for the former appellation "spindle and epithelioid cell nevus." That is but one of several predecessors to the term "Spitz's nevus," including melanomas of childhood, juvenile melanomas, and benign juvenile melanomas. In brief, this neoplasm illustrates different architectural patterns and cytologic features in a single Spitz's nevus. The benign character of the neoplasm is determined by its silhouette.

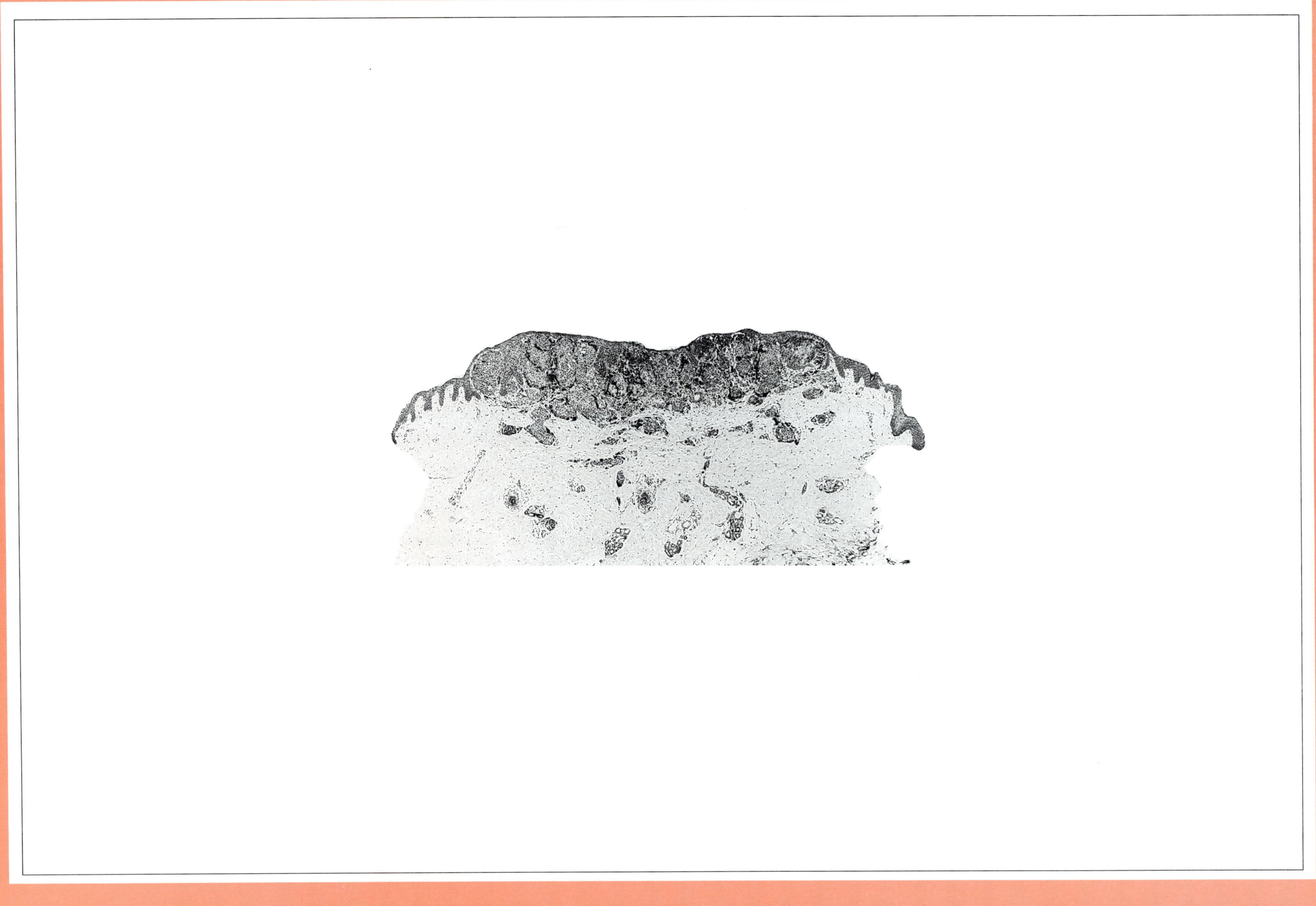

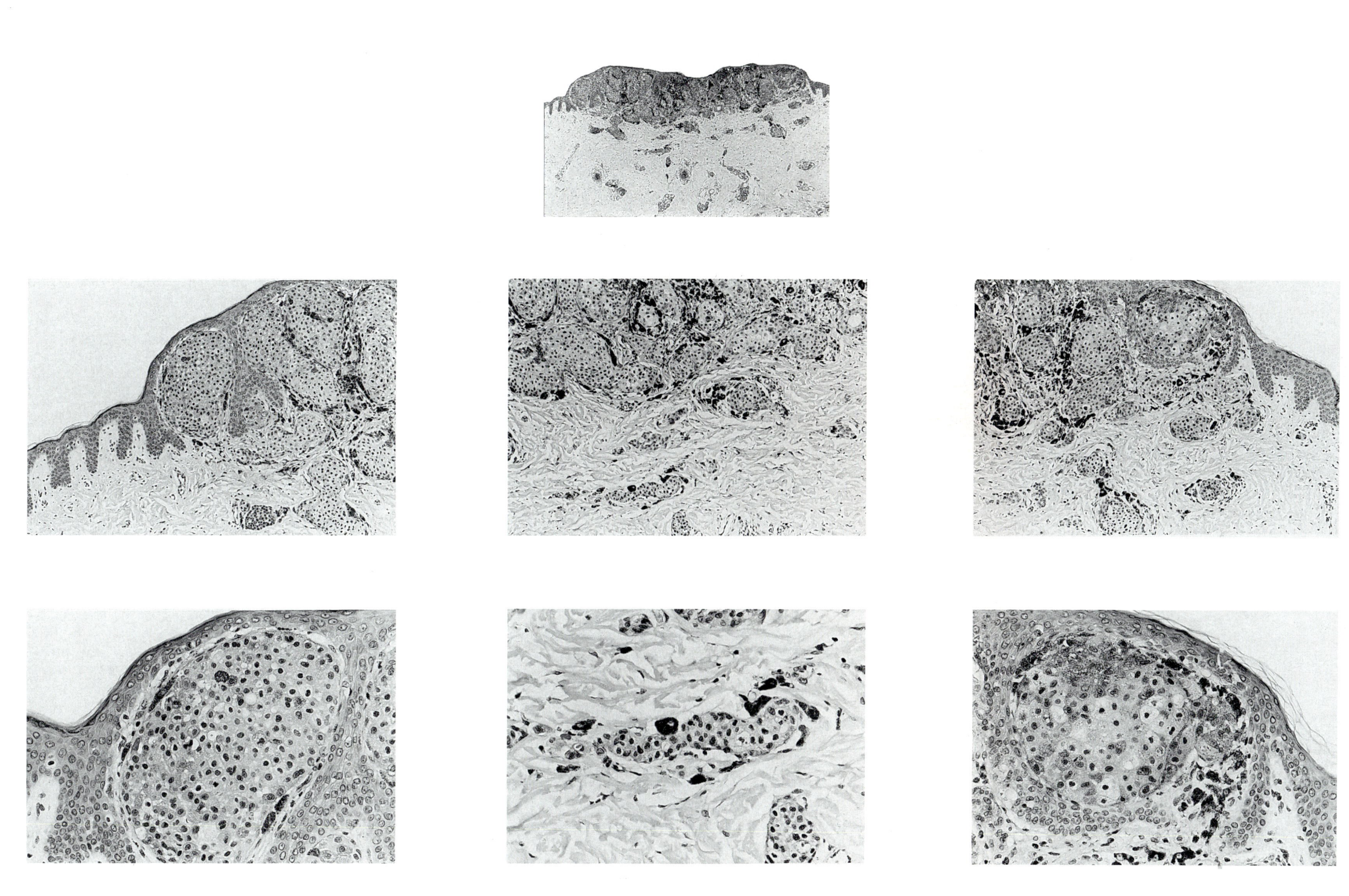

68. What is your diagnosis?

Pigmented lesion on the right side of the chest of an infant boy. Clinical diagnosis: nevus. No follow-up data were available.

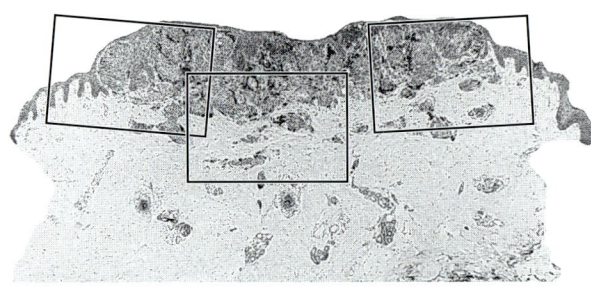

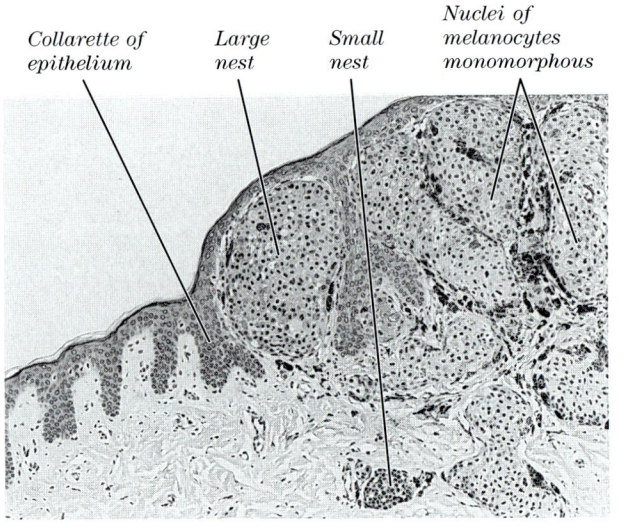

Collarette of epithelium | *Large nest* | *Small nest* | *Nuclei of melanocytes monomorphous*

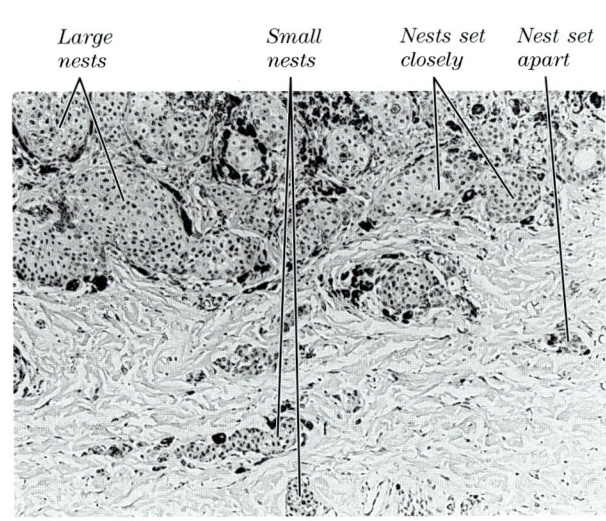

Large nests | *Small nests* | *Nests set closely* | *Nest set apart*

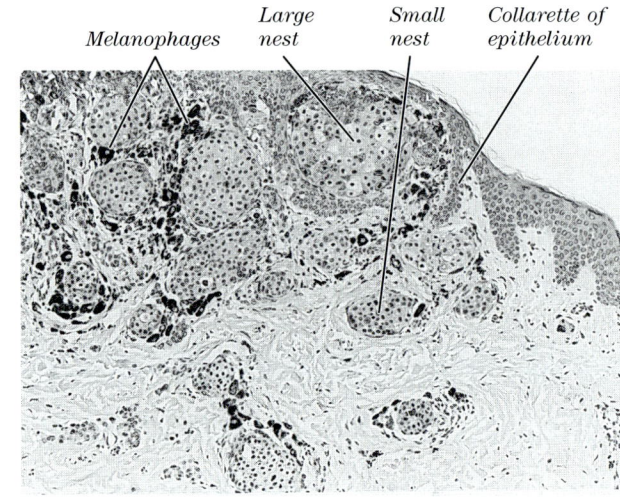

Melanophages | *Large nest* | *Small nest* | *Collarette of epithelium*

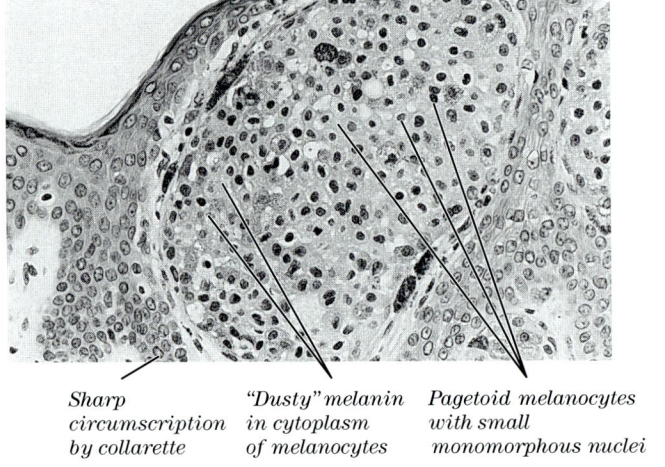

Sharp circumscription by collarette | *"Dusty" melanin in cytoplasm of melanocytes* | *Pagetoid melanocytes with small monomorphous nuclei*

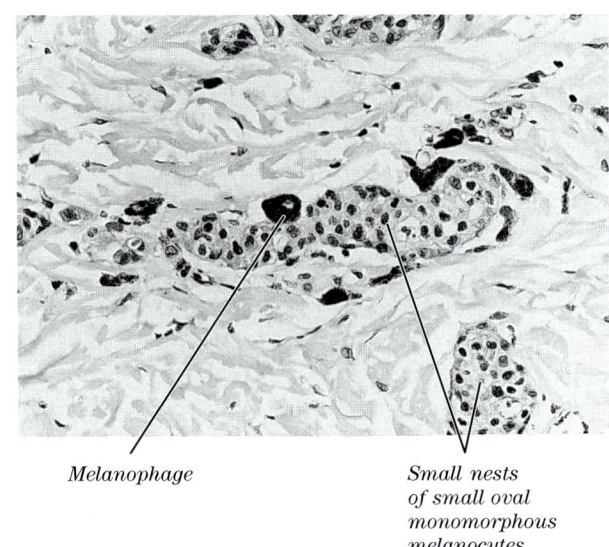

Melanophage | *Small nests of small oval monomorphous melanocytes*

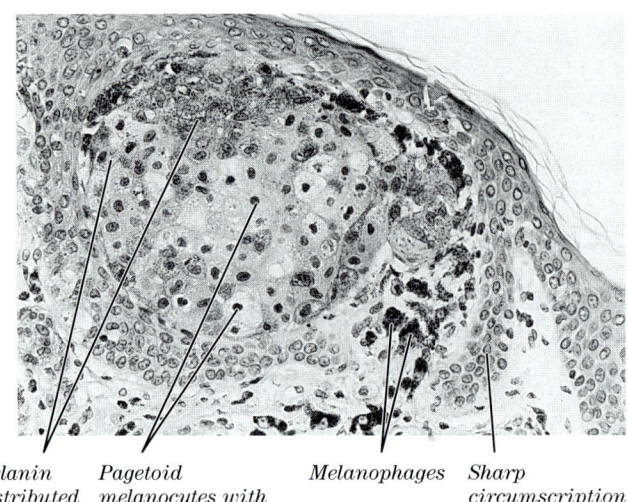

Melanin distributed unevenly | *Pagetoid melanocytes with small round and oval monomorphous nuclei* | *Melanophages* | *Sharp circumscription by collarette*

68 • Congenital Nevus *(superficial type)* Biopsied Shortly After Birth

Criteria for diagnosis of this congenital nevus (superficial type) biopsied soon after birth

This is a superficial congenital nevus because:

1. It is symmetric.

2. It is sharply circumscribed.

3. Melanocytes show maturation with progressive descent into the reticular dermis, and nests also become smaller with descent.

4. Melanin is distributed in uniform fashion.

5. Melanocytes within the epidermis are situated at the dermo-epidermal junction and not above it.

6. Nuclei of pagetoid melanocytes are small, round, or oval, and mostly monomorphous.

Pitfall in diagnosis

This superficial congenital nevus could be misread as a metastasis of melanoma because:

1. Many pagetoid melanocytes are dispersed in the upper part of the lesion.

2. Nests of melanocytes in the upper part of the lesion are large, vary in size and shape, and have become confluent.

3. Adnexocentricity and angiocentricity of melanocytes simulates multifocality of metastases.

4. Some melanocytes of the nevus appear to be situated within endothelium-lined spaces.

5. Melanin is not distributed evenly.

That pagetoid melanocytes are not necessarily synonymous with melanoma is illustrated in this neoplasm. The neoplasm is benign because of its architectural pattern, and the pagetoid melanocytes are not those of melanoma because their nuclei are monomorphous. Pagetoid melanocytes such as these are common in congenital nevi in biopsies shortly after birth, in congenital combined nevi of one type, in nevi on genitalia of young adults, in "deep penetrating" nevi, and sometimes at the shoulders of Clark's nevi.

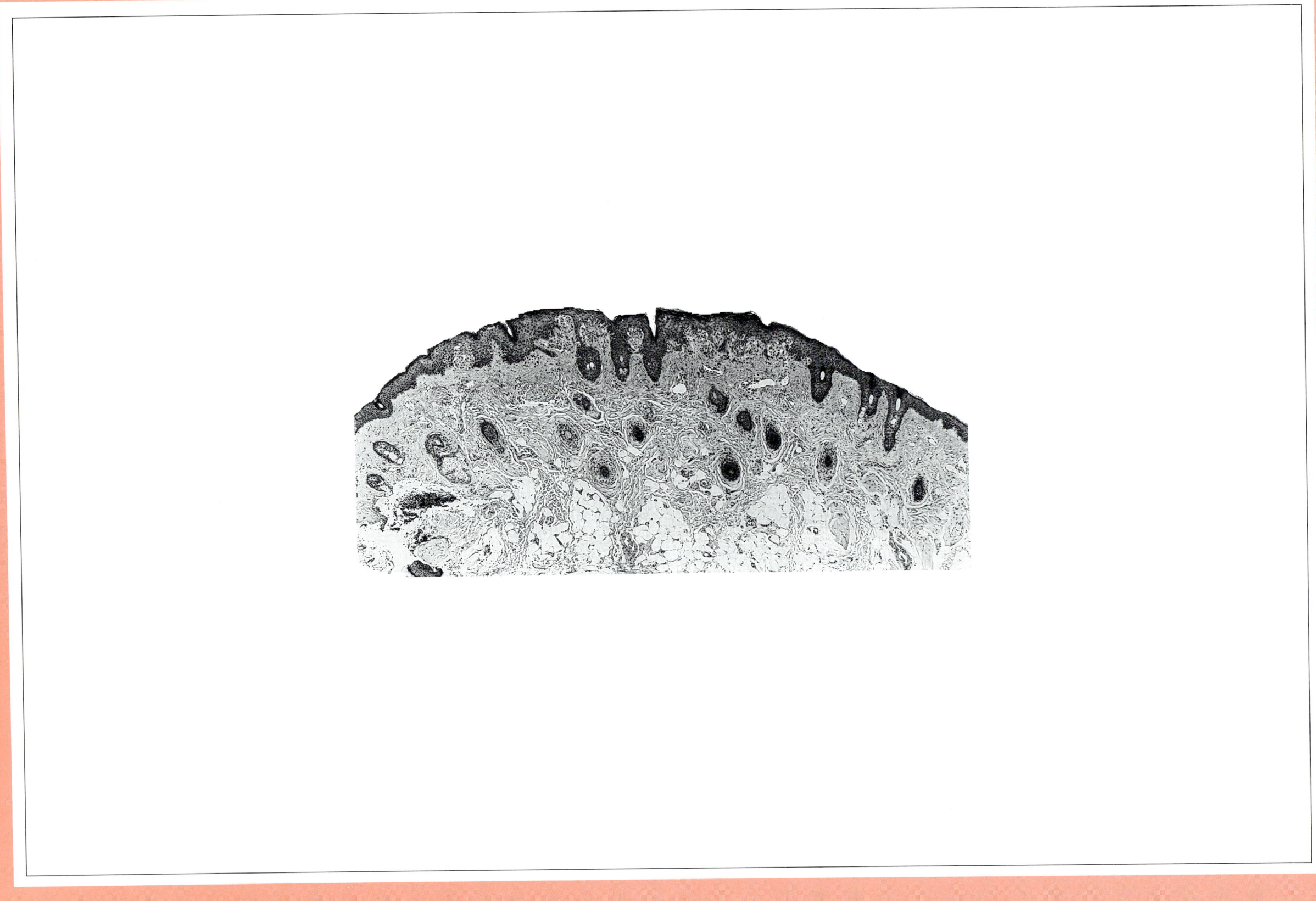

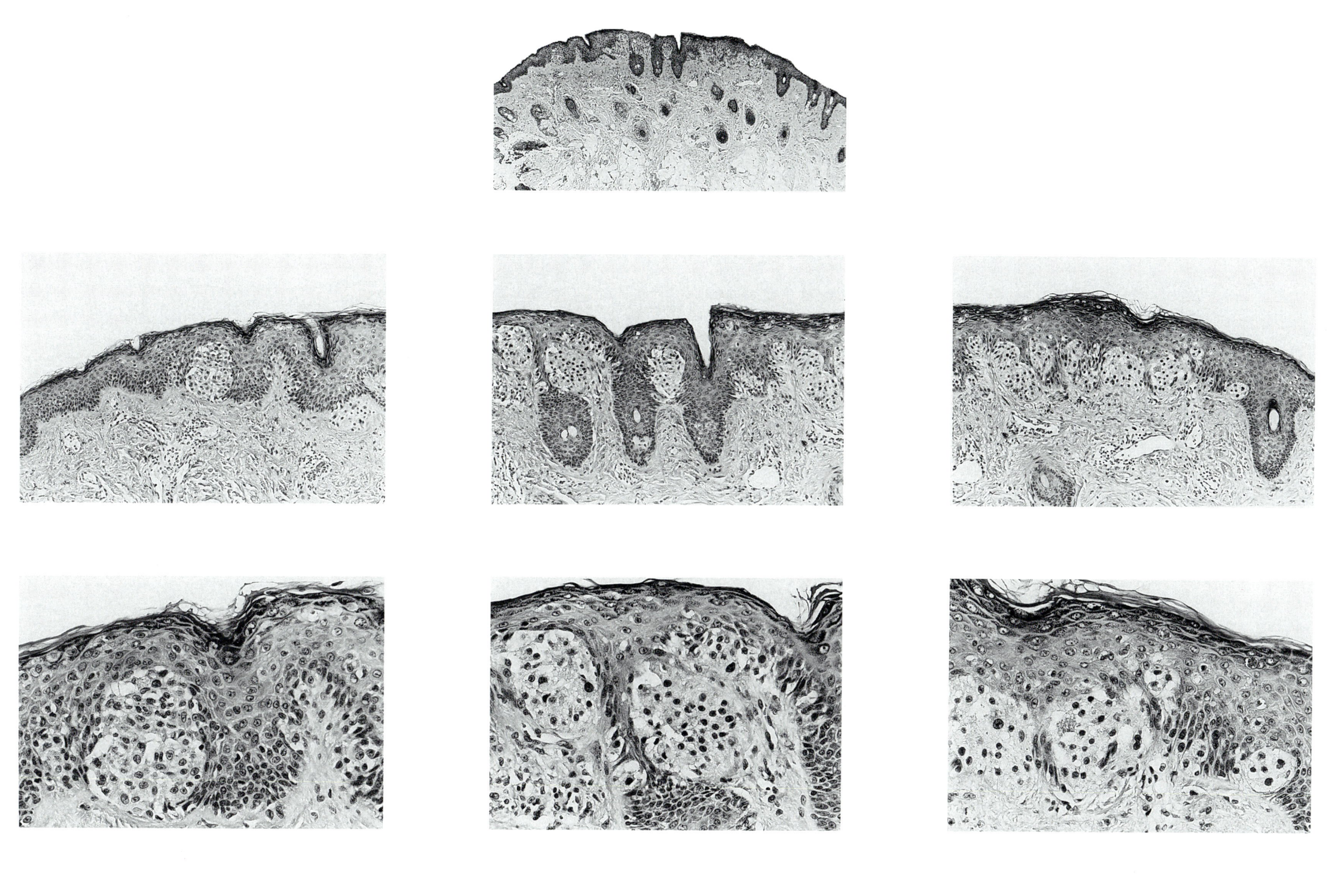

69. What is your diagnosis?

Brown-black lesion on the left earlobe of a 40-year-old woman came to be accompanied by a brown rim during the preceding year. Clinical diagnosis: melanoma. Patient was free of disease after 1 year.

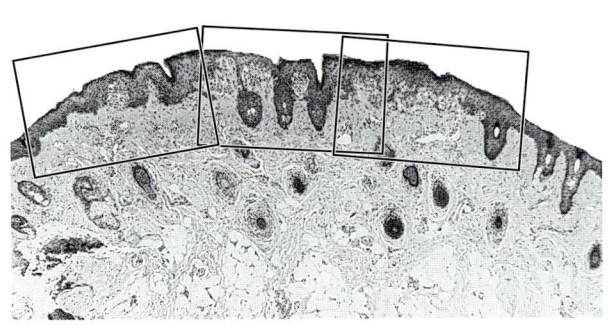

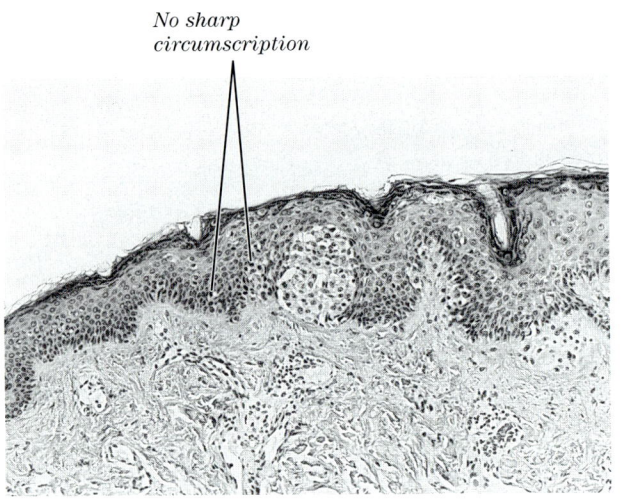

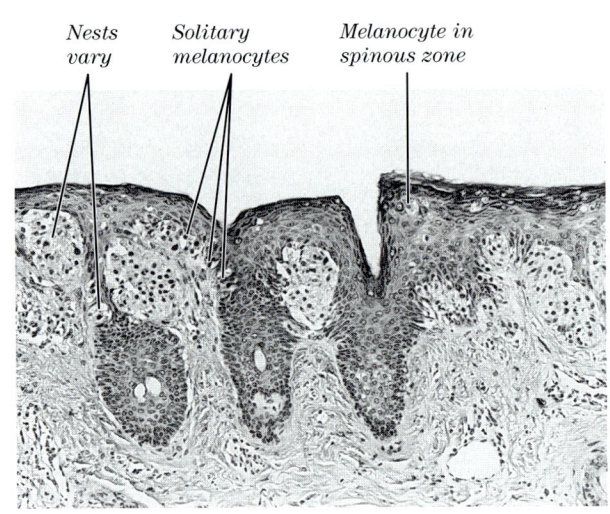

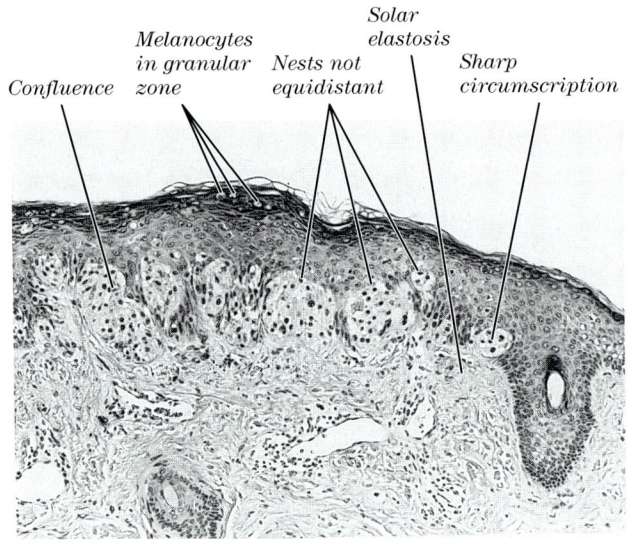

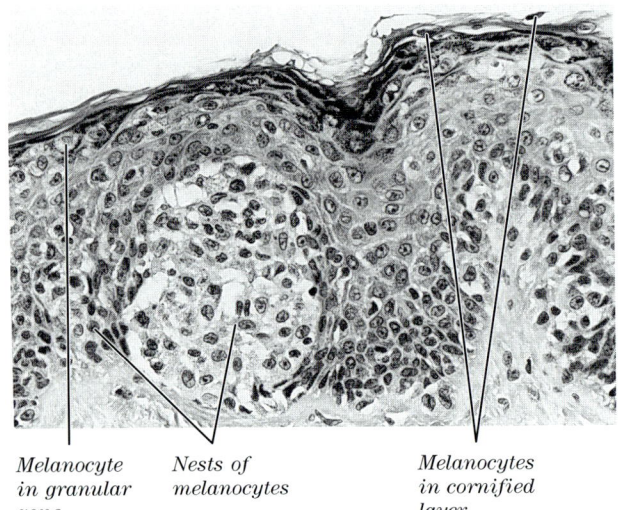

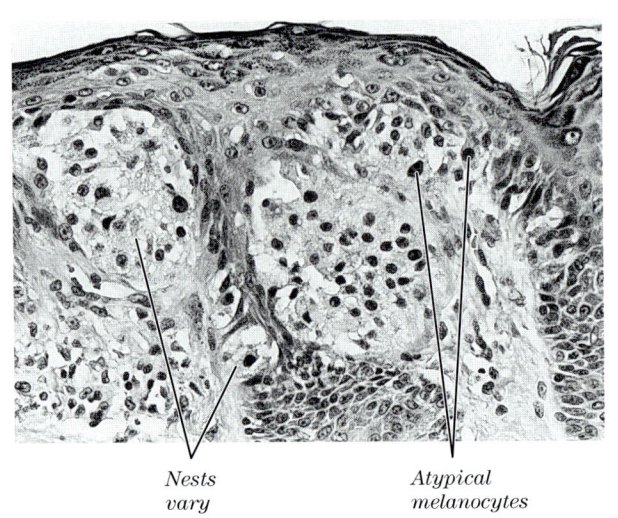

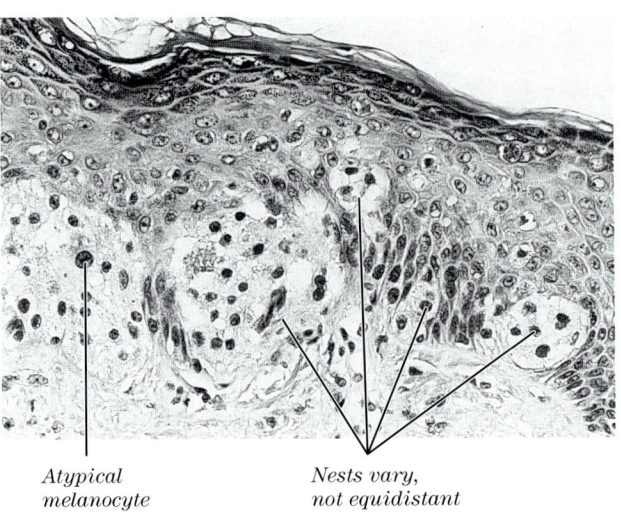

69 • Melanoma in situ

Criteria for diagnosis of this melanoma in situ on skin damaged severely by sunlight

This is a melanoma in situ because:

1. Nests of melanocytes within the epidermis are not equidistant from one another.

2. Nests of melanocytes vary in size and shape.

3. Some nests of melanocytes have become confluent.

4. Some melanocytes arranged as solitary units and in nests are present far above the dermo-epidermal junction and even in the cornified layer.

5. Melanocytes disposed as solitary units predominate over nests in some high-power fields.

6. Nuclear atypia of melanocytes is striking.

7. The changes within the epidermis, just listed, are present also within epithelial structures of adnexa.

Pitfall in diagnosis

This melanoma in situ on sun-damaged skin could be misinterpreted as a junctional "dysplastic" nevus because:

1. Melanocytes within the epidermis across the entire front of the lesion are arranged mostly in nests, rather than as solitary units.

2. Most of the nests of melanocytes are situated at the dermo-epidermal junction and not above it.

3. Melanocytes arrayed as solitary units and in nests are present not only within the epidermis, but also within epithelial structures of adnexa.

4. The melanocytes themselves have round and oval nuclei with abundant pale cytoplasm.

5. The neoplasm is well-circumscribed on one side.

These histopathologic findings are those of melanoma in situ. They are the same criteria that are applied to melanoma, unmodified, i.e., within the epidermis and the dermis, on any anatomic site. The neoplasm is not a nevus of any kind and surely not a "dysplastic" one. In our view, no nevus is "dysplastic," and, furthermore, there is no place for the flawed concept of "dysplasia" anywhere in dermatopathology.

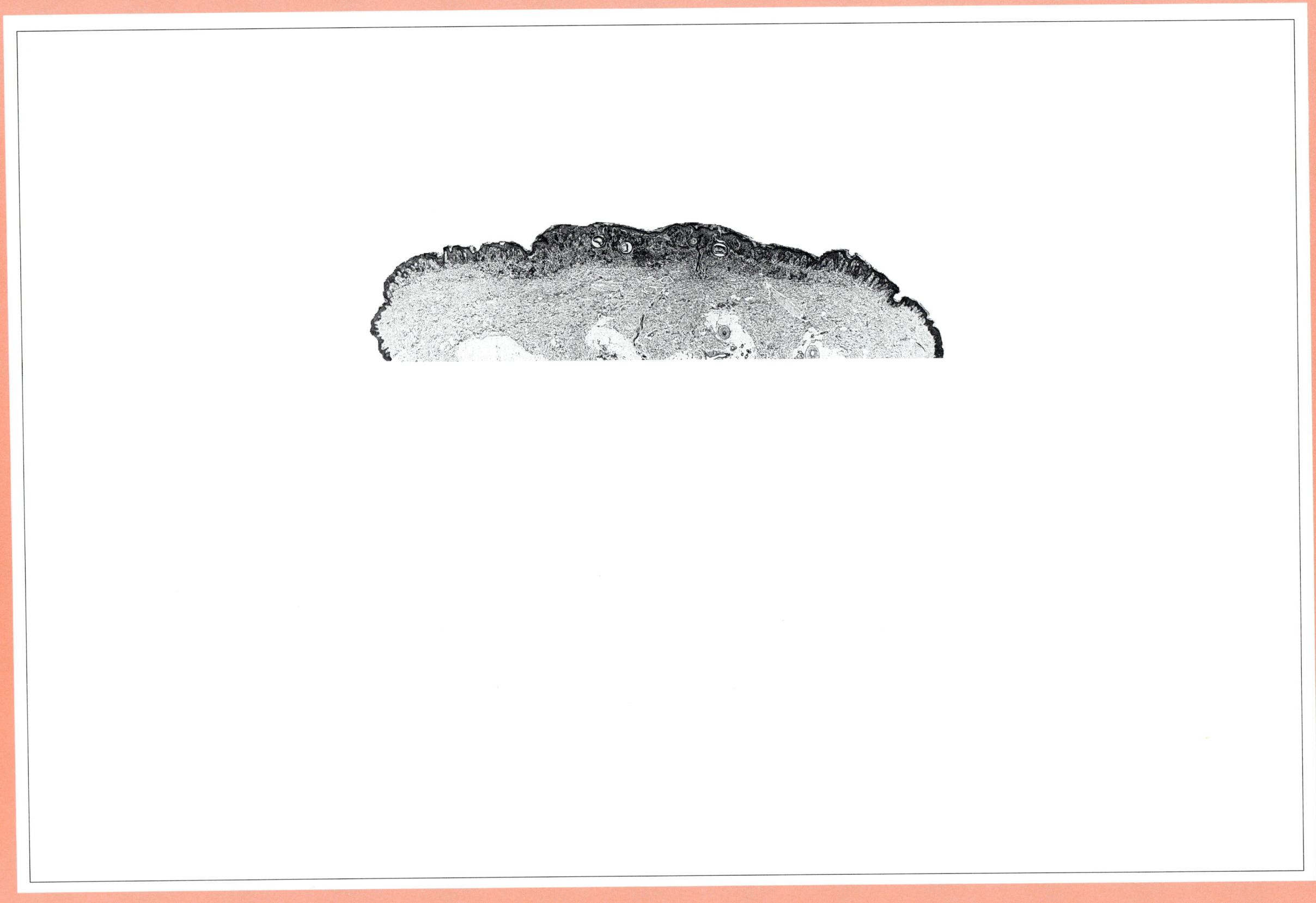

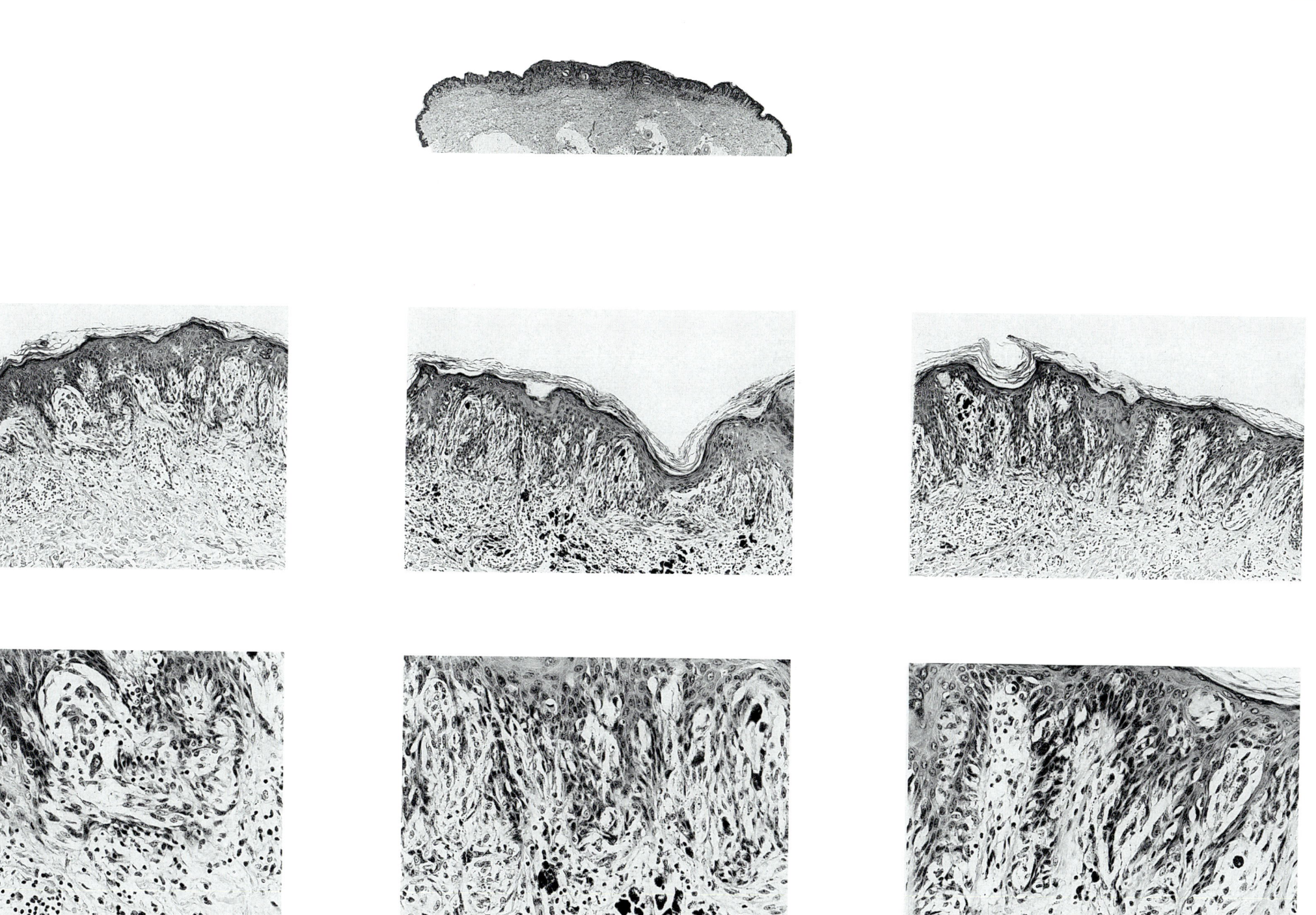

70. What is your diagnosis?

Pigmented papule on the lateral aspect of the left thigh of a 23-year-old woman. Clinical diagnosis: dysplastic nevus vs. melanoma. The patient was free of disease after 3 years.

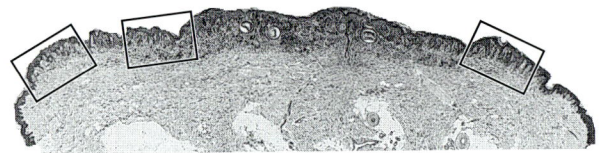

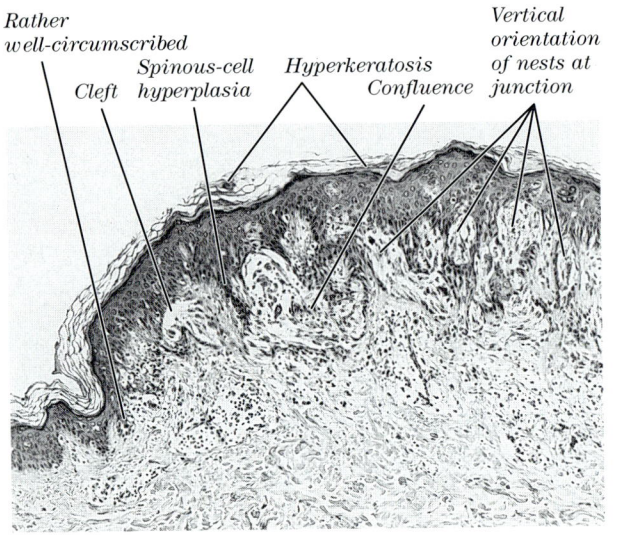
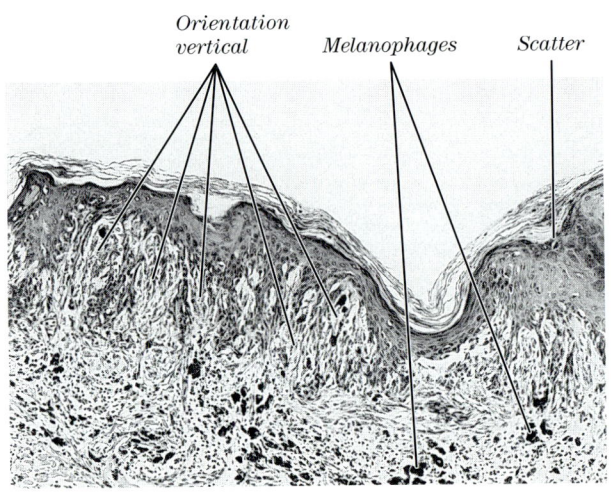
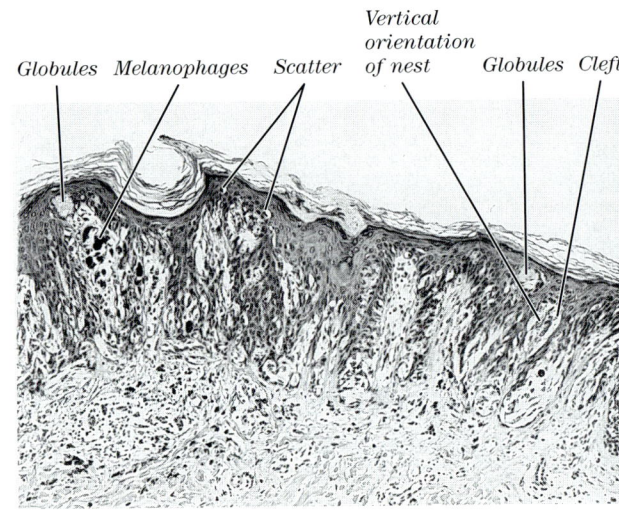
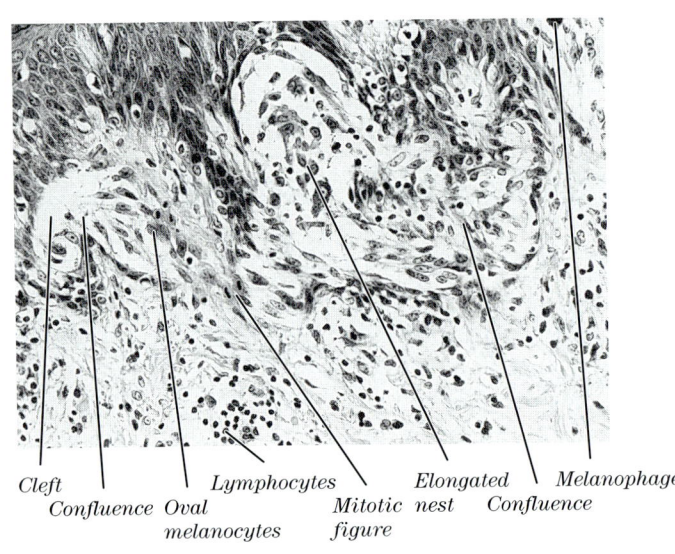
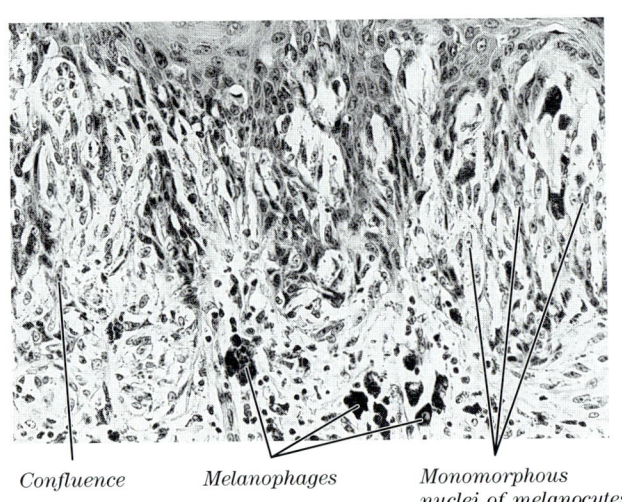
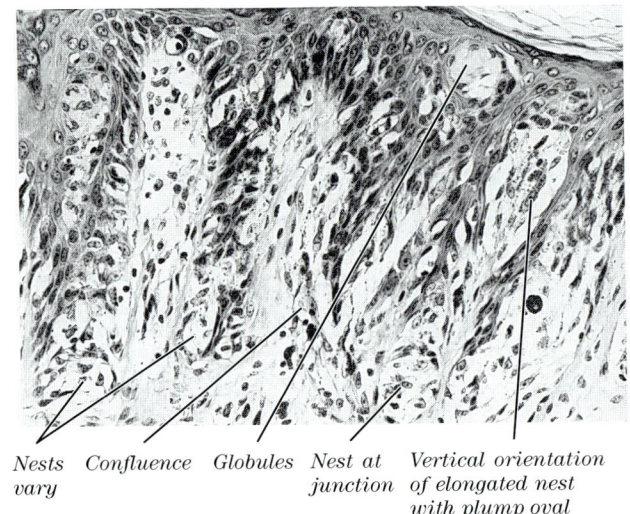

70 • Spitz's Nevus ("*pigmented spindle-cell*" *type*)

Criteria for diagnosis of this Spitz's nevus ("pigmented spindle-cell" type)

This is a nevus because:

1. The neoplasm is symmetric.
2. It is well-circumscribed.
3. Melanocytes within the epidermis are organized mostly in nests, rather than as solitary units.
4. Nests of melanocytes are present mostly at the dermo-epidermal junction, rather than above it.
5. Nuclei of melanocytes are relatively monomorphous.
6. Melanocytes mature.

This is a Spitz's nevus because:

1. The melanocytes have largish nuclei, abundant cytoplasm, and plump oval shape.
2. There is slight hyperkeratosis, hypergranulosis, and irregular hyperplasia of spinous cells.
3. Some nests of melanocytes are perpendicular to the skin surface.
4. Clefts are present between some nests of melanocytes and adjacent keratinocytes.
5. Numerous globules are present within the epidermis.

Pitfall in diagnosis

This Spitz's nevus could be misread as a melanoma because:

1. Nests of melanocytes vary in size and shape.
2. Many nests of melanocytes have become confluent.
3. Some melanocytes disposed as solitary units are present above the dermo-epidermal junction.
4. Lymphocytes are dispersed within intra-epidermal nests of melanocytes.

A particular Spitz's nevus may have more features in common with a melanoma than it has differences with it. Despite that reality, the architectural pattern of this nevus differs dramatically from that of melanoma, to wit, it is symmetric, is well-circumscribed, and shows maturation of melanocytes with progressive descent. Furthermore, in this instance, the nuclei of melanocytes are oval and monomorphous, and there are globules within the epidermis that are colored dull pink by hematoxylin and eosin. This constellation of findings marks this neoplasm as an indubitable Spitz's nevus. Parenthetically, this variant of Spitz's nevus also has been termed "pigmented spindle-cell tumor."

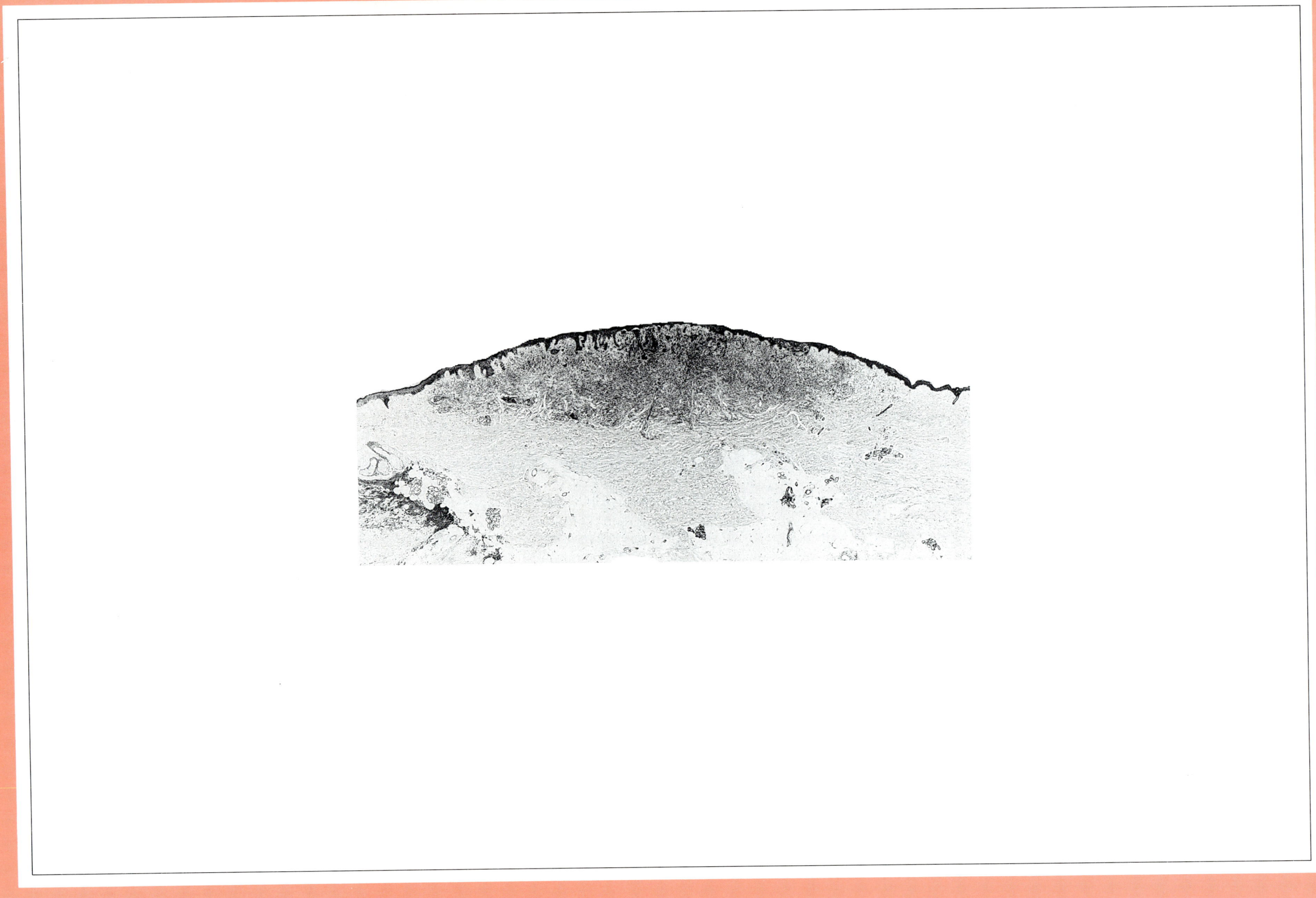

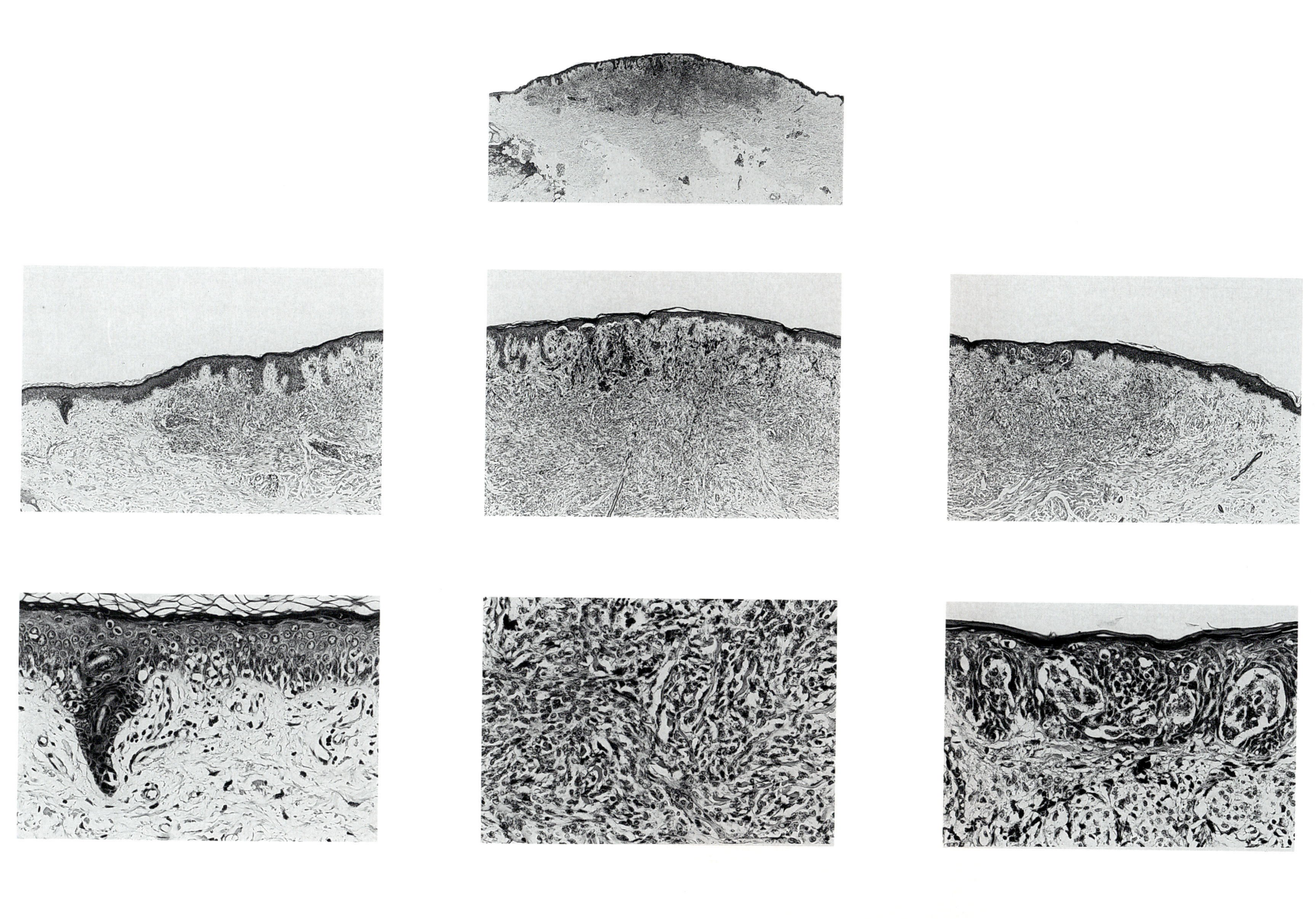

71. What is your diagnosis?

Lesion of 6 to 8 years duration on the left arm of a 53-year-old woman. Clinical diagnosis: melanoma. Site was excised 3 months later. No nodes were palpable in the left axilla. Patient was in good health 7 years later.

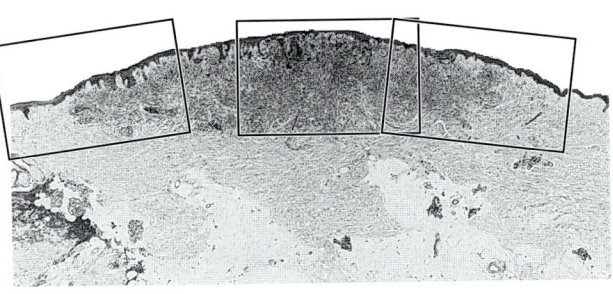

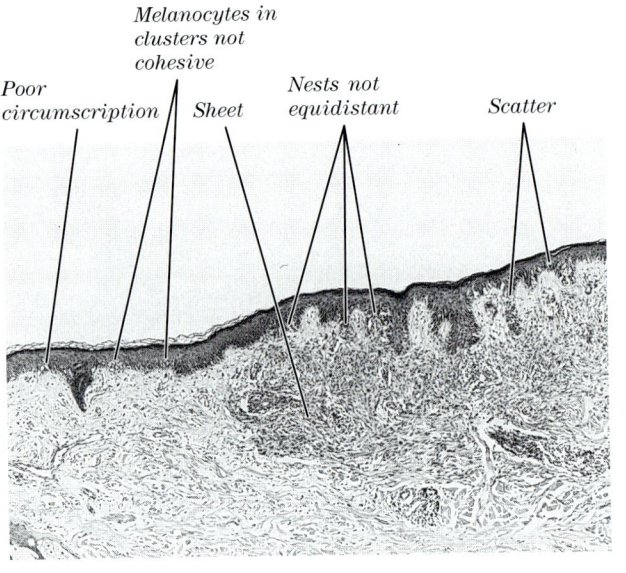
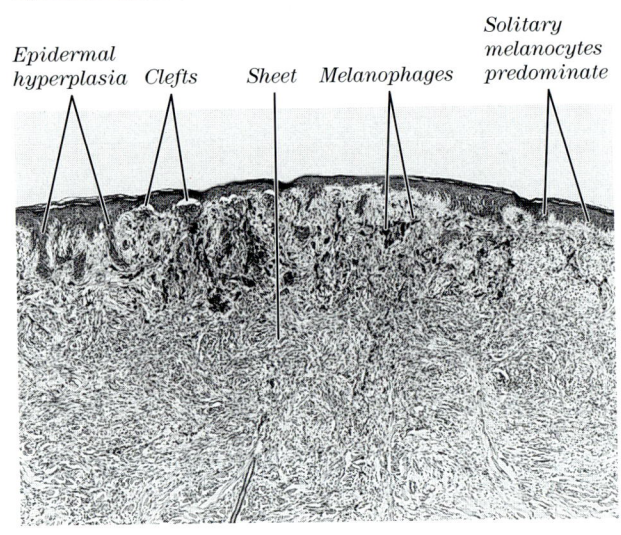
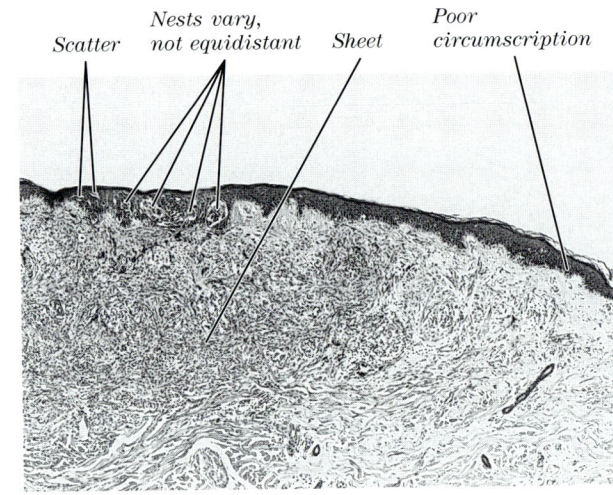

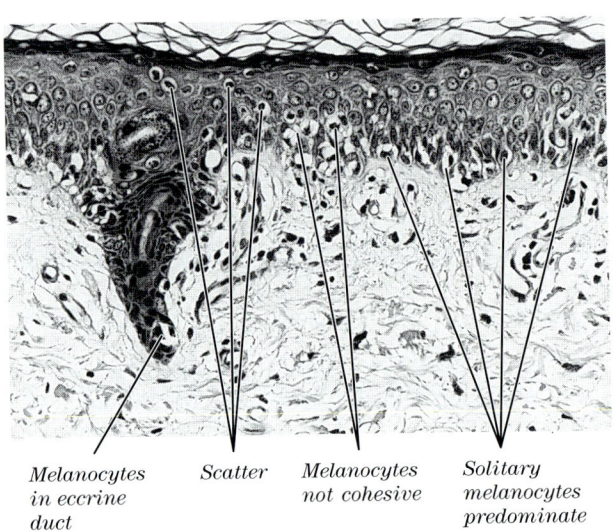
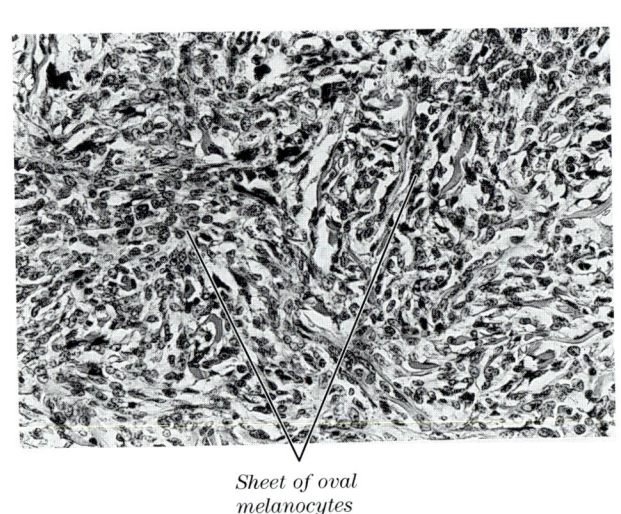
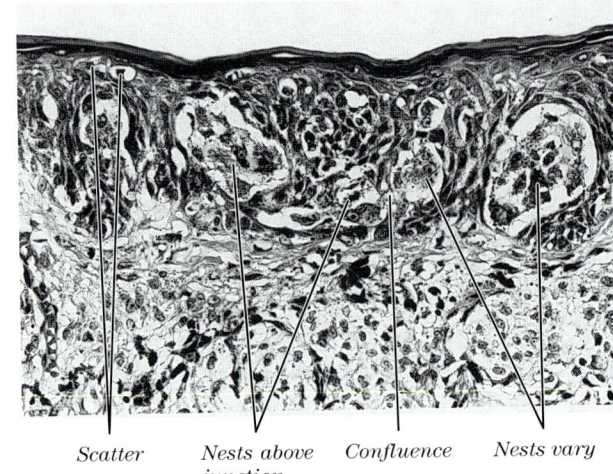

71 • Melanoma

Criteria for diagnosis of this melanoma

This is a melanoma because:

1. Circumscription of the neoplasm is poor.
2. Melanocytes disposed as solitary units within the epidermis predominate over nests of melanocytes in some high-power fields.
3. Nests of melanocytes are not equidistant from one another.
4. Nests of melanocytes vary in size and shape.
5. Some nests of melanocytes have become confluent.
6. Melanocytes arrayed as solitary units are scattered far above the dermo-epidermal junction.
7. Melanocytes arranged as solitary units extend far down epithelial structures of adnexa.
8. Some atypical pagetoid melanocytes are situated in the upper part of the dermis.

Pitfall in diagnosis

This melanoma could be misinterpreted as a pigmented Spitz's nevus because:

1. The neoplasm is relatively symmetric, at first glance at scanning magnification.
2. The neoplasm is wedge-shaped.
3. The epidermis is hyperkeratotic and irregularly hyperplastic.
4. Some elongated nests of melanocytes are perpendicular to the skin surface.
5. Clefts have formed between some nests of melanocytes and adjacent keratinocytes.
6. Melanin is distributed in relatively uniform fashion throughout the neoplasm.
7. Melanocytes mature somewhat with progressive descent into the dermis.

This neoplasm demonstrates how difficult it may be to assess symmetry and asymmetry accurately. At scanning magnification, the neoplasm appears to be symmetric. At higher magnifications, however, it becomes apparent that within the epidermis on the left side, melanocytes arranged as solitary units predominate overwhelmingly over nests of them, whereas in the epidermis on the right side, nests of melanocytes predominate over melanocytes disposed as solitary units in many high-power fields. Furthermore, on the left side, there is much more melanin within the dermis than there is on the right side. In short, this neoplasm is strikingly asymmetric and is a melanoma.

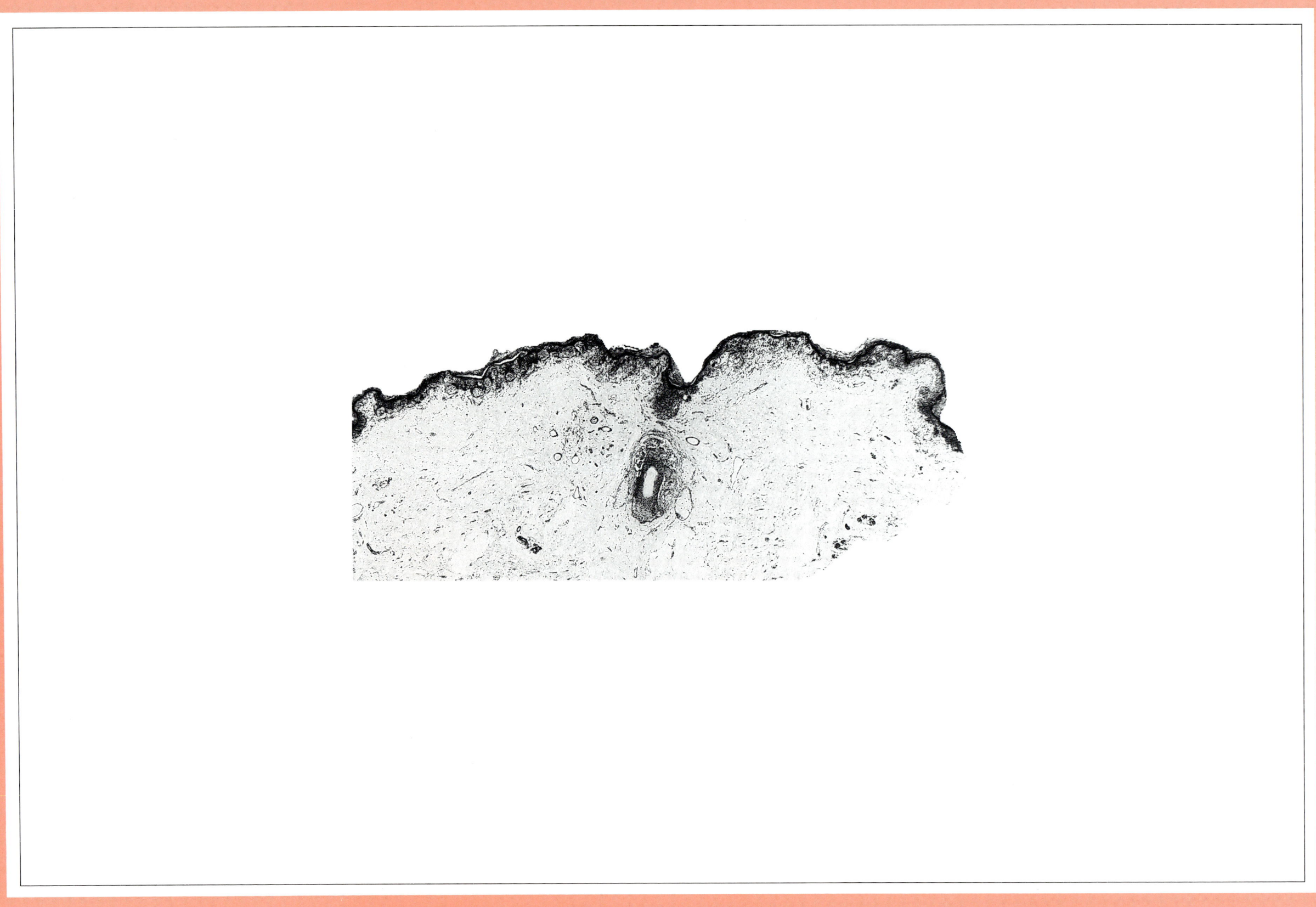

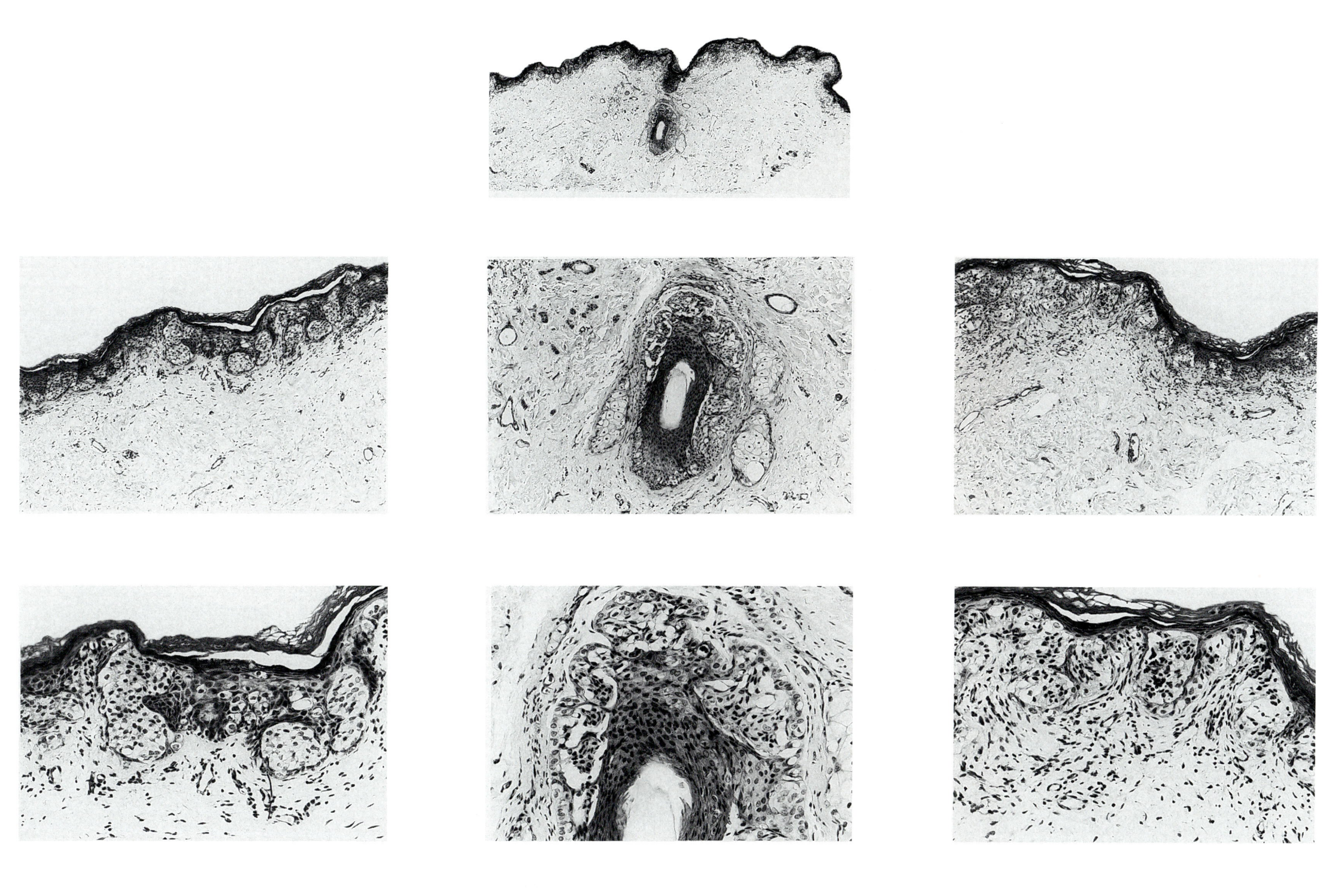

72. What is your diagnosis?

Erythematous lesion on the left labium majus of a 74-year-old woman. Clinical diagnosis: seborrheic dermatitis. No follow-up data were available.

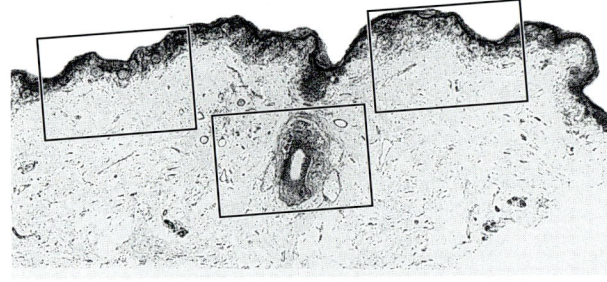

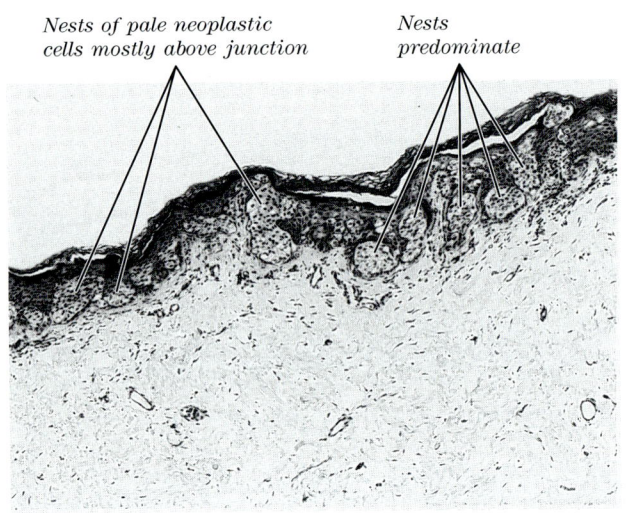
Nests of pale neoplastic cells mostly above junction — Nests predominate

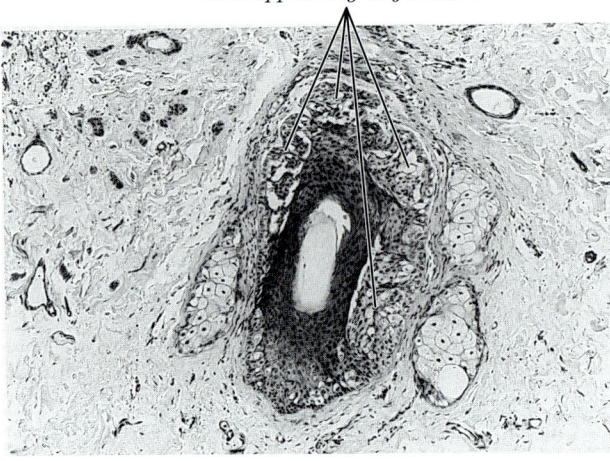
Nests of pale neoplastic cells within infundibulum, some apparently at junction

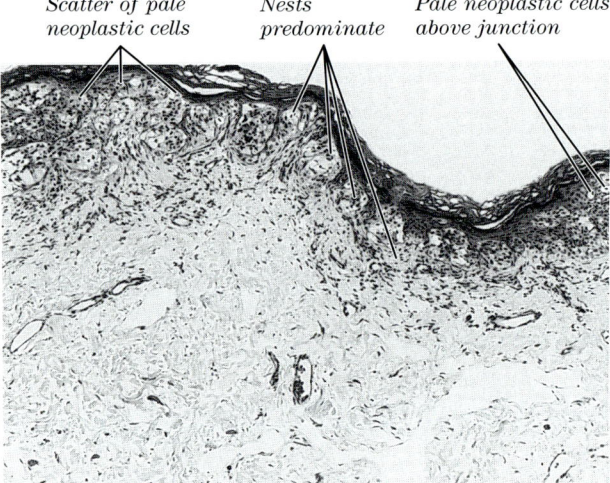
Scatter of pale neoplastic cells — Nests predominate — Pale neoplastic cells above junction

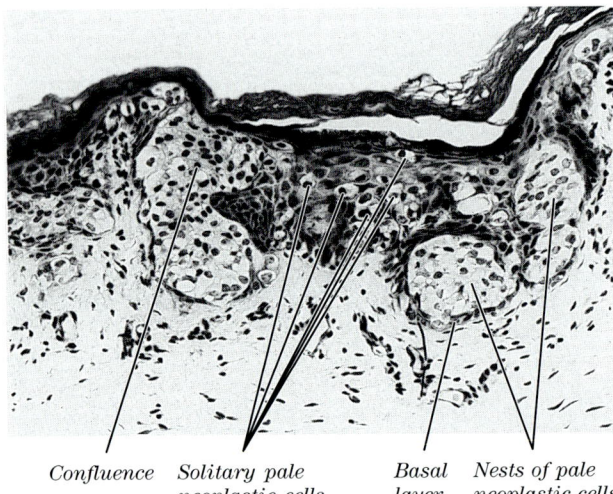
Confluence — Solitary pale neoplastic cells scattered throughout epidermis — Basal layer — Nests of pale neoplastic cells above junction

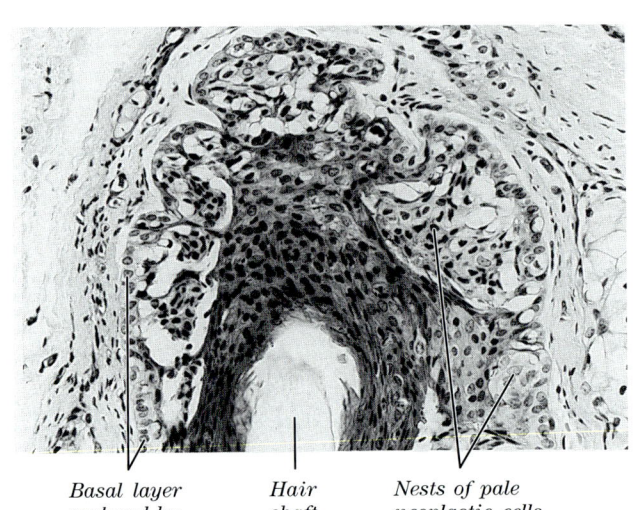
Basal layer replaced by neoplastic cells — Hair shaft — Nests of pale neoplastic cells within infundibulum

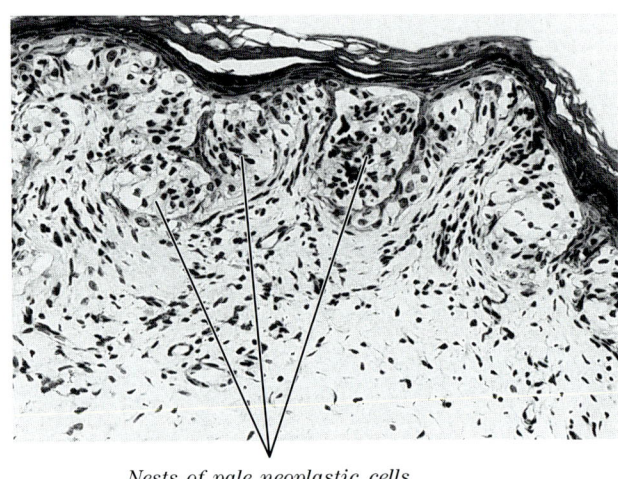
Nests of pale neoplastic cells, mostly above junction

72 • Extramammary Paget's Disease

Criteria for diagnosis of this lesion of extramammary Paget's disease

This is extramammary Paget's disease because:

1. Paget cells are present within the surface and adnexal epithelium.

2. Paget cells are positioned mostly above the basal layer, i.e., in the spinous, granular, and cornified layers.

3. Nests of Paget cells are not equidistant from one another.

4. Many nests of Paget cells have become confluent.

5. Some nests of Paget cells have jagged peripheries.

Superimposed on this lesion of extramammary Paget's disease is lichen simplex chronicus in the form of compact orthokeratosis, hypergranulosis, and spinous-cell hyperplasia. On the vulva especially, lesions of extramammary Paget's disease are severely pruritic and are rubbed vigorously.

Pitfall in diagnosis

This lesion of extramammary Paget's disease could be misread as melanoma in situ because:

1. Nests of pale cells are present within the epidermis.

2. Many of the nests seem to be situated at the dermo-epidermal junction, although in reality they are above it.

3. Nests vary in size and shape.

4. Nests have become confluent.

5. Pale cells disposed as solitary units are scattered above the junction, some of them in the upper reaches of the epidermis.

6. Nests of pale cells and solitary pale cells are present far down adnexal epithelial structures in the same pattern as they are distributed within the epidermis.

7. Nuclei of pale cells are atypical.

Differentiation of extramammary Paget's disease, as pictured here, from melanoma in situ is accomplished by ascertaining the relationship of solitary neoplastic cells and nests of them to the dermo-epidermal junction. In extramammary Paget's disease, virtually all of the neoplastic cells are situated above the junction, whereas in melanoma in situ many of the neoplastic cells are seated at the junction. In some instances, as illustrated, some nests of neoplastic cells in extramammary Paget's disease, such as those in the hair follicle shown, appear to be present at the junction; that usually is an illusion. Nests of Paget cells, as a rule, are not positioned at the junction, but above it. When doubt remains, differentiation between Paget's disease and melanoma can be accomplished by histochemical and immunohistochemical methods.

The neoplastic cells in extramammary Paget's disease are authentic Paget cells that show apocrine differentiation, whereas the cells that simulate Paget cells in melanoma are pagetoid melanocytes.

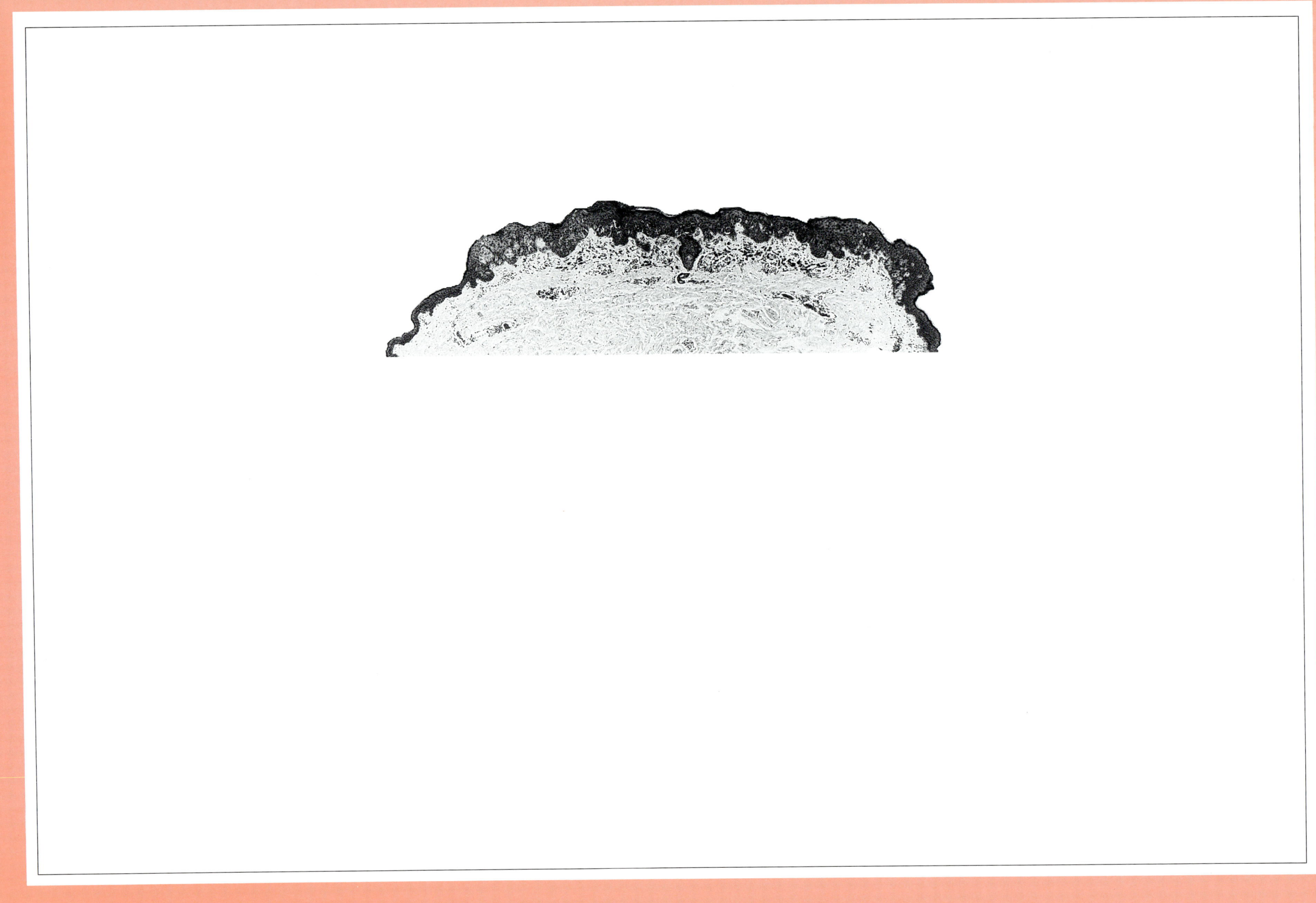

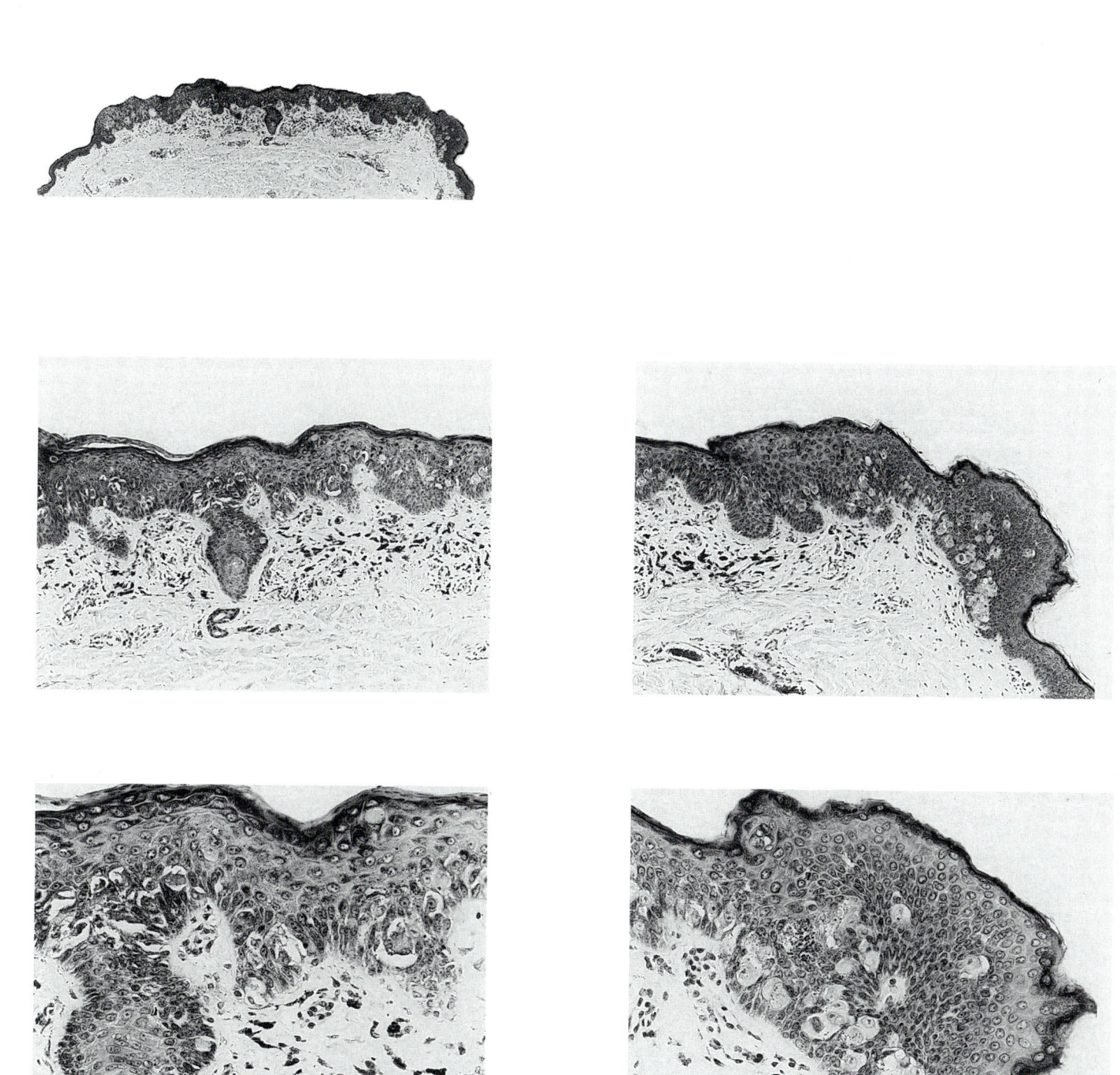

73. What is your diagnosis?

Pigmented lesion on the right lateral thigh of a 27-year-old woman with a history of Spitz's nevi and melanoma. Clinical diagnosis: Spitz's nevus. Patient had several Spitz's nevi excised 3 years later. No additional follow-up information was available.

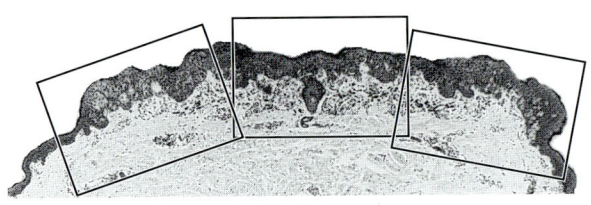

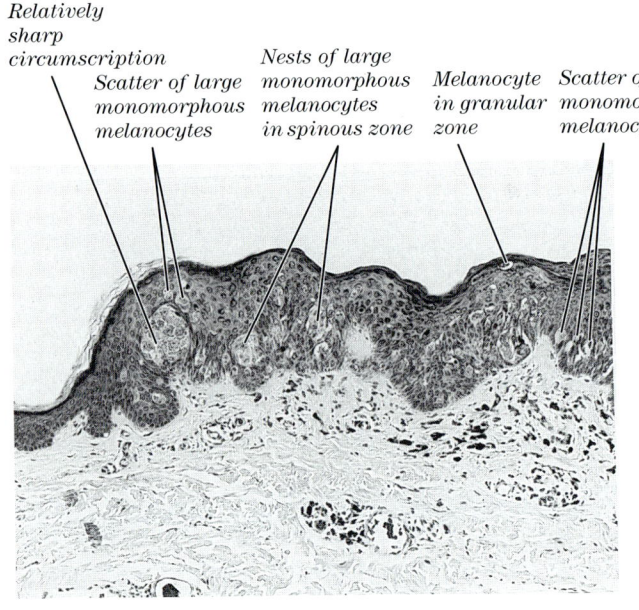
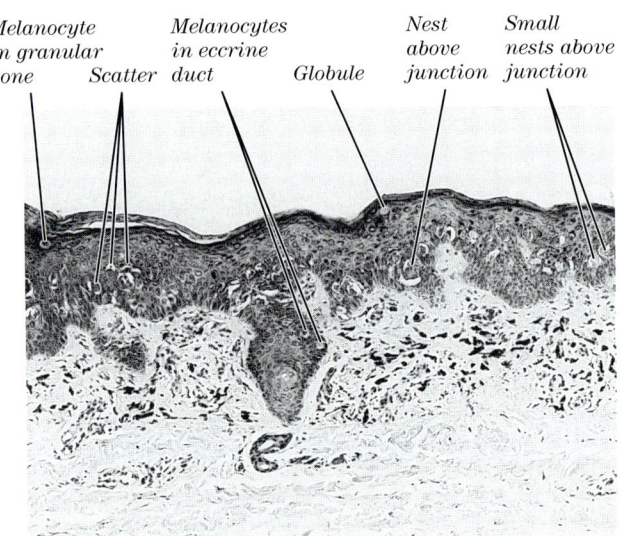
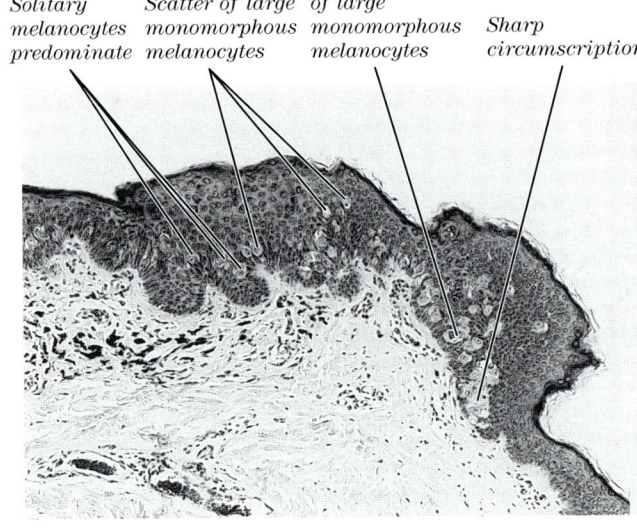
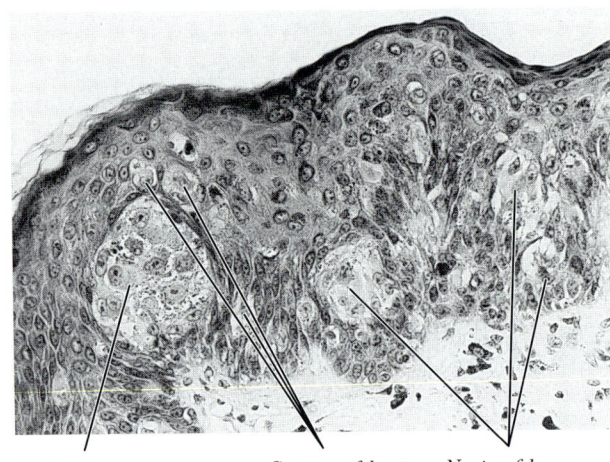
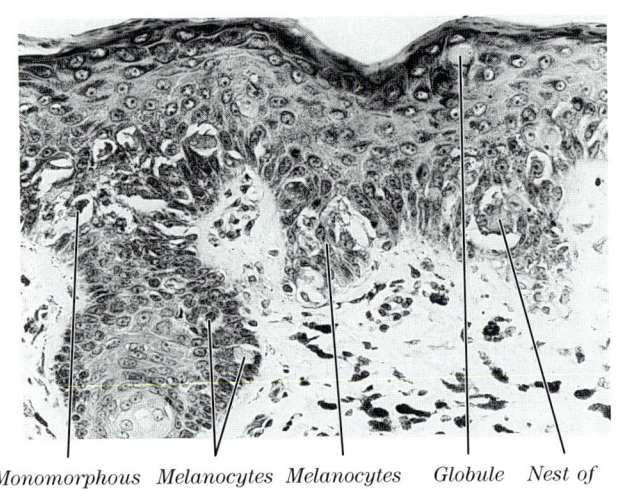
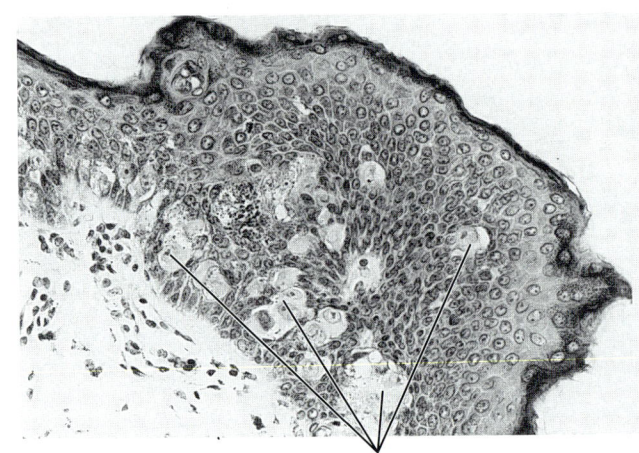

73 • Spitz's Nevus

Criteria for diagnosis of this Spitz's nevus (junctional type)

This is a Spitz's nevus because:

1. It is relatively symmetric.
2. Circumscription is relatively sharp.
3. Melanocytes are arranged mostly in nests, rather than mostly as solitary units, in a small lesion, i.e., one that measures less than 2.5 mm in diameter.
4. Monomorphous melanocytes have large, roundish nuclei and abundant, pale cytoplasm.
5. Melanin is distributed in relatively uniform fashion within the epidermis and epithelial structures of adnexa.

Pitfall in diagnosis

This junctional Spitz's nevus could be misinterpreted as a melanoma in situ because:

1. Melanocytes are large.
2. Melanocytes are present throughout most of the thickness of the epidermis.
3. Melanocytes are disposed mostly as solitary units within the epidermis and within epithelial structures of adnexa.
4. Nests of melanocytes are not equidistant from one another.
5. Melanocytes arrayed as solitary units are not equidistant from one another.

The single most important criterion for differentiating a junctional Spitz's nevus, such as this one, from melanoma in situ is the remarkably monomorphous quality of the melanocytes in Spitz's nevus. Not only are the nuclei, but also the cytoplasm is monomorphous. In short, the monomorphous appearance of melanocytes, some of which resemble histiocytes in granulomas, makes this a Spitz's nevus and not a melanoma.

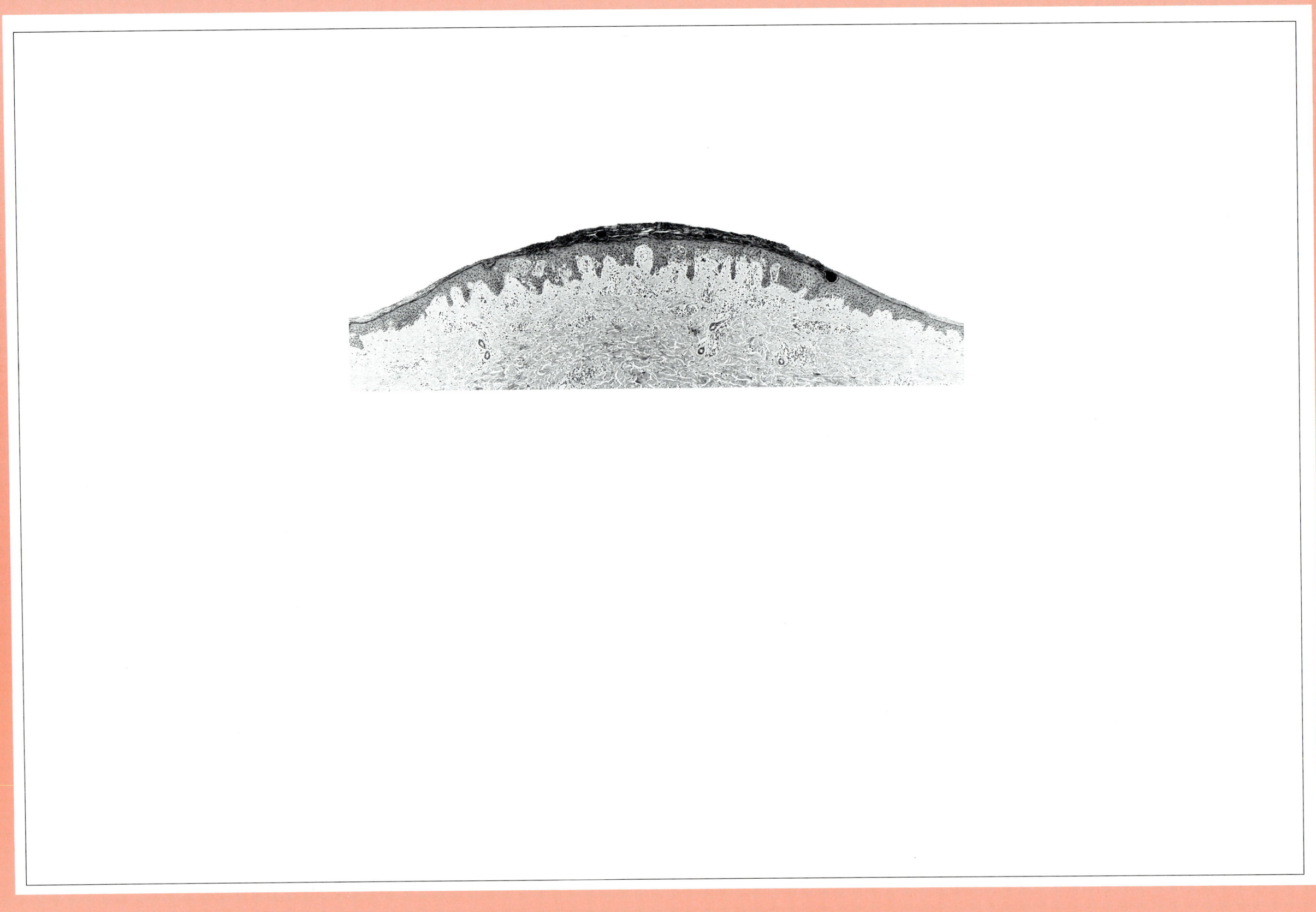

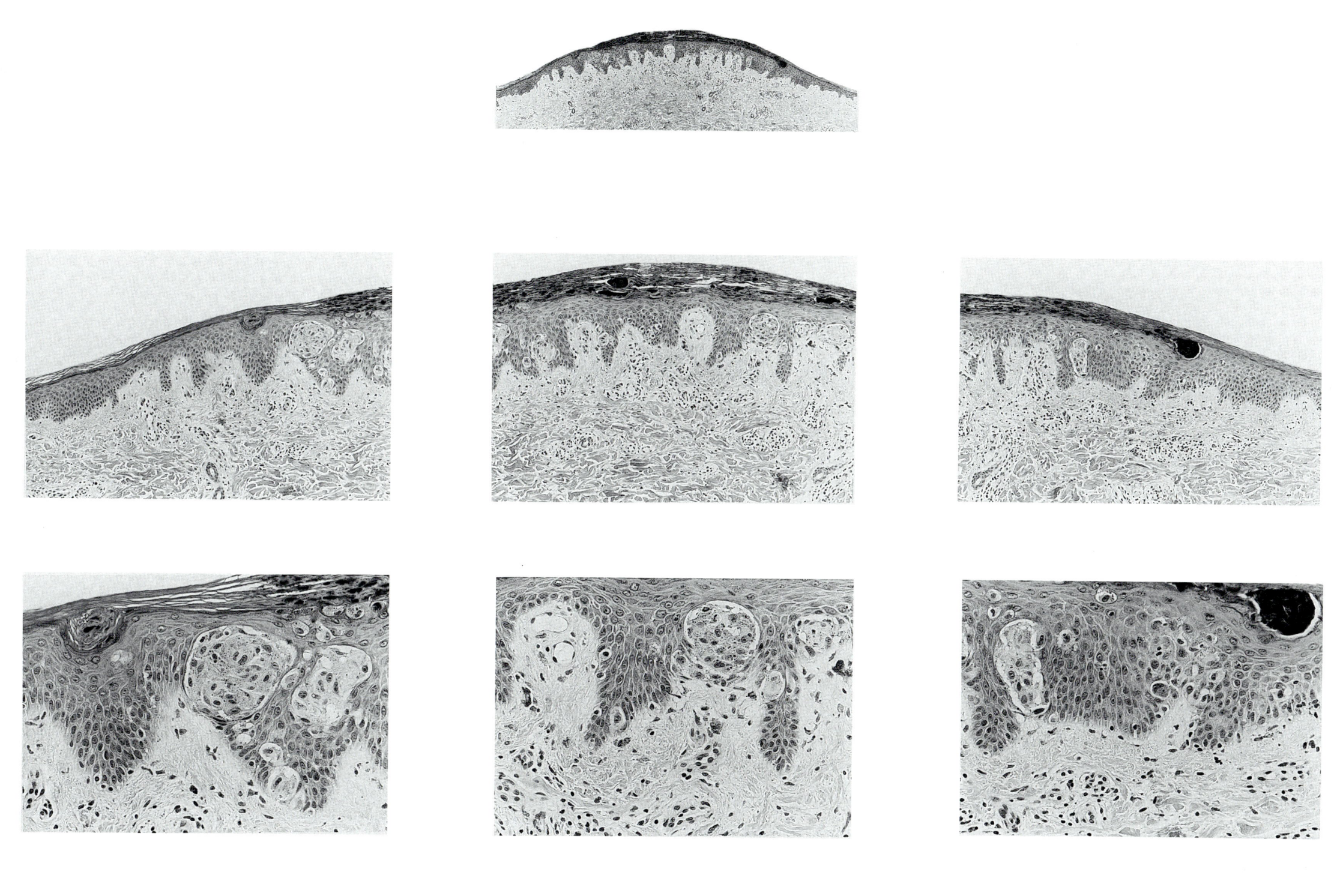

74. What is your diagnosis?

Pigmented lesion on the lower part of the right leg of a 27-year-old woman. Clinical diagnosis: nevus vs. melanoma. The site was excised completely and the patient was free of disease after 1 year.

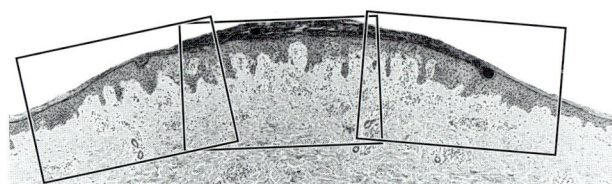

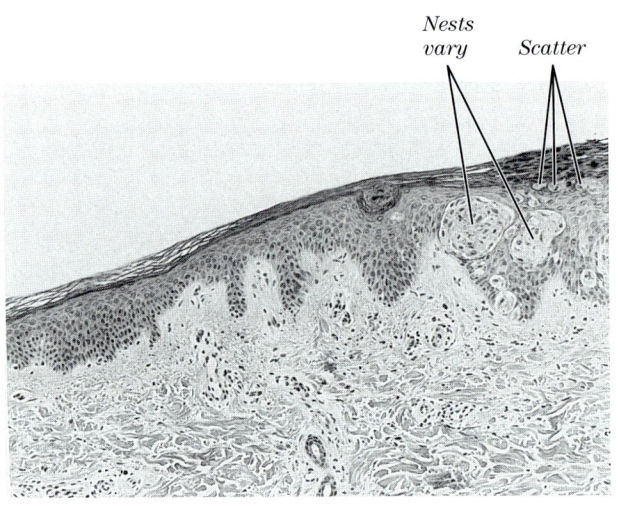
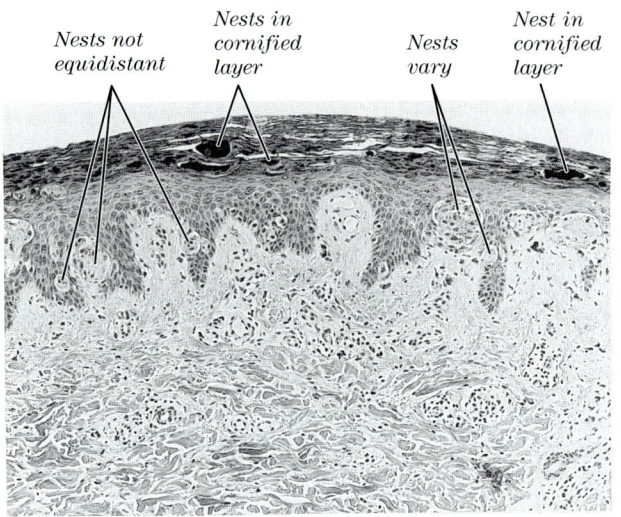
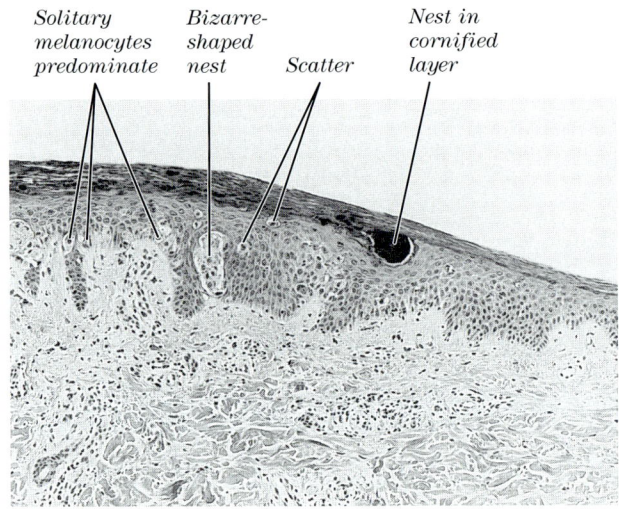

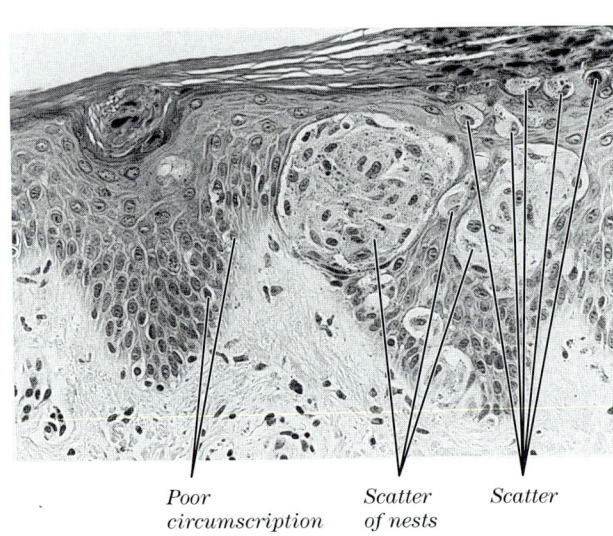
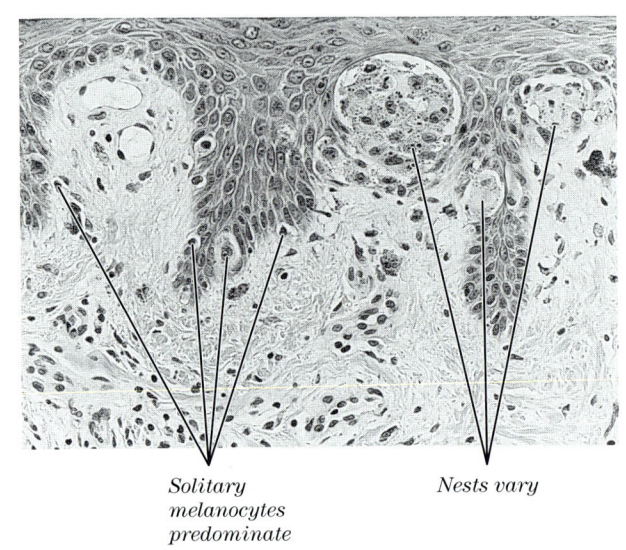
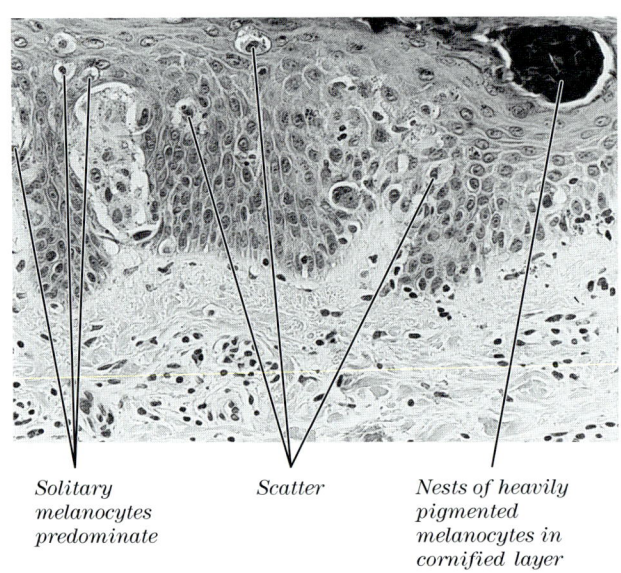

74 • Melanoma in situ

Criteria for diagnosis of this small melanoma in situ

This is a melanoma in situ because:

1. The neoplasm is asymmetric (a large clump of melanocytes is present in the cornified layer on the left side of the neoplasm, but not on the right).

2. The neoplasm is not sharply circumscribed.

3. Nests of melanocytes within the epidermis are not equidistant from one another.

4. Nests of melanocytes vary in size and shape.

5. Melanocytes arranged both as solitary units and in nests are scattered at all levels of the epidermis, including the cornified layer.

6. Melanin is not distributed in uniform fashion throughout the epidermis.

7. Abundant pigment is present within the cornified layer, but it is not distributed in discrete columns.

Pitfall in diagnosis

This small melanoma in situ could be misinterpreted as a junctional Spitz's nevus because:

1. There are hyperkeratosis and irregular spinous-cell hyperplasia.

2. Some nests of melanocytes within the epidermis are elongated.

3. Clefts separate some elongated nests of melanocytes from adjacent keratinocytes.

4. Melanocytes within the epidermis are arranged both as solitary units and in nests.

5. Some nests of melanocytes and melanocytes disposed as solitary units are present above the dermo-epidermal junction.

6. Nuclei of melanocytes are large, pleomorphic, and mostly round and oval.

It is extremely difficult sometimes to differentiate a small melanoma from a Spitz's nevus. When, however, nests of melanocytes are not equidistant from one another, nests vary in size and shape, and melanocytes arranged as solitary units predominate over nests in high-power fields, the neoplasm must be a melanoma, as is this one.

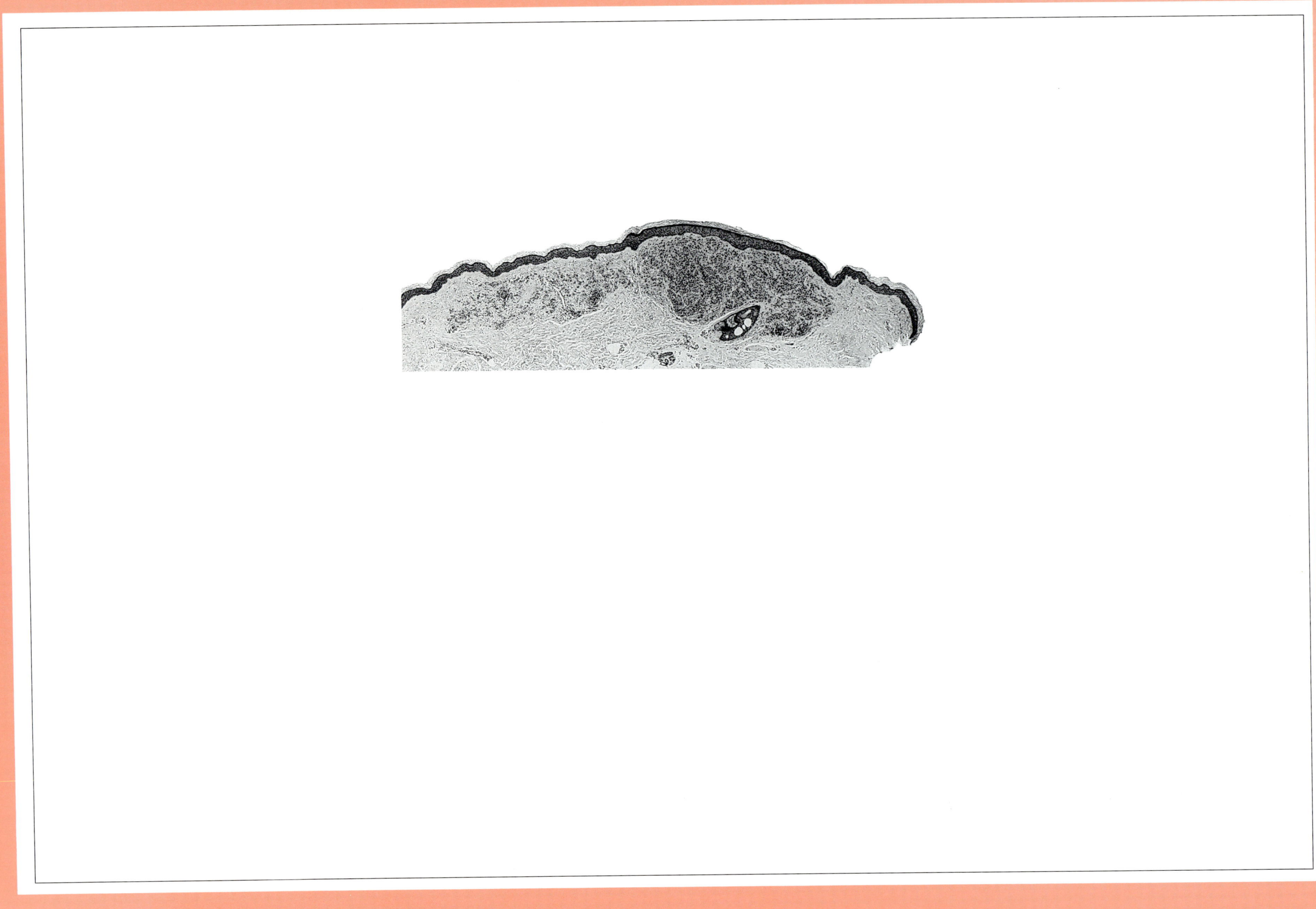

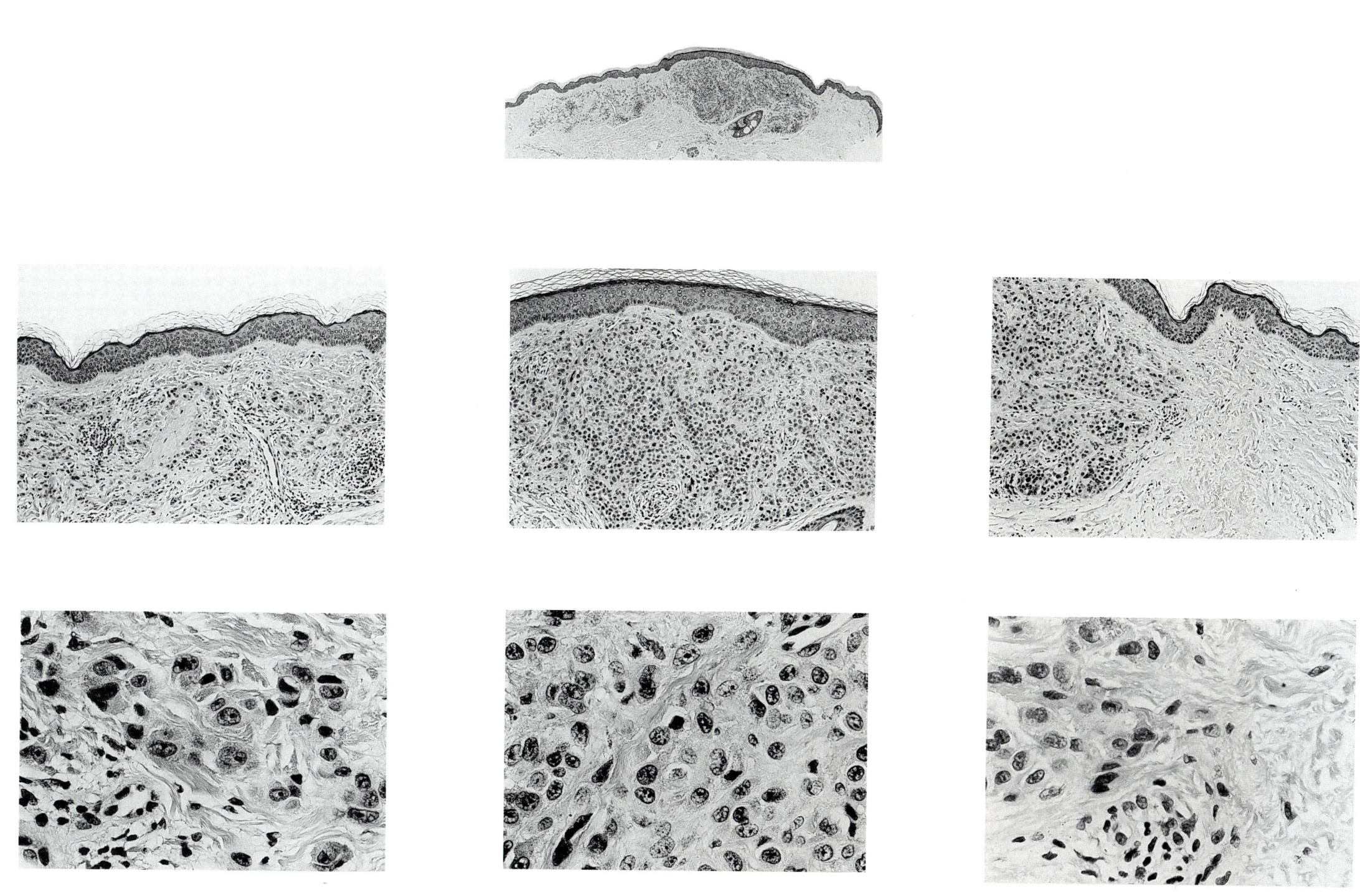

75. What is your diagnosis?

Pigmented papule appeared at a site of cryosurgery, performed 3 years previously, on the right arm of a 74-year-old woman. Clinical diagnosis: melanoma. Subsequent excision revealed no residuum of the neoplasm. No follow-up data were available.

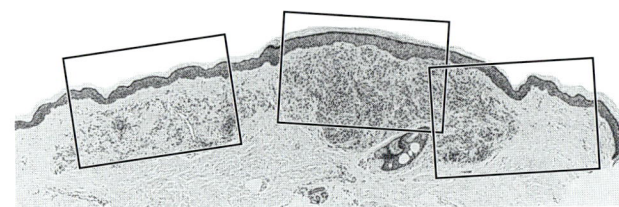

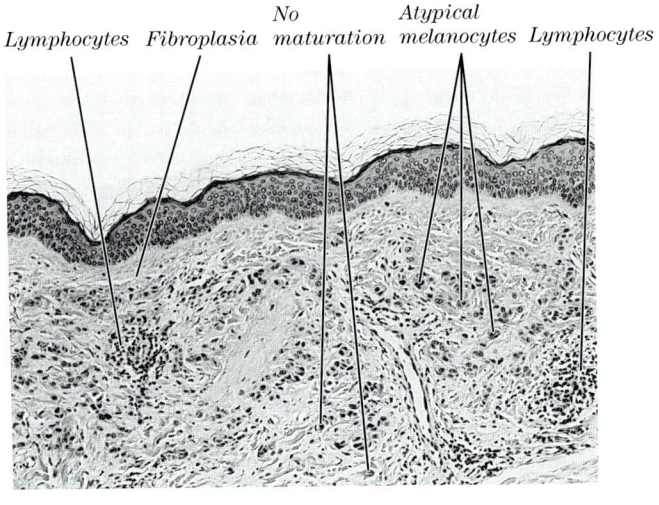
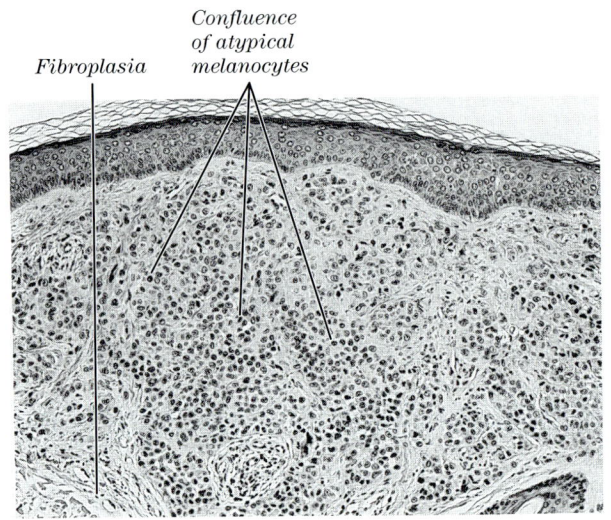
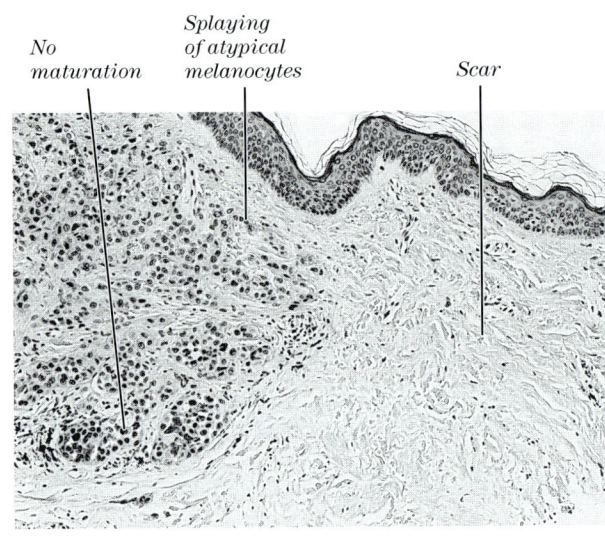

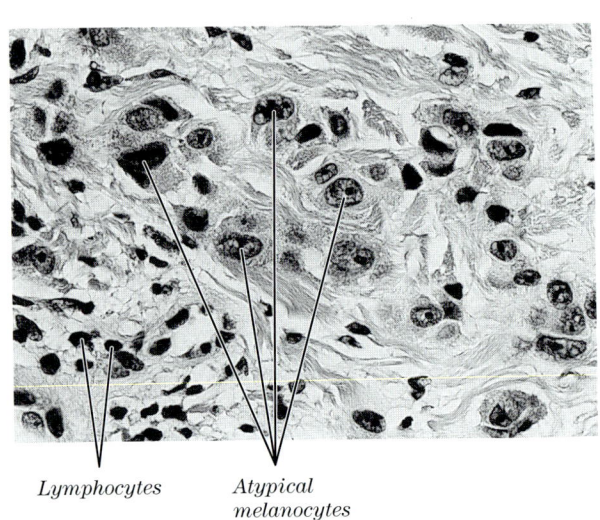
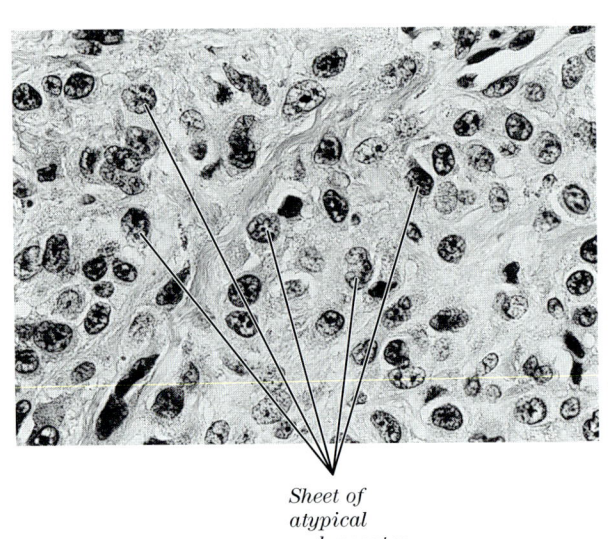
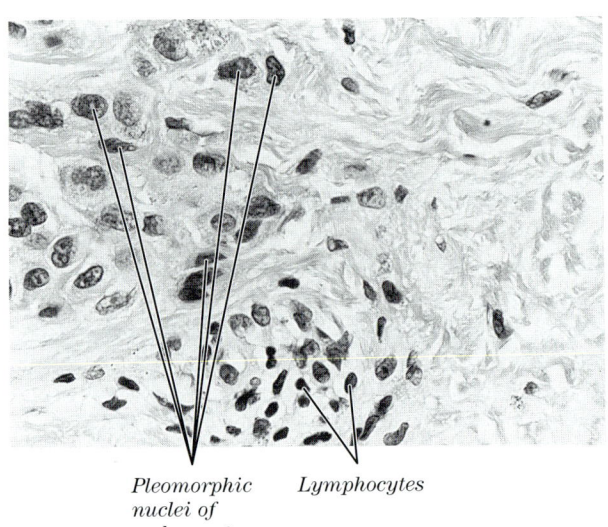

75 • Melanoma (persistent)

Criteria for diagnosis of this persistent melanoma

This is a persistent melanoma because:

1. The neoplasm is confined, in somewhat band-like fashion, to the upper part of the dermis.

2. Prominent fibrosis is apparent in the upper part of the dermis on the right side of the neoplasm, a sign of a previous surgical procedure at this site.

3. Lymphocytes are present around blood vessels in the upper part of the dermis of this relatively superficial neoplasm.

Pitfall in diagnosis

This persistent melanoma could be misinterpreted as a metastasis of melanoma because:

1. The neoplasm is confined entirely to the dermis; there are no evidences of melanoma in situ.

2. The neoplastic cells are strikingly atypical.

3. Aggregations of melanocytes have indistinct boundaries.

4. Many aggregations of melanocytes have become confluent.

5. Melanocytes do not mature.

6. The neoplasm is asymmetric.

Whenever a histopathologist sees a neoplasm that is thought to be either a persistent (recurrent) nevus or a persistent (recurrent) melanoma, sections from the original biopsy specimen should be reviewed. In the case presented here, such review revealed a primary melanoma.

It is far easier to diagnose accurately persistent lesions confined to the dermis, as in this instance, than those confined to the epidermis in which recurrent junctional nevi so often simulate recurrent melanomas.

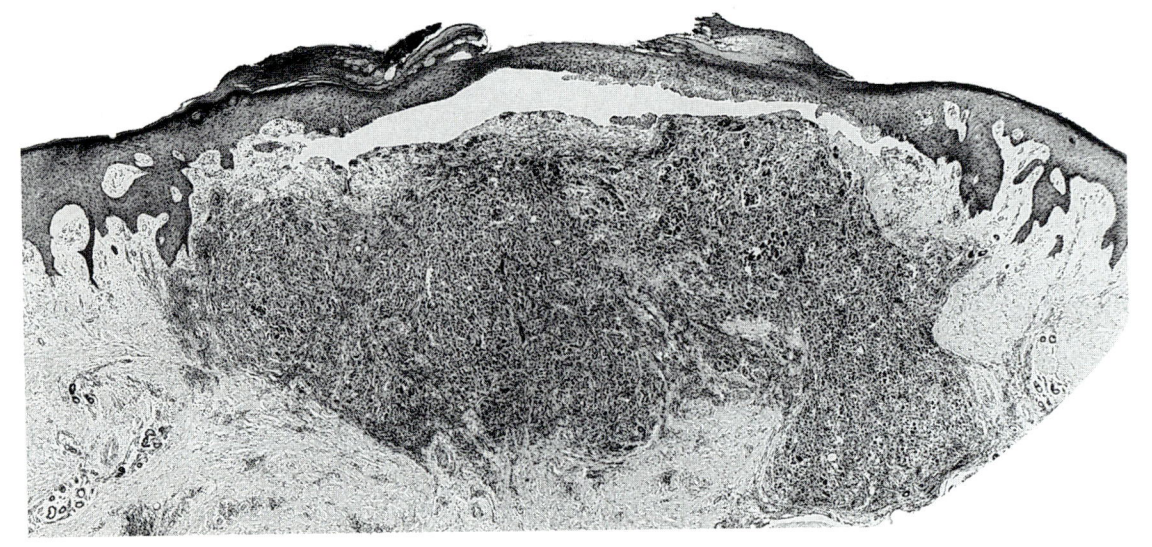

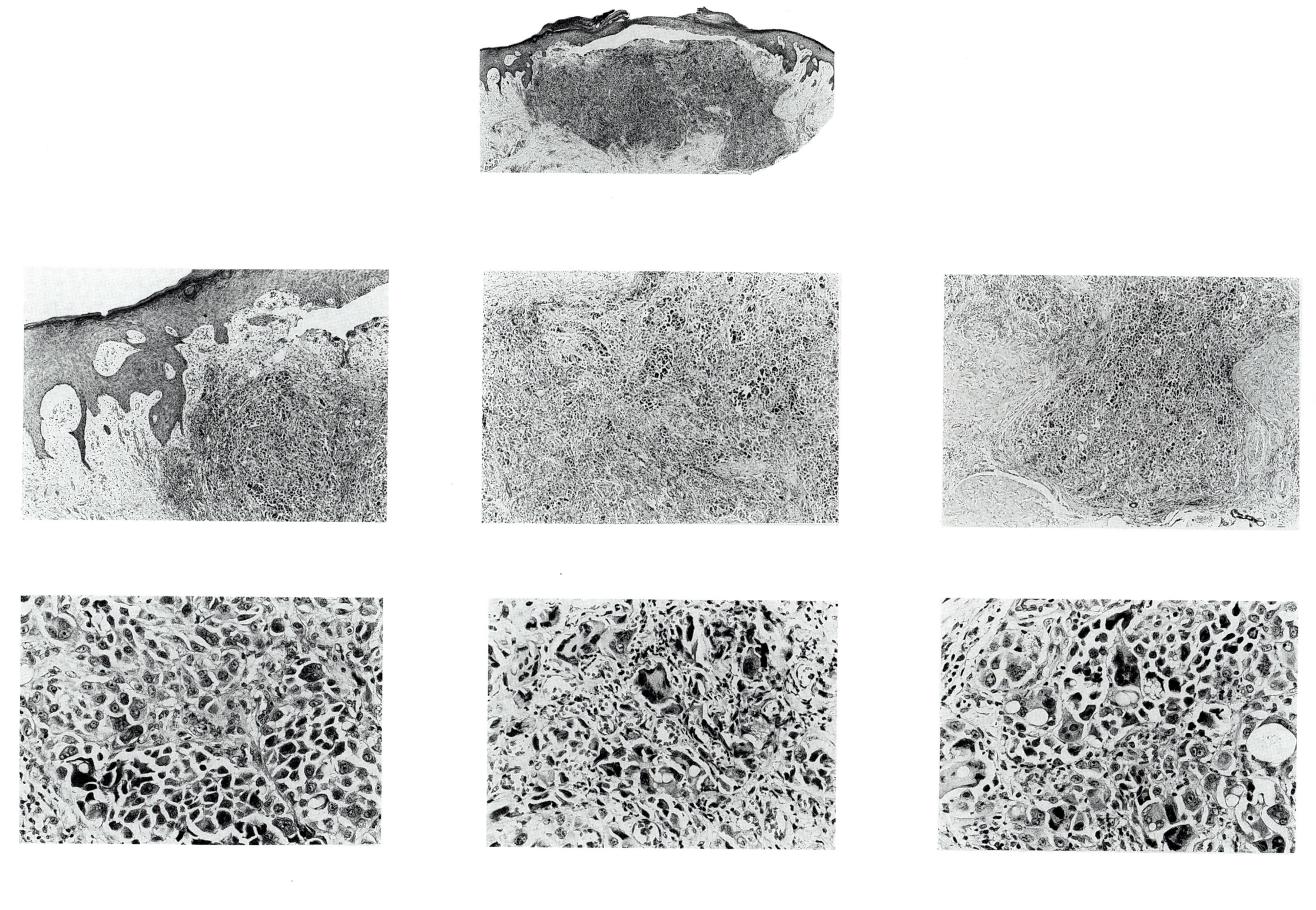

76. What is your diagnosis?

Skin-colored lesion that appeared suddenly on the left leg of a 4-year-old girl. Clinical diagnosis: rule out malignant neoplasm. No evidence of disease was present after 1 year.

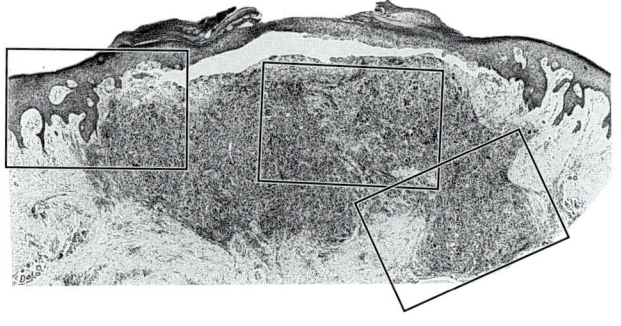

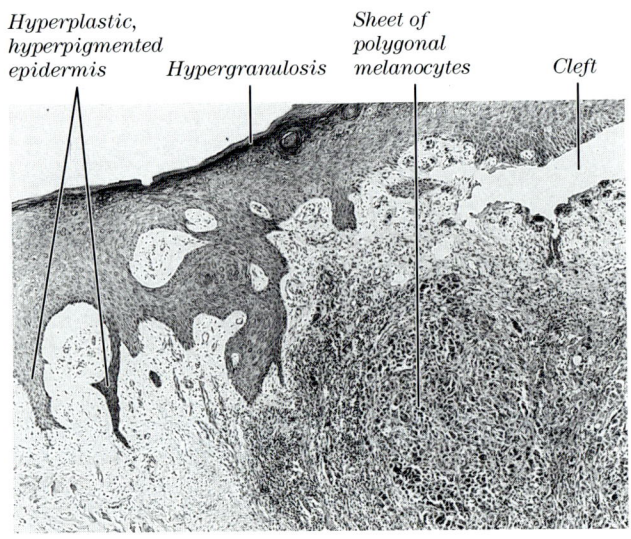

Hyperplastic, hyperpigmented epidermis — Hypergranulosis — Sheet of polygonal melanocytes — Cleft

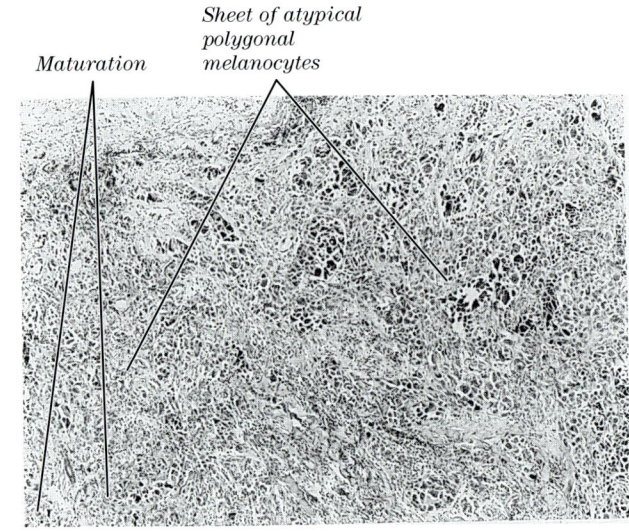

Maturation — Sheet of atypical polygonal melanocytes

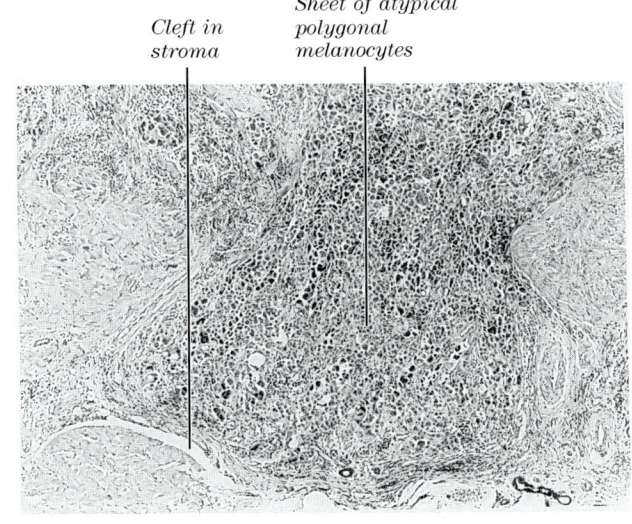

Cleft in stroma — Sheet of atypical polygonal melanocytes

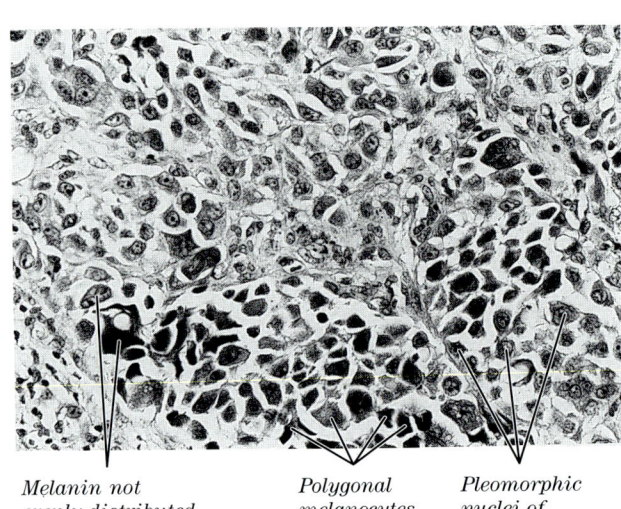

Melanin not evenly distributed — Polygonal melanocytes — Pleomorphic nuclei of melanocytes

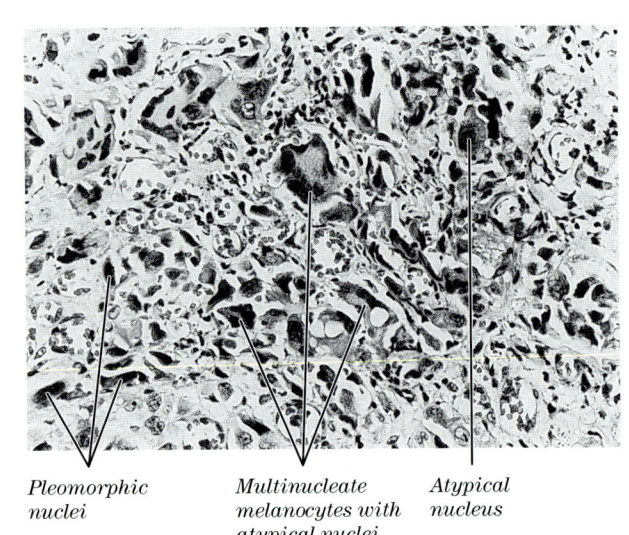

Pleomorphic nuclei — Multinucleate melanocytes with atypical nuclei — Atypical nucleus

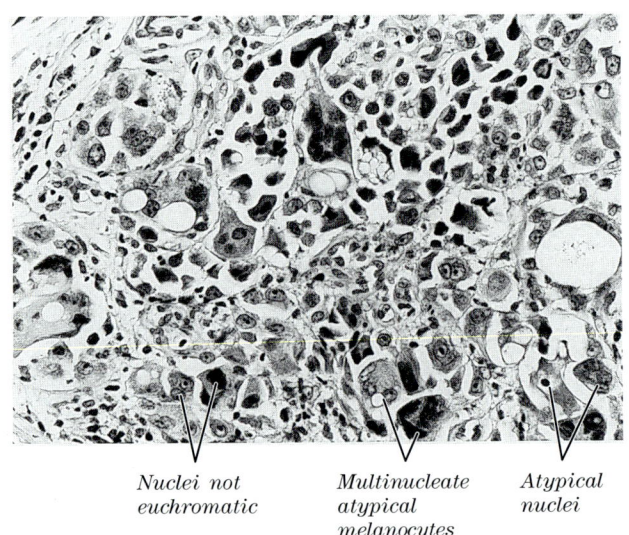

Nuclei not euchromatic — Multinucleate atypical melanocytes — Atypical nuclei

76 • Spitz's Nevus *(persistent)*

Criteria for diagnosis of this persistent Spitz's nevus

This neoplasm is benign because:

1. It is small, yet neoplastic cells extend far into the reticular dermis.
2. It is well-circumscribed.
3. At the base of it, on the right, clefts separate compressed fibrous tissue contiguous with the neoplasm from adjacent normal dermis.
4. Melanocytes mature.

This is a Spitz's nevus because:

1. There are hyperkeratosis, hypergranulosis, and irregular spinous-cell hyperplasia.
2. The polygonal melanocytes are relatively monomorphous.
3. In some high-power fields, many of the melanocytes are multinucleate.

Pitfall in diagnosis

This persistent (recurrent) Spitz's nevus could be misinterpreted as a persistent (recurrent) melanoma because:

1. The neoplasm is asymmetric.
2. There are sheets of melanocytes within the dermis.
3. Some of the melanocytes have atypical nuclei.
4. The base of the neoplasm is irregular.

A major hazard for histopathologists impressed overly with cytologic features is equation of extraordinary cytologic atypia of melanocytes with melanoma. That thesis is given the lie in this Spitz's nevus. The neoplasm is benign, despite striking cytologic atypia, because of its silhouette, namely, it is narrow but thick, and it is very well-circumscribed.

That this neoplasm is persistent can be inferred from the presence of a scar and of a subepidermal cleft which represents faulty adhesion between the fibrotic dermis and the newly re-formed epidermis.

The terms "persistent" and "recurrent" in this context are interchangeable because the neoplasms are truly persistent, but they also are recurrent.

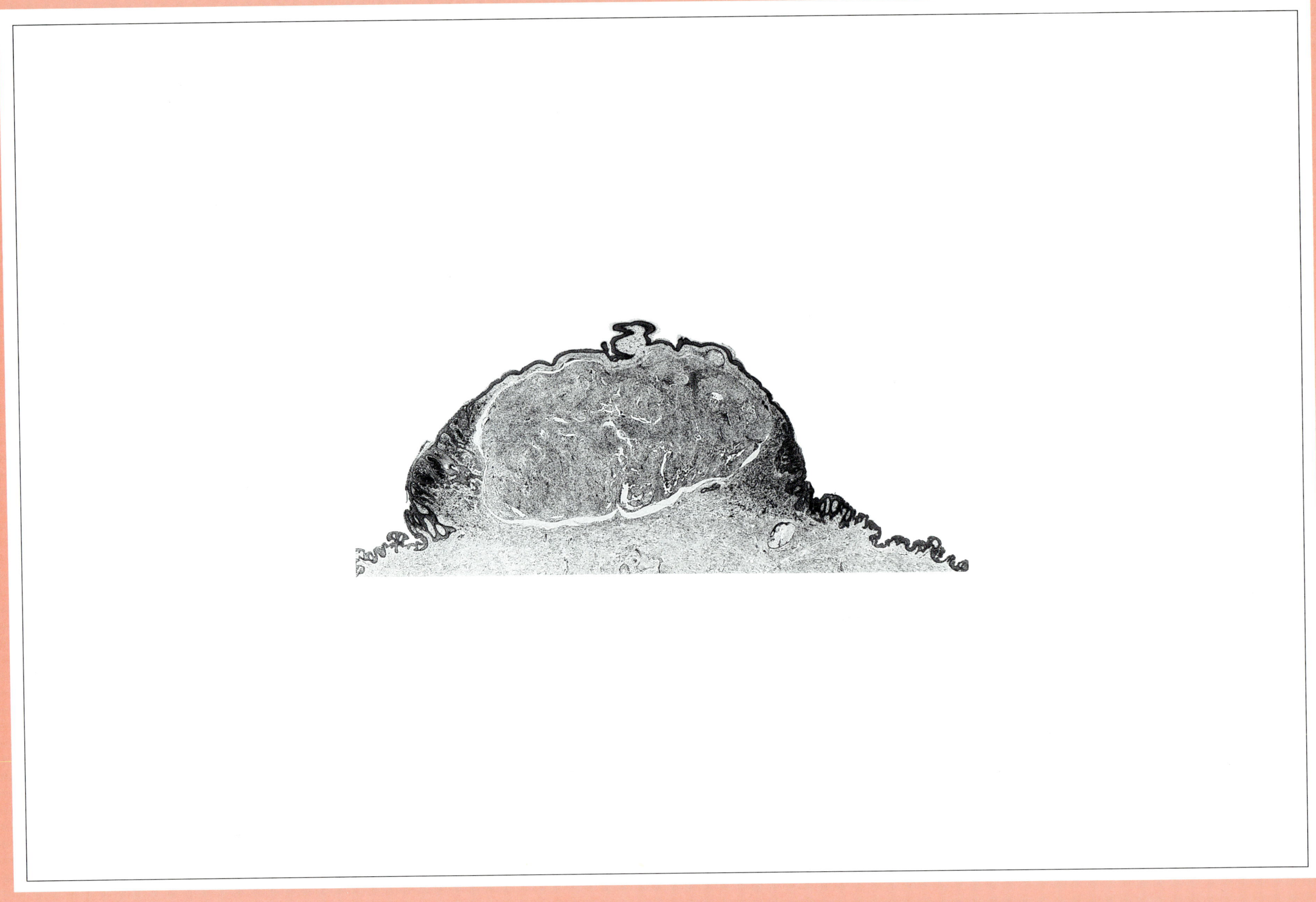

572

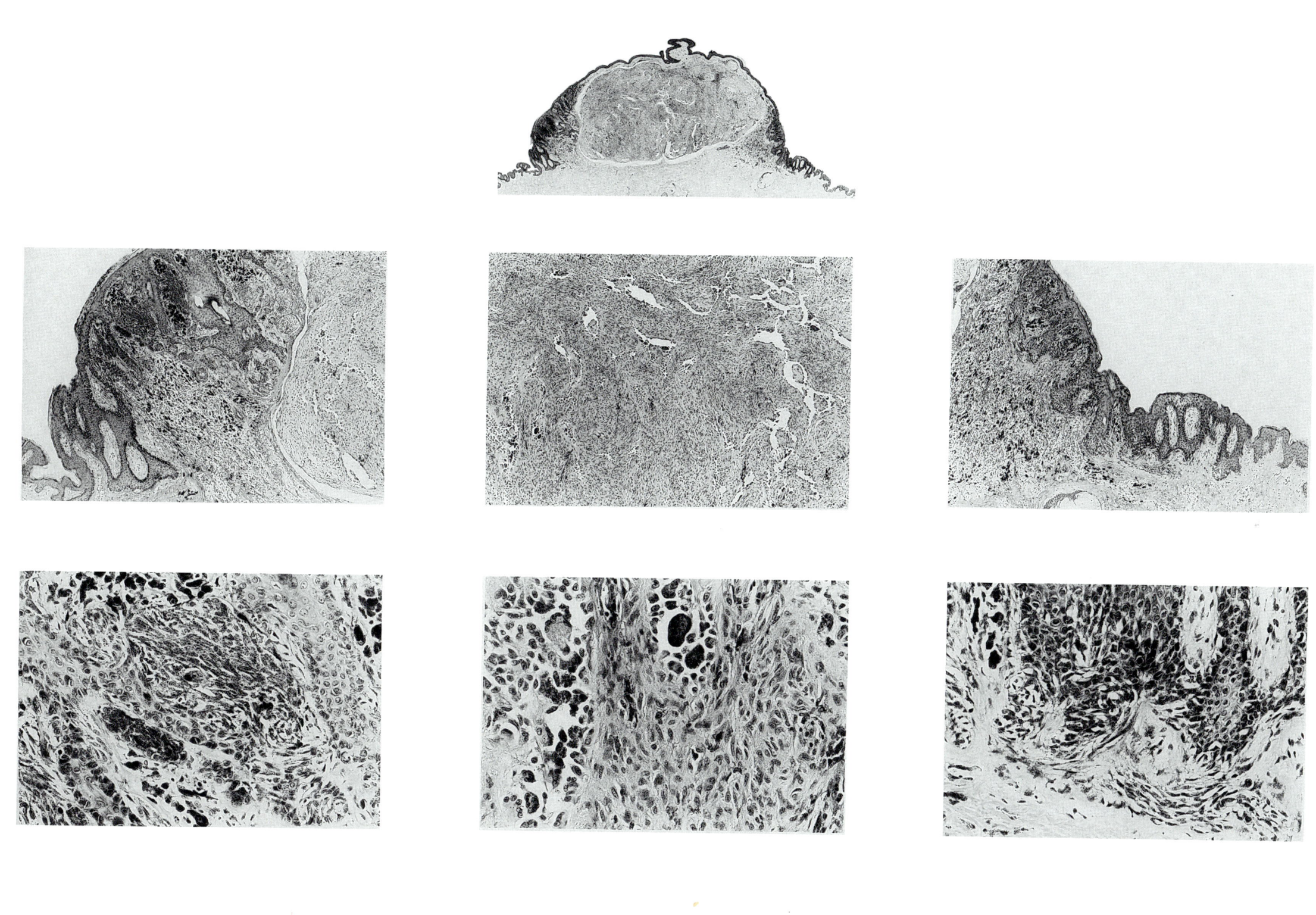

77. What is your diagnosis?

Pigmented macule on the right flank of a 24-year-old woman was present since childhood. No clinical diagnosis or follow-up data were available.

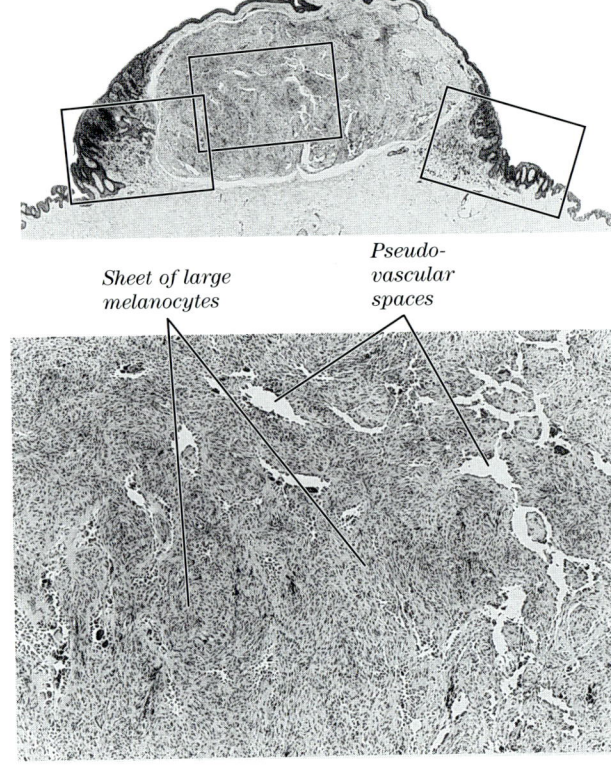

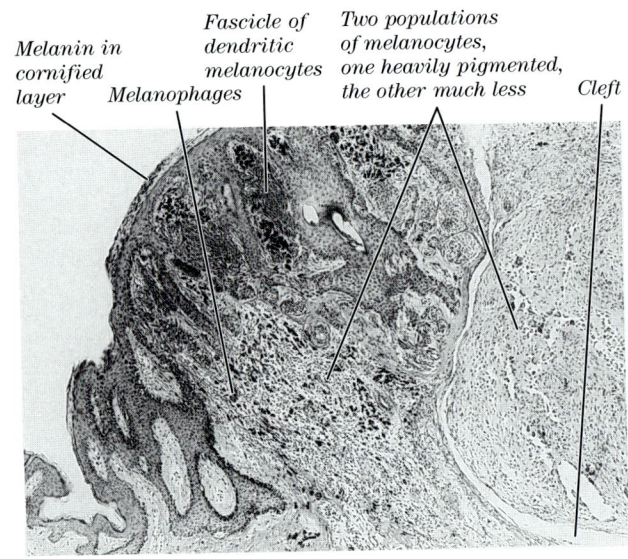

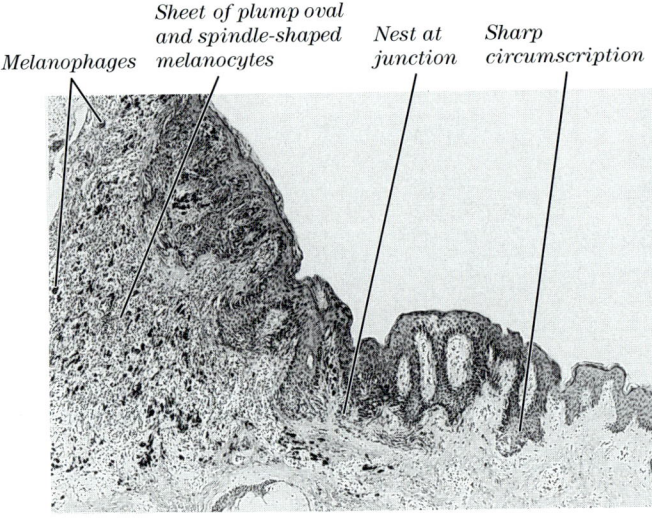

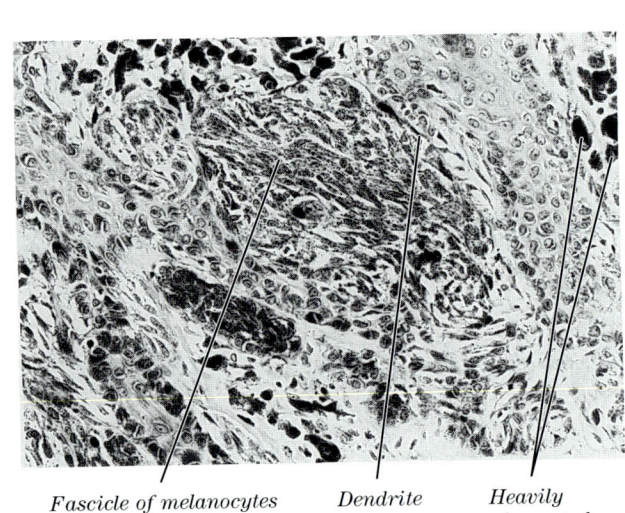

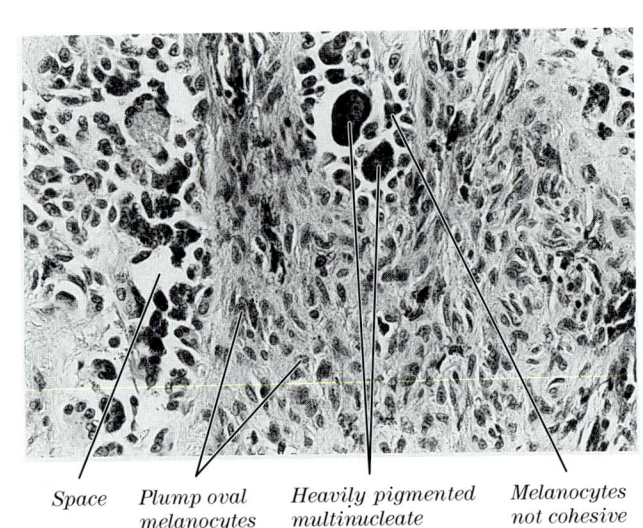

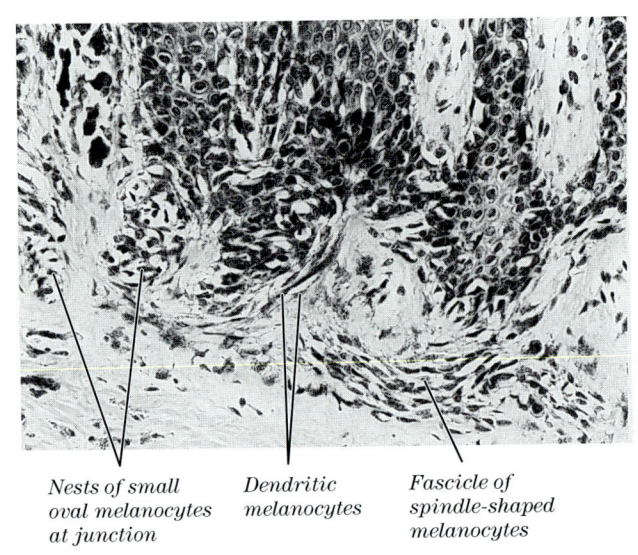

77 • Blue Nevus (combined type)

Criteria for diagnosis of this blue nevus (combined type)

This lesion is benign because:

1. The neoplasm is symmetric topographically.
2. The neoplasm is well-circumscribed.
3. Melanocytes mature.

This neoplasm is a combined blue nevus because:

1. There are two distinct components, one markedly pigmented at the periphery and one much less pigmented in the center, and both have the architectural character of a benign neoplasm—sharp circumscription and maturation of melanocytes.
2. In the strikingly pigmented zone, the nuclei of melanocytes are monomorphous; those in the less pigmented zone are monomorphous also.
3. Pigment is distributed relatively uniformly both in the heavily pigmented zone and in the much less pigmented one.
4. Prominent clefts separate the less pigmented central zone from the heavily pigmented peripheral one.
5. Prominent clefts with jagged outlines are present throughout the central portion of the neoplasm.

Pitfall in diagnosis

This combined blue nevus could be misinterpreted as a melanoma that developed within a pre-existing nevus because:

1. The silhouette of the central component is asymmetric, and so, too, is the peripheral pigmented component.
2. The character of the neoplastic melanocytes in zones of different pigmentation differ.
3. The quantity of melanin in the two components of the neoplasm differs.
4. The deeply pigmented multinucleate melanocytes in the less pigmented zone could be misconstrued as atypical melanocytes.

This unusual melanocytic nevus consists mostly of darkly pigmented dendritic melanocytes at its periphery and of lightly pigmented non-dendritic melanocytes, many of which are binucleate and multinucleate, in its center. These features are most consonant with a blue nevus comprising two populations of melanocytes, analogous to the situation in Masson's blue neuro-nevus.

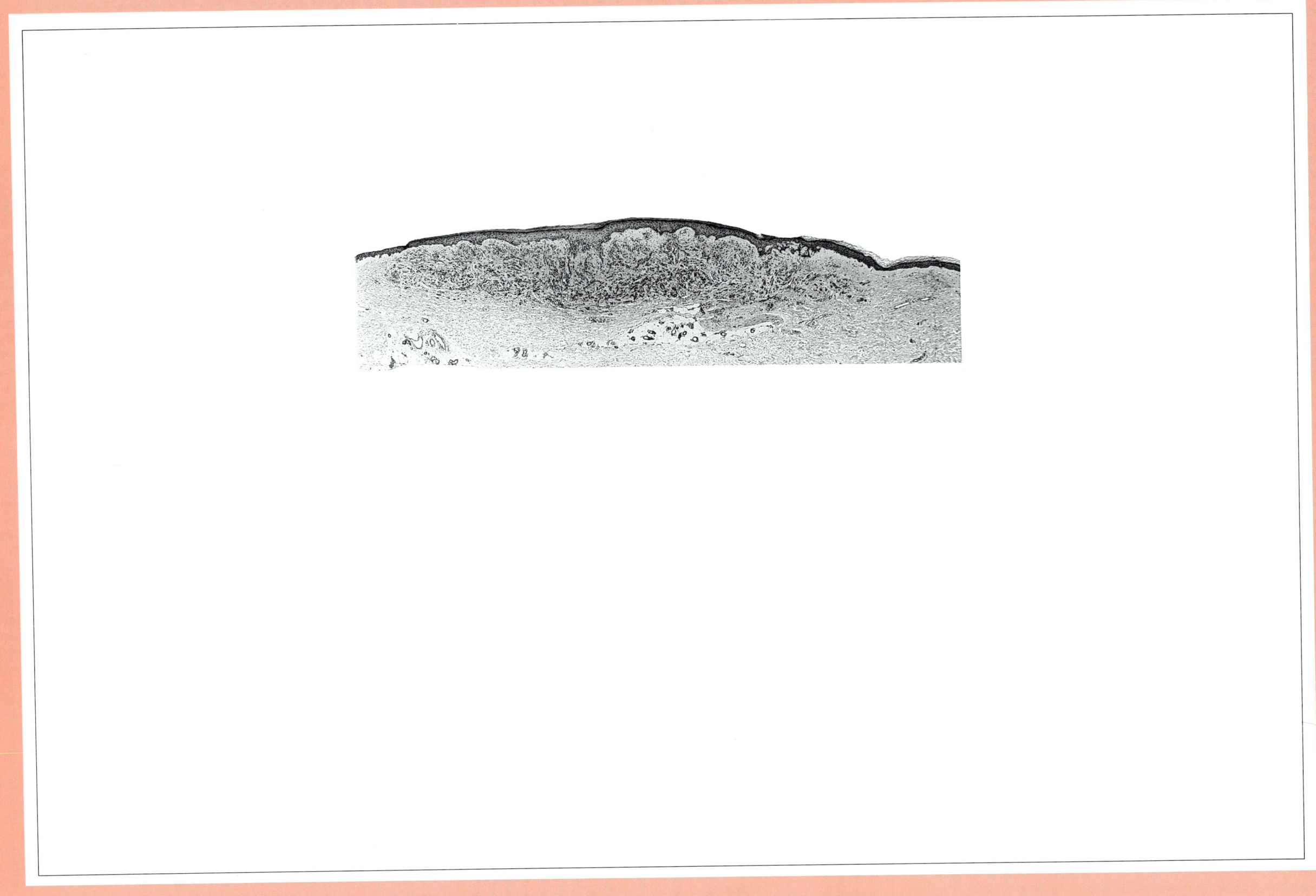

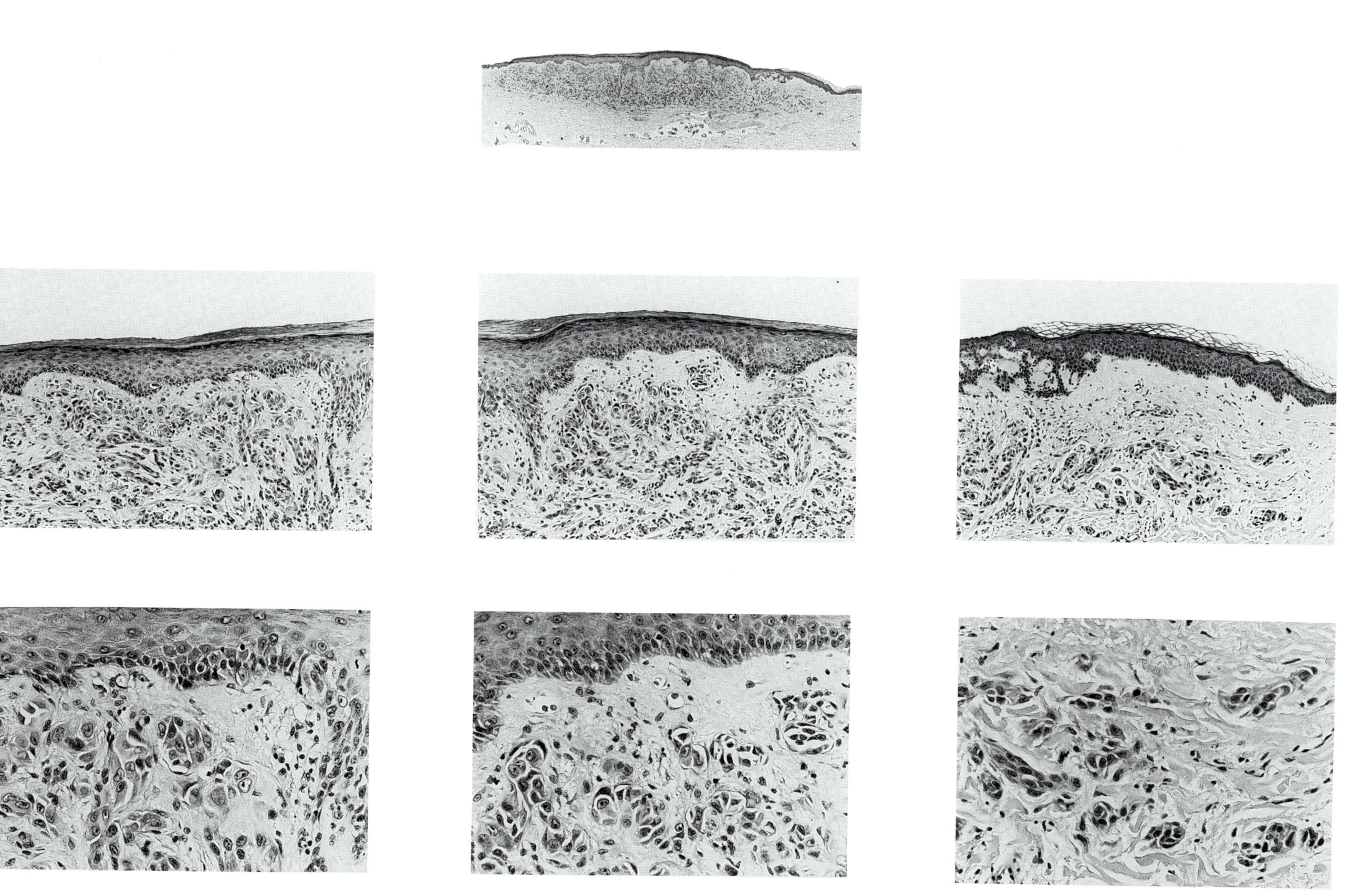

78. What is your diagnosis?

Pink papule on the lateral aspect of the right leg of a 68-year-old woman. Clinical diagnosis: metastatic melanoma. Patient was alive and well after 2 years.

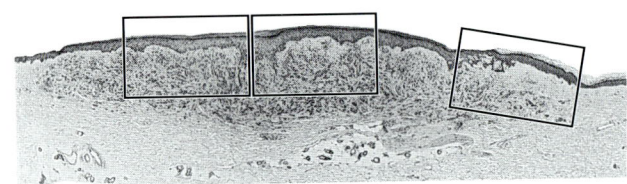

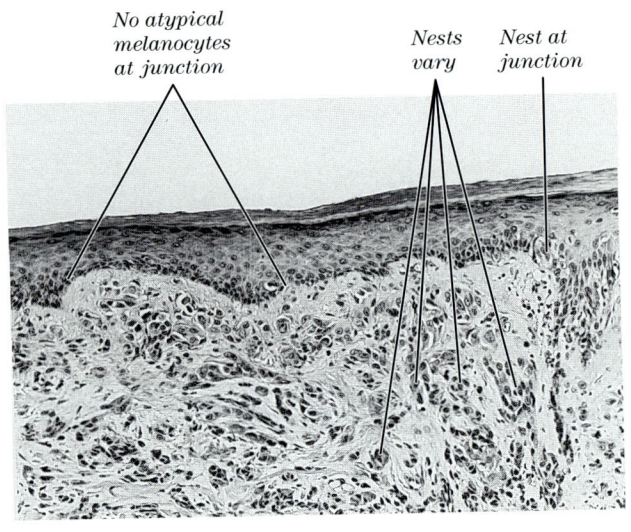

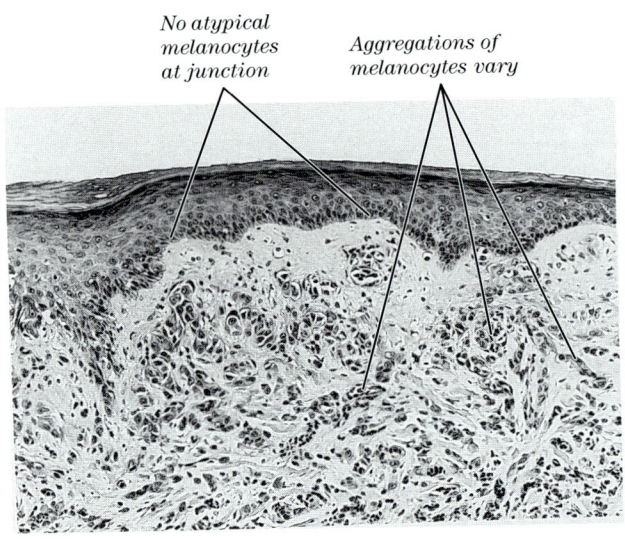

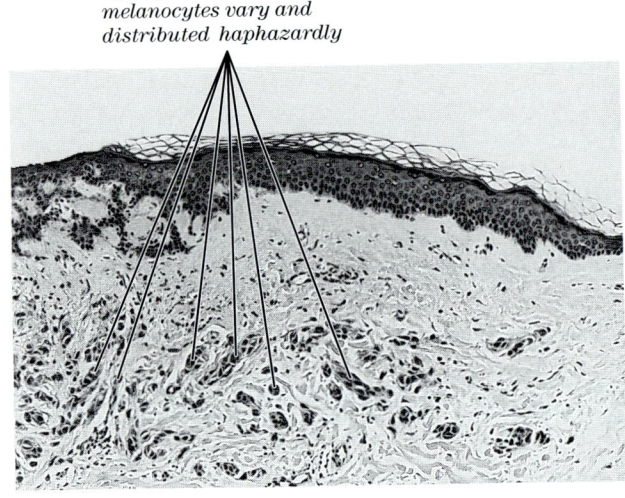

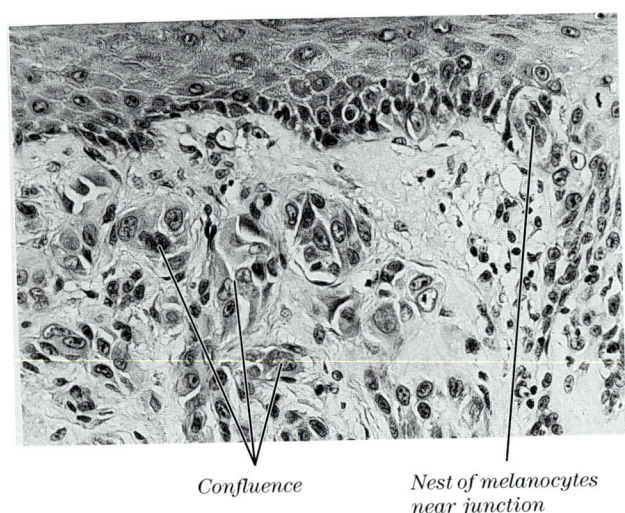

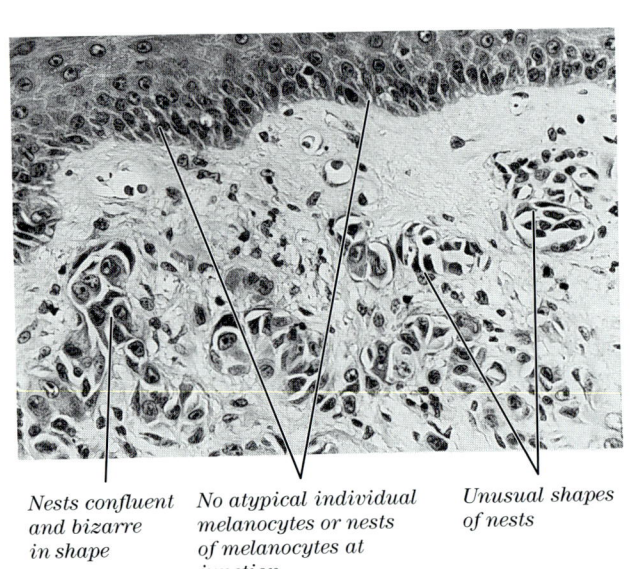

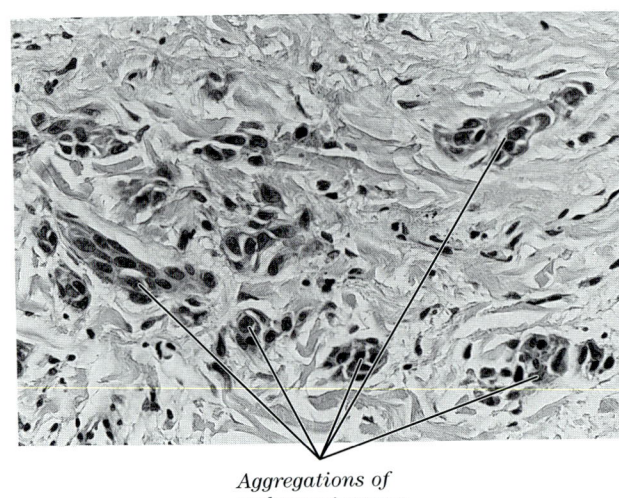

78 • Metastasis of Melanoma

Criteria for diagnosis of this metastasis of melanoma

This is a metastasis of melanoma because:

1. The neoplasm is asymmetric.

2. Across the entire front of the neoplasm, only a single nest of melanocytes is present within the epidermis.

3. Aggregations of neoplastic cells differ in size and shape.

4. Aggregations of neoplastic cells are arranged haphazardly.

5. Some neoplastic cells are arrayed in very elongated fascicles.

6. Hardly any infiltrate of lymphocytes is seen.

Pitfall in diagnosis

This metastasis of melanoma could be misinterpreted as a compound Spitz's nevus because:

1. The neoplasm is slightly wedge-shaped.

2. Hyperkeratosis, hypergranulosis, and epidermal hyperplasia are evident in foci.

3. Nuclei of melanocytes are atypical.

4. Melanocytes are mostly polygonal and oval.

5. Within nests, discrete clefts are present among polygonal melanocytes.

6. Some melanocytes at the base of the neoplasm are smaller than those above them.

This epidermotropically metastatic melanoma simulates a compound Spitz's nevus. In some foci, it is virtually impossible to distinguish cytologically between atypical polygonal cells of Spitz's nevus and their analogues in melanoma. An important clue to distinguishing a Spitz's nevus constituted of polygonal melanocytes from a metastasis of melanoma of similar composition is relative absence in the metastasis of melanocytes arranged as solitary units and in nests at the dermo-epidermal junction, unlike the situation in primary melanomas and in Spitz's nevi where these findings are expected. Absence of neoplastic melanocytes of melanoma from the dermo-epidermal junction indicates that this neoplasm is a metastasis.

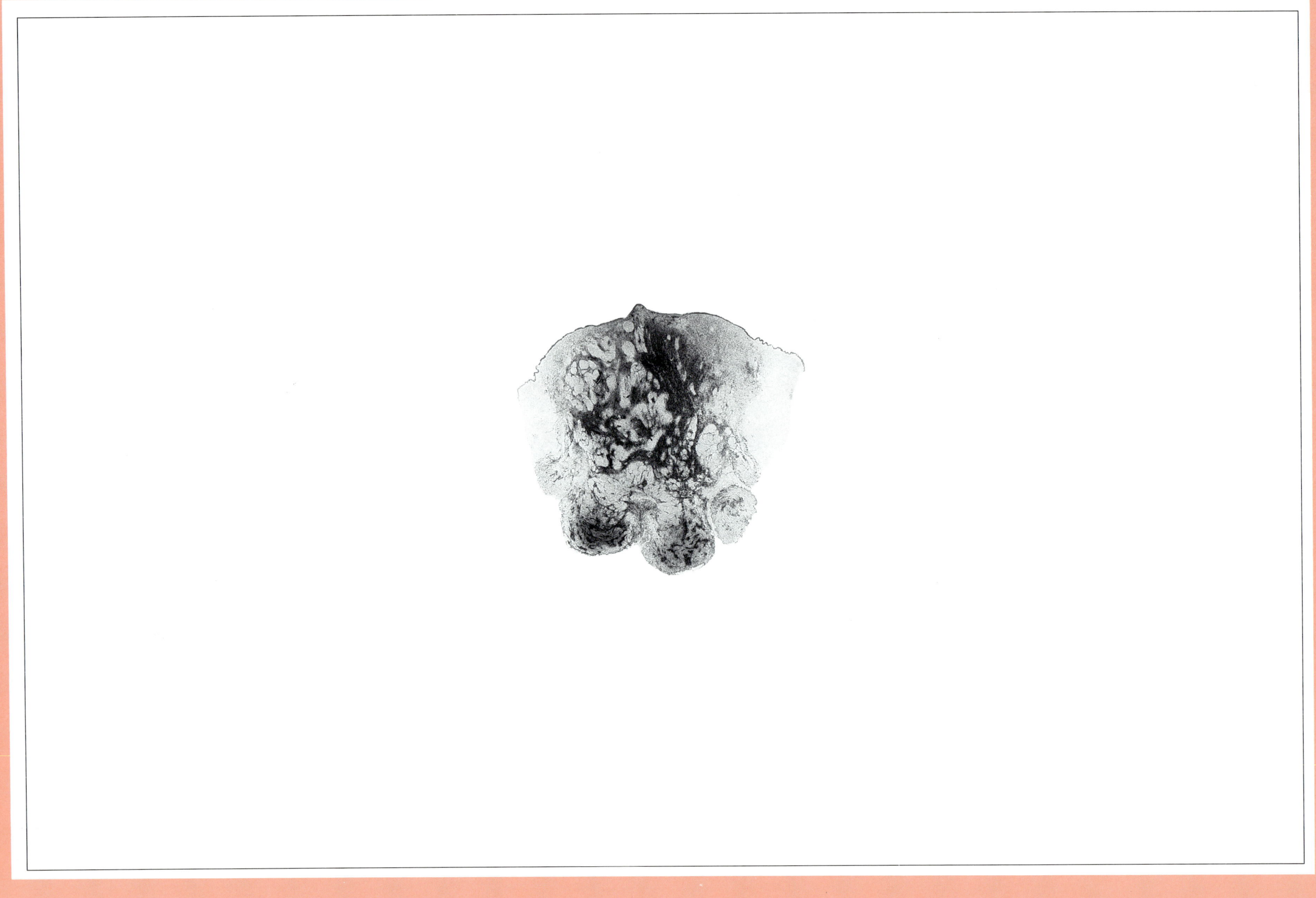

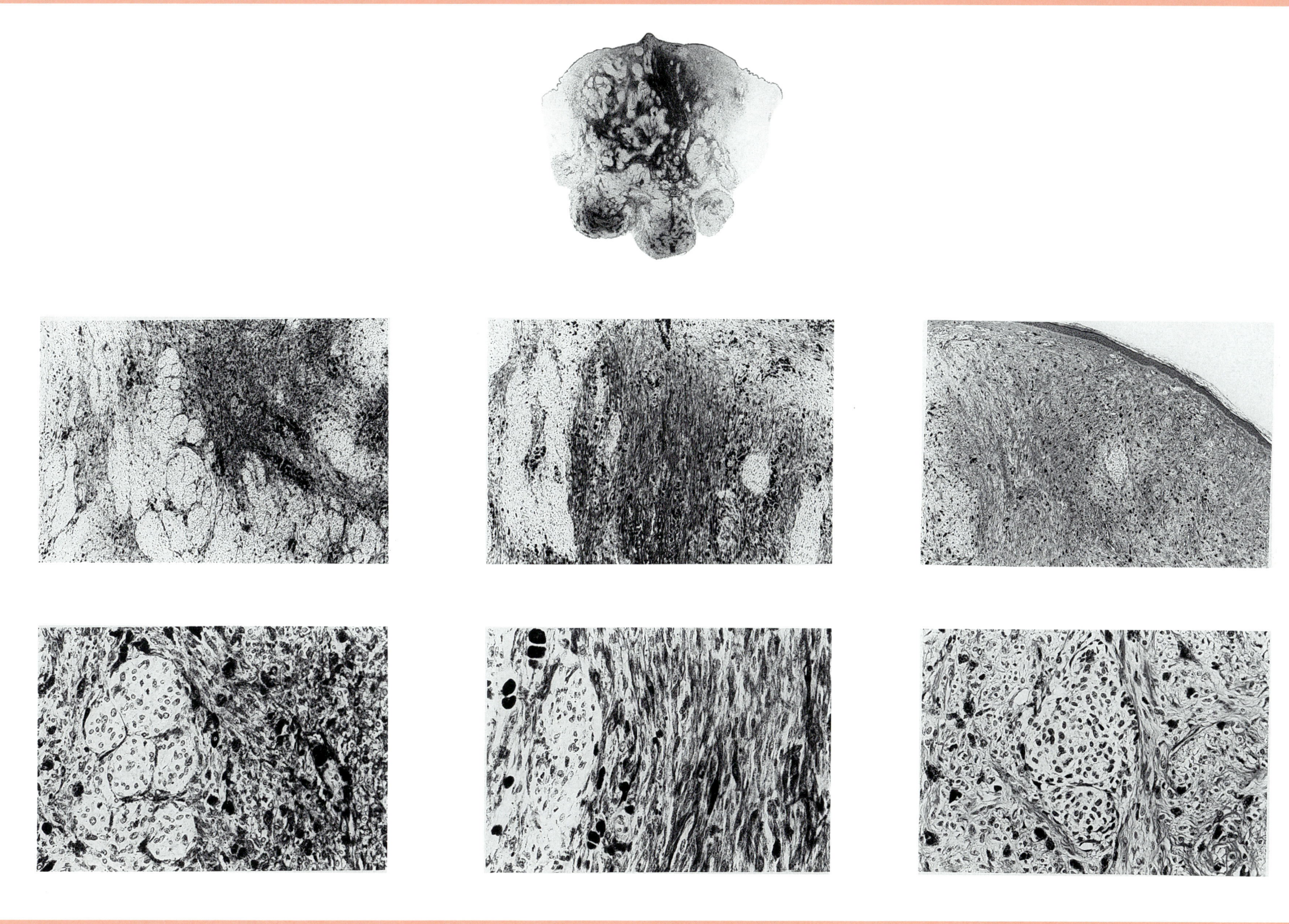

79. What is your diagnosis?

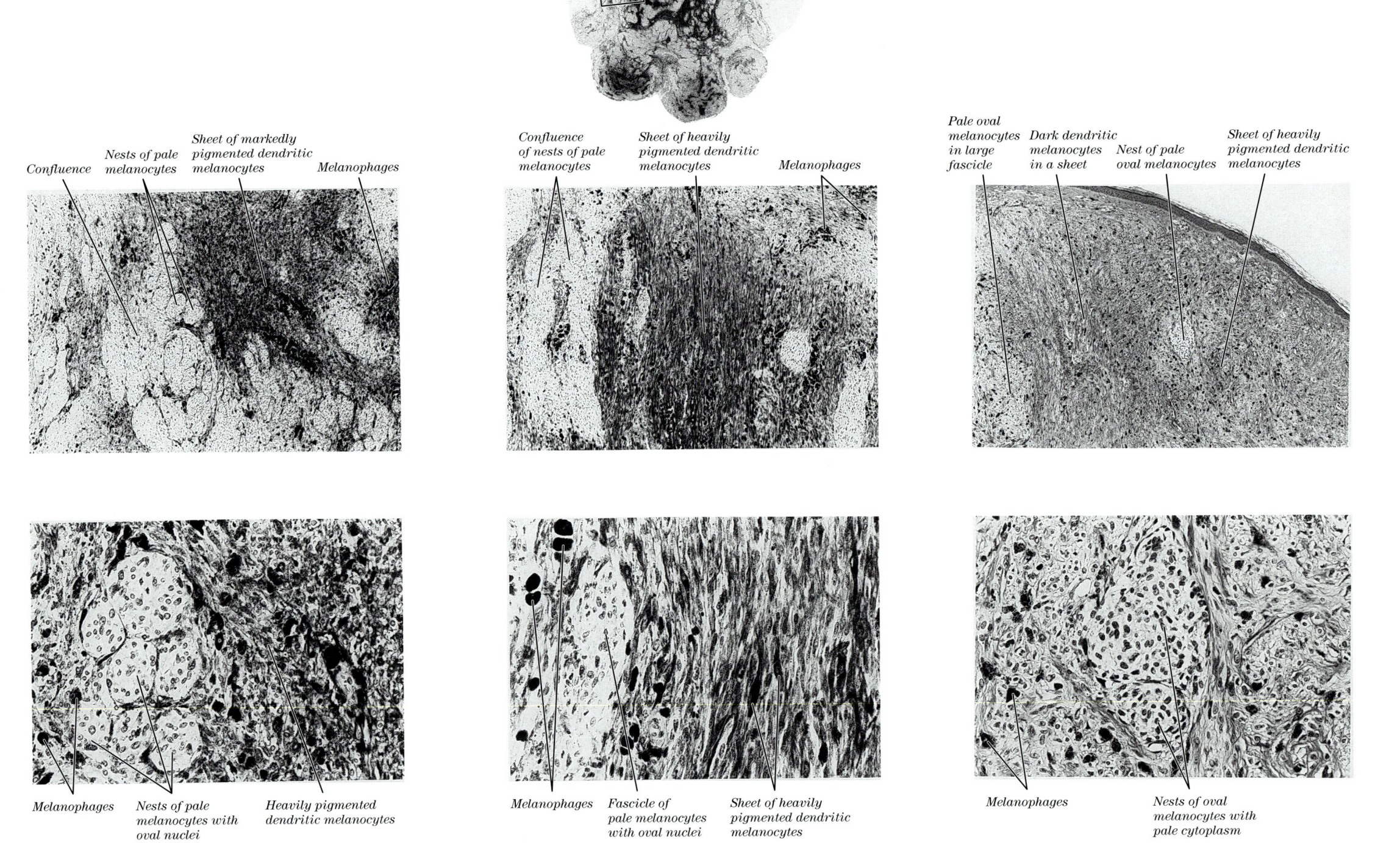

79 • Blue Nevus of Masson (deep dendritic and non-dendritic type)

Criteria for diagnosis of this blue nevus (deep dendritic and non-dendritic type)

This lesion is benign because:

1. The neoplasm is oriented vertically.
2. It is well-circumscribed.
3. Nests of melanocytes within the dermis are discrete and well-circumscribed.

This is a blue nevus because:

1. There are two populations of melanocytes: darkly pigmented dendritic ones and lightly pigmented, non-dendritic round and oval ones.
2. Nuclei of both types of melanocytes are typical.
3. There are no mitotic figures in melanocytes.

Pitfall in diagnosis

This blue nevus of Masson could be misdiagnosed as a so-called malignant blue nevus because:

1. The neoplasm is asymmetric.
2. Melanin is distributed in uneven fashion within the neoplasm.
3. Neoplastic melanocytes extend far into the subcutaneous fat.
4. Many nests of melanocytes have become confluent.

For the aforementioned reasons, this lesion represents one type of blue nevus. Parenthetically, we do not accept the concept of "malignant blue nevus," because all malignant neoplasms of melanocytes are melanomas. A melanoma may arise in a blue nevus, and exceedingly rarely at that, but a blue nevus cannot be malignant; it always is benign.

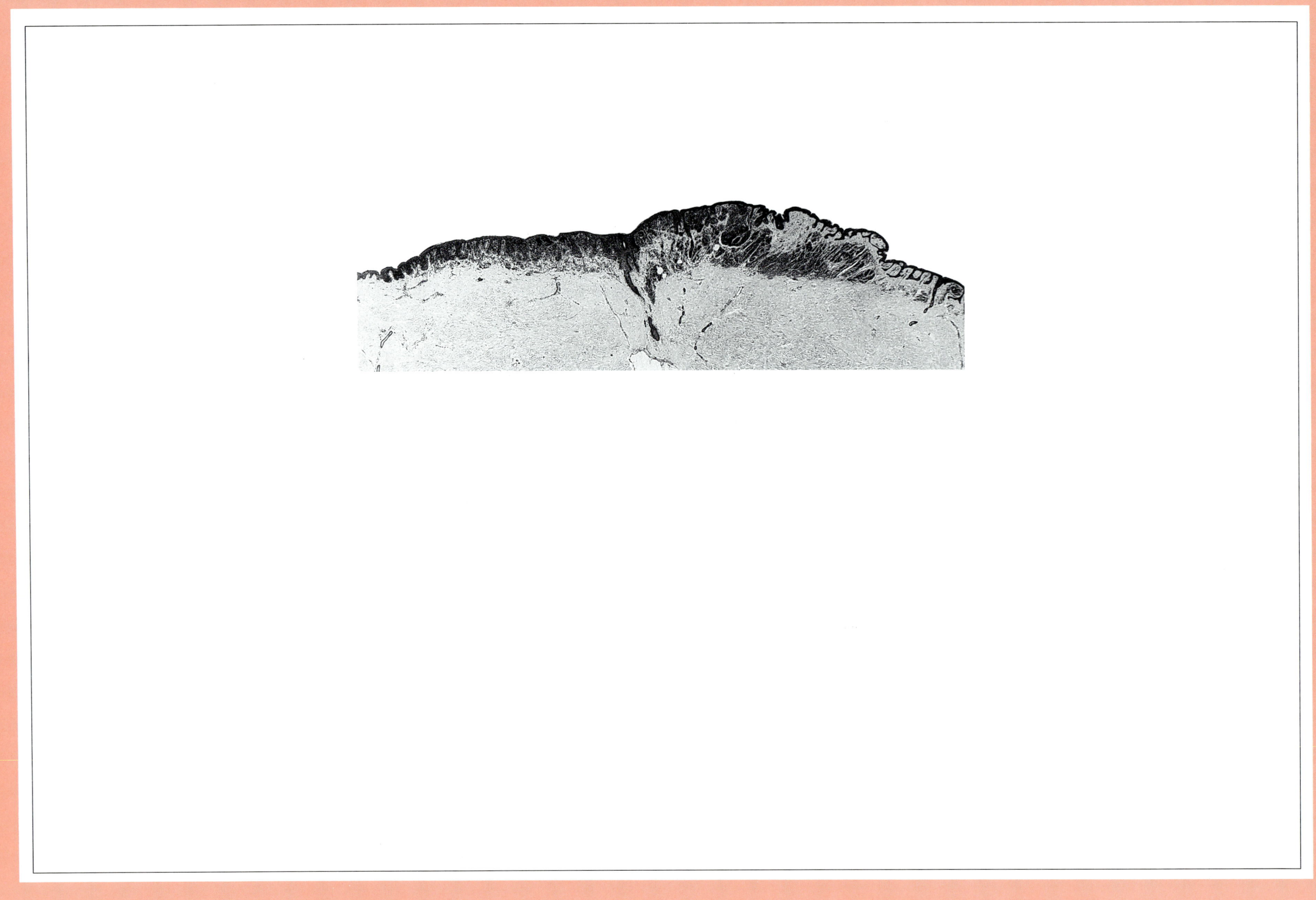

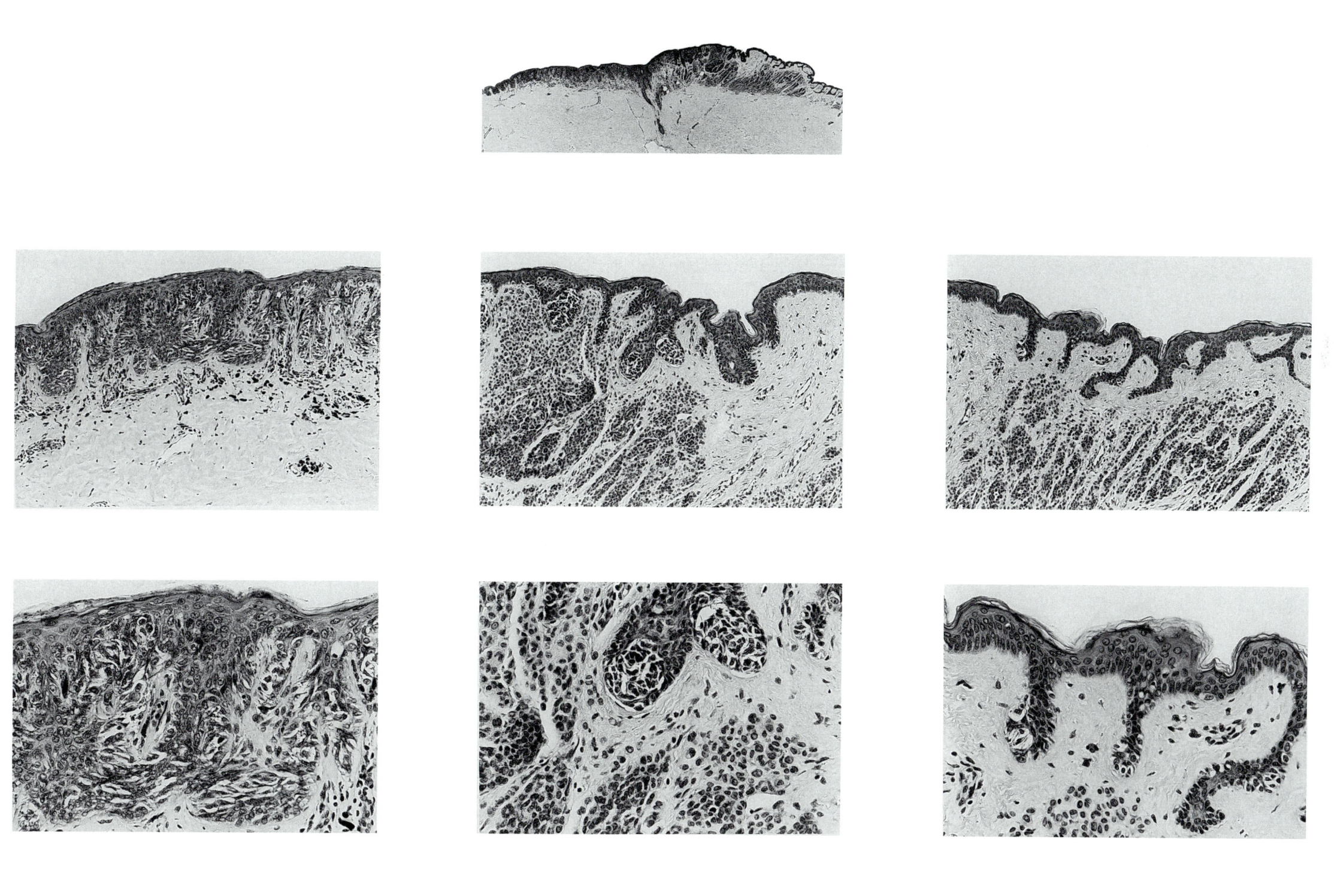

80. What is your diagnosis?

Long-standing, unevenly pigmented lesion on the back of a 45-year-old woman. Clinical diagnosis: compound nevus. Patient was free of disease after 3 years.

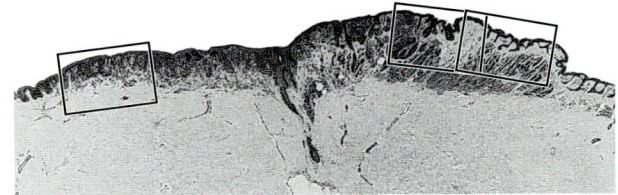

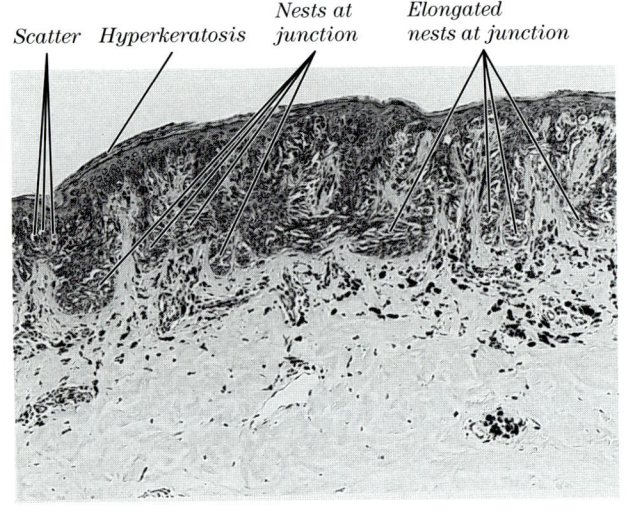
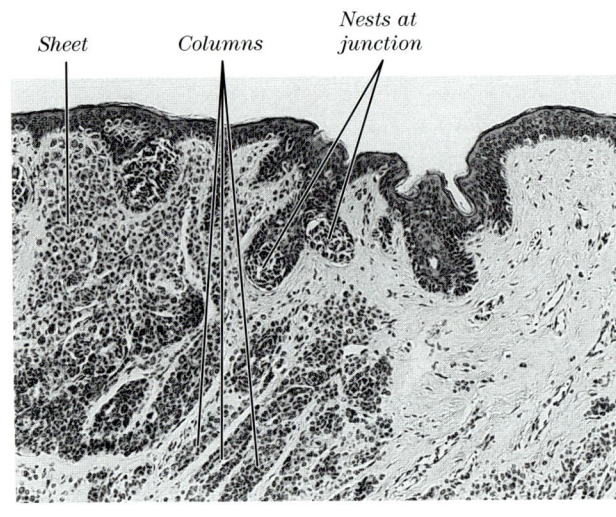
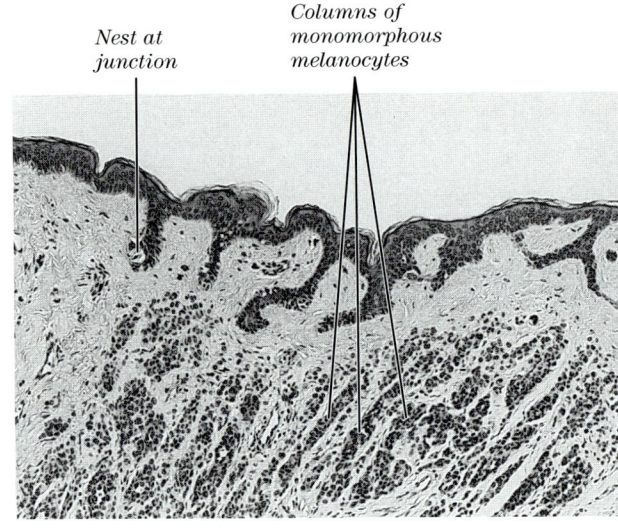
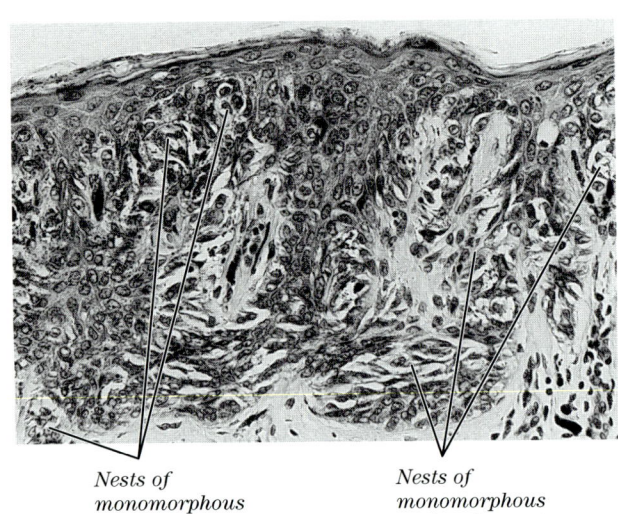
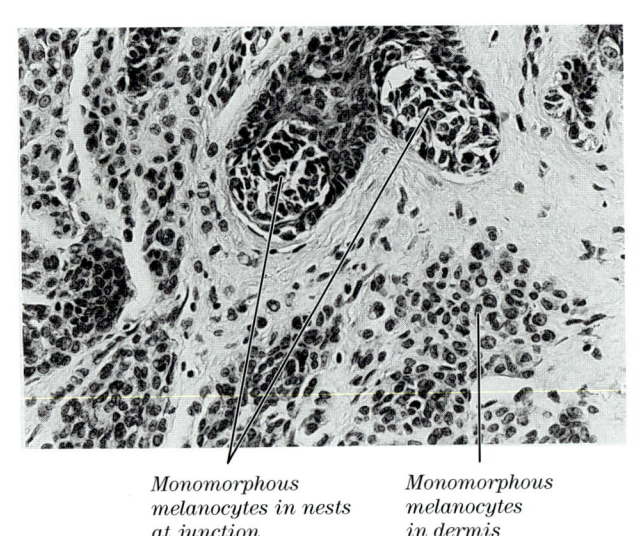
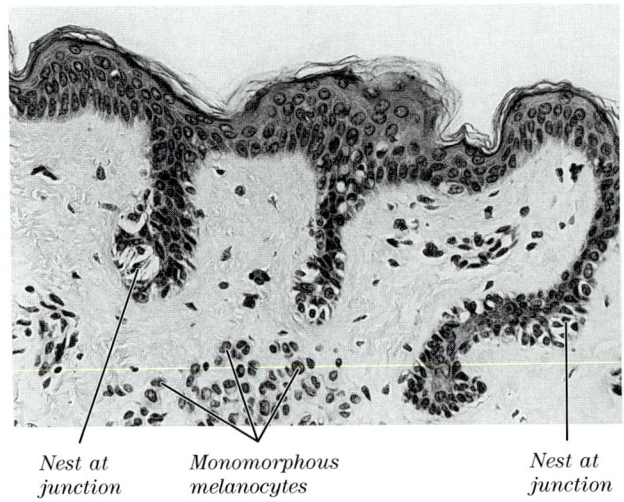

80 • Combined Nevus *(Spitz's and Clark's)*

Criteria for diagnosis of this combined nevus (Spitz's and Clark's)

This is a nevus because:

1. The neoplasm is well-circumscribed.
2. It has a flat bottom that rests upon the reticular dermis.
3. Melanocytes within the epidermis, both those arranged as solitary units and those in nests, are situated mostly at the dermo-epidermal junction.
4. Melanocytes mature.
5. Melanocytes in each component of the neoplasm have monomorphous nuclei.

This is a combined nevus because:

1. The pattern of the neoplasm on the left is different from that on the right (on the left the surface is a near plateau with gentle mammillations, whereas on the right it is more elevated and more papillated).
2. Cytologic features in the component on the left are different from those on the right (those on the left are plump oval and arranged in fascicles, whereas those on the right are roundish and arranged in nests).
3. The component on the left is confined to the epidermis, whereas that on the right is located in both the epidermis and the dermis.
4. The component on the left is heavily pigmented by melanin within melanocytes, keratinocytes, and macrophages, whereas the component on the right has hardly any melanin.
5. No fibroplasia accompanies the component on the left, whereas notable fibroplasia and telangiectases join the component on the right.

Pitfall in diagnosis

This combined nevus with features of Spitz's nevus and Clark's nevus could be confused with a melanoma in situ that began in association with a pre-existing compound Clark's nevus because:

1. The neoplasm is asymmetric.
2. Melanin is not distributed in uniform fashion throughout it.
3. Some melanocytes that reside in the Spitz's nevus component are present above the dermo-epidermal junction.
4. Fibroplasia is present focally.

Combined nevi, like melanomas, are asymmetric and often are constituted of more than one population of melanocytes. If the components of a neoplasm such as this one are studied separately, it becomes apparent that the component on the right is a Clark's nevus and the one on the left is a pigmented spindle-cell variant of Spitz's nevus.

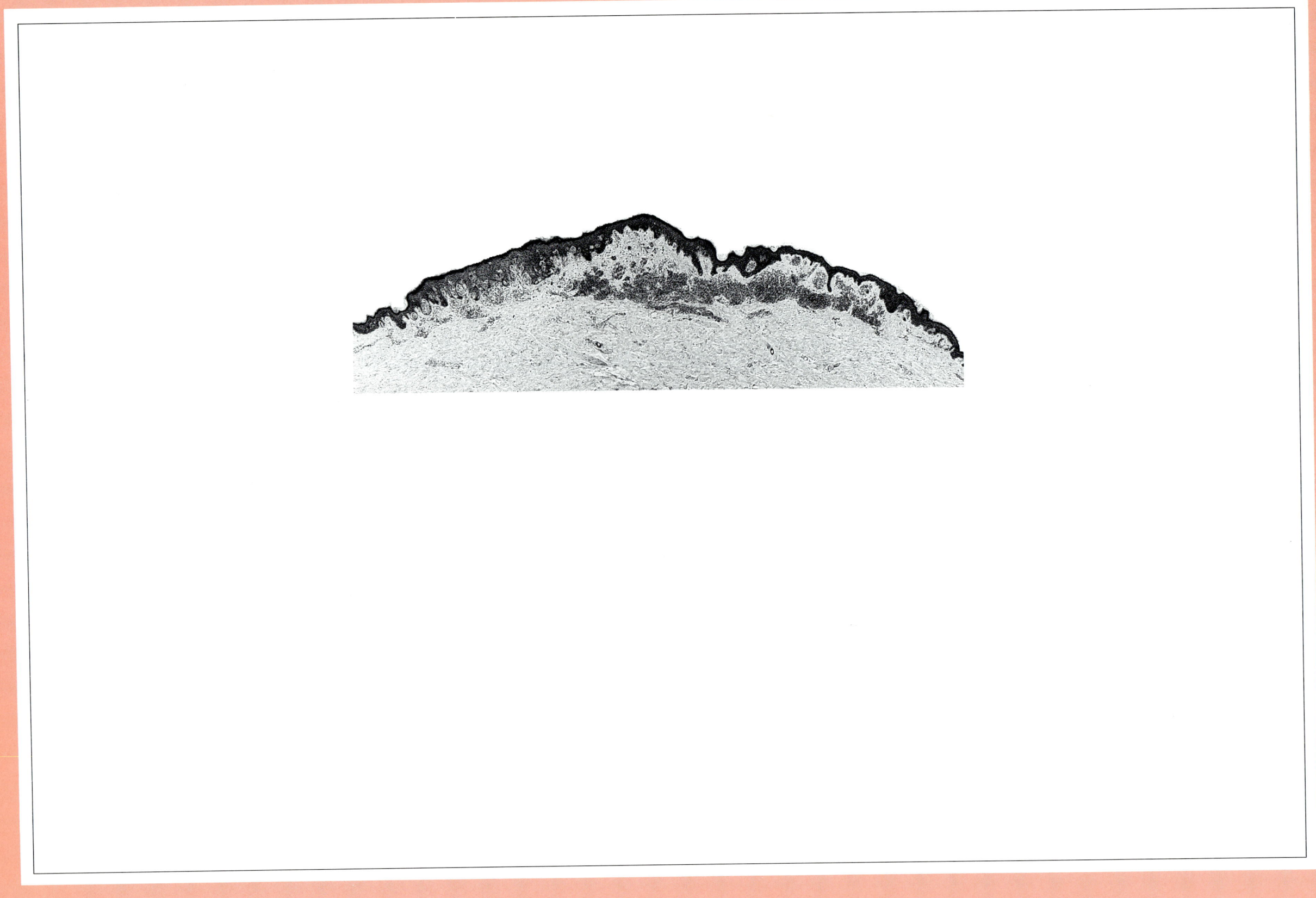

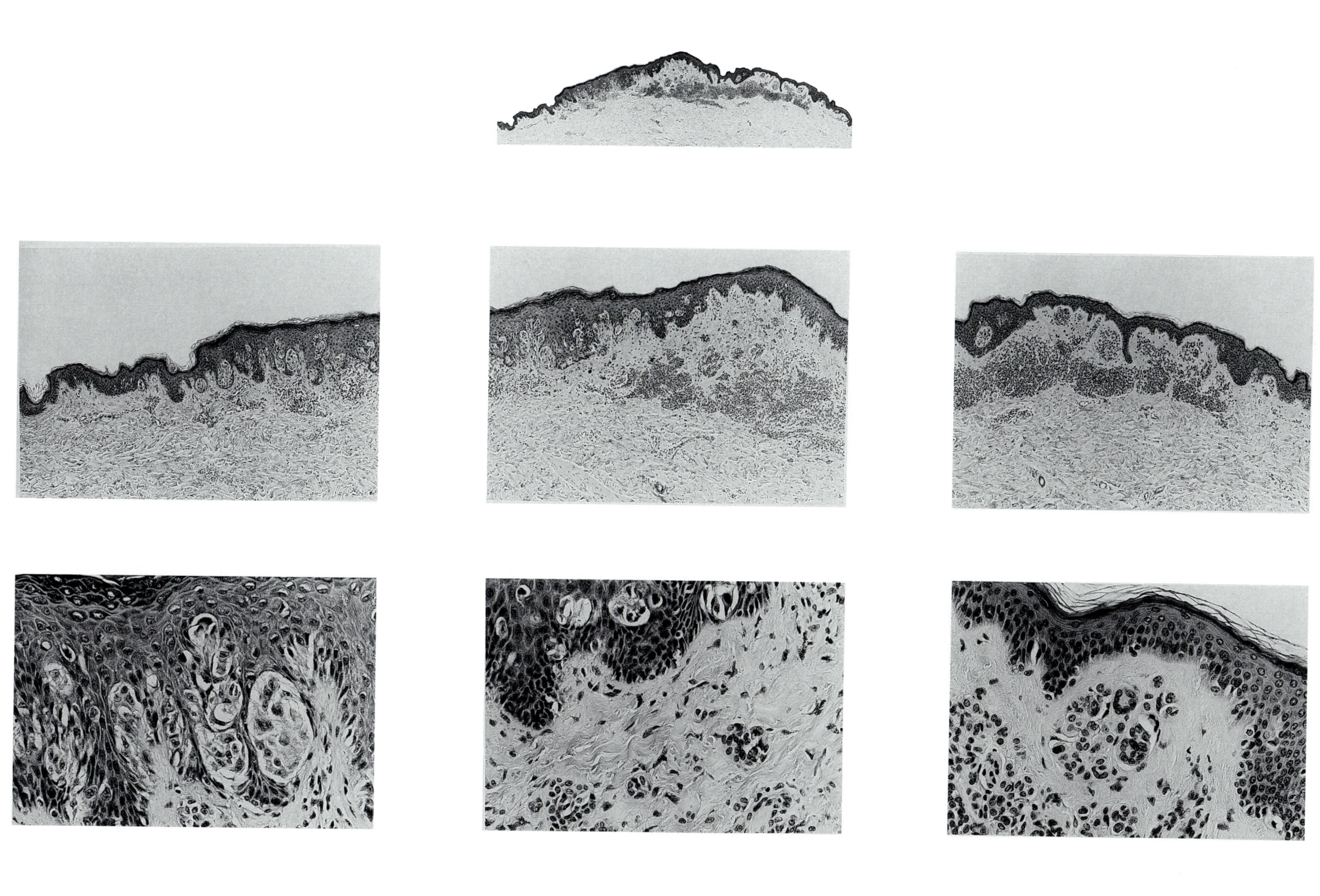

81. What is your diagnosis?

Pigmented lesion of unknown duration on the left anterior thigh of a 19-year-old woman. Clinical diagnosis: pigmented nevus. No follow-up data were available.

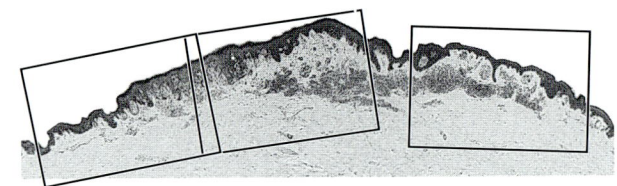

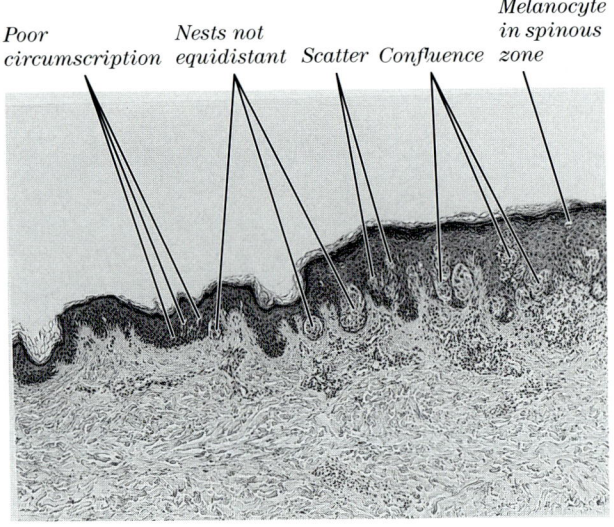

Poor circumscription — Nests not equidistant — Scatter — Confluence — Melanocyte in spinous zone

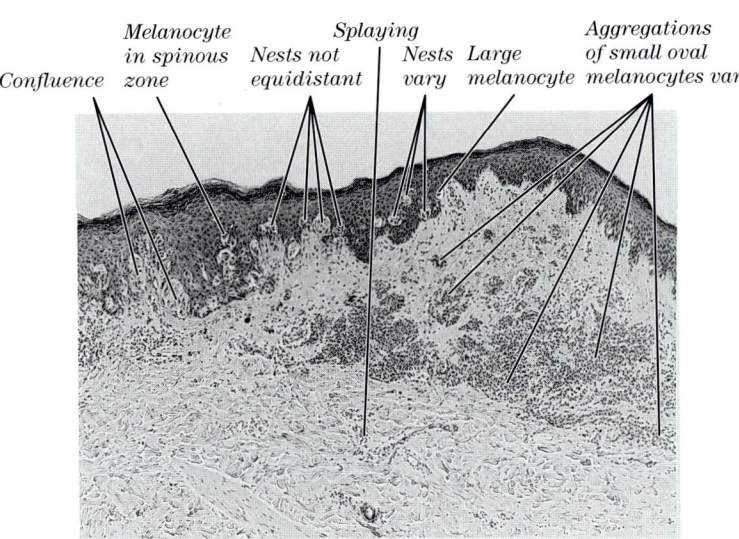

Confluence — Melanocyte in spinous zone — Nests not equidistant — Nests vary — Splaying — Large melanocyte — Aggregations of small oval melanocytes vary

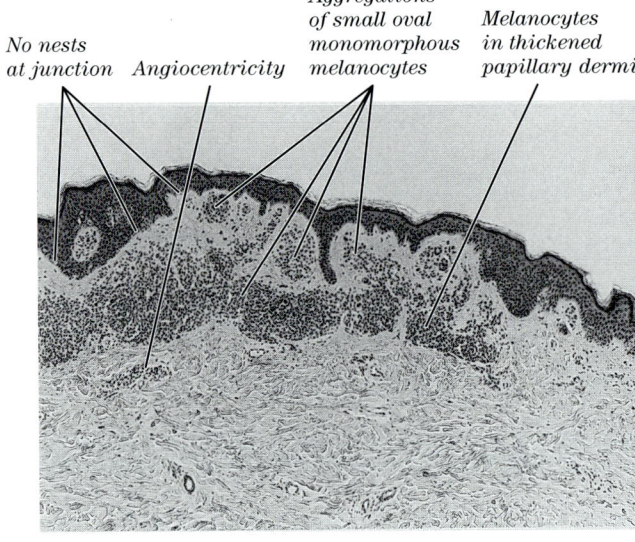

No nests at junction — Angiocentricity — Aggregations of small oval monomorphous melanocytes — Melanocytes in thickened papillary dermis

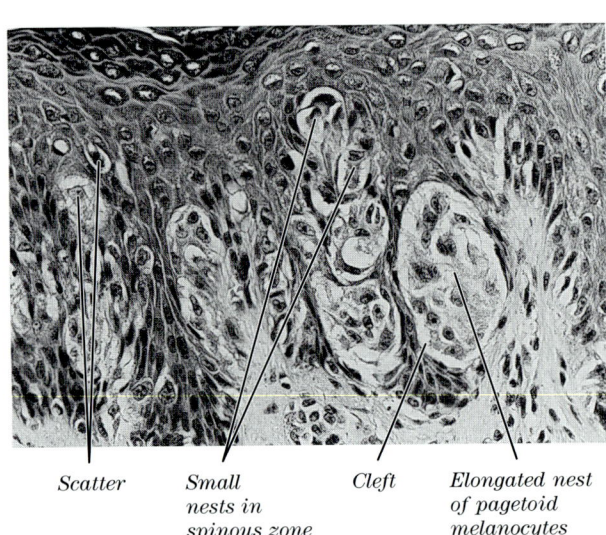

Scatter — Small nests in spinous zone — Cleft — Elongated nest of pagetoid melanocytes

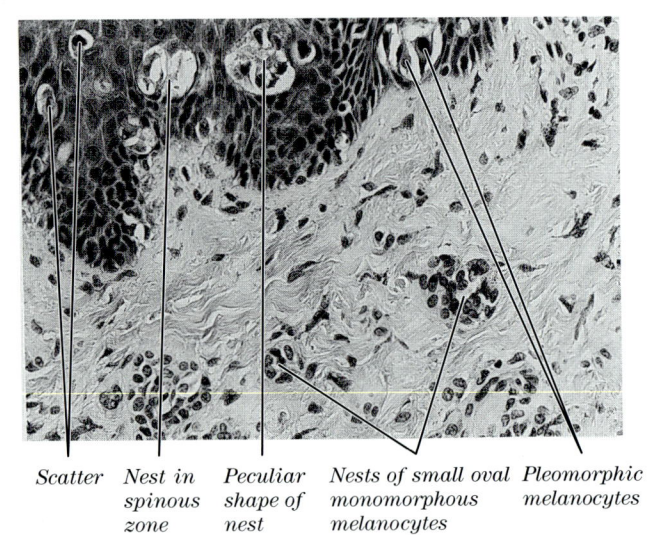

Scatter — Nest in spinous zone — Peculiar shape of nest — Nests of small oval monomorphous melanocytes — Pleomorphic melanocytes

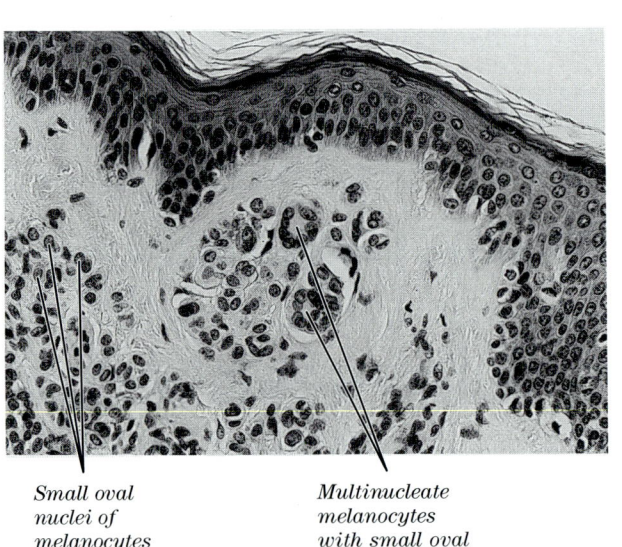

Small oval nuclei of melanocytes — Multinucleate melanocytes with small oval nuclei

81 • Melanoma in situ and Congenital Nevus (superficial type)

Criteria for diagnosis of this melanoma in situ in association with a superficial congenital nevus

The neoplasm on the left is a melanoma because:

1. It is poorly circumscribed.
2. Nests of melanocytes within the epidermis are not equidistant from one another.
3. Nests of melanocytes within the epidermis vary in size and shape.
4. Some nests of melanocytes within the epidermis have become confluent.
5. Melanocytes within the epidermis arranged as solitary units predominate over nests of melanocytes in some high-power fields
6. Pagetoid melanocytes are arrayed in pagetoid pattern.
7. Nuclei of melanocytes are atypical.

The neoplasm on the right is a nevus because:

1. The nests, which are entirely intradermal, consist of melanocytes with small, oval, monomorphous nuclei.
2. Melanocytes mature.
3. No nuclei of melanocytes are atypical.

The nevus is a superficial congenital one because:

1. Melanocytes are situated in the reticular dermis, but only in the upper half of it.
2. Melanocytes in the uppermost portion of the reticular dermis are distributed in angiocentric fashion.
3. Some melanocytes are splayed between collagen bundles in the upper part of the reticular dermis.

Pitfall in diagnosis

This melanoma in association with a superficial congenital nevus could be misconstrued as a combined nevus (Spitz's and Clark's) because:

1. At first glance, the lesion on the left appears to be a Clark's nevus, confined as it seems to be to a thickened papillary dermis.
2. At first blush, the lesion on the left also resembles a Spitz's nevus because so many nests of melanocytes are elongated and oriented perpendicularly to the skin surface, nuclei of those melanocytes are large, cytoplasm is abundant, and shapes of melanocytes are oval, round, and polygonal. Furthermore, there are hyperkeratosis, hypergranulosis, and irregular spinous-cell hyperplasia, and clefts separate elongated nests of melanocytes from adjacent keratinocytes.
3. Indubitable melanocytes of a nevus are present in the upper part of the dermis beneath a second population of melanocytes on the left.

In actuality, the lesion on the right is a superficial congenital nevus because melanocytes are splayed between collagen bundles in the reticular dermis. The lesion on the left is a melanoma in situ for reasons enumerated under "Criteria for diagnosis." The presence of atypical pagetoid melanocytes in pagetoid pattern stamps a neoplasm as a melanoma and excludes a Spitz's nevus.

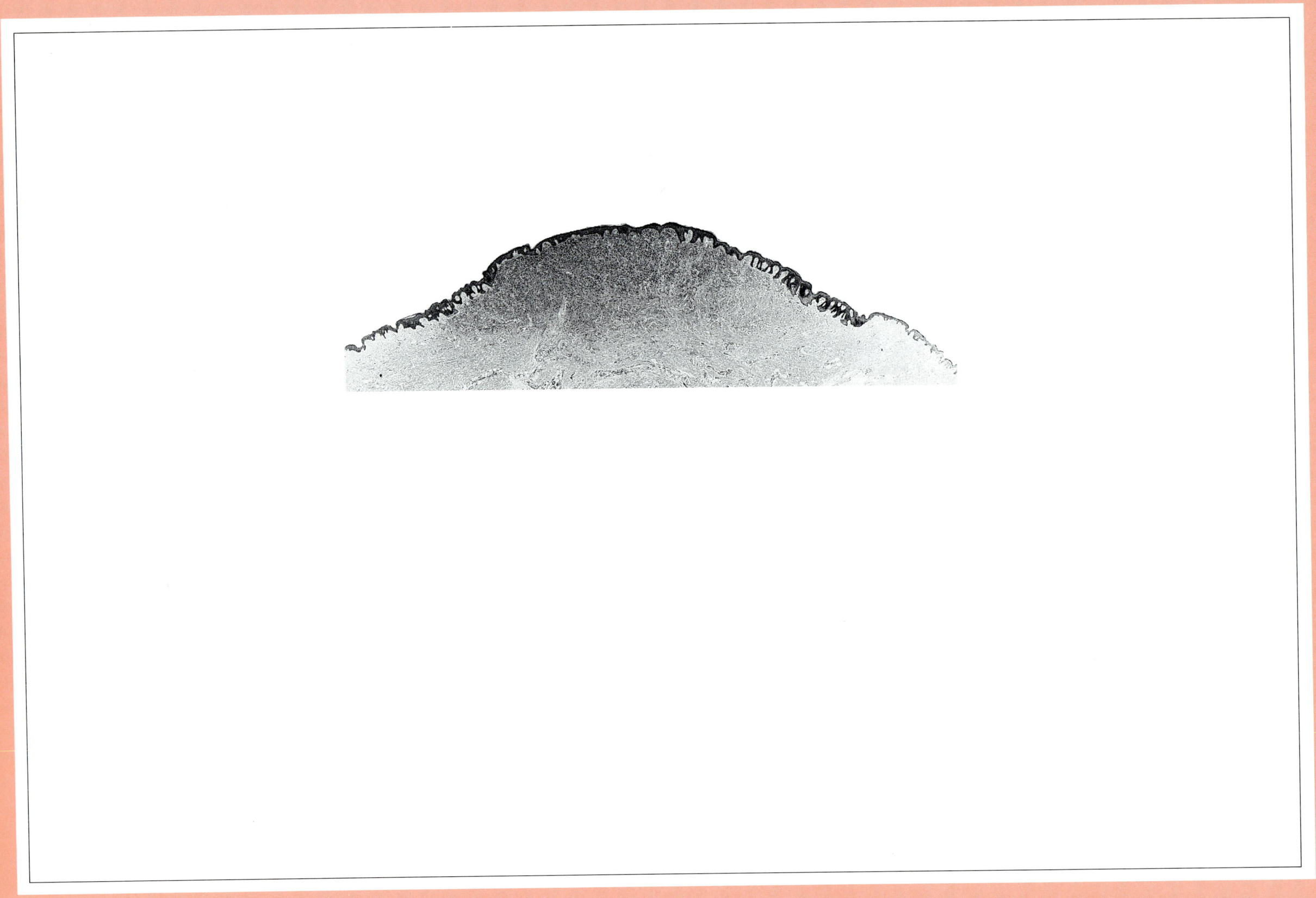

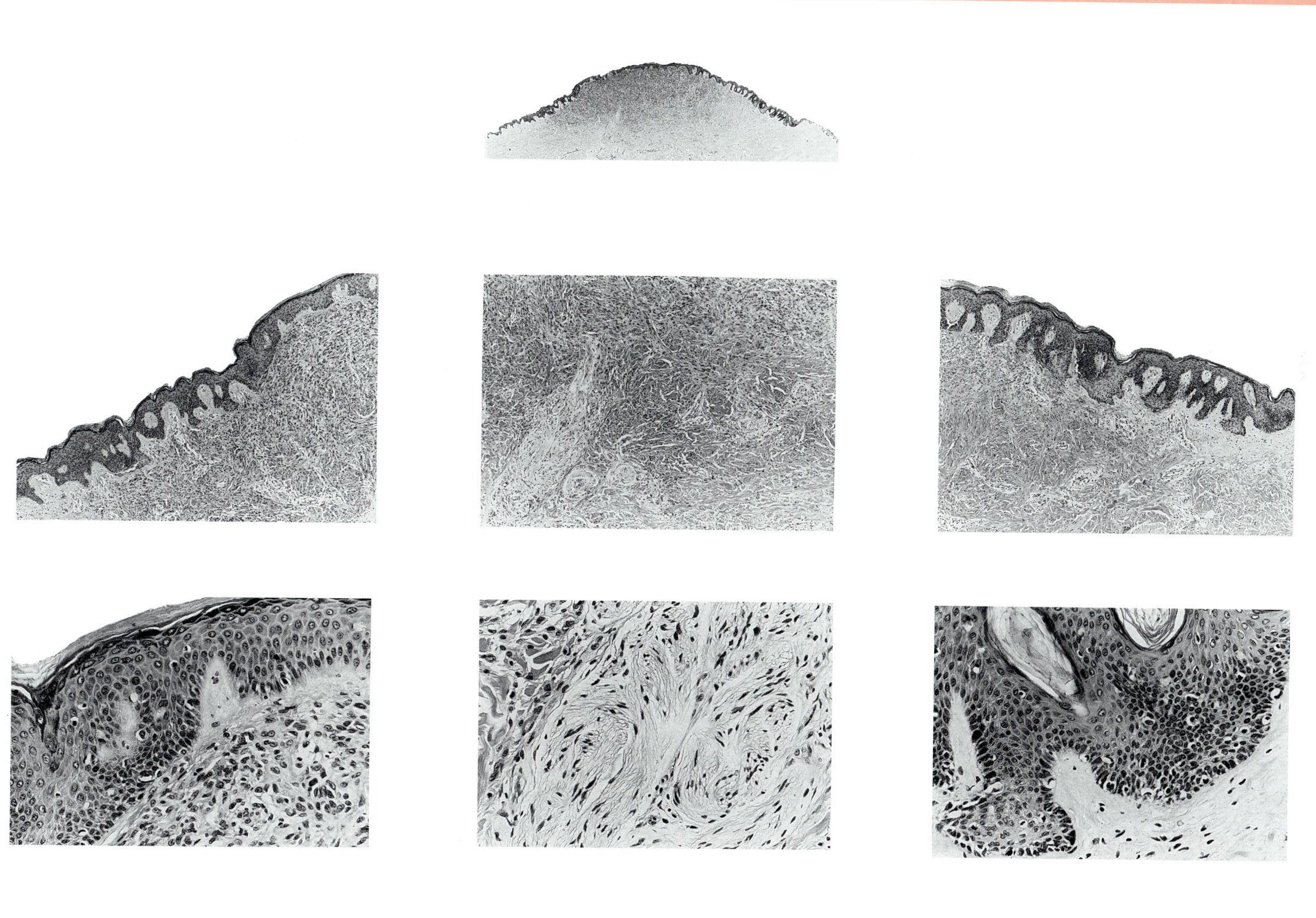

82. What is your diagnosis?

Brown nodule on the right buttock of a 71-year-old woman. Clinical diagnosis: histiocytoma. The patient was free of disease after 1 year.

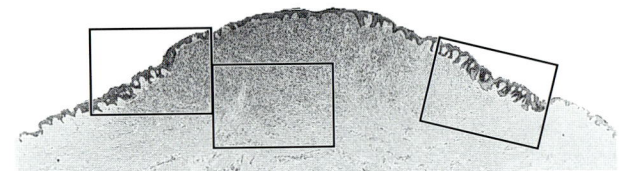

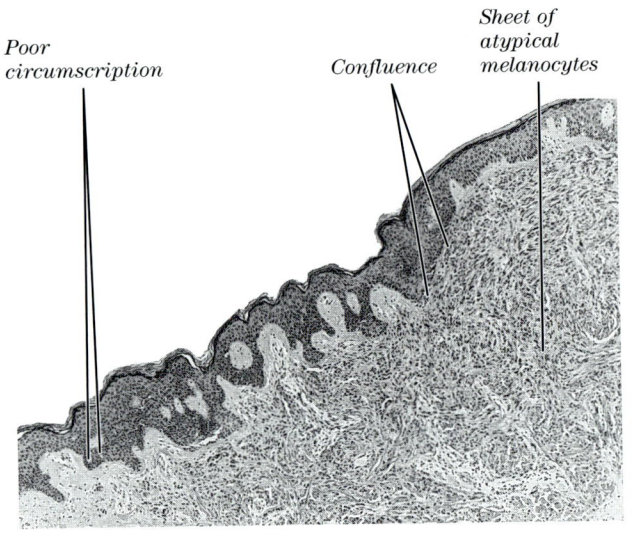

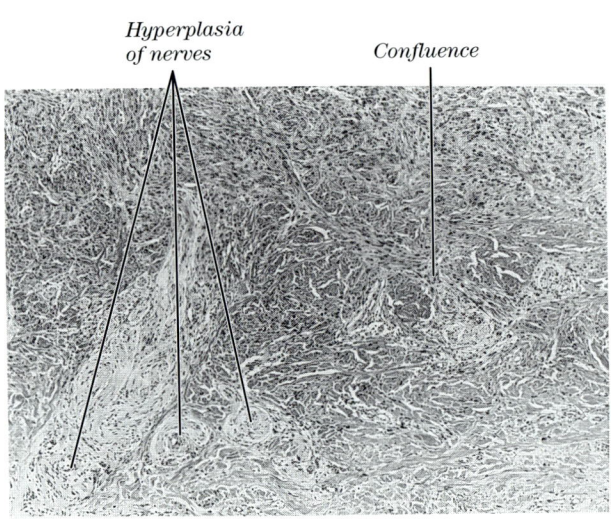

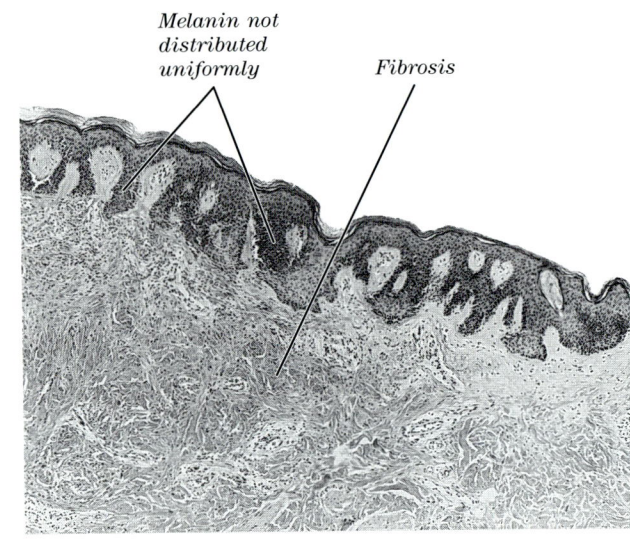

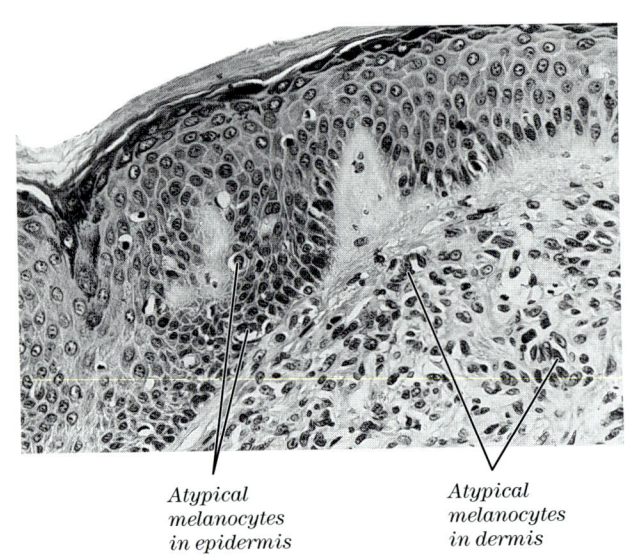

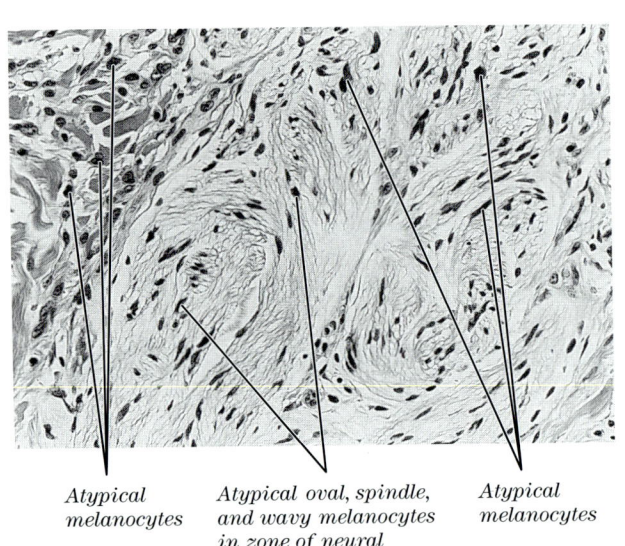

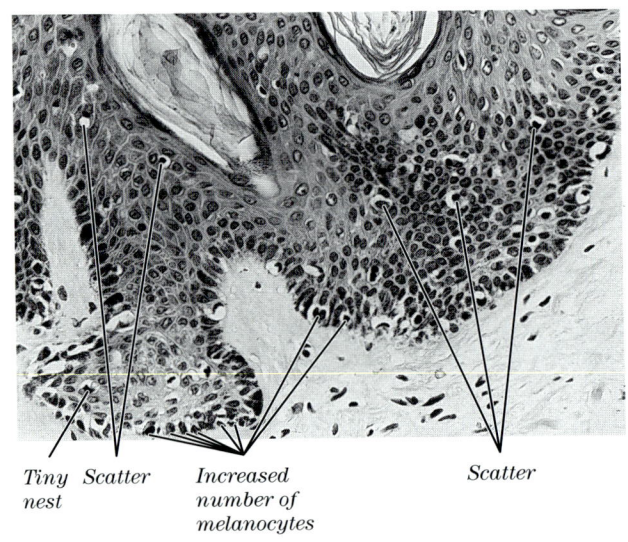

82 • Melanoma *(with neurotropism and neural hyperplasia)*

Criteria for diagnosis of this melanoma
(with neurotropism and neural hyperplasia)

This is a melanoma because:

1. It is asymmetric.

2. It is poorly circumscribed.

3. Melanocytes are scattered as solitary units far above the dermo-epidermal junction.

4. Melanin is not distributed in uniform fashion throughout the epidermis.

5. There are dense diffuse infiltrates of atypical melanocytes within the dermis.

There is neurotropism because:

Neoplastic melanocytes are present within hyperplastic nerve fascicles.

There is neural hyperplasia because:

1. Caricatures of nerve fascicles are scattered throughout the neoplasm.

2. Atypical melanocytes with wavy nuclei are present within faulty nerve fascicles.

Pitfall in diagnosis

This melanoma with hyperplastic nerve fascicles could be mistaken for a compound nevus with neural differentiation because:

1. Melanocytes disposed as solitary units and in nests are present within the epidermis and the dermis.

2. Melanocytes mature with progressive descent.

3. Many melanocytes within the epidermis and the dermis have small oval nuclei.

4. The neural hyperplasia simulates neural differentiation as is seen commonly in Unna's and Miescher's nevi.

What seems to be neural differentiation in this melanocytic neoplasm actually is neural hyperplasia secondary to neurotropism by neoplastic melanocytes of melanoma. Neural differentiation usually signifies a nevus rather than a melanoma, but in this neoplasm, the changes resemble neural differentiation, but are not. In sum, it may be exceedingly difficult to distinguish neural differentiation from neural hyperplasia, but recognition of neurotropism of melanocytes is decisive, as it is in this instance of melanoma. Regardless of considerations of neural differentiation and neural hyperplasia, the silhouette of this neoplasm is that of melanoma, not a nevus.

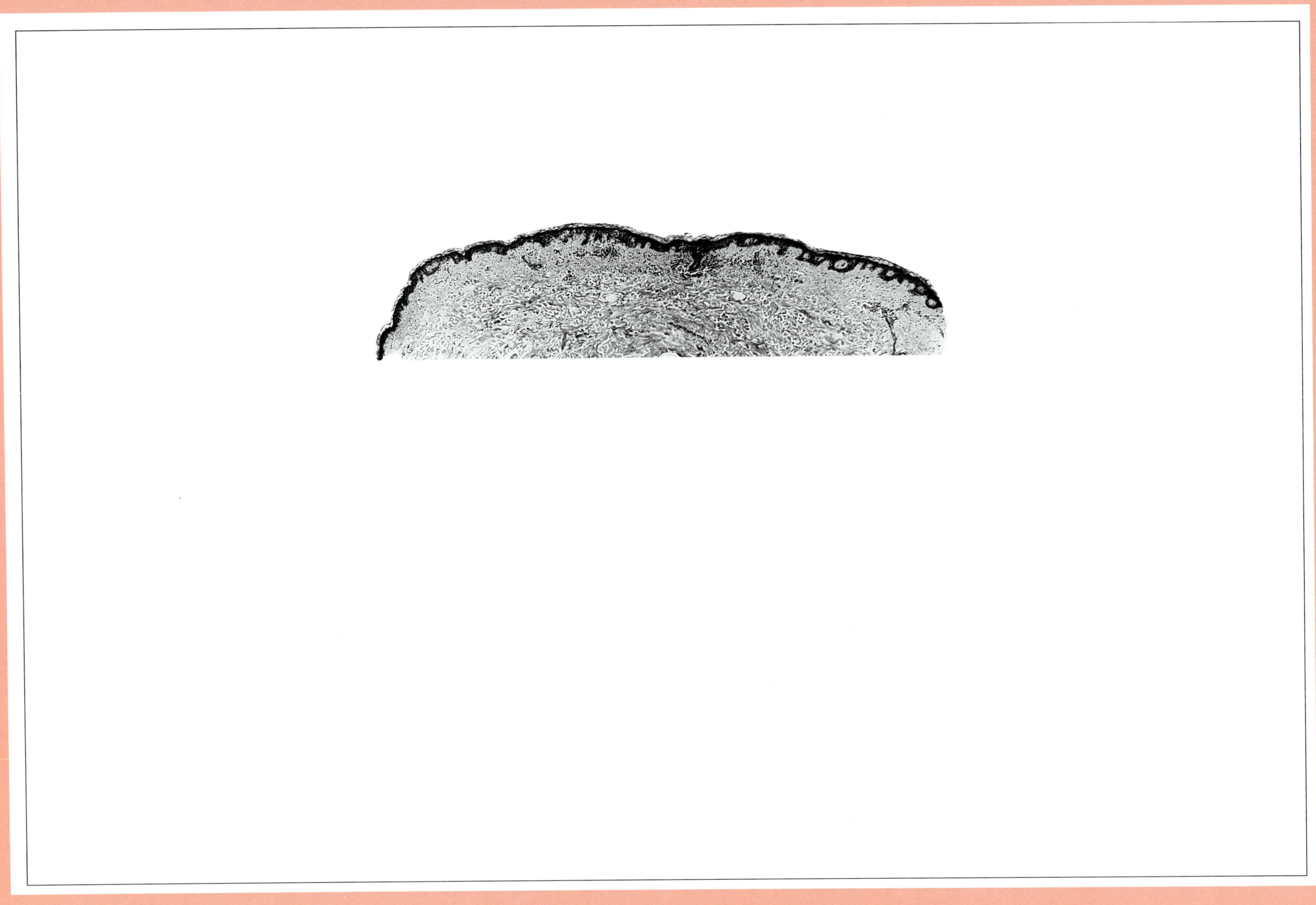

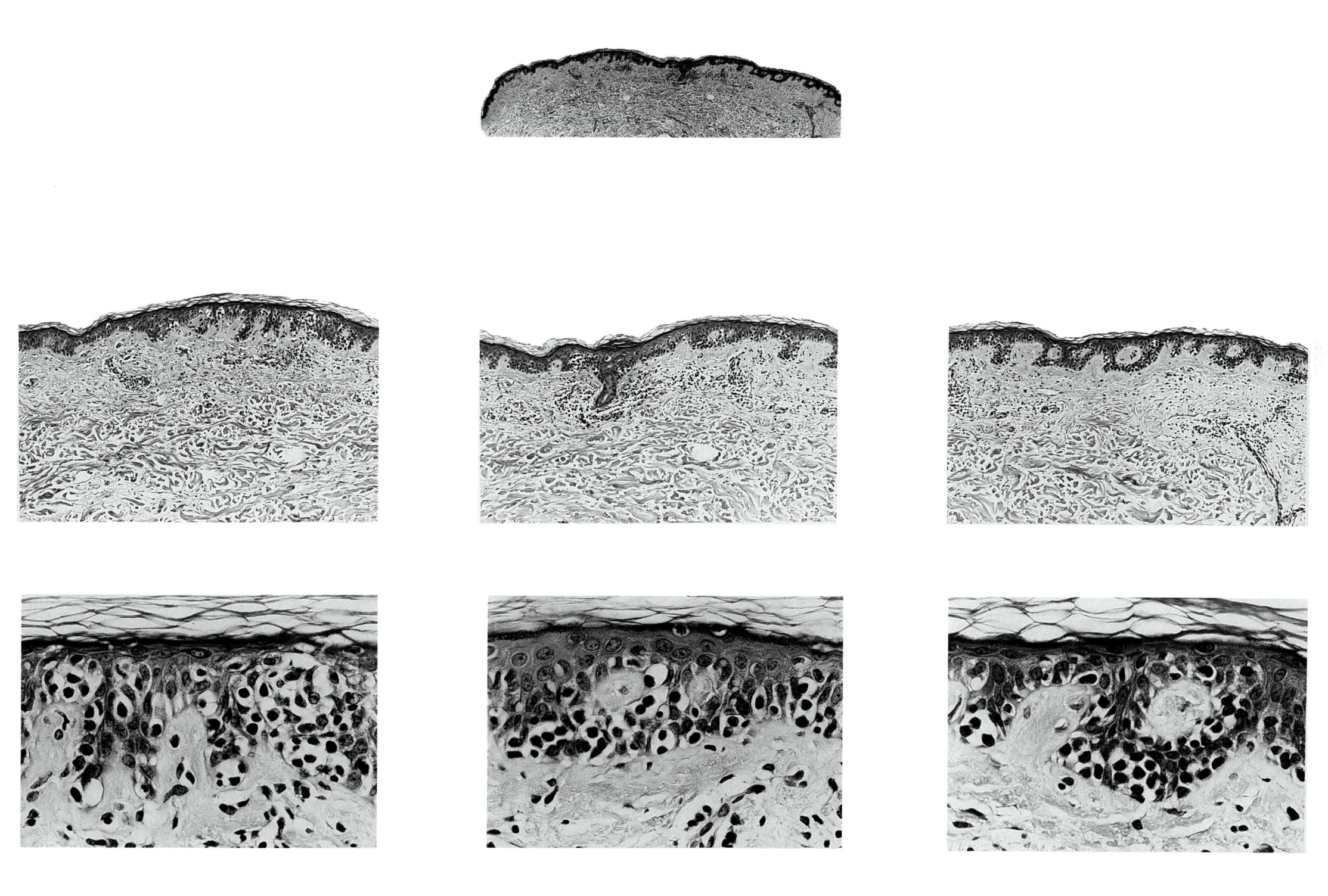

83. What is your diagnosis?

Asymptomatic, atrophic, violaceous lesion on the lower part of the abdomen of a 60-year-old woman. Clinical diagnosis: tick bite vs. lichen sclerosus et atrophicus. After 1 year of topical application of corticosteroids, the skin disease was reputed to be under control.

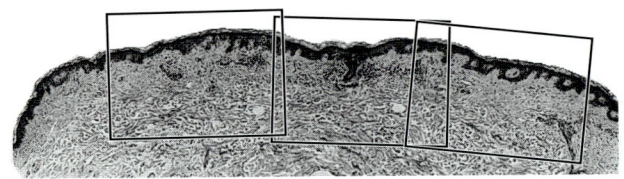

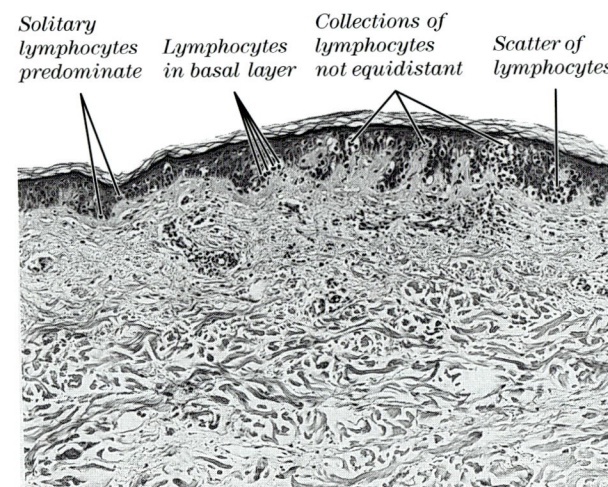
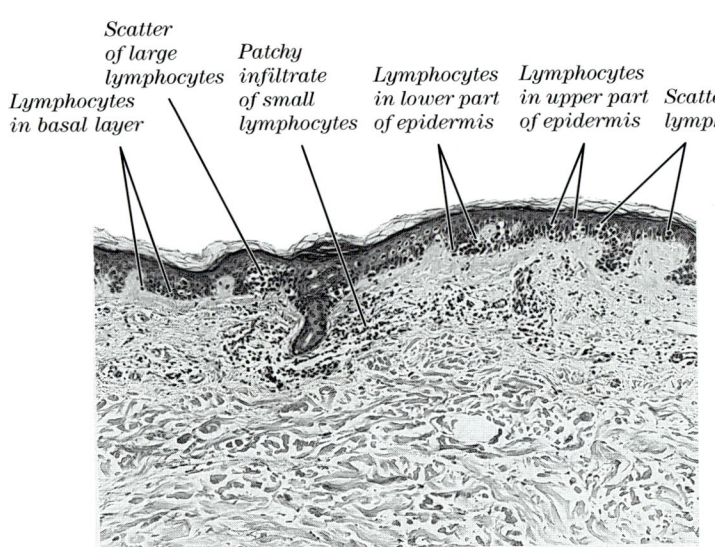
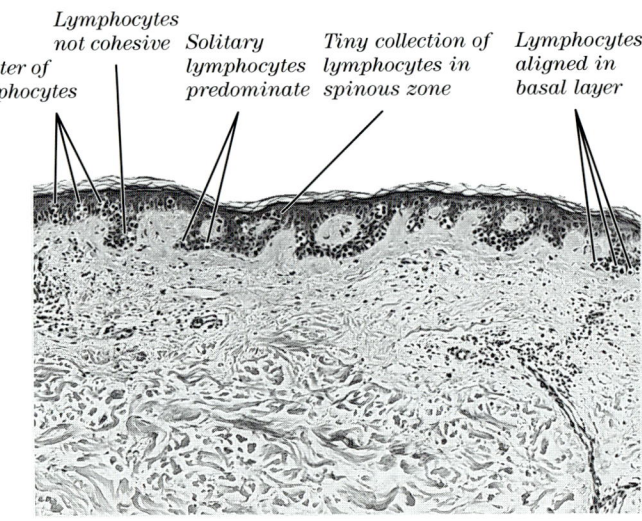

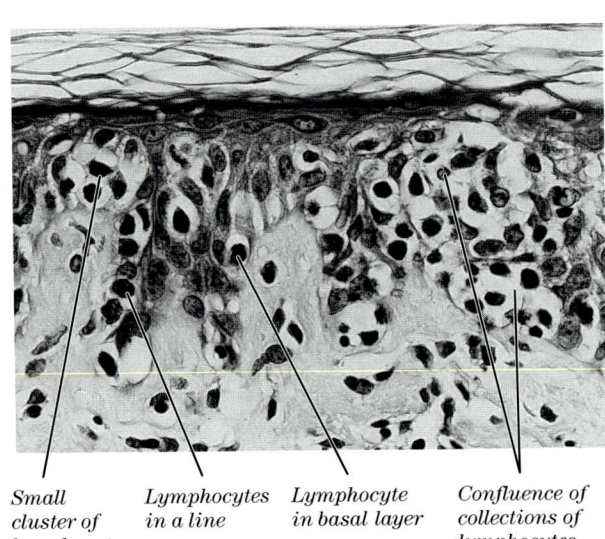
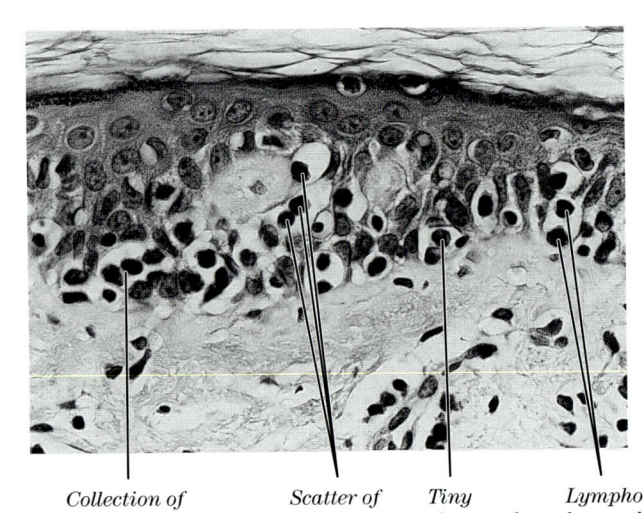
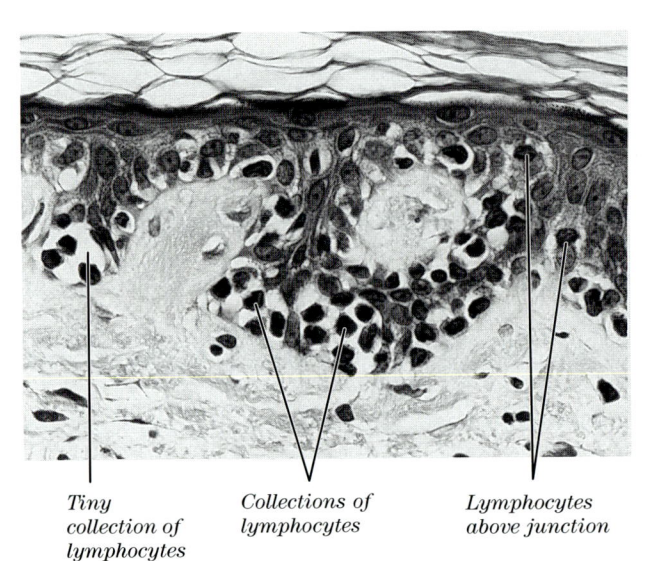

83 • Mycosis Fungoides

Criteria for diagnosis of this patch of mycosis fungoides

This is mycosis fungoides because:

1. Individual neoplastic cells and collections of them are found mostly in the basal row of keratinocytes and above it, rather than mostly at the dermo-epidermal junction.

2. Where neoplastic cells disposed as solitary units predominate in foci, virtually all of them are present above the dermo-epidermal junction.

3. Neoplastic cells within the upper part of the dermis are of the same family as those within the epidermis, and those in the dermis are clearly lymphocytes.

4. A few neoplastic cells possess cerebriform nuclei.

Pitfall in diagnosis

This lesion of mycosis fungoides could be misinterpreted as that of melanoma in situ because:

1. Neoplastic cells are arrayed both as solitary units and in nests within the epidermis.

2. Neoplastic cells, both those arranged as solitary units and those in nests, are present throughout most of the epidermis.

3. A few neoplastic cells seem to be situated at the dermo-epidermal junction.

4. Nuclei of some neoplastic cells are atypical.

5. Nests of neoplastic cells are not equidistant from one another.

6. Nests of neoplastic cells vary in size and shape.

7. Some nests of neoplastic cells have become confluent.

8. Neoplastic cells disposed as solitary units predominate over nests of neoplastic cells in some high-power fields.

9. A patchy lymphocytic infiltrate is present in the upper part of the dermis.

Mycosis fungoides, in fully developed patch and early plaque lesions, may resemble melanoma in situ, as these photomicrographs illustrate. Unlike the melanocytes of melanoma in situ, nearly all lymphocytes of mycosis fungoides, both those disposed as solitary units and those in nests, are present above the dermo-epidermal junction. Those arranged as solitary units, in some high-power fields, tend to be aligned in the basal layer. In short, nests of lymphocytes in mycosis fungoides, in contrast to melanocytes in melanoma in situ, do not cluster at the dermo-epidermal junction itself. This difference in distribution of neoplastic cells enables distinction to be made readily between melanoma in situ and mycosis fungoides.

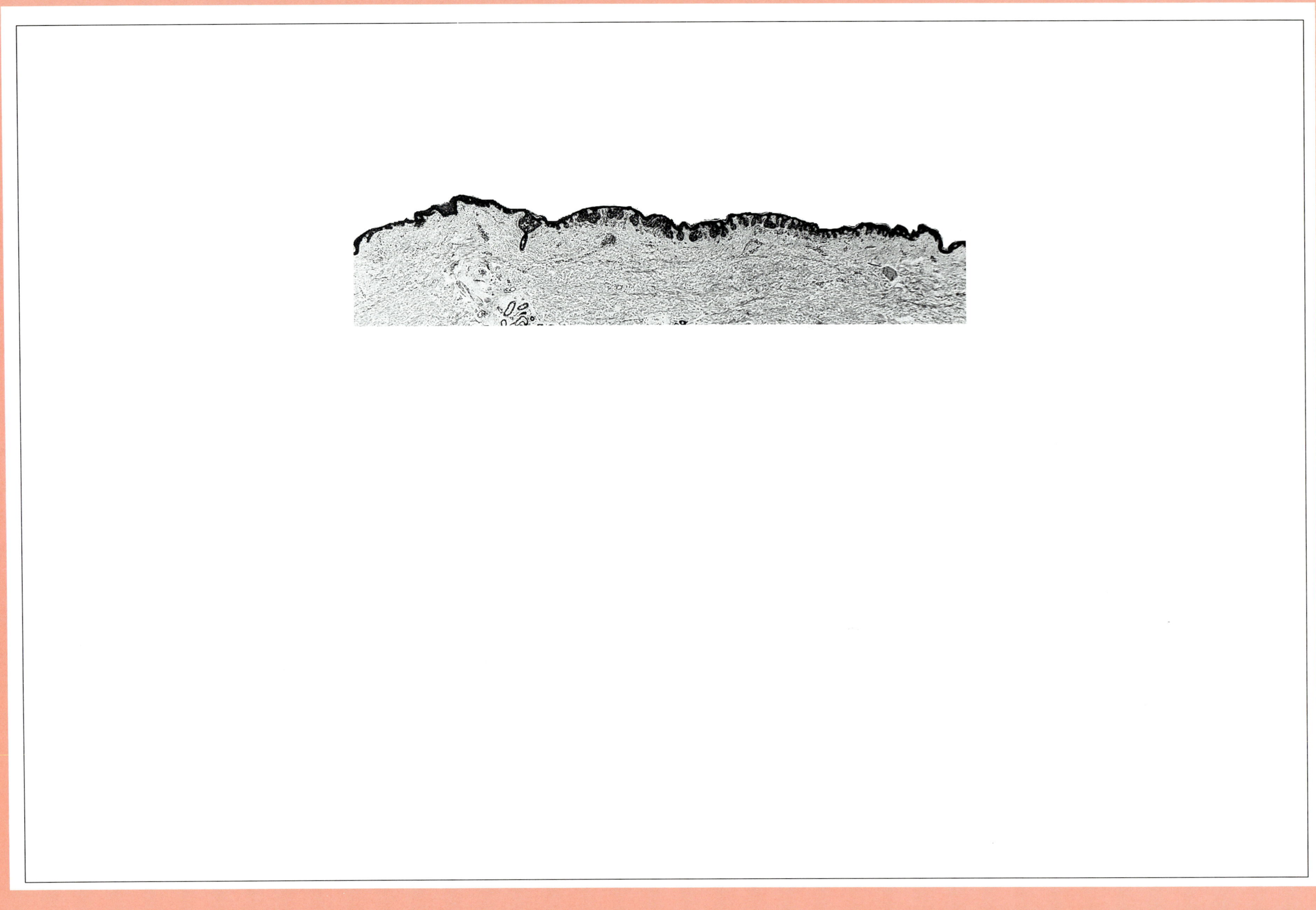

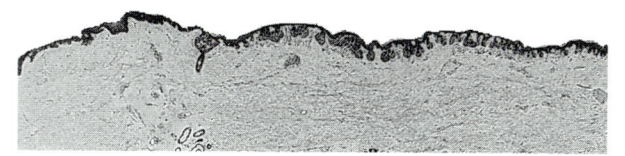
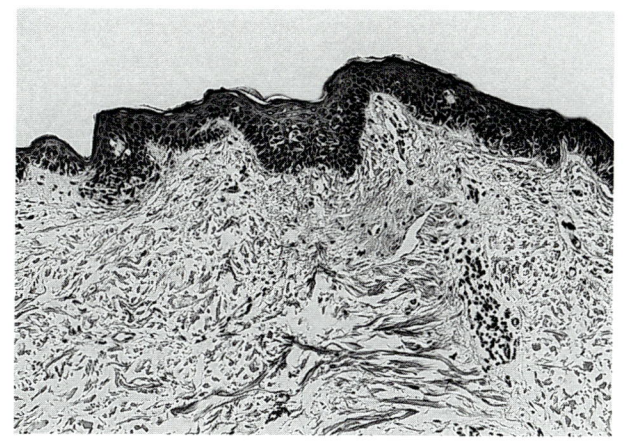
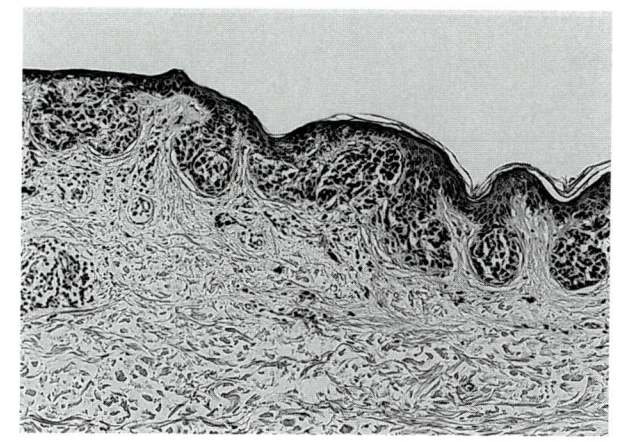
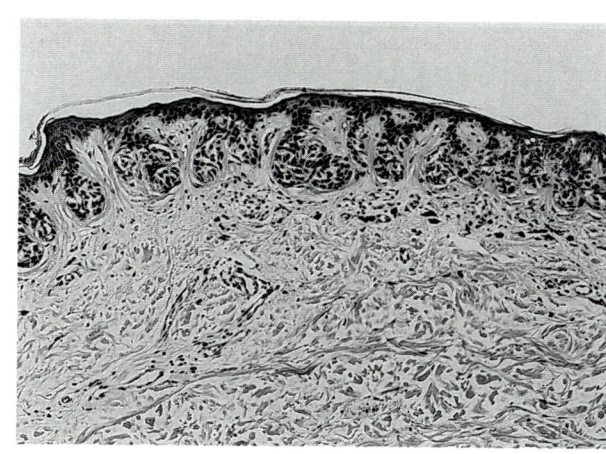
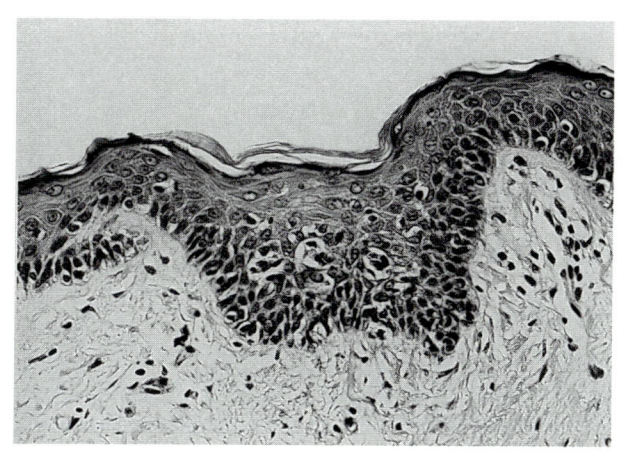
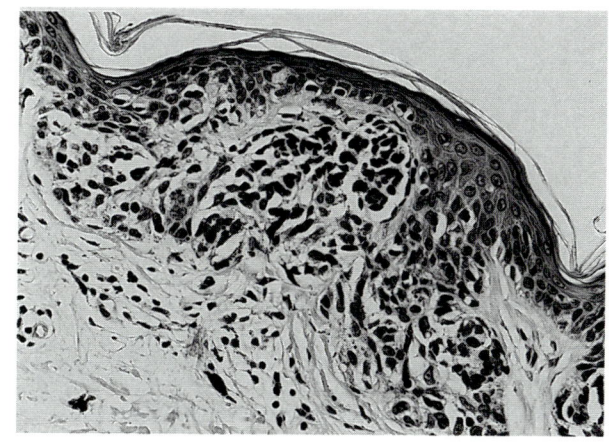
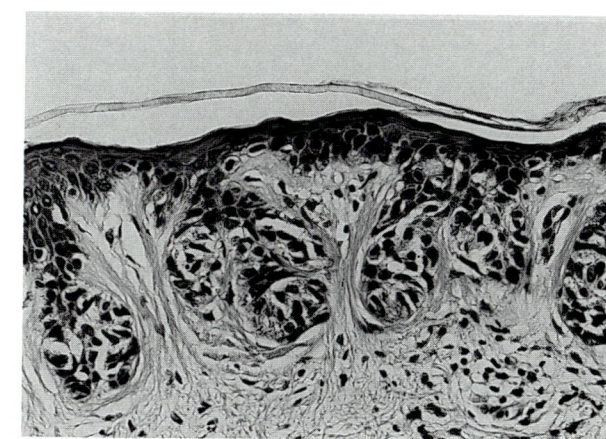

84. What is your diagnosis?

Lesion from the right side of the chest of a 66-year-old man. Clinical diagnosis: dysplastic nevus. Patient had no evidence of a melanocytic neoplasm 5 years later.

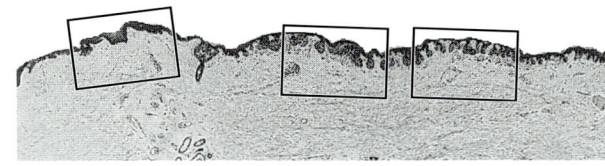

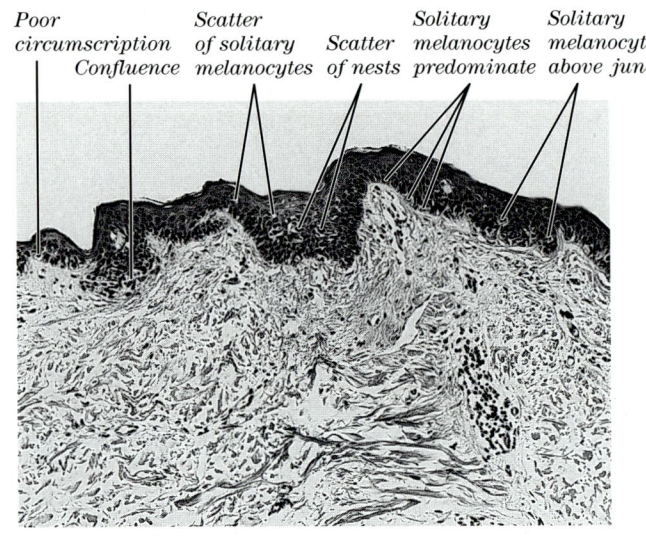

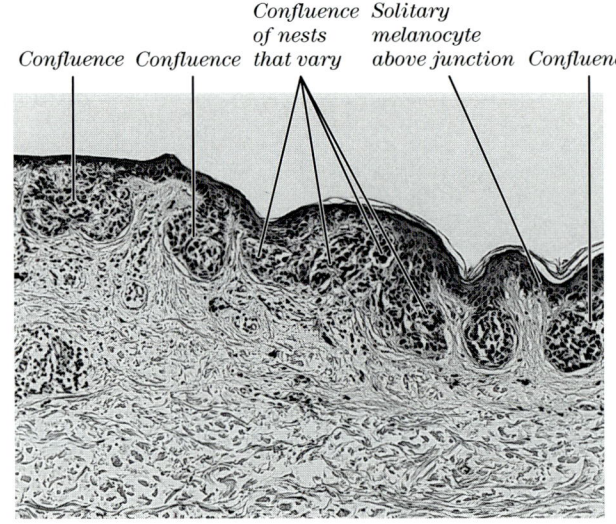

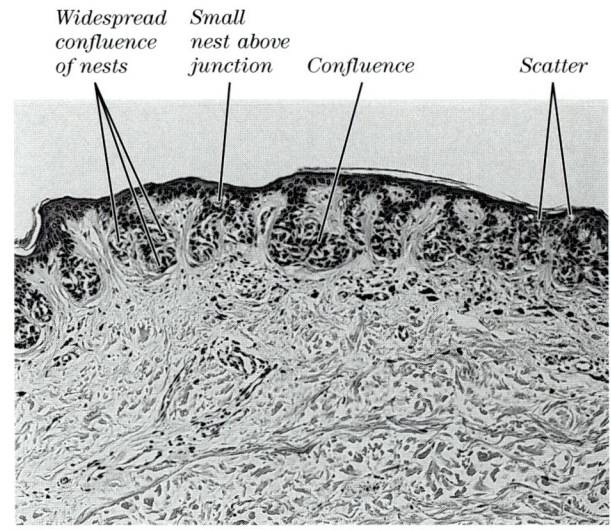

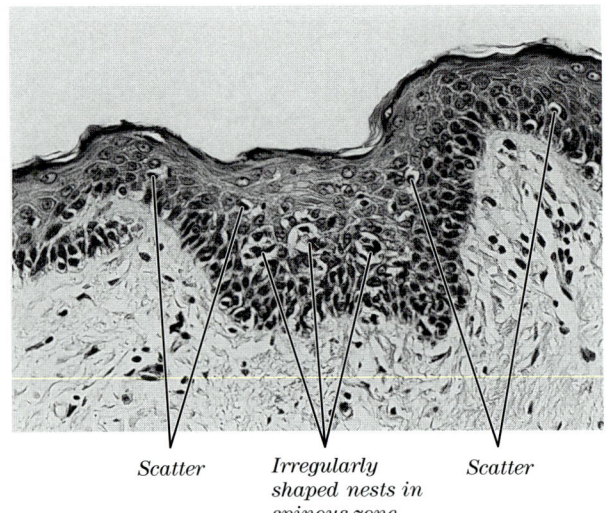

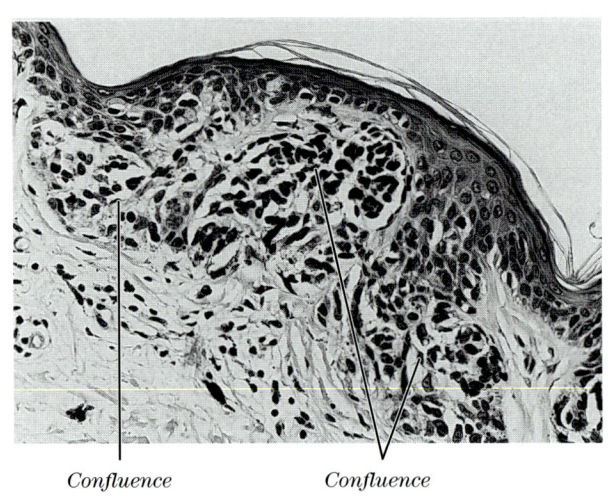

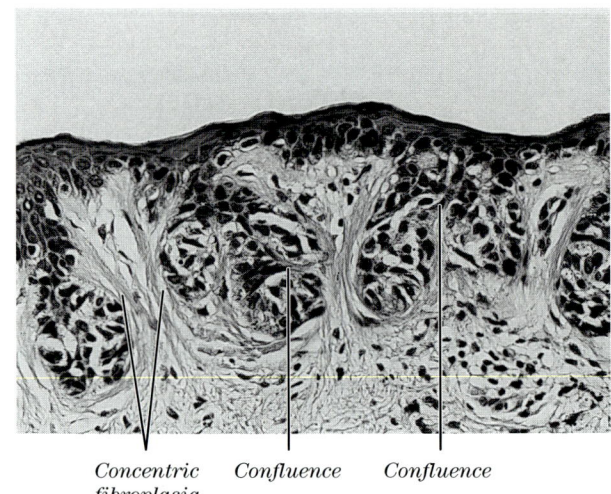

84 • Melanoma in situ

Criteria for diagnosis of this melanoma in situ

This is a melanoma in situ because:

1. Nests of melanocytes are not equidistant from one another.
2. Nests of melanocytes vary in size and shape.
3. Some nests of melanocytes have become confluent.
4. Some nests of melanocytes have peculiar shapes, i.e., they are neither round nor oval.
5. Melanocytes are present above the dermo-epidermal junction in some high-power fields.
6. Nuclei of melanocytes in nests are atypical.

Pitfall in diagnosis

This melanoma in situ could be misread as a melanoma in situ in association with a pre-existing junctional Clark's nevus because:

1. There is an indubitable melanoma in situ on the left side of the neoplasm in the form of scatter of atypical melanocytes as solitary units.
2. Melanocytes in nests, rather than solitary units of them are apparent throughout most of the front of the neoplasm.
3. Most nests of melanocytes are seated at the dermo-epidermal junction.
4. Concentric fibroplasia, sparse lymphocytic infiltrates, and melanophages are recognizable in the upper part of the dermis.

Proponents of the concept of "melanocytic dysplasia" might contend that the changes on the right of this neoplasm are those of a "dysplastic" nevus and those on the left are those of "severe dysplasia," i.e., a "precursor" of melanoma. In our view, the changes throughout this neoplasm are those of a single neoplasm, i.e., melanoma in situ, for reasons stated in the section "Criteria for diagnosis."

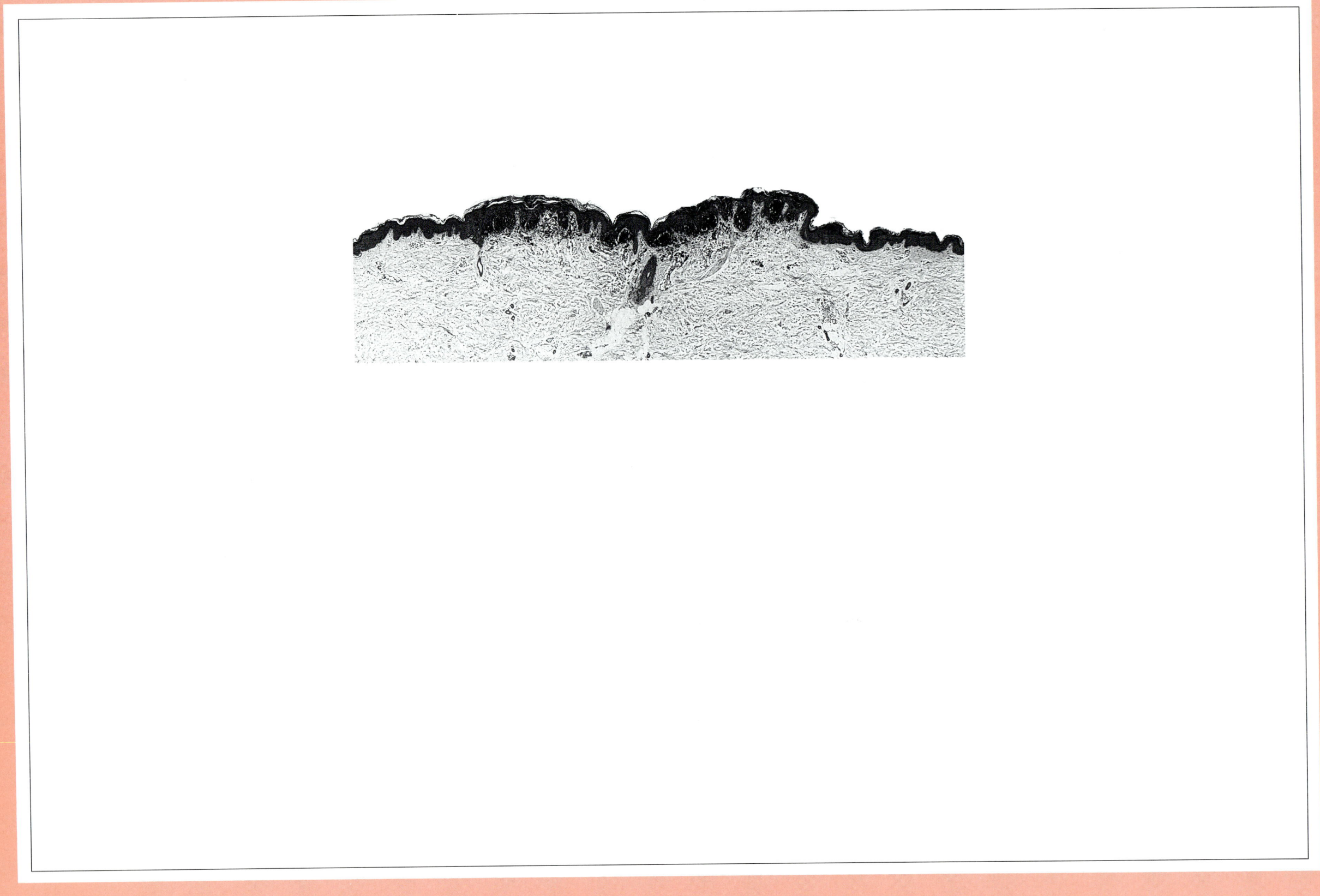

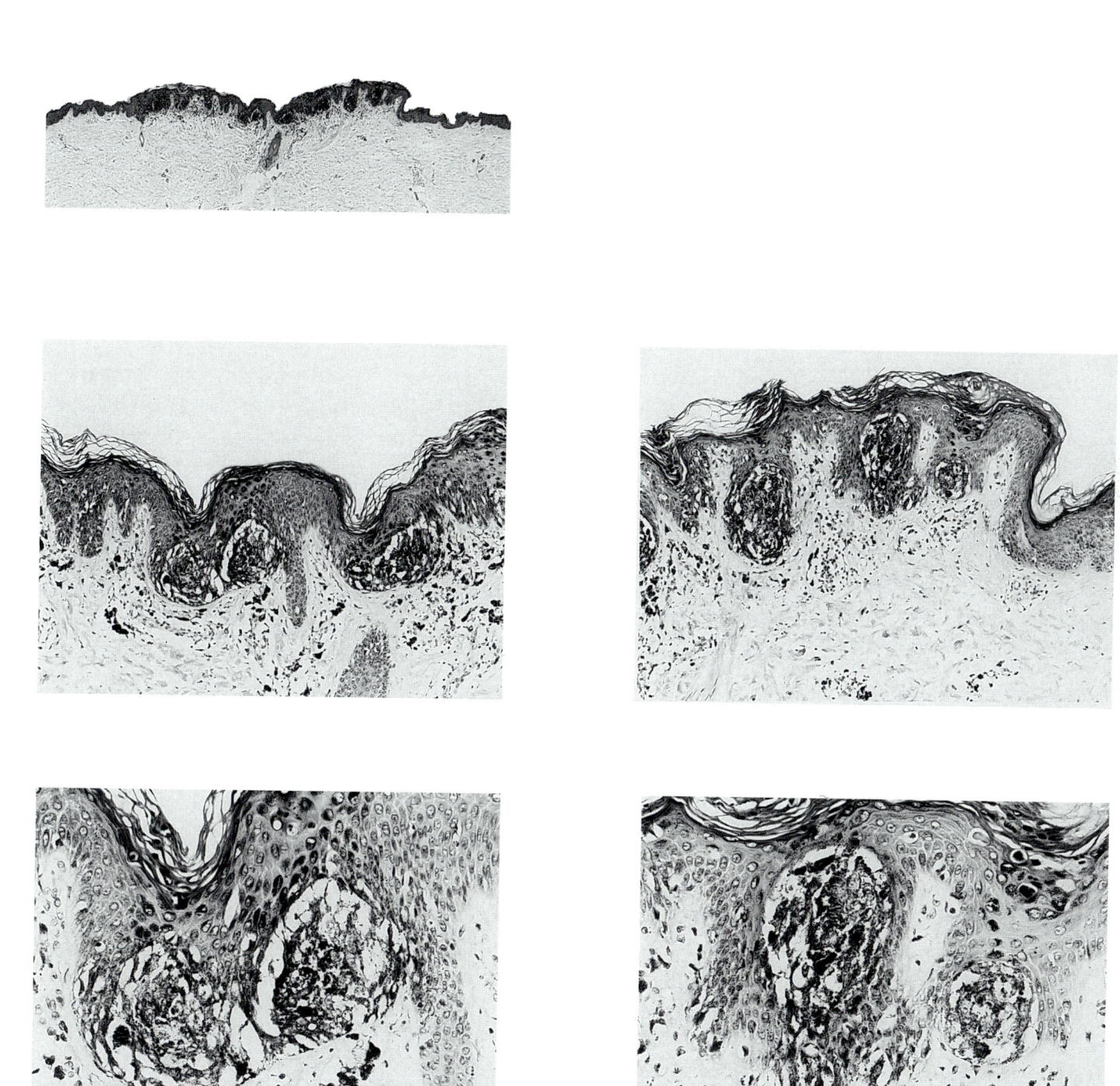

85. What is your diagnosis?

Deeply pigmented, flat, irregularly shaped lesion on the left calf of a 3-year-old girl. Clinical diagnosis: Spitz's nevus vs. melanoma. No follow-up information was available.

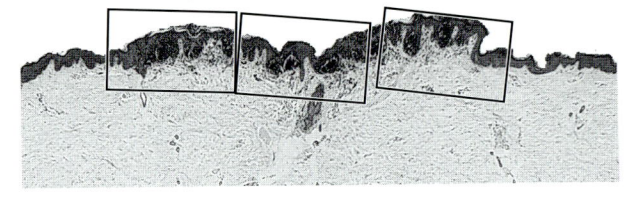

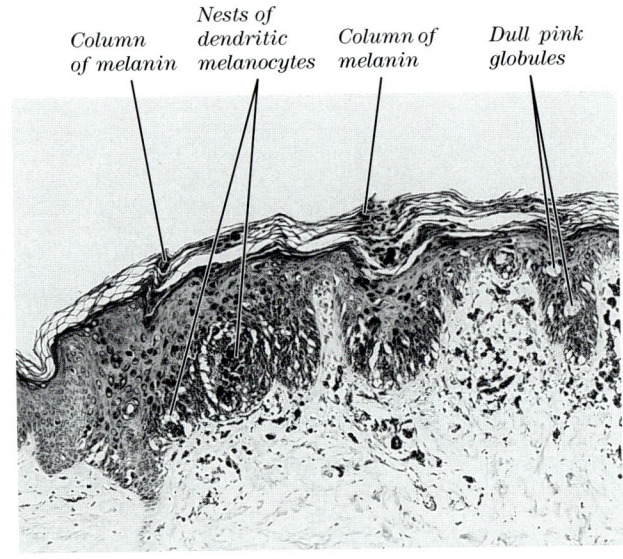

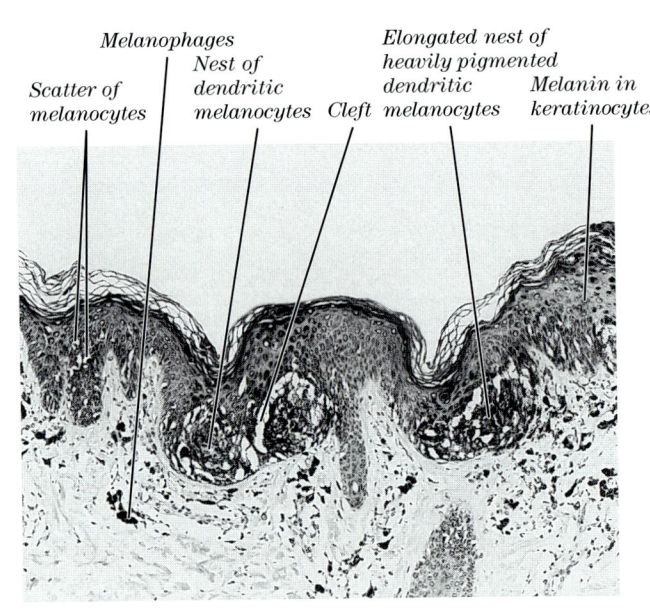

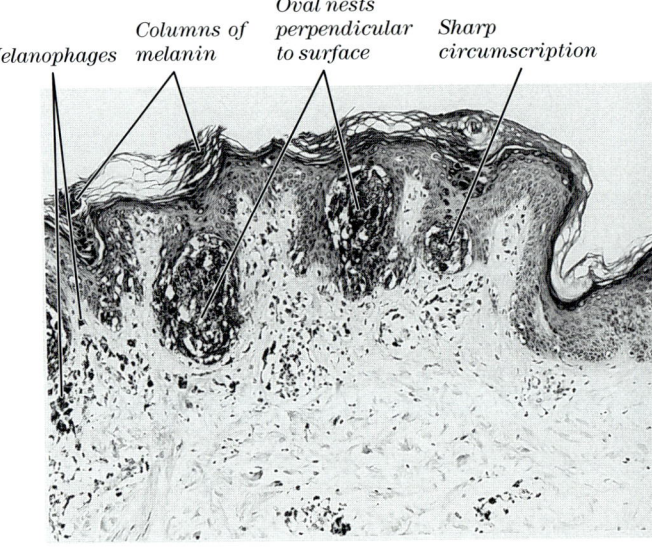

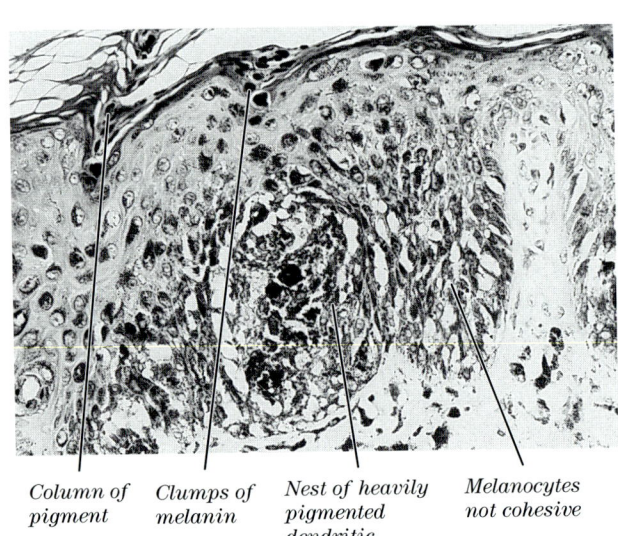

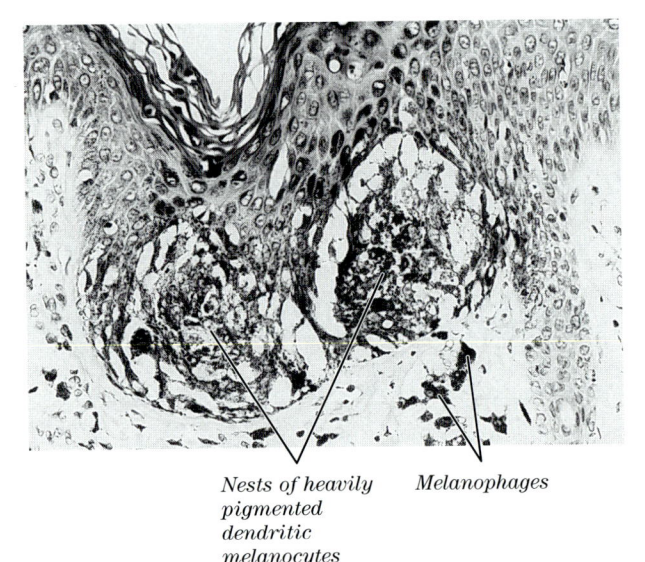

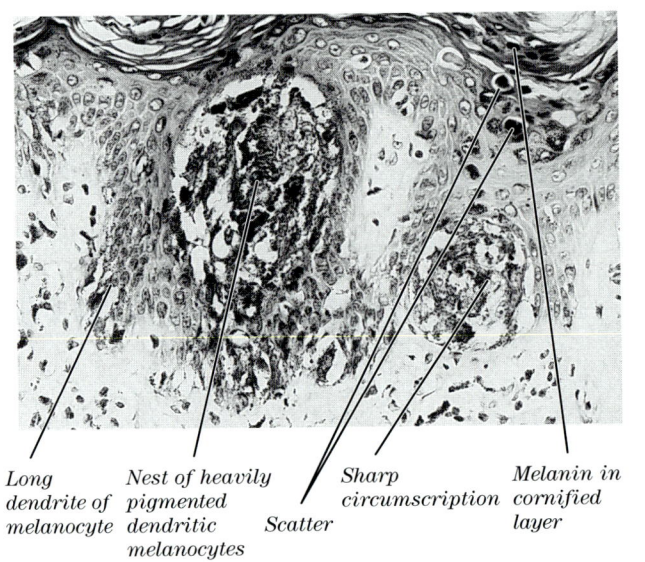

85 • Spitz's Nevus

Criteria for diagnosis of this Spitz's nevus (junctional type)

This is a nevus because:

1. The neoplasm is relatively symmetric.
2. It is quite well-circumscribed.
3. Nests of melanocytes within the epidermis predominate overwhelmingly over melanocytes arranged as solitary units.
4. Most nests of melanocytes are discrete.
5. Discrete columns of melanin are present within the cornified layer.
6. Nests of melanocytes are pigmented in relatively even fashion.
7. The melanocytes themselves have large oval monomorphous nuclei and dendritic cytoplasm.

This is a Spitz's nevus because:

1. Melanocytes are large and oval.
2. A few globules are present within the epidermis.
3. There are foci of hyperkeratosis and hypergranulosis.
4. The epidermis is hyperplastic.
5. Nests of melanocytes tend to be ellipsoid and mostly perpendicular to the skin surface.
6. Clefts are present between some nests of melanocytes and adjacent keratinocytes.

Pitfall in diagnosis

This junctional Spitz's nevus could be misinterpreted as a melanoma in situ because:

1. Melanin is not distributed uniformly throughout the entire epidermis.
2. Some nests of melanocytes have become confluent.
3. Melanocytes in some foci are clustered, but are not cohesive.
4. Some melanocytes disposed as solitary units are scattered in the upper reaches of the epidermis.
5. Some nests of melanocytes are not equidistant from one another.

This melanocytic neoplasm confined to the epidermis should not be construed a melanoma in situ simply because of scatter of melanocytes above the dermo-epidermal junction, abundant melanin within neoplastic melanocytes and keratinocytes, and confluence of nests of melanocytes. All three are expected findings in Spitz's nevi, too. Furthermore, discrete columns of melanin in the cornified layer are compelling indications of a nevus, not a melanoma.

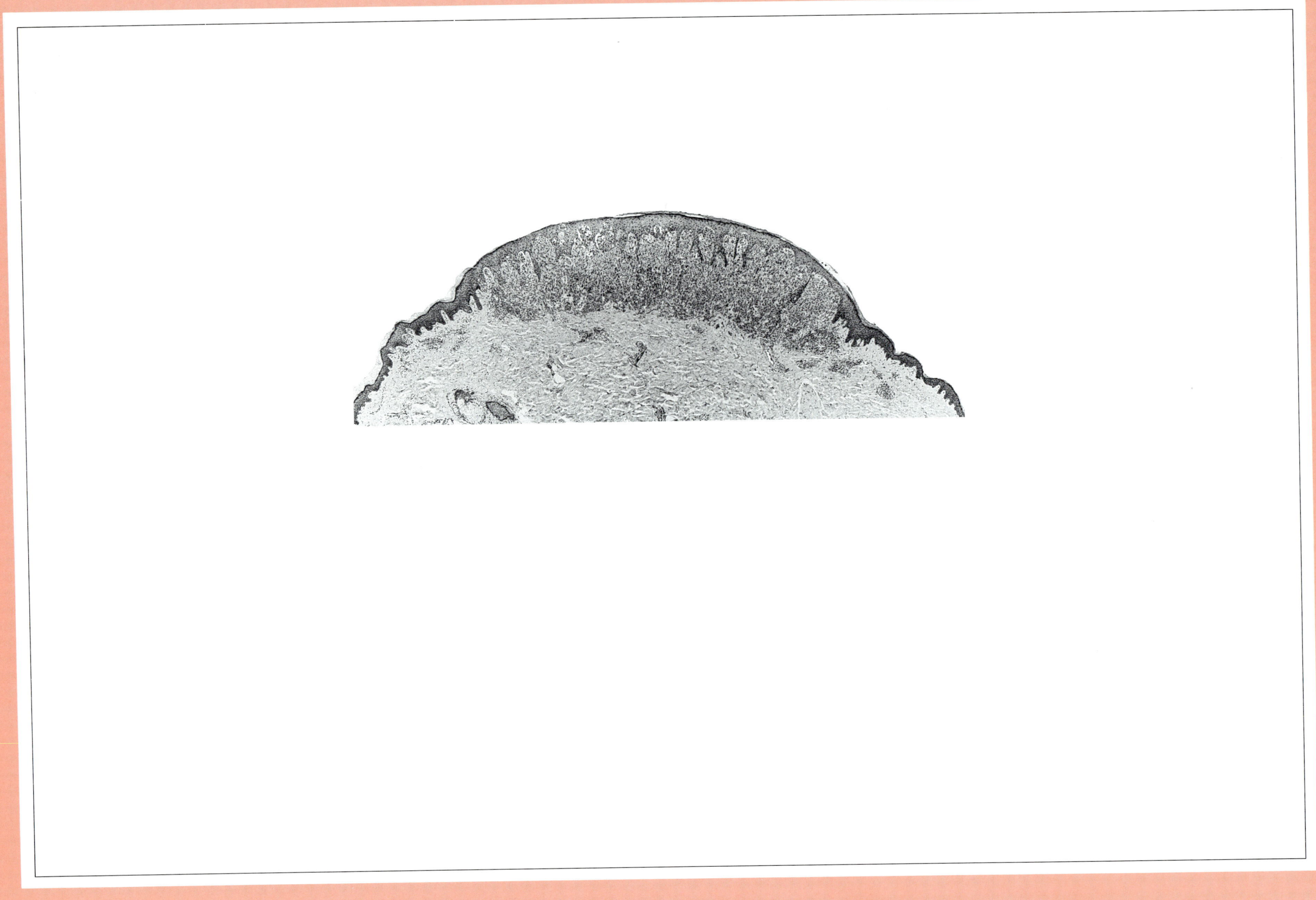

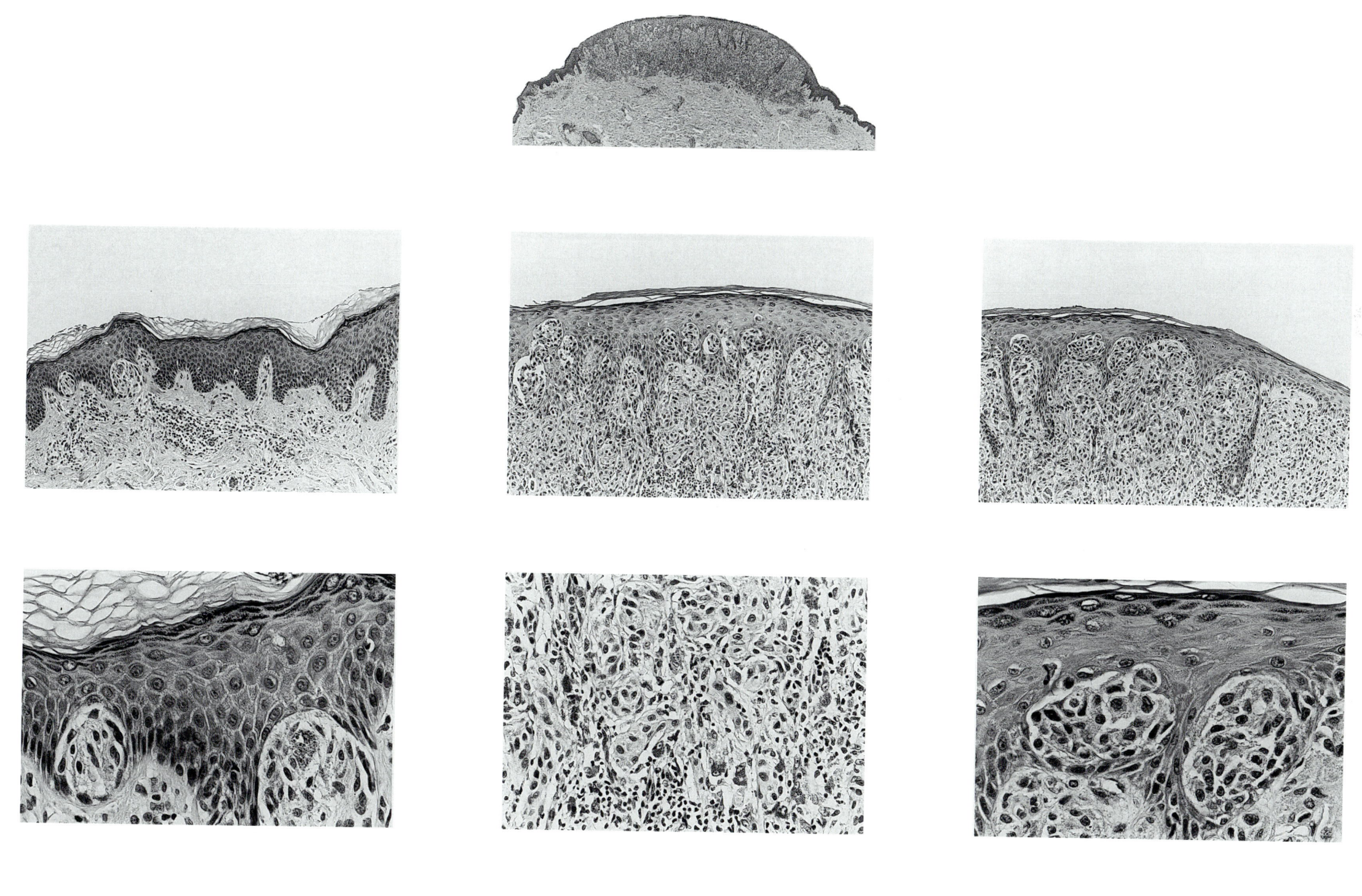

86. What is your diagnosis?

Dark brown nodule of 2 months duration on the right calf of a 23-year-old woman. Clinical diagnosis: nevus vs. melanoma. Re-excision was performed, and no residual neoplasm was found. Patient had no evidence of disease after 1 year. No additional follow-up information was available.

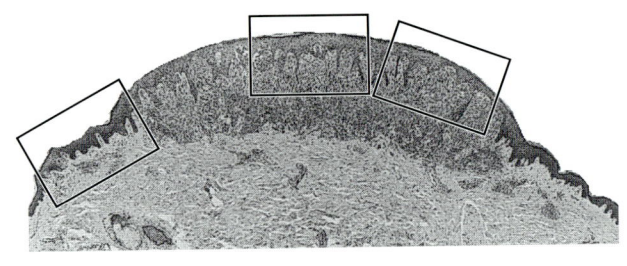

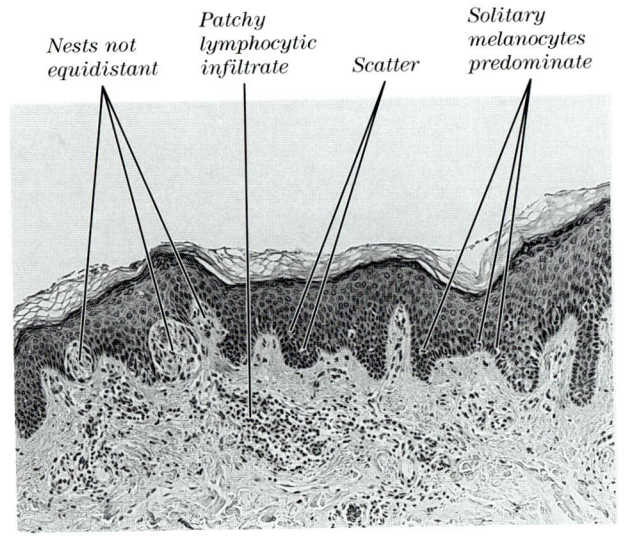

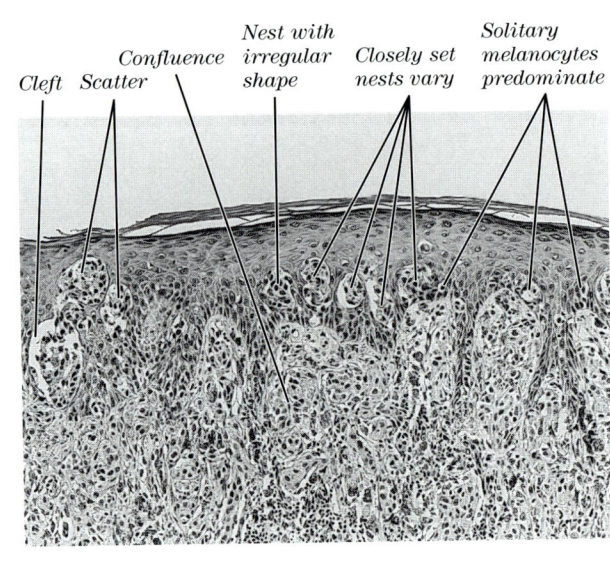

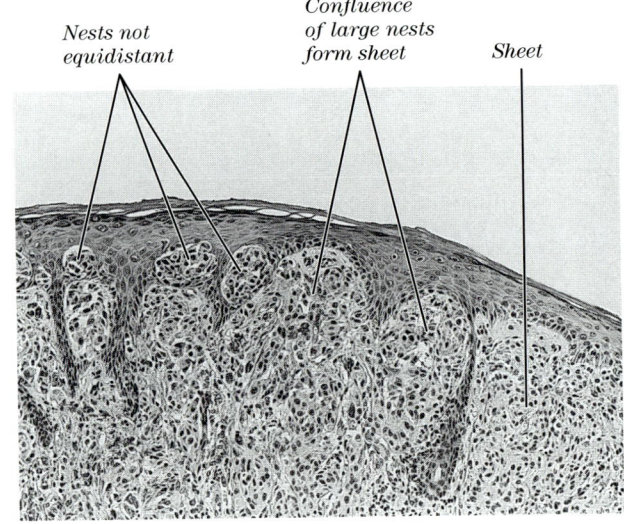

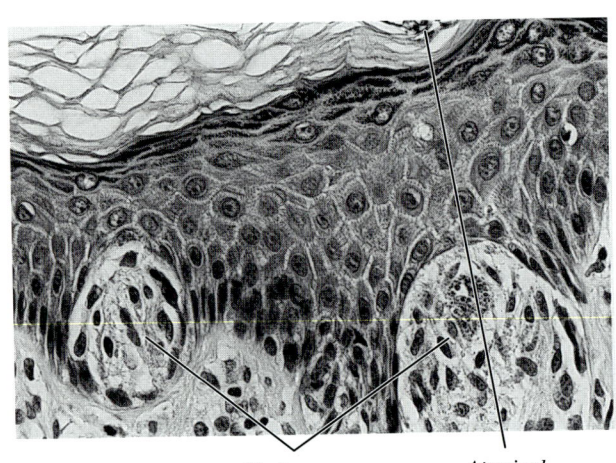

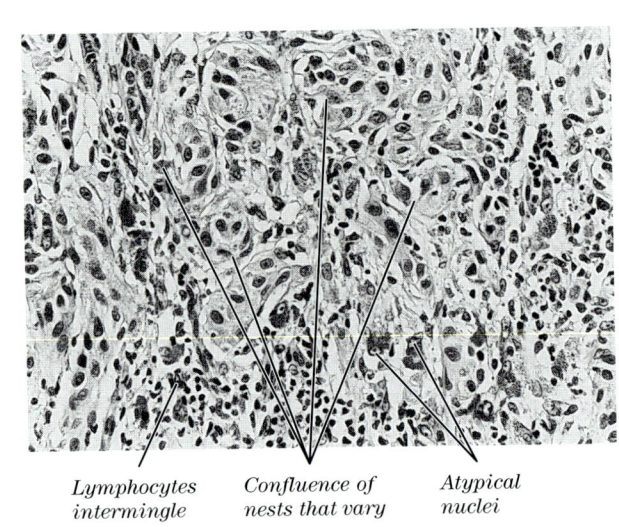

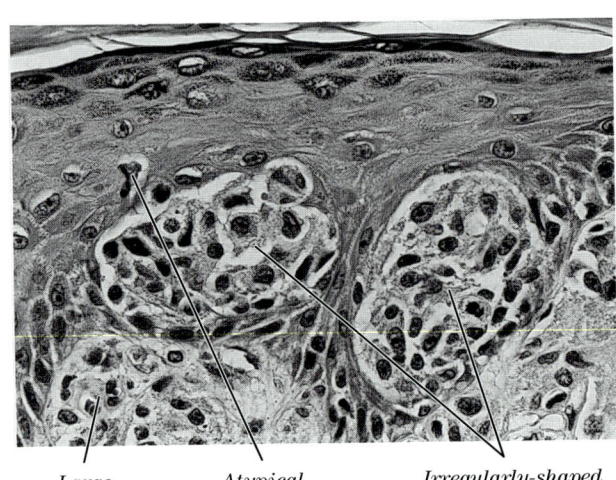

86 • Melanoma

Criteria for diagnosis of this melanoma

This is a melanoma because:

1. It is asymmetric.
2. Circumscription is poor.
3. Nests of melanocytes within the epidermis are not equidistant from one another.
4. Nests of melanocytes within the epidermis differ in size and shape.
5. Melanocytes disposed as solitary units within the epidermis outnumber nests of melanocytes in some high-power fields.
6. Nests of melanocytes within the dermis have become confluent to form sheets.
7. Melanocytes fail to mature.
8. Lymphocytic infiltrates are placed mostly at the base of the neoplasm.

Pitfall in diagnosis

This melanoma could be misinterpreted as a compound Spitz's nevus because:

1. The lesion is domed.
2. The size is small.
3. Hyperkeratosis, hypergranulosis, and epidermal hyperplasia are present.
4. Clefts occur between some nests of melanocytes and adjacent keratinocytes.
5. Some elongated nests of melanocytes within the epidermis are oriented somewhat vertically to the skin surface.
6. Neoplastic melanocytes have large nuclei, abundant cytoplasm, and mostly oval shape.
7. Some melanocytes are dispersed as solitary units and in nests above the dermo-epidermal junction.

In the differentiation of some melanomas from Spitz's nevi, a helpful sign for recognition of the melanomas is tendency of nests of melanocytes within the dermis to become confluent and form sheets. That finding, in the context of all the other features of melanoma present in these sections, enables diagnosis of melanoma to be made with confidence.

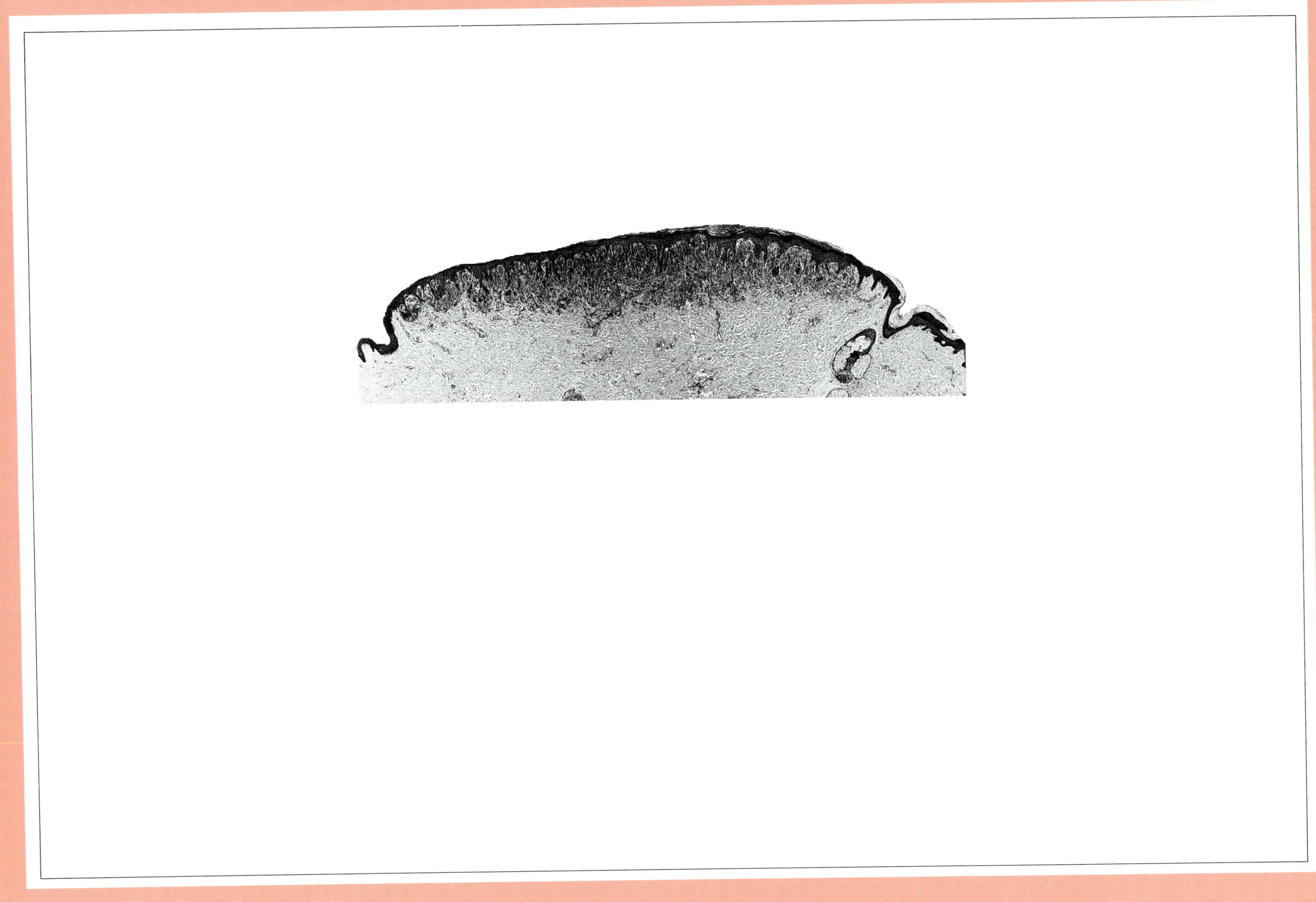

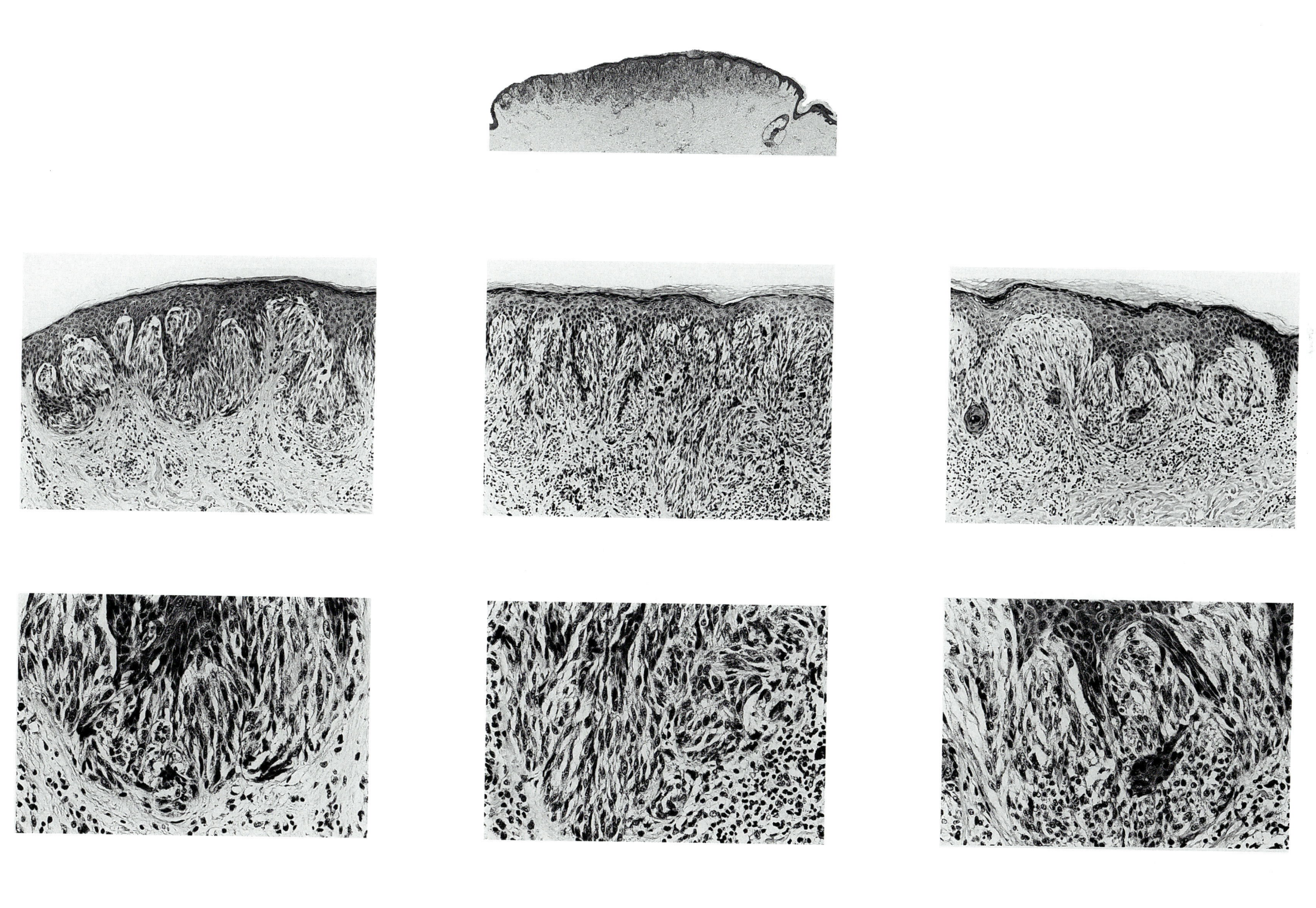

87. What is your diagnosis?

Slightly raised black "mole" on the midback of a 20-year-old man. Clinical diagnosis: atypical mole vs. melanoma. Excision was performed with narrow margins. No persistence of the melanocytic neoplasm was noted.

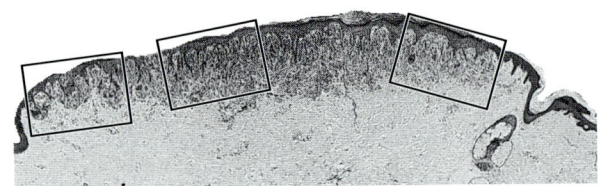

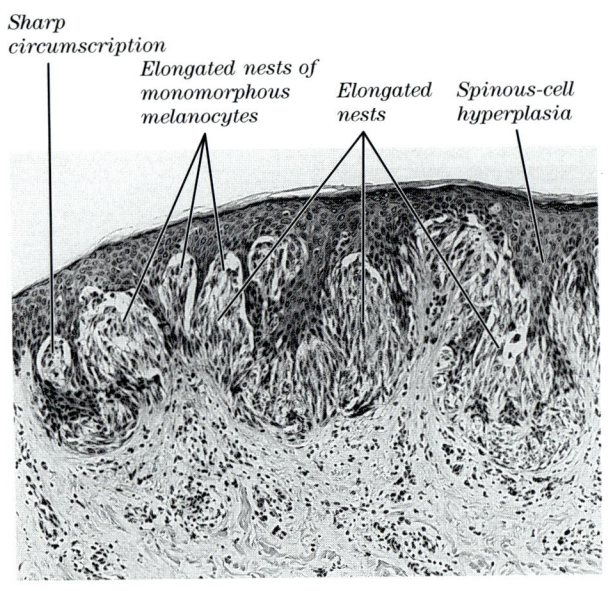

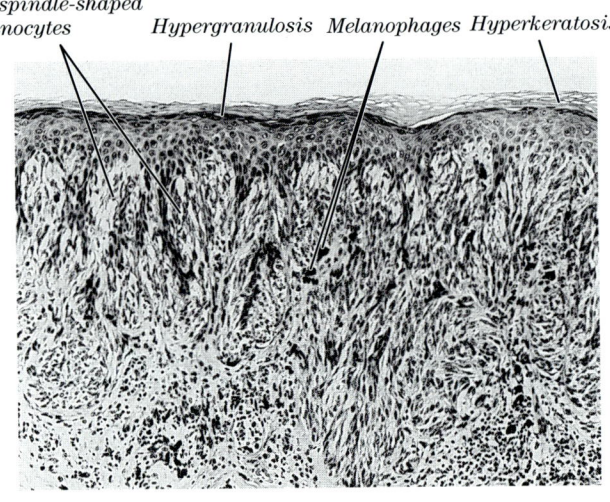

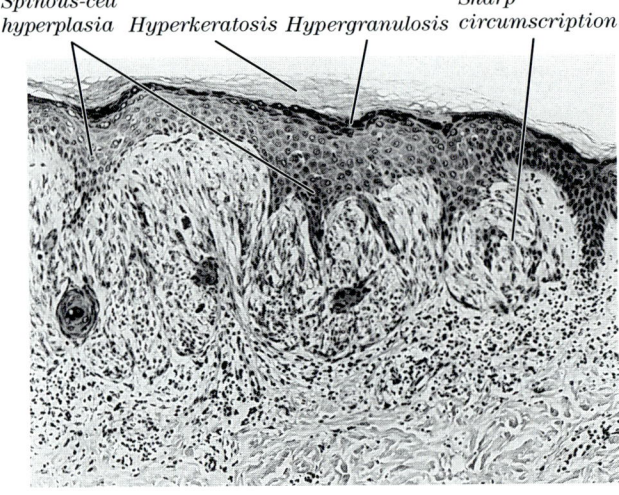

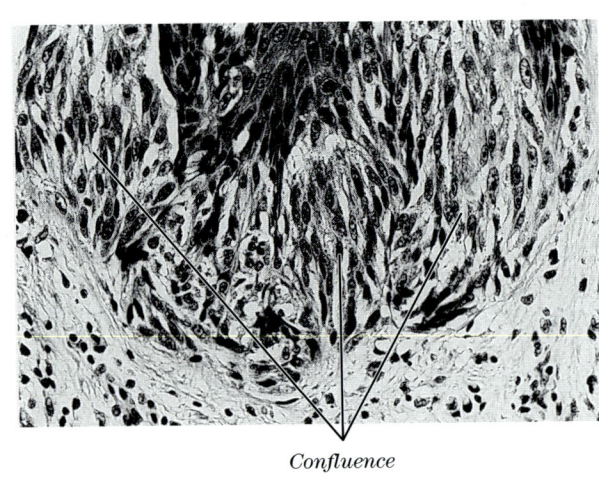

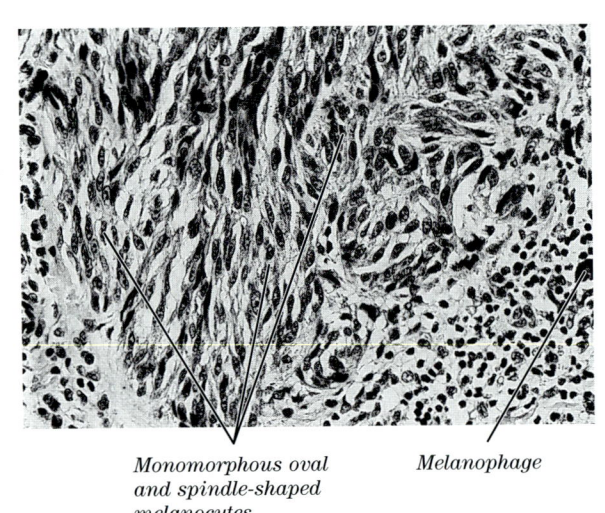

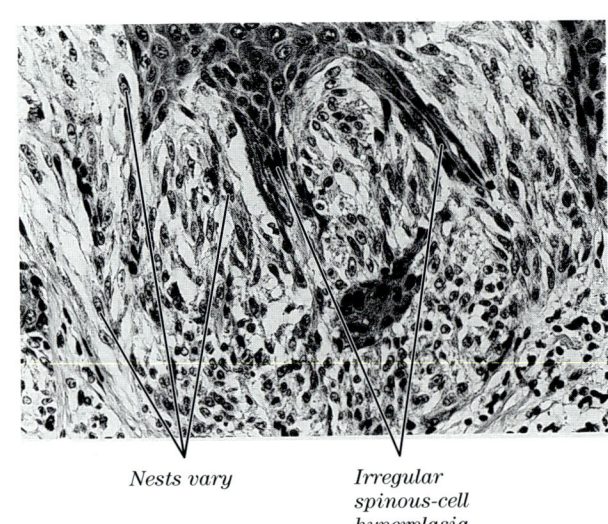

87 • Spitz's Nevus ("pigmented spindle-cell" type)

Criteria for diagnosis of this Spitz's nevus ("pigmented spindle-cell" type)

This is a nevus because:

1. The neoplasm is relatively symmetric.
2. It is well-circumscribed.
3. The base of it is relatively flat.
4. There is maturation of melanocytes.
5. Melanocytes within the epidermis are arranged mostly in nests, rather than as solitary units.
6. The melanocytes have monomorphous nuclei.

This is a Spitz's nevus because:

1. Many melanocytes have largish nuclei, abundant cytoplasm, and oval and spindle shape.
2. There are hyperkeratosis, hypergranulosis, and irregular spinous-cell hyperplasia.

3. Clefts are present between some elongated nests of melanocytes and adjacent keratinocytes.
4. Nests of melanocytes at the dermo-epidermal junction are mostly perpendicular to the skin surface.

This is a "pigmented spindle-cell" variant of Spitz's nevus because:

1. Nearly all melanocytes within the epidermis have oval or spindle shapes.
2. Abundant melanin is distributed in relatively uniform fashion throughout the neoplasm, both in melanocytes and macrophages.

Pitfall in diagnosis

This Spitz's nevus could be misinterpreted as a melanoma because:

1. Nests of melanocytes within the epidermis and the dermis vary in size and shape.
2. Some nests of melanocytes in the epidermis and the dermis have become confluent.
3. Some melanocytes have large nuclei and prominent nucleoli.

The architectural pattern of this neoplasm is that of a nevus because of symmetry and sharp circumscription. Furthermore, melanocytes mature with progressive descent into the dermis. Last, virtually all of the melanocytes organized in nests are situated at the dermo-epidermal junction, not above it. For these reasons, this lesion is a nevus.

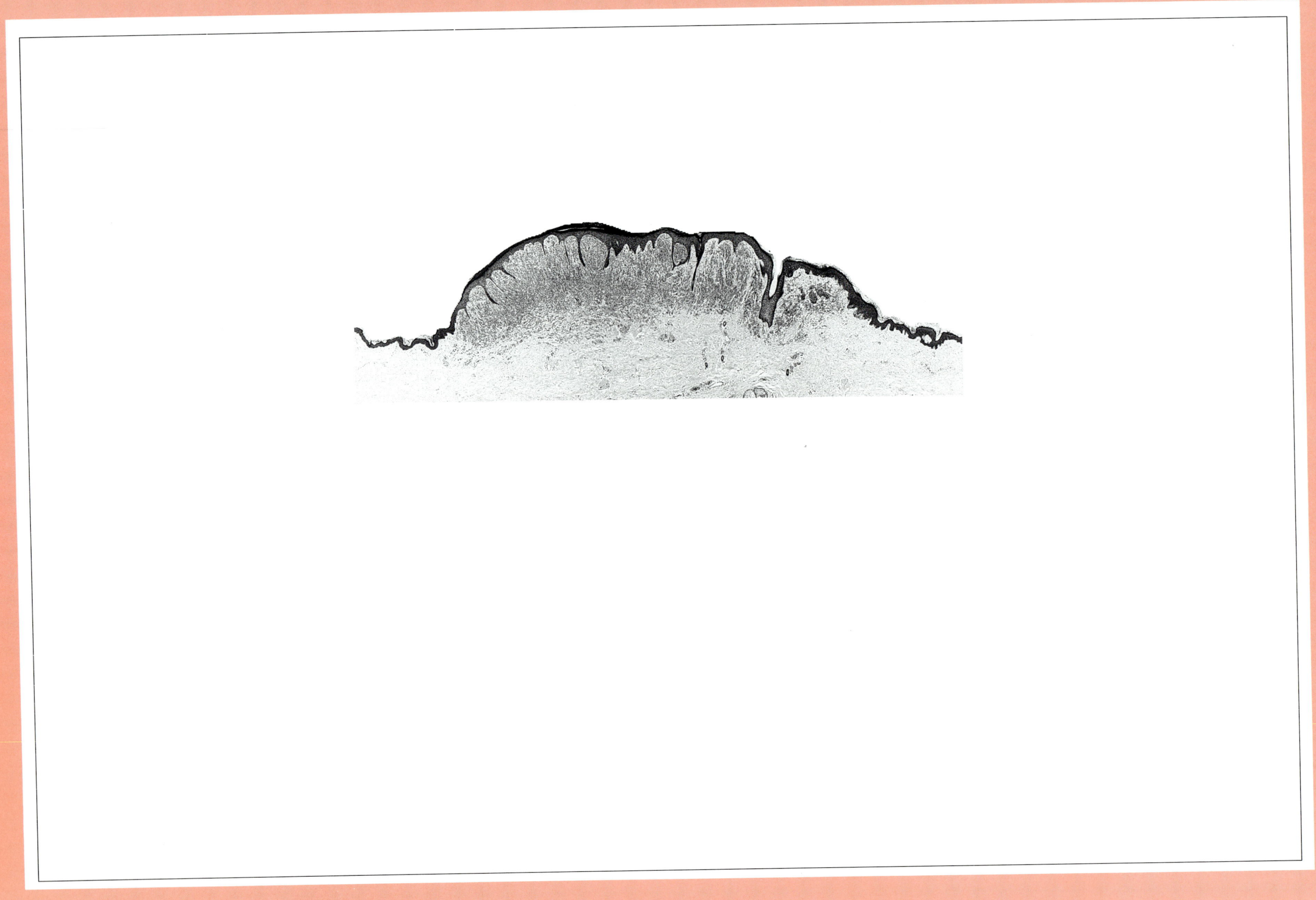

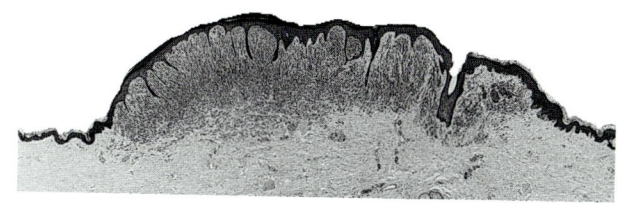
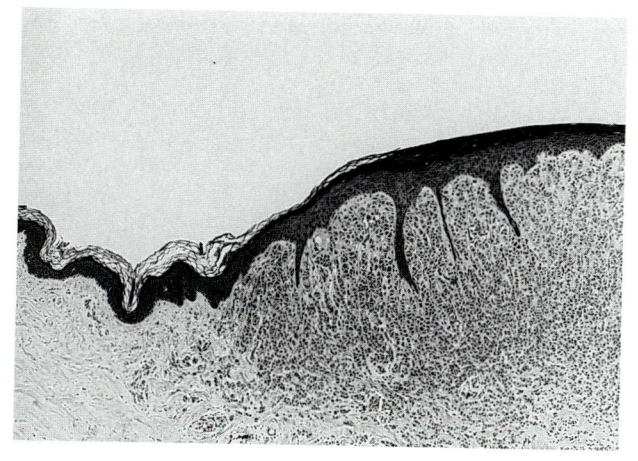
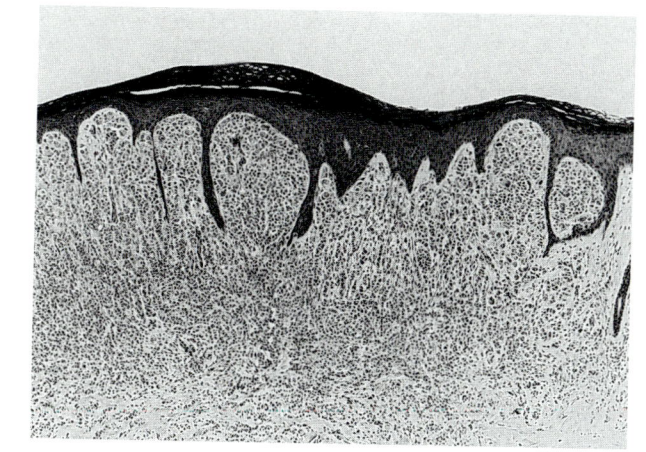
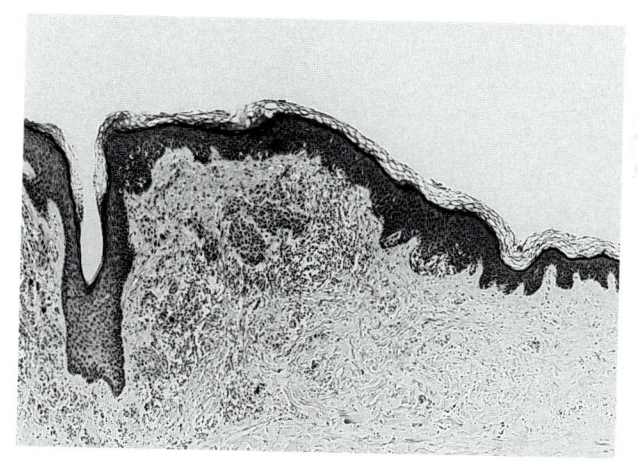
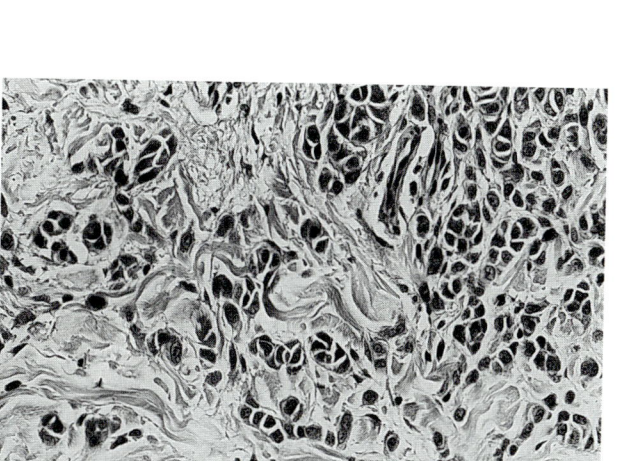
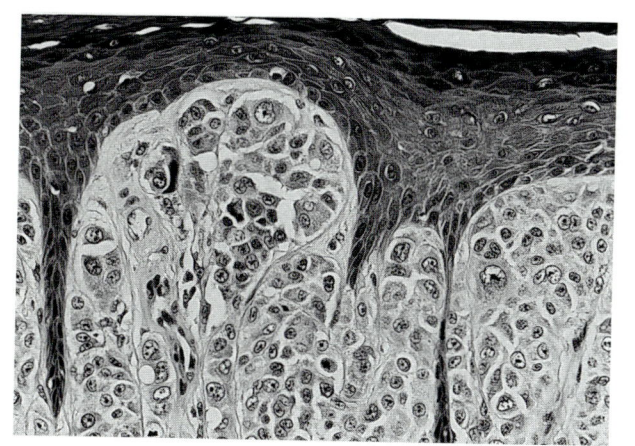
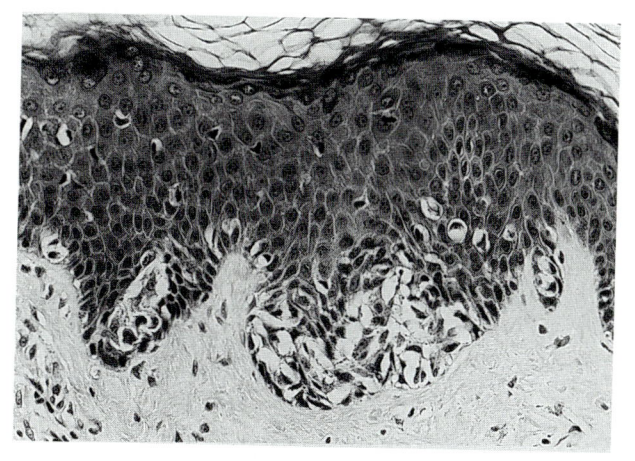

88. What is your diagnosis?

A cluster of papules appeared on the right shin of a 40-year-old man. Originally they were brown "freckles," but in 1 year they came to range in color from that of normal skin to red brown. Clinical diagnosis: amelanotic melanoma. Wide excision of the site with skin graft, superficial groin dissection, and isolation perfusion were performed. All lymph nodes removed were negative for signs of metastasis. No additional follow-up information was available.

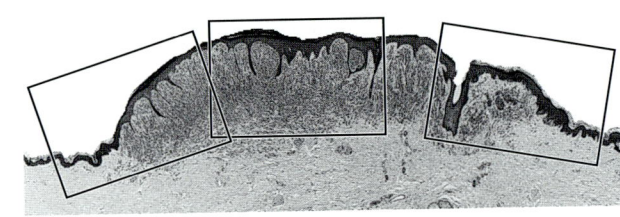

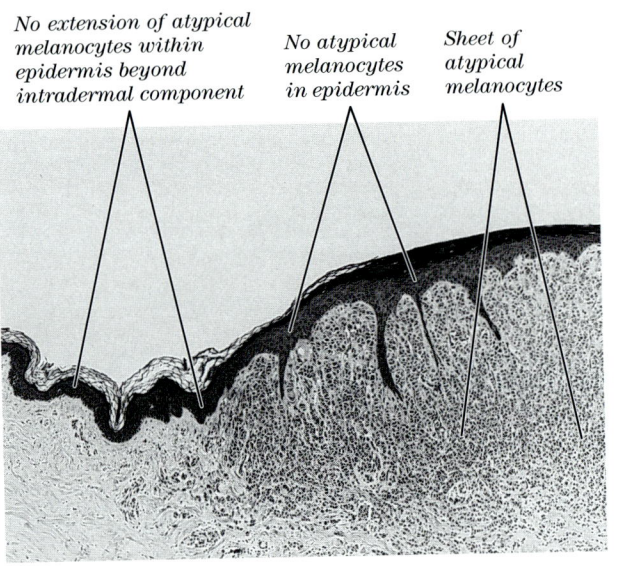

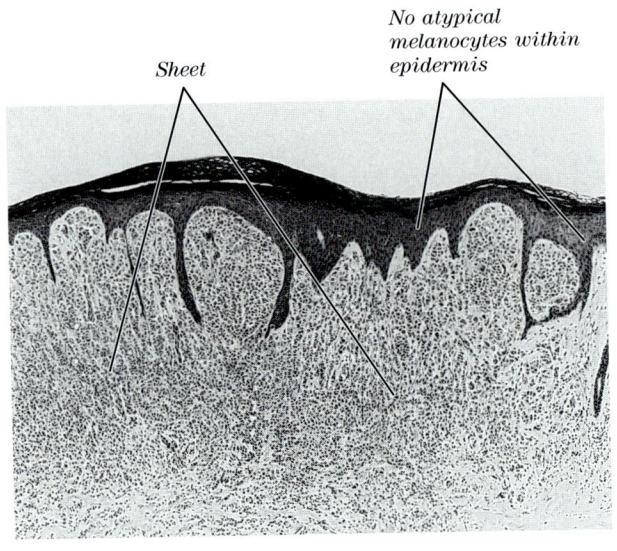

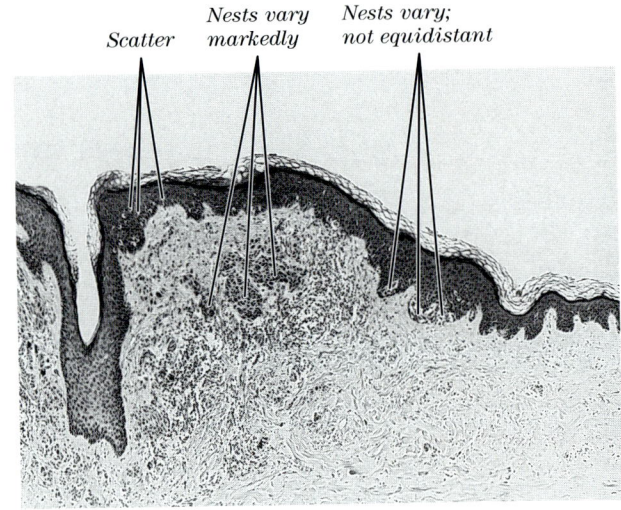

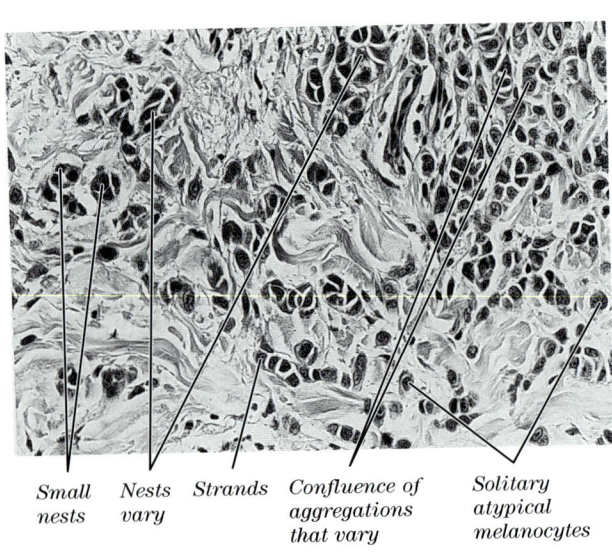

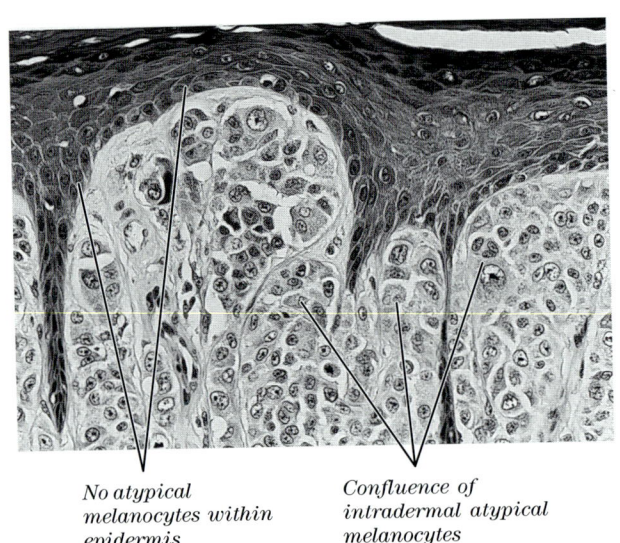

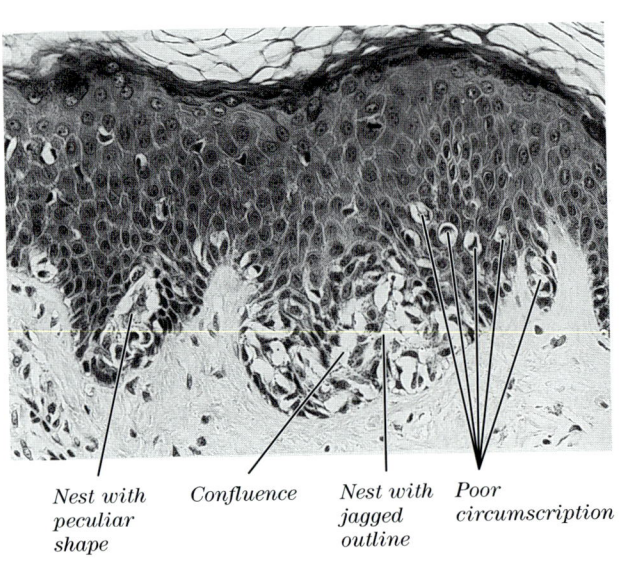

88 • Metastasis of Melanoma *(epidermotropic)*

Criteria for diagnosis of this epidermotropically metastatic melanoma

This is a metastatic melanoma because:

1. On the left side, the intradermal component of the neoplasm extends far beyond the intra-epidermal component of it.

2. The overwhelming majority of neoplastic melanocytes reside within the dermis; relatively few neoplastic melanocytes are positioned within the epidermis.

3. Neoplastic melanocytes within the epidermis are situated mostly above the dermo-epidermal junction, rather than precisely at it.

Pitfall in diagnosis

This epidermotropically metastatic melanoma could be misinterpreted as a primary cutaneous melanoma because:

1. Atypical melanocytes, both those disposed as solitary units and those in nests, are arrayed at the dermo-epidermal junction and above it.

2. Atypical melanocytes are arranged both in discrete nests and sheets within the dermis.

3. Atypical melanocytes disposed as solitary units are distributed between bundles of collagen in the reticular dermis.

4. Melanocytes do not mature.

5. The intra-epidermal component on the right side of the neoplasm appears to extend beyond the intradermal component.

This metastasis of melanoma has many features in common with primary melanoma, including proliferation of melanocytes as solitary units and in nests at all levels of the epidermis. Those changes, however, are present only on the right side of the neoplasm. The remainder of the dermo-epidermal junction is devoid of a proliferation of melanocytes, either as solitary units or in nests. That finding militates against primary melanoma. In short, for the aforementioned reasons, this is an epidermotropically metastatic melanoma.

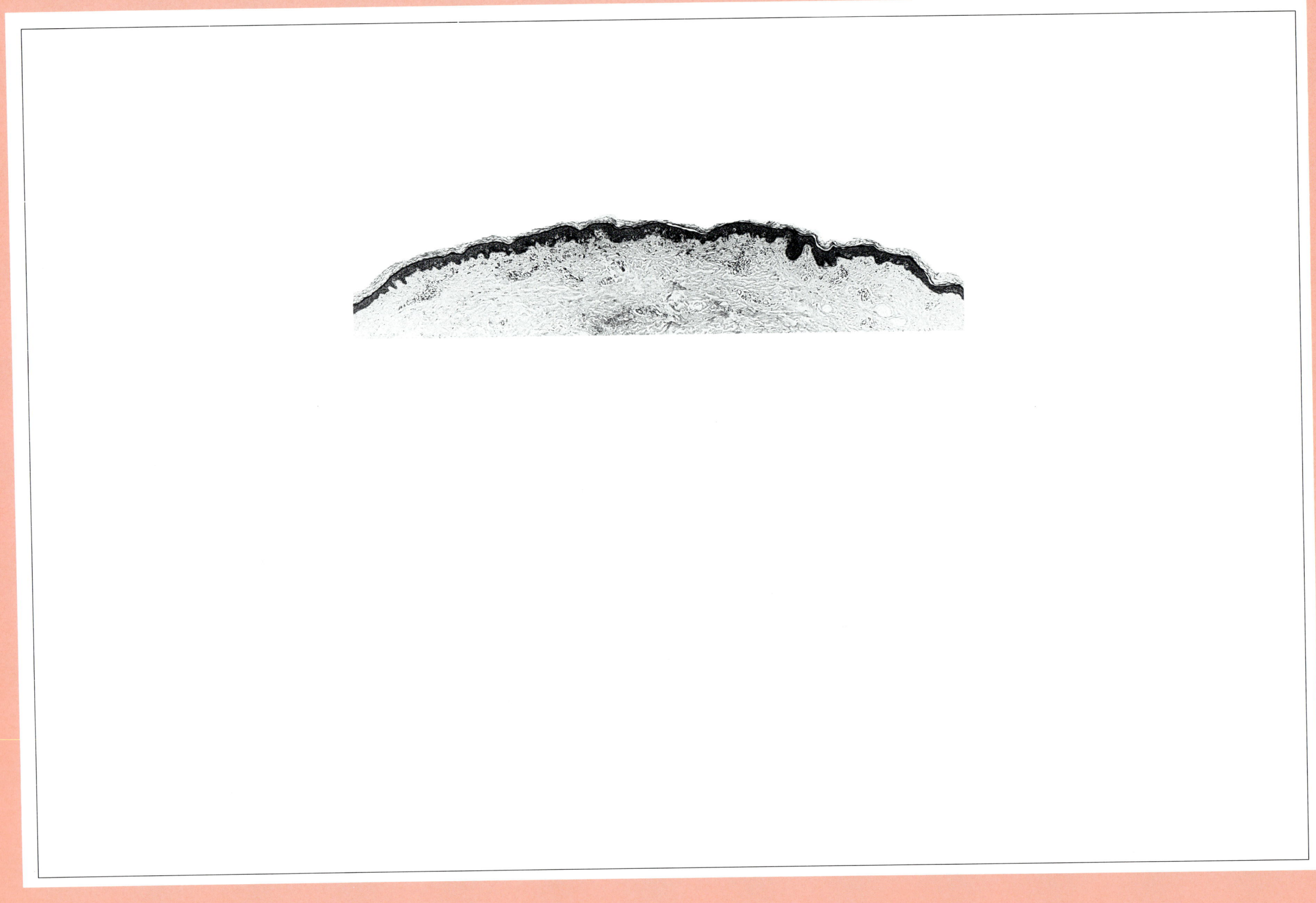

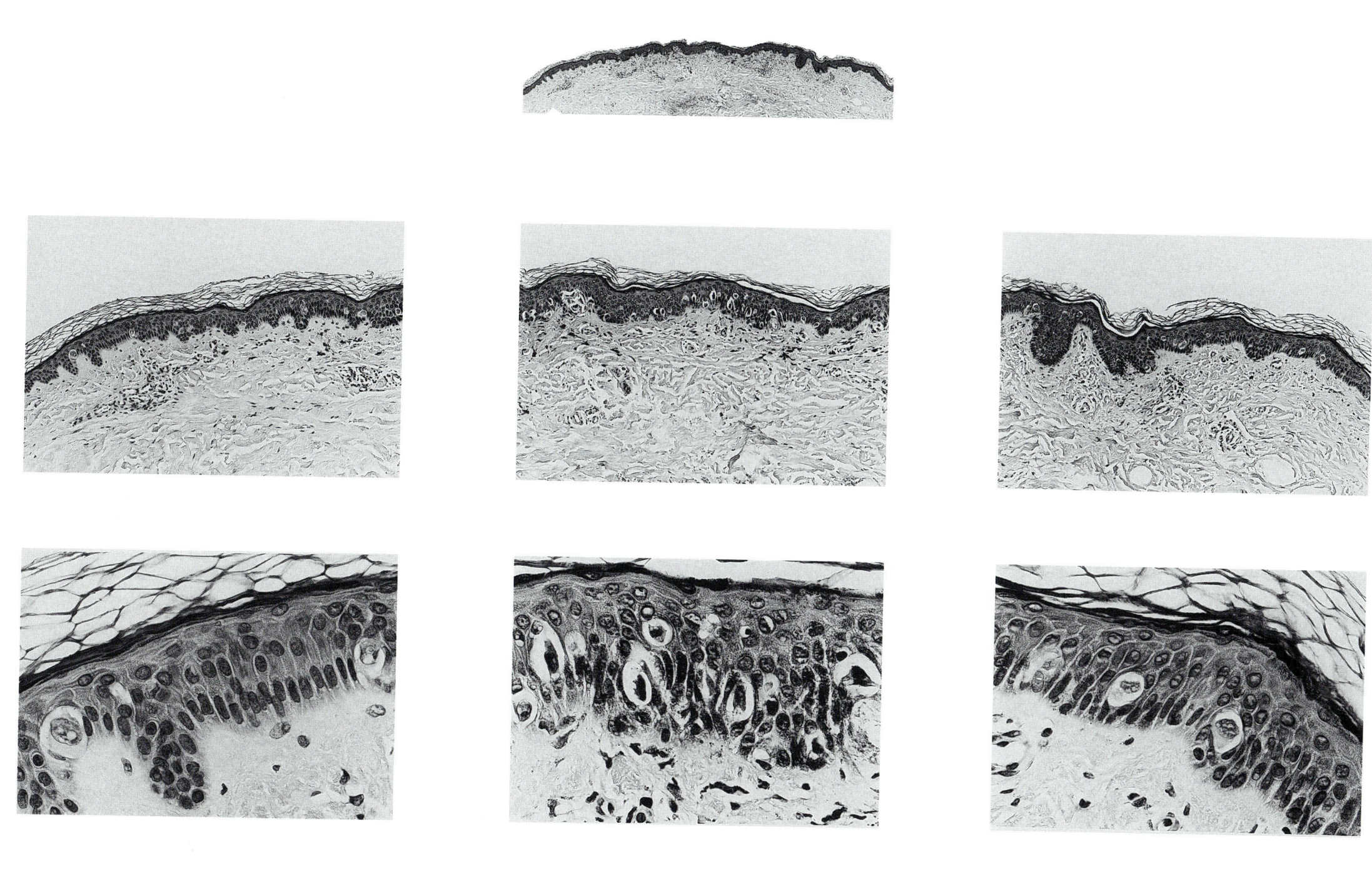

89. What is your diagnosis?

Pigmented lesion from the right thigh of a 25-year-old woman. Clinical diagnosis: dysplastic nevus. No follow-up data were available.

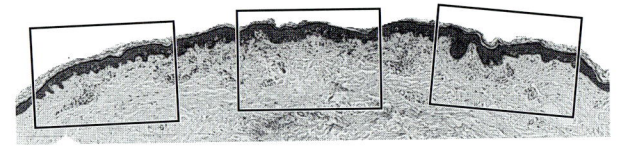

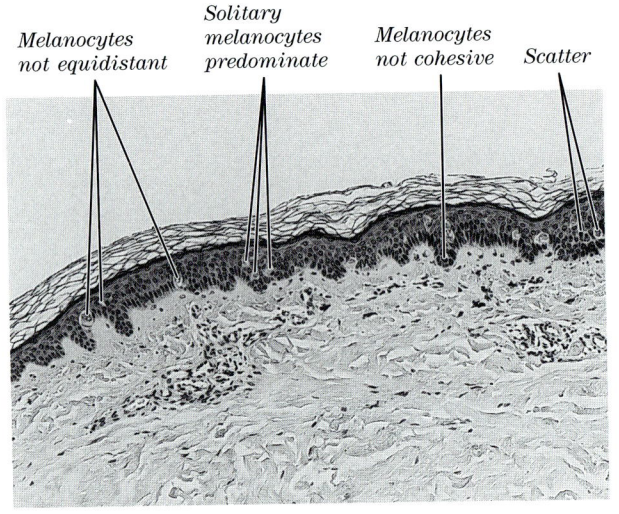

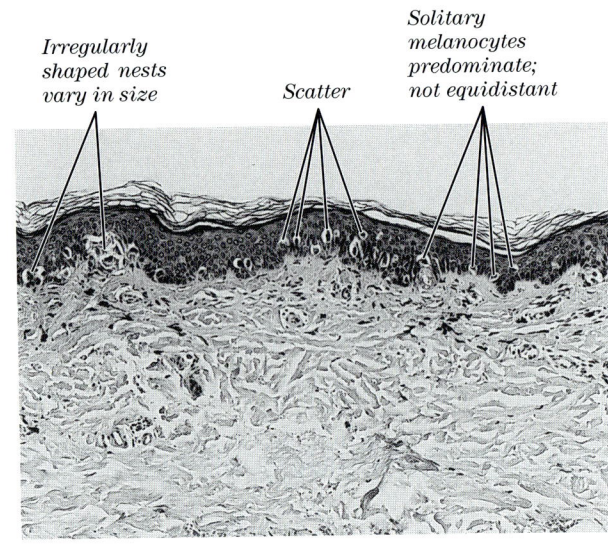

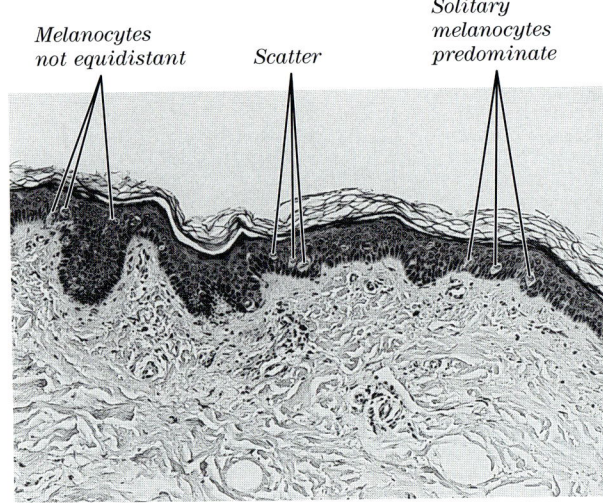

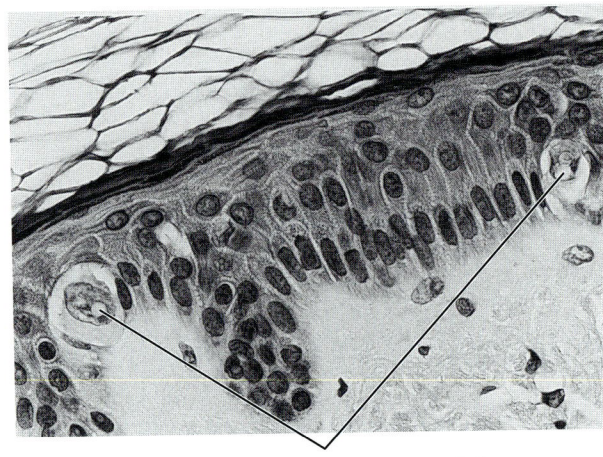

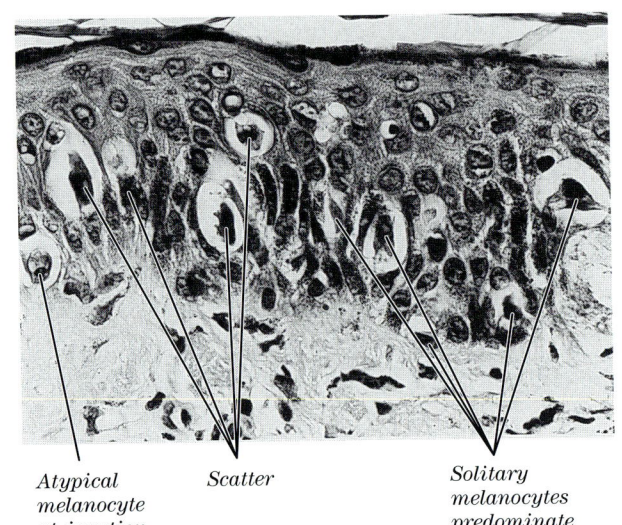

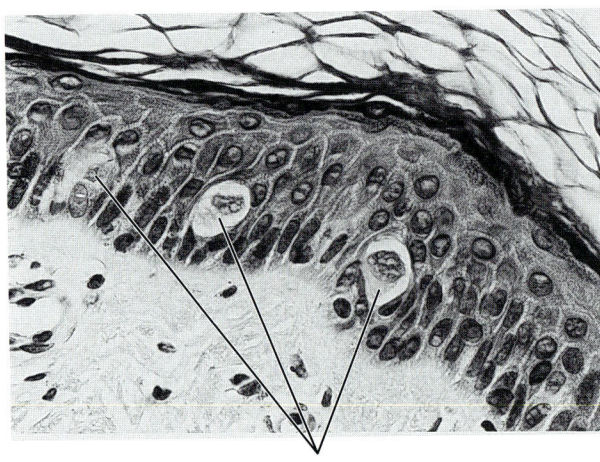

89 • Melanoma in situ

Criteria for diagnosis of this melanoma in situ

This is a melanoma in situ because:

1. Melanocytes arranged as solitary units within the epidermis predominate overwhelmingly over melanocytes arranged in nests there.

2. Melanocytes disposed as solitary units are not equidistant from one another.

3. Melanocytes arrayed as solitary units are scattered throughout the lower half of the epidermis.

4. Nuclei of melanocytes are atypical.

5. Melanin is not distributed in uniform fashion throughout the neoplasm.

Pitfall in diagnosis

This melanoma in situ could be misread as a junctional Spitz's nevus because:

1. The neoplasm is small.

2. Most melanocytes are positioned in the lower portion of the epidermis.

3. Melanocytes at the periphery of the neoplasm have relatively monomorphous nuclei.

The differential diagnosis of this melanoma in situ is junctional Spitz's nevus at an early stage of its development. Unlike Spitz's nevus, however, this melanoma in situ is characterized by individual melanocytes that are not equidistant from one another and by marked pleomorphism of melanocytes. This combination of findings enables definitive diagnosis of the neoplasm as melanoma in situ.

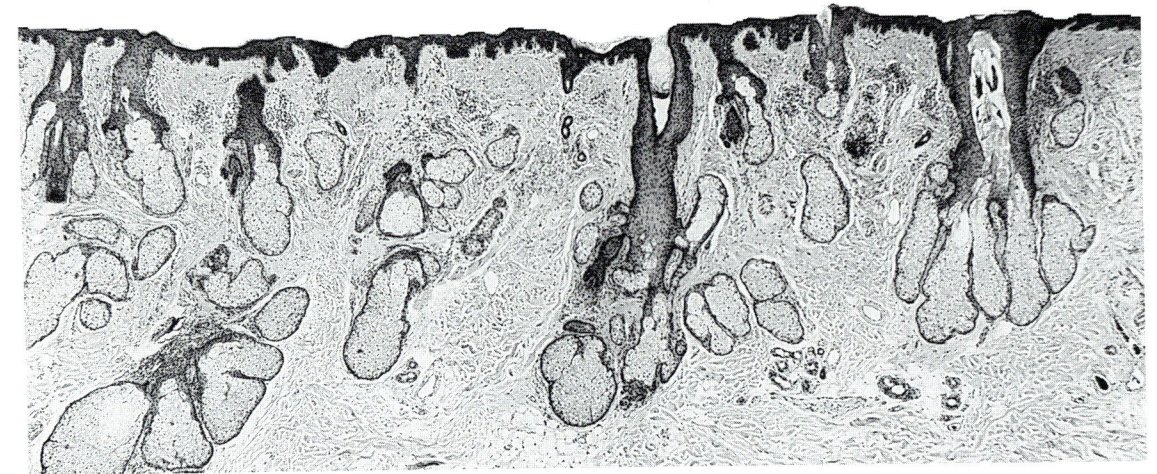

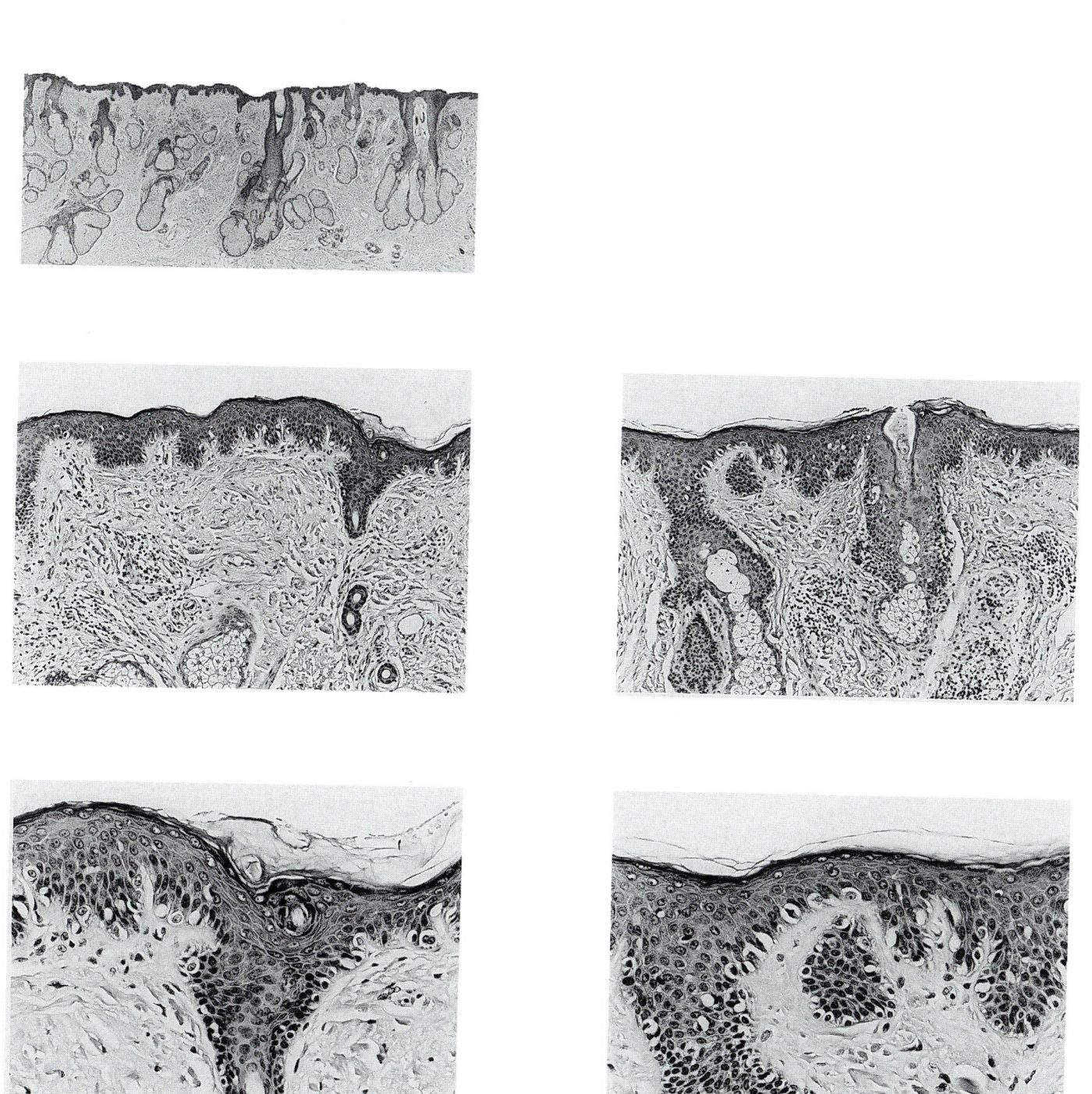

90. What is your diagnosis?

Specimen of a blephoroplasty performed on a 46-year-old white woman.

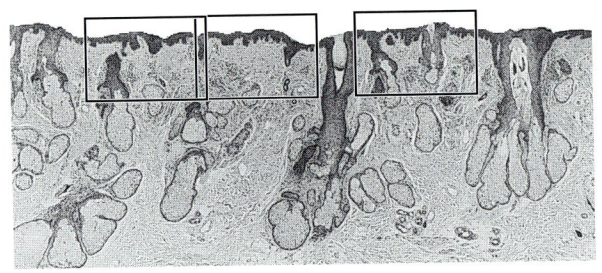

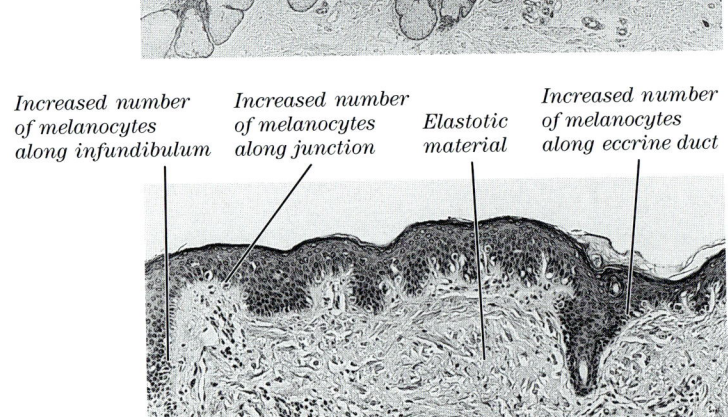

Increased number of melanocytes — *Sparse infiltrate of lymphocytes* — *Abundant solar elastosis* — *Increased number of melanocytes*

Increased number of melanocytes along infundibulum — *Increased number of melanocytes along junction* — *Elastotic material* — *Increased number of melanocytes along eccrine duct*

Melanocytes at junction of infundibulum and dermis — *Lymphocytes* — *Increased number of melanocytes at junction* — *Extensive solar elastosis*

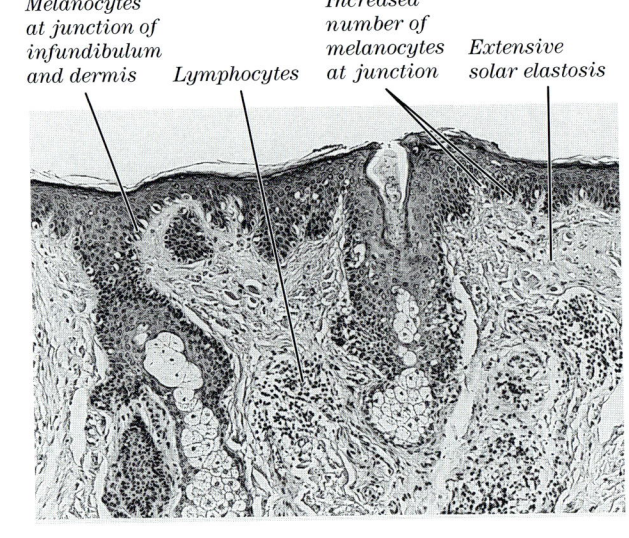

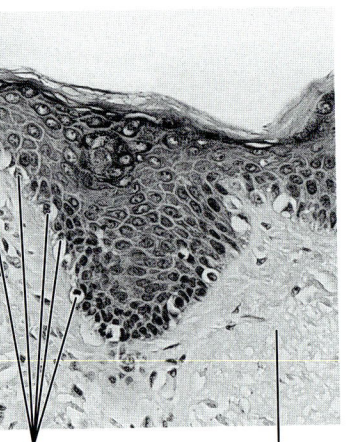

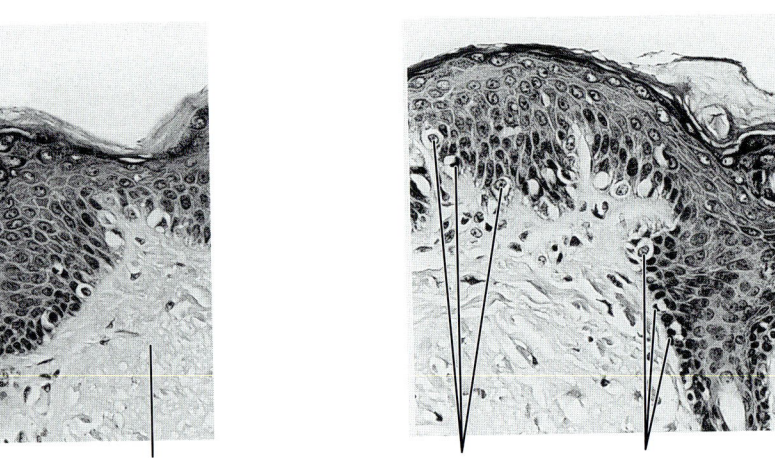

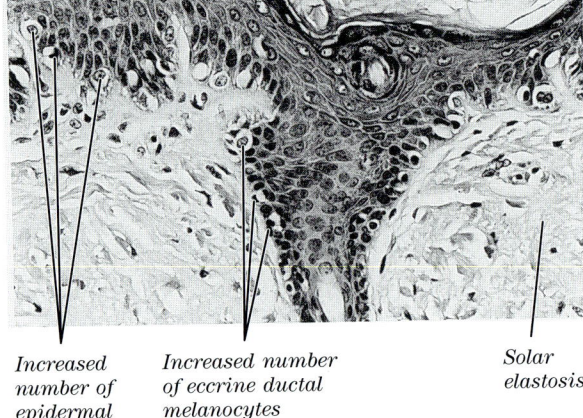

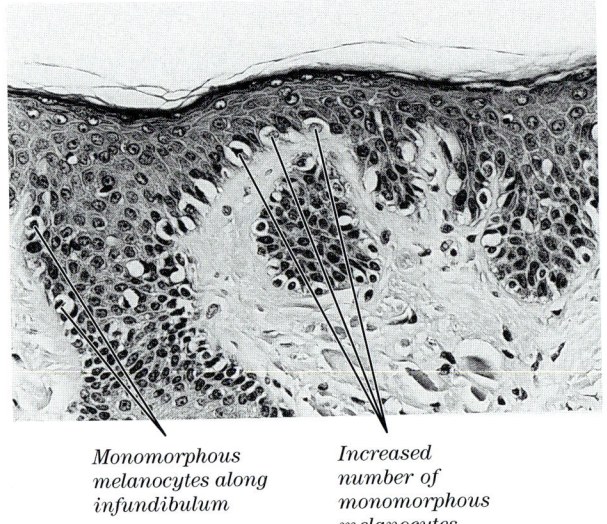

Increased number of monomorphous melanocytes — *Copious elastotic material*

Increased number of epidermal melanocytes — *Increased number of eccrine ductal melanocytes* — *Solar elastosis*

Monomorphous melanocytes along infundibulum — *Increased number of monomorphous melanocytes*

90 • Normal Skin of Eyelid

Criteria for diagnosis of this section of normal skin of an eyelid

This is normal skin of an eyelid because:

1. The melanocytes are nearly equidistant from one another.

2. The nuclei of melanocytes are small, oval, and monomorphous.

3. No melanocytes are present above the dermo-epidermal junction.

4. There are no nests of melanocytes, even tiny ones.

5. None of the melanocytes are multinucleate.

6. Melanin is hardly noticeable and what little there is, is distributed uniformly.

7. Most nuclei of melanocytes are not hyperchromatic.

Pitfall in diagnosis

This specimen from normal skin of an eyelid could be misread as an early lesion of melanoma in situ (so-called lentigo maligna) because:

1. What seems to be an increased number of melanocytes at the dermo-epidermal junction is actually normal for an eyelid.

2. The presence of melanocytes within the upper reaches of epithelial structures of adnexa is within expected normal limits for a normal eyelid.

3. Nuclei of melanocytes are slightly large, but not pleomorphic.

4. The "clear cells" just above the mid-spinous zone are Langerhans' cells, not melanocytes.

Histopathologists must be alert to the pitfall of overdiagnosing a "normal" proliferation of melanocytes at the dermo-epidermal junction of skin of a normal eyelid or skin badly damaged by sunlight as melanoma in situ. As a rule, unless melanocytes arranged as solitary units are not equidistant from one another and at least a few melanocytes are not present above the dermo-epidermal junction, a diagnosis of melanoma in situ should not be made without equivocation when solitary melanocytes monopolize. Nuclear atypia is not a sine qua non for diagnosis of melanoma in situ, although that finding is common. If, in this same setting, one or more nests of melanocytes were present within the epidermis, then a diagnosis of melanoma in situ should be considered seriously. Last, it should be noted that, in some instances, especially on sun-damaged skin of a face, a diagnosis of melanoma in situ can be made when melanocytes are disposed only as solitary units seated entirely at the dermo-epidermal junction. In those instances, however, criteria for diagnosis of melanoma in situ must be fulfilled strictly.

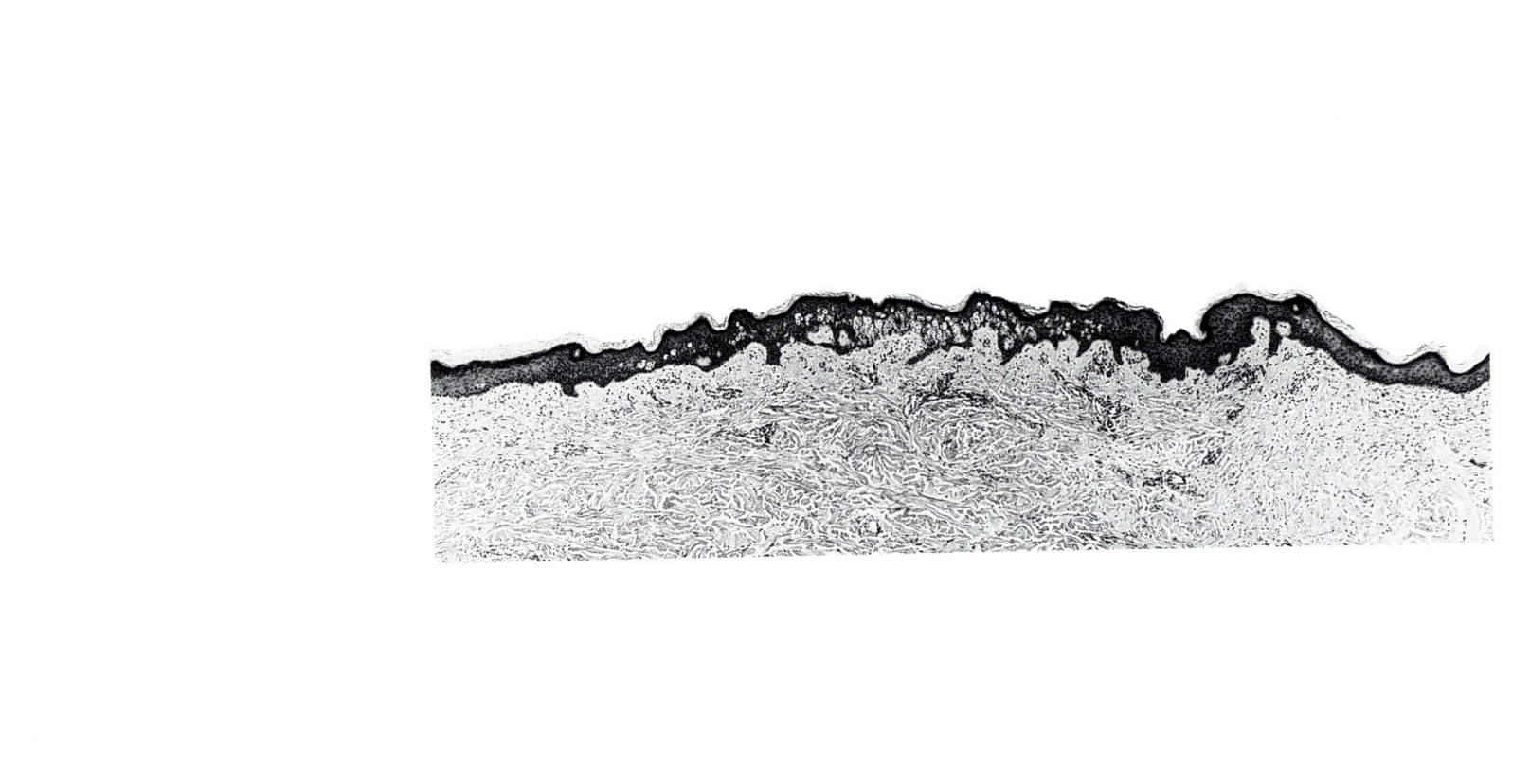

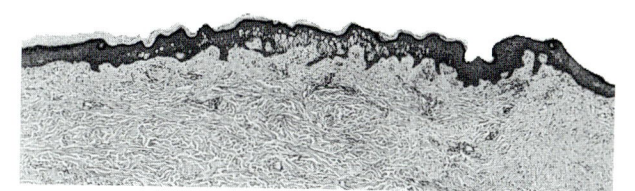
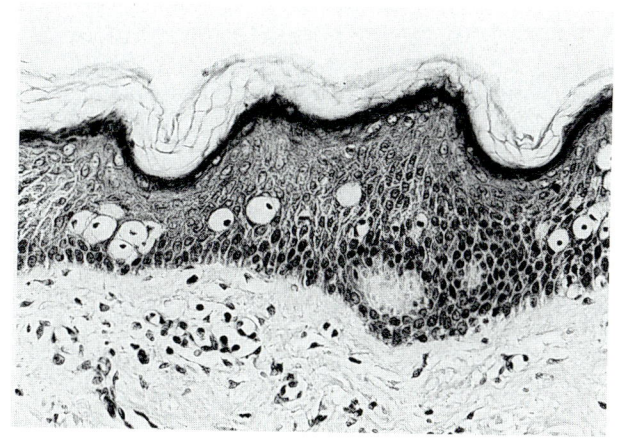
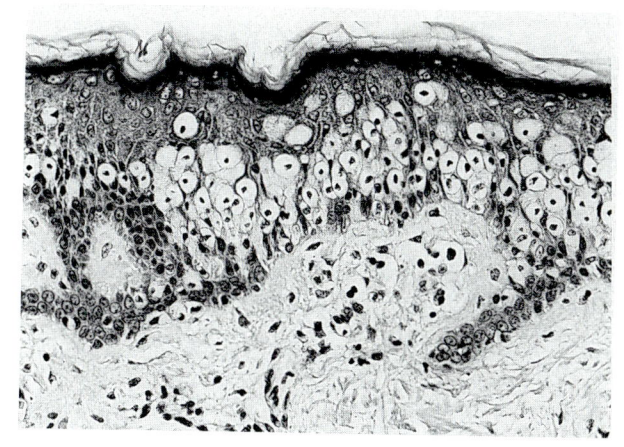
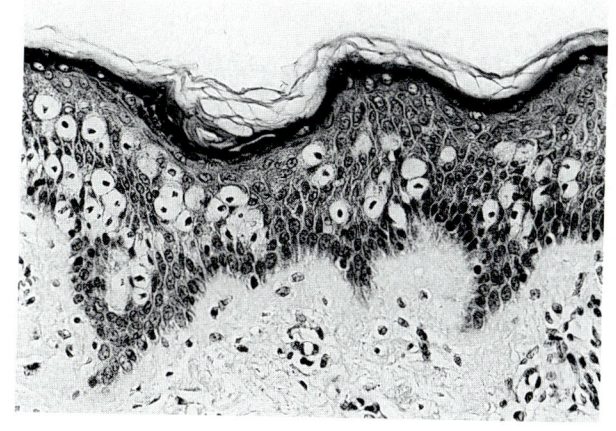
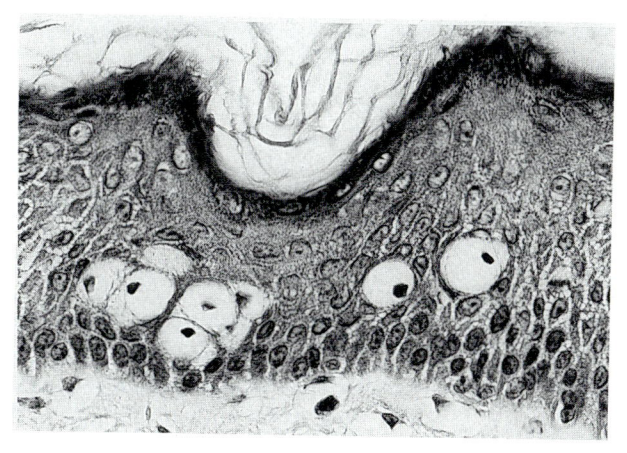
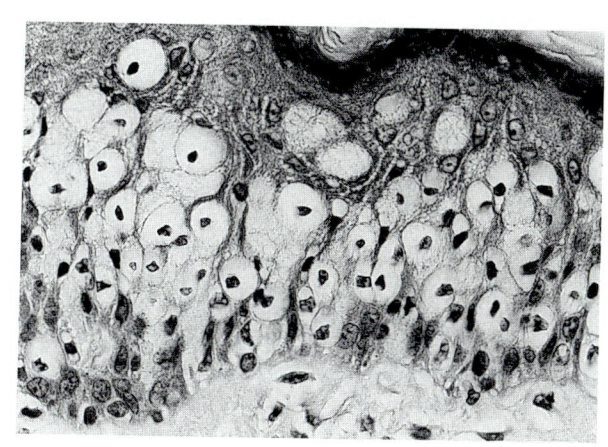
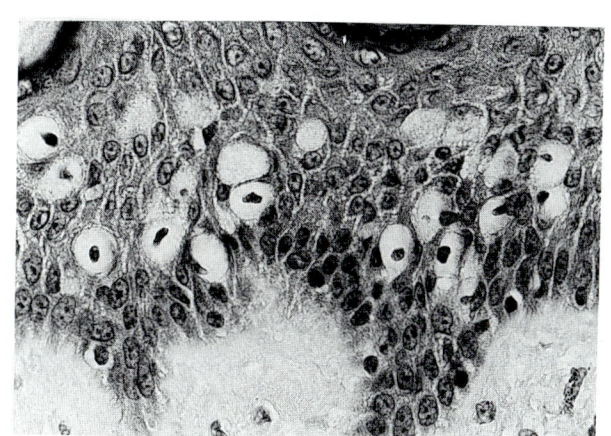

91. What is your diagnosis?

Apparently normal skin from the margin of a specimen that contained basal-cell carcinoma was removed from the trunk of a 52-year-old white man.

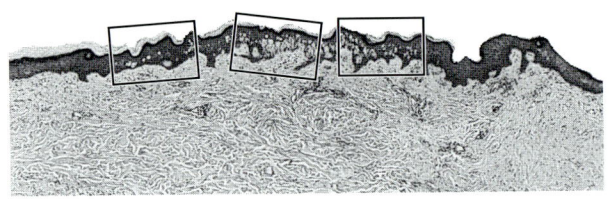

Large spaces around nuclei of keratinocytes

Large spaces around nuclei of contiguous keratinocytes

Clear cell keratinocytes in upper part of epidermis

Large halos around nuclei of keratinocytes

No spaces around nuclei of keratinocytes in lower part of epidermis

Normal melanocytes

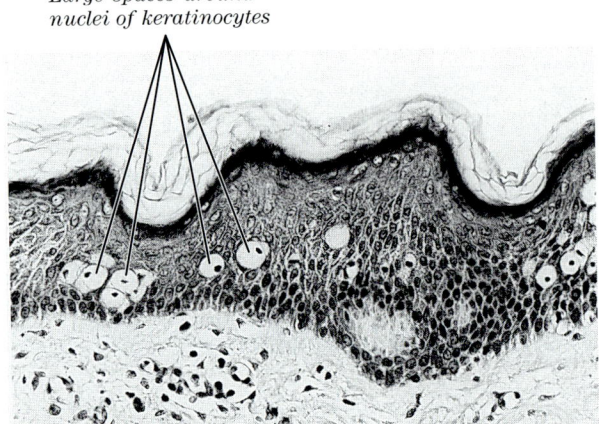
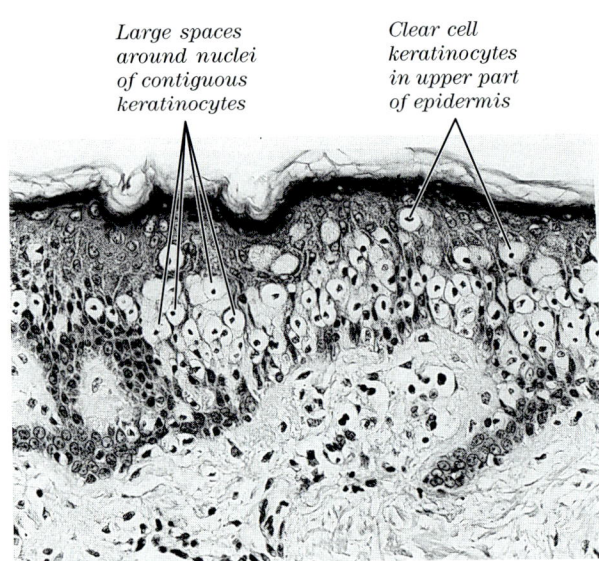
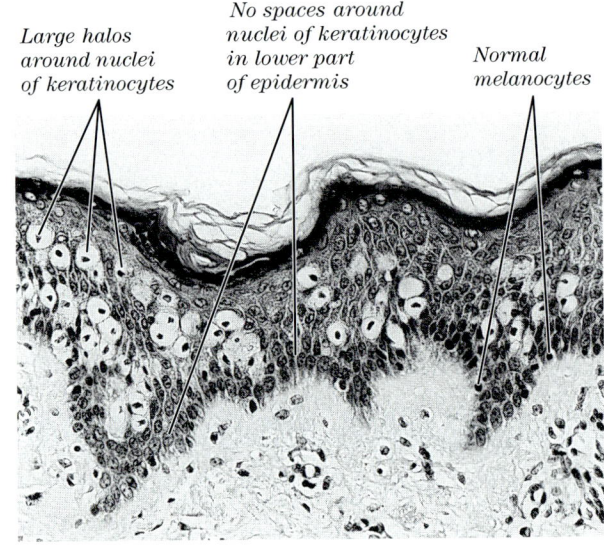

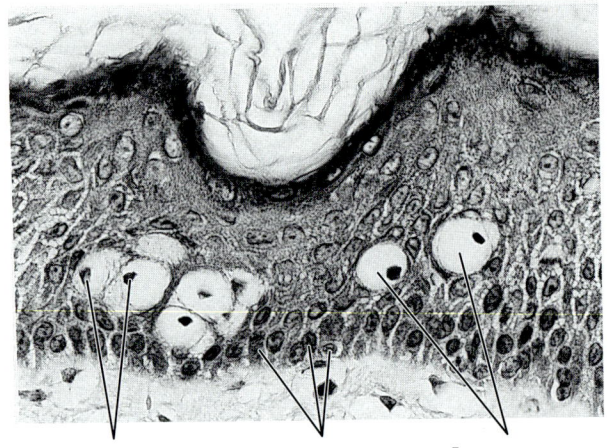
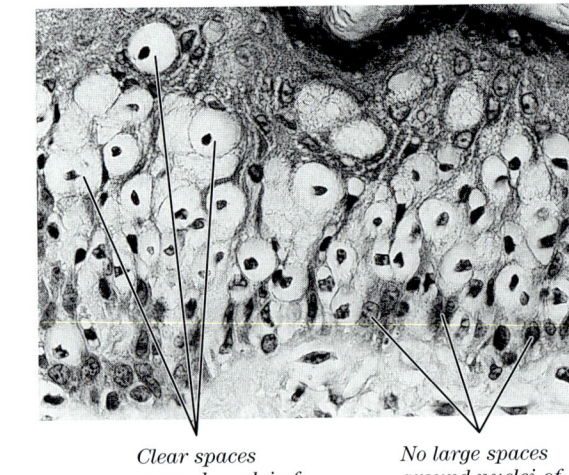
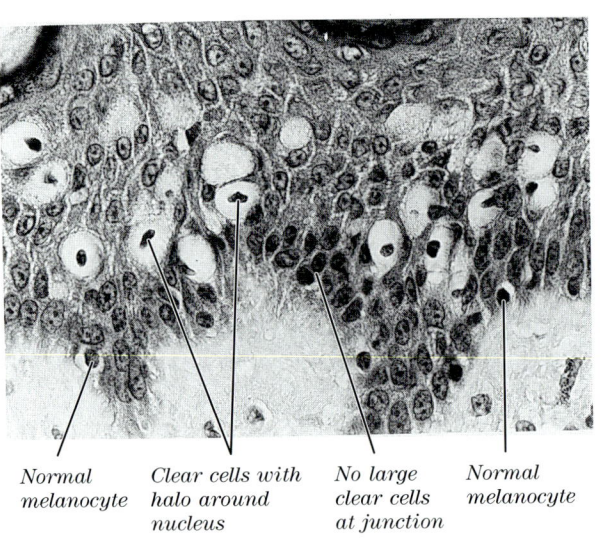

Large spaces around nuclei of spinous keratinocytes

No large spaces around basal keratinocytes or melanocytes

Large spaces around nuclei of spinous keratinocytes

Clear spaces around nuclei of keratinocytes

No large spaces around nuclei of cells in basal layer

Normal melanocyte

Clear cells with halo around nucleus

No large clear cells at junction

Normal melanocyte

91 • Artifactual Changes in Keratinocytes

Criteria for diagnosis of these artifactual changes in keratinocytes

This is an artifact in keratinocytes, not a proliferation of melanocytes, because:

1. The spaces are present around nuclei, not around cytoplasm.

2. No proliferation of melanocytes is present at the dermo-epidermal junction.

3. The nuclei surrounded by clear spaces are small and relatively monomorphous.

4. Some nuclei are distorted and shrunken.

5. Some intercellular bridges can still be identified around the "clear cells."

Pitfall in diagnosis

The keratinocytes associated with artifactual halos within the epidermis could be misconstrued as pagetoid or balloon melanocytes of melanoma in situ because:

1. Pale and clear cells are present throughout the epidermis.

2. Pale and clear cells have become confluent and appear to have formed aggregations that vary in size and shape.

3. Pale and clear cells are not equidistant from one another.

The finding crucial to differentiation of pale and clear keratinocytes from melanocytes of melanoma is absence of them from the dermo-epidermal junction. In order for a diagnosis of melanoma in situ to be made, some neoplastic melanocytes must be present at the junction. Furthermore, artificial spaces occur around the nuclei of keratinocytes and around the shrunken cytoplasm of melanocytes.

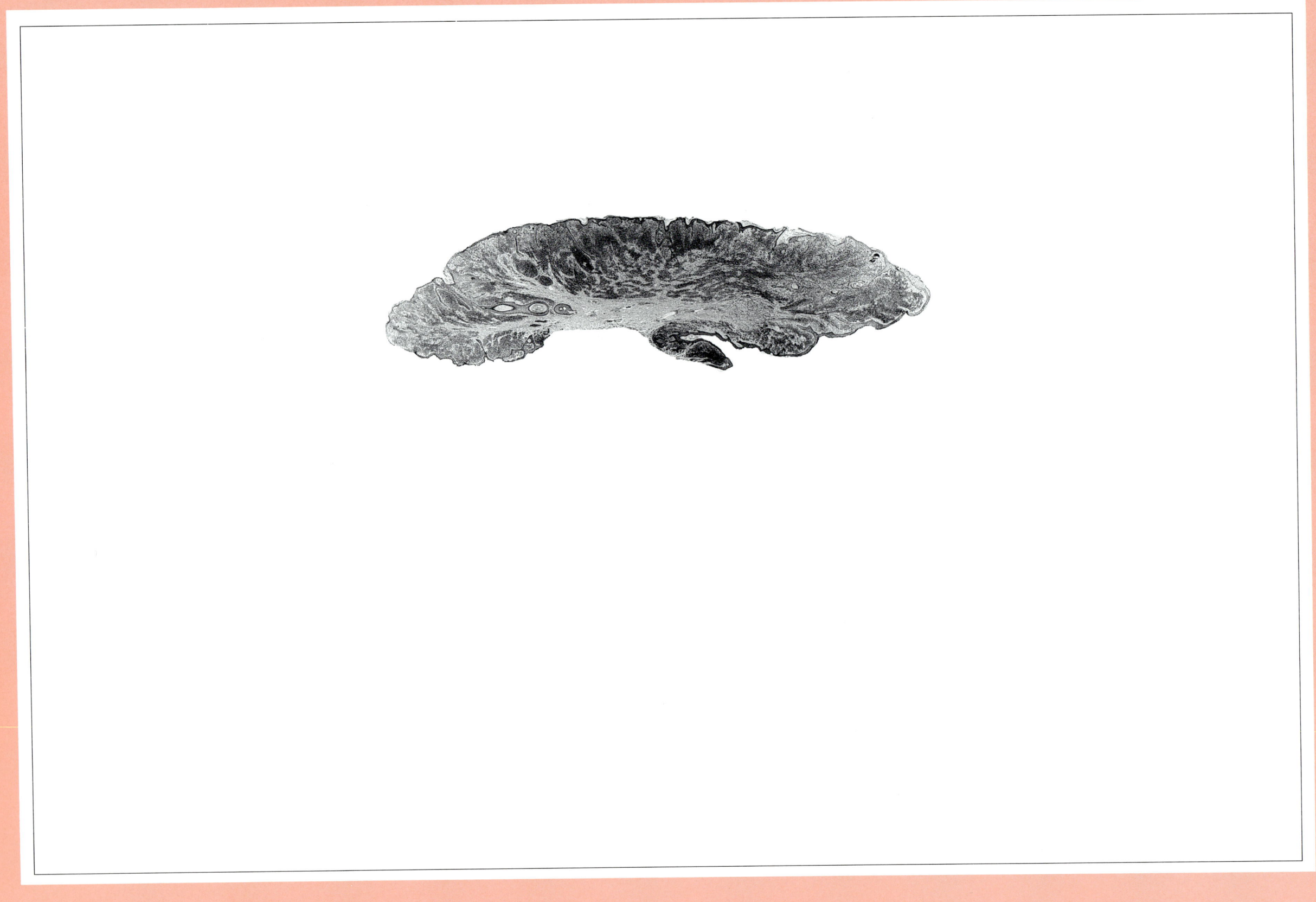

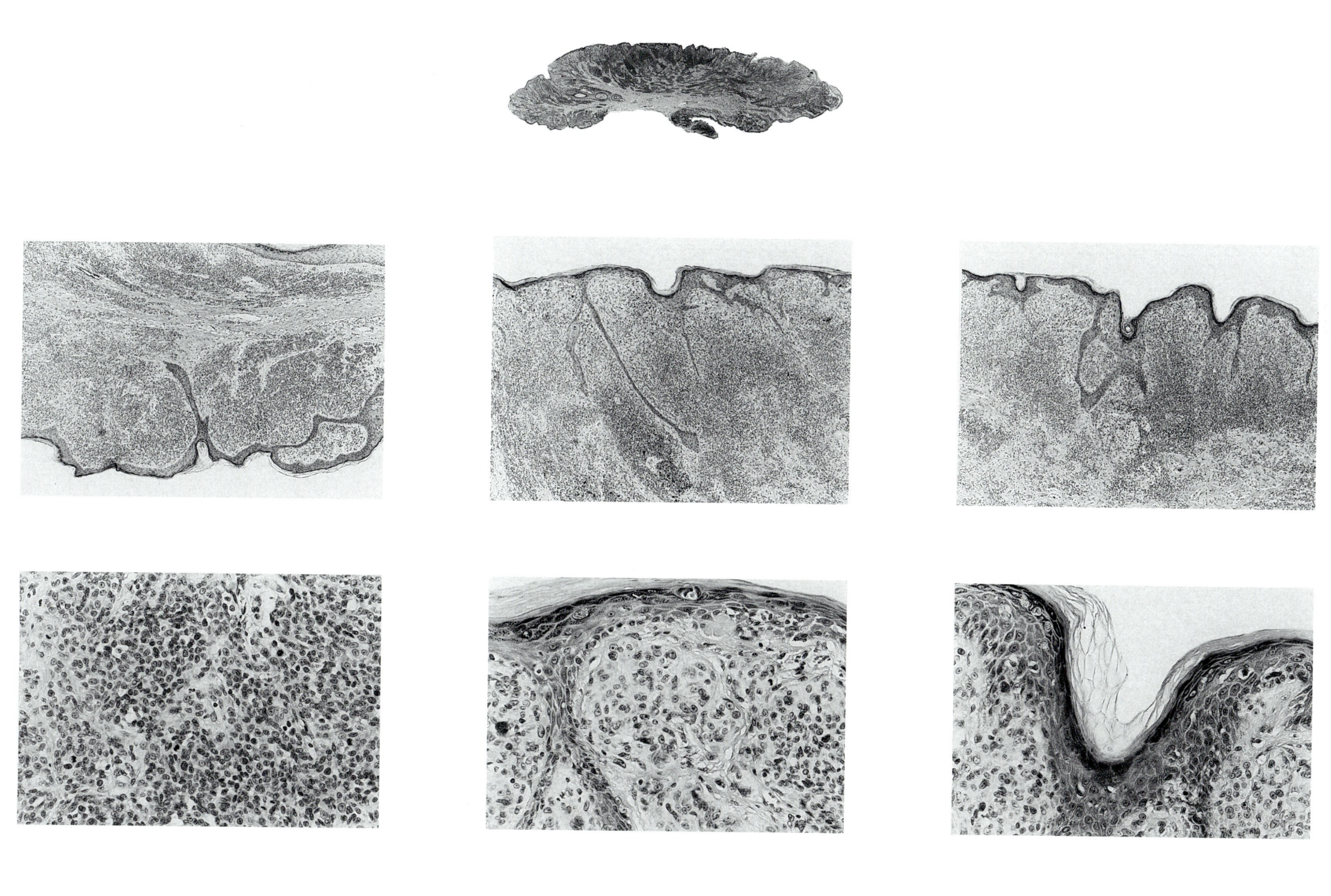

92. What is your diagnosis?

Pigmented lesion on the forearm of a 63-year-old man. Clinical diagnosis: basal-cell carcinoma. No follow-up data were available.

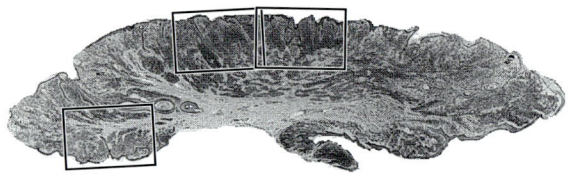

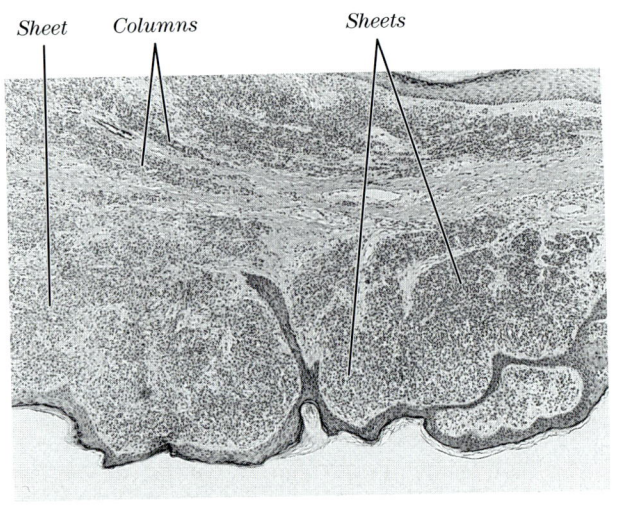

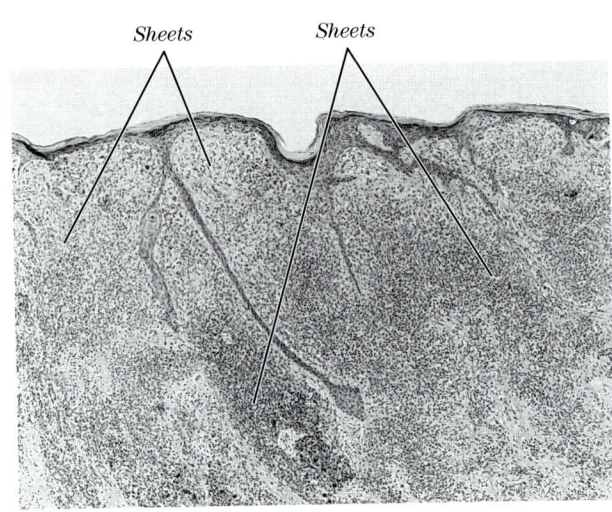

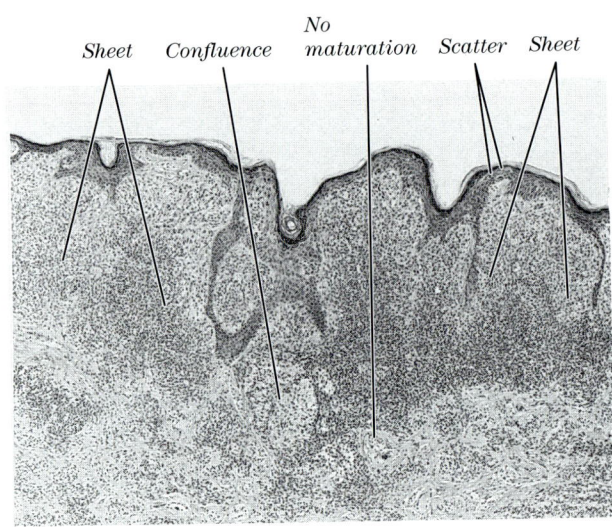

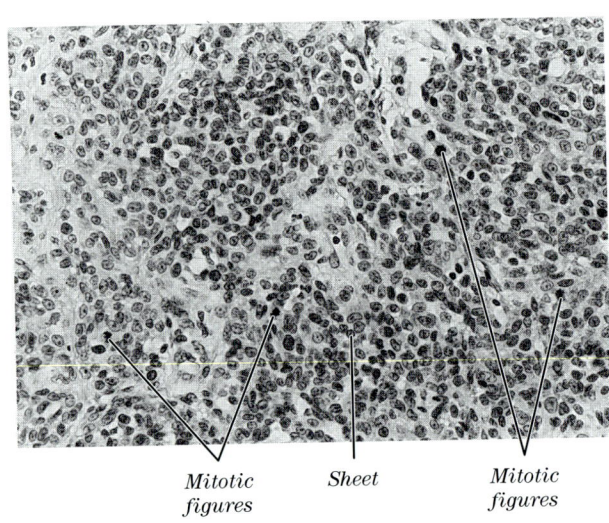

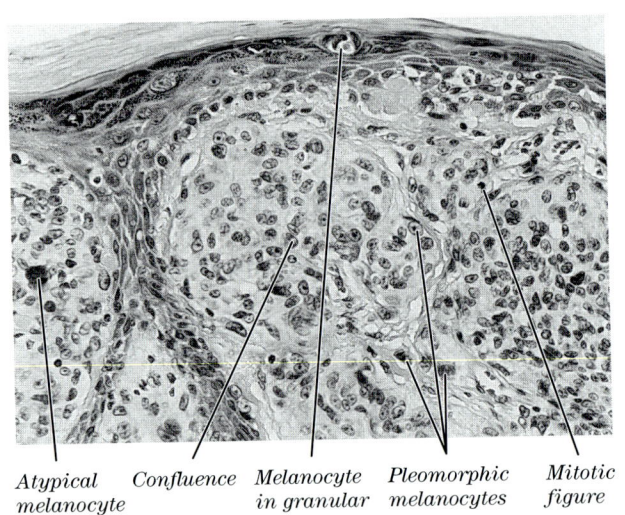

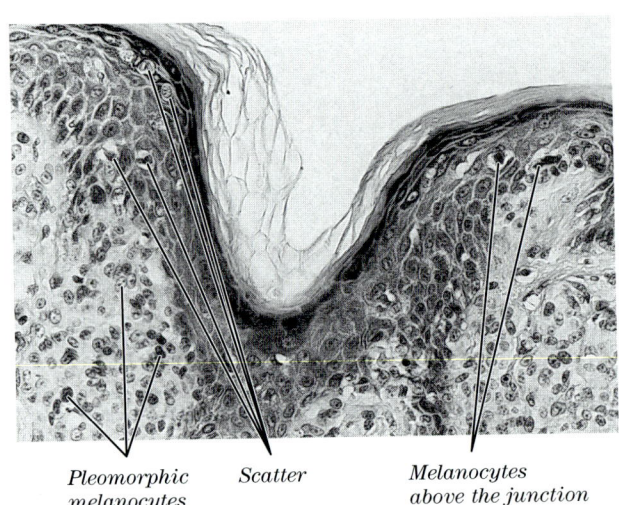

92 • Melanoma

Criteria for diagnosis of this melanoma

This is a melanoma because:

1. The neoplasm is asymmetric.
2. Melanocytes within the dermis are arranged in sheets.
3. Some melanocytes disposed as solitary units are present in the upper reaches of the epidermis.
4. Many neoplastic melanocytes within the dermis have atypical nuclei.
5. Many nuclei of melanocytes within the dermis are in mitosis.

Pitfall in diagnosis

This melanoma could be misconstrued as Unna's nevus because:

1. The neoplasm is mostly exophytic.
2. It is papillated.
3. Melanocytes of the neoplasm involve both the epidermis and the dermis.
4. Hyperplastic epithelial structures of adnexa, namely, eccrine ducts and infundibula, interweave to form reticulated and fenestrated patterns.
5. Nuclei of melanocytes are monomorphous in some foci.
6. There is practically no infiltrate of lymphocytes.

At scanning magnification, this polypoid lesion looks very much like Unna's nevus. That illusion is precisely why it is imperative to study all melanocytic neoplasms at higher magnification, despite the undisputed value of scanning magnification in the assessment of silhouette. When that was done here, sheets of melanocytes became apparent, as did many mitotic figures in those melanocytes. That combination of findings indicates melanoma.

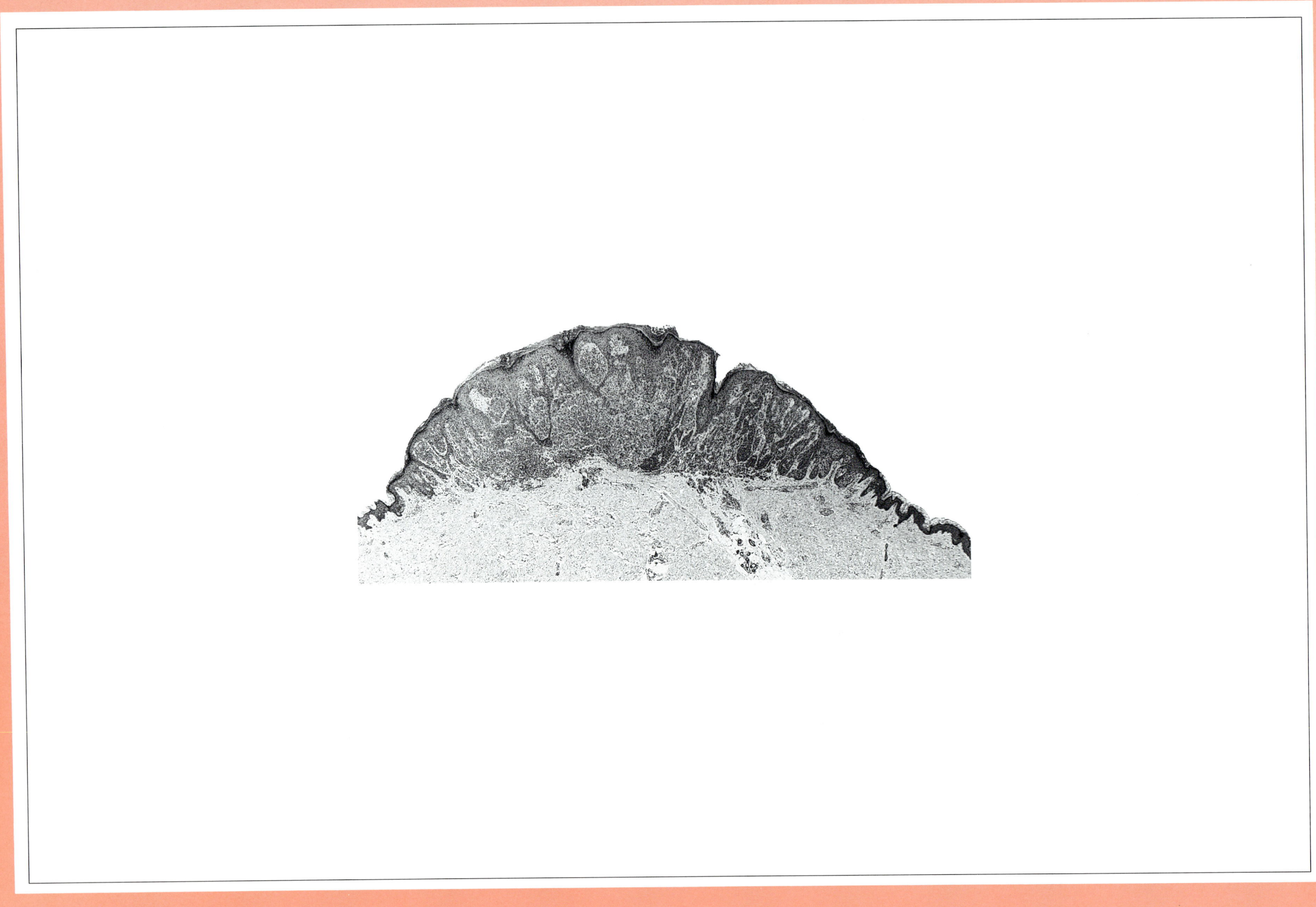

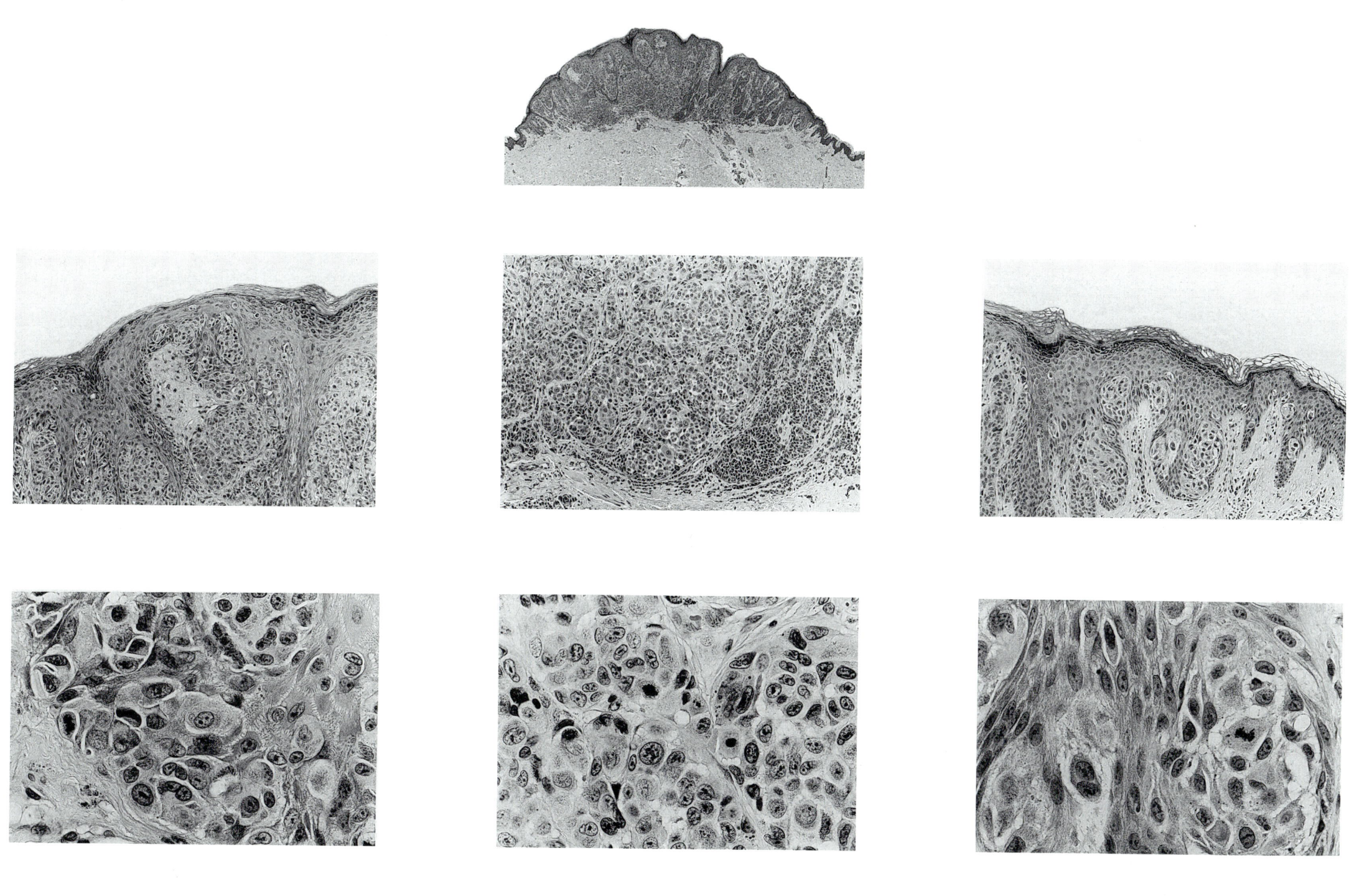

93. What is your diagnosis?

Lesion on the right knee of a 24-year-old woman. Clinical diagnosis: "active nevus." Patient was well after 1 year.

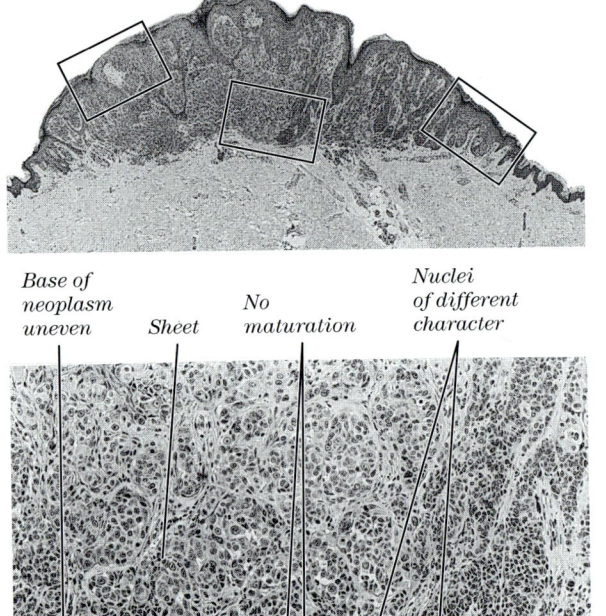

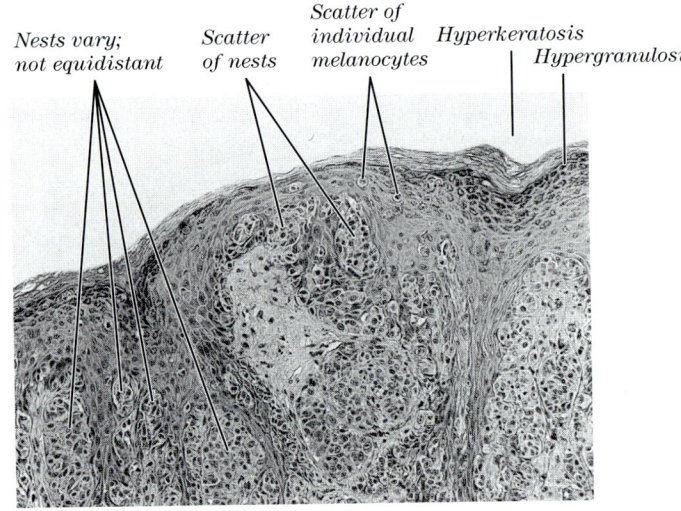
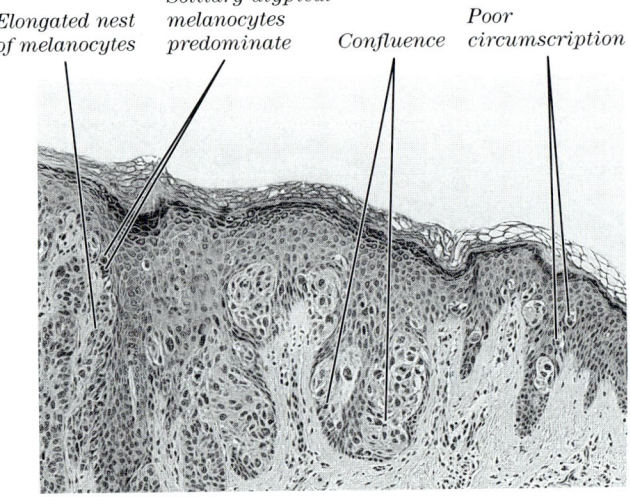

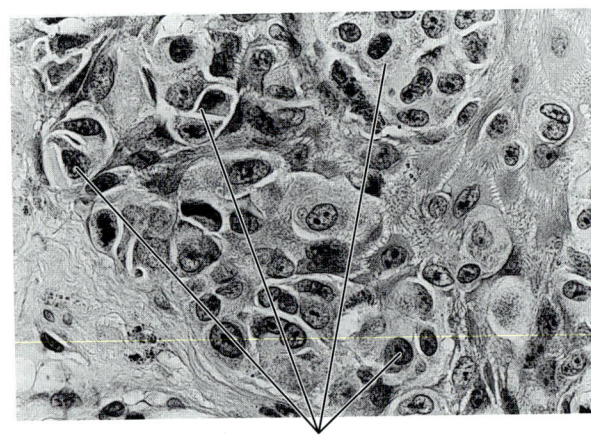
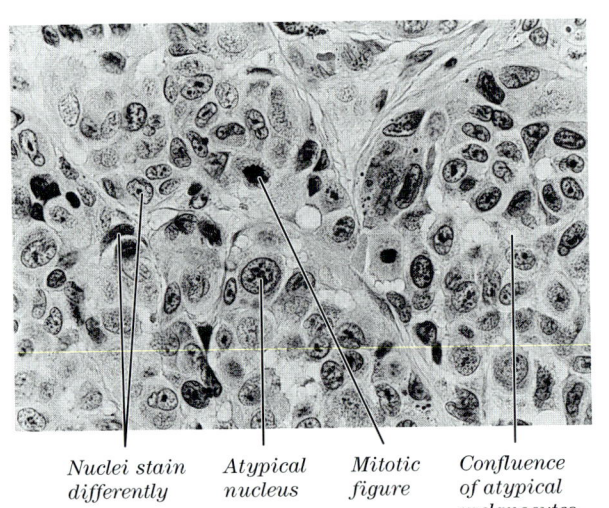
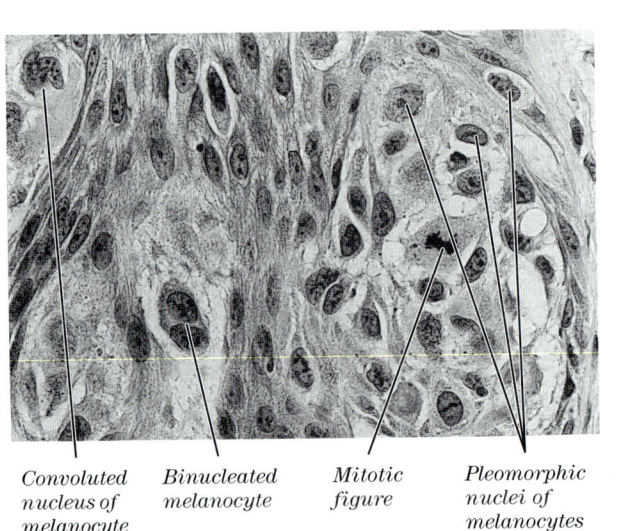

93 • Melanoma

Criteria for diagnosis of this melanoma

This is a melanoma because:

1. The neoplasm is asymmetric.//
2. Circumscription on one side of the neoplasm is poor.
3. Nests of melanocytes within the epidermis are not equidistant from one another.
4. Nests of melanocytes vary in size and shape.
5. Melanocytes disposed as solitary units within the epidermis predominate over nests of melanocytes in some high-power fields.
6. Many nests of melanocytes have become confluent and have formed sheets in the dermis.
7. In some foci, melanocytes fail to mature with progressive descent into the dermis.
8. Nuclei are pleomorphic and variable in staining quality.

Pitfall in diagnosis

This melanoma could be misjudged as a compound Spitz's nevus because:

1. The neoplasm is well-circumscribed on one side.
2. The bottom of the neoplasm is relatively flat.
3. Melanocytes mature somewhat with progressive descent into the dermis.
4. There are hyperkeratosis, hypergranulosis, and irregular epidermal hyperplasia.
5. Some nests of melanocytes are elongated and oriented perpendicularly to the skin surface.
6. Many melanocytes have large nuclei, abundant cytoplasm, and oval or round shapes.

The three cardinal histopathologic signs of melanoma are asymmetry, poor circumscription, and failure of maturation of melanocytes with progressive descent into the dermis. All three are present in this neoplasm.

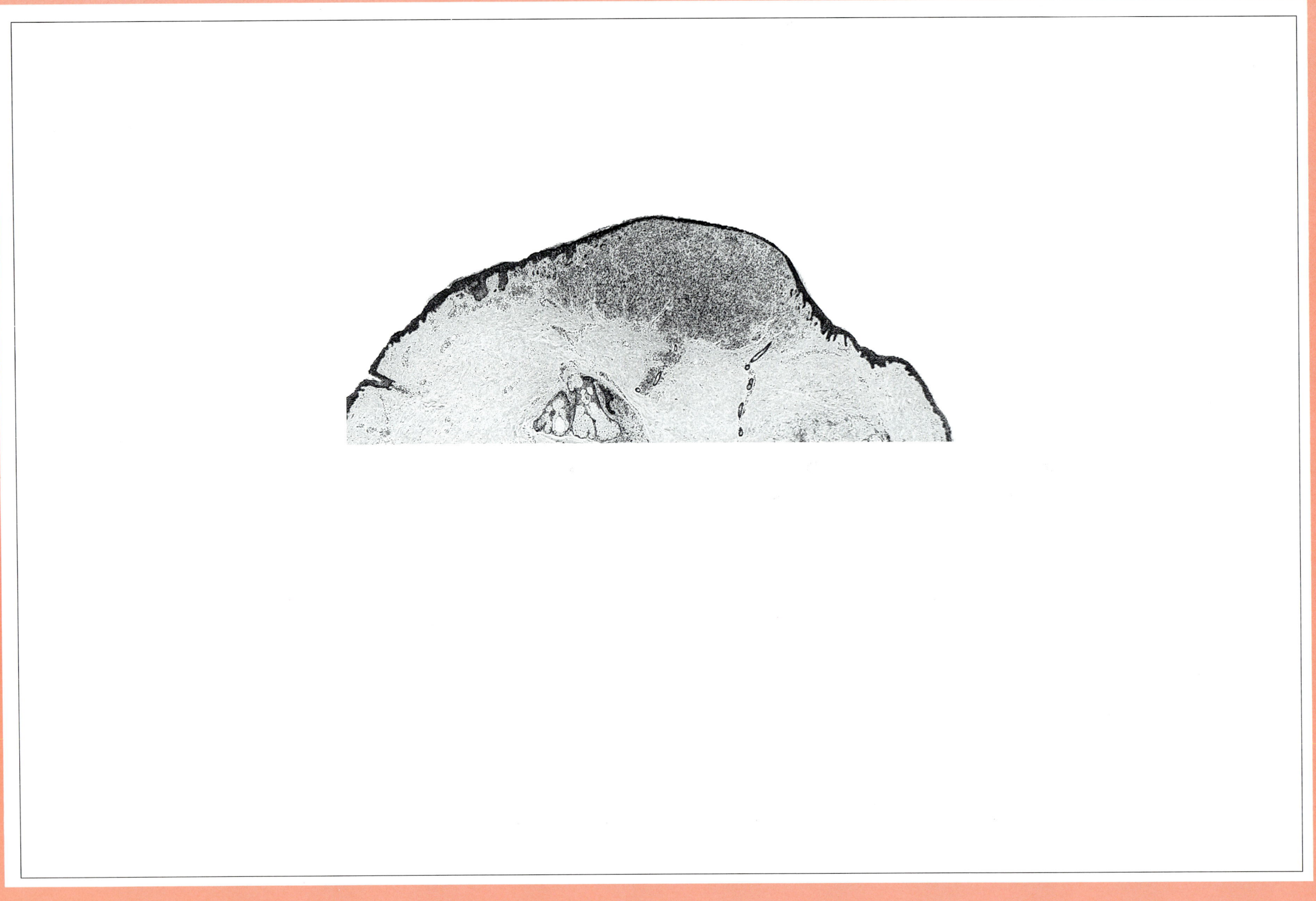

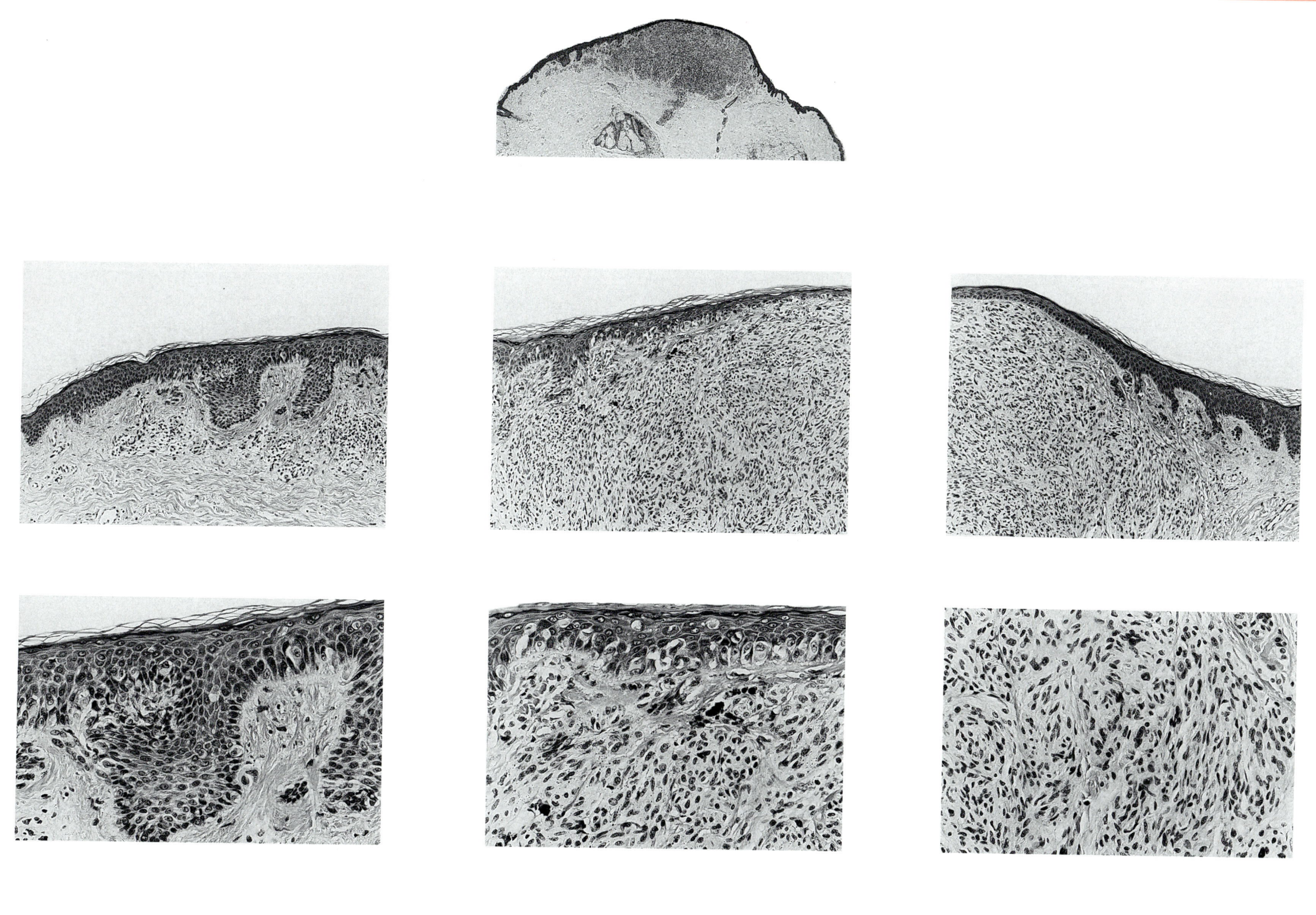

94. What is your diagnosis?

Domed, pink-brown papule on the left forearm of a 32-year-old man. Clinical diagnosis: dysplastic nevus. The site was excised and the patient was well after 1 year.

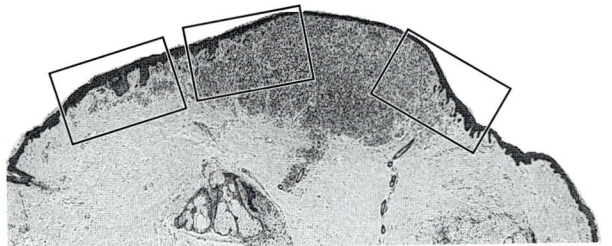

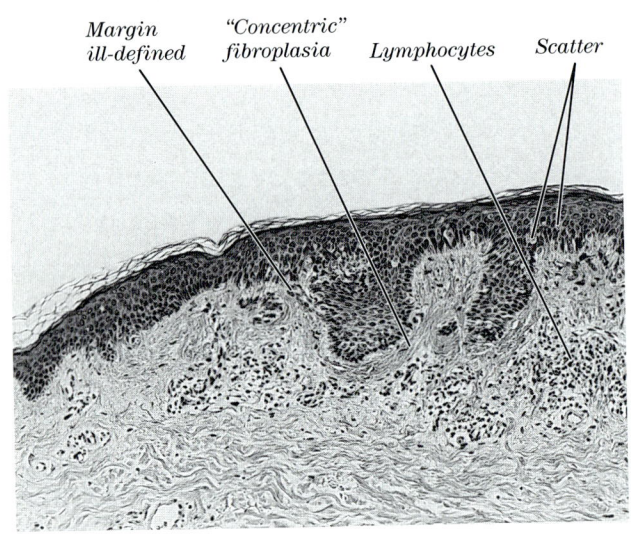

Margin ill-defined *"Concentric" fibroplasia* *Lymphocytes* *Scatter*

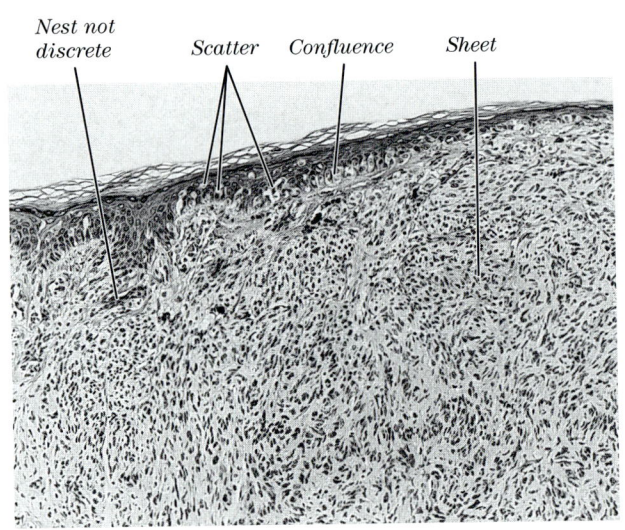

Nest not discrete *Scatter* *Confluence* *Sheet*

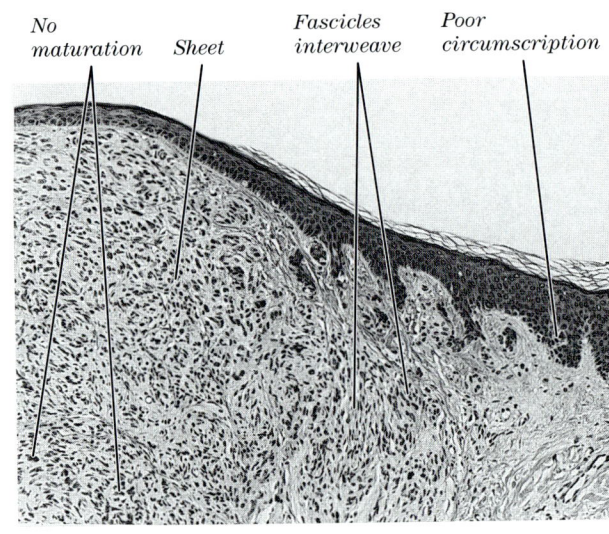

No maturation *Sheet* *Fascicles interweave* *Poor circumscription*

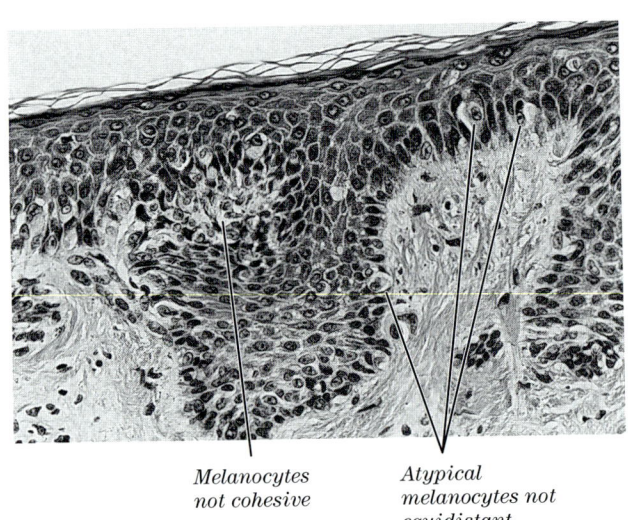

Melanocytes not cohesive *Atypical melanocytes not equidistant*

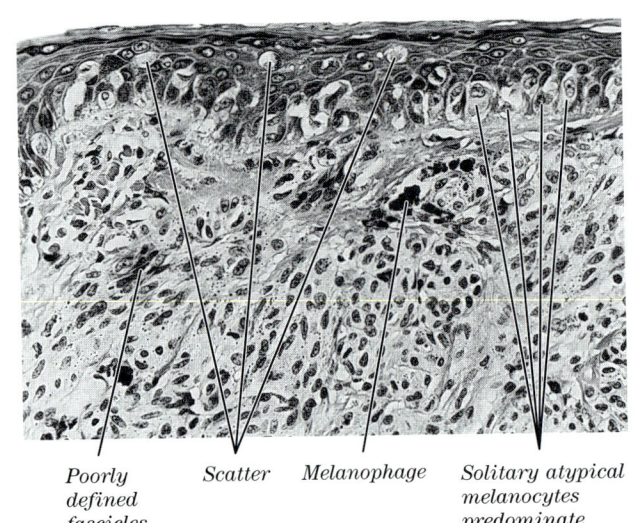

Poorly defined fascicles *Scatter* *Melanophage* *Solitary atypical melanocytes predominate*

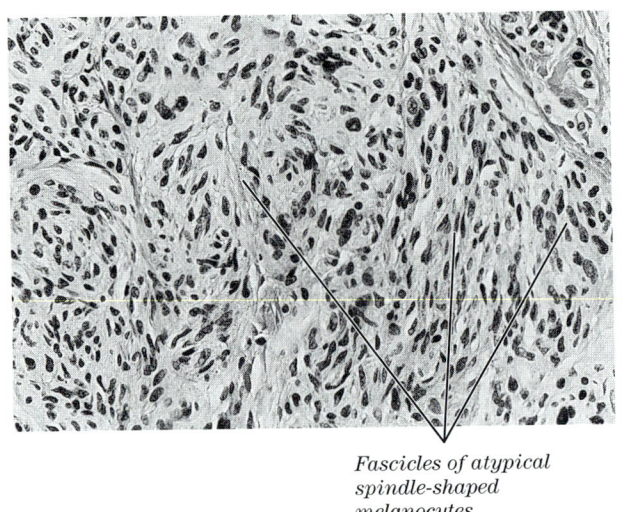

Fascicles of atypical spindle-shaped melanocytes

94 • Melanoma

Criteria for diagnosis of this small melanoma

This is a melanoma because:

1. The neoplasm is asymmetric.
2. The neoplasm is poorly circumscribed.
3. Melanocytes arranged as solitary units predominate over nests of melanocytes within some high-power fields.
4. There is scatter of melanocytes above the dermo-epidermal junction.
5. Some nests of melanocytes within the dermis have become confluent.
6. Maturation of melanocytes is not striking.

Pitfall in diagnosis

This melanoma could be misread as a compound Clark's nevus because:

1. The neoplasm is small.
2. It is confined to the epidermis and upper part of the dermis.
3. A "shoulder" of intra-epidermal melanocytes extends beyond the intradermal component.
4. Many of the melanocytes within the dermis have small, oval, and wavy nuclei.
5. Lamellar and concentric fibroplasia are apparent at the "shoulder."

This neoplasm is a melanoma. It should not be called "dysplastic," "borderline," or "minimal deviation." Melanoma suffices.

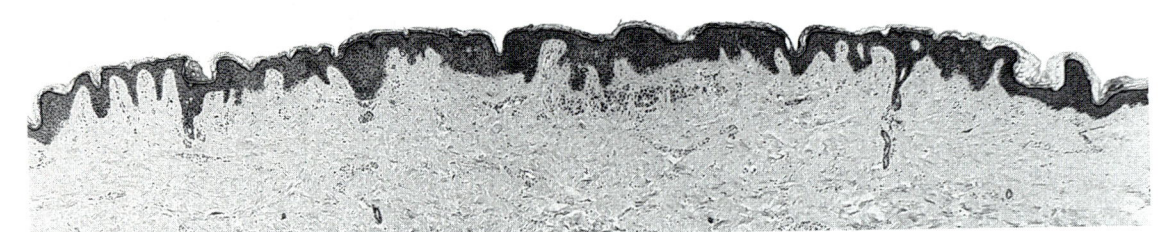

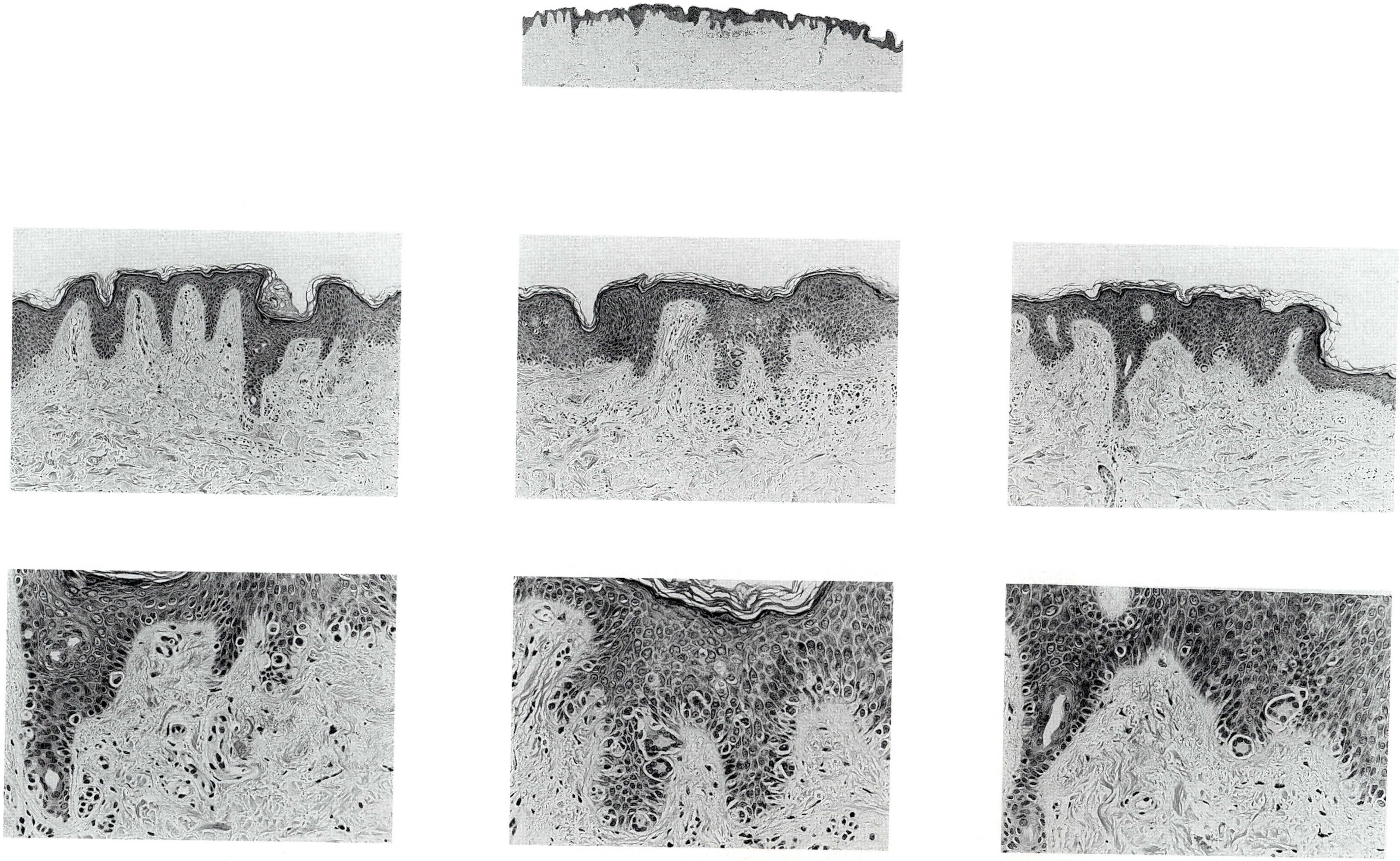

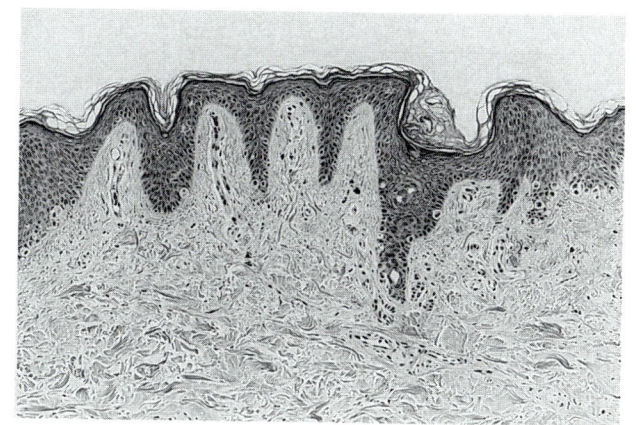
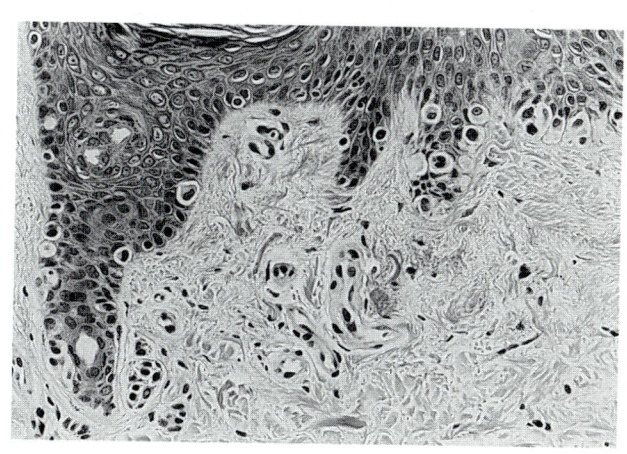
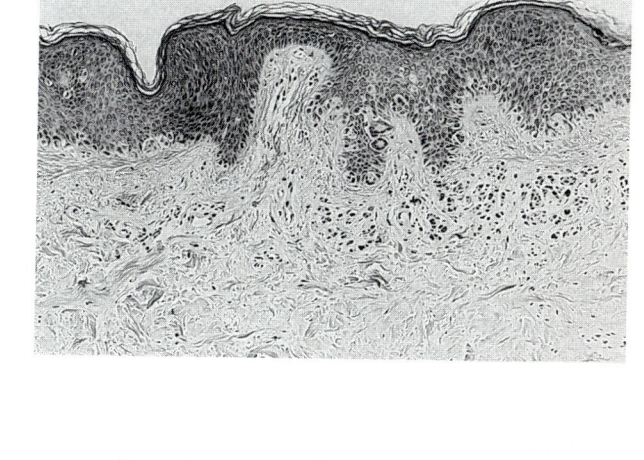
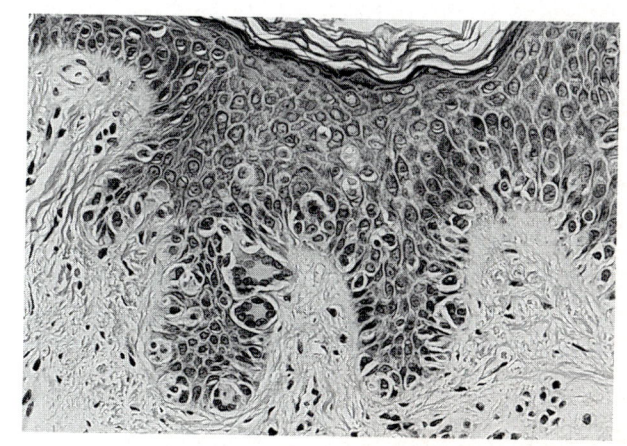

95. What is your diagnosis?

Pigmented lesion on the left ankle of a 38-year-old woman. It was said to have been present since birth, but recently to have changed in size. Clinical diagnosis: "benign or melanoma?" Site was re-excised. Patient was free of disease after 1 year.

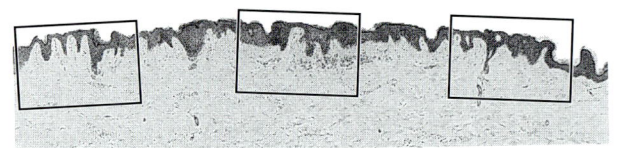

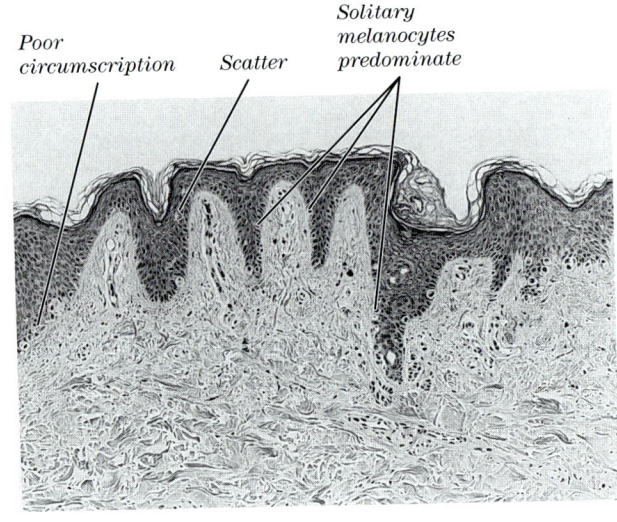

Poor circumscription — *Scatter* — *Solitary melanocytes predominate*

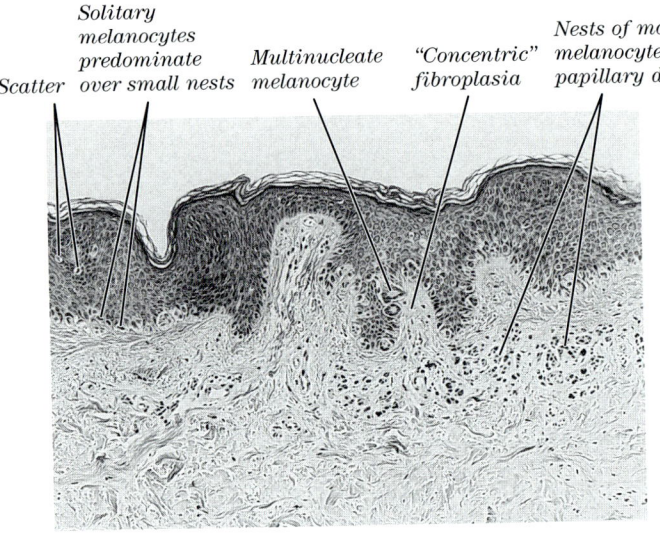

Scatter — *Solitary melanocytes predominate over small nests* — *Multinucleate melanocyte* — *"Concentric" fibroplasia* — *Nests of monomorphous melanocytes in the papillary dermis*

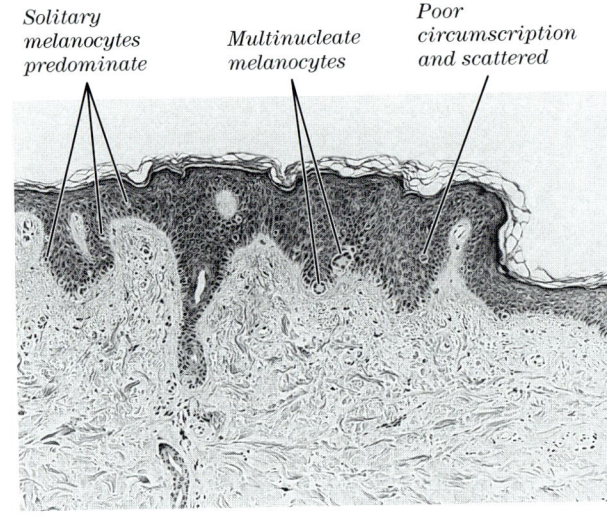

Solitary melanocytes predominate — *Multinucleate melanocytes* — *Poor circumscription and scattered*

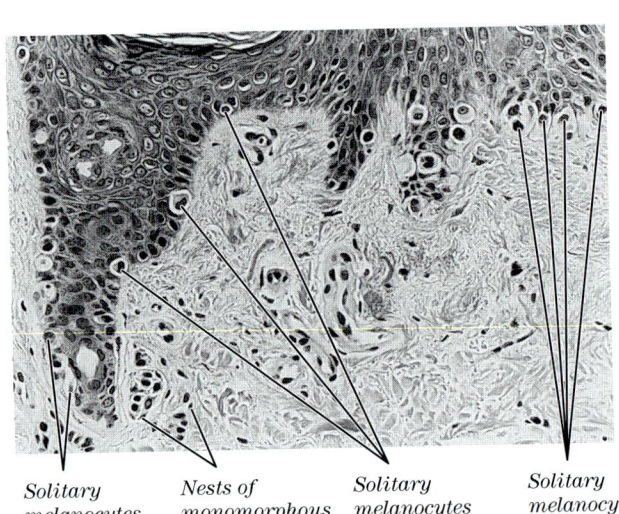

Solitary melanocytes only in an acrosyringium — *Nests of monomorphous melanocytes* — *Solitary melanocytes not equidistant* — *Solitary melanocytes predominate in epidermis*

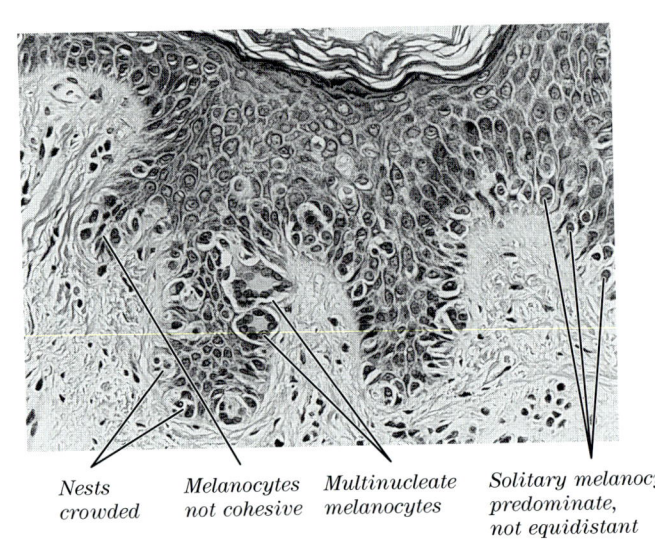

Nests crowded — *Melanocytes not cohesive* — *Multinucleate melanocytes* — *Solitary melanocytes predominate, not equidistant*

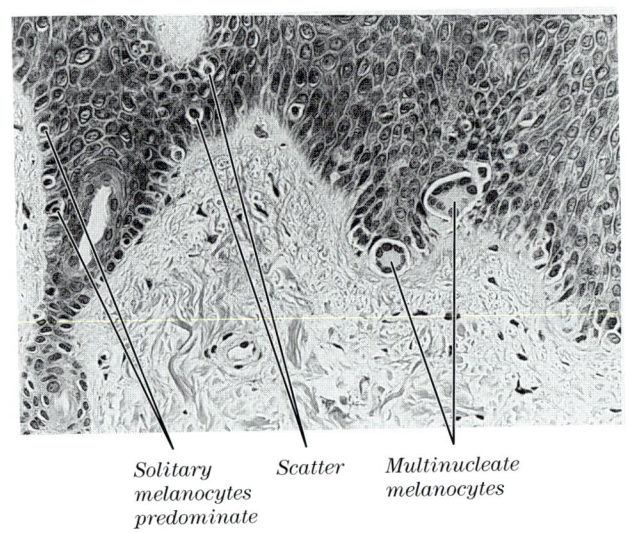

Solitary melanocytes predominate — *Scatter* — *Multinucleate melanocytes*

95 • Melanoma in situ and Clark's Nevus

Criteria for diagnosis of melanoma in situ in association with a Clark's nevus (intradermal type)

This is a melanoma in situ because:

1. Melanocytes within the epidermis disposed as solitary units predominate overwhelmingly over melanocytes arranged in nests.

2. Melanocytes arrayed as solitary units within the epidermis are not equidistant from one another.

3. Melanocytes within the epidermis, especially those that appear as solitary units, are scattered far above the dermo-epidermal junction.

4. Melanocytes arranged as solitary units predominate over nests of melanocytes within epithelial structures of adnexa.

5. Nests of melanocytes within the epidermis are not equidistant from one another.

6. Numerous melanocytes within the epidermis are multinucleate.

7. Neoplastic melanocytes within the epidermis have atypical nuclei.

Pitfall in diagnosis

This melanoma in situ in association with an intradermal Clark's nevus could be misinterpreted as a compound Clark's nevus because:

1. The neoplasm is but slightly elevated.

2. The surface of the neoplasm is gently mammillated.

3. Nests of melanocytes are confined to the epidermis and thickened papillary dermis.

4. There is an indubitable intradermal nevus in the thickened papillary dermis.

5. Most of the melanocytes within the epidermis, both those disposed as solitary units and those in nests, are situated a the dermo-epidermal junction.

6. "Concentric" fibroplasia is seen focally in dermal papillae.

The principle that melanocytes arranged as solitary units predominate over melanocytes in nests in some high-power fields within melanoma is illustrated beautifully in this neoplasm. This neoplasm also has features in common with Spitz's nevus, e.g., many multinucleate melanocytes. The finding of overwhelming predominance of melanocytes arranged as solitary units, however, marks this neoplasm as melanoma.

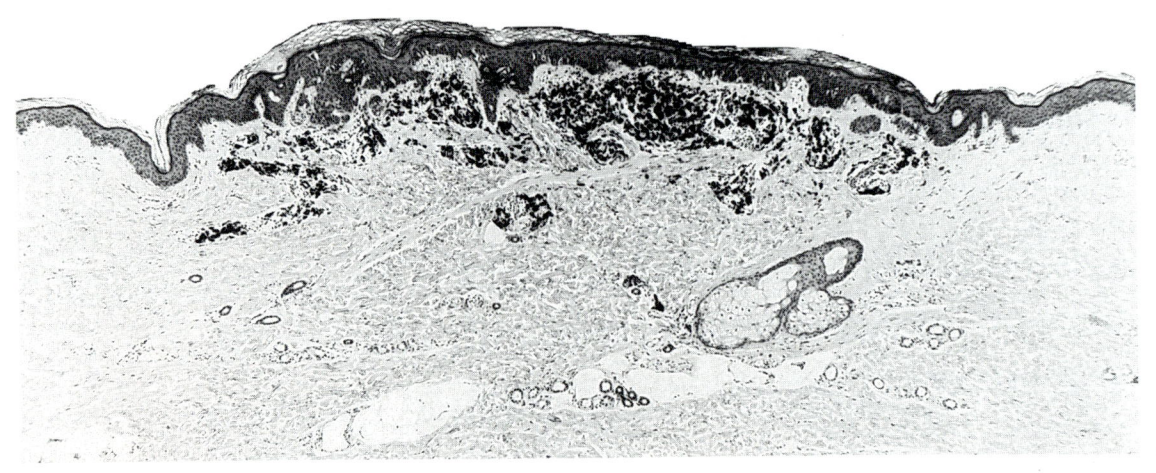

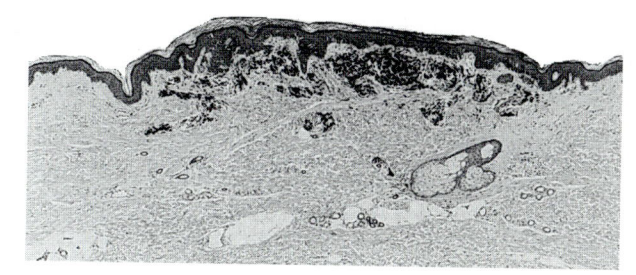
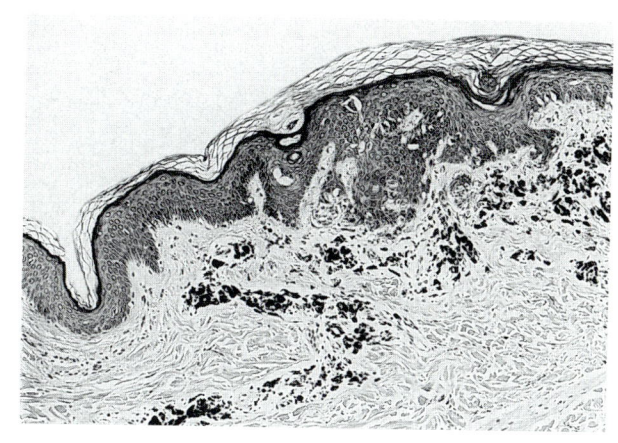
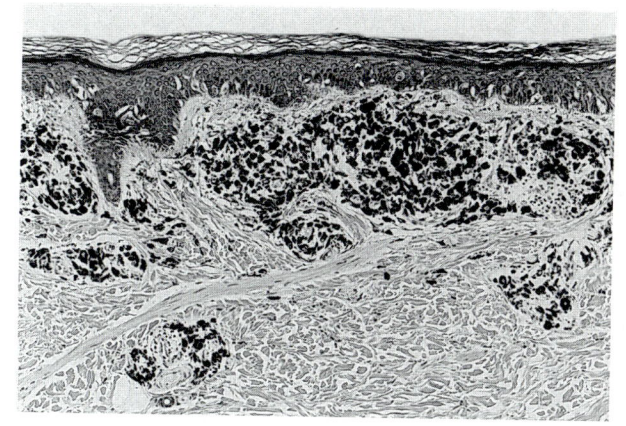
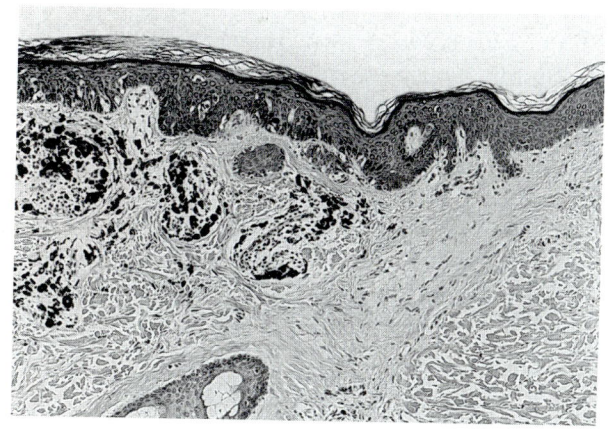
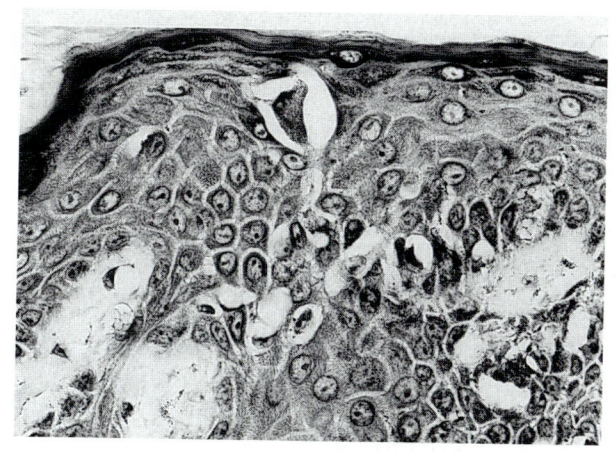
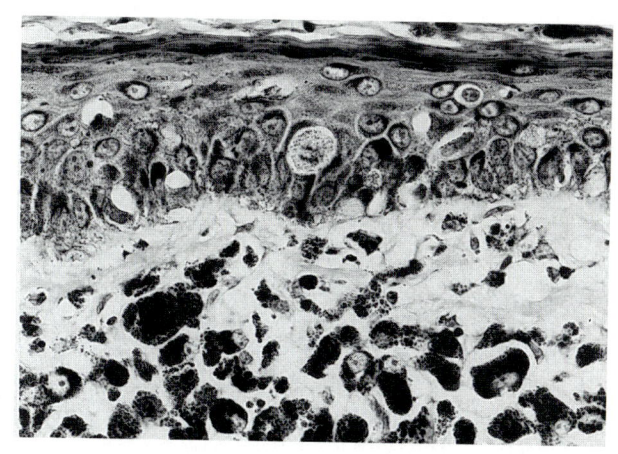
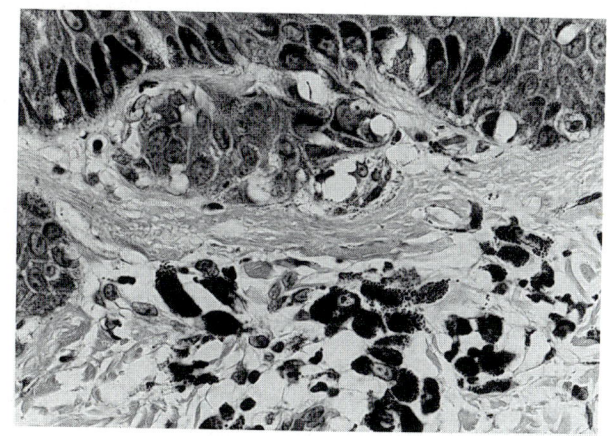

96. What is your diagnosis?

Brownish-black lesion of 1 year duration on the lower part of the right arm of a 48-year-old woman. Clinical diagnosis: atypical nevus vs. melanoma. Patient was free of disease 4 years after complete excision.

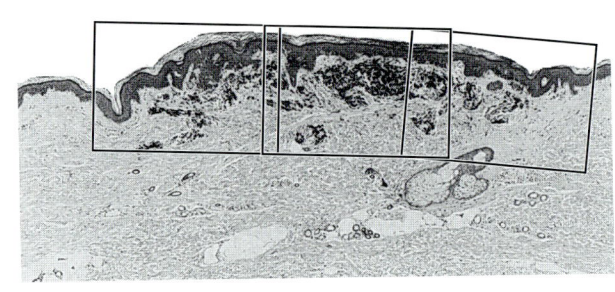

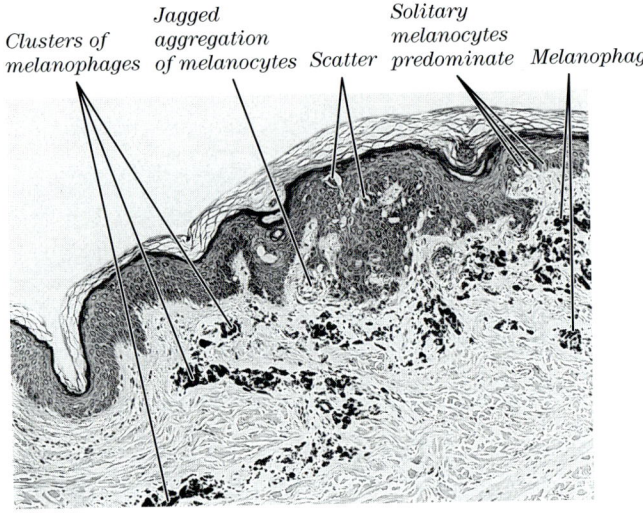
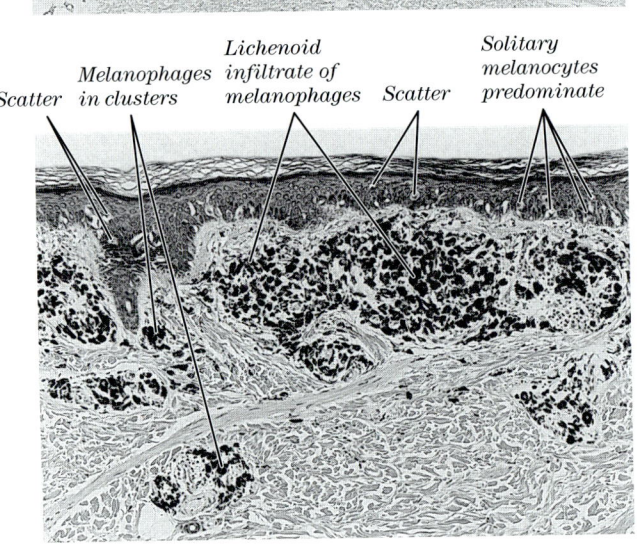
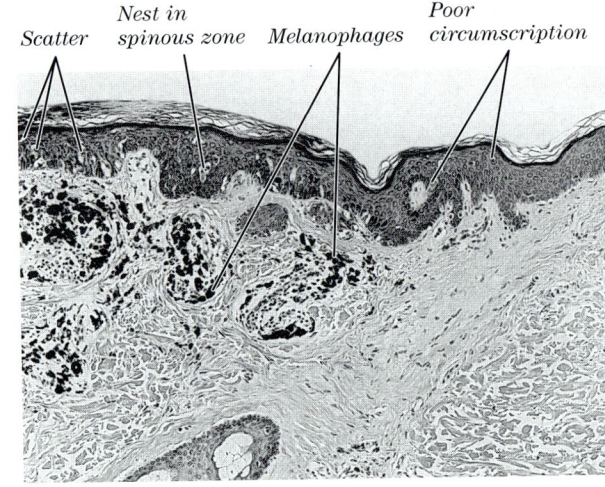

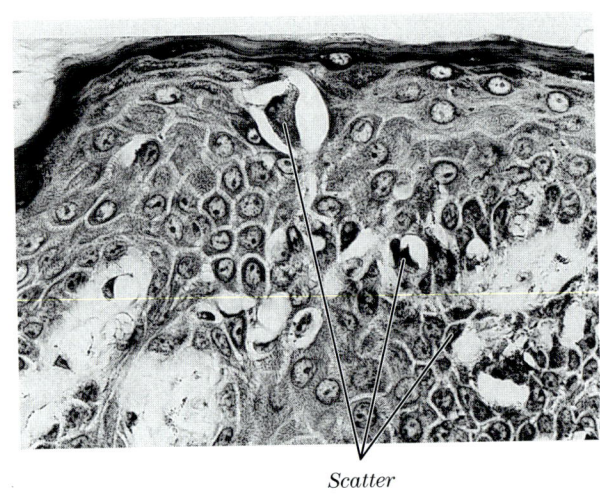
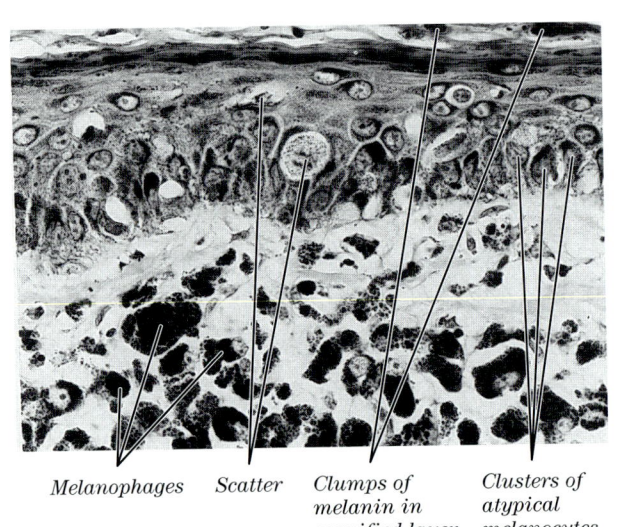
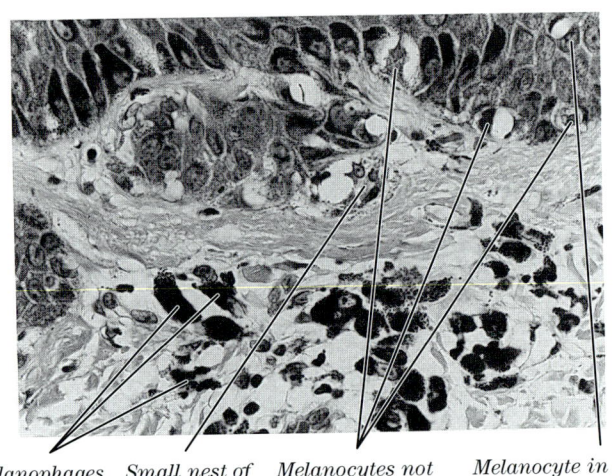

96 • Melanoma in situ

Criteria for diagnosis of this melanoma in situ

This is a melanoma in situ because:

1. Signs of melanoma in situ, namely, scatter of melanocytes arranged as solitary units at all levels of the epidermis and within epithelial structures of adnexa, are present.

2. Melanophages are positioned mostly around vessels of the superficial plexus, but also in lichenoid foci in the thickened papillary dermis.

Pitfall in diagnosis

This melanoma in situ with numerous melanophages could be misinterpreted as a melanoma with partial regression, as manifested by melanosis, because:

1. Melanophages are distributed in patchy, predominantly perivascular distribution, rather than as a band across a thickened papillary dermis.

2. Rete ridges are not preserved across much of the breadth of the lesion.

3. No fibrosis accompanies the infiltrate of melanophages.

The proliferation of atypical melanocytes within the epidermis of this melanoma in situ is responsible for the presence of melanophages in the dermis. In regression of melanoma, destruction of intraepidermal and intradermal melanocytes by lymphocytes is responsible for the presence of melanophages in the dermis. It may be assumed that no neoplastic melanocytes of melanoma ever were situated in the papillary dermis of this neoplasm, in contrast to the situation in regression of melanoma where the presence of some neoplastic melanocytes in the papillary dermis is thought to be requisite for the initiation of that phenomenon. In melanoma in situ accompanied by enormous numbers of melanophages, neoplastic melanocytes are present within the epidermis across the entire front of those melanophages. In regression of melanoma typified by melanosis, neoplastic melanocytes are absent from the epidermis above the zone of melanophages.

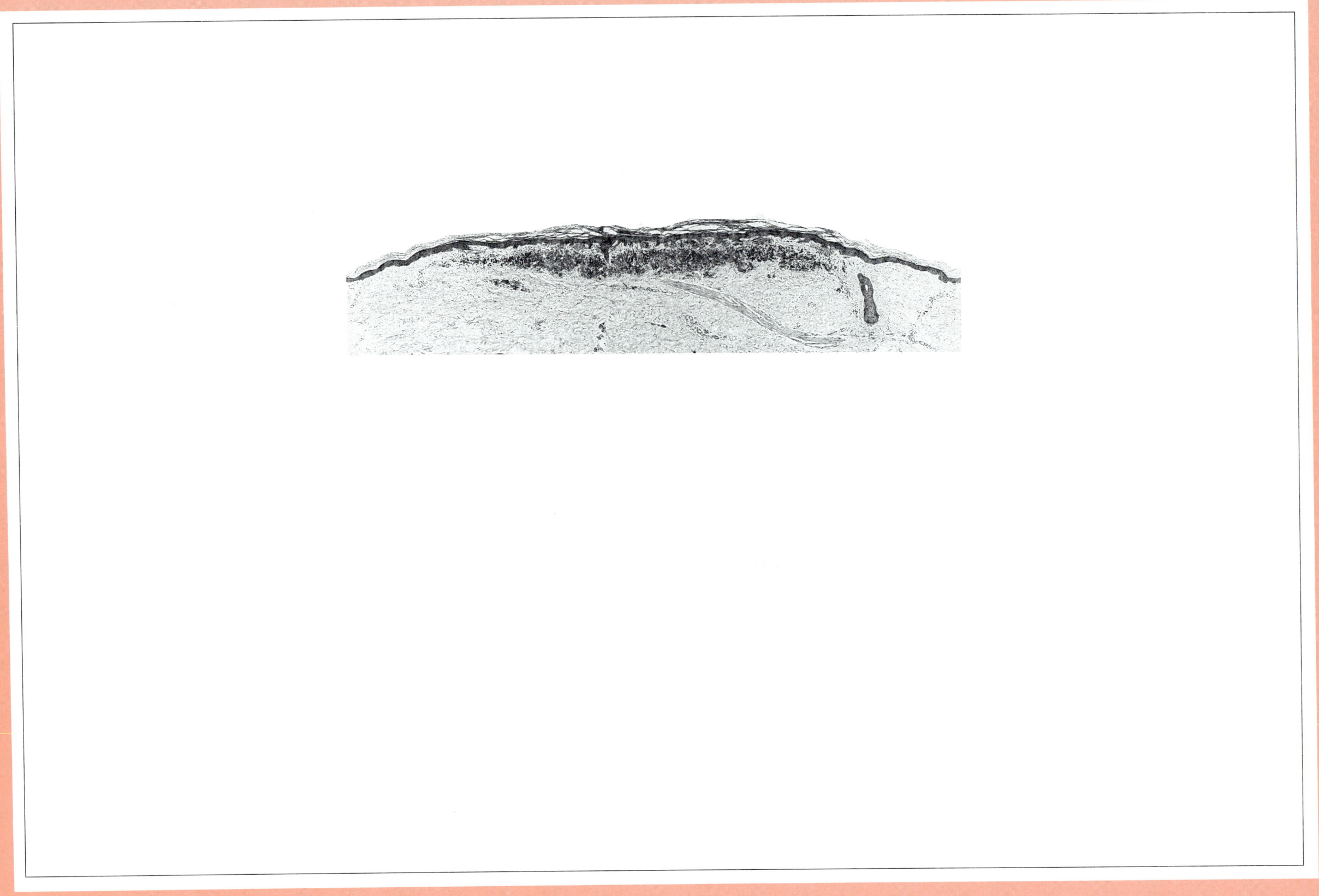

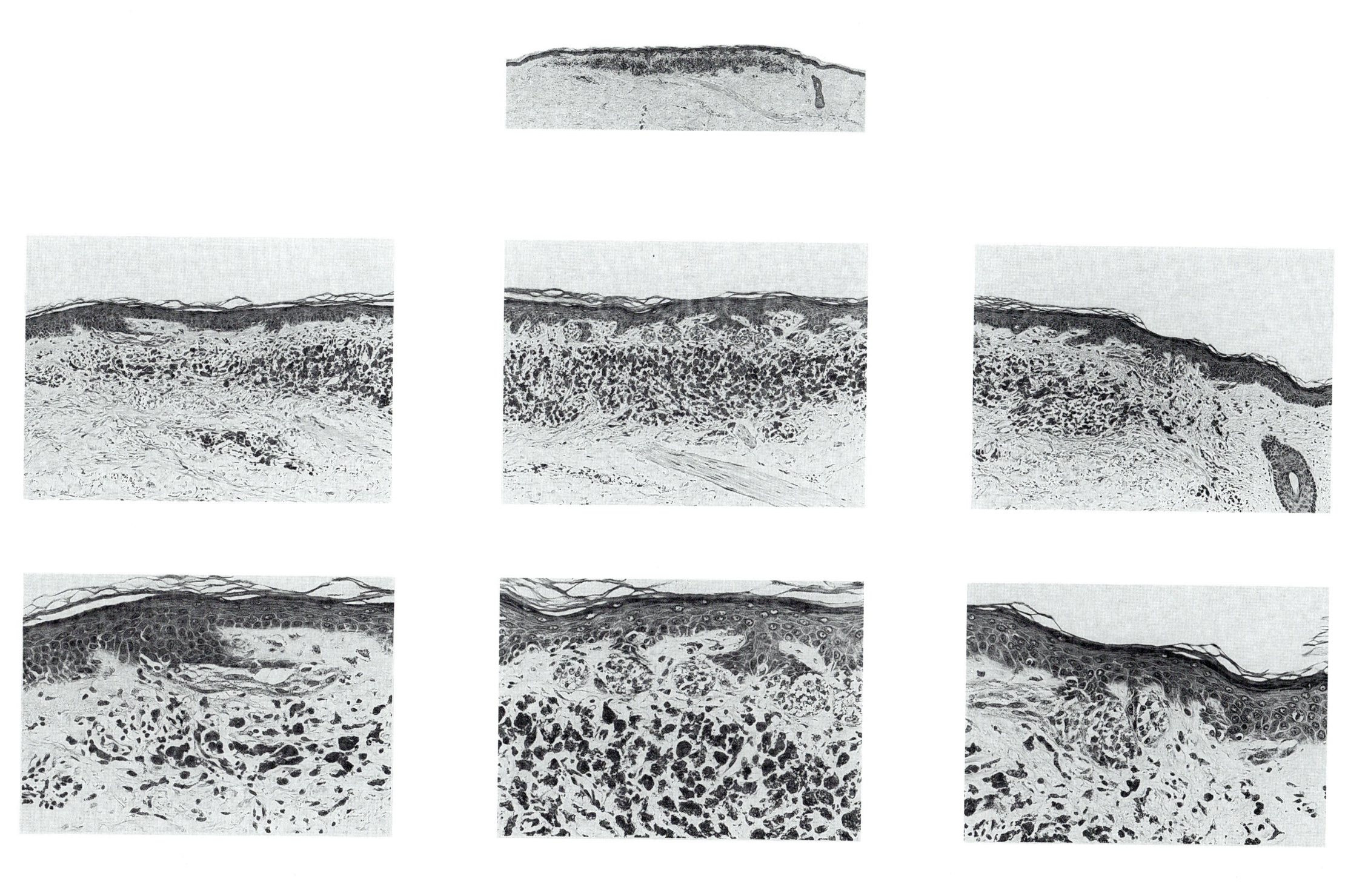

97. What is your diagnosis?

Lesion on the left arm of a 53-year-old woman. Clinical diagnosis: seborrheic keratosis. The site was excised completely. Patient was free of disease after 7 years.

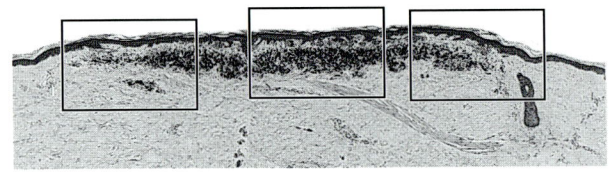

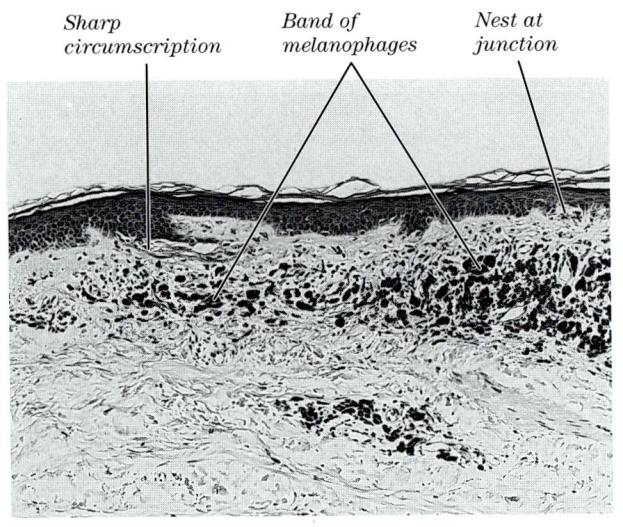
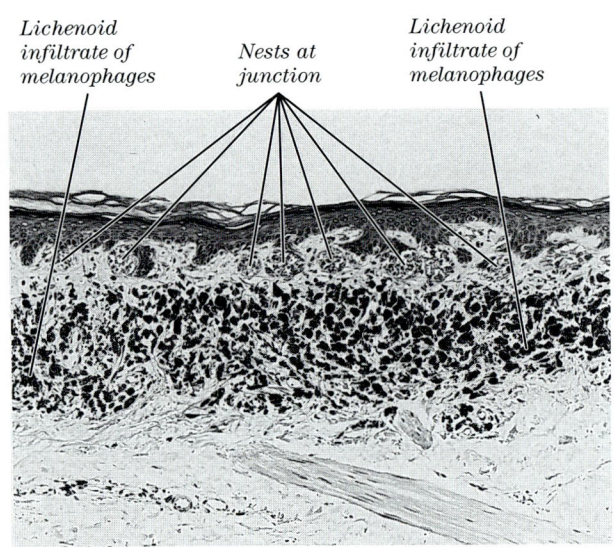
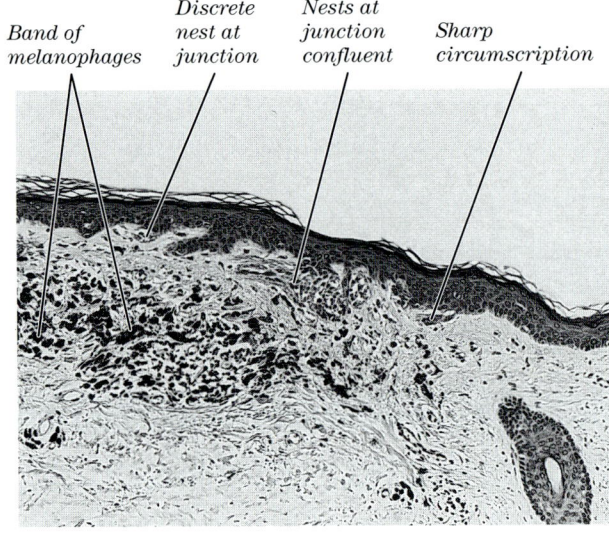

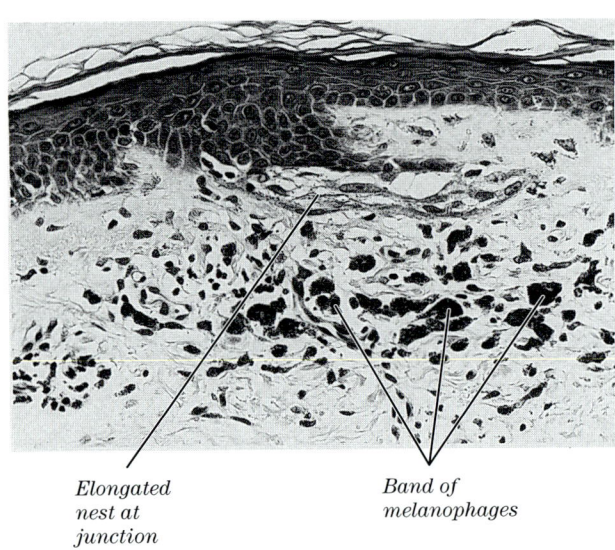
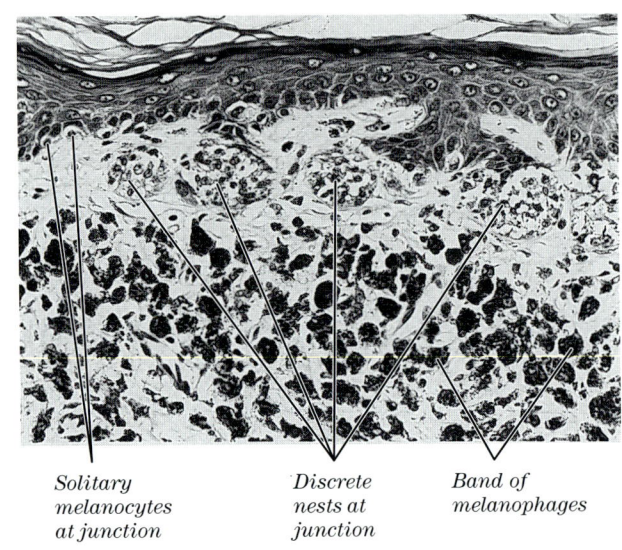
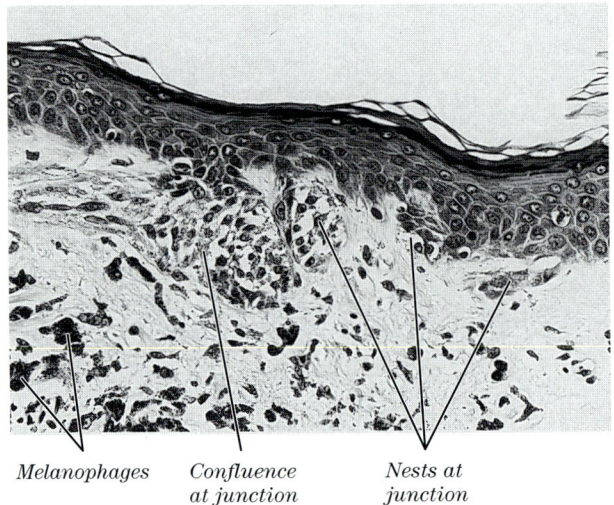

97 • Clark's Nevus

Criteria for diagnosis of this junctional Clark's nevus

This is a Clark's nevus because:

1. The lesion is symmetric.

2. It is well-circumscribed.

3. Nests of melanocytes are situated at the dermo-epidermal junction, not above it.

4. Melanocytes within the epidermis are arranged mostly in nests, rather than as solitary units.

5. Nests of melanocytes are relatively equidistant from one another.

6. Most nests of melanocytes are discrete.

7. Nuclei of melanocytes are typical.

Pitfall in diagnosis

This junctional Clark's nevus could be misinterpreted as a melanoma that has undergone partial regression because:

1. A dense band-like infiltrate of melanophages is present in a markedly thickened papillary dermis.

2. Clusters of melanophages are present around venules in the upper portion of the reticular dermis.

A dense band of melanophages in a thickened papillary dermis does not necessarily signify regression of melanoma in the form of melanosis. Melanosis results from destruction, by effects of lymphocytes, of neoplastic melanocytes in the epidermis and the papillary dermis. But a band of melanophages in a thickened papillary dermis also may result from exuberant production of melanin by melanocytes in nests situated at the dermo-epidermal junction. That is the case in the junctional nevus pictured here.

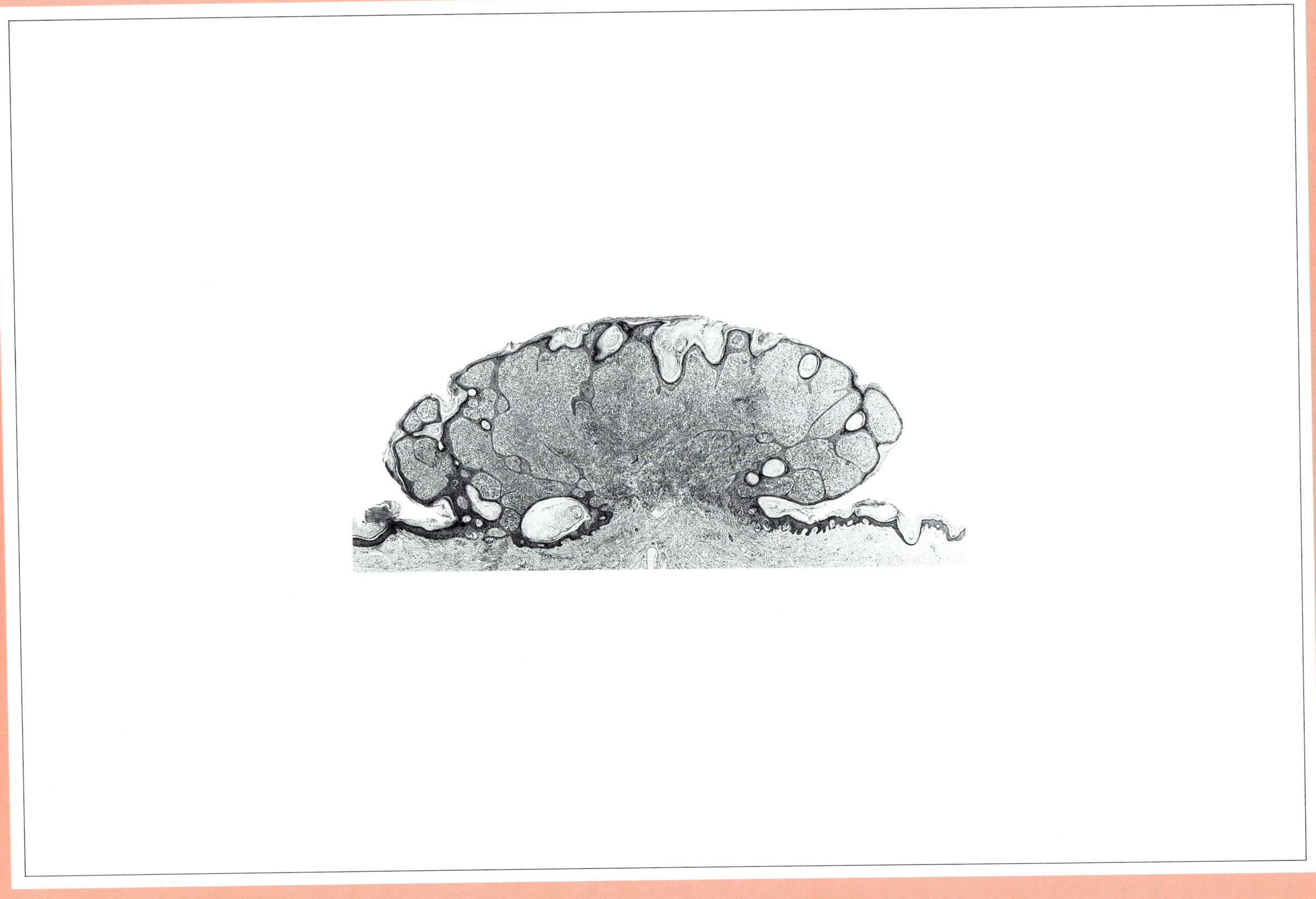

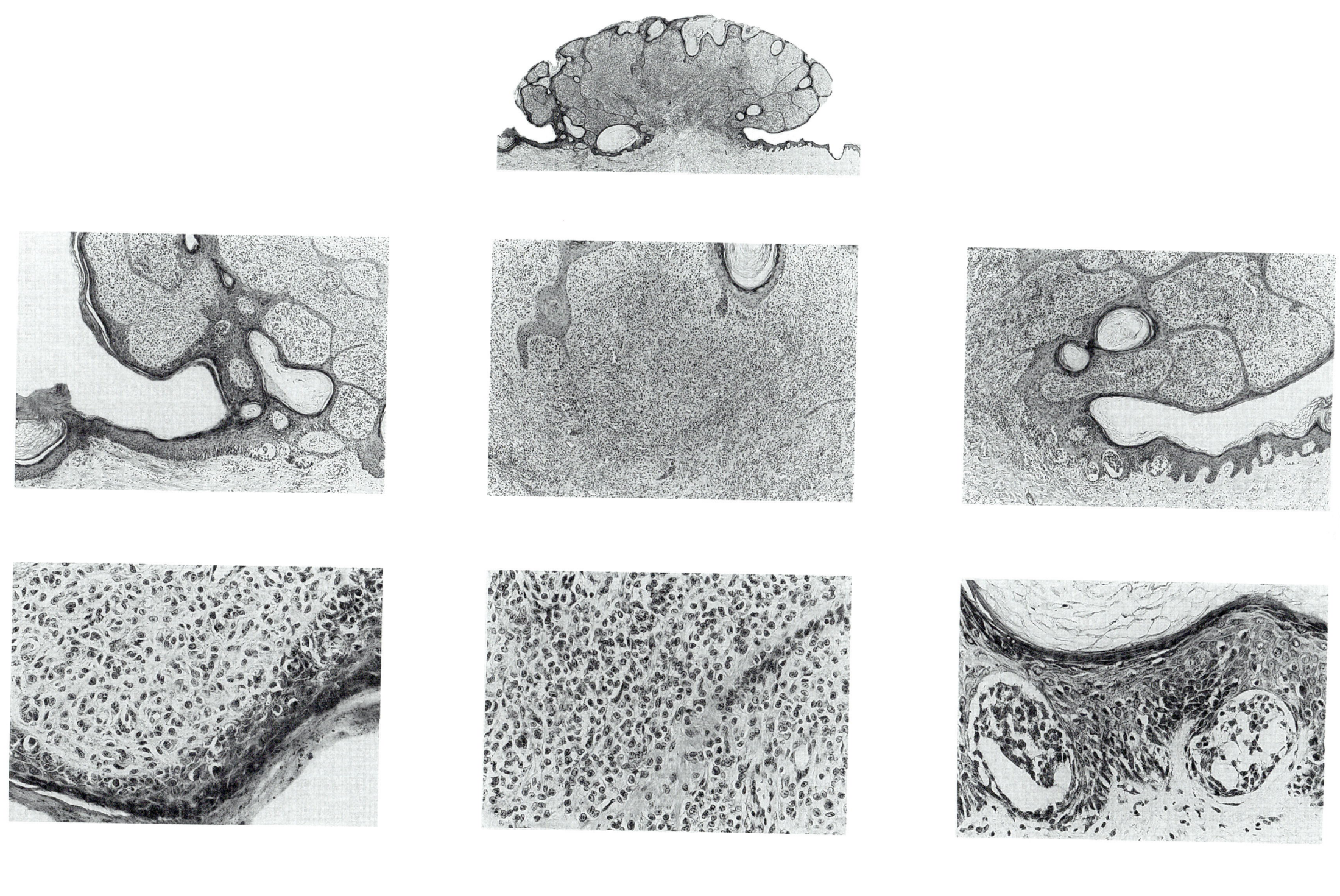

98. What is your diagnosis?

Pigmented lesion on the upper part of the right leg of a 52-year-old man. Clinical diagnosis: nevus vs. melanoma. The site was excised completely. Patient was free of disease after 2 years.

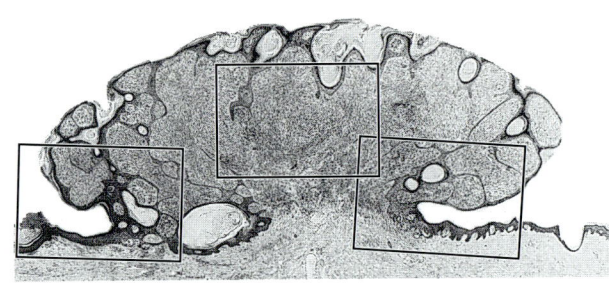

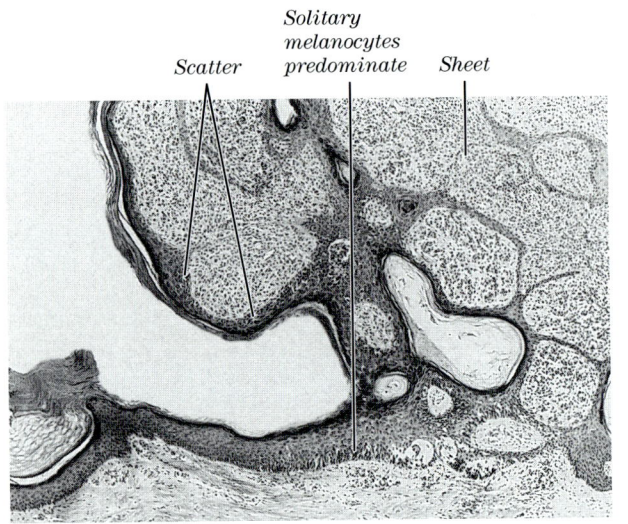

Scatter — *Solitary melanocytes predominate* — *Sheet*

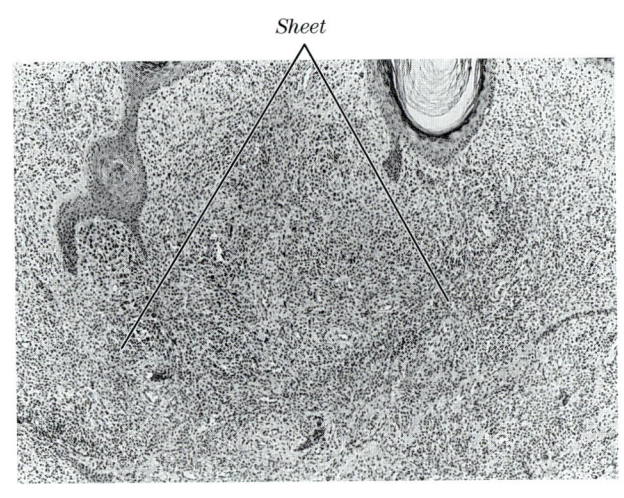

Sheet

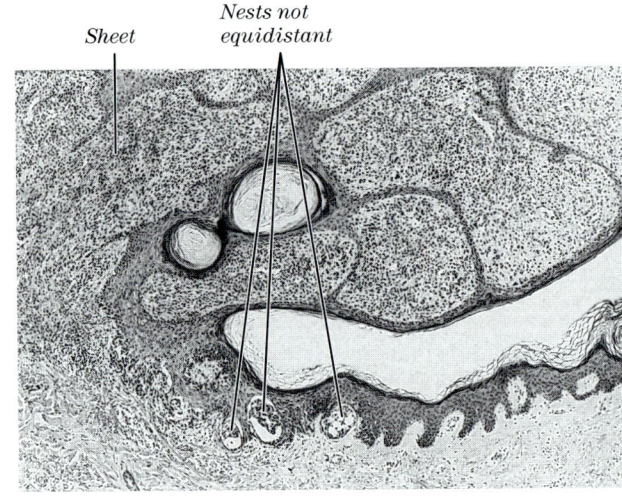

Sheet — *Nests not equidistant*

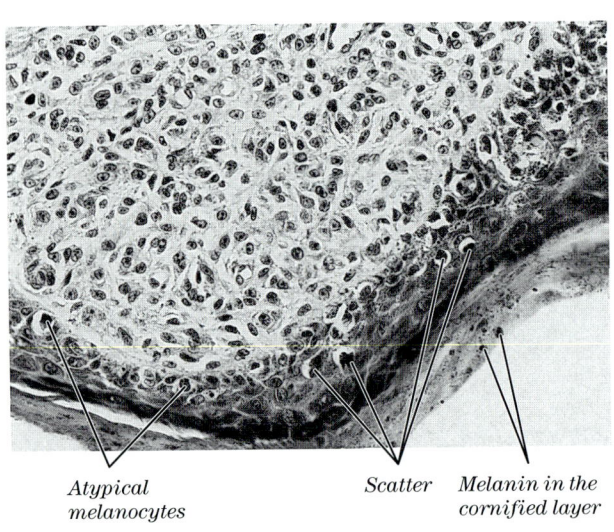

Atypical melanocytes — *Scatter* — *Melanin in the cornified layer*

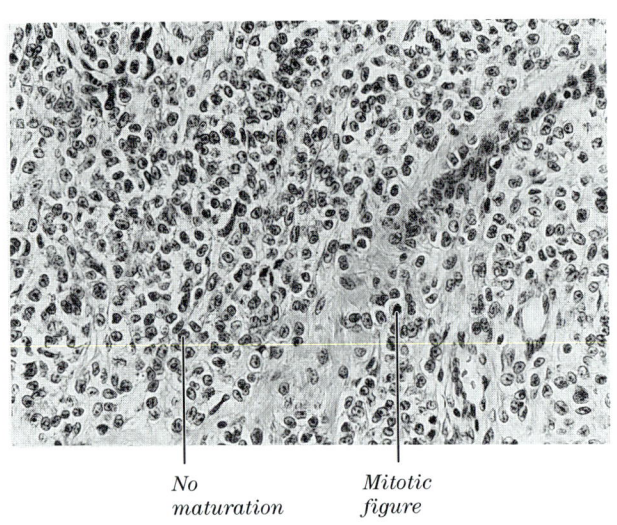

No maturation — *Mitotic figure*

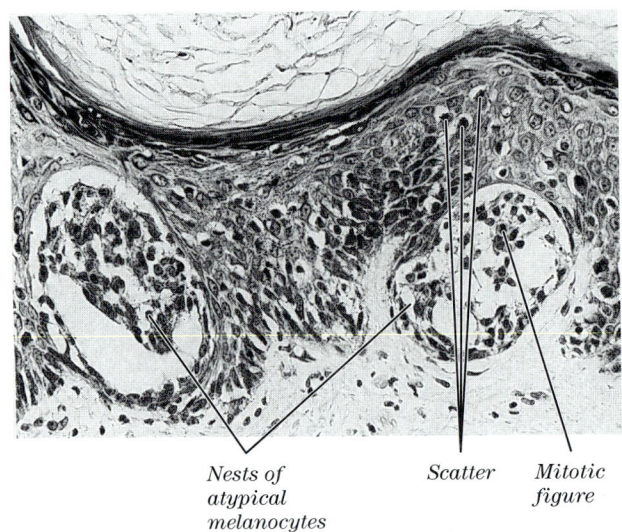

Nests of atypical melanocytes — *Scatter* — *Mitotic figure*

98 • Melanoma

Criteria for diagnosis of this melanoma

This is a melanoma because:

1. The lesion is poorly circumscribed.
2. There are sheets of melanocytes throughout the markedly thickened papillary dermis.
3. Melanocytes disposed mostly as solitary units are scattered throughout the epidermis, especially at the periphery of the neoplasm.
4. Melanocytes arranged as solitary units predominate over nests of melanocytes in many high-power fields.
5. Nests of melanocytes are not equidistant from one another.
6. Nests of melanocytes vary in size and shape.
7. Some nests of melanocytes have become confluent.
8. Some melanocytes are in mitosis, even at the base of the neoplasm.
9. Some melanocytes are necrotic.

Pitfall in diagnosis

This papillomatous melanoma could be misinterpreted as Unna's nevus because:

1. The neoplasm is exophytic.
2. The lesion is papillomatous.
3. The lesion is relatively symmetric.
4. Cords of adnexal epithelial cells form fenestrated patterns within which reside tiny cysts that contain cornified cells.
5. There are collarettes of adnexal epithelium at the periphery of the lesion.

Although this sessile melanocytic neoplasm resembles closely an Unna's nevus by silhouette, the poor circumscription of melanocytes within the epidermis, scatter of melanocytes above the dermo-epidermal junction, and sheets of melanocytes throughout the thickened papillary dermis mark it as a melanoma.

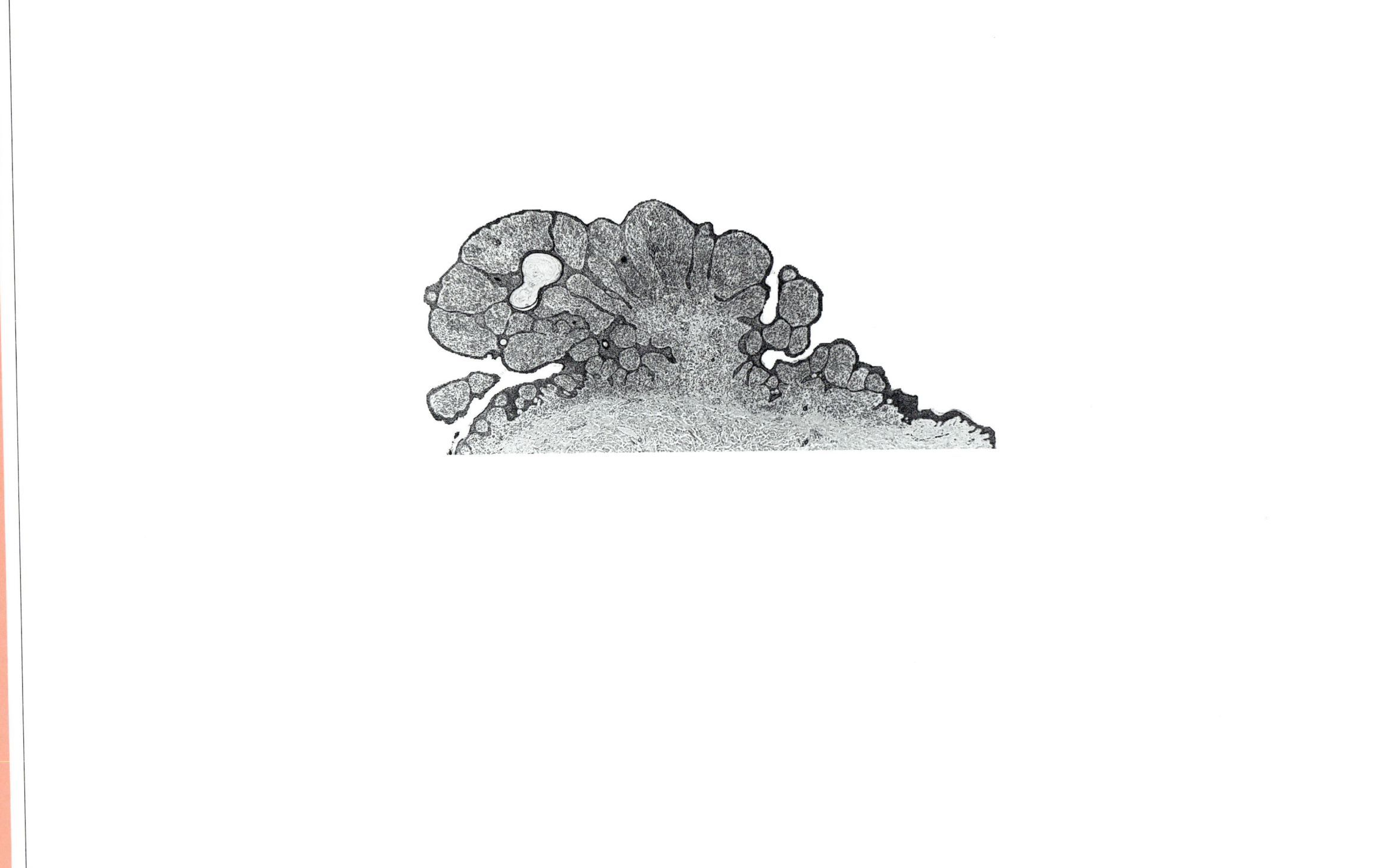

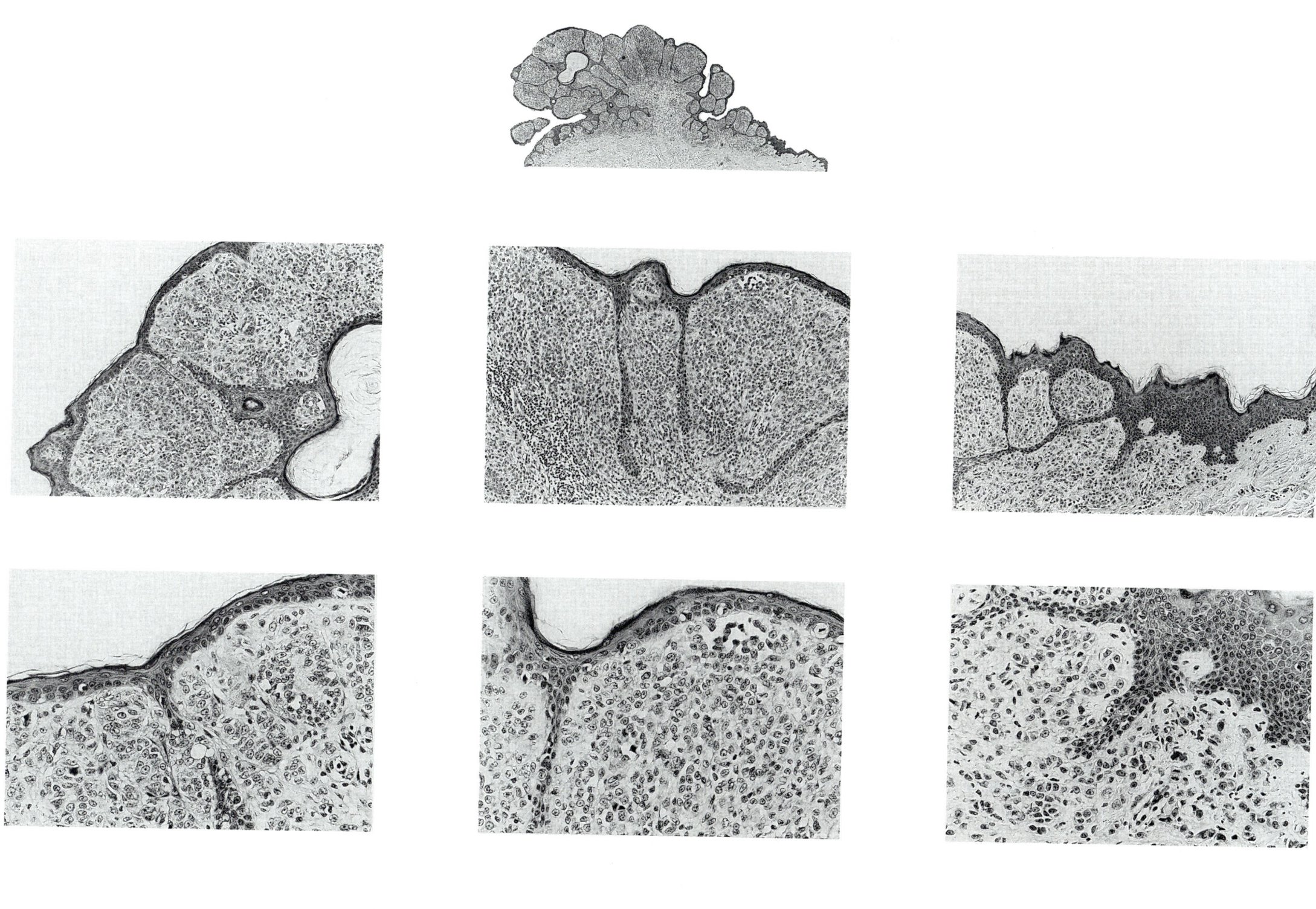

99. What is your diagnosis?

Pigmented lesion on the back of a 67-year-old woman. Clinical diagnosis: melanoma. Patient was given a series of injections of melanoma vaccine, but developed widespread metastases.

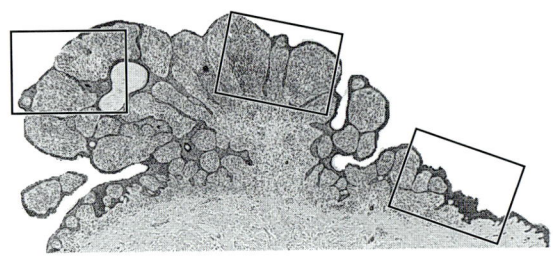

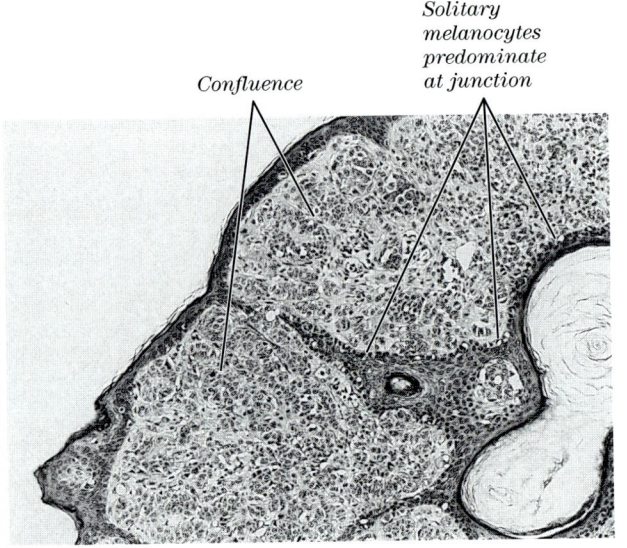

Confluence — *Solitary melanocytes predominate at junction*

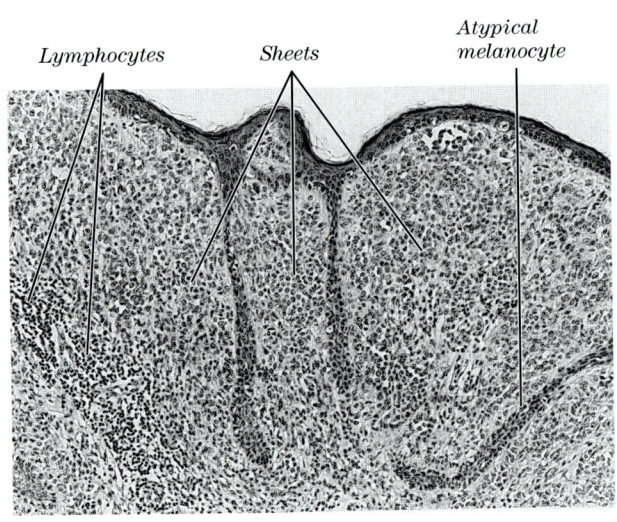

Lymphocytes — *Sheets* — *Atypical melanocyte*

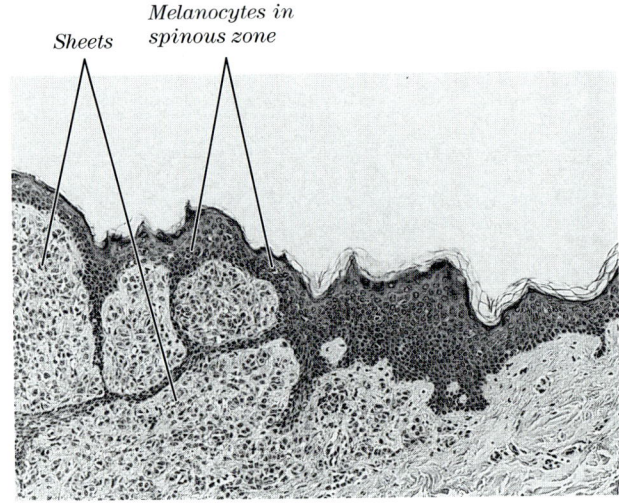

Sheets — *Melanocytes in spinous zone*

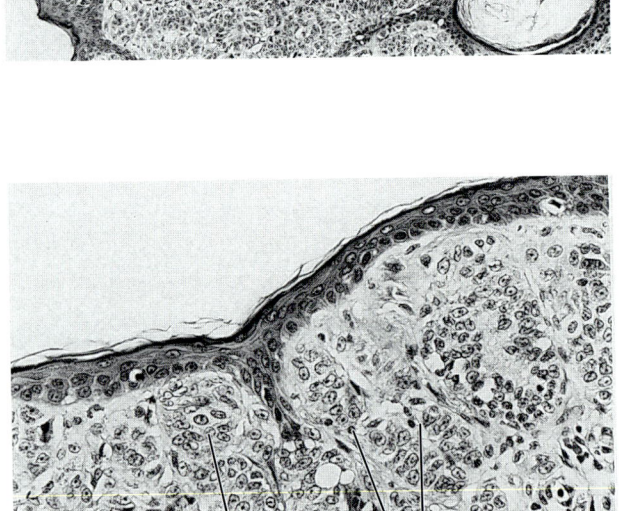

Atypical melanocytes — *Confluence of nests that vary* — *Confluence*

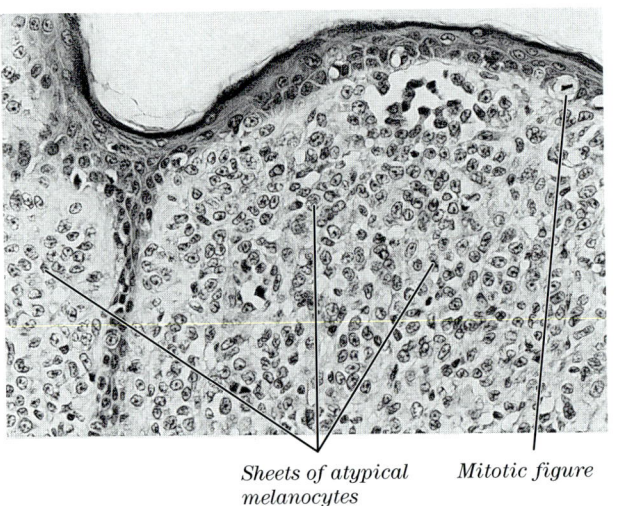

Sheets of atypical melanocytes — *Mitotic figure*

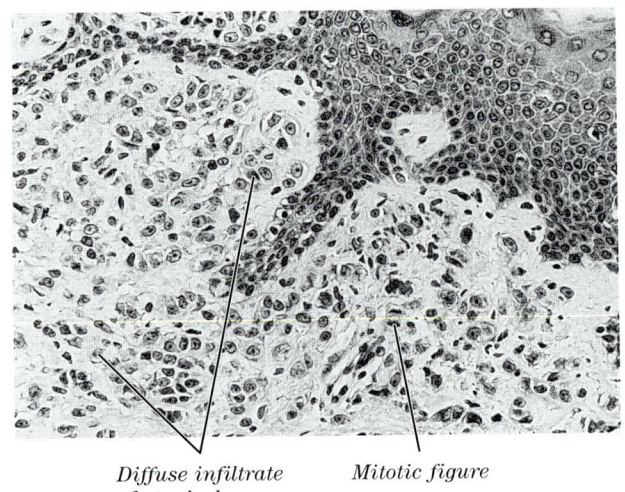

Diffuse infiltrate of atypical melanocytes — *Mitotic figure*

99 • Melanoma

Criteria for diagnosis of this melanoma

This is a melanoma because:

1. The neoplasm is asymmetric.

2. Sheets of neoplastic cells monopolize in the absence of any nests, cords, or strands of melanocytes.

3. Atypia of nuclei, particularly pleomorphism, is evident.

4. Mitotic figures are present in some neoplastic melanocytes lodged within the epidermis and the dermis.

5. A perivascular infiltrate of lymphocytes punctuates the neoplasm itself.

Pitfall in diagnosis

This melanoma could be misdiagnosed as Unna's nevus because:

1. The neoplasm is exophytic.

2. The neoplasm is papillated.

3. The base of the neoplasm is flattish.

4. Nuclei of neoplastic cells are small.

5. Hardly any scatter of melanocytes is noted above the dermo-epidermal junction.

Unlike Unna's nevus, this papillated melanocytic neoplasm is asymmetric, an observation that indicates the neoplasm probably is not a nevus, but a melanoma. The judgment can be confirmed at scanning magnification by recognizing sheets of melanocytes, and, at higher magnification, by identifying atypical melanocytes and melanocytes in mitosis.

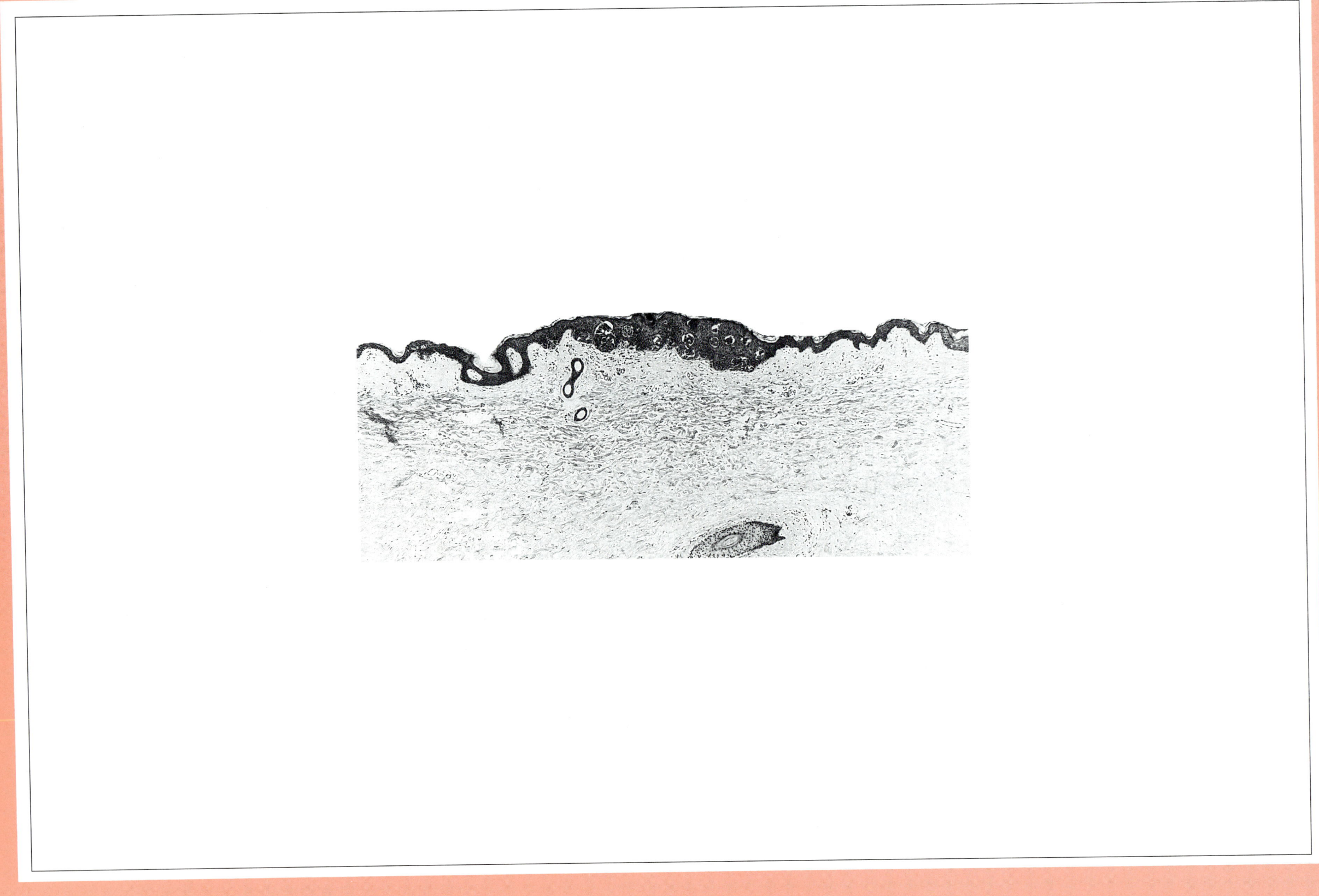

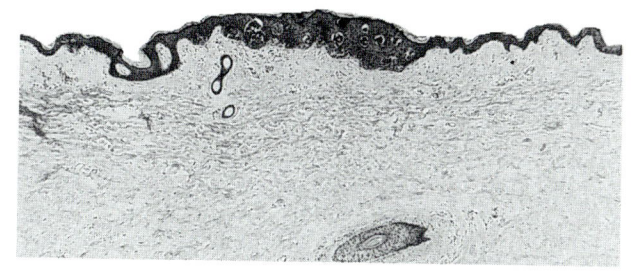
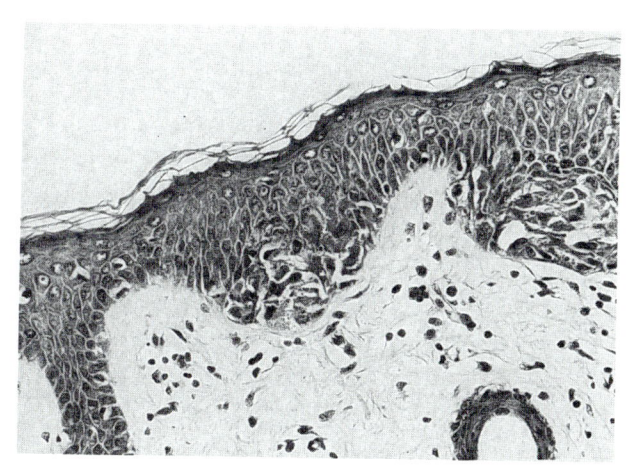
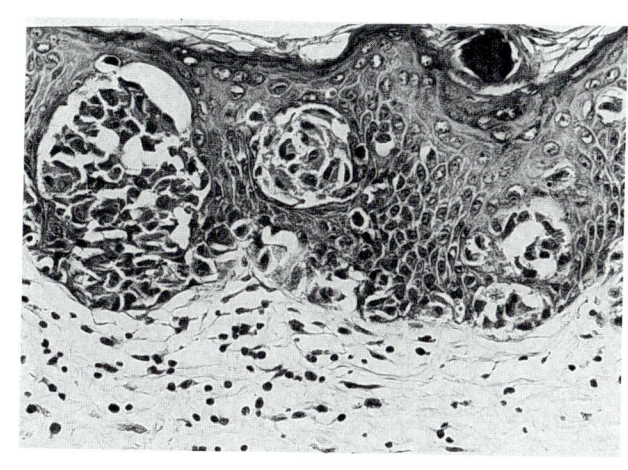
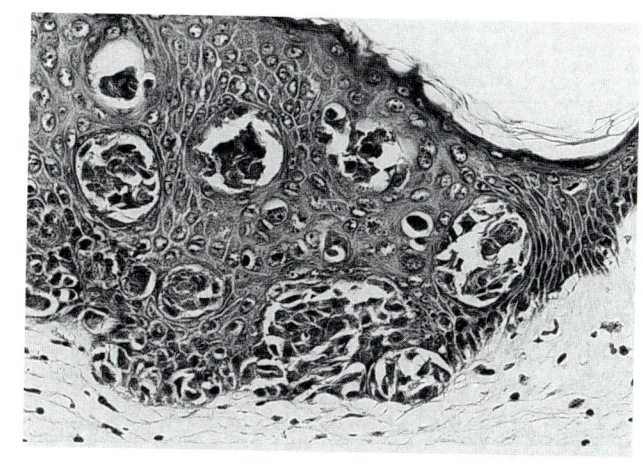
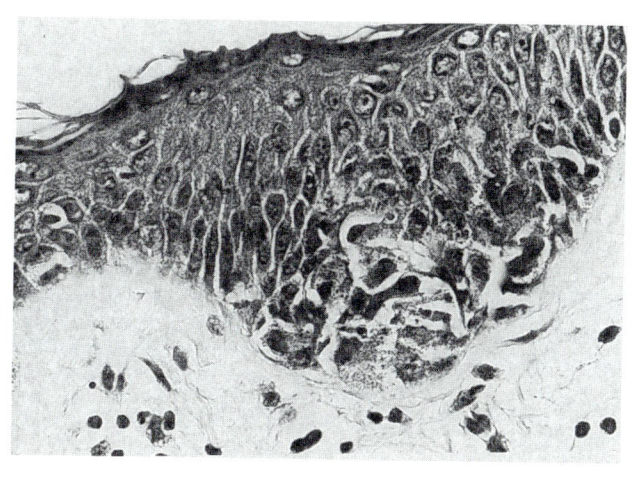
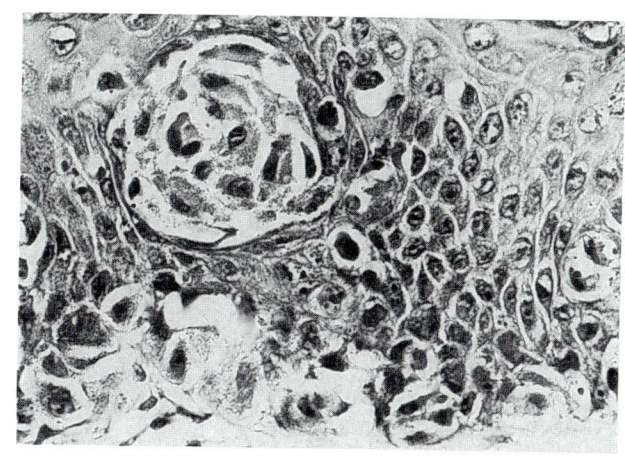
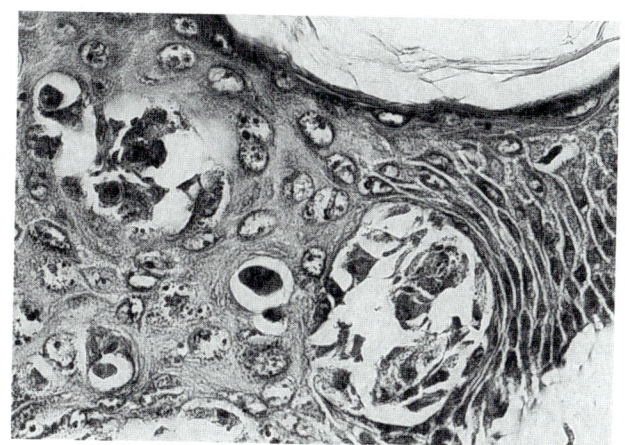

100. What is your diagnosis?

Pigmented macules developed on the head and trunk of a 67-year-old man. No clinical diagnosis was submitted. A primary melanoma had been excised from a shoulder 2 years previously.

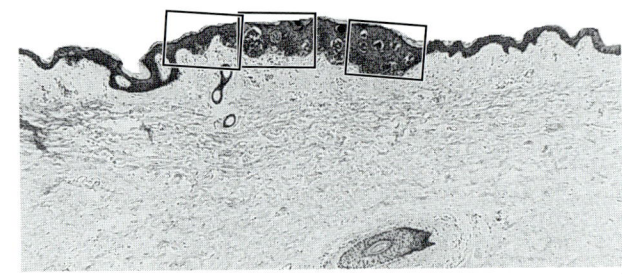

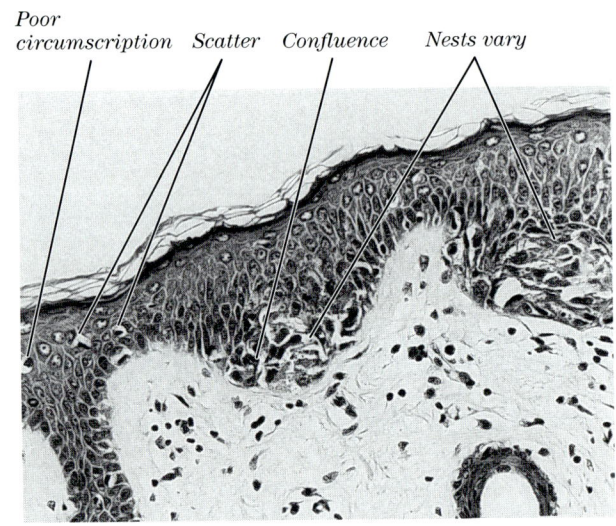

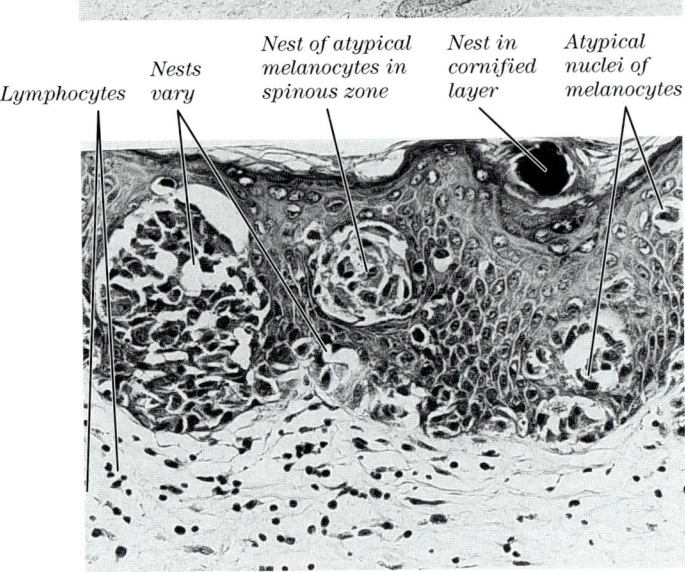

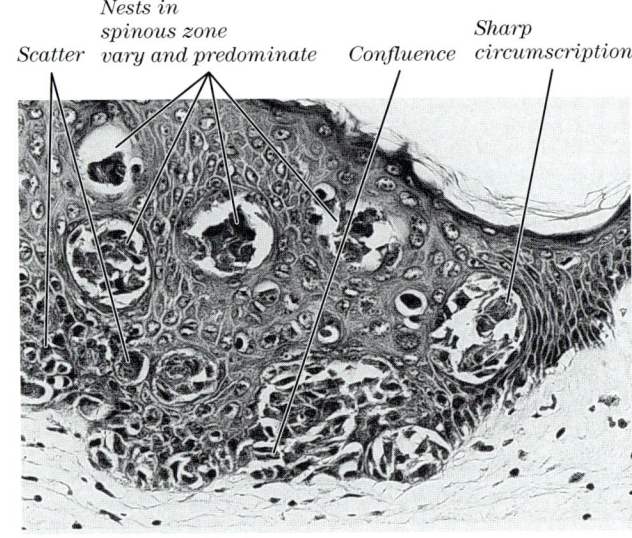

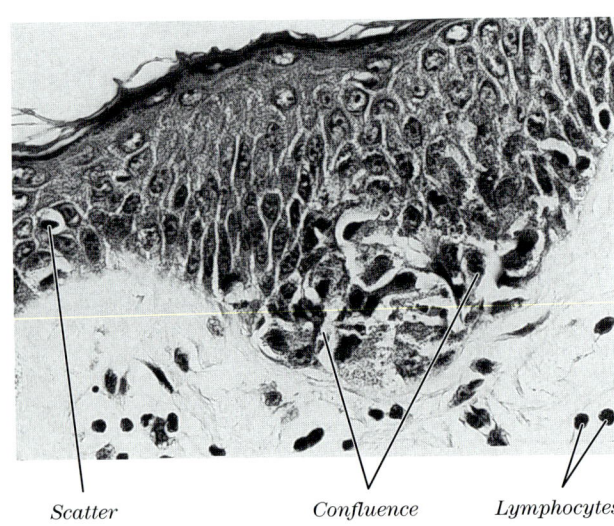

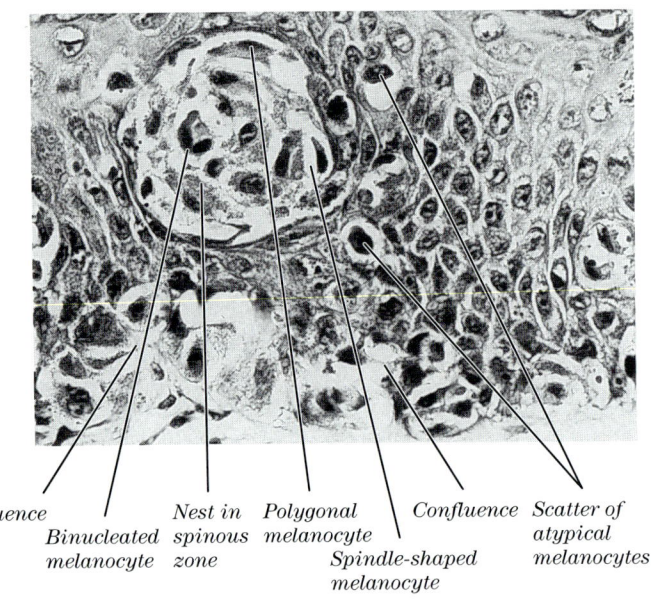

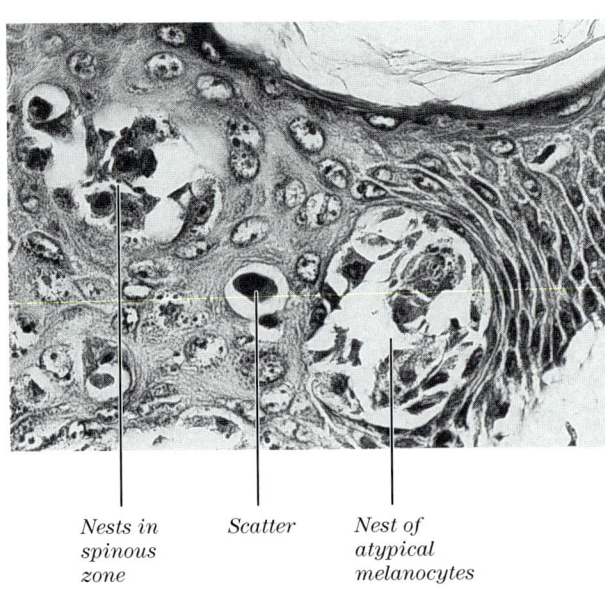

100 • Melanoma in situ

Criteria for diagnosis of this melanoma in situ

This appears to be a melanoma in situ because:

1. Atypical melanocytes arranged as solitary units and in nests are present throughout the entire thickness of the epidermis, including the cornified layer.

2. Nests of melanocytes are not equidistant from one another.

3. Nests of melanocytes vary in size and shape.

4. Some nests of melanocytes have become confluent.

5. Melanin is not distributed in uniform fashion throughout the neoplasm.

6. No neoplastic melanocytes are detectable in the dermis.

Pitfall in diagnosis

This melanoma in situ could be misinterpreted as a junctional Spitz's nevus because:

1. The neoplasm is extremely small, less than 3.0 mm in greatest diameter, but consists mostly of nests of melanocytes.

2. Nests of melanocytes predominate over melanocytes arranged as solitary units.

3. Many of the atypical melanocytes have oval, spindle, and polygonal shapes.

4. Some atypical melanocytes are binucleate and multinucleate.

5. The lesion is relatively well-circumscribed.

The major pitfall in diagnosis of this neoplasm derives from the clinical history. In short, a 65-year-old man had an indubitable, thick melanoma on the right shoulder. Within 2 years, showers of small flattish pigmented lesions developed on the scalp and trunk, and in the larynx. Biopsy of numerous skin lesions revealed changes of melanoma in situ like those shown here. On the basis of the clinical history and the clinical findings, the diagnosis should be epidermotropically metastatic melanoma rather than melanoma in situ. However, in none of the apparent metastases were any neoplastic melanocytes found within the dermis itself or within vascular lumina there. In the context of this reality, we are forced to conclude that this patient has innumerable primary cutaneous melanomas. Despite the seeming logic of this conclusion, we remain unsatisfied by it.

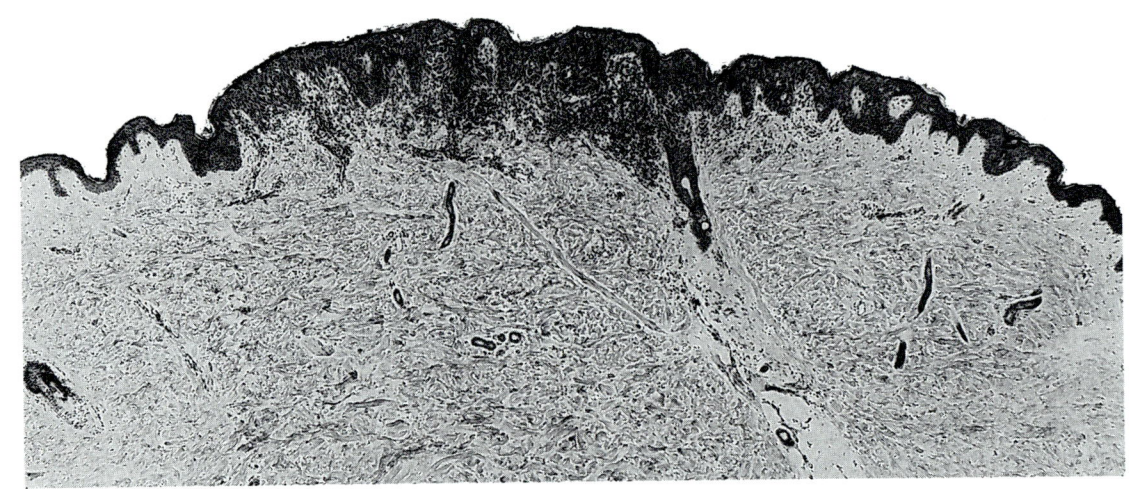

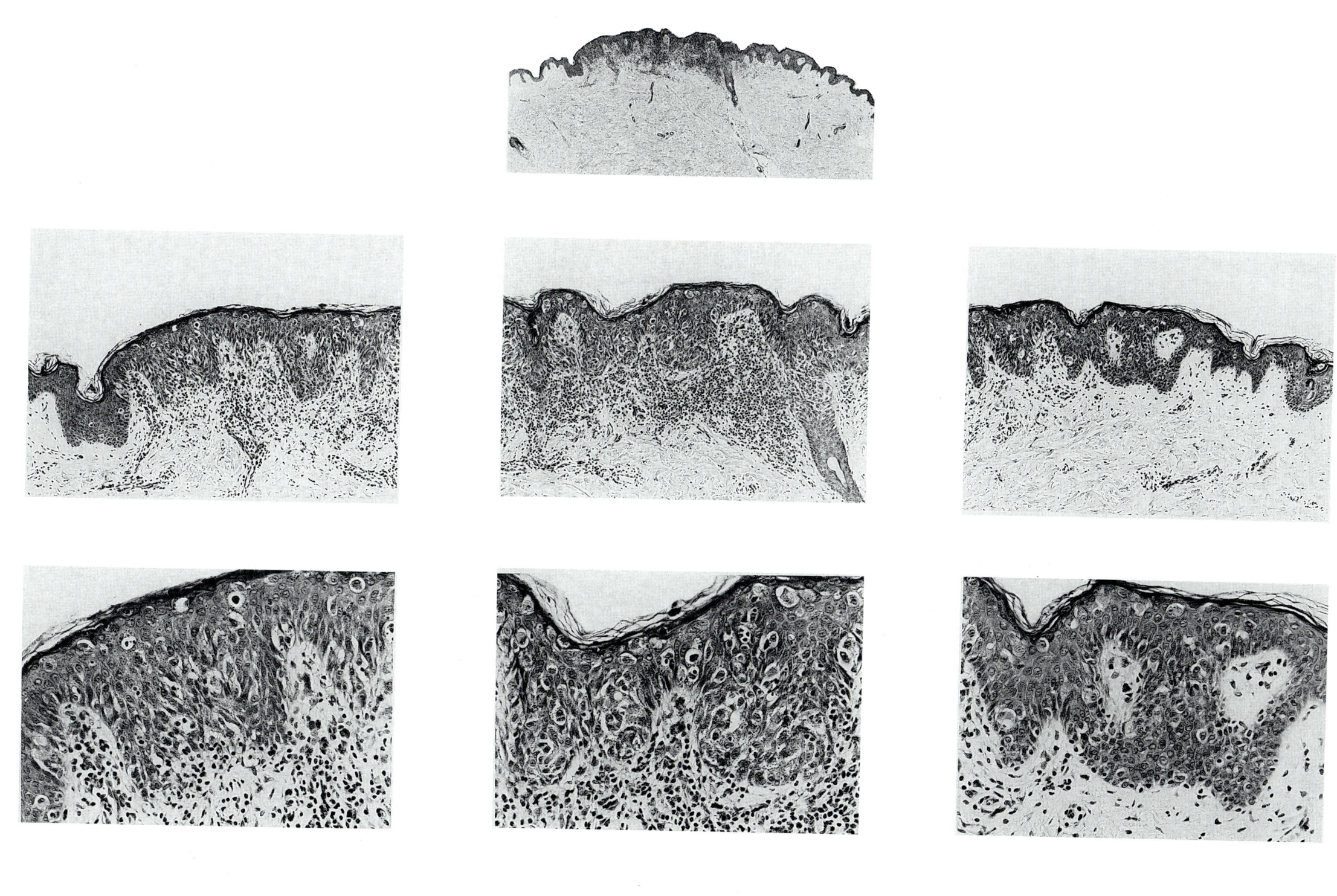

101. What is your diagnosis?

Small pigmented lesion on the back of a 5-year-old boy. Clinical diagnosis: melanoma. The lesion was removed completely. Patient was free of disease after 18 months.

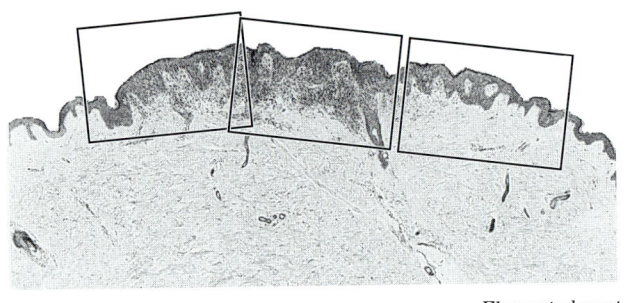

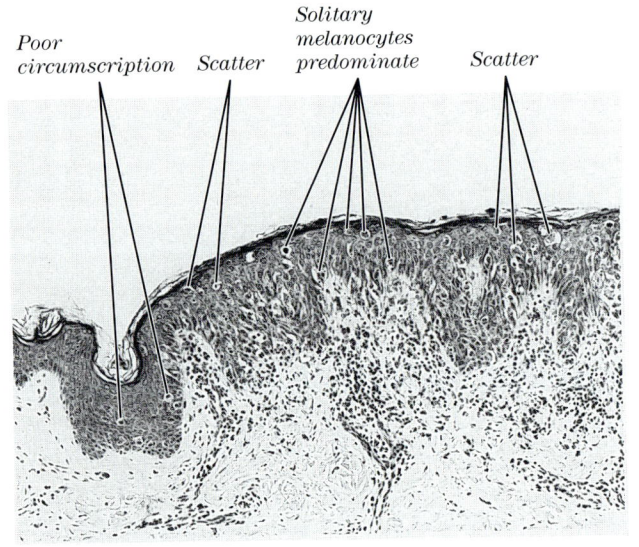
Poor circumscription — Scatter — Solitary melanocytes predominate — Scatter

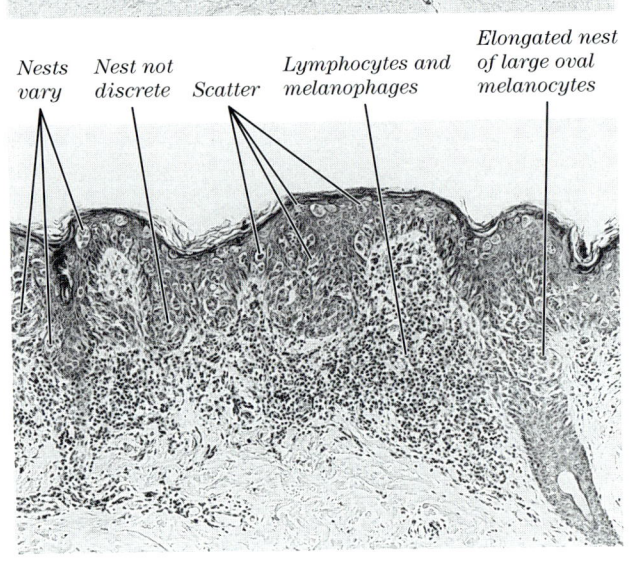
Nests vary — Nest not discrete — Scatter — Lymphocytes and melanophages — Elongated nest of large oval melanocytes

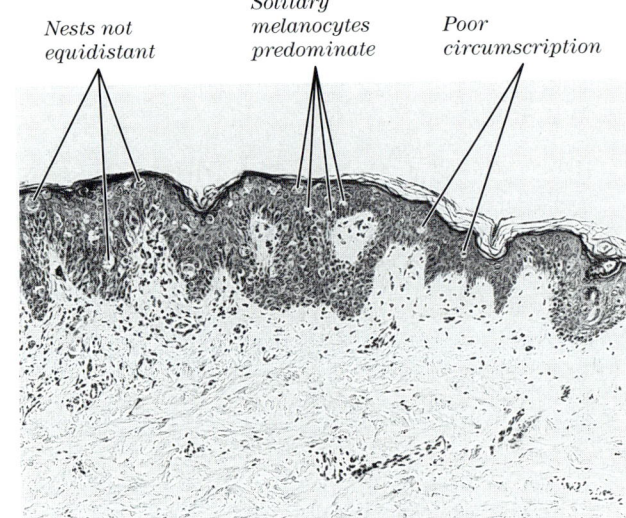
Nests not equidistant — Solitary melanocytes predominate — Poor circumscription

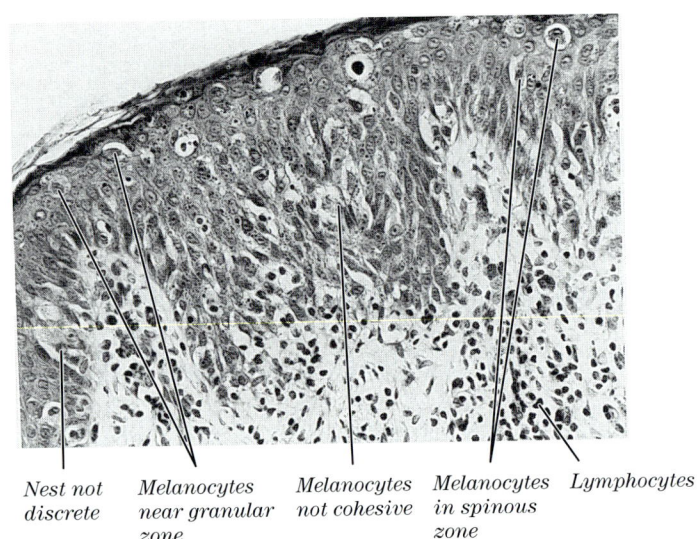
Nest not discrete — Melanocytes near granular zone — Melanocytes not cohesive — Melanocytes in spinous zone — Lymphocytes

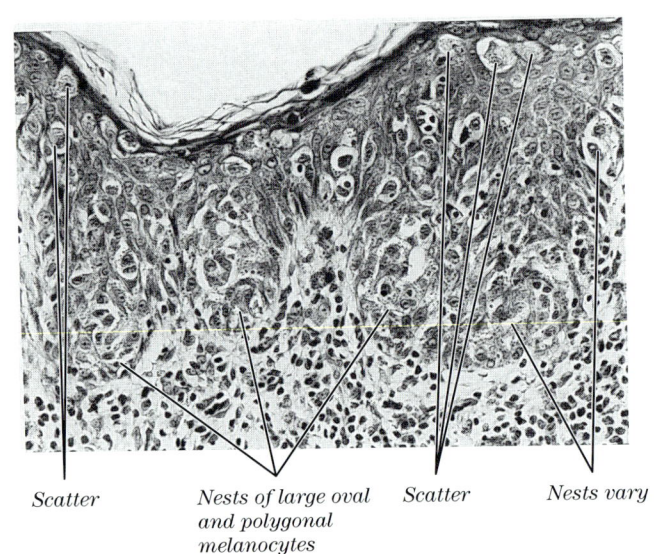
Scatter — Nests of large oval and polygonal melanocytes — Scatter — Nests vary

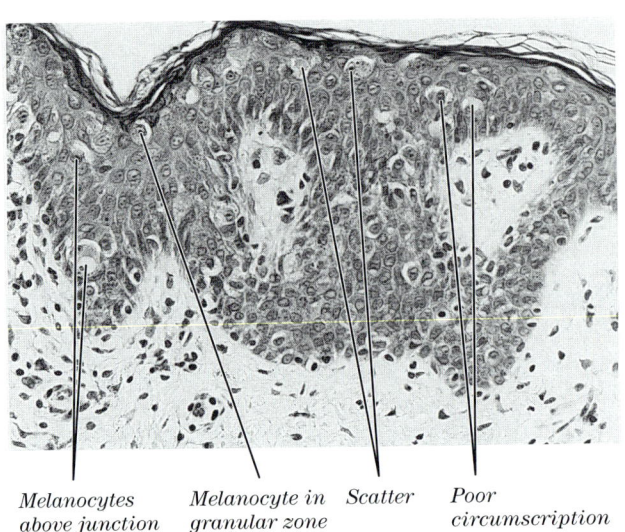
Melanocytes above junction — Melanocyte in granular zone — Scatter — Poor circumscription

101 • Spitz's nevus? Melanoma?

Criteria that favor Spitz's nevus are:

1. Monomorphous largish nuclei of melanocytes that contain abundant cytoplasm.
2. Shapes of melanocytes mostly oval and round.
3. Nests of melanocytes mostly at the dermo-epidermal junction, rather than above it.
4. Some large nests of melanocytes in a neoplasm that is small, i.e., less than 3.0 mm in greatest diameter.
5. There are epidermal hyperplasia and hypergranulosis.

Criteria that favor melanoma are:

1. The lesion is asymmetric.
2. It is poorly circumscribed.
3. There is extensive involvement of the upper half of the epidermis by neoplastic melanocytes.
4. Melanocytes disposed as solitary units within the epidermis are more numerous than nests of melanocytes in several high-power fields.

Pitfall in diagnosis

This melanocytic neoplasm exhibits features of a compound Spitz's nevus and a melanoma, to wit:

1. Melanocytes are disposed both as solitary units and in collections within the epidermis.
2. Melanocytes have large nuclei and abundant cytoplasm.
3. Melanocytes are dispersed at all levels of the epidermis.
4. There is epidermal hyperpigmentation.
5. Infiltrates of lymphocytes are present in the upper part of the dermis and even within the epidermis.
6. Melanophages are numerous in the dermis.

This neoplasm engendered considerable and spirited debate. Some histopathologists who studied it were adamant about its being a melanoma. Only a few averred that it was a Spitz's nevus. We favor a Spitz's nevus in this youngster because the lesion was small, about 3.0 mm in greatest diameter, and consisted, in part, of many large nests of melanocytes, in addition to melanocytes arranged as solitary units. It is unbiologic for such large nests to form in a 3.0-mm melanoma. The poor circumscription of the neoplasm could be explained by the dynamic of its evolution. The melanocytes themselves are remarkably monomorphous. This constellation of findings compels us to the conclusion that this lesion is benign. The history also helps in that regard. In truth, however, although we favor a diagnosis of Spitz's nevus, we are not completely certain of it.

Index

Note: Page numbers followed by D indicate diagrams and silhouettes; page numbers followed by M indicate micrographs; page numbers followed by T indicate tables.

Acquired nevi
  Clark's. *See* Clark's nevus
  combined. *See* Combined nevi
  discussion, 46, 51, 67, 86–89
  Miescher's nevi. *See* Miescher's nevus
  Spitz's nevus. *See* Spitz's nevus
  Unna's nevus. *See* Unna's nevus
"Acrolentiginous melanoma", discussion, 257, 260
Anogenital region. *See also* Genitalia
  nevi in association with lichen sclerosus et atrophicus, 218M
    criteria for diagnosis of, 219
    discussion, 212
  discussion, 212
Artifacts
  around keratinocytes. *See* Keratinocytes, artifacts around
  in extramammary Paget's disease, 236M
    criteria for diagnosis of, 237
    discussion, 228–229
"Atypical mole." *See also* Clark's nevus
  discussion, 89, 256

BANS areas, discussion, 257
Basal-cell carcinoma, with partial regression, 456M–458M
  criteria for diagnosis of, 459
  pitfall in diagnosis of, 459
Becker's nevus, discussion, 3
"Benign" cells, discussion, 248
Blue nevi
  combined. *See* Combined nevi, blue nevi
  deep, 10T
    dendritic, 22M, 26M, 36M, 484M–486M
      criteria for diagnosis of, 23, 27, 37, 487
      multifocal, 38M
        criteria for diagnosis of, 39
      pitfall in diagnosis of, 487
    discussion, 10

    non-dendritic, 24M, 40M, 42M, 44M
      criteria for diagnosis of, 25, 41, 43, 45
  definition, discussion, 5, 10
  discussion, 5, 10, 15, 32–33
  histopathologic classification of, 10T
    discussion, 10
  Masson's nevus. *See* Masson's blue nevus
  mongolian spot (patch), discussion, 15, 32
  of Ito, discussion, 10, 15, 32
  of Ota, discussion, 10, 15, 32
  superficial, 10T
    dendritic, 20M, 28M, 34M
      criteria for diagnosis of, 21, 29, 35, 359
      pitfall in diagnosis of, 359
    discussion, 10
Bowen's disease, pagetoid type, 238M
  criteria for diagnosis of, 239
  discussion, 229

Carbon, in tattoos. *See* Tattoos, carbon in
Carcinoma, basal-cell, with partial regression, 456M–458M
  criteria for diagnosis of, 459
  pitfall in diagnosis of, 459
Clark's nevus, 88D
  combined. *See* Combined nevi, Clark's nevus
  compound, 90M, 92M, 94M, 96M, 400M–402M
    criteria for diagnosis of, 91, 93, 95, 97, 403
    discussion, 87
    melanoma in association with, 148M, 152M
      criteria for diagnosis of, 149, 153
      discussion, 142
    on genitalia, 214M, 368M–370M
      criteria for diagnosis of, 215, 371
      discussion, 212
      pitfall in diagnosis of, 371
    on volar skin, 216M, 372M–374M
      criteria for diagnosis of, 217, 375
      discussion, 212
      pitfall in diagnosis of, 375
    pitfall in diagnosis of, 403
  discussion, 5, 86–88, 89
  halo type, 200M, 324M–326M
    criteria for diagnosis of, 201, 327

    discussion, 194, 199
    pitfall in diagnosis of, 327
    with nearly complete regression, 202M
      criteria for diagnosis of, 203
      discussion, 194
  histopathologic diagnosis of, 86T
    discussion, 86–87
  intradermal, 100M
    criteria for diagnosis of, 101
    discussion, 87
    melanoma in association with, 150M
      criteria for diagnosis of, 151
      discussion, 142
    melanoma in situ, 396M–398M, 644M–646M
      criteria for diagnosis of, 399, 647
      pitfall in diagnosis of, 399, 647
  junctional, 98M, 104M, 652M–654M
    above band of melanophages, 220M
      criteria for diagnosis of, 221
      discussion, 212–213
    criteria for diagnosis of, 99, 105, 655
    discussion, 87
    pitfall in diagnosis of, 655
  lichen sclerosus et atrophicus in anogenital region in association with, 218M
    criteria for diagnosis of, 219
    discussion, 212
  melanoma in association with. *See* Melanoma, in situ, nevi in association with; Melanoma, nevi in association with, Clark's nevus
  melanoma with regression, 292M–294M
    criteria for diagnosis of, 295
    pitfall in diagnosis of, 295
Combined nevi
  blue nevi, 572M–574M
    Clark's nevus and, 30M
      criteria for diagnosis of, 31
      discussion, 15, 32
    criteria for diagnosis of, 575
    Miescher's nevus and, 472M–474M
      criteria for diagnosis of, 475
      pitfall in diagnosis of, 475
    pitfall in diagnosis of, 575
  Clark's nevus, 106M

Combined nevi (Continued)
   blue nevi and, 30M
      criteria for diagnosis of, 31
      discussion, 15, 32
   criteria for diagnosis of, 107
   discussion, 88
   Spitz's nevus and, 82M, 269M–270M, 332M–334M, 448M–450M, 584M–586M
      criteria for diagnosis of, 83, 271, 335, 451, 587
      discussion, 67
      pitfall in diagnosis of, 271, 335, 451, 587
   Unna's nevus and, melanoma in situ in association with, 344M–346M
      criteria for diagnosis of, 347
      discussion, 183
      pitfall in diagnosis of, 347
   Miescher's nevus
      blue nevi and, 472M–474M
         criteria for diagnosis of, 475
         pitfall in diagnosis of, 475
      Spitz's nevus and, 188M
         criteria for diagnosis of, 189
         discussion, 183
      non-blue nevi, superficial, 190M
         criteria for diagnosis of, 191
         discussion, 183
   Spitz's nevus, 532M–534M
      Clark's nevus and, 82M, 269M–270M, 332M–334M, 448M–450M, 584M–586M
         criteria for diagnosis of, 83, 271, 335, 451, 587
         discussion, 67
         pitfall in diagnosis of, 271, 335, 451, 587
      criteria for diagnosis of, 535
      Miescher's nevus and, 188M
         criteria for diagnosis of, 189
         discussion, 183
      pitfall in diagnosis of, 535
      Unna's nevus and, 186M
         criteria for diagnosis of, 187
         discussion, 183
   Unna's nevus
      Clark's nevus and, melanoma in situ in association with, 344M–346M
         criteria for diagnosis of, 347
         pitfall in diagnosis of, 347
      Spitz's nevus and, 186M
         criteria for diagnosis of, 187
         discussion, 183
   with balloon melanocytes, 528M–530M
      criteria for diagnosis of, 531
      discussion, 183
      Miescher's nevus, 192M
         criteria for diagnosis of, 193
         pitfall in diagnosis of, 531
   with pagetoid melanocytes, discussion, 183
Compound nevi
   Clark's nevus. See Clark's nevus, compound
   discussion, 5
   Spitz's nevus, 58M, 62M, 68M, 70M, 78M, 80M, 84M
      criteria for diagnosis of, 59, 63, 69, 71, 79, 81, 85
      discussion, 51, 67
Congenital nevi
   blue. See Blue nevi
   classification by size, discussion, 5
   combined. See Combined nevi
   deep, 14D, 16M. See also specific types of congenital nevi
      discussion, 10, 15
      melanoma in association with, 146M
         criteria for diagnosis of, 147
         discussion, 142
   discussion, 5, 9D, 10, 15, 32–33
   garment, discussion, 15
   giant hairy, discussion, 15
   in newborns and infants
      discussion, 199
      non-blue, deep, 206M, 208M, 210M
         criteria for diagnosis of, 207, 209, 211
         discussion, 199
      superficial, 280M–282M, 348M–350M, 536M–538M
         criteria for diagnosis of, 283, 351, 539
         pitfall in diagnosis of, 283, 351, 539
      junctional, 420M–422M
         criteria for diagnosis of, 423
         pitfall in diagnosis of, 423
   nevus spilus (congenital speckled lentiginous nevus), discussion, 15
   non-blue. See Non-blue nevi
   "satellite", discussion, 15
   superficial, 11D, 12M. See also specific types of congenital nevi
      discussion, 10, 15
      melanoma in association with, 144M, 154M
         criteria for diagnosis of, 145, 155
         discussion, 142
      melanoma in situ, 588M–590M
         criteria for diagnosis of, 591
         pitfall in diagnosis of, 591
      persistent (recurrent), 196M, 312M–314M, 460M–462M
         criteria for diagnosis of, 197, 315, 463
         discussion, 194
         pitfall in diagnosis of, 315, 463
   with balloon melanocytes. See Combined nevi, with balloon melanocytes

Dermatofibroma, 404M–406M
   criteria for diagnosis of, 407
   pitfall in diagnosis of, 407
"Dysplasia", discussion, 88–89, 256
"Dysplastic cells", discussion, 88–89
"Dysplastic nevi." See also Clark's nevus
   discussion, 88–89, 256
"Dysplastic nevus syndrome", discussion, 88–89, 256

Epidermis, melanocytic proliferation in. See Melanocytes, proliferation of, in epidermis
Epidermotropic metastases, of melanoma. See Melanoma, metastases to skin, epidermotropic
"Epithelioid dysplastic nevi", discussion, 256
Eyelid, normal skin of, 624M–626M
   criteria for diagnosis of, 627
   melanocytic proliferation in epidermis of, 232M
      criteria for diagnosis of, 233
      discussion, 228
   pitfall in diagnosis of, 627

"Familial dysplastic nevi", discussion, 256
Fibrosis, partial regression of melanoma by, 166M
   criteria for diagnosis of, 167
   discussion, 167
Fibrous papule, of face, melanocytic proliferation in epidermis above, 224M
   criteria for diagnosis of, 225
   discussion, 213

Garment nevi, discussion, 15
Genitalia. See also Anogenital region
   labial lentigo and, 258M
      criteria for diagnosis of, 259
      discussion, 257
   melanosis of, 222M
      criteria for diagnosis of, 223
      discussion, 213
   nevi on
      Clark's compound nevus. See Clark's nevus, compound, on genitalia
      discussion, 212
Giant hairy nevus, discussion, 15

Halo nevi
    Clark's nevus. *See* Clark's nevus, halo type
    discussion, 194, 198D, 199
    regression of, 202M
        criteria for diagnosis of, 203
        discussion, 159, 194
Hamartoma, discussion, 3

In-transit metastases, of melanoma, discussion, 171
Infants, congenital nevi in. *See* Congenital nevi, in newborns and infants
Intradermal nevi
    Clark's nevus. *See* Clark's nevus, intradermal
    discussion, 5
    Miescher's nevus, melanocytic proliferation in epidermis above, discussion, 213
    Spitz's nevus, 64M
        criteria for diagnosis of, 65
        discussion, 51
    Unna's nevus, 48M
        criteria for diagnosis of, 49
"Invasive" neoplasms, discussion, 248
Ito, nevus of, discussion, 10, 15, 32

Junctional nevi
    above band of melanophages, discussion, 212–213
    Clark's nevus. *See* Clark's nevus, junctional
    congenital, 420M–422M
        criteria for diagnosis of, 423
        pitfall in diagnosis of, 423
    discussion, 3, 5, 89
    Spitz's nevus. *See* Spitz's nevus, junctional

Keratinocytes, artifacts around, 234M, 628M–630M
    criteria for diagnosis of, 235, 631
    discussion, 228
    pitfall in diagnosis of, 631
Keratosis, lichen planus-like. *See* Lichen planus-like keratosis

Lentigines, solar, melanocytic proliferation in epidermis of, 230M
    criteria for diagnosis of, 231
    discussion, 228
"Lentiginous dysplastic nevi", discussion, 256
Lentiginous nevus, speckled, congenital (nevus spilus), discussion, 15
Lentigo
    labial, 258M
        criteria for diagnosis of, 259
        discussion, 257
    simple, 102M
        criteria for diagnosis of, 103
        discussion, 87
"Lentigo maligna melanoma", discussion, 257, 260
Lichen planus-like keratosis, 244M
    complete regression of, 246M
        criteria for diagnosis of, 247
        discussion, 229
    criteria for diagnosis of, 245
    discussion, 229
    regression of, discussion, 159
Lichen sclerosus et atrophicus, in anogenital region, nevi in association with
    Clark's nevus, 218M
        criteria for diagnosis of, 219
        discussion, 212
    discussion, 212

"Malignant" cells, discussion, 248, 249
Masson's blue nevus, 42M, 44M
    criteria for diagnosis of, 43, 45
    deep dendritic and non-dendritic, 580M–582M
        criteria for diagnosis of, 583
        pitfall in diagnosis of, 583
    discussion, 33
Melanocytes
    balloon, combined nevi with, 192M
        criteria for diagnosis of, 193
        discussion, 183
    in normal skin
        cytologic features of, 2D
            discussion, 1
        distribution of, discussion, 1, 3
        location of, 4D
            discussion, 3
    of nevi and melanomas, criteria for differentiation of, 110T
        discussion, 108
    pagetoid, combined nevi with, discussion, 183
    proliferation of
        at dermo-epidermal junction, 6D, 7D
            discussion, 3, 5
        in epidermis
            above fibrous papules of face, 224M
                criteria for diagnosis of, 225
                discussion, 213
            above intradermal Miescher's nevi, discussion, 213
            of normal skin of eyelid, 232M
                criteria for diagnosis of, 233
                discussion, 228
            of solar lentigines, 230M
                criteria for diagnosis of, 231
                discussion, 228
            of sun-damaged skin, 226M
                criteria for diagnosis of, 227
                discussion, 213, 228
        mostly within dermis from outset, 8D
            discussion, 5
Melanoma, 109D, 124M, 128M, 138M, 140M, 284M–286M, 288M–290M, 308M–310M, 320M–322M, 364M–366M, 376M–378M, 384M–386M, 392M–394M, 408M–410M, 412M–414M, 424M–426M, 436M–438M, 452M–454M, 468M–470M, 496M–498M, 500M–502M, 508M–510M, 516M–518M, 520M–522M, 548M–550M, 608M–610M, 632M–634M, 636M–638M, 640M–642M, 656M–658M, 660M–662M, 668M–670M
    "acrolentiginous", discussion, 257, 260
    balloon-cell type, 388M–390M
        criteria for diagnosis of, 391
        pitfall in diagnosis of, 391
    "borderline", discussion, 249, 256
    criteria for diagnosis of, 125, 129, 139, 141, 287, 291, 311, 323, 367, 379, 387, 395, 411, 415, 427, 439, 455, 471, 499, 503, 511, 519, 523, 551, 611, 635, 639, 659, 663, 671
    definition, discussion, 108
    desmoplastic, 336M–338M, 464M–466M
        criteria for diagnosis of, 339, 467
        neurotropic, 130D, 134M
            criteria for diagnosis of, 135
            discussion, 120–121
        pitfall in diagnosis of, 339, 467
    discussion, 108, 110
    epidemic of, discussion, 260
    histopathologic diagnosis of, 108T
        discussion, 108, 110
    in situ, 111D, 112M, 114M, 116M, 118M, 126M, 272M–274M, 316M–318M, 352M–354M, 440M–442M, 444M–446M, 476M–478M, 492M–494M, 512M–514M, 560M–562M, 600M–602M, 620M–622M, 648M–650M, 664M–666M
        criteria for diagnosis of, 113, 115, 117, 119, 127, 275, 319, 355, 443, 447, 479, 495, 515, 563, 603, 623, 651, 667

Melanoma, in situ *(Continued)*
   discussion, 110, 120
   in volar skin, 122M
     criteria for diagnosis of, 123
   nevi in association with
     Clark's intradermal nevus, 396M–398M, 644M–646M
       criteria for diagnosis of, 399, 647
       pitfall in diagnosis of, 399, 647
     combined, 344M–346M
       criteria for diagnosis of, 347
       pitfall in diagnosis of, 347
     congenital, superficial, 588M–590M
       criteria for diagnosis of, 591
       pitfall in diagnosis of, 591
     on skin damaged by sunlight, 540M–542M
       criteria for diagnosis of, 543
       pitfall in diagnosis of, 543
     partial regression by fibrosis, 166M
       criteria for diagnosis of, 167
       discussion, 158
     pitfall in diagnosis of, 275, 319, 355, 443, 447, 479, 495, 515, 563, 603, 623, 651, 667
   "intra-epidermal", discussion, 110
   "intra-epithelial", discussion, 110, 120
   "lentigo maligna", discussion, 257, 260
   melanocytes of, criteria for differentiation from melanocytes of nevi, 110T
     discussion, 108
   melanocytic simulators of, discussion, 182–183, 194, 199, 212, 228
   metastases to skin, 172M, 174M, 176M, 304M–306M, 480M–482M, 576M–578M
     completely regressed, 296M–298M, 360M–362M
       criteria for diagnosis of, 299, 363
       pitfall in diagnosis of, 299, 363
       satellite metastases, 360M–362M
         criteria for diagnosis of, 363
         pitfall in diagnosis of, 363
     criteria for diagnosis of, 173, 175, 177, 307, 483, 579
     discussion, 170–171, 248
     epidermotropic, 178M, 416M–418M, 616M–618M
       criteria for diagnosis of, 179, 419, 619
       discussion, 170
       histopathologic differentiation of, 170T
         discussion, 170
       pitfall in diagnosis of, 419, 619
     in-transit, discussion, 171
     pitfall in diagnosis of, 307, 483, 579
     regional, discussion, 171
     satellite, 180M, 254M
       criteria for diagnosis of, 181, 255
       discussion, 171, 249
       with complete regression, 360M–362M
         criteria for diagnosis of, 363
         pitfall in diagnosis of, 363
   "minimal deviation", discussion, 249, 256
   nevi in association with, 156M. *See also* Melanoma, in situ, nevi in association with
     Clark's nevus
       compound, 148M, 152M
         criteria for diagnosis of, 149, 153
         discussion, 142
       intradermal, 150M
         criteria for diagnosis of, 151
         discussion, 142
       melanoma in regression and, 292M–294M
         criteria for diagnosis of, 295
         pitfall in diagnosis of, 295
     congenital
       deep, 146M
         criteria for diagnosis of, 147
         discussion, 142
       superficial, 144M, 154M
         criteria for diagnosis of, 145, 155
         discussion, 142
     criteria for diagnosis of, 157
     discussion, 142–143
   "nodular", discussion, 257
   nonmelanocytic simulators of, discussion, 228–229
   persistent, 564M–566M
     criteria for diagnosis of, 567
     pitfall in diagnosis of, 567
   pitfall in diagnosis of, 287, 291, 311, 323, 367, 379, 387, 395, 411, 415, 427, 439, 455, 471, 499, 503, 511, 519, 523, 551, 611, 635, 639, 643, 659, 663, 671
   criteria for diagnosis of, 643
   regression of, 160M
     Clark's nevus in association with, 292M–294M
       criteria for diagnosis of, 295
       pitfall in diagnosis of, 295
     complete
       by fibrosis, 162M
         criteria for diagnosis of, 163
         discussion, 158
       by melanosis, 168M
         criteria for diagnosis of, 169
         discussion, 158–159
       discussion, 257
       satellite metastases, 360M–362M
         criteria for diagnosis of, 363
         pitfall in diagnosis of, 363
     criteria for diagnosis of, 161
     discussion, 158–159
     focal
       by fibrosis, 164M
         criteria for diagnosis of, 165
         discussion, 158
       by melanosis, 360M–362M
         criteria for diagnosis of, 363
         pitfall in diagnosis of, 363
     partial
       by fibrosis, 166M
         criteria for diagnosis of, 167
         discussion, 158
     discussion, 257
   simulators of
     melanocytic, discussion, 182–183, 194, 199, 212, 228
     nonmelanocytic, discussion, 228–229
   "superficial spreading", discussion, 257
   thickness as measure of prognosis of, discussion, 121
   with abundant mucin, 136M
     criteria for diagnosis of, 137
     discussion, 121
   with neural differentiation, 328M–330M
     criteria for diagnosis of, 331
     pitfall in diagnosis of, 331
   with neurotropism and neural hyperplasia, 592M–594M
     criteria for diagnosis of, 595
     pitfall in diagnosis of, 595
Melanosis
   of genitalia, 222M
     criteria for diagnosis of, 223
     discussion, 213
   regression of melanoma by. *See* Melanoma, regression of
Metastases, of melanoma, to skin. *See* Melanoma, metastases to skin
Miescher's nevus, 50D, 52M
   ancient, 276M–278M
     criteria for diagnosis of, 279
     discussion, 199
     pitfall in diagnosis of, 279
   combined
     with balloon melanocytes, 192M
       criteria for diagnosis of, 193
     with blue nevus, 472M–474M
       criteria for diagnosis of, 475

pitfall in diagnosis of, 475
with Spitz's nevus, 188M
criteria for diagnosis of, 189
discussion, 183
criteria for diagnosis of, 53
discussion, 46, 51
follicular cysts developing in, discussion, 143
intradermal, melanocytic proliferation in epidermis above, discussion, 213
with collagenization, 56M
criteria for diagnosis of, 57
discussion, 51
with neurotization, 54M
criteria for diagnosis of, 55
discussion, 51
Mole, "atypical." *See also* Clark's nevus
discussion, 89, 256
Mongolian spot (patch), discussion, 15, 32
Mycosis fungoides, 240M, 596M–598M
criteria for diagnosis of, 241, 599
discussion, 229
pitfall in diagnosis of, 599

Nevi. *See also specific types of nevi*
definition of, discussion, 3, 5, 257
Nevus spilus (congenital speckled lentiginous nevus), discussion, 15
Newborns, congenital nevi in. *See* Congenital nevi, in newborns and infants
"Nodular melanoma", discussion, 257
Non-blue nevi
combined, superficial, 190M
criteria for diagnosis of, 191
discussion, 183
deep, 14D, 16M
criteria for diagnosis of, 17
discussion, 10
in newborns and infants, 206M, 208M, 210M
criteria for diagnosis of, 207, 209, 211
discussion, 199
discussion, 10, 15
histopathologic classification of, 10T
discussion, 10
superficial, 11D, 12M, 18M
combined, 190M
criteria for diagnosis of, 191
discussion, 183
criteria for diagnosis of, 13, 19
discussion, 10

Ota, nevus of, discussion, 10, 15, 32

Paget's disease, extramammary, 236M, 552M–554M
criteria for diagnosis of, 237, 555
discussion, 228–229
pitfall in diagnosis of, 555
Palms. *See* Volar skin
"Penetrating" nevus, deep, 250M, 524M–526M
criteria for diagnosis of, 251, 527
discussion, 249
pitfall in diagnosis of, 527
Persistent melanoma, 564M–566M
criteria for diagnosis of, 567
pitfall in diagnosis of, 567
Persistent (recurrent) nevi, 195D
congenital, superficial. *See* Congenital nevi, superficial, persistent (recurrent)
discussion, 194
Spitz's nevus, 568M–570M
criteria for diagnosis of, 571
pitfall in diagnosis of, 571
Pregnancy, Unna's nevus during, 261M
criteria for diagnosis of, 262
discussion, 260

"Radial growth phase", discussion, 248–249
Recurrent nevi. *See* Persistent (recurrent) nevi
Regional metastases, of melanoma, discussion, 171
Regression. *See specific lesions*

Satellite metastases, of melanoma. *See* Melanoma, metastases to skin, satellite
"Satellite" nevi, discussion, 15
Skin
melanocytic proliferation in. *See* Melanocytes, proliferation of, in epidermis
metastases of melanoma to. *See* Melanoma, metastases to skin
normal, of eyelid. *See* Eyelid, normal skin of
sun-damaged. *See* Solar lentigines; Sun-damaged skin
volar. *See* Volar skin
Solar lentigines, melanocytic proliferation in epidermis of, 230M
criteria for diagnosis of, 231
discussion, 228
Soles. *See* Volar skin
Speckled lentiginous nevus, congenital (nevus spilus), discussion, 15

Spitz's nevus, 65D, 66D, 72M, 184M, 252M, 340M–342M, 380M–382M, 504M–506M, 668M–670M
combined. *See* Combined nevi, Spitz's nevus
compound, 58M, 62M, 68M, 70M, 78M, 80M, 84M
criteria for diagnosis of, 59, 63, 69, 71, 79, 81, 85
discussion, 51, 67
criteria for diagnosis of, 73, 185, 253, 343, 383, 507, 671
desmoplastic, 428M–430M
criteria for diagnosis of, 431
pitfall in diagnosis of, 431
discussion, 51, 67, 86, 89, 121, 182–183, 248, 249
histopathologic features in common between melanoma and, 182T
discussion, 182
intradermal, 64M
criteria for diagnosis of, 65
discussion, 51
junctional, 60M, 300M–302M, 556M–558M, 604M–606M
criteria for diagnosis of, 61, 303, 559, 607
discussion, 51
pitfall in diagnosis of, 303, 559, 607
persistent, 568M–570M
criteria for diagnosis of, 571
pitfall in diagnosis of, 571
"pigmented spindle-cell" type, 72M, 74M, 76M, 544M–546M, 612M–614M
criteria for diagnosis of, 73, 75, 77, 547, 615
discussion, 51, 67
pitfall in diagnosis of, 547, 615
pitfall in diagnosis of, 343, 383, 507, 671
"Sporadic dysplastic nevi", discussion, 256
Sun-damaged skin. *See also* Solar lentigines
melanocytic proliferation in epidermis of, 226M
criteria for diagnosis of, 227
discussion, 213, 228
melanoma in situ on, 540M–542M
criteria for diagnosis of, 543
pitfall in diagnosis of, 543
"Superficial spreading melanoma", discussion, 257

Tattoos, carbon in, 242M, 488M–490M
criteria for diagnosis of, 243, 491
discussion, 229
pitfall in diagnosis of, 491

Ultraviolet light, skin damaged by. *See* Solar lentigines; Sun-damaged skin

Unna's nevus, 47D
  ancient, 204M, 432M–434M
    criteria for diagnosis of, 205, 435
    discussion, 199
    pitfall in diagnosis of, 435
  combined. *See* Combined nevi, Unna's nevus
  discussion, 46
  during pregnancy, 261M
    criteria for diagnosis of, 262
    discussion, 260
  intradermal type, 48M
    criteria for diagnosis of, 49

"Vertical growth phase", discussion, 248–249

Volar skin
  melanoma in situ in, 122M
    criteria for diagnosis of, 123
  nevi on
    Clark's compound nevus. *See* Clark's nevus, compound, on volar skin
    discussion, 212